Surgical Treatment of
Digestive Disease

Surgical Treatment of Digestive Disease

Frank G. Moody, M.D.
Professor and Chairman
Department of Surgery
The University of Texas Medical School at Houston
Surgeon-in-Chief
Hermann Hospital
Houston, Texas

Larry C. Carey, M.D.
Robert M. Zollinger Professor of Surgery
Chairman, Department of Surgery
The Ohio State University
Columbus, Ohio

R. Scott Jones, M.D.
Stephen H. Watts Professor and Chairman
Department of Surgery
Surgeon-in-Chief
University of Virginia Medical Center
Charlottesville, Virginia

Keith A. Kelly, M.D.
Roberts Professor of Surgery
Mayo Medical School
Mayo Clinic
Rochester, Minnesota

David L. Nahrwold, M.D.
Loyal and Edith Davis Professor of Surgery
Chairman, Department of Surgery
Northwestern University Medical School
Surgeon-in-Chief
Northwestern Memorial Hospital
Chicago, Illinois

David B. Skinner, M.D.
Dallas B. Phemister Professor of Surgery
The University of Chicago
Chairman, Department of Surgery
The University of Chicago Medical Center
Chicago, Illinois

YEAR BOOK MEDICAL PUBLISHERS, INC.
CHICAGO

0   9   8   7   6   5   4   3   2   1

Library of Congress Cataloging-in-Publication Data

Main entry under title:

Surgical treatment of digestive disease.

Includes bibliographies and index.
1.   Gastrointestinal system—Surgery.   I.   Moody, Frank G.   [DNLM: 1.   Digestive System—surgery. WI 900 S9615]
RD540.S95 1986   617'.43   85-11760
ISBN 0-8151-5943-9

Sponsoring editor: Daniel J. Doody
Manager, copyediting services: Frances M. Perveiler
Production project manager: Sharon W. Pepping
Proofroom supervisor: Shirley E. Taylor

Contributors

DAVID H. AHRENHOLZ, M.D.
Instructor in Surgery, University of Minnesota Medical School, Assistant Director of Burn Center, St. Paul–Ramsey Medical Center, St. Paul, Minnesota

STANLEY W. ASHLEY, M.D.
Fellow, Department of Surgery, Washington University School of Medicine, St. Louis, Missouri

RONALD BELSEY, M.B., F.R.C.S.
Emeritus Consulting Cardiothoracic Surgeon, Bristol University Hospital, Bath, Avon, England

KIRBY I. BLAND, M.D.
Professor and Vice Chairman, Department of Surgery, University of Florida College of Medicine, Gainesville, Florida

SCOTT J. BOLEY, M.D.
Professor of Surgery, Chief, Pediatric Surgical Services, Albert Einstein College of Medicine–Montefiore Medical Center, Bronx, New York

EDWARD B. BORDEN, M.D.
Assistant Professor of Surgery, Assistant Attending, Albert Einstein College of Medicine–Montefiore Medical Center, Bronx, New York

ROBERT H. BOWER, M.D.
Assistant Professor of Surgery, University of Cincinnati College of Medicine, Director, Nutritional Support Service, University of Cincinnati Medical Center, Cincinnati, Ohio

MURRAY F. BRENNAN, M.D.
Chief, Gastric and Mixed Tumor Service, Memorial Sloan-Kettering Cancer Center, New York, New York

JOHN G. BULS, M.D., F.R.C.S., F.A.C.S.
Clinical Instructor, Department of Surgery (Colon and Rectal), University of Minnesota, Rochester, Minnesota

JOHN L. CAMERON, M.D.
Professor and Chairman, Department of Surgery, The Johns Hopkins University School of Medicine, Chief of Surgery, The Johns Hopkins Hospital, Baltimore, Maryland

LARRY C. CAREY, M.D., F.A.C.S.
Robert M. Zollinger Professor of Surgery, Chairman, Department of Surgery, The Ohio State University, Columbus, Ohio

THOMAS A. CASTILLE, M.D.
Department of Surgery, Louisiana State University School of Medicine, New Orleans, Louisiana

LAURENCE Y. CHEUNG, M.D.
Professor of Surgery, Washington University School of Medicine, General Surgeon, Barnes Hospital, St. Louis, Missouri

JAMES CHRISTENSEN, M.D.
Professor and Acting Director, Division of Gastroenterology-Hepatology, Department of Internal Medicine, University of Iowa, University of Iowa Hospitals and Clinics, Iowa City, Iowa

ISIDORE COHN, JR., M.D.
Professor and Chairman, School of Medicine in New Orleans, Louisiana State University Medical Center, New Orleans, Louisiana

DANIEL G. COIT, M.D.
Assistant Clinical Instructor in Surgery, Cornell Medical School, Chief Surgical Fellow, Memorial Sloan-Kettering Cancer Center, New York, New York

ROBERT E. CONDON, M.D., F.A.C.S.
Ausman Foundation Professor and Chairman, Department of Surgery, Medical College of Wisconsin, Milwaukee, Wisconsin

EDWARD M. COPELAND III, M.D.
Professor and Chairman, Department of Surgery, University of Florida College of Medicine, Chief of Surgery, Shands Hospital, Gainesville Florida

RICHARD DAVIES, M.D.
Chief, Surgical Oncology, Veterans Administration Medical Center, Assistant Professor of Surgery, University of California, San Diego Medical Center, San Diego, California

TOM R. DeMEESTER, M.D.
Professor and Chairman of Surgery, Creighton University School of Medicine, Chief of Surgery, St. Joseph Hospital, Veterans Administration Hospital, Omaha, Nebraska

LAWRENCE DenBESTEN, M.D.
Professor of Surgery, UCLA School of Medicine, Professor and Chief of the Gastrointestinal Surgery Section, UCLA Medical Center, Los Angeles, California

THOMAS L. DENT, M.D.
Professor of Surgery, Temple University School of Medicine, Chairman, Department of Surgery, Abington Memorial Hospital, Abington, Pennsylvania

ARTHUR J. DONOVAN, M.D.
Professor of Surgery, University of Southern California, Director of Surgery, L.A. County–USC Medical Center, Los Angeles, California

JEFFREY E. DOTY, M.D.
Assistant Professor of Surgery, UCLA School of Medicine, Los Angeles, California

ROGER R. DOZOIS, M.D., F.A.C.S.
Associate Professor of Surgery, Mayo Medical School, Consultant Surgeon, St. Mary's Hospital, Rochester Methodist Hospital, Rochester, Minnesota

E. CHRISTOPHER ELLISON, M.D.
Assistant Professor of Surgery, The Ohio State University, The Ohio State University Hospitals, Columbus, Ohio

PETER J. FABRI, M.D.
Associate Professor, The Ohio State University, Chief, General Surgery, The Ohio State University Hospitals, Columbus, Ohio

VICTOR W. FAZIO, M.B., F.R.A.C.S., F.A.C.S.
Chairman, Department of Colon and Rectal Surgery, The Cleveland Clinic Foundation, Cleveland, Ohio

JOSEF E. FISCHER, M.D., F.A.C.S.
Christian R. Holmes Professor and Chairman, Department of Surgery, University of Cincinnati College of Medicine, Cincinnati, Ohio

HERBERT R. FREUND, M.D.
Associate Professor of Surgery, Hebrew University, Hadassah University Medical Center, Jerusalem, Israel

DAVID FROMM, M.D.
Professor and Chairman of Surgery, State University of New York at Syracuse, University Hospital, Syracuse, New York

FREDERICK C. GOETZ, M.D.
Professor of Medicine and Physiology, Department of Surgery, University of Minnesota Hospital, Minneapolis, Minnesota

STANLEY M. GOLDBERG, M.D.
Clinical Professor of Surgery, Director of Colon and Rectal Surgery, Department of Surgery, University of Minnesota Medical School, Minneapolis, Minnesota

JOHN C. GOLIGHER, M.B., CH.B., CH.M., F.R.C.S.
Consultant in General and Colorectal Surgery, Emeritus Professor of Surgery, University of Leeds, Leeds, England, Consulting Surgeon, St. Mark's Hospital for Diseases of the Rectum and Colon, London, England

JIN GONGLIANG, M.D.
Department of Surgery, Zhejiang Medical College, People's Republic of China, No. 2 Hospital, Hangzhov, Zhejiang

ROBERT D. GORDON, M.D.
Assistant Professor of Surgery, University of Pittsburgh, Attending Surgeon, Presbyterian-University Hospital, Children's Hospital, Pittsburgh, Pennsylvania

WILLIAM R. GOWER, JR., PH.D.
Assistant Professor of Surgery, The Ohio State University Hospital, Columbus, Ohio

HERBERT B. GREENLEE, M.D.
Professor and Vice Chairman, Department of Surgery, Loyola University Stritch School of Medicine, Maywood, Illinois, Chief, Surgical Service, Veterans Administration Hospital, Hines, Illinois

WARD O. GRIFFIN, JR., M.D., PH.D.
Executive Director, The American Board of Surgery, Professor of Surgery, Temple University School of Medicine, Philadelphia, Pennsylvania

GERALD M. HAASE, M.D.
Assistant Clinical Professor of Surgery, University of Colorado Health Science Center, Chairman, Department of Pediatric Surgery, Children's Hospital, Denver, Colorado

ROBERT E. HERMANN, M.D.
Chairman, Department of General Surgery, The Cleveland Clinic Foundation, Cleveland, Ohio

JOHN M. HOWARD, M.D.
Professor of Surgery, Department of Surgery, Division of General Surgery, Medical College of Ohio, Toledo, Ohio

SHUNZABURO IWATSUKI, M.D.
Assistant Professor of Surgery, University of Pittsburgh, Pittsburgh, Pennsylvania

RAYFORD SCOTT JONES, M.D.
Stephen H. Watts Professor and Chairman, Department of Surgery, Surgeon-in-Chief, University of Virginia Medical Center, Charlottesville, Virginia

FREDERICK M. KARRER, M.D.
Instructor in Surgery, Pediatric Surgical Research Fellow, University of Colorado, Denver, Colorado

KEITH A. KELLY, M.D.,
Roberts Professor of Surgery, Mayo Medical School, Mayo Clinic, Rochester, Minnesota

DAVID KENDALL, B.A.
Medical Student, University of Minnesota, Minneapolis, Minnesota

JOSEPH K. T. LEE, M.D.
Associate Professor of Radiology, Co-Director, Computed Body Tomography Section, Mallinckrodt Institute of Radiology, Washington University School of Medicine, St. Louis, Missouri

JOHN R. LILLY, M.D.
Professor of Surgery, Chief, Pediatric Surgery, University of Colorado School of Medicine, University Hospital, Denver, Colorado

DONALD C. MCILRATH, M.D.
Professor of Surgery, Mayo Medical School, Chairman, Department of Surgery, Mayo Clinic, Rochester, Minnesota

THOMAS A. MILLER, M.D.
Associate Professor of Surgery, University of Texas Medical School, Houston, Texas

FRANK G. MOODY, M.D.
Professor and Chairman, Department of Surgery, The University of Texas Medical School at Houston, Surgeon-in-Chief, Hermann Hospital, Houston, Texas

A. RAHIM MOOSSA, M.D., F.R.C.S., F.A.C.S.
Professor and Chairman, Department of Surgery, University of California, San Diego, California

TAKUO MURAKAMI, M.D.
Visiting Clinician, Mayo Clinic, Rochester, Minnesota, Assistant Professor, 2nd Surgical Division of Yamaguchi University School of Medicine, Ube, Japan

DAVID L. NAHRWOLD, M.D.
Loyal and Edith Davis Professor of Surgery, Chairman, Department of Surgery, Northwestern University Medical School, Surgeon-in-Chief, Northwestern Memorial Hospital, Chicago, Illinois

JOHN S. NAJARIAN, M.D.
Professor and Chairman, Department of Surgery, University of Minnesota Hospitals, Minneapolis, Minnesota

LLOYD M. NYHUS, M.D.
Warren H. Cole Professor and Head, Department of Surgery, University of Illinois College of Medicine at Chicago, Surgeon-in-Chief, University of Illinois Hospital, Chicago, Illinois

W. SPENCER PAYNE, M.D.
James C. Masson Professor of Surgery, Mayo Medical School, Consultant in Thoracic Surgery, Mayo Clinic, Rochester Methodist Hospital, St. Marys Hospital, Rochester, Minnesota

ALICE R. PEREZ, M.D.
Fellow, Gastrointestinal Research, Department of Surgery, Temple University Hospital, Philadelphia, Pennsylvania

HENRY A. PITT, M.D.
Associate Professor of Surgery, UCLA School of Medicine, Los Angeles, California

JOHN H. C. RANSON, B.M., B.CH.
Professor of Surgery, New York University Medical School, Attending Surgeon, New York University Hospital, New York, New York

JONATHAN E. RHOADS, M.D.
Professor of Surgery, Department of Surgery, University of Pennsylvania School of Medicine, Philadelphia, Pennsylvania

HARRY M. RICHTER III, M.D.
Department of Surgery, Cook County Hospital, Chicago, Illinois

LAYTON F. RIKKERS, M.D.
Professor and Chairman, Department of Surgery, University of Nebraska College of Medicine, Omaha, Nebraska

WALLACE P. RITCHIE, JR., M.D., PH.D.
Professor and Chairman, Department of Surgery, Temple University Hospital, Philadelphia, Pennsylvania

JOEL J. ROSLYN, M.D.
Assistant Professor of Surgery, UCLA School of Medicine, Los Angeles, California

JOHN L. SAWYERS, M.D.
John Clinton Foshee Distinguished Professor of Surgery and Chairman, Department of Surgery, Vanderbilt University School of Medicine, Surgeon-in-Chief, Vanderbilt University Hospital, Nashville, Tennessee

KENNETH W. SHARP, M.D.
Assistant Professor of Surgery, Vanderbilt School of Medicine, Attending Physician, Vanderbilt University Hospital, Veterans Administration Medical Center, Nashville, Tennessee

BYERS W. SHAW, JR., M.D.
Assistant Professor of Surgery, University of Pittsburgh, Attending Physician, Presbyterian-University Hospital, Children's Hospital, Pittsburgh, Pennsylvania

CHARLES M. SHEAFF, M.D., PH.D.
Clinical Assistant Professor of Surgery, University of Illinois Medical Center, Associate Attending in Surgery, Northwest Community Hospital, Arlington Heights, Illinois

RICHARD L. SIMMONS, M.D.
Professor of Surgery, University of Minnesota, Rochester, Minnesota

DAVID B. SKINNER, M.D.
Dallas B. Phemister Professor of Surgery, The University of Chicago, Chairman, Department of Surgery, The University of Chicago Medical Center, Chicago, Illinois

THOMAS C. STARZL, M.D., PH.D.
Professor of Surgery, University of Pittsburgh, Pittsburgh, Pennsylvania

ROSS E. J. STIMPSON, M.D., F.R.C.S.(C)
Fellow in Gastrointestinal Surgery, University of California, San Francisco, San Francisco, California

WILLIAM E. STRODEL, M.D.
Associate Professor of Surgery, University of Michigan, Ann Arbor, Michigan

DAVID E. R. SUTHERLAND, M.D., PH.D.
Associate Professor of Surgery, University of Minnesota, Minneapolis, Minnesota

RONALD K. TOMPKINS, M.D., M.SC., F.A.C.S.
Professor of Surgery, UCLA School of Medicine, Chief, Division of General Surgery, UCLA Medical Center, Los Angeles, California

VICTOR F. TRASTEK, M.D.
Instructor, Cardiovascular and Thoracic Surgery, Mayo Medical School, Rochester, Minnesota

ERIC vanSONNENBERG, M.D.
Assistant Professor of Radiology and Medicine, University of California, San Diego, Assistant Professor in Residence, Department of Radiology and Medicine, USCD Medical Center, V.A. Medical Center, San Diego, California

ALEXANDER J. WALT, M.B., CH.B., F.R.C.S., F.R.C.S(C), F.A.C.S.
Penberthy Professor of Surgery and Chairman, Department of Surgery, Wayne State University School of Medicine, Chief of Surgery, Harper-Grace Hospitals, Attending Surgeon, Detroit Receiving Hospital, Detroit, Michigan

W. DEAN WARREN, M.D.
Joseph Brown Whitehead Professor and Chairman, Department of Surgery, Emory University School of Medicine, Atlanta, Georgia

ANDREW L. WARSHAW, M.D.
Associate Professor of Surgery, Harvard Medical School, Associate Visiting Surgeon, Massachusetts General Hospital, Boston, Massachusetts

LAWRENCE W. WAY, M.D.
Professor of Surgery, University of California, San Francisco, Chief, Surgical Service, Veterans Administration Medical Center, San Francisco, California

JOHN P. WELCH, M.D., F.A.C.S.
Associate Professor of Surgery, University of Connecticut School of Medicine, Adjunct Assistant Professor of Surgery, Dartmouth Medical School, Associate Surgeon, Hartford Hospital, Hartford, Connecticut, Consultant Surgeon, Newington V.A. Hospital, Newington, Connecticut

GERHARD R. WITTICH, M.D.
Assistant Professor of Radiology, University of California, San Diego, Department of Radiology, San Diego, California

ALBERT E. YELLIN, M.D.
Professor of Surgery, University of Southern California School of Medicine, Chief Physician and Director, Vascular Surgery Service, Los Angeles County–USC Medical Center, Hospital of the Good Samaritan, Kenneth Norris Jr. Cancer Hospital, Los Angeles, California

Foreword

DISEASES of the digestive tract have concerned physicians since the dawn of history. Surgeons are recent participants, for their important contributions have occurred only in the past century. However, modern surgery, fueled by an enormous increase in knowledge, is a product chiefly of the past two decades. The editors' intent is to collate and assess this pertinent material—material that is so extensive that they believe a new type of specialist must be recognized.

Digestive Surgeons describe this new breed. The term may be awkward but at least it is brief. This brevity should not deceive the reader; the concept is far more inclusive. Study of this book will elucidate the characteristics of the digestive surgeon, detail the subsidiary disciplines with which he must be familiar, and, for every reader, present the fascinating material that suggests this specialty actually is mature enough to merit special designation.

The past decade has witnessed further blurring of the boundaries between gastroenterology and digestive surgery. Both groups have espoused endoscopy with great enthusiasm. The fruits of clinical and experimental research that arise from all laboratories immediately become common knowledge. On the other hand, if a degree of chauvinism may be permitted, the surgeon holds the ultimate weapons against many types of gastrointestinal disease. But to wield this awesome power, he must be familiar with all the benefits other disciplines can offer.

Judging from this book, from the editors' choice of contributors, and from the content of the chapters, this new type of surgeon actually is emerging. The leaders are those who are equally at home in the operating room or in the laboratory. They pay relatively little attention to historical references, and opinions recorded more than two decades ago often fail to pass muster. Certainly older surgeons relied heavily on empiricism, tended to magnify impressions into facts, and blindly followed courses that had outlived their usefulness. Today, prospective controlled clinical studies that preferably are based on successful experiments in the laboratory are recognized as the most likely means by which truths may be identified.

The contributors, who are teachers and often serve as models for this new type of surgeon, conform to this mold and display a wide variety of interests. Gastroenterology, radiology, and endoscopy emerge as the most important related disciplines. Gastroenterologists have been stimulated by many new drugs, of which the H2 antagonists are the most important. Radiologists, both diagnostic and therapeutic, have developed body scans, computerized tomography, interventional radiology, angiography, and nuclear magnetic resonance. Endoscopists probe the entire gastrointestinal tract except for the mid small intestine, and from information they have acquired, they rewrite statistics, simplify therapeutic decisions, and promise to exert a tremendous influence on the mortality of colorectal cancer. Nor have surgeons remained static; major advances are apparent in the surgery of nearly every digestive organ.

In addition, etiology, epidemiology, and medical economics vie with the usual subjects for attention. Descriptive pathology bows to physiology of the normal and abnormal. Surgical procedures and techniques are considered in only a few chapters, for the book is not an atlas.

The knowledge provided by all of these disciplines must be synthesized by every surgeon who chooses to employ his skills in each individual case. The task is formidable even for the established surgeon because discoveries occur every day. Younger surgeons and medical students will find these decisions more difficult and often frustrating; to reduce this confusion the editors stress the overuse of laboratory examinations and suggest methods by which they can be reduced in number. It is well to remember that an excellent history and physical examination are far more valuable than many laboratory tests.

Finally, this book, though designed primarily for surgeons, deserves a far wider audience. It is no secret that the benefits of operative procedures often are not recognized by many physicians. The editors and contributors have demonstrated that no one need remain ignorant of the advantages of modern day gastrointestinal surgery or of the factual foundation upon which surgical decisions must be made.

CLAUDE E. WELCH, M.D.
EMERITUS CLINICAL PROFESSOR OF SURGERY
HARVARD MEDICAL SCHOOL
BOSTON, MASSACHUSETTS

Preface

FOR OVER a hundred years, the abdominal cavity and its contents has been the spawning ground for surgeons. Many of the early advances in anesthesia, fluid and electrolyte therapy, control of sepsis, and principles of surgical technique are derivative from the demands of surgically treating the gastrointestinal tract and its appendages, the liver and pancreas. New and advancing technology allows precise diagnosis and treatment of diseases of the digestive organs by methods that do not require formal surgical intervention by thoracotomy or laparotomy. This has generated a higher standard for precision and quality for surgeons who work in this area.

Surgical Treatment of Digestive Disease is designed to be an authoritative source of current knowledge and techniques applicable to the diagnosis, treatment, and prevention of surgically amenable diseases of the digestive organs. Emphasis has been placed on the presentation of alternative approaches to complex problems in the treatment of digestive disease, with a focus on efficacy and safety. The details of surgical technique are provided when appropriate to the topic. In the opinion of the editors, technique continues to be the single most important component of therapy once a precise diagnosis has been made. The section editors, expert in their own right, have selected authors who are not only authorities in their field, but known to be articulate and timely communicators of their knowledge and skills. Only you, the reader, will know whether we have succeeded in serving your needs in digestive surgery.

I wish to acknowledge the tireless efforts of the section editors and their editorial assistants, and the authors and their staffs. A special word of appreciation to my colleague, Maryalice Hoogland, who deserves the credit for the high editorial standard achieved in this book. And to Daniel J. Doody and his staff at Year Book Medical Publishers, our heartfelt thanks for providing us with the opportunity to preach our gospel.

On behalf of the Editors: Larry C. Carey, R. Scott Jones, Keith A. Kelly, David L. Narhwold, and David B. Skinner.

FRANK G. MOODY, M.D.

Contents

PART VIII. INVITED COMMENTARIES

PART I

Special Considerations in Digestive Disease

1

Surgical Consultation in Digestive Disease

Frank G. Moody, M.D.

The board-certified* general surgeon is often called on during the diagnosis and treatment of digestive disease to render an appropriate course of action. Consultation is sometimes requested during the acute or late stages of an illness, when prompt operative intervention is essential for a successful outcome. More commonly, the patient requiring a surgical opinion has a chronic problem that may benefit from an operative approach. The recommendation of a surgical procedure in this situation will depend on the relative safety and efficacy of the proposed operation as compared to other less aggressive therapeutic interventions.

Until recently, the question of appropriateness of a surgical option involved primarily an assessment of the risk-benefit ratio. Contemporary therapeutic decisions however, include a cost-benefit factor that as yet has not been clearly defined in either economic or ethical terms. In 1982, Congress passed a law enacting DRGs—diagnosis-related groups. Will Medicare fees based on DRGs control hospital costs? There has been much written, both pro and con, on this issue.[1-4] (See also the editorial by P. Drucker, *Wall Street Journal*, July 5, 1984.) The public's interest in this matter dictates that it will continue to be important in this country. This book addresses these economic issues in only a peripheral manner. Rather, the focus is on the current state of knowledge and technology for the surgical treatment of digestive disease. The validity of its contents must be borne by the credibility of the authors, all of whom are well-known experts in their fields. They have been asked to express their opinions and preferences, supported by their own experience and that reported by others.

The following discussion concerns four issues: (1) the qualifications of the digestive surgeon; (2) the ingredients of a proper consultation; (3) the sequencing of tests; and (4) the timing and selection of operative interventions. A more generic discussion is offered as a stimulus for thought and future discussions as to how surgical services might best be provided to patients with gastrointestinal (GI) illness.

THE DIGESTIVE SURGEON

For the most part, surgeons who treat diseases of the digestive tract are trained in the discipline of general surgery. Such surgeons may have received a year or more of training in a specialized area of esophageal, GI, hepatobiliary, pancreatic, or colorectal surgery, but the majority of board-certified general surgeons have gained their knowledge of digestive disease during their five years of surgical residency. This experience is usually sufficient for the surgical management of about 80% of digestive illnesses that are amenable to surgical therapy. More complex problems, such as esophageal disease, biliary stricture, hepatic and pancreatic neoplasms, pancreatitis, portal hypertension, and inflammatory bowel disease, are examples in which arriving at a valid opinion may require consulting an expert in the treatment of the specific disease in question. General surgeons, as is true for physicians in general, should seek out the very best opinion and care for their patients. This is easy to accomplish, with the availability of almost instantaneous communication by telephone with those who are known to have experience with the disease in question. It is difficult, however, to identify those who are expert in GI surgery, since training programs devoted to the digestive tract, except for colorectal surgery, do not exist in this country.

Should there be training programs specifically designed for the development of a specialist in digestive surgery? Surgical gastroenterology is a specialty in one third of the European countries, where two to five years of additional training are required after a general surgical residency.[5] Further delineation of specialization in this area has not been well received in the United States in view of the potential for further fragmentation of general surgery. Unfortunately, digestive surgery is already fragmented—from within by the disciplines of thoracic, vascular, oncologic, and trauma surgery, and from without by gastroenterologists, endoscopists, and radiologists. One might argue that there remains a need for surgeons who are knowledgeable in the diagnosis and treatment of those digestive diseases that are diagnosed or treated by operative means. This point of view may provoke the specialists who view the surgeon as a technical participant in the treatment of disorders of the GI tract. On the other hand, with advanced education and training in this area, surgeons might contribute a great deal to the knowledge base of gastroenterology, since they have the opportunity to view the disturbed organ directly and to remove it if the situation demands. Furthermore, the digestive disease surgeon with special knowledge and skills may provide more effective and safer therapy the first time around in patients with complex problems. In

---

*"Board-certified" refers to standards established by the American Board of Surgery. Throughout this book, "general surgeon" will mean "board certified."

fact, there has been an evolution toward the identification of the well-skilled individuals in each community to whom the "tough" cases are referred. They usually are surgeons who by practice or by training have gained special expertise and knowledge in this field. Silen,[6] in discussing this matter, has stated: ". . . Surgery and gastroenterology are so intimately entwined as to be often inextricable from each other . . . Small attempts have been made [in the U.S.] to combine training efforts in these areas, and these should certainly be encouraged." My own personal view is that the field of general surgery would clearly benefit from the development of accredited educational programs in surgical gastroenterology.

THE SURGICAL CONSULTATION

Most patients who need an operative approach to their problem are seen and evaluated initially by their family physician. This is an appropriate starting point. But it should not be a stopping point if the problem is not quickly identified and resolved. Gastrointestinal symptoms are common, often bland, and ill defined. Unfortunately, the most serious of digestive problems may present as vague complaints of indigestion or change in bowel habit. It is commonplace for weeks or months to pass before a diagnosis of gastric or pancreatic cancer is made. Occasionally, years will go by before colon cancer, a potentially curable GI neoplasm, is detected. For these reasons patients with persistent GI complaints should be carefully evaluated and referred to a specialist in the treatment of digestive disorders if the initial work-up is nonrevealing but the symptoms persist.

Now, for the key question: Who should the patient be referred to, and who is qualified to render an opinion? Obviously, the case should be referred to the individual who has an established reputation of knowing the most about the disease in question. For example, the GI surgeon is best qualified to diagnose and treat acute pancreatitis. This is a disease that requires hospitalization, critical care, and occasionally intervention for the treatment of gallstones or the life-threatening complications of acute pancreatitis. Obstructive jaundice also falls into the area of competence of the digestive surgeon, as do bleeding esophageal varices, the complications of peptic ulcer, inflammatory bowel disease, intestinal obstruction, and neoplasms of the esophagus, GI tract, hepatobiliary tree, and the pancreas. What of appendicitis, acute cholecystitis, traumatic visceral injury, or diverticulitis? Well-trained general surgeons who have kept up their skills and knowledge in these areas are capable of handling such acute surgical problems. It is the complex problems that present the therapeutic dilemma of selecting and performing an appropriate, safe intervention. The skilled digestive surgeon should have no need for special recognition by certification. These individuals would be easily recognized by their results as a consequence of their special training. Nor would there be a need for large numbers of such professionals, since their superior skills and knowledge would cater to relatively rare diseases in the general community.

The preceding discussion reveals my bias: formal training programs should be established for surgeons who plan to devote their careers to digestive surgery. These individuals, true surgical gastroenterologists, should be expert in the diagnostic techniques of imaging and endoscopy and highly skilled in operating on the digestive system. They would do their work in large community hospitals or academic medical centers where complex cases even now tend to be concentrated.

TIMING OF THE SURGICAL CONSULTATION

When should the surgeon's opinion be obtained? The answer to this question would vary according to the urgency of the problem and the expertise of the family physician or internist. For example, a patient with a perforated ulcer or massive upper GI bleeding may bypass their physician and present immediately to an emergency center. A surgical consultation should be obtained early in all acute GI emergencies that involve perforation, obstruction, bleeding, or inflammation of the intra-abdominal viscera. When a patient presents with signs of peritonitis, the GI surgeon is not likely to be consulted primarily. Most general surgeons can effectively manage the problem of the acute abdomen, as well as massive bleeding from the GI tract. The definitive treatment of bleeding esophageal varices, however, might best be conducted by a surgeon with special knowledge and training in the treatment of cirrhosis and complications of portal hypertension.

A referring physician usually consults a surgeon for a specific opinion about whether surgical intervention will either help to clarify the diagnosis or contribute to an improvement or cure of the patient's condition. The opinion rendered by the surgical consultant must therefore be both specific and precise, for the recommendation is most likely to form the basis of definitive therapy. In acute illness, an aggressive management plan may have to be formulated quickly. It is important to initiate resuscitative efforts early, even when the diagnosis is obscure. Most referring physicians appreciate the consultant's involvement in supportive or preparative therapy at the time of consultation.

In less acute situations, especially when the digestive tract has been previously operated on, it is important to obtain as much of the prior operative and hospital record as possible. Telephone communication with the referring physician is often most helpful in gaining relevant bits of information. The consultant has the responsibility of either making the diagnosis and initiating therapy or sending the patient along to someone who can. It is a mistake, and possibly unethical, to pursue a problem with which one has little knowledge or experience. Surgical meddling has unfortunately been a negative legacy of our concern with maintaining the prerogatives of the broadly competent but less than expert generalist in American medicine. Further definition of expected outcomes and the establishment of high standards of care in digestive disease should, in the years ahead, catalyze the formal training of the surgical gastroenterologist.

DIAGNOSTIC SEQUENCING

The rapid proliferation of ways to assess the structure and function of the digestive system has provided an excess of diagnostic options that have led to inconvenience for the patient and inordinate expense for the health care system in America. This new technology, however, offers a precision in diagnosis previously not available to those who treat digestive disease. Identification of the pathologic process and its associated anatomical deformity is of vital importance to the surgeon who plans an operative intervention. Detailed knowledge of the primary and associated diseases allows for a planned operation with few surprises and a predictable outcome. The comments below focus on two areas of the organization of a diagnostic approach: (1) the availability and sequencing of tests and (2) the process of decision making.

Organizing the Diagnostic Work-Up

The case history remains one of the most useful tools in diagnosis of digestive disease. A surgical consultant should carefully review with the patient every detail of the illness.[7] Consider a patient referred with jaundice and gallstones. A case of this type brings up numerous questions. Are the gallstones symptomatic? Is the jaundice related to the gallstones? Does the patient have hepatitis and, if so, from what cause? A carefully directed history will provide answers not only to these questions, but also will lead to the appropriate diagnostic plan. Furthermore, it will help to avoid the performance of an ill-advised or harmful surgical intervention. For example, in a jaundiced patient, a history of chronic alcoholism may lead to a completely different conclusion than a history of chills and fever in association with a severe episode of upper abdominal pain.

The art of physical examination is also of great importance in the diagnosis of diseases of the intra-abdominal viscera. The quality of bowel sounds or their absence may serve to distinguish intestinal obstruction from an adynamic ileus. Palpitation for visceral or peritoneal tenderness may be a lifesaving maneuver in such a mundane disease as acute appendicitis. It is not my intent to belabor the issue. The message is clear and simple; to be successful, the digestive surgeon must perfect his or her skills in the art of physical diagnosis. This is an important discipline in the process of evaluation, since it sets the stage for selection of appropriate tests and timing of therapy. The sampling of blood, GI secretions, and feces, and endoscopy, diagnostic imaging, manometry, and histologic examination represent techniques that help to make a specific diagnosis of digestive disease, and they also provide information on the general health of the patient. An abbreviated list of helpful blood studies with their unique area of usefulness is shown in Table 1–1. I have found the hemogram and liver-related serum analyses to be the most helpful in determining the acuity of illness (white blood cell count) and the general state of nutrition (hemoglobin, albumin). Stool guaiac analysis is an essential component of a physical examination. Analysis of gastric and pancreatic secretions and bile are not used except in special cases where unique diseases of the respective organ systems are suspected. Examples of diseases in which secretory tests might be helpful are listed in Table 1–2.

Endoscopy of either the upper or lower GI tract has emerged as a prime diagnostic tool. In fact, it is so precise in the detection of lesions of the gut epithelium (ulcers and neoplasms) that it may currently be overutilized in the search for an explanation of commonplace symptoms. The value of en-

TABLE 1–1.—SPECIFIC DIAGNOSTIC BLOOD STUDIES IN SURGICAL TREATMENT OF DIGESTIVE DISEASE

TEST	DISEASE
Alkaline phosphatase	Mechanical cholestasis
Albumin	Chronic liver disease
α-Fetoprotein	Hepatoma
Amylase	Pancreatitis
Antinuclear antibodies	Primary biliary cirrhosis
Carcinoembryonic antigen	Colon cancer
Gastrin	Zollinger-Ellison syndrome
Glucagon	Glucagonoma
Hemogram	Gastrointestinal bleeding
Indirect bilirubin	Hemolytic anemia
Insulin	Insulinoma
Transaminase	Hepatitis
Vasoactive polypeptide	Vipoma
White blood cell count	Inflammation

TABLE 1–2.—SAMPLING OF BODY FLUIDS IN DIGESTIVE DISEASE

TEST	DISEASE
Gastric analysis	Peptic ulcer
Duodenal drainage (Melzer-Lyons)	
Cholecystokinin	Gallstones
Secretin	Chronic pancreatitis
Stool analysis	
Volume and electrolytes	Secretory diarrhea
White blood cells	Inflammatory bowel disease
Ova and parasites	Infectious diarrhea
Guaiac	Colon cancer
Urine analysis	
5-HIAA	Carcinoid
(5-hydroxyindoleacetic acid)	

doscopy in the detection and treatment of hepatobiliary and pancreatic disease will be discussed in chapter 3. I recommend its use early in patients with dysphagia, upper GI bleeding, and vague upper GI complaints that persist and are associated with weight loss. Furthermore, endoscopic contrast visualization (ERCP) in suspected biliary and pancreatic disease is essential in the evaluation of chronic upper abdominal pain.

The array of techniques available for imaging the digestive tract and its appendages is shown in Table 1–3. Ultrasound has emerged as one of the most useful and risk-free tests for evaluation of the hepatobiliary tree, the pancreas, and other retroperitoneal organs. Computed tomography, while quite precise for evaluation of the liver and the peripancreatic area, is more expensive, requires radiation, and is generally less available. Radionuclide scanning has also emerged as a sensitive means for assessing the patency of the biliary tract in the jaundiced patient, as well as the mechanisms of gastroesophageal reflux, duodenogastric reflux, and the rate of gastric emptying. Manometric techniques have provided ways to assess sphincter function from the cricopharyngeus to the anus. What then is the role of conventional barium contrast radiography of the gut? Clearly, a carefully performed barium swallow, or barium enema, remains the most convenient, simplest, and safest way to assess the configuration of the gut. The major problem is sensitivity. Barium studies often fail to

TABLE 1–3.—Imaging Techniques
in Digestive Disease

Barium roentgenogram	Intraluminal and adjacent diseases of the esophagus and gastrointestinal tract
Upright chest roentgenogram	Perforated viscus Subdiaphragmatic abscess
Plain abdominal roentgenogram	Intra-abdominal abscess Intestinal obstruction Biliary enteric fistula Calcific pancreatitis Opaque gallstones
Biliary scan	Acute cholecystitis Biliary obstruction Biliary fistula Duodenogastric reflux

Radionuclide scan
  Esophageal
  Gastric
  Hepatic
	
	Reflux esophagitis
	Gastric anatomy
	Liver tumors

Percutaneous transhepatic cholangiogram	Biliary obstruction Biliary lithiasis
Ultrasound	Gallstones Biliary obstruction Pancreatic disease Intra-abdominal abscess
Computed tomography	Liver abscess Liver tumors Pancreatic disease Intra-abdominal tumors
Endoscopic retrograde cholangiopancreatography	Biliary-pancreatic disease
Oral cholecystogram	Gallbladder disease

TABLE 1–4.—Histologic Sampling
Techniques in Digestive Disease

Percutaneous thin-needle biopsy
  Ultrasound guided
  CT scan guided
  Peritoneoscope, direct or guided
Percutaneous thin-needle aspiration
  (guided as above)
Transendoscopic biopsy or aspiration
Direct biopsy or aspiration
Brush cytology (transendoscopic, percutaneous, or direct)
Gastric washings (cytology)
Special stains
Immunofluorescence
Ultrastructural analysis
"Touch" preparations
Histochemical analysis
Radioactography

detect the early or subtle lesion. Possibly double contrast barium radiography will improve the reliability of GI evaluation by this means in the future.

Histologic diagnosis of digestive disease has been greatly enhanced by the techniques listed in Table 1–4. Direct transendoscopic biopsy has evolved as a most precise way to diagnose intraluminal lesions of the gut. Cytology by either aspiration or brushing through the endoscope, or percutaneous thin-needle or transhepatic catheter, provides the most sensitive means for making a diagnosis of bile duct cancer. Direct percutaneous thin-needle aspiration cytology under CT control is currently the most precise way to obtain a tissue diagnosis of hepatobiliary or pancreatic cancer. These indeed are remarkable technical advances that provide essential information for the treatment of complex lesions of the GI tract.

Diagnostic Sequencing

The sequencing of tests is an important issue in this age of cost awareness in medicine. In fact, seeking the most direct route to diagnosis has always been a prime goal of the concerned physician. Medical folklore is replete with apocryphal stories of the professor diagnosing a difficult case after listening to the history and uncovering a previously overlooked finding on physical examination. Modern clinical practice demands confirmation of even the most informed, presumed diagnosis. As a rule of thumb, perform the simplest, least invasive, and least costly tests first, and select by deduction. By that, I mean select the test or combination of tests that are

most likely to confirm your diagnosis. For example, if you suspect acute cholecystitis, a WBC count, serum amylase and liver chemistries, and an ultrasound of the gallbladder, pancreas, and biliary tree will usually suffice to reveal gallstones and the status of the pancreas and biliary tree. The next step is surgery. Barium studies should be delayed in cases of chronic abdominal pain, where percutaneous transhepatic retrograde endoscopic or CT imaging of the hepatobiliary tree or pancreas is anticipated. The same is true for patients with massive lower GI bleeding who may require angiography for identification of the source of bleeding. Barium can be especially difficult to clear from the GI tract of the elderly, or in those patients who have an ileus as a component of their underlying disease.

Barium studies of the GI tract are most helpful in assessing vague GI symptoms that may or may not have an organic basis. For example, patients with a chronic complaint of constipation should have three sequential heme-occult stool examinations, a sigmoidoscopy, and a barium enema. I prefer a barium upper GI examination when patients complain of chronic dyspepsia, heartburn, or dysphagia. A carefully performed barium examination of the small bowel can be most helpful in cases of chronic midabdominal pain, diarrhea, and weight loss where Crohn's disease or neoplasm of the small bowel is suspected.

Difficult problems in diagnosis or management may require a full array of diagnostic procedures. For example, a patient with obstructive jaundice may receive an ultrasound to assess the gallbladder and bile ducts, CT scan to view the liver and pancreas, and an ultrasonic or CT-guided thin-needle aspiration cytologic examination or biopsy. Endoscopic retrograde cholangiopancreatography with aspiration and brush cytology may be performed if the diagnosis is still in doubt. Visceral angiography may help to determine operability vis-à-vis vessel encasement if a lesion in the pancreas is identified. One might argue that information derived from the above studies can be more easily obtained at operation, but this is contrary to my experience. It is often difficult to distinguish neoplastic lesions from inflammatory lesions of the hepatobiliary tree and pancreas. Furthermore, a precise histologic diagnosis and preoperative staging allows a more expeditious performance of biliary drainage by a percutaneous or transendoscopic endoprosthesis, internal biliary-enteric fistula, or reconstruction following a curative resection. A diagnostic-procedure matrix for several common disease states is provided in Table 1–5.

Therapeutic Options

The selection of appropriate therapy requires an understanding of the normal function of the afflicted organ and its unique role in the process of digestion. Knowledge of the natural history of the disease process is of equal importance in the timing and selection of the optimum intervention. This selection process must include a consideration of associated diseases and of the effect on the patient's occupation and future role in the community at large. As a general rule, an operation with a low risk-benefit ratio and minimal sequelae should be selected. This adage assumes that the risk as well as the benefit is well defined. Cholecystectomy for acute cholecystitis is a good example of an operation with a low risk-benefit ratio and few postoperative sequelae when the operation is performed by an experienced surgeon. On the contrary, pancreaticoduodenectomy is an operation with a high mortality and postoperative morbidity, with questionable benefit to most patients with pancreatic cancer even when performed by a master surgeon.

The background, training, and experience of the surgeon play a critical role in the outcome following an operation. Unfortunately, there is a tendency on the part of the public and the nonsurgeon physician to assume that all surgeons are equally competent. This generalization is close to the truth, in the management of many common GI problems. Most board-certified general surgeons have had an adequate didactic and technical background in the care of digestive problems by operative means. But successful resolution of complex problems within the GI system requires the skills of those who have been taught or who have acquired a unique experience with the recalcitrant disease process. A partial list of problems that require special care is shown in Table 1–6.

The decision-making process is therefore complex—dependent on the disease to be treated, the precision of diagnosis,

TABLE 1–5.—DIAGNOSIS—THERAPEUTIC
OPTION MATRIX

PROCEDURE	TREATMENT
Angiography	Pharmacologic or mechanical hemostasis
Percutaneous transhepatic techniques	Cholangiography External drainage Endoprosthesis Removal of biliary stones
T-Tube manipulation (Burhenne technique)	Removal, biliary stones
Endoscopy	Polypectomy Hemostasis Sclerotherapy, varices Vaterian papillotomy Removal, biliary stones
Percutaneous catheter drainage	Gastrostomy Abscesses Pseudocyst
Hydrostatic barium enema	Reduction-intussusception

TABLE 1–6.—COMPLEX SURGICAL PROBLEMS
IN DIGESTIVE DISEASE

Esophagus
  Cancer
  Dysmotility
  Stricture
  Varices
Stomach
  Cancer
  Zollinger-Ellison syndrome
  Postgastrectomy syndrome
Liver
  Tumors
  Abscess
Bile ducts
  Cancer
  Choledochal cysts
  Intrahepatic stones
  Stenosing papillitis
Pancreas
  Cancer
  Pancreatitis
Gut
  Cancer
  Inflammatory bowel disease
  Pseudo-obstruction
  Fecal incontinence
Morbid obesity

the knowledge and skill of the surgeon, and the general physical and social well-being of the patient. Careful thought must also be given to the risk of the procedure and the disability that may follow. For example, an antrectomy and truncal vagotomy is a sure way to minimize the persistence or risk of recurrence of peptic duodenal ulcer. The possibility of incurring a postgastrectomy syndrome, however, has relegated this effective operation to a secondary role in the treatment of peptic ulcer. Proximal gastric vagotomy, with a nearly nil mortality and morbidity, has emerged as the procedure of choice in medically refractory peptic ulcer disease, even though recurrence rates are in the range of 10%. Modern surgery for peptic ulcer provides an important principle in the management of benign diseases of the digestive system: be conservative! One should select the operative procedure that will provide for the majority of patients a safe return to good health with minimal side effects. This philosophy is especially relevant to the treatment of inflammatory diseases of the bile ducts, pancreas, and small bowel, in which an effort should be made to conserve organ function as long as possible.

It is not my intent to preempt the opinions of the digestive surgeons who have contributed to the authoritative communications within this book. Rather, I have expressed a personal belief of how to approach the diagnosis and how to render an opinion on the appropriate therapy for diseases of the digestive system. The contributions that follow will provide insight into how highly skilled surgeons apply their knowledge and expertise to restore patients with digestive problems to good health. Several chapters deal with methods of preventing the complications of disease elsewhere in the body (morbid obesity) or within the GI tract (postgastrectomy syndromes). The variety and complexity of digestive problems have provided a supreme challenge to the collective wisdom of these authors. From my highly biased point of view, they have achieved their goal of providing an informed, readable, authoritative text on the surgical therapy of digestive disease.

REFERENCES

1. Blendon R.J., Altman D.W.: Special report: Public attitudes about health care costs: A lesson in national schizophrenia. *N. Engl. J. Med.* 311(9):613, 1983.
2. Wennberg J.E., McPherson K., Caper P.: Will payment based on diagnosis-related groups control hospital costs? *N. Engl. J. Med.* 311(5):295, 1983.
3. Carey L.C.: The new ball game (editorial). *Surg. Gastroenterol.* 2(1):3, 1983.
4. Grimaldi P.L., Micheletti J.A.: *Diagnosis Related Groups: A Practitioner's Guide.* Chicago, Pluribus Press, 1983.
5. Emas S.: Gastroenterology in Europe 1983. *Dig. Dis. Sci.* 29(8):758, 1984.
6. Silen W.: Presidential Farewell Address: A surgeon looks at training in gastroenterology. *Gastroenterology* 77:429, 1979.
7. Drossman D.A.: The physician and patient: Review of the psychosocial gastrointestinal literature with an integrated approach to the patient, in Sleisenger M.H., Fordtran J.S. (eds.): *Gastrointestinal Disease: Pathophysiology, Diagnosis, Management.* Philadelphia, W.B. Saunders Co., 1964, pp. 3–20.

2

Special Diagnostic Techniques

Laurence Y. Cheung, M.D.
Joseph K. T. Lee, M.D.

Radiologic procedures have played a large part in the diagnosis of gastrointestinal (GI) disease since the turn of the century. Over the past decade, the development of a host of new diagnostic techniques has greatly extended the importance of radiography in the management of GI disorders. In 1972, Hounsfield announced the development of a CT scanner for clinical radiologic studies, and Hublitz first reported the use of ultrasonography in the detection of gallstones. In 1974, gray-scale ultrasound became commercially available, the same year that thin-needle transhepatic cholangiography was introduced from Japan. Endoscopic retrograde cholangiopancreatography (ERCP) came of age over the same period. Biliary scintiscanning using the technetium 99m-labeled N-substituted iminodiacetic acid compound has been a development of the past ten years. Refinement of these techniques appeared at an astonishing rate. Because of these new diagnostic procedures, many of the older techniques were modified, adapted to new roles, or abandoned.

Although these new diagnostic techniques represent a significant advance, they are expensive, and some involve risks. It will continue to be the clinicians' task, often after consultation with their radiology colleagues, to pick the proper sequence of available tests to arrive at a diagnosis in the most rapid, efficient, and safe manner. To achieve this goal, it is essential that the surgeon, faced with the patient with GI disease, fully understand the capability of each new procedure. He must be able to order the appropriate test(s) with enough confidence in the results not to require a subsequent study solely for confirmation. This chapter will attempt to present the advantages and limitations of selected new diagnostic techniques. A brief description of the clinical use of these procedures in some common GI disorders follows. The objective of these discussions is to provide a rationale for deciding which procedures to use and in what sequence. This is by no means a comprehensive review but is intended to provide the surgeon with a broad conceptual framework within which to develop his diagnostic approaches to these problems.

ULTRASONOGRAPHY

Largely because of its lower cost, ease of performance, and wide availability, ultrasonography has become the procedure of choice in many clinical situations. Ultrasound is based on the electrical production of high-frequency sound waves which, when directed at an anatomical area, are reflected back from tissue-tissue interfaces. The strength of this reflection is based primarily on the relative elasticity and content of collagen of the two tissues. The returning reflected waves are converted into voltage images for graphic display.

Major improvements of this technique have been made in the last few years. From the initial one dimensional A-mode scanners, the technology has progressed through two-dimensional B-mode machines to the gray-scale imager, which provides multiple shades of intensity, and finally to real-time ultrasound or sonofluoroscopy, which allows continuous imaging and display of moving structures. Several recent studies have demonstrated real-time ultrasound to be faster and more convenient than static imaging. In addition, it seems to be more sensitive and specific.[1, 2] The technique is easier to learn and therefore it partially eliminates one of the shortcomings of sonography—its dependence on examiner's experience.[3]

Within the energy range used for diagnostic studies, ultrasonography has no known deleterious biological side effects and causes no genetic damage. Because it uses no ionizing radiation, the technique can be safely employed in pregnant women and children. Patient acceptance is also high, because there is no special preparation required and no discomfort is experienced during the procedure. Ultrasound equipment is relatively inexpensive, and examinations are less costly than CT scans. These advantages make ultrasonography a valuable and useful diagnostic method.

There are several disadvantages of ultrasonography in the diagnosis of GI disease. First, the abdomen cannot be adequately studied when the intestine is full of gas. Therefore, many acutely ill patients are poor subjects for ultrasound studies. Obese patients may also be difficult to study with ultrasound because of the limited penetration of high-frequency sound beams. It may be impossible to use on some surgical patients because of the presence of bulky dressings, open wounds, or drainage tubes. Unlike CT, contrast mediums have not been developed to widen the application of ultrasound study. Although to a lesser degree with the more recent technology, considerable skill is required of the examiner. Therefore, its accuracy depends to some extent on the examiner's experience.

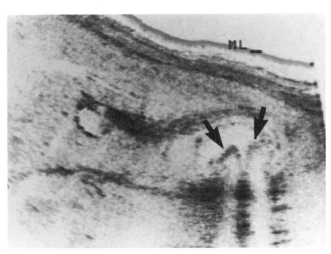

Fig 2–1.—Longitudinal B-mode ultrasound of the gall-bladder from a patient with cholelithiasis. The *arrows* indicate two echogenic gallbladder calculi with strong acoustic shadowing.

Ultrasound is well suited for the evaluation of biliary tract disorders. Oral cholecystography can no longer be considered the "gold standard" in the diagnosis of gallbladder disease. Real-time ultrasonography, being able to visualize the entire gallbladder in most patients, has recently been recommended by many radiologists as the screening procedure of choice (Fig 2–1).[1, 2] Currently, it is indicated in patients with a nonvisualized gallbladder on the oral cholecystogram or in any condition which might result in jaundice, pancreatitis, vomiting, or diarrhea. It is also the procedure of choice for diagnosis of gallbladder disease in children and during pregnancy. Review of a recent series reveals a sensitivity, specificity, and accuracy of greater than 99% in the detection of cholelithiasis.[4] Although biliary scintigraphy is more specific than ultrasound in the diagnosis of acute cholecystitis, its many limitations have allowed sonography to remain an important diagnostic tool for this entity (Fig 2–2).[5] The ability simultaneously to examine other organs, such as the kidneys and pancreas, is a distinct advantage of ultrasound when evaluating patients with right upper quadrant pain suspected of having acute cholecystitis.

Because of its high degree of accuracy in detecting biliary dilatation (Fig 2–3), ultrasound is now the screening procedure of choice for evaluating the jaundiced patient.[6–10] The accuracy of sonography in diagnosing surgical jaundice approaches at least 90%, though false-negatives may occur in partial or early obstruction.[6]

Ultrasound is quite accurate in the detection of focal hepatic lesions (Fig 2–4). Hepatic cysts can be easily differentiated from hepatic abscesses and metastases. Ultrasound is less accurate in the diagnosis of diffuse hepatocellular disease. Although hepatitis, cirrhosis, and fatty infiltration all may cause alterations in hepatic echogenicity, these diseases are often far advanced before they become apparent on sonography.

Ultrasonography is a useful diagnostic method for evaluating both diffuse and focal pancreatic disease. Both a true cyst and a pseudocyst can be identified (Fig 2–5). However, bowel gas may prevent the transmission of the ultrasound beam and obscure a portion of the pancreas. This is especially true in patients with acute pancreatitis, because the associated paralytic ileus increases the amount of bowel gas and the chance of a technically inadequate examination. Ultrasonography is also quite accurate in the detection of intra-abdominal abscesses and other postoperative fluid collections (Fig 2–6).

COMPUTED TOMOGRAPHY

Computed tomography (CT) of the abdomen vies with ultrasonography as the first-line procedural choice in many GI disorders. The machine utilizes multiple fan-shaped, tightly collimated x-ray beams which, after traversing a human body, are collected by an array of scintillation detectors. The data obtained are entered into a computer, which utilizes mathematical algorithms to reconstruct an image based on attenuation coefficients. The CT body scanner allows examination of body tissue as a series of cross-sectional slices of varying thickness (0.2–1.0 cm). The scanning time for one slice has

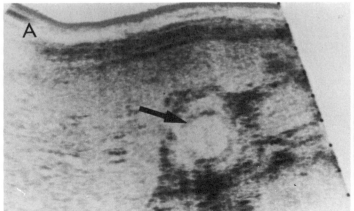

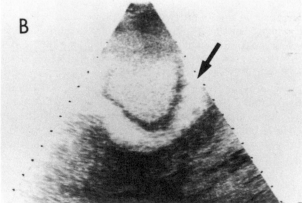

Fig 2–2.—Cholecystitis. **A,** transverse B-mode scan from a patient with acute cholecystitis revealing gallbladder wall thickening to 5 mm *(arrow)*. This was associated with tenderness over the gallbladder fossa. **B,** real-time scan from a patient with acute acalculous disease demonstrating a pericholecystic fluid collection *(arrow)*.

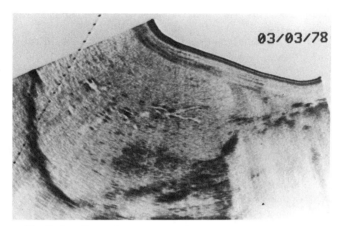

Fig 2–3.—B-mode sonogram from a patient with obstructive jaundice demonstrating intrahepatic biliary dilatation.

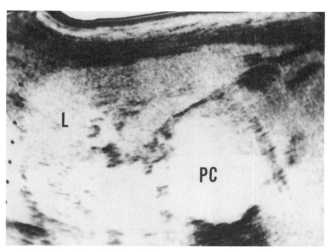

Fig 2–5.—Longitudinal B-mode scan of the upper abdomen demonstrates a large pseudocyst *(PC)* in the head of the pancreas. *L* = liver.

varied from five minutes in the earliest scanners to less than five seconds in recently introduced equipment. This technical improvement not only reduces time for examination but also avoids motion artifacts.

There are several advantages of CT scanning over ultrasonography.[11, 12] One of its most appealing characteristics to surgeons is its reproduction of a concrete, real-to-life anatomical projection that the surgeon can identify and interpret in the operating room. It is not limited by bowel gas, obesity (in fact, it is impaired by extreme cachexia), ascites, or dressings. Resolution is generally excellent, and there is little, if any, artifact in most patients. The use of IV contrast material further increases its ability to detect and characterize many of the intra-abdominal lesions.

Compared with other imaging techniques such as ultrasound, CT also has some disadvantages. It is more expensive and therefore less widely available than ultrasonography. Standard abdominal examinations are about twice as expensive as ultrasonography, and the machine itself is ten times more costly. In addition, it requires a specially shielded room. CT is hampered by dense barium contrast medium and by metallic objects such as clips. It is limited to the transverse

plane and exposes the patient to some radiation (3–5 rad/study).

CT is not used as a screening procedure for evaluating gallbladder disease because ultrasonography is both accurate and easy to perform. Although CT is only slightly more accurate than ultrasound in detecting biliary obstruction, CT is much more accurate than ultrasound in defining the level and etiology of obstruction (Fig 2–7).

CT is not sensitive to the textural change seen with many forms of hepatitis. However, it is accurate in identifying fatty infiltration and changes associated with advanced cirrhosis and in characterizing cysts, abscesses, and neoplasms. These focal hepatic lesions can be identified and often differentiated on the basis of their attenuation value. On the relative scale,

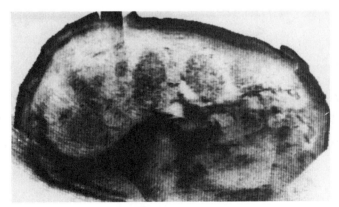

Fig 2–4.—Transverse B-mode scan of the liver revealing multiple hyperechoic lesions compatible with metastases in this patient with known breast cancer.

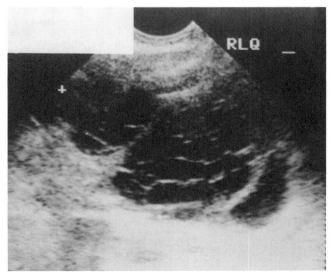

Fig 2–6.—Longitudinal B-mode scan of the right lower quadrant shows a multiloculated fluid collection compatible with an abscess.

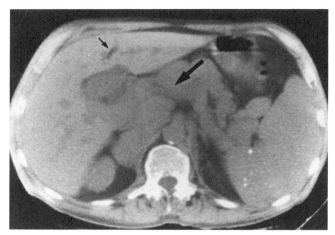

Fig 2–7.—CT of biliary obstruction from a patient with lymphoma demonstrating intrahepatic biliary dilatation *(small arrow)* as a result of obstruction by massive hilar and retroperitoneal adenopathy *(large arrow)*.

0–3 (where 0 is the density of water and 3 is the density of normal liver parenchyma), cysts have a value of 0, abscesses a value about 1, and neoplasm about 2. Primary and metastatic neoplasms appear as focal areas of slightly diminished density within the liver (Fig 2–8). They can be either well circumscribed or poorly marginated. Identification of these lesions may be facilitated after IV administration of water-soluble contrast medium. One recent study by Snow et al.[13] found CT to be the most specific study for detecting hepatic neoplasm, with a reported accuracy and sensitivity greater than 90%. While ultrasound can detect solid lesions of about 2 cm and cystic lesions of 5 mm, CT is sensitive to focal abnormality in the range of 3–5 mm. In addition, like ultrasonography, CT has the advantage over other studies such as liver scintigraphy in providing information about organs and anatomical areas other than the liver. It is also helpful in the evaluation of suspected hepatic trauma (Fig 2–9).

CT is an accurate method for evaluating pancreatic disease, with an overall accuracy ranging from 85% to 95% in most large series.[14–16] The sensitivity of CT for detecting pancreatic carcinomas is higher (88%–94%) than for detecting pancreatitis (9%–81%). This is especially true in patients with chronic pancreatitis, where the pancreas can appear normal on a CT scan. Although the number of reported pseudocysts has been relatively small, the detection rate has been high owing to the ease with which CT can demonstrate low-density cystic masses, regardless of the presence of retroperitoneal fat.

CT has proved useful in the evaluation of intra-abdominal abscess. An abscess cavity appears as an area of low density, often with a rim of enhanced density following IV contrast medium injection. A collection of a gas bubble outside the expected bowel lumen is a more specific CT sign of an abscess.

The retroperitoneal space, one of the least accessible parts of the body to conventional radiography, is displayed with remarkable clarity by CT. CT is extremely helpful in delineating retroperitoneal tumors, abscesses, and diseases arising from the retroperitoneum lymph nodes or blood vessels.

CT evaluation of the spleen should include both pre- and post-contrast scans. Subcapsular hematomas, rupture, abscesses, cysts, and neoplasms all can be identified by CT.

RADIONUCLIDE HEPATOBILIARY SCINTIGRAPHY

Nuclear medicine studies have played an important role in the evaluation of hepatobiliary disorders. With the development of some new radionuclides, their role has been rapidly evolving in the past few years. Although sulfur colloid liver scanning has been available for many years, the use of the new N-substituted iminodiacetic acid agents for biliary imaging is a development of the 1970s. Both of these agents utilize

Fig 2–8.—Postcontrast CT scan demonstrates multiple hypodense hepatic metastases in this patient with a primary colon carcinoma. Splenic metastases were also present.

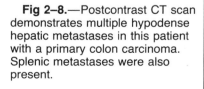
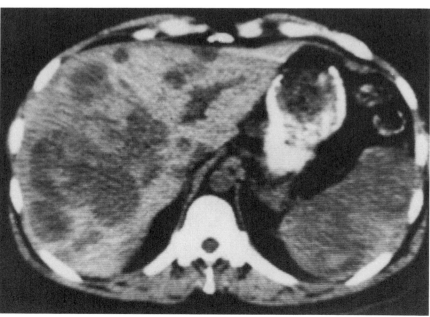

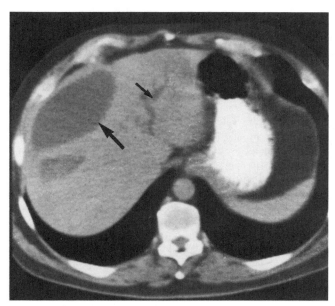

Fig 2–9.—Third-generation CT scan from a jaundiced patient with a traumatic hepatic fracture which extended into the biliary tree. The *large arrow* identifies a hematoma. The *small arrow* points to segmental dilatation of the secondarily obstructed left intrahepatic bile ducts.

organ. Sulfur colloid liver scanning depends on the uptake of sulfur colloid by the reticuloendothelial system of the liver. Biliary imaging studies involve the extraction of the iminodiacetic acid compounds from the blood and the excretion into the biliary tree by the hepatocyte. In recent years, various derivatives of the initial iminodiacetic acid (IDA) prototype have been developed and tested; e.g., HIDA, PIPIDA, DISIDA, and BIDA. These agents vary in the rate and the quantity of their extraction by the hepatocyte, the liver washout time, and the percentage of dose eliminated by the kidney. Search for the ideal biliary contrast agent continues. Currently, the diisopropyl derivative (DISIDA) seems to have the greatest liver uptake and the highest bile concentration at all serum bilirubin levels.[17]

Hepatobiliary scintigraphy studies are rapid, accurate, and less affected by hyperbilirubinemia or pancreatitis than IV cholangiography. The sensitivity of the study in the presence of marked jaundice has not yet been determined, but demonstration of the biliary tree is possible even in patients with serum bilirubin levels up to 30 mg/dl.[18] Although the interpretation of hepatobiliary scintigraphy does depend on the rate of this visualization, marked jaundice most certainly will slow the excretion of the radionuclide. Acute pancreatitis does not seem to influence the study as it does in oral cholecystography. It involves a very low radiation dose. It costs approximately twice oral cholecystography, one and a half times ultrasonography, and slightly less than CT.

The efficacy of these newer agents for hepatobiliary scintigraphy in demonstrating acute cholecystitis has been documented.[19] Visualization of the biliary tree, gallbladder, and duodenum normally occurs within one hour following the injection of contrast agents. Acute cholecystitis is usually accompanied by cystic duct obstruction, which results in nonvisualization of the gallbladder (Fig 2–10). The overall

technetium 99m as the radionuclide. This isotope has a half-life of only six hours, an emission range ideal for gamma camera counting, and an absence of particulate emissions, reducing the overall radiation dosage. For these reasons, this isotope has been found to be particularly useful. Unlike most other imaging procedures, the scintigraphic study provides functional information rather than anatomical display of the

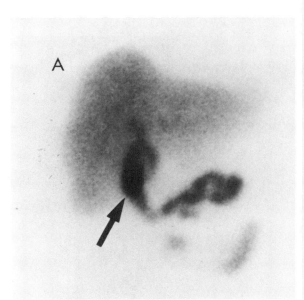
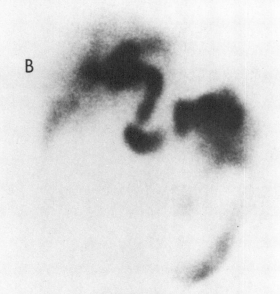

Fig 2–10.—DISIDA biliary scans. **A,** a normal scan at 40 minutes demonstrating the biliary tree, duodenum and gallbladder *(arrow).* **B,** a similar scan at 45 minutes in a patient with acute cholecystitis. There is complete failure to visualize the gallbladder, a finding consistent with cystic duct obstruction.

accuracy for diagnosis of acute cholecystitis has been reported at approximately 95%. The study can occasionally be misleading in cases of acalculous gallbladder disease. Chronic disease is reported to produce delayed visualization. The significance and specificity of delayed visualization in the diagnosis of cholelithiasis and chronic cholecystitis remain problematic. Nonvisualization of the gallbladder occasionally occurs in alcoholics and in patients receiving parenteral nutrition and therefore results in a falsely positive interpretation. Furthermore, hepatobiliary scintigraphy does not provide information regarding other organs as does ultrasonography or CT. Although controversy regarding the choice between ultrasonography and biliary scintigraphy continues for the diagnosis of acute cholecystitis, both techniques are highly accurate, and either can be used for this purpose.

Because radionuclide scintigraphy provides functional information about the biliary tree, it also can be used to assess postoperative bile leaks, traumatic injuries to the biliary system and the patency of biliary enteric anastomosis.

For determining the presence or absence of biliary obstruction, ^{99m}Tc-IDA scintigraphy is not as accurate as ultrasonography or CT. It has a reported accuracy of no more than 85% owing to its failure to identify some instances of partial obstruction. After an initial period of enthusiasm, the role of IDA scintigraphy for the diagnosis of neonatal jaundice has been questioned, and ^{131}I-rose bengal, the older biliary agent, remains the radionuclide of choice for the diagnosis of biliary atresia.

Sulfur colloid liver-spleen scan is used for detecting focal hepatic disease (Fig 2–11). It is able to detect focal lesions of 1–2 cm in diameter near the surface and lesions of 2 cm within the central parenchyma of the liver. Overall, its sensitivity for focal disease is in the range of 80%–90%. Snow et al.[13] recently reported a sensitivity of 94% and a specificity of 67% in detecting hepatic neoplasm. It is a sensitive but nonspecific study for diffuse hepatocellular disease.

PERCUTANEOUS TRANSHEPATIC CHOLANGIOGRAPHY

Although percutaneous transhepatic cholangiography (PTC) was initially introduced in the mid-1930s, it has not gained wide popularity until the last decade because of concern over its complication rate and the poor success in visualizing nondilated biliary ducts.[21] In 1974, Okuda and associates[22] from Chiba University in Japan described their results with a technique using a "skinny" needle. The Chiba needle, a 23-gauge, 15-cm, flexible needle, has significantly reduced the complications of the procedure. The needle is passed transcutaneously deep into the hepatic parenchyma under fluoroscopic guidance. Water-soluble iodinated contrast medium is injected as the needle is withdrawn until a biliary duct is visualized. As many as 12 to 15 passes can be made per examination. Broad-spectrum antibiotics should be given immediately before and after the procedure to prevent cholangitis. The reported success rates are greater than 90% in the presence of dilated intrahepatic ducts and 70% when the ducts are not dilated.

The primary role of PTC is to evaluate obstructive jaundice.[23, 24] One recent review by Mueller and associates described four main advantages for the use of this procedure.[23] First, it can accurately define the site and etiology of the biliary obstruction (Figs 2–12 and 2–13). It has a higher accuracy (approximately 95%) than CT and ultrasonography in ascertaining the site of obstruction. In addition, a specific diagnosis can often be made by examining the pattern of termination (i.e., gradual tapering vs. abrupt termination). Second, PTC provides an excellent view of the proximal biliary tree.[13] This is extremely useful to the surgeon planning some form of surgical intervention. The third advantage of PTC is its ability to determine the cause of obstruction in the jaundiced patient with nondilated ducts.[25] This entity, which has been described in the radiology literature with increasing frequency, has been proposed as the major basis for the occasional failures of ultrasound and CT in differentiating medical from surgical jaundice. It is usually the result of low-grade, partial intermittent obstruction in patients with choledocholithiasis, ampullary stenosis, or sclerosing cholangitis. The fourth major advantage of PTC is to establish drainage subsequent to the cholangiogram. It has been suggested that preoperative drainage may be helpful in the preparation for surgical intervention. It also offers an alternative to surgical drainage in patients with an inoperable lesion.[26] Simultaneous therapeutic interventions with maneuvers such as transhe-

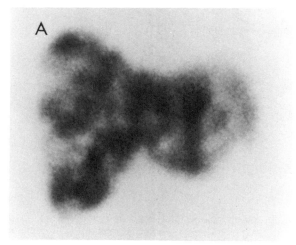
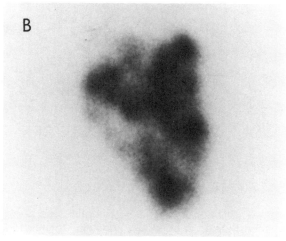

Fig 2–11.—Sulfur colloid liver scan from a patient with metastatic breast cancer demonstrating multiple space-occupying lesions in the anterior **(A)** and lateral **(B)** views.

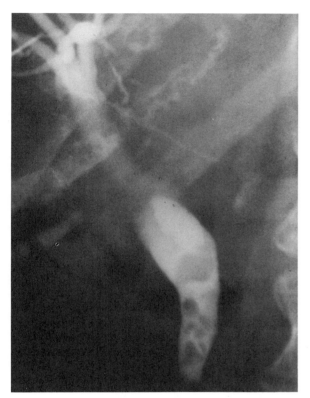

Fig 2–12.—PTC from a patient with choledocholithiasis demonstrating biliary dilatation as a result of obstruction by multiple distal common bile duct stones.

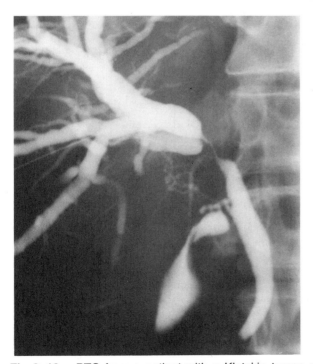

Fig 2–13.—PTC from a patient with a Klatskin tumor, a bile duct carcinoma at the junction of the right and left hepatic ducts. The needle is in the right lobe ductal system, and the contrast fails to visualize the left duct, which is totally obstructed by tumor.

patic stone extraction and balloon dilatation of biliary strictures have made PTC even more attractive.

Complications, though reduced by use of the Chiba needle, still occur in approximately 5% of the patients. These include biliary sepsis, bile peritonitis, hemorrhage, cholangitis, contrast reaction, and pneumothorax. The mortality is approximately 0.2%. Percutaneous cholangiography is contraindicated in the presence of marked ascites or an uncorrectable coagulopathy.

ENDOSCOPIC RETROGRADE CHOLANGIOPANCREATOGRAPHY

Endoscopic retrograde cholangiopancreatography (ERCP) was first described in 1968 by McCune,[27] though the procedure was not widely used until the 1970s, when flexible, side-viewing endoscopes became available.[28–31] The technique sounds relatively simple—the scope is passed into the duodenum, the papilla is located, and the catheter is passed into the common bile duct and the pancreatic duct for injection of iodinated contrast medium (Fig 2–14). However, it requires somewhat more technical skill than the transhepatic cholangiogram. For optimal results, it is best performed in the x-ray suite with a team consisting of an endoscopist, a radiologist, and a technical assistant. Image intensification with television monitor is necessary to control properly the degree of ductal filling. Immediate spot filming capability is essential to record portions of the ductal system that tend to empty rapidly. The procedure is usually more time consuming than PTC, although this is highly variable depending on the expertise of the endoscopist. Visualization of the pancreatic and biliary duct is usually successful in 80%–90% of the patients regardless of the presence or absence of ductal dilatation. In approximately 5%, complications occur, including pancreatitis, a pseudocyst, pancreatic abscess, instrumental injury, sepsis, cholangitis, and aspiration pneumonia. The success and complication rate have been related more closely to the experience of the endoscopist than to any other single factor. The entire procedure costs approximately three times that of per-

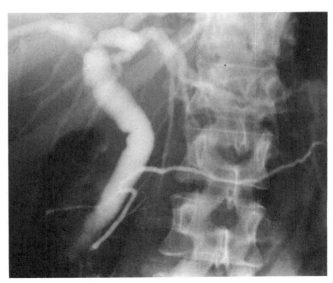

Fig 2–14.—ERCP from a postcholecystectomy patient showing normal biliary anatomy and a clear pancreatogram.

cutaneous cholangiography. ERCP is not contraindicated in patients with coagulopathy or ascites; however, it is contraindicated in patients with hepatitis, because of inherent problems with cleaning the scope, and in patients with pancreatitis.

Prospective analysis has revealed an accuracy rate comparable to that of PTC in the detection of bile duct obstruction and in the localization and identification of its cause (Fig 2–15). Although there is disagreement about which procedure is more valuable (PTC or ERCP), both techniques offer distinct advantages. ERCP permits endoscopic visualization and biopsy of lesions in the upper GI tract. Ampullary carcinoma may be seen and biopsied directly. The visualization of the pancreatic duct is a valuable adjunct to cholangiography because of the close anatomical relationship of the distal common bile duct to the head of the pancreas. The collection of pure pancreatic juice for physiologic and cytologic studies during the course of ERCP can be critical to diagnosis. Finally, endoscopic sphincterotomy with stone removal is a therapeutic vehicle of increasing importance. ERCP does not at all depend on the presence of dilated ducts and therefore is usually the procedure of choice for direct biliary visualization in patients without intrahepatic ductal dilatation. The choice between PTC and ERCP depends on its availability in any given institution, in addition to the advantages and limitations as described above.

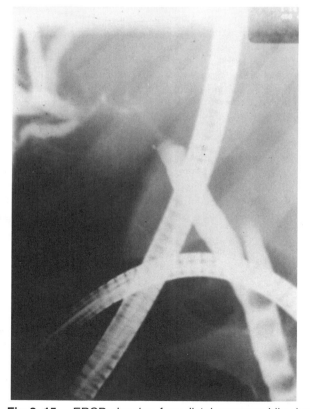

Fig 2–15.—ERCP showing four distal common bile duct stones, the cystic duct remnant, and a more proximal biliary stricture in a postcholecystectomy patient. The intrahepatic biliary tree could not be adequately visualized in this patient.

MAGNETIC RESONANCE IMAGING (MRI)

Since the initial application of magnetic resonance imaging (MRI) of the body, a great deal of enthusiasm and hope has developed within the medical community. While its superiority over existing imaging methods, including CT, in the diagnosis of intracranial and spinal diseases has been established, its utility for the diagnosis of intra-abdominal diseases is not yet proved.

MRI is based on radiowaves emitted by protons which, when they are within a magnetic field, can be excited by the absorption of energy from radiofrequency (RF) pulses. Most of the protons in the human body are within water molecules, and their properties differ from tissue to tissue. The important difference between MRI and other imaging techniques is that it depends not on one single parameter but on multiple parameters, some of which carry a great deal of information. These parameters are: (1) proton density, (2) the tissue relaxation characteristics, and (3) proton bulk motion, which provides information about blood flow.

The advantages of MRI over CT include superior contrast sensitivity, direct multiplaner imaging capability, and the potential for in vivo biochemical studies. The disadvantages include inferior spatial resolution, long imaging time, and patient exclusion owing to claustrophobia or the presence of pacemakers or intracranial aneurysm clips.

Our initial experience with MRI suggests that it is slightly more sensitive than CT for detecting focal hepatic lesions. While hepatic cysts can be differentiated from solid hepatic neoplasms, differentiation between benign and malignant hepatic neoplasms is not yet possible based on MRI criteria. To date, MRI has not proved to be superior to existing imaging techniques in the diagnosis of gallbladder disease, biliary obstruction, and pancreatic and GI pathology. The definitive role of MRI in abdominal imaging awaits further clinical studies.

APPROACHES TO SOME SPECIFIC PROBLEMS

The clinician is faced with the responsibility of choosing the proper procedure for each patient. Each situation is different, and no simple formula can be applied in every case. However, general guidelines for the approach to some of the common surgical problems will be suggested.

Cholelithiasis and Chronic Cholecystitis

In patients with suspected cholelithiasis and chronic cholecystitis, oral cholecystography and ultrasound are the procedures of choice. Oral cholecystography is simple, inexpensive, and easy to perform. All radiology departments possess the capability. It is very accurate when the gallbladder is opacified and stones are seen. However, a second-day study is often required in patients with a nonvisualized gallbladder on the first-day examination. Ultrasound is slightly more expensive and requires more elaborate equipment and a skilled technician. With the development of real-time scanners, the procedure is less operator dependent and faster. It is equal in accuracy to oral cholecystography. The use of either procedure as the diagnostic choice can be justified in most patients.

Ultrasound would be the procedure of choice in pregnant women and in children.

Most surgeons occasionally see a patient with clinically suspected gallbladder disease but in whom both oral cholecystography and ultrasonography are normal. As emphasized by Cole,[32] insufficient attention has been given to these occasional patients. On the other hand, cholecystectomy should not be recommended on clinical grounds alone, since so many other diseases, such as duodenal ulcer, pancreatitis, hiatal hernia, arthritis of spine, liver disease, and irritable bowel, may produce symptoms similar to those of biliary colic. Therefore, other tests are needed to verify gallbladder disease prior to the recommendation of cholecystectomy in these patients. From the information reported in the literature, it seems reasonable to recommend ERCP if a patient's episode of "gallbladder pain" is associated with mild, transient abnormal liver function tests. Venu and colleagues[33] attempted ERCP in 206 patients who had symptoms suggestive of biliary tract disease and had normal results of oral cholecystography and ultrasonography. Of the 195 patients who had successful ERCP, 32 patients had mild and transient abnormalities in liver function tests during an episode of abdominal pain, and 163 had normal liver function tests. Small gallstones were demonstrated on ERCP examination in 25 of the 32 patients in the former group and in 4 of the 163 patients in the latter group. These findings seem to support the recommendation that ERCP examination should be considered for definitive diagnosis in patients with associated abnormal liver function tests. In patients without associated abnormality on liver function tests, it may not be justified to do ERCP, since the incidence of gallstones demonstrated by ERCP in this group of patients is extremely low. For such patients, cholecystokinin cholecystography or analysis of duodenal bile may provide some circumstantial evidence of gallbladder disease.[34–37] One may consider cholecystectomy if the patient's symptoms are characteristic of biliary colic and the results of these tests are positive.

Acute Cholecystitis

In the patient with suspected acute cholecystitis, sonography or cholescintigraphy should be the procedure of choice. Several factors influence the clinician's decision about these techniques. The clinician needs to keep abreast of the availability of each procedure and the skill of the sonographer in the radiology department. The IDA scans have the advantage of providing a specific radiologic diagnosis of cystic duct obstruction. However, chronic cholecystitis may lead to a false positive interpretation. Sonography is less specific. It detects the presence or absence of stones with great accuracy but must rely on the ancillary findings of wall thickness, hypoechoic rim and gas, pericholecystic abscess, and focal tenderness to render such a diagnosis. There has been considerable controversy over significance of wall thickening, the classic finding in acute disease.[38] In one recent study, only 45% of patients with acute cholecystitis had walls thicker than 5 mm.[39] On the other hand, ascites and hypoalbuminemic states can result in increased wall thickness. Sonography is the procedure of choice in the jaundiced patient with suspected acute cholecystitis because sonography also offers a means of assessing ductal dilatation and because scintigraphy is less reliable in the presence of an elevated bilirubin.

Controversy continues in the radiology literature over which procedure should be used in a nonjaundiced patient.[40, 41] Most reports seem to favor sonography, but the use of either examination, with the other as a backup for evaluation of an equivocal result, cannot be criticized. With the availability of sonography and scintigraphy, there is no role for oral cholecystogram or CT scan in the evaluation of acute gallbladder disease. Plain radiographs can reveal emphysematous cholecystitis but otherwise are not very helpful. Intravenous cholangiography has been almost completely replaced by scintigraphy and ultrasound in the evaluation of acute cholecystitis.

Jaundice

Usually, a careful history and physical examination combined with liver function tests will suggest whether jaundice is caused by intrahepatic cholestasis or extrahepatic obstruction. However, these clinical assessments in the differentiation of medical vs. surgical jaundice are not infallible. It is in this diagnostic arena that most of the newer techniques are helpful. Most clinicians and radiologists currently recommend ultrasound as the first procedure in demonstrating ductal dilatation. A prospective study from our institution demonstrated that ultrasound is as accurate as CT in determining the presence or absence of ductal dilatation.[6] CT scan, on the other hand, is more sensitive to isolated dilatation of the extrahepatic system and is clearly more accurate for delineating the level and etiology of the obstruction. Either test is helpful in instances where the other is equivocal. CT is usually recommended if the suspicion of malignancy is high, since it will be helpful for a surgeon to know the level of obstruction and the extent of the tumor. Biliary scintigraphy is useful in evaluating suspected obstruction in the postsurgical patient with a biliary enteric anastomosis. Otherwise, it has no value in the evaluation of jaundice.

In most patients, findings on ultrasound or CT permit a definitive diagnosis. Direct opacification of the bile ducts by one of the invasive methods may be necessary in some patients. The choice between the ERCP and percutaneous cholangiogram is no simpler than that between ultrasound and CT. They have comparable success rates. ERCP is more expensive and requires a somewhat more skillful operator, but offers the additional value of upper endoscopy and the pancreatogram. PTC is somewhat more invasive and cannot be safely performed in patients with coagulopathy. Even when PTC is unsuccessful, it provides indirect evidence for the absence of biliary dilatation. The decision ultimately depends on the clinical suspicion and what portion of the biliary tree is most important to visualize. For a surgeon, a "road map" of the proximal bile duct may be critical in planning surgery. For example, it is frequently necessary to determine the length of common duct proximal to a stricture available for an anastomosis. In this instance, PTC is the most desirable study. It also offers the possibility of percutaneous decompression preoperatively or even as an alternative to surgical drainage. ERCP, on the other hand, allows visualization of the ampulla and pancreatic head region. Therapeutic sphincterotomy and stone extraction may be performed through ERCP.

Focal Hepatic Lesions

Liver scintigraphy with ^{99m}Tc-labeled sulfur colloid has been accepted as the initial radiologic examination for the detection of focal hepatic lesions. It is relatively inexpensive, quick, and widely available. It has a sensitivity of at least 80% for lesions larger than 2 cm.[42] Small, deeply seated lesions may result in false negative radionuclide scans. The overall accuracy of the radionuclide scan in detecting focal hepatic lesions is approximately 80%–85%. The major limitation of radionuclide hepatic imaging is that it cannot evaluate other areas in the abdomen for tumor involvement.

With modern equipment, hepatic sonography is at least as accurate as radionuclide imaging in the detection of focal hepatic lesions.[43] It is comparable in cost and widely available. However, approximately 10% of hepatic sonograms are suboptimal owing to the overlying ribs or occasionally interposed intestinal loops, both of which interfere with transmission of the sonic beam. Ultrasonography also has the advantage of being able to evaluate other portions of the abdomen, including the retroperitoneum, although diagnostic images of these regions are not produced as reliably as by CT.

Computed tomography with a state-of-the-art scanner is the most accurate, noninvasive way of detecting focal hepatic lesions. CT can detect liver metastasis with an accuracy exceeding 95%,[44] although careful attention to technique is required to achieve this level of accuracy. All scans of the liver must be evaluated at several CT window settings. Narrowing the CT window enhances visual perception of small differences in attenuation and thus increases detectability of hepatic lesions. Intravenous administration of contrast medium, preferably as a bolus or a rapid infusion, generally helps in the detection of hepatic lesions. Intravenous contrast medium is used to increase the density difference between normal and abnormal liver parenchyma.

Both CT and ultrasound can differentiate a cystic from a solid lesion. Abscesses may be localized and aspirated with the guidance of either technique. Cavernous hemangioma, the most common benign hepatic tumor, has characteristic CT findings. Focal nodular hyperplasia, hematoma, and other benign lesions can also be imaged by these techniques. CT is considered to be the most effective study for the diagnosis of hepatoma.

Diffuse Liver Disease

In general, radiologic procedures are less helpful in determining the etiology of diffuse liver disease, which are apparent only in far advanced disease. Liver scintigraphy and ultrasound are helpful in confirming hepatomegaly. Liver spleen scan can demonstrate a decrease in functional activity with a shift of colloid to the spleen and marrow. It may be helpful in differentiating hepatitis from cirrhosis. Fatty infiltration causes a characteristic decrease in hepatic density and is readily demonstrated by CT. CT can also review areas of increased density and may assist in the diagnosis of hemochromatosis and glycogen storage disease.

Pancreatic Diseases

Both ultrasound and CT scan are useful diagnostic methods for evaluating the pancreas. The two imaging methods are competitive in some cases, but complementary in others. In general, the success rate for delineation of a normal pancreas in its entirety is higher with CT because bowel gas prevents the transmission of the ultrasound beam and obscures a portion of the pancreas. Furthermore, an ultrasound examination often is suboptimal in patients with acute pancreatitis because the associated paralytic ileus increases the amount of bowel gas and thereby the chance of a technically unsatisfactory examination. Neither examination is capable of reliably detecting a small intrapancreatic tumor that does not alter the size and shape of the pancreas.

Neither imaging method is indicated for patients with good clinical evidence of acute or chronic pancreatitis. Diagnostic studies should be reserved for patients with suspected complication from pancreatitis, such as pseudocyst or pancreatic abscess. CT is the method of choice in patients with acute pancreatitis because of the high incidence of gaseous abdomen in these patients. Ultrasound is the method of choice in pregnant women and in children because it does not depend on ionizing radiation. Ultrasound is also used in patients who are extremely emaciated or unable to hold still for the duration of the CT scan. However, the choice of examination for a given institution depends strongly on the local experience and the available expertise in addition to the relative advantages and disadvantages of each imaging method. This is especially true in ultrasound, where a relatively high degree of technical skill is required to obtain the images, as well as experience and expertise in interpretation.

ERCP may be indicated for establishing the diagnosis of pancreatitis when such a diagnosis is suspected but not confirmed by other means. Assessment of the pancreatic ductal system in chronic pancreatitis or after acute pancreatitis has subsided may be helpful for a surgeon, particularly if pancreatic surgery is under consideration. Evaluation of the ductal system after pancreatic surgery is another indication. ERCP may also be performed for suspected carcinoma of the pancreas. In such cases, the pancreatic fluid may be collected for cytology. Although there are no strict contraindications for ERCP, there are circumstances in which they should be avoided, if possible. These include acute pancreatitis and pancreatic pseudocyst because of the risk of exacerbation of the pancreatitis.

Intra-abdominal Abscesses

CT and ultrasound have proved to be useful in the evaluation of intra-abdominal abscesses. There is no general consensus which imaging method should be used first, since both examinations are capable of yielding useful information. A recent study by Korobkin et al.[45] showed similar diagnostic accuracy in the detection of abscesses among ^{67}Ga, ultrasound, and CT. Since gallium scanning is easy to perform and offers a unique view of the entire body in a single image, it may be performed first in patients with no localizing signs and symptoms, when a 24- to 48-hour delay is not critical. If the gallium scan is normal, no further radiologic evaluation is necessary. If an abnormality is present on the gallium study, CT or ultrasound is used for better delineation of the lesion. With localized signs and symptoms, CT or ultrasound should be performed initially, and a gallium study may follow if the CT and ultrasound are negative. CT is a better imaging method in patients with open wounds or surgical dressings and those with a large amount of bowel gas. Ultrasound might be better suited in patients who are unable to suspend respiration and are suspected of having subdiaphragmatic abscess.

Staging of GI Neoplasm

Barium studies have been and remain the diagnostic studies of choice for detecting malignant neoplasms of the GI tract. However, they provide little information regarding the stage of the GI neoplasms. In fact, until recently, preoperative radiologic staging of GI neoplasms was not commonly performed because accurate noninvasive imaging methods were not available. In most instances, radionuclide hepatic imaging has been the only diagnostic method performed to assess distant metastases prior to surgical intervention.

Several noninvasive imaging methods such as ultrasound and CT are capable of delineating not only local but also distant metastases. However, ultrasonography is often hampered by overlying bowel gas or adjacent bony structures. In many centers CT has now become the procedure of choice for staging GI malignancies.

At our institution, patients with proved esophageal carcinoma routinely undergo CT studies to determine the extent and the resectability of the tumors.[46] The esophagus is usually seen throughout its entire course, being separated from adjacent vascular cardiac structures by a periesophageal fat plane, which is present in all but the very thin or emaciated patient. Obliteration of the fat plane between the esophagus and the adjacent structure indicates extraesophageal spread of the tumor. Other CT signs of local spread of tumor include sinus tract or fistula formation to the tracheal bronchial tree and regional adenopathy. In the upper third of the esophagus, dissemination through the lymphatic system may lead to lymphadenopathy in the anterior jugular chain or in the supraclavicular region. Tumors of the middle third may metastasize to the mediastinum and subdiaphragmatic lymph nodes. Tumors of the lower third metastasize predominantly to the left gastric nodes, which lie within the gastrohepatic ligament. All of these groups can be easily visualized on CT scans. A CT diagnosis of malignant lymphadenopathy depends on the identification of enlargement of the involved node; a normal-sized lymph node that has been replaced by a tumor will not be recognized as abnormal by CT.

After the initial diagnosis of primary malignant gastric neoplasm is made, the most accurate information concerning regional spread of tumor or lymphadenopathy is also obtained by CT.[47-49] Gastric adenocarcinoma appears as an intraluminal mass or as focal or concentric wall thickening on CT. The gastric wall is normally less than 1 cm thick. In some cases, if the gastric lumen is inadequately distended, the collapsed gastric rugae may simulate wall thickening. Obliteration of perigastric fat plane is a reliable indicator of extragastric spread of tumor. Difficulty in interpretation arises in patients with paucity of intra-abdominal fat. Direct extension of tumor into the esophagus or pancreas, down the gastric colic liga-

ment to the colon, along the gastrohepatic ligament to the liver, or along the gastrosplenic ligament to the spleen can be identified on CT. Enlargement of the regional nodes in the left gastric, gastroepiploic, celiac, peripancreatic, and splenic hilar nodal chains can also be identified. In patients with gastric lymphoma or leiomyosarcoma, CT is valuable in delineating the extent of the extraluminal component of the tumor as well as in detecting concomitant retroperitoneal and mesenteric lymphadenopathy.

Although the experience in radiologic staging of malignant neoplasms of the duodenum and small bowel is limited, owing to the rarity of these tumors, CT is playing an ever-increasing role in the staging of colonic and rectal carcinoma because of its ability to delineate accurately the extent of the tumor mass. Obliteration of the pericolonic or perirectal fat suggests local extension of tumor.[50] Tumor extension into the urinary bladder, prostate, seminal vesicles, ovaries, other visceral organs, and pelvic musculature may be identified on CT, although it is occasionally difficult to distinguish between frank invasion and mere contiguity. Lymphatic spread from colorectal cancer along the mesenteric vessels can also be detected by CT. However, lymphatic metastases can be diagnosed by CT only when they have caused nodal enlargements.

Both CT and ultrasound can detect omental, mesenteric or peritoneal masses directly and therefore can document intraperitoneal metastasis earlier than conventional radiologic methods.[51] In patients with adequate intra-abdominal fat, CT can detect masses as small as 1 cm. Mesenteric tumor deposits appear as masses of soft tissue attenuation, often with central areas of low density representing tumor necrosis.

Although barium examinations and endoscopy are used to detect mucosal recurrence from tumors of the GI tract, recurrent tumors may be primarily extraluminal and therefore escape detection by these methods. In this setting, CT plays a valuable role in the detection of recurrent lesions.[52] CT has been shown to be accurate in the detection and restaging of recurrent rectosigmoid carcinoma. It is particularly useful for detection and staging of a recurrent tumor in patients who have undergone an abdominal perineal resection for a rectal carcinoma. Except by physical examination through the vaginal canal in females, the operative site cannot be accurately evaluated by physical examination. CT is therefore the method of choice for detecting early recurrences in these patients. Recurrent tumor following abdominal perineal resection usually appears as a homogeneous, globular soft tissue mass situated anterior to the sacrum.

SUMMARY

The abdominal organs have become increasingly accessible to the clinician through these new diagnostic techniques as described above. Already the new techniques, such as ultrasonography, computed tomography, and magnetic resonance imaging, have enabled us to visualize hepatobiliary, pancreatic, and intestinal pathology. There will undoubtedly be more developments and refinements in the years ahead.

However, it would be unrealistic to expect any one of these techniques to become the single procedure of choice for diagnosis in all types of GI disease. The clinician should be well versed in the strengths and weaknesses of each imaging technique. In some instances, no single test is really the best, and choices should be made on the basis of the resources available. If the clinician is able to make an accurate assessment of the diagnostic capability of his own institution, and approaches each individual problem with a logical progression from the initial screening technique to second-line invasive procedures, fewer unnecessary mistakes will be made. The challenge to the clinician is to minimize the risk, expense, and time involved in obtaining sufficient information for a definitive diagnosis and treatment.

REFERENCES

1. Raptopoulos V., Moss L., Reuter K., et al.: Comparison of real-time cholecystosonography and oral cholecystography. *Radiology* 140:153, 1981.
2. Cooperberg P.L., Burhenne H.J.: Real-time ultrasonography: diagnostic technique of choice in calculous gallbladder disease. *N. Engl. J. Med.* 302:1277, 1980.
3. Berk R.N., Ferrucci J.T. Jr., Fordtran J.S., et al.: The radiologic diagnosis of gallbladder disease: An imaging symposium. *Radiology* 141:49, 1981.
4. Filly R.A., Laing F.C., Callen P.W., et al.: Liver and biliary tract: Ultrasonography, in Margulis A.R., Burhenne H.J. (eds.): *Alimentary Tract Radiology*, ed. 3. St. Louis: C.V. Mosby, 1983, pp. 1479–1510.
5. Laing F.C., Federele M.P., Jeffrey R.B., et al.: Ultrasonic evaluation of patients with acute right upper quadrant pain. *Radiology* 140:449, 1981.
6. Baron R.L., Stanley R.J., Lee J.K.T., et al.: A prospective comparison of the evaluation of biliary obstruction using computed tomography and ultrasonography. *Radiology* 145:91, 1982.
7. Stanley R.J.: Liver and biliary tract, in Lee J.K.T., Sagel S.S., Stanley R.J. (eds.): *Computed Body Tomography*. New York, Raven Press, 1983, pp. 167–211.
8. Scharschmidt B.F., Goldberg H.I., Schmid R.: Approach to the patient with cholestatic jaundice. *N. Engl. J. Med.* 308:1515, 1983.
9. Berk R.N., Cooperberg P.L., Gold R.P., et al.: Radiography of the bile ducts. *Radiology* 145:1, 1982.
10. McPhee M.S., Schapiro R.H.: Biliary obstruction: Current approaches to diagnosis and treatment, in Isselbacher K.J., et al. (eds.): *Update I. Harrison's Principles of Internal Medicine*, ed. 9. New York, McGraw-Hill, 1981, pp. 1–22.
11. Stanley R.J., Sagel S.S., Levitt R.G.: Computed tomography of the body: Early trends in application and accuracy of the method. *A.J.R.* 127:53, 1976.
12. Melson G.L., Biello D.R., Lee J.K.T.: Comparative imaging, in Lee J.K.T., Sagel S.S., Stanley R.J. (eds.): *Computed Body Tomography*. New York, Raven Press, 1983, pp. 535–545.
13. Snow J.H. Jr., Goldstein H.M., Wallace S.: Comparison of scintigraphy, sonography, and computed tomography in the evaluation of hepatic neoplasms. *A.J.R.* 132:915, 1979.
14. Haaga J.R., Alfidi R.J.: Computed tomographic scanning of the pancreas. *Radiol. Clin. North Am.* 15:367, 1977.
15. Levitt R.G., Stanley R.J., Sagel S.S., et al.: Computed tomography of the pancreas: 3 second scanning vs 18 second scanning. *J. Comput. Assist. Tomogr.* 6:259, 1982.
16. Sheedy P.F. II, Stephens D.H., Hattery R.R., et al.: Computed tomography of the pancreas. *Radiol. Clin. North Am.* 15:349, 1977.
17. Hernandez M., Rosenthall L.: A crossover study comparing the kinetics of ^{99m}Tc-labeled diethyl and diisopropyl-IDA. *Clin. Nucl. Med.* 5:159, 1980.
18. Ram M.D., Hagihara P.T., Kim E.E., et al.: Evaluation of biliary disease by scintigraphy. *Am. J. Surg.* 141:77, 1981.
19. Rosenthall L.: Nuclear medicine of the biliary tract, in Margulis A.R., Burhenne H.J. (eds.): *Alimentary Tract Radiology*, ed. 3. St. Louis: C.V. Mosby, 1983, pp. 1554–1564.
20. Collier B.D., Treves S., McAffee J., et al.: Simultaneous Tc-99m parabutyl-IDA and 131-I-rose bengal examination in jaundiced neonates (abstract). *J. Nucl. Med.* 20:637, 1979.
21. Hines C. Jr., Ferrante W.A., Davis W.D., et al.: Percutaneous transhepatic cholangiography: Experience with 102 procedures. *Am. J. Dig. Dis.* 17:868, 1972.
22. Okuda K., Tanikawa K., Emura T., et al.: Non-surgical percutaneous transhepatic cholangiography—diagnostic significance in medical problems of the liver. *Am. J. Dig. Dis.* 19:21, 1974.
23. Mueller P.R., van Sonnenberg E., Simeone J.F.: Fine-needle transhepatic cholangiography: Indications and usefulness. *Ann. Intern. Med.* 92:567, 1982.
24. Thomas M.J., Pelligrini C.A., Way L.W.: Usefulness of diagnostic tests for biliary obstruction. *Am. J. Surg.* 144:102,1982.
25. Beinart C., Efremidis S., Cohen B., et al.: Obstruction without dilatation: Importance in evaluating jaundice. *J.A.M.A.* 245:353, 1981.
26. McLean G.K., Ring E.J., Freiman D.B.: Therapeutic alternatives in the treatment of intrahepatic biliary obstruction. *Radiology* 145:289, 1982.
27. McCune W.S., Shorb P.E., Moscovitz H.: Endoscopic cannulation of the ampulla of Vater: A preliminary report. *Ann. Surg.* 167:752, 1968.
28. Vennes J.A., Silvis S.E.: Endoscopic visualization of bile and pancreatic ducts. *Gastrointest. Endosc.* 18:149, 1972.
29. Kasugai T., Kuno N., Kobayashi S., et al.: Endoscopic pancreatocholangiography: I. The normal endoscopic pancreatocholangiogram. *Gastroenterology* 63:217, 1972.
30. Kasugai T., Kuno N., Kizu M., et al.: Endoscopic pancreatocholangiography: II. The pathological endoscopic pancreatocholangiogram. *Gastroenterology* 63:227, 1972.
31. Ogoshi K., Niwa M., Hara Y., et al.: Endoscopic pancreatocholangiography in the evaluation of pancreatic and biliary disease. *Gastroenterology* 64:210, 1973.
32. Cole W.H.: The false-normal oral cholecystogram. *Surgery* 81:121, 1977.
33. Venu R.P., Geenen J.E., Toouli J., et al.: Endoscopic retrograde cholangiopancreatography: Diagnosis of cholelithiasis in patients with normal gallbladder x-ray and ultrasound studies. *J.A.M.A.* 249:758, 1983.
34. Freeman J.B., Cohen W.N., DenBesten L.: Cholecystokinin cholangiography and analysis of duodenal bile in the investigation of pain in the right upper quadrant of the abdomen without gallstones. *Surg. Gynecol. Obstet.* 140:371, 1975.
35. Griffen W.O. Jr., Bivins B.A., Rogers E.L., et al.: Cholecystokinin cholecystography in the diagnosis of gallbladder disease. *Ann. Surg.* 191:636, 1980.
36. Porterfield G., Cheung L.Y., Berenson M.: Detection of occult gallbladder disease by duodenal drainage. *Am. J. Surg.* 134:702, 1977.
37. Nora P.F., Davis R.P., Fernandez M.J.: Chronic acalculous gallbladder disease: A clinical enigma. *World J. Surg.* 8:106, 1984.
38. Sanders R.C.: The significance of sonographic gallbladder wall thickening. *J. Clin. Ultrasound* 8:143, 1980.
39. Ralls P.W., Colleti P.M., Halls J.M., et al.: Prospective evaluation of ^{99m}Tc-IDA cholescintigraphy and gray-scale ultrasound in the diagnosis of acute cholecystitis. *Radiology* 144:369, 1982.
40. Shuman W.P., Mack L.A., Rudd T.G., et al.: Evaluation of acute right upper quadrant pain: Sonography and ^{99m}Tc-PIPIDA cholescintigraphy, *A.J.R.* 139:61, 1982.
41. Worthen N.J., Uszler J.M., Funamura J.L.: Cholecystitis: Prospective evaluation of sonography and ^{99m}Tc-HIDA cholescintigraphy. *A.J.R.* 137:973, 1981.
42. Ostfeld D.A., Meyer J.E.: Liver scanning in cancer patients with short-interval autopsy correlation. *Radiology* 138:671, 1981.
43. Bernardino M.E., Thomas J.L., Maklad N.: Hepatic sonography: Technical considerations, present applications and possible future. *Radiology* 142:249, 1982.
44. Knopf D.R., Torres W.E., Fajman W.J., et al.: Liver lesions: Comparative accuracy of scintigraphy and computed tomography. *A.J.R.* 138:623, 1982.
45. Korobkin M., Callen P.W., Filly R.A., et al.: Comparison of computed tomography, ultrasonography, and gallium-67 scanning

in the evaluation of suspected abdominal abscess. *Radiology* 129:89, 1978.

46. Picus D., Balfe D.M., Koehler R.E., et al.: Computed tomography in the staging of esophageal carcinoma. *Radiology* 146:433, 1983.

47. Balfe D.M., Koehler R.E., Karstaedt N., et al.: Computed tomography of gastric neoplasms. *Radiology* 140:431, 1981.

48. Lee K.R., Levine E., Moffat R.E., et al.: Computed tomographic staging of malignant gastric neoplasms. *Radiology* 133:151, 1979.

49. Buy J.N., Moss A.A.: Computed tomography of gastric lymphoma. *A.J.R.* 138:859, 1982.

50. Thoeni R.F., Moss A.A., Schnyder P., et al.: Detection and staging of primary rectal and rectosigmoid cancer by computed tomography. *Radiology* 141:135, 1981.

51. Levitt R.G., Sagel S.S., Stanley R.J.: Detection of neoplastic involvement of the mesentery and omentum by computed tomography. *A.J.R.* 131:835, 1978.

52. Lee J.K.T., Stanley R.J., Sagel S.S., et al.: CT appearance of the pelvis after abdomino-perineal resection for rectal carcinoma. *Radiology* 141:737, 1981.

3

Endoscopic Diagnosis and Treatment

THOMAS L. DENT, M.D.
WILLIAM E. STRODEL, M.D.

THE REVOLUTIONARY development of flexible fiberoptic endoscopes has changed and expanded the role of endoscopy in all surgical disciplines, but none as much as gastrointestinal (GI) surgery. The improvement in flexibility and length of endoscopes now makes it possible to examine directly, with minimal morbidity and mortality, the upper GI tract to the distal duodenum and the lower GI tract to the terminal ileum.

Diagnostic flexible GI endoscopy has become essential to the overall evaluation of GI tract symptoms. In many centers in Europe and Japan, esophagogastroduodenoscopy (EGD) and colonoscopy have replaced barium contrast studies as the initial diagnostic screening procedures for any GI complaint. In the United States, flexible endoscopy already has replaced barium contrast studies in the evaluation of acute GI hemorrhage. The major reasons for still choosing barium contrast studies for the initial evaluation of GI symptoms, despite the clearly superior diagnostic capability of flexible endoscopy, are the higher costs and the lack of adequate numbers of physicians trained to perform flexible endoscopy. When costs are reduced to those of comparable diagnostic studies, more physicians are educated in endoscopic techniques, and better endoscopes are developed, flexible fiberoptic endoscopy will become the study of choice for diagnosing mucosal lesions of the GI tract.

As experience with flexible endoscopy accumulates, the indications for and limitations of endoscopic examination have become better defined. As with any new diagnostic technique, overutilization has occurred. Many thoughtful authors have tried to define the place of endoscopy in our diagnostic armamentarium. Although highly accurate and useful, flexible endoscopy is only one method for evaluating selected diseases of the GI tract.

In addition to diagnostic uses, an increasing number of surgical procedures can be performed through flexible endoscopes without the morbidity and mortality of laparotomy and general anesthesia. Many of these procedures are similar or identical to traditional operations, such as electrocautery of mucosal lesions and vaterian sphincterotomy, or are refinements of techniques previously performed through rigid endoscopes, such as snare polypectomy and sclerotherapy of esophageal varices. Clearly, the future of endoscopy will involve the development of additional surgical techniques.

Despite the entry into the marketplace of many manufacturers of endoscopes, the high cost of these instruments has not decreased. Perhaps with increasing competition among manufacturers, their cost will decrease, allowing a reduction in cost for each diagnostic and therapeutic endoscopic procedure. Physician fees for performing diagnostic endoscopy are also frequently excessive and must decrease.

Endoscopy has always been an integral part of the training and practice of surgeons. The esophagoscope and bronchoscope in thoracic surgery, the cystoscope in urologic surgery, and the esophagoscope and the proctoscope in GI surgery all greatly aided the diagnosis and therapy of surgical diseases of the esophagus, bronchi, urinary tract, and rectum. The importance of modern flexible fiberoptic endoscopy to the training and practice of surgeons treating patients with diseases of the GI tract was recognized early by some.[1, 2] Few surgical training programs, however, provided formal training in flexible fiberoptic endoscopy until very recently. The American Board of Surgery now requires candidates for certification to have a knowledge of flexible endoscopic techniques and, it is hoped, will require them to be proficient in flexible endoscopy.

Using modern instruments, the techniques of fiberoptic endoscopy are learned easily, especially by the surgical resident whose entire training constantly emphasizes the gentle manipulation of tissue, eye-hand coordination, and decision-making based on visual inspection of gross pathology. The description of a surgeon as "an internist who operates" is especially applicable to the practice of flexible endoscopy as an integral part of gastroenterological surgery.

For the past eight years, the Section of General Surgery at the University of Michigan has included two months of concentrated didactic and practical endoscopic experience for each third-year general surgery resident. They are taught by eight full-time GI surgeons who are proficient in endoscopy. We have found that this experience, coupled with continuing senior-level experience, has increased our residents' understanding of GI pathology and has prepared them well when they have chosen to incorporate flexible endoscopy into their surgical practices.

This chapter will emphasize modern endoscopic techniques as they apply to the surgical treatment of diseases of the GI tract. Some endoscopic applications, such as polypectomy, sclerotheraphy, and colon decompression, will be particularly emphasized because of their importance to surgical practice. Other applications, such as the assessment of inflammatory bowel disease and duodenal ulcer, will be discussed less extensively.

HISTORY

Although rigid endoscopy of the GI tract[1] has been an integral part of the diagnosis and therapy of GI diseases for over 100 years, the revolutionary development of flexible fiberoptic endoscopy is recent. A semiflexible gastroscope, designed by Schindler and Wolf, was used in 1932. A fully flexible fiberoptic gastroscope, designed by Curtiss at the University of Michigan, was used clinically at University Hospital in Ann Arbor in 1957. In 1961, a flexible fiberoptic sigmoidoscope was developed and first used by Overholt, also at the University of Michigan. Operative flexible endoscopy began when Shinya and Wolff developed the technique of snare polypectomy in 1969. Endoscopically assisted cannulation of the papilla of Vater was performed by Oi in 1970, and endoscopic sphincterotomy with stone extraction was reported from both Japan and Germany in 1974.

Continual technological improvements of the endoscopes by the manufacturers have aided in the clinical application and safety of these instruments. Brighter light sources, more slender, durable endoscopes with greater tip flexibility, and better optics are but a few of these technological achievements.

DOCUMENTATION

We believe that the surgeon who plans to operate on a patient for a GI lesion should personally examine the lesion with the endoscope. Accurate documentation of the endoscopic findings is essential. Endoscopists are convinced that the flexible endoscope is the most accurate way to define mucosal lesions of the upper and lower GI tract. Nonendoscopists have been slower to accept endoscopy as the best diagnostic tool. A major reason for this reluctance is that the physician who is not present during the endoscopic examination must rely on the oral or written description of the endoscopic findings rather than being shown an x-ray film or a high-quality photograph that corroborates the endoscopist's findings. Barium contrast studies, arteriograms, CT scans, ultrasonography, and radioisotope scanning all have an instant permanent visual record to document the examination and help the clinician better understand their interpretation. The development of endoscopic photography has lagged behind other technological advances in endoscopy, and much improvement is necessary.

ESOPHAGOGASTRODUODENOSCOPY (EGD)

Instrumentation

A variety of endoscopes and accessories are available for performing routine and specialized diagnostic studies as well as therapeutic procedures. Forward-viewing instruments, large and small diameter (Fig 3–1), are used for routine EGD, and side-viewing instruments are used primarily for

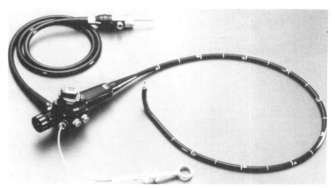

Fig 3–1.—End-viewing gastroscope with biopsy forceps.

duodenoscopy and endoscopic retrograde cholangiopancreatography (ERCP). Injection sclerotherapy, foreign-body retrieval, and large-particle biopsy are usually performed with dual channel endoscopes.

Preparation

An appropriate history and physical examination are essential parts of the preparation for an endoscopic examination. In addition, if a barium contrast study has been performed, knowledge of the results and a review of the films may direct the endoscopic procedure. Informed consent to the procedure should be obtained. In elective cases, patients should fast overnight. Inpatients receive premedication with IM atropine, meperidine, and secobarbital and supplemental sedation with IV diazepam. Outpatients receive only IV diazepam sedation. A simethicone solution is administered orally to prevent obscuration of the view by foam. We also use topical pharyngeal anesthesia by spray or gargle.

Indications for Esophagogastroduodenoscopy (EGD) (Table 3–1)

The indications for upper GI endoscopy have expanded as new instruments and techniques have been introduced, and the safety, accuracy, and patient acceptability of EGD have been amply demonstrated. The past decade has provided data comparing the value, in specific situations, of radiographic contrast studies and endoscopy as the sole diagnostic modality or used together as complementary studies. Elective barium contrast studies are inaccurate and misleading in nearly 25% of cases.[4, 5] Endoscopic examination clearly is the better method for detecting mucosal lesions, while radiographic studies are preferred to demonstrate motility disorders and extrinsic defects.

When EGD is performed for diagnostic purposes, the entire upper GI tract is usually surveyed, unless an obstructing lesion prevents passage of the endoscope. In symptomatic postgastrectomy patients, 50% of radiographic contrast studies are inaccurate owing to misinterpretation of normal postoperative and anastomotic deformities.

With the advent of EGD a more precise end point in the evaluation of therapeutic agents for the treatment of peptic ulcer disease has been established, but the clinical applicability of this role remains undefined.

Jaundice alone does not appear to be an indication for rou-

TABLE 3–1.—INDICATIONS FOR
ESOPHAGOGASTRODUODENOSCOPY (EGD)

Diagnostic
  Abnormal barium contrast study requiring biopsy
    or additional information
  Persistent symptoms despite, or in place of,
    normal barium contrast study
    Dysphagia
    Heartburn
    Vomiting
    Abdominal pain
    Symptoms after gastric operations
  Gastrointestinal bleeding
  Ingestion of corrosive material
  Cancer surveillance
  Assessment of therapy
Therapeutic
  Dilation of strictures
  Foreign-body extraction
  Polypectomy
  Hemostasis
  Percutaneous gastrostomy

tine forward-viewing upper GI panendoscopy. Our experience demonstrates an overall low specificity of diagnosis in obstructive jaundice. The discovery of unsuspected synchronous lesions did not change our diagnostic or therapeutic planning in any case. Duodenoscopy during ERCP is more productive than panendoscopy in this group of patients.

The disadvantages of EGD are few. They include discomfort to the patient, inability to detect extrinsic lesions, and the small but real incidence of false negative examinations.

Contraindications to EGD

Absolute Contraindications

SUSPECTED PERFORATION OR PERITONITIS.—Maneuvering the endoscope and insufflation of air may cause an area of impending perforation to perforate or may cause widespread peritoneal contamination through a perforation. Air may be forced through a perforation, causing massive pneumoperitoneum and respiratory compromise.

UNCOOPERATIVE PATIENT.—Because virtually all EGD is performed with topical anesthesia and sedation, it is important that the patient be cooperative. An uncooperative patient may increase the risk of perforation or pulmonary aspiration.

Relative Contraindications

The risk of EGD may be increased in patients with prior myocardial infarction, severe angina, or a coagulopathy.

Diagnostic Esophagogastroduodenoscopy

Esophagus

HIATUS HERNIA.—An asymptomatic hiatus hernia is not an indication for EGD, which should be used to evaluate only patients with symptoms of dysphagia or gastroesophageal reflux. The relation of the squamous-columnar mucosal junction to the diaphragmatic hiatus is the primary endoscopic criterion for determining the presence of a hiatus hernia. When the mucosal junction is more than 2 cm above the hiatus, a hernia is present. Frequently in patients with a hiatus hernia,

a Valsalva maneuver, increasing the abdominal pressure, or turning the patient will result in the junction's ascending 2–3 cm, making the diagnosis of hernia unequivocal. In addition, when a hernia is present, retroflexed viewing of the esophagogastric junction demonstrates a distinct recess with an upper and lower border.

REFLUX ESOPHAGITIS.—Esophagitis is considered to be a reliable guide to the presence of gastroesophageal reflux. Although ulceration and stricture are clear manifestations of esophageal disease, there is some variability and disagreement among endoscopists as to the significance of erythema alone.[6] Additionally, only half of those patients who have severe symptoms of gastroesophageal reflux show any endoscopic evidence of esophagitis.[7] With long-standing reflux, mucosal nodularity, ulceration, and eventually stricture may occur. When a stricture is identified, carcinoma must be strongly considered and multiple biopsies and brushings performed to evaluate this diagnosis.

Barrett's esophagus, a segment of the distal esophagus lined with columnar epithelium, is being reported with increasing frequency and has been observed in up to 10% of patients with symptomatic reflux esophagitis who undergo endoscopic examinations.[8] The incidence of Barrett's esophagus in 20,000 endoscopic examinations was 0.05%, and the incidence of adenocarcinoma of the esophagus in patients with Barrett's esophagus is 10%.[9] Biopsy is necessary to confirm the diagnosis.

INFECTIOUS ESOPHAGITIS.—An extensive mucous coating of an inflamed esophagus suggests mycotic infection, and brushings and biopsies will usually reveal fungal organisms. Symptoms referable to candidiasis are uncommon, and radiography is usually not helpful in diagnosis. Candidiasis occurs more frequently in patients with esophageal cancer, gastric cancer, benign gastric ulcers, or esophagitis.[10] Monilial esophagitis occurs frequently in immunosuppressed patients and must be considered if dysphagia or esophageal bleeding is present.

NEOPLASMS.—Benign neoplasms including leiomyoma, lipoma, neurofibroma, and lymphangioma are usually covered by normal-appearing esophageal mucosa, and small endoscopic biopsies usually demonstrate only normal mucosa. Further endoscopic differentiation is impossible.

A patient with an esophageal stricture and/or dysphagia should *always* be evaluated endoscopically for the presence of esophageal carcinoma. Dysphagia in an individual over 40 years of age should be assumed to be due to cancer until proven otherwise. Many squamous cell carcinomas stimulate a fibrous reaction at the advancing margins of the tumor, and false negative biopsies are not uncommon. Seven to ten biopsies should be obtained to ensure adequate sampling. Squamous cell carcinomas notoriously extend intramurally far beyond the level of the mucosal lesion. Endoscopic examination is therefore of limited value in determining the extent of the tumor. Early diagnosis with improved survival is possible if patients with minimal symptoms undergo thorough visual assessment as well as with endoscopic brushings and biopsies. Screening endoscopy is appropriate for patients with premalignant conditions of the esophagus, such as Plummer-Vinson syndrome, tylosis, achalasia, Barrett's esophagus, prior lye burn, and previous carcinoma.

Adenocarcinomas comprise fewer than 10% of esophageal cancers. Adenocarcinomas of the esophagogastric junction are difficult to diagnose endoscopically, and retroflexed viewing is usually necessary to detect small tumors and to obtain adequate biopsies.

VARICES.—The endoscopic diagnosis of esophageal varices is much more accurate than the radiographic assessment.[11] Varices appear as longitudinal, tortuous columns and have been compared to a "string of beads" (Fig 3–2). Overdistention of the esophagus by air insufflation may compress the varices and mask their presence. Frequently the columns look blue, but if the mucosa is thick, the color will be that of normal esophageal mucosa. A blood clot or mucosal erosion on a varix is a sign of recent hemorrhage. Active bleeding can also be observed. Patients with known varices who develop upper GI hemorrhage should undergo endoscopic study, because the incidence of the bleeding originating from other synchronous upper GI lesions has been reported to be as high as 40%.[12]

Dilated small vessels or microtelangiectasias on the surface of the varix and large, blue varices accurately predict subsequent or recurrent bleeding.[13] When microtelangiectasias are absent, bleeding occurs in fewer than 10% of patients, but nearly 60% of patients with these vessels will bleed. The incidence of bleeding in patients with blue varices is nearly 80%, but is less than 50% in patients with white varices. Other factors, such as the configuration, location, or proximal extent of varices, are of minor significance in predicting bleeding.

MALLORY-WEISS LESIONS.—The increased number of reports of Mallory-Weiss lesions is clearly related to the widespread use of fiberoptic endoscopy in the evaluation of GI hemorrhage. Mallory-Weiss tears constitute 8%–11% of up-per GI bleeding lesions.[14] Approximately 24 hours after acute bleeding from a Mallory-Weiss laceration, the lesion appears as a superficial linear ulcer. Complete healing usually occurs in 48–72 hours.

Stomach

GASTRIC ATROPHY AND SUPERFICIAL GASTRITIS.—Gastric atrophy is frequently present following gastric resection, as a diffuse process involving particularly the body and fundus of the stomach. Large veins may be visible in these areas. Occult bleeding from atrophic mucosa may occur and raises the possibility of malignancy. Biopsy will establish the diagnosis of atrophic gastritis. Of patients with atrophic gastritis, nearly 10% will develop gastric cancer or neoplastic polyps over 10–15 years.[15] Superficial gastritis appears as localized vascular engorgement, intramural hemorrhage, and tiny erosions covered with fibrin. Symptoms of superficial gastritis and atrophic gastritis are variable and do not correlate with endoscopic findings.

ACUTE MUCOSAL EROSIONS.—Endoscopic examination in patients with acute upper GI hemorrhage demonstrates erosive gastritis as the cause of bleeding in nearly 30% of cases.[16] The mucosa may appear edematous and hyperemic, with surface erosions and mucosal hemorrhage. Recovery and mucosal healing are usually rapid.

Stress ulceration may occur throughout the stomach or in discrete areas. The location and degree of development correlate with the causative factors of the stress.[17] Lesions associated with trauma and sepsis occur more frequently in the proximal stomach and have a dark brown to black appearance. Those lesions caused by acute alcohol ingestion also occur in the proximal stomach but appear as confluent petechiae. Aspirin-induced acute mucosal lesions occur more frequently in the distal stomach and appear as clusters of petechiae. Lesions associated with burns are larger, deeper, and usually in the distal stomach or duodenum.

EGD performed prospectively in critically ill patients frequently shows clinically silent acute lesions.[18] Although asymptomatic, gastric erosions have been found within a few hours or days in all patients after severe trauma,[19] in nearly 90% of patients with large burns,[20] and in all patients with severe sepsis and positive blood cultures.[21]

In our experience, 15% of patients receiving selective hepatic artery infusion chemotherapy have patchy gastric erythema, diffuse erosions, or discrete ulcers, mainly on the lesser curvature.[22]

ANGIODYSPLASIA.—Lesions of angiodysplasia appear as friable, flat, or slightly raised lesions that are bright red and usually 5–10 mm in diameter. A small central umbilication may be present. These lesions may also appear as reddened folds and linear erythema and may be mistaken for gastritis or trauma from endoscopy or nasogastric suction. Gastric angiodysplasia is the cause of bleeding in 1.5% of cases of upper GI hemorrhage.[23] Treatment is primarily by local excision or suture ligation. Endoscopic electrocautery has also been successful. In cases of hereditary hemorrhagic telangiectasia, the numerous lesions appear as discrete reddened areas 5 mm in diameter, with small vascular channels that resemble spider angiomas.

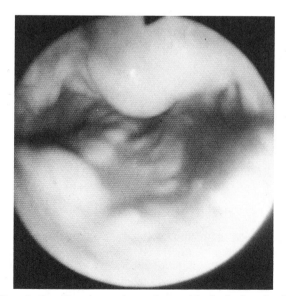

Fig 3–2.—Esophageal varices. Typical longitudinal "string-of-beads" appearance representing dilated submucosal veins encroaching on the esophageal lumen.

GASTRIC ULCER (Fig 3–3).—Benign chronic gastric ulcers are usually single and located on the lesser curvature of the stomach at the gastric angulus or within 2 cm of the pylorus (prepyloric and channel ulcers). These lesions are sharply demarcated, punched-out defects with distinct borders and a clean, gray-white base. Among a large group of patients with abdominal pain, bleeding, or anemia, and a normal upper GI radiograph, nearly 15% had significant lesions found at endoscopy, including gastric ulcer (7%) and gastric cancer.[4]

Gastroscopic examination, including biopsy and cytology, is indicated in every patient with a demonstrated gastric ulcer. Ten percent of benign-appearing gastric ulcers will be malignant, and the incidence of cancer increases when the ulcer is atypical in location or appearance. Although much has been written about visual differentiation between benign and malignant gastric ulcers, it is frequently impossible to distinguish between the two. Cytologic brushings and a minimum of seven biopsies of the ulcer margin are mandatory.[24]

Of patients who receive medical treatment for benign gastric ulcer, 15% experience healing at 1 month, 30% at 2 months, 40% at 3 months, and 80% at 12 months.[25] The recurrence rate after complete healing is nearly 45% at 12 months. If gastric resection is not performed, repeated endoscopy with biopsy and cytology is indicated at periodic intervals until complete healing occurs.

BENIGN NEOPLASMS.—In the United States, most polypoid lesions of the stomach are hyperplastic or inflammatory. Mucosal adenomas are believed to be premalignant, and the incidence of carcinoma within the polyp is directly proportional to the size of the lesion. Malignant polyps have an irregular surface, are sessile, and usually 3.5 cm or greater in diameter.[26] Fractional biopsy or cytology of mucosal polypoid lesions is inadequate unless positive. Endoscopic snare excision of smaller lesions and partial gastrectomy for larger lesions are indicated.

Submucosal tumors appear as smooth, raised lesions covered by normal gastric mucosa. They include leiomyomas, fibromas, neurofibromas, lipomas, and nodules of aberrant pancreas. Multiple endoscopic diagnostic techniques have been described, including large-particle biopsy, needle-aspiration cytology, and multiple deep biopsies, but their yield is low. Individualized treatment is recommended, but surgical excision should be considered for tumors greater than 1 cm in diameter in good-risk patients.

GASTRIC CANCER.—Flexible endoscopy has greatly improved the ability to diagnose mucosal malignancies of the stomach. An accurate histologic diagnosis can be established in more than 95% of exophytic cancers of the stomach but in less than half of infiltrating lesions. Large-particle biopsy, cytology, and lift-and-cut techniques improve the diagnostic accuracy of flexible endoscopy, but complementary single and double contrast barium radiography also increase the diagnostic yield. This is especially true in early gastric cancer, limited to the mucosa, and in benign-appearing gastric ulcers.[27] The only way to improve the dismal cure rate of gastric cancer in the United States is to subject all patients over 40 years of age with unrelieved symptoms of dyspepsia to gastroscopy and directed mucosal biopsy. With a combination of a high index of suspicion, double contrast radiography, and gastroscopy with biopsy and brush cytology, an accurate diagnosis of cancer can be made in 97% of cases.

SYMPTOMS FOLLOWING GASTRIC OPERATIONS.—Endoscopy of the stomach, duodenum, and jejunum should be performed in the symptomatic patient who has undergone prior gastric resection or pyloroplasty and may be performed safely as early as a few hours following operation.[28] Findings include suture line bleeding, diffuse or focal gastritis, recurrent peptic ulcer, stomal ulcer, anastomotic edema or stricture, and gastric remnant cancer and bezoars.

Nonspecific gastritis occurs in nearly 90% of postgastrectomy patients and appears as mild hyperemia with diffuse radial bands close to the stoma.[29] Stomal ulcers appear on either the jejunal or gastric side of the gastrojejunal anastomosis. Severe and extensive hyperemia, bile staining of the gastric mucosa, and superficial ulceration are more commonly observed in symptomatic patients.

Carcinoma of the stomach developing after gastric resection and Billroth II reconstruction for peptic ulcer disease occurs in fewer than 5% of patients but may be detected at an early stage even in symptomatic patients.

Duodenum

The duodenum may be examined with either side-viewing or forward-viewing instruments, and on occasion both may be desirable. In the majority of patients the forward-viewing endoscope can be used alone, permitting a coordinated examination of the esophagus, stomach, pyloric channel, and duodenum with a single intubation. Increased motility of the duodenum occasionally hampers examination but may be arrested by administering glucagon as a single IV (0.2–1.0 mg) dose.

DUODENAL ULCER.—When radiography and endoscopy are compared, 25%–40% of duodenal ulcers are detectable only by endoscopy.[30] Associated duodenal deformity makes x-ray interpretation even more difficult.

Most duodenal ulcers occur within 3 cm of the pylorus, but 10% occur beyond the duodenal bulb. They are uniformly distributed around the circumference of the lumen and are usually smaller than 1 cm in diameter. Larger ulcers tend to

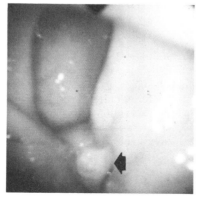

Fig 3–3.—1.5-cm benign ulcer *(arrow)* located on the greater curvature of the gastric antrum.

be deep, and smaller ulcers are often superficial and irregular. Some ulcers may acutely distort the duodenal bulb, and as they heal produce permanent deformity, stenosis, or pseudodiverticula. Ulcers of the pyloric channel are usually located superiorly and produce longitudinal contraction and eccentricity of the pyloric opening.

DUODENITIS.—Duodenitis may be part of the pathophysiologic spectrum of duodenal ulceration, but the clinical importance of acute duodenal inflammation in the absence of chronic ulceration remains controversial.[31] Duodenitis may occur alone, in association with chronic duodenal ulcer, or with Crohn's disease. Resolution of duodenitis does not always accompany complete healing of an ulcer, despite an overall improvement in histologic and endoscopic features.

Reactive inflammatory changes of the descending duodenum are frequently noted at endoscopy in patients with pancreatitis. These usually appear as enlargement, hyperemia, and friability of the papilla of Vater and mucosal folds of the descending duodenum. Occasionally, mass-like deformities of this area are noted, especially in patients with chronic pancreatitis and pseudocysts.

Crohn's disease of the duodenum is uncommon, occurring in approximately 2% of patients with Crohn's disease. Endoscopy allows better visualization of mucosal defects, but other features, such as a diminished pliability and the presence of contiguous lesions, are better demonstrated by barium contrast studies. The mucosal lesions are heterogeneous, irregularly shaped ulcers and erosions, and may have a patchy distribution.[32] Histologic examination of endoscopic biopsies permits a conclusive diagnosis based on the presence of granulomas in 70% of cases.

POLYPS AND NEOPLASMS.—Polyps of the duodenum include inflammatory lesions, adenomas, villous tumors, Brunner gland hyperplasia, lymphomas, carcinoids, leiomyomas, lipomas, hemangiomas, or heterotopic gastric or pancreatic lesions. Biopsy of polyps of mucosal origin will usually establish the diagnosis, and snare polypectomy may also be useful. Histologic verification of submucosal polyps is difficult, and diagnosis is usually based on radiographic or operative demonstration.

Villous adenomas, though rare, have been found in all portions of the duodenum and are usually solitary. Malignant transformation can occur.

Leiomyomas of the duodenum (Fig 3–4) usually occur immediately distal to the papilla of Vater, appear as a firm, spherical bulge under the intact mucosa, and frequently have a central ulcer. Lipomas and carcinoids resemble leiomyomas but usually do not have a central ulcer.

Primary carcinoma of the duodenum may be missed if the entire duodenum is not examined. Fifty percent of duodenal carcinomas occur at or near the papilla and the remainder more distally.

STRICTURES AND DIVERTICULA.—Strictures may be postinflammatory, postoperative, neoplastic, or congenital. Associated ulceration may make endoscopic interpretation or localization difficult. A combination of direct visualization, biopsy, and complementary barium radiography should establish the diagnosis in almost all cases.

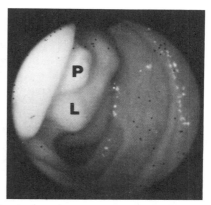

Fig 3–4.—Leiomyoma *(L)* of the second portion of the duodenum located just distal to the papilla of Vater *(P)*. This tumor bled 3,000 ml one day prior to endoscopy.

Reports of duodenal diverticula have stressed their juxtapapillary localization.[33] Most of these diverticula are found in the medial wall of the descending part of the duodenum close to the papilla, where passage of the ductal system presumably may cause a weakness of the wall.

Therapeutic Esophagogastroduodenoscopy

Dilation of Strictures

With the advent of flexible endoscopy, there has been renewed interest in stricture dilation. Endoscopic dilation has been described for esophageal stricture, achalasia, pyloric stenosis, and narrowed anastomoses. Both metal and balloon dilators have been used. The metal dilators are usually threaded over a guide wire that is passed through the endoscope and introduced through the narrowed segment to be dilated. Balloon dilators may be passed alongside or through the endoscope and inflated under direct vision. The benefit of dilation in cases of achalasia remains in dispute. Experience is accumulating with other uses of endoscopic dilation.

Foreign-Body Extraction

Foreign bodies, including tubing, toothbrushes, thermometers (Fig 3–5), safety pins, sewing needles, wire coat hangers, razor blades, dentures, and spoons, have been removed by endoscope. Most swallowed foreign bodies pass per rectum without incident. Indications for endoscopic removal are danger of perforation (owing to the type of object) and failure of the object to progress. Complications occur in up to 12% of cases with sharp objects; the most frequent is perforation.[34] Various methods have been devised to remove foreign bodies from the GI tract, each method often as ingenious as the ingestion of the object. The most frequent site of lodgment is in the cervical esophagus. Other common sites include the stomach, terminal ileum, and cecum. Impaction of a foreign body in the pharynx or upper esophagus requires immediate localization and removal. Impaction in the mid- or distal esophagus suggests the prior existence of an esophageal stricture. The endoscope may be used to remove certain foreign bodies from the esophagus and stomach without the use of general anesthesia or laparotomy and with minimal discomfort to the patient.

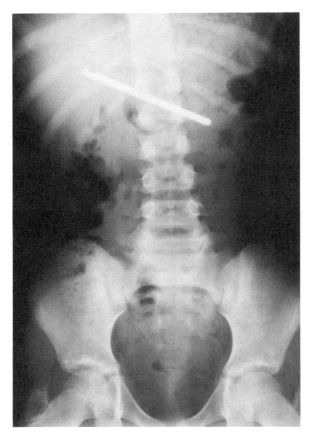

Fig 3–5.—Accidentally swallowed thermometer in the stomach of a 12-year-old girl. It was retrieved easily using a gastroscopic snare.

Polypectomy

Polyps occur less commonly in the upper GI tract than in the colon. Most are submucosal or inflammatory, and true neoplastic polyps are rare. Biopsy specimens may not be representative of a polyp greater than 5 mm in diameter, and snare excision or partial gastrectomy should be performed. The techniques of polypectomy are similar to those described for the colon.[35] Many gastric polyps do not have a stalk; thus, the lift-and-cut method via the dual channel gastroscope may be necessary.

Hemostasis

ENDOSCOPIC INJECTION SCLEROSIS (EIS).—Esophageal variceal hemorrhage is a serious problem for which there is occasionally no satisfactory solution. Bleeding resumes after discontinuance of balloon tamponade in 60% of patients, with an in-hospital mortality rate of 60%.[36]

During the early 1970s, Johnston and Rodgers[37] described a 15-year experience of 217 EIS procedures performed through a rigid endoscope using ethanolamine oleate. Bleeding initially was controlled in 93% of patients, with a complication rate of 0.9% per procedure. Many different approaches have been used in adapting EIS to the flexible endoscope, including tamponade with or after injection, a variety of sclerosing agents, and different schedules of injections. Some en-

doscopists still use a rigid endoscope and general anesthesia. In a survey of the membership of the American Society for Gastrointestinal Endoscopy (ASGE) conducted in 1981, a total of 610 patients had undergone 1,305 procedures, and bleeding was controlled in 75%.[38] The mean follow-up, however, was only 3.75 months. EIS was usually performed with fiberoptic instruments and sedation was favored over general anesthesia.

The indications for EIS are not yet defined. Generally, injections are begun in response to confirmed variceal hemorrhage in patients who are not good operative candidates. Some advocate EIS for any patient who has bled from varices, but no published data support this indication. It has not been demonstrated that EIS results in less bleeding or improved survival in Child's class A or B patients compared with those who undergo shunting procedures. Except for controlled trials, we currently believe that EIS should be reserved for patients for whom surgical treatment is not indicated, including those for whom shunts are technically impossible, those who have undergone shunting procedures but continue to bleed, and those with poor liver function (Child's class C). Acute bleeding can be controlled by EIS 80%–95% of the time.[39] Since the incidence of rebleeding following an initial EIS is reportedly reduced 50% by repeated treatments, repeated treatments may be useful, but the most effective and safe schedule has not yet been defined.[40] EIS also can be used to stop acute bleeding until improvement in the patient's general condition permits a shunting procedure. EIS is probably contraindicated in cases of severe mucosal ulceration caused by previous injections, severe coagulopathy, and severe esophagitis caused by prolonged esophageal intubation with the Sengstaken-Blakemore tube.

A variety of sclerosants are in use, including sodium morrhuate, sodium tetradecyl sulfate, ethanolamine oleate, hypertonic glucose, thrombin, cephalothin sodium, and combinations of agents. Most endoscopists in this country currently use a 5% solution of sodium morrhuate. The sclerosing agent is usually injected directly into a varix, although some prefer paravariceal injection. A slow, steady injection over 10–15 seconds may be effective without the necessity for venous compression. Paravariceal injection produces an intense submucosal inflammatory response that may result in occlusion of the varix. Some paravariceal injections certainly occur even when intravariceal injection is intended.

Complications of EIS include precipitation or worsening of hemorrhage, esophageal necrosis and ulcer formation with or without perforation, and esophageal stricture. In the ASGE survey, 118 complications were noted in 610 patients (19% per patient, 9% per procedure).[38] Substernal discomfort often develops after the procedure. Low-grade fever may occur, and can persist for as long as 36 hours. Death attributable to EIS occurred in 0.7% of cases. The most common complication is ulceration, which represented nearly half of all complications. The ulcer usually develops within 7–10 days, and although it may heal completely, it may take months. Precipitation of hemorrhage accounts for one third of all complications. Slight bleeding, frequently encountered on withdrawal of the needle, will stop spontaneously. More serious hemorrhage usually can be controlled with repeated injections and IV vasopressin. Delayed hemorrhage during the first 24 hours after the procedure is rare. Strictures are thought to be due to sclerosant damage and account for 3% of all complications.

ELECTROCAUTERY AND HEATER PROBES.—Much has been written about the uses of heater probes and electrocautery treatment of acute bleeding lesions of the upper GI tract. The benefits of endoscopic control of bleeding lesions remain unproven. Many studies are under way, but more data and controlled studies must be accumulated before recommending this as a standard form of treatment. Most GI hemorrhage will stop spontaneously without specific therapy.

LASERS.—Laser photocoagulation is a promising endoscopic modality for treating GI hemorrhage and is in the developmental stage. The recognition that argon and Nd:YAG laser energy could be transmitted through a small flexible quartz fiber led to the endoscopic application of this technique to the treatment of GI bleeding. More the 2,500 patients with GI bleeding have been treated with lasers with a reported 80%–90% success in achieving initial hemostasis.[41] Laser perforation of the gastric or duodenal wall has been reported in 1%–2% of patients.

Endoscopic Percutaneous Gastrostomy (EPG)

Ponsky and Gauderer[42] developed a method for percutaneous gastrostomy tube placement that is performed with local anesthesia with endoscopic control. Precise placement of the tube can be attained, and approximation of the stomach to the abdominal wall can be accomplished by traction on the gastrostomy tube. We have performed EPG in 110 adult patients who were poor risks for laparotomy and/or general anesthesia owing to head and neck cancer, stroke, or closed head injury. The procedure can be performed at the bedside or in the endoscopy suite and takes only 10–15 minutes to complete. Since ileus occurs rarely, we initiate enteral feedings 24 hours following tube insertion. The few complications associated with this procedure included stomal infection, intraperitoneal leakage of gastric contents, and gastrocolonic fistula; most occurred early in our experience. Contraindications to EPG include ascites, esophageal and/or gastric varices, marked obesity, and esophageal obstruction. Prior gastric and other upper abdominal surgery is a relative contraindication to EPG. Gastroesophageal reflux does not preclude the performance of EPG placement. The gastrostomy can later be changed to a transpyloric jejunostomy using endoscopic techniques.[43] Currently, we believe that EPG is a rapid, safe, and perhaps the preferred technique for gastrostomy tube placement in most patients.

Complications of EGD[44]

Perforation of a viscus, bleeding, and pulmonary aspiration are the most common complications of EGD. Perforation occurs in 0.03%–0.1% of cases and usually requires laparotomy or thoracotomy. Bleeding occurs in 0.03% of cases but rarely requires operation. Aspiration has been reported in 0.08% of cases and is especially high in patients with GI hemorrhage and those who are heavily sedated.

Less common complications of EGD include prolonged ileus, transient megacolon, chylothorax, benign air dissection of the esophagus and stomach, strangulated small-bowel obstruction, cardiac arrhythmias, respiratory arrest, and septicemia. Transient bacteremia has been identified in 8% of patients examined,[45] but clinical symptoms are rare. Prophylactic antibiotic therapy is recommended in patients with vascular or cardiac prostheses, rheumatic valvular disease, or mitral valve prolapse. Transmission of viral hepatitis is of concern but has not been reported.

Electrocardiographic recordings during EGD[46] have shown that 40% of patients have ECG changes, including sinus tachycardia, ST-T changes, ventricular and atrial premature beats, atrial premature beats with aberrant conduction, and coronary sinus rhythm. These changes disappear spontaneously, and only 5 of 267,175 patients suffered acute myocardial infarction during EGD. ECG changes are not seen as frequently if premedication has been given.

SMALL-BOWEL ENDOSCOPY

Endoscopes 135–180 cm long can be passed orally into the upper jejunum, and most standard colonoscopes can be advanced nearly 50 cm proximal to the ileocecal valve into the terminal ileum. The major portion of the small intestine, however, is not easily accessible to standard endoscopic instrumentation. Fortunately, the majority of significant abnormalities of the GI tract are located within the range of the gastroscope or colonoscope.

Fiberoptic endoscopy and retrograde pyelography of ileal urinary conduits have been performed with ease and without complication in patients who are suspected of having abnormalities of their ureteroileal conduit.[47] The indications for examination include bleeding, postoperative urinary leakage, stone formation, and ureteric stenosis.

Endoscopes can also be introduced through an ileostomy to assess suspected bleeding from the small bowel or to diagnose recurrent Crohn's disease.

ENDOSCOPY OF THE BILIARY TRACT AND PANCREAS

Choledochoscopy

The incidence of overlooked stones following bile duct exploration and postexploration cholangiography is 2%–10%. Unsuspected stones may be identified by the addition of choledochoscopy to ductal exploration in 5%–24% of cases.[48] Despite this, choledochoscopy has not yet become a routine part of common bile duct exploration.

Postoperative percutaneous flexible fiberoptic choledochoscopy has been performed through the tract formed by a T tube.[49] Stones may be crushed or extracted under direct visualization and mucosal biopsies obtained. Similarly, the gallbladder can be cleared of calculi after cholecystostomy.

The reported complications of choledochoscopy are few and include posterior ductal injury and cholangitis caused by high-pressure injection of saline solution.

Endoscopic Retrograde Cholangiopancreatography (ERCP)

ERCP enables fluoroscopic visualization and radiographic documentation of the biliary tree and the main pancreatic duct. It must be performed with a side-viewing endoscope and high-resolution radiographic equipment. The success rates for visualization of the pancreatic duct and the biliary system in expert hands are 95% and 85%, respectively.[50]

ERCP may detect correctable causes of biliary and pancreatic disease without diagnostic laparotomy. In addition, ERCP provides information about the pancreatic duct that would be difficult to obtain even at laparotomy. A successful ERCP almost always detects extrahepatic biliary obstruction. The site and etiology of the obstruction are also correctly determined in nearly 90% of studies.

Cholangiography is indicated in the jaundiced patient suspected of having surgically treatable bile duct obstruction. Preoperative visualization of the biliary tree may direct surgical management or may obviate operative therapy in patients with hepatocellular disease or surgically untreatable disease. Cholangiography also may be indicated in patients without jaundice who have clinical features and laboratory studies that strongly suggest biliary disease. Cholangiography probably is not indicated for evaluation of obscure abdominal pain without objective evidence of biliary tract disease. The choice between ERCP and percutaneous transhepatic cholangiography (PTC) for visualization of the biliary ductal system depends on several factors, including the availability, quality, safety, and cost of each study at a particular institution.

Pancreatography is indicated in patients with symptoms suggestive of pancreatic adenocarcinoma when ultrasound and CT scan results are normal or nondiagnostic. It is also indicated in patients with recurrent pancreatitis of uncertain etiology and in patients with chronic alcoholic pancreatitis as a guide for operative treatment. In patients with pancreatic ascites from chronic pancreatitis and a pancreaticoperitoneal fistula, ERCP may localize the point of leakage of pancreatic juice and may direct operative treatment.[51] ERCP also permits direct visualization and biopsy of the duodenal papilla, pancreatic fluid cytology and chemical analysis, bile microscopy for occult gallbladder disease, and sphincter of Oddi manometry. An uncooperative patient and acute pancreatitis are generally contraindications to ERCP.

The biliary ductal system must be filled adequately for an accurate assessment. Narrowing of the distal bile duct can be the result of chronic pancreatitis, carcinoma of the pancreas, primary bile duct carcinoma, metastatic carcinoma, and ampullary or papillary stenosis. Tumors usually cause tapered occlusion of the common bile duct, but may show a meniscus above a filling defect. Bile duct stones can coexist with either carcinoma or benign strictures. Obstruction that is complete or nearly complete with irregular margins suggests malignancy. Smooth contours may appear in both benign and malignant processes.

Chronic pancreatitis with fibrosis or pseudocyst formation can cause narrowing and incomplete obstruction of the distal common duct. Ampullary carcinoma is difficult to distinguish radiographically, but direct visualization and endoscopic biopsy of the papilla may be diagnostic. The ductal changes of chronic pancreatitis include irregularities of the side branches, narrowing and dilation of the main duct, and marked "chain-of-lakes" beading (Fig 3–6).

Pancreatic pseudocysts are common in chronic pancreatitis and communicate with the pancreatic ductal system in 75% of

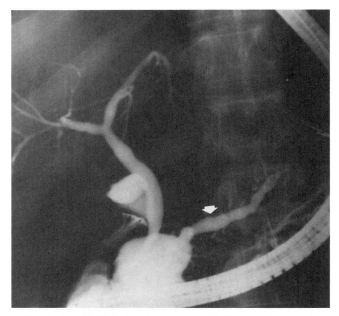

Fig 3–6.—ERCP showing a normal biliary system and an irregular pancreatic duct *(arrow)* with the "chain-of-lakes" appearance associated with chronic pancreatitis. Several radiolucent filling defects are seen in the distal pancreatic duct.

patients. If the pseudocyst is filled, the patient should be treated with IV antibiotics and operated on promptly within 24 hours, unless the cyst is very small and drains rapidly.[52]

In pancreas divisum, the dominant dorsal duct of Santorini empties through an accessory papilla and requires separate cannulation. Changes of chronic pancreatitis may be found either in the attenuated duct of Wirsung or in the dorsal duct of Santorini with dilatation, segmentation, and beading of secondary branches. Pancreas divisum occurs in 3%–4% of patients.[53]

Carcinoma of the pancreas is implied by simultaneous bile duct and pancreatic duct obstruction, segmental disruption of the pancreatic duct, or normal segment of pancreatic duct distal to an obstructing lesion. Pancreatic duct obstruction in the absence of associated biliary duct lesions is not diagnostic of carcinoma and may be the result of pancreatitis. When ductal strictures suggest but are not diagnostic of carcinoma, a cytologic study of secretin-stimulated pancreatic juice may be helpful.

Complications of ERCP include pancreatitis, pancreatic abscess, and cholangitis.[54] The number and diversity of pharmacologic agents used during ERCP increases the likelihood of medication-related reactions compared with colonoscopy and gastroscopy. Choledocholithiasis, pseudocysts, bile duct and pancreatic strictures or tumors increase the risk of developing pancreatitis or biliary sepsis following ERCP. The most important factor in avoiding these problems is recognition of the underlying biliary or pancreatic pathology before or during ERCP and avoidance of overfilling with contrast material. Although the use of prophylatic antibiotics has not been proven, their use when dealing with obstruction of either ductal system is logical.

Sphincterotomy

The development of endoscopic stone removal originated in Germany and Japan in 1974.[55, 56] The indications for sphincterotomy are still evolving. Most retained common duct stones following choledochotomy and cholecystectomy are probably best managed by endoscopic sphincterotomy, unless the stone can be extracted through the T-tube tract. Common duct stones occurring in poor-risk patients whose gallbladder has not been removed may be managed by endoscopic sphincterotomy alone or, in better-risk patients, prior to cholecystectomy. In European centers, as many as 40% of patients undergoing endoscopic sphincterotomy have not had a cholecystectomy. Both benign and malignant strictures of the distal common bile duct have been treated by endoscopic sphincterotomy. Emergency sphincterotomy has been advocated to relieve acute gallstone pancreatitis caused by stone impaction in the distal bile duct.[57] Relative contraindications to endoscopic sphincterotomy include irreversible coagulation disorders and very large stones. A small number of patients will require urgent surgical intervention because of complications or failure to clear the duct.

ERCP is performed in the standard manner. Once the presence of ductal stricture or stones is confirmed, a diagnostic catheter is replaced by one containing a diathermy wire. Stones may be removed by basket forceps or irrigation. Stones smaller than 1 cm will pass spontaneously within a few weeks following sphincterotomy.

For common bile duct stones, sphincterotomy can be successful in 95% of attempts, and all stones are removed in over 90%.[58] Failure of sphincterotomy is usually due to poor access (Billroth II gastrectomy, large diverticula), and failure to extract stones is almost always due to their large size.

Complication rates vary from 7%–10%, with a mortality of 0.5%–2%.[59] Two percent of patients require emergency laparotomy, most frequently for bleeding. Cholangitis occurs only when the technique has failed to provide adequate drainage. Retroperitoneal perforation is a rare complication. Transient hyperamylasemia is common after sphincterotomy, but symptomatic pancreatitis is uncommon. Severe pancreatitis usually means that the orifice of the pancreatic duct has been damaged inadvertently. Impaction of the stone at the sphincterotomy site may occur spontaneously or during attempted basket extraction and can usually be managed endoscopically.

Of 1,000 patients reported, 95% were free of significant biliary symptoms between one and six years following successful sphincterotomy.[59] Papillary stenosis and new stone formation rarely occur and can usually be treated by endoscopic techniques.

FLEXIBLE FIBEROPTIC SIGMOIDOSCOPY (FFS)

In our practice, the flexible fiberoptic sigmoidoscope has replaced the rigid proctoscope. This also has been the experience of others who perform a high volume of rectosigmoid examinations either in the hospital or the office.[60] The rectum and sigmoid colon harbor more than 50% of colonic neoplasms and are the most difficult areas for radiologists to examine with a barium enema. Not surprisingly, FFS yields twice the number of polyps and three times the number of cancers compared with rigid proctoscopy.[61] Preparation is accomplished by two 800–1,000-ml tap water or phosphate enemas. No sedation is required for the examination, and patient comfort is equal to that experienced with rigid proctoscopy. Experienced endoscopists can examine two thirds of patients to 55 cm and 95% of the examinations can be completed in less than ten minutes.[61] The technique is relatively simple to learn and has gained widespread acceptance and use.

We believe that the indications for FFS are the same as those for rigid proctosigmoidoscopy. FFS is safe in the hands of well-trained people, but occasional complications occur, as with rigid proctosigmoidoscopy. Complications of FFS are identical to those of colonoscopy.

COLONOSCOPY

Since its introduction in 1968, the flexible fiberoptic colonoscope has become the most accurate method for the diagnosis of mucosal diseases of the colon. Although the technological advances necessary for the development of the colonoscope were enormous, it is simply a longer, flexible proctoscope.

Preparation

A thorough understanding of the indications and anticipated benefits of the colonoscopic examination are essential. Appropriate history and physical examination and a knowledge of the results of any previous barium enema studies are part of the preparation. Informed consent should be obtained from the patient.

An empty, clean colon can be achieved by a variety of methods.[62] We premedicate our inpatients with meperidine and secobarbital, but this is impractical in an outpatient setting. Additional sedation, as needed, is achieved with IV diazepam and/or meperidine. Both diagnostic and therapeutic colonoscopy can be performed safely on an outpatient basis.[63] We admit only patients in whom therapeutic colonoscopy may be unusually dangerous or difficult, such as patients with large or multiple polyps or elderly patients. For convenience we perform most colonoscopic examinations in an ambulatory surgery unit, but colonoscopy can be performed in a treatment room, office, or at the bedside.

Technique

There are several very good descriptions of the techniques of colonoscopy.[64] Gentleness and a willingness to terminate the examination are essential. We do not employ fluoroscopy. Manual pressure to the abdomen applied by an assistant can be very helpful. Because the colon may be stretched in length during the examination, the centimeter markings on the colonoscope do not reliably measure distances from the anus to points in the colon. The internal landmarks of the colonic segments combined with abdominal wall transillumination will give the best indication of the location of the tip of the colonoscope.

Indications for Colonoscopy (Table 3–2)

Although barium enema and diagnostic colonoscopy are said to be complementary studies, some European centers

TABLE 3–2.—INDICATIONS FOR COLONOSCOPY

Diagnostic
  Barium enema abnormality requiring additional information
  Colon carcinoma
  Cancer surveillance
  Unexplained colonic bleeding
  Unexplained and persistent diarrhea
  Inflammatory bowel disease—selected patients
    Mass
    Stricture
    Preoperative definition of extent of disease
    Nonspecific colitis
    Surveillance for cancer
Therapeutic
  Polypectomy
  Foreign-body removal
  Decompression of acute colon dilatation
  Hemostasis

now perform colonoscopy as the initial diagnostic study in all patients with lower GI symptoms. Until colonoscopy becomes less expensive and more endoscopists are trained to perform the examination, we believe that a barium enema is a better initial diagnostic procedure. If the barium enema is abnormal but more information such as histologic confirmation is required, or if the barium enema is normal but significant symptoms such as diarrhea or bleeding remain unexplained, colonoscopy is indicated. We do not obtain an initial barium enema in screening patients at high risk for colon cancer, but proceed directly to colonoscopy. We also are beginning to use colonoscopy to evaluate any lower GI bleeding that is not explained by proctoscopy. In addition, selected patients with inflammatory bowel disease will benefit from a screening colonoscopic examination.

Contraindications to Colonoscopy

Absolute Contraindications

SUSPECTED PERFORATION OR PERITONITIS.—Manipulation of the endoscope and increased intracolonic pressure may cause a weak area to perforate or spread the contents of a localized perforation to the entire peritoneal cavity.

ACUTE FULMINATING INFLAMMATORY DISEASE.—Perforation of the colon may result from colonscopy in cases of toxic megacolon, acute ulcerative colitis, acute diverticulitis, and appendicitis.

SEVERE COAGULOPATHY.—This may occur during a difficult diagnostic examination in patients with coagulopathy. Small vessels may be torn, resulting in major bleeding or obstruction. Ideally, patients should have a negative bleeding history or a normal blood coagulation profile before undergoing either diagnostic or therapeutic colonoscopy.

Relative Contraindications

The risk of colonoscopy may be increased in patients with prior myocardial infarction, severe angina, and abdominal aortic or iliac aneurysms because of the usually minor, but real, stress of the examination and the necessary manipulations of the colonoscope causing direct trauma to the aneurysm wall.

Diagnostic Colonscopy

Barium Enema Abnormality Requiring Additional Information

The barium enema is an indirect examination, often resulting in equivocal findings that must be evaluated by direct visualization and biopsy of the mucosa. Lesions suggestive of cancer or polyps on barium enema require endoscopic examination; polyps can be removed. It is important to remember that *a negative fractional biopsy of a colon lesion is inadequate,* and excisional biopsy is indicated for most mucosal lesions.

Strictures of the colon always require examination and biopsy because of the possibility of malignancy.[65] In cases of inflammatory bowel disease, especially ulcerative colitis, a stricture should be considered malignant until proven otherwise. Anastomotic narrowing following colon resection for cancer might indicate a suture line recurrence. Following a resection for colon cancer, we routinely examine the anastomosis endoscopically every six months for two years; more than 90% of suture line recurrences will occur during this interval. Submucosal lesions cannot be biopsied with current techniques, but direct visualization of these lesions will at least exclude a mucosal abnormality.

A colonic fistula to another organ (bladder, stomach, small intestine, uterus, vagina), to the retroperitoneum, or to the skin usually has an obvious cause, such as diverticulitis, cancer, or Crohn's disease. However, if the differential diagnosis includes colon cancer, colonoscopy and biopsy will significantly aid in preoperative planning.

Colon Carcinoma

If a lesion has the obvious appearance of cancer by barium enema, biopsy is unnecessary and costly (Fig 3–7). However, we believe that it is extremely important to *clear* the rest of the colon, especially the part that will remain following cancer resection, of synchronous lesions. The incidence of synchronous colon cancers is 3%–7%,[66] and the incidence of synchronous neoplastic polyps, believed to be premalignant lesions, is 20%–40%.[67] "Clearing" colonoscopy ideally is done preoperatively, but in the case of a near-obstructing cancer, it can

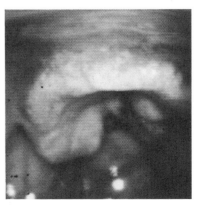

Fig 3–7.—Typical annular carcinoma of the sigmoid colon with heaped-up edges and ulcerated center.

be performed postoperatively or even intraoperatively. After all neoplastic colon lesions have been removed or excluded, a schedule for future surveillance can be determined.

Cancer Surveillance for High-Risk Patients

Patients with a prior colon cancer or neoplastic polyp, a ureterosigmoidostomy, a less than subtotal colectomy for familial polyposis, and those with chronic ulcerative colitis are at greater risk for the future development of colon cancer. There is debate about how frequently, or even whether, colonoscopic surveillance is indicated for these patients. Firm data are not available, and the following recommendations are based on the best information presently available.

PREVIOUS COLON CANCER.—Since more than 90% of suture line recurrences appear within two years, we examine the anastomosis every six months for two years with either sigmoidoscopy or colonscopy, depending on the level of the anastomosis. The incidence of metachronous polyps is 10%–20%[67] and that of metachronous colonic cancer is 1.6%–4.6%[68]; therefore, we perform clearing colonoscopy every two to three years for the remaining life of the patient. A combination of flexible sigmoidoscopy and air contrast barium enema is an acceptable alternative if the patient is especially difficult to examine with the colonoscope or finds the examination particularly uncomfortable.

PREVIOUS NEOPLASTIC POLYP(S) (TUBULAR ADENOMA, VILLOUS ADENOMA, OR CARCINOMA IN SITU).—Because removal of polyps may prevent subsequent cancer[69] and because of the 20%–30%[67] incidence of subsequent polyps, we perform colonscopy, and excision of newly discovered polyps every two to three years.

PREVIOUS URETEROSIGMOIDOSTOMY.—There is a known increased incidence of colon cancer at or very near stomas of long-standing ureterosigmoidostomies.[70] Flexible endoscopic examination of the sigmoid colon every two to three years is probably indicated, beginning 5–10 years after construction of a ureterosigmoidostomy. There have also been reports (including two cases in our series) of snare excision of a prolapsed ureter that was mistaken for a pedunculated polyp. We therefore recommend initial biopsy prior to snare excision of pedunculated lesions in such patients.

LONG-STANDING ULCERATIVE COLITIS.—There is clear evidence that the incidence of colon cancer is markedly increased in patients who have had ulcerative pancolitis for at least 8–10 years. If colectomy is not contemplated, screening colonoscopy and biopsy are performed every 6–12 months. This type of surveillance is not infallible, and cancers can be missed.[71] There is good evidence that rectal biopsies containing severe mucosal dysplasia frequently accompany cancer in other parts of that colon.[72] Many centers sample the mucosa of the entire colon annually, but it is unclear whether this sampling will detect more colon cancers earlier than will simple rectal biopsy and barium enema.

Unexplained Colonic Bleeding[73]

In our practice, flexible endoscopy and arteriography have totally replaced barium contrast studies in the initial evaluation of patients with GI hemorrhage.

ACUTE ACTIVE BLEEDING.—After resuscitation of the bleeding patient, it is important first to determine whether the bleeding originates from the upper or lower GI tract. Red blood per rectum is more likely to originate from the more common lesions of the upper GI tract (ulcers, esophageal varices, gastritis). If the nasogastric tube aspirate of the stomach is clear, we recommend rapid esophagogastroduodenoscopy to eliminate an upper GI source of bleeding. In cases of acute massive bleeding from the colon, urgent colonoscopy may be performed following a gavage preparation. A precise diagnosis can be made in at least 50% of patients.[74] If colonoscopy is unrewarding, we proceed with emergency visceral arteriography to attempt to localize the bleeding site.

INTERMITTENT BLEEDING.—Fortunately, even the most massive lower GI bleeding usually stops. Colonoscopy is the most accurate method for localizing lower GI hemorrhage. It is the preferred diagnostic study when the history suggests colonic bleeding from above the rectum and the proctoscopy is negative. Several large series of patients undergoing colonoscopy after a negative barium enema and sigmoidoscopy showed a 10%–13% incidence of colon cancer, a 14%–16% incidence of neoplastic polyps, and a 7%–10% incidence of inflammatory bowel disease.[75–77]

OCCULT BLEEDING.—Most often occult bleeding originates in the lower GI tract. Although some centers continue to evaluate such patients with rigid sigmoidoscopy, barium enema, and barium upper GI examination, we have replaced these studies with more accurate and rapid endoscopic examinations. If colonscopy is nondiagnostic, esophagogastroduodenoscopy is indicated to eliminate a chronic upper GI bleeding source.

Unexplained and Persistent Diarrhea

Surgeons rarely see patients for this complaint, but there is a place for colonoscopic examination and mucosal biopsy in selected patients.

ISCHEMIC COLITIS.—Elderly patients can present with hematochezia, abdominal pain, and diarrhea suggestive of acute ischemia without systemic intoxication. Operation is indicated for patients with signs of peritoneal irritation, but colonscopy may be useful in accurately establishing the diagnosis of segmental mucosal ischemic colitis in less ill patients.[78]

At least 7% of patients will develop mucosal or even full-thickness ischemic necrosis of a part of the rectosigmoid colon during the first week following aortic reconstruction.[79] Flexible fiberoptic examination of the left colon can demonstrate mucosal changes of ischemia and can guide the surgeon in subsequent therapy. If normal mucosa is seen, the diagnosis of ischemia can be eliminated. It is important to remember that only the mucosa is visualized endoscopically, but the necrosis may be partial or full thickness. Our experience includes more than 15 patients who have had mucosal ischemic necrosis of the mucosa that has healed totally without the need for colostomy or colectomy.

Pseudomembranous colitis.—Antibiotic-induced colitis is being seen more frequently. A precise diagnosis can be made by visualization of mucosal inflammation, by the classic pseudomembrane, and by mucosal biopsy.

Inflammatory Bowel Disease

Colonoscopy should not be a routine procedure for the evaluation of patients with inflammatory bowel disease. The diagnostic study of choice remains single or double contrast barium enema.[80] Patients with the following specific indications may benefit from colonoscopic examination.

Mass.—The possibility of colon cancer must be eliminated, and if the barium enema suggests a neoplasm, colonoscopy and biopsy are indicated.

Stricture.—If a stricture is found during barium enema, it should be evaluated by direct visualization and biopsy to eliminate the possibility of a malignant stricture.

Nonspecific colitis.—As more specific forms of therapy are developed, it becomes important to differentiate among Crohn's, ulcerative, and other forms of colitis. Because barium enema and sigmoidoscopy may fail to provide a specific diagnosis, colonoscopy and directed biopsies may be helpful.

Therapeutic Colonoscopy

Polypectomy

Developed by Wolff and Shinya in the early 1970s,[81] colonoscopic polypectomy has changed the excision of colon polyps from a major procedure requiring laparotomy to a simple outpatient procedure. This change has also been associated with a significant reduction in cost, morbidity, and mortality.

Polyp-cancer sequence.—Almost all colon cancers develop in preexisting adenomas.[82] The removal of neoplastic (tubular adenoma, tubulovillous adenoma, villous adenoma, carcinoma in situ) polyps will therefore decrease the incidence of colon cancer.[69] Because adenomatous polyps may contain random small areas of invasive cancer, complete excision rather than fractional biopsy is essential for all neoplastic colon lesions.

Guidelines for polypectomy.[83]—Generally the colon should be completely cleared, and any polyp greater than 0.5 cm in diameter should be totally excised and submitted for histologic examination. Large polyps that appear sessile on barium enema may have a stalk and should be visualized endoscopically. If final histology reveals a neoplastic polyp with no evidence of invasion of the muscularis mucosa, polypectomy alone has been adequate therapy. If focally invasive adenocarcinoma is confined to the head of a pedunculated adenoma, polypectomy alone is controversial treatment.[83, 84] If there is invasive cancer in a sessile adenoma or if there is cancer at the line of polyp resection, a colon resection is indicated. Piecemeal excision of large sessile polyps, snare removal of polyps with a stalk 1 cm or greater in diameter, and snare removal of submucosal polyps are not recommended for the occasional colonoscopist.

Foreign-Body Removal

Although most foreign objects that pass the pylorus rarely lodge in the colon, dental crowns, dental drills, intestinal tubes, and sutures are some of the objects that have been removed colonoscopically.

Decompression of Acute Colon Dilatation

With untreated volvulus or dilatation of the colon, ischemia of the wall and/or perforation are common sequelae. The colonoscope has been used successfully to correct these conditions.

Volvulus.—For many years, rigid proctoscopy and the insertion of a rectal tube have been used to treat acute sigmoid volvulus. After acute detorsion and decompression of the colon, the patient may undergo elective sigmoid resection. Treatment of transverse colon and cecal volvulus with the colonoscope have also been described, but most clinicians agree that colon resection is indicated for these segments of colon instead of, or soon after, acute decompression.

Nonobstructive colonic dilatation (NCD) (Fig 3–8, A and B).—This entity, also called Ogilvie's syndrome, adynamic ileus of the colon, and pseudo-obstruction, is uncommon in severely ill patients. If untreated, NCD may progress to cecal perforation or rupture. Operative tube cecostomy has been advocated for these critically ill patients but has been associated with a high operative mortality. In 1977 we described five patients in whom the colon was decompressed successfully using the colonoscope.[85] Others have also reported successful colonoscopic decompression for patients with NCD.[86] Our recent experience shows that 38 of 44 patients (86%) were successfully treated by this method with few complications.[87] Colonoscopic examination is also helpful to eliminate obstructing carcinoma, volvulus, or ischemic disease as the cause of acute colonic dilatation. In addition, we have been able to assess the viability of the cecal mucosa in these patients. In patients who were noted to have patchy areas of mucosal necrosis, cecectomy was performed before perforation occurred. Colonoscopy in an unprepared colon is difficult and should be attempted only by an experienced colonoscopist.

Hemostasis

Endoscopic snare polypectomy will eliminate polyps as possible sources of bleeding. The results of electrocoagulation and laser photocoagulation of arteriovenous malformations and other bleeding lesions of the colon are promising, but these techniques are still in an experimental stage and are not now recommended for general use.

Complications

As with any invasive diagnostic or therapeutic procedure, complications of colonoscopy and flexible fiberoptic sigmoidoscopy are inevitable. Nevertheless, these procedures are surprisingly safe, and complications can be minimized by technical expertise, a gentle and careful technique, clear in-

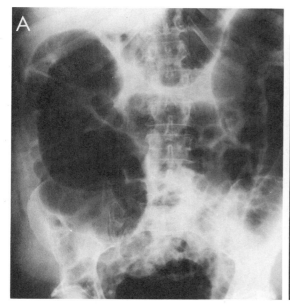
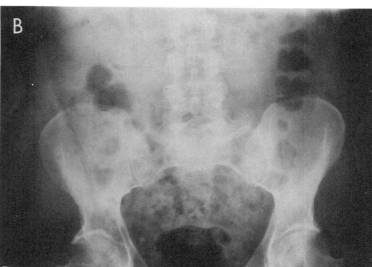

Fig 3–8.—A, patient with nonobstructive cecal dilatation. The cecum measures 14 cm in transverse diameter. **B,** same patient following colonoscopic decompression. Normal bowel function returned within 48 hours.

dications for the procedure, and a knowledge of potential complications and their prevention. Complications should be recognized and dealt with quickly and appropriately. As with any surgical procedure, the incidence of complications varies inversely with the experience of the endoscopist.

Death rarely results from colonoscopy but is usually a consequence of perforation of the colon. In a survey of the membership of the American Society for Gastrointestinal Endoscopy, the mortality rate for colonoscopy was 0.3%.[88]

Perforation occurs rarely after flexible fiberoptic sigmoidoscopy, but the incidence after diagnostic colonoscopy is 0.2%–0.3% and 0.5%–1.9% after therapeutic colonscopy.[89] Causes of perforation during diagnostic colonoscopy include rupture of a diverticulum due to increased intraluminal pressure, forcing the scope through a narrowed colonic segment, improper use of the alpha or other manuevers, using a splinting device without fluoroscopy, and forceful advancement without a view of the colon lumen. During therapeutic colonscopy, perforation may occur because of deep electrocautery damage to the colon wall or laceration or penetration of the colon wall by the particular instrument. Immediate perforations are recognized by sudden severe abdominal pain, signs of peritonitis, and shock. After fluid resuscitation and antibiotic administration, immediate laparotomy is required. Delayed perforations are more common and usually occur within 72 hours. The onset of symptoms may be insidious and mimic flu-like syndromes, with abdominal pain and diarrhea. Laparotomy and resection or colostomy are usually necessary for delayed perforations. After polypectomy, an occasional patient may develop abdominal pain and tenderness without generalized peritonitis and may be managed conservatively. Asymptomatic pneumoperitoneum occurs, presumably due to air dissection through the colon wall, and may not require specific therapy.

Bleeding occurs in 0.07%–0.5% of diagnostic examinations and in 1%–1.8% of therapeutic examinations.[89] The bleeding usually is self-limited, and laparotomy is rarely necessary. Regrasping and/or recoagulating the transected polyp stalk and arteriographic vasopressin infusion may induce hemostasis. Most bleeding occurs immediately, but delayed hemorrhage can occur up to two weeks following polypectomy.

Miscellaneous complications include adverse reactions to medication, dehydration from cathartics, cardiac arrhythmias, gangrenous cecal volvulus, splenic rupture and incarceration of an inguinal hernia. Bacteremia occurs occasionally, but prophylactic antibiotics are recommended only when a patient is immunosuppressed; has a cardiac, vascular, bone, or other prosthesis; or has valvular heart disease.

SPECIAL PROBLEMS

Gastrointestinal Hemorrhage

Our approach to GI hemorrhage has become very straightforward.[73] Most patients who have acute, intermittent, or even chronic blood loss are ideal candidates for direct endoscopic examination of their GI mucosa. Endoscopy will provide an immediate diagnosis with minimal morbidity, and therapeutic measures can be instituted promptly. Barium contrast studies now are rarely used in the evaluation of GI hemorrhage. Endoscopy and visceral angiography have virtually eliminated exploratory laparotomy followed by "blind" gastrectomy and colectomy, which, as recently as 15 years ago, were common operations for GI hemorrhage.

For those few patients with truly massive bleeding, visceral angiography is probably a better initial diagnostic procedure, although emergent laparotomy occasionally may be necessary if vital signs cannot be maintained by vigorous resuscitation with fluids and blood.

The patient with active GI hemorrhage should have rapid resuscitation, a complete history and physical examination, appropriate laboratory studies, and nasogastric tube aspiration. If the stomach contains blood, saline lavage is used to clear the stomach, and esophagogastroduodenoscopy is performed. If the lavage fluid remains bloody with clots, visceral arteriography should be considered. However, a limited EGD examination might be useful to determine whether or not esophageal varices are present. Even if the initial nasogastric aspirate is clear, EGD should be performed to eliminate the possibility of intermittent bleeding from statistically more common upper GI lesions. If EGD is negative, colonoscopy is indicated if proctoscopy is unrewarding. Stool and blood can be rapidly eliminated by a 4–6 L gavage by nasogastric tube. If urgent EGD and/or colonoscopy are unrewarding, arteriography and red cell scans may be helpful in some cases of mild to moderately active bleeding (0.5 ml/min or greater). EGD is at least 90% accurate in determining the source of acute upper GI hemorrhage. Colonoscopy has revealed significant lesions in 50% with active colonic hemorrhage.[74]

For patients with intermittent hemorrhage of unknown origin, we follow the same sequence of EGD, proctoscopy, colonoscopy, and then arteriography. Obviously, this diagnostic sequence is stopped when a convincing source of hemorrhage is found. Appropriate treatment is instituted. We believe that barium studies are inaccurate and delay appropriate therapy in patients with intermittent bleeding. Colonoscopy has revealed significant lesions in 40% of patients with intermittent rectal bleeding and negative barium contrast studies.[75]

In patients with occult chronic GI blood loss, screening barium contrast studies may be useful. However, we frequently proceed with endoscopic examination because of their rapidity and accuracy, reserving barium contrast studies for those with unrewarding endoscopic examinations.

Intraoperative Endoscopy

Endoscopic examination of the GI tract during an operative abdominal procedure occasionally is helpful. A 185-cm endoscope can be passed either orally or anally and manipulated through the entire alimentary tract, allowing visualization of the mucosa and transillumination of the small bowel in search of obscure bleeding lesions. When preoperative colonoscopy has been prevented by sharp kinking of the colon and adhesion formation, the scope can be manipulated intraoperatively, allowing a safe examination.[90] Colonoscopic clearing of the proximal colon can be accomplished by passing the endoscope through a colostomy made above an obstructing rectal or sigmoid colon cancer.

REFERENCES

1. Dent T.L.: The surgeon and fiberoptic endoscopy. *Surg. Gynecol. Obstet.* 137:278, 1973.
2. Wolff W.I., Shinya H.: Modern endoscopy of the alimentary tract. *Curr. Probl. Surg.* Chicago, Year Book Medical Publishers Inc., January 1974.
3. Sugawa C., Schuman B.M.: *Primer of Gastrointestinal Fiberoptic Endoscopy.* Boston, Little, Brown & Co., 1981.
4. Schuman B.M.: The gastroscopic yield from the negative upper gastrointestinal series. *Gastrointest. Endosc.* 19:79, 1972.
5. Tedesco F.J.: Endoscopy in the evaluation of patients with upper gastrointestinal symptoms: Indications, expectations, and interpretation. *J. Clin. Gastroenterol.* 3:67, 1981.
6. Strawn T., Knutson C.O., Max M.H.: The role of endoscopy in patients with suspected esophageal reflux. *Am. Surg.* 46:95, 1980.
7. DeMeester T.R., Lafontaine E., Joelsson B.E., et al.: Relationship of a hiatal hernia to the function of the body of the esophagus and the gastroesophageal junction. *J. Thorac. Cardiovasc. Surg.* 92:547, 1981.
8. Stadelmann O., Elster K., Kuhn H.A.: Columnar-lined oesophagus (Barrett's syndrome)—congenital or acquired? *Endoscopy* 13:140, 1981.
9. Naef A.T., Savary M., Ozzello L.: Columnar-lined lower esophagus: An acquired lesion with malignant predisposition. *J. Thorac. Cardiovasc. Surg.* 70:826, 1975.
10. Scott B.B., Jenkins D.: Gastro-oesophageal candidiasis. *Gut* 23:137, 1982.
11. Dagradi A.E., Rodiles D.H., Cooper E., et al.: Endoscopic diagnosis of esophageal varices. *Am. J. Gastroenterol.* 60:371, 1973.
12. Mitchell C.J., Jewell D.P.: The diagnosis of the site of upper gastrointestinal hemorrhage in patients with established portal hypertension. *Endoscopy* 9:131, 1977.
13. Beppu K., Inokuchi K., Koyanagi N., et al.: Prediction of variceal hemorrhage by esophageal endoscopy. *Gastrointest. Endosc.* 27:213, 1981.
14. Hixon N.D., Burns R.P., Britt L.G.: Mallory-Weiss syndrome: Restrospective review of eight years' experience. *South. Med. J.* 72:1249, 1979.
15. Whitehead R., Truelove S.C., Gear M.W.L.: The histological diagnosis of chronic gastritis in fiberoptic gastroscope biopsy specimens. *J. Clin. Pathol.* 25:1, 1972.
16. Op Den Orth J.O., Dekker W.: Gastric erosions: Radiological and endoscopic aspects. *Radiol. Clin.* 45:88, 1976.
17. Moody F.G., Cheung L.Y.: Stress ulcers; their pathogenesis, diagnosis, and treatment. *Surg. Clin. North Am.* 56:1469, 1976.
18. Lucas C.E., Sugawa C., Friend W., et al.: Therapeutic implications of disturbed gastric physiology in patients with stress ulcerations. *Am. J. Surg.* 123:25, 1972.
19. Kamada T., Fusamoto H., Kawano S., et al.: Acute gastroduodenal lesions in head injury. *Am. J. Gastroenterol.* 68:249, 1977.
20. Rosenthal A., Czaja A.J., Pruitt B.A.: Gastrin levels and gastric acidity in the pathogenesis of acute gastroduodenal disease after burns. *Surg. Gynecol. Obstet.* 144:232, 1977.
21. Le Gall J.R., Mignon F.C., Rapin M., et al.: Acute gastroduodenal lesions related to severe sepsis. *Surg. Gynecol. Obstet.* 142:377, 1976.
22. Wells J.J., Nostrant T.T., Wilson J.A.P., et al.: Gastroduodenal ulcerations in patients receiving selective hepatic artery infusion chemotherapy. *Gastrointest. Endosc.* 29:169, 1983.
23. Partyke E.K., Sanowski R.A., Kozarek R.A.: Endoscopic diagnosis of gastric angiodysplasis. *Gastrointest. Endosc.* 26:151, 1980.
24. Graham D.Y., Schwartz J.T., Cain G.D., et al.: Prospective evaluation of biopsy number in the diagnosis of esophageal and gastric carcinoma. *Gastroenterology* 82:228, 1982.
25. Halse S.A., Kristensen E., Jensen O.M., et al.: Prognosis of medically treated gastric ulcer: A prospective endoscopic study. *Scand. J. Gastroenterol.* 12:489, 1977.
26. ReMine S.G., Hughes R.W., Weiland L.H.: Endoscopic gastric polypectomies. *Mayo Clin. Proc.* 56:371, 1981.
27. Okui K., Tejima H.: Minute gastric cancers found by gastric mass surveys. *Gastroenterol. Jpn.* 15:108, 1980.
28. Bowden T.: Fiberoptic endoscopy of the stomach after gastrectomy. *Am. Surg.* 43:287, 1977.
29. Geboes K., Rutgeerts P., Broekaert L., et al.: Histologic appearances of endoscopic gastric mucosal biopsies 10–20 years after partial gastrectomy. *Ann. Surg.* 192:179, 1980.
30. Kiil J., Andersen D.: X-ray examination and/or endoscopy in the diagnosis of gastroduodenal ulcer and cancer. *Scand. J. Gastroenterol.* 15:39, 1980.
31. Gelzayd E.A., Gelfand D.W., Rinaldo J.A.: Nonspecific duodenitis: A distinct clinical entity. *Gastrointest. Endosc.* 19:131, 1973.
32. Rutgeerts P., Onette E., Vantrappen G., et al.: Crohn's disease of the stomach and duodenum: A clinical study with emphasis on the value of endoscopy and endoscopic biopsies. *Endoscopy* 12:288, 1980.
33. Hajiro K., Yamamoto H., Matsui H., et al.: Endoscopic diagnosis

and excision of intraluminal duodenal diverticulum. *Gastrointest. Endosc.* 25:151, 1979.

34. Gelzayd E.A., Jetly K.: Fiberendoscopy: Removal of a retained sewing needle from the stomach. *Gastrointest. Endosc.* 18:161, 1972.

35. Asaki S., Nishimura T., Sato M., et al.: Endoscopic gastric polypectomy using high frequency current; its significance for total biopsy of gastric polyp. *Tohoju J. Exp. Med.* 135:309, 1981.

36. Smith J.L., Graham D.Y.: Variceal hemorrhage: A critical evaluation of survival analysis. *Gastroenterology* 82:968, 1982.

37. Johnston G.W., Rodgers H.W.: A review of 15 years' experience in the use of sclerotherapy in the control of acute haemorrhage for oesophageal varices. *Br. J. Surg.* 60:797, 1973.

38. Sivak M.V.: Letter to the editor. *Gastrointest. Endosc.* 28:116, 1982.

39. Terblanche J., Yakoob H.I., Bornman P.C., et al.: Acute bleeding varices: A five-year prospective evaluation of tamponade and sclerotherapy. *Ann. Surg.* 194:521, 1981.

40. Hennessy T.P.J., Stephens R.B., Keane F.B.: Acute and chronic management of varices by injection sclerotherapy. *Surg. Gynecol. Obstet.* 154:375, 1982.

41. Fleischer D.E.: The current status of gastrointestinal laser activity in the United States. *Gastrointest. Endosc.* 28:157, 1982.

42. Ponsky J.L., Gauderer M.W.L.: Percutaneous endoscopic gastrostomy: A non-operative technique for feeding gastrostomy. *Gastrointest. Endosc.* 27:9, 1981.

43. Strodel W.E., Eckhauser F.E., Dent T.L. et al.: Gastrostomy to jejunostomy conversion. *Gastrointest. Endosc.* 30:35, 1984.

44. Shahmir M., Schuman B.M.: Complications of fiberoptic endoscopy. *Gastrointest. Endosc.* 26:86, 1980.

45. Stephenson P.M., Dorrington L., Harris O.D., et al.: Bacteraemia following oesophageal dilatation and oesophago-gastroscopy. *Aust. N.Z. J. Med.* 7:32, 1977.

46. Levy N., Abinader E.: Continuous electrocardiographic monitoring with Holter electrocardiocorder throughout all stages of gastroscopy. *Dig. Dis. Sci.* 22:1091, 1977.

47. Ramsburgh S.R., Dent T.L., Herwig K.R.: Flexible fiberoscopy of urinary conduits. *J. Urol.* 116:166, 1976.

48. Shore J.M., Berci G., Morgenstern L.: The value of biliary endoscopy. *Surg. Gynecol. Obstet.* 140:601, 1975.

49. Jakimowicz J.J., Mak B., Carol E.J., et al.: Postoperative choledochoscopy. *Arch. Surg.* 118:810, 1983.

50. Cotton P.B.: ERCP. *Gut* 18:316, 1977.

51. Levine J.B., Warshaw A.L., Falchuk K.R., et al.: The value of endoscopic retrograde pancreatography in the management of pancreatic ascites. *Surgery* 81:360, 1977.

52. Sugawa C., Walt A.S.: Endoscopic retrograde pancreatography in the surgery of pancreatic pseudocysts. *Surgery* 86:639, 1979.

53. Gregg J.A., Monaco A.P., McDermott W.V.: Pancreas divisum. *Am. J. Surg.* 145:488, 1983.

54. Ihre T., Hellers G.: Complications and endoscopic retrograde cholangio-pancreatography: A review of the literature and presentation of a duodenal perforation. *Acta Chir. Scand.* 143:167, 1977.

55. Kawai K., et al.: Endoscopic sphincterotomy of the ampulla of Vater. *Gastrointest. Endosc.* 20:148, 1974.

56. Classen M., Demling L.: Endoskopisch sphincterotomie der papilla Vateri. *Dtsch. Med. Wochenschr.* 99:496, 1974.

57. Zimmon D.S., Clemett A.R.: Endoscopic stents and drains in the management of pancreatic and bile duct obstruction. *Surg. Clin. North Am.* 62:837, 1982.

58. Cotton P.B., Villon A.G.: British experience with duodenoscopic sphincterotomy for treatment of bile duct stones. *Br. J. Surg.* 68:1373, 1982.

59. Safrany L., Cotton P.B.: Endoscopic management of choledocholithiasis. *Surg. Clin. North Am.* 62:825, 1982.

60. Traul D.G., Davis C.B., Pollock J.C., et al.: Flexible fiberoptic sigmoidoscopy—the Monroe Clinic experience. *Dis. Colon Rectum* 26:161, 1983.

61. Marks G., Boggs H.W., Castro A.F., et al.: Sigmoidoscopic examinations with rigid and flexible fiberoptic sigmoidoscopes in the surgeon's office: A comparative prospective study of effectiveness in 1,012 cases. *Dis. Colon Rectum* 22:162, 1979.

62. Thomas G., Brozinsky S., Isenberg J.I.: Patient acceptance and effectiveness of a balanced lavage solution (Golytely) versus the standard preparation for colonoscopy. *Gastroenterology* 82:435, 1982.

63. Norfleet R.G.: Colonoscopy and polypectomy in nonhospitalized patients. *Gastrointest. Endosc.* 28:15, 1982.

64. Cotton P., Williams C.: *Practical Gastrointestinal Endoscopy.* St. Louis, Blackwell Scientific Publications, 1980.

65. Forde K.A., Lebwohl O., Seaman W.B.: Colonoscopy as an adjunctive technique in evaluating acquired colonic narrowing. *Surgery* 87:243, 1980.

66. Kronborg O., Hage E., Deichgraeber E.: The remaining colon after radical surgery for colorectal cancer: The first three years of a prospective study. *Dis. Colon Rectum* 26:172, 1983.

67. Shinya H.: *Colonoscopy, Diagnosis and Treatment of Colonic Diseases.* New York, Igaku-Shoin Medical Publishers Inc., 1982.

68. Nava H.R., Pagana T.J.: Postoperative surveillance of colorectal carcinoma. *Cancer* 49:1043, 1982.

69. Gilbertson V.A.: Proctosigmoidoscopy and polypectomy in reducing the incidence of rectal cancer. *Cancer* 34:936, 1974.

70. Tank E.S., Karsch D.N., Lapides J.: Adenocarcinoma of the colon associated with ureterosigmoidoscopy: Report of a case. *Dis. Colon Rectum* 16:300, 1973.

71. Butt J.H., Konishi F., Morson B.C., et al.: Macroscopic lesions in dysplasia and carcinoma complicating ulcerative colitis. *Dig. Dis. Sci.* 28:18, 1983.

72. Gewertz B.L., Dent T.L., Appleman H.D.: Implications of precancerous rectal biopsy in patients with inflammatory bowel disease. *Arch. Surg.* 111:326, 1976.

73. Dent T.L.: Evaluation of the bleeding patient. *Surg. Gynecol. Obstet.* 151:817, 1980.

74. Forde K.A.: Colonoscopy in acute rectal bleeding. *Gastrointest. Endosc.* 27:219, 1981.

75. Swarbrick E.T., Fevre D.I., Hunt R.H., et al.: Colonoscopy for unexplained rectal bleeding. *Br. Med. J.* 2:1685, 1978.

76. Teague R.H., Thornton J.R., Manning A.P., et al.: Colonoscopy for investigation of unexplained rectal bleeding. *Lancet* 1:1350, 1978.

77. Knutson C.O., Max M.H.: Value of colonoscopy in patients with rectal blood loss unexplained by rigid proctosigmoidoscopy and barium contrast enema examinations. *Am. J. Surg.* 139:84, 1980.

78. Forde K.A., Lebwohl O., Wolff M., et al.: Reversible ischemic colitis—correlation of colonoscopic and pathologic changes. *Am. J. Gastroenterol.* 72:182, 1979.

79. Hagihara P.F., Ernst C.B., Griffen W.O. Jr.: Incidence of ischemic colitis following abdominal aortic reconstruction. *Surg. Gynecol. Obstet.* 149:571, 1979.

80. Hogan W.J., Hensley G.T., Geenen J.E.: Endoscopic evaluation of inflammatory bowel disease. *Med. Clin. North Am.* 64:1083, 1980.

81. Wolff W.I., Shinya H.: Polypectomy via the fiberoptic colonoscope. *N. Engl. J. Med.* 288:329, 1973.

82. Fenoglio C.M., Pascal R.R.: Colorectal adenomas and cancer: Pathologic relationships. *Cancer* 50:2601, 1982.

83. Shinya H., Cooperman A., Wolff W.I.: A rationale for the endoscopic management of colonic polyps. *Surg. Clin. North Am.* 62:861, 1982.

84. Colacchio T.A., Forde K.A., Scantlebury V.P.: Endoscopic polypectomy: Inadequate treatment for invasive colorectal carcinoma. *Ann. Surg.* 194:704, 1981.

85. Kukora J.S., Dent T.L.: Colonoscopic decompression of massive nonobstructive cecal dilation. *Arch. Surg.* 112:512, 1977.

86. Nivatvongs S., Vermeulen F.D., Fang D.T.: Colonoscopic decompression of acute pseudo-obstruction of the colon. *Ann. Surg.* 196:598, 1982.

87. Strodel W.E., Nostrant T.T., Eckhauser F.E., et al.: Therapeutic and diagnostic colonoscopy in nonobstructive colonic dilatation. *Ann. Surg.* 197:416, 1983.

88. Rodgers B.H.G., Silvis S.E., Nebel O.T., et al.: Complications of flexible fiberoptic colonoscopy and polypectomy. *Gastrointest. Endosc.* 22:73, 1975.

89. Smith L.E.: Fiberoptic colonoscopy: Complications of colonoscopy and polypectomy. *Dis. Colon Rectum* 19:407, 1976.

90. Bowden T.A. Jr., Hooks V.H. III, Mansberger A.R. Jr.: Intraoperative gastrointestinal endoscopy. *Ann. Surg.* 191:680, June 1980.

4

Interventional Radiology in Gastrointestinal Disease

Eric vanSonnenberg, M.D.
Gerhard R. Wittich, M.D.

BACKGROUND AND PHILOSOPHY

It has long been appreciated that draining an abscess, extracting a stone, relieving pressure, and abating hemorrhage have been major goals of surgical and medical care. Radiologists now do or contribute to each of these interventions. Few fields in medicine have had the extraordinary recent innovations of radiology. Ten years ago, ultrasound, CT, interventional radiology, and MNR either were in their infancy or did not exist. The developments in machinery and instrumentation have been applied to clinical situations, opening up new vistas. Radiology has evolved from its use only in diagnosis into an experimental science and an active therapeutic field. The latter aspect will be the focus of this chapter.

Interventional radiology is an amalgamation of various techniques and skills, a union of technology and practical application. Cross-sectional imaging—ultrasound and CT—have demonstrated the abdomen in a manner heretofore beyond expectation: bile ducts are seen routinely, and the pancreas no longer is a hidden organ. Diagnostic specificity of liver lesions has taken a quantum leap, and detection of abscess and fluid no longer requires potentially harmful delays in diagnosis.

Landmark radiologic advances in the early 1970s permitted the radiologist to become conversant with surgical procedures.[1, 2] The combination of this knowledge with new machine technology and needle and catheter skills provided new opportunities for diagnosis and treatment. The inherent safety of the fine needle under ultrasound and CT guidance permitted needles to be placed in structures previously never considered—pancreatic ducts, the gallbladder, through bowel, into the celiac ganglia, and into portal veins—as well as providing greater safety in placement into bile ducts, abscesses, and tumor masses. Guide wire and catheter techniques, originally utilized in angiography in the 1950s and '60s, were adapted for biliary drainage, stone removal, renal tracts (nephrostomy), the GI system (intubation, stricture dilatation), and for fluids and abscesses (percutaneous drainage). As these techniques developed, a new breed of radiologist emerged, the interventional radiologist. Angiography itself evolved in other therapeutic dimensions—bleeding control, tumor ablation, infusion therapy, and angioplasty.

One final ingredient has been the *sine qua non* of the growth and continued development of interventional radiology—the surgical interaction. The understanding of the disease processes for which interventional radiology is used and the principles of therapy come from surgical experience. The care of patients pre- and postprocedure mirrors surgical tenets. Conversely, the diagnostic and therapeutic information provided by interventional radiology often reduced the surgeon's guesswork, and led to appropriate surgical intervention, and palliation or cures when operation was not optimal.

As much as any other major change in radiology, interventional radiology has thrust the radiologist into becoming a clinician. Thus, radiologists must preoperatively prepare their patients, care for their catheters (as surgeons do their drains), and manage postprocedure problems. Ward rounds and even occasional admission of patients have become integral parts of interventional radiology.

PERCUTANEOUS GUIDED BIOPSY

Guided percutaneous biopsy of tumors is now a standard procedure yielding high specificity. It is one of the most widely available of the procedures in interventional radiology and one of the least hazardous. The major values of percutaneous biopsy are preoperative diagnosis, staging, proof of postoperative recurrence, and oncologic planning. Virtually all abdominal masses, palpable or not, are amenable to safe biopsy with current guidance systems and appropriate needles.[3–6]

Guidance Systems

Generally three guidance systems are used for percutaneous biopsy: (1) ultrasound, (2) CT, and (3) fluoroscopy. For the general interventional radiologist, each modality has advantages and disadvantages.

Fluoroscopy for Biopsy

Fluoroscopy, the original guidance system, currently is used the least. Fluoroscopic guidance is reserved for cases in which an internal body landmark is opacified by contrast ma-

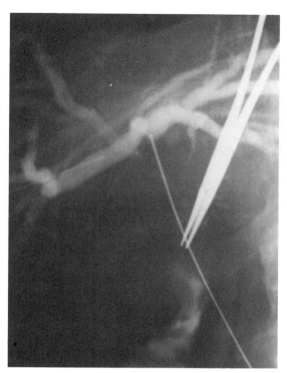

Fig 4–1.—Fluoroscopic guidance for percutaneous biopsy: PTC demonstrates an obstructed common hepatic duct high in the portahepatis. A second 20-gauge needle for biopsy is placed at the site of obstruction. Diagnosis was cholangiocarcinoma, consistent with Klatskin tumor.

terial. Structures which may be filled with contrast and define the suspected tumor are (1) bile ducts (at percutaneous transhepatic cholangiography or through a percutaneous biliary drainage catheter) (Fig 4–1), (2) the GI tract (barium study), (3) the pancreatic duct (by ERCP or percutaneous pancreatic ductography), and (4) lymph node (by lymphangiography). Fluoroscopic control also serves as guidance for brush biopsy, typically for stenosing tumors of the bile duct (Fig 4–2).

Advantages of fluoroscopy are its relative simplicity, its availability, and that it may be done expeditiously. Drawbacks are the use of radiation (for the patient and the operator), its limitation in seeing only one dimension (rather than numerous dimensions of cross-sectional imaging), and its reliance on contrast media to demonstrate tumor location.

Ultrasound Guidance for Biopsy

The popularity of radiologically guided biopsy received its impetus from ultrasound-controlled puncture techniques. The procedure was initiated in Europe and soon spread to the United States. Ultrasound offers the following advantages over fluoroscopy:[7–9] (1) lesions which are seen at cross-sectional imaging may be biopsied as a next step (another advantage over radionuclide techniques); (2) ultrasound depicts structures in a multitude of planes and therefore is adaptable to a variety of lesions (liver, pancreas, spleen, pelvis, retroperitoneum, superficial masses); (3) no ionizing radiation is needed; (4) ultrasound is relatively inexpensive and less time-consuming than CT.

The major indications for sonographic-guided biopsy are: (1) relatively superficial lesions (e.g., liver lesions near the surface of the liver); (2) relatively large lesions (greater than or equal to 4 cm); (3) biopsy in children or pregnant females. Limitations of ultrasound-guided biopsy are: (1) the inherent limitations of sonographic visibility (i.e., lesions in and around bowel frequently are obscured by gas); (2) small or deep lesions, since ultrasound does not demonstrate the needle tip as reliably as CT; (3) lesions too small to be resolved (which may be visualized by CT). Marked improvements in resolution have occurred with continuous real-time sonographic monitoring (see Fig 4–2). However, for small or relatively inaccessible lesions, we, as do most interventional radiologists, choose CT guidance.

CT Guidance for Biopsy

By virtue of its precise resolution, CT is used for difficult biopsies.[10–12] CT is the modality of choice when needle visualization within the lesion is imperative, since it best demonstrates the needle tip. Indications for CT-guided biopsy are: (1) small lesion (less than 3–4 cm); (2) relatively hazardous structures juxtaposed to the target lesion, i.e., aorta, inferior vena cava, or ureter (CT depicts these structures and decreases risk of their puncture); (3) failed initial biopsy with fluoroscopy or ultrasound—thus the certainty of needle tip localization within the lesion (Fig 4–3); (4) to assess vascularity of the lesion at the time of biopsy; IV contrast during CT depicts vascularity and helps determine appropriate needle size and design; (5) for lesions that are not visible at fluoroscopy or ultrasound (obscured by bowel gas).

Drawbacks to CT-guided biopsy are: (1) the most costly of the guidance systems; (2) the most time-consuming; (3) thin patients—lesions may be seen better by ultrasound in some patients who have minimal body fat, since CT depends on inherent fat planes for visualization of structures; (4) rarely, ultrasound may detect a small lesion not seen by CT; and

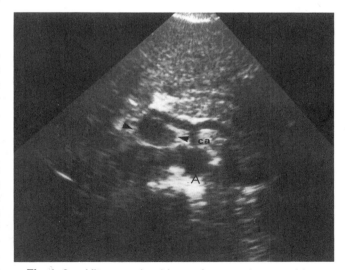

Fig 4–2.—Ultrasound guidance for percutaneous biopsy. Under real-time sonographic guidance, this 3 × 2-cm lymph node *(arrowheads)* to the right of the celiac axis was biopsied. The biopsy was positive for metastatic pancreatic carcinoma. A = aorta, ca = celiac axis.

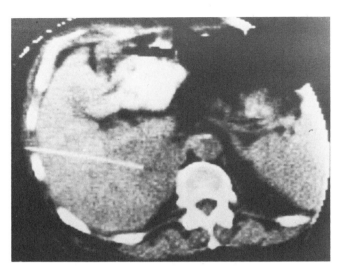

Fig 4–3.—Value of CT guidance for percutaneous biopsy. CT demonstrates the needle tip clearly within this irregular 5-cm liver metastasis. Previous ultrasound-guided biopsy had been negative.

(5) availability—CT and CT scheduling time is the least available of the three systems, although still quite popular in the United States.

Instruments and Technique for Guided Biopsy

The fine needle (Chiba needle, thin needle, 22-gauge needle) revolutionized percutaneous biopsy. The combination of the safety of the fine needle, the refinements in technique and guidance systems, and cytopathologists' gaining comfort and expertise with specimens[10, 13] have made percutaneous biopsy procedures commonplace. Cytologic evaluation used to be the goal of biopsy; histology frequently can be obtained as well with the improved methods, even utilizing 22- and 20-gauge needles.[5, 14] One series showed a 14% increase in diagnostic information with histology in addition to cytology (Fig 4–4). Gradual use of larger needles (20- and 18-gauge)

with cutting edges has further improved diagnosis without significantly increasing complications.[15, 16]

The technique of percutaneous biopsy initially involves localization of the lesion in at least two planes by the particular guidance system. The next step is measurement of depth. Actual needle insertion is performed by continuous monitoring with fluoroscopy or real-time sonography. With static ultrasound scanning and CT, needle localization accurately marks the lesion; needle introduction itself is not followed moment by moment. However, particularly with CT, needle visibility is clearly portrayed, and there is virtually no uncertainty as to position. When the needle is correctly localized, it is left in place as the marker needle for the "tandem biopsy technique." Biopsy passes are taken around the marker needle, which permits a wide sampling zone and multiple passes without having to relocalize each needle. Another biopsy method is the "coaxial technique," used with smaller lesions or those adjacent to vessels. The initial marker needle is replaced coaxially by a larger outer needle, which then serves as the conduit for coaxial needle passes to retrieve the specimen.[17]

Handling of the Specimen

Close cooperation among the referring physician, the radiologist, and the cytopathologist increases the yield from the biopsy. Clinical information is required to optimize the specific information needed for further treatment. Which lesion to biopsy, the exact location of biopsy, whether to biopsy the primary or secondary lesion, and needle size are all decisions the radiologist makes which are influenced by the clinical situation. Similarly, the radiologist conveys to the cytopathologist the area of biopsy, whether the lesion is likely to be a primary or secondary, and whether he is certain the needle tip is in the lesion. The cytopathologist accordingly determines optimal staining technique (variable even within the hospitals at the University of California at San Diego medical complex), the appropriateness of special stains, electron microscopy, and immunologic markers.[18]

The use of the quick-stain technique has simplified and

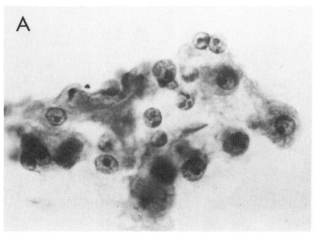

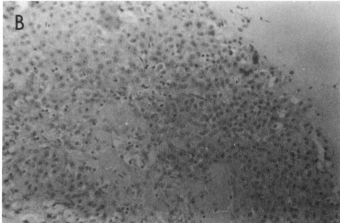

Fig 4–4.—**A** and **B,** cytologic and histologic diagnoses achieved by fine-needle (20-gauge) biopsy. Ultrasound guidance permitted core biopsy samples, showing **(A)** cytologically malignant cells and **(B)** characteristic of hepatocellular carcinoma.

shortened biopsy procedure,[10, 13] during which the cytopathologist is in attendance when the biopsy specimen is actually obtained. The specimen is collected and fixed immediately and run through a five-minute staining sequence. Within ten minutes, information is provided as to adequacy of tissue and usually whether there is malignancy (although specific type may not be apparent without further stains). By this method, the number of passes generally is reduced, as no extra biopsies need be taken. This technique reduces patient discomfort and provides same-day diagnosis.

Indications and Results of Biopsy in Various Organs

Liver biopsy is performed under ultrasound or CT guidance, depending on lesion size and position. Metastatic lesions and hepatoma may be diagnosed accurately by percutaneous biopsy. Bile duct and gallbladder cancer may be biopsied as well, although more frequently the associated adenopathy is biopsied. Primary biliary lesions or those causing biliary obstruction may be diagnosed by opacifying the biliary tract (PTC, PBD), by direct biopsy under fluoroscopy, or by brush biopsy through the catheter. CT or ultrasound guidance is used if fluoroscopic techniques are unsuccessful.

Benign liver tumors (hemangioma, adenoma, focal nodular hyperplasia) frequently can be distinguished by their ultrasound and/or CT appearance. Dynamic scanning with contrast infusion or adjunctive tests (radionuclide and angiographic) may be diagnostic. Generally, biopsy is unnecessary. In equivocal cases these lesions have been biopsied safely, but only 22-gauge needles are recommended in these equivocal cases. Results in several large series have shown an accuracy of 82%–98% for percutaneous biopsy of liver lesions.[4–8, 10, 11] Ultrasound and CT results are not always comparable, since CT is used for more difficult lesions.

Pancreatic biopsy is performed with ultrasound or CT guidance. Results have shown 86%–95% accuracy with fine-needle biopsy.[4, 10] CT is more apt to be used, since lesions are often relatively small or the pancreas is obscured by overlying gas during ultrasound (Fig 4–5). Fine needles (22-gauge and occasionally 20-gauge) may be passed through stomach and small intestine for tumor biopsy without harmful sequelae; care is taken to avoid puncturing the large intestine, however. An initial negative biopsy prompts repeated biopsy; this adds approximately 5%–10% accuracy.

Lymph nodes and adrenal glands are frequently sampled for tissue confirmation of metastatic disease. Lymph node biopsy may be performed fluoroscopically if a lymphangiogram has been performed previously. Owing to time, technical expertise required, and limited visualization of high abdominal nodes, CT biopsy has substituted for lymphangiogram in many centers. Adrenal lesions usually are biopsied with CT guidance, as they frequently do not exceed 3–4 cm. To avoid puncturing the pleura, with the attendant risk of pneumothorax, adrenal and posterior liver lesions frequently are biopsied with the patient in the prone position from below the 12th rib, in an angled fashion[19] (Fig 4–6).

With GI lesions, biopsy is more useful for diagnosis of local lymph nodes or distant disease than of the primary lesion itself. However, primary gastric or enteric lesions may be biopsied by any of the guidance modalities.[9]

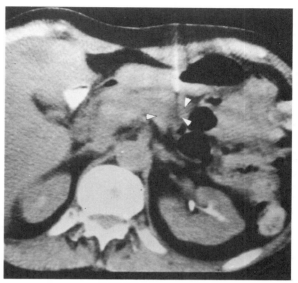

Fig 4–5.—CT-guided percutaneous biopsy of small pancreatic carcinoma. A slightly low-density 2 cm lesion is noted in the body of the pancreas *(arrowheads).* The fine needle has traversed the stomach wall and is at the anterior margin of the tumor. Diagnosis: pancreatic carcinoma.

Lymphoma presents a special problem for percutaneous biopsy.[20] The large amount of tissue necessary for classification of primary disease frequently is not obtained with 22-gauge needles. Accuracy rates of diagnosis of primary lymphoma in early studies were only 64%.[20] Biopsy of recurrent lymphoma is accurate in a much larger percentage, especially when the tissue may be compared to previously obtained material. Blind biopsy of the spleen for lymphoma is not efficacious; however, biopsy of focal splenic lesions with 22-gauge needles is safe and may be diagnostic.

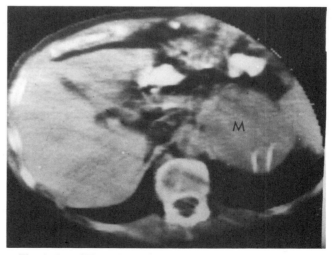

Fig 4–6.—CT-guided prone biopsy of metastatic adrenal lesion. The needle is angled cephalad from below the 12th rib to avoid the lung and pleura. Two needles are in the adrenal mass *(M),* and the posterior lung is avoided. Diagnosis: metastatic carcinoma, colon primary.

Pelvic biopsy is more appropriate in the context of possible recurrence of rectal carcinoma. Presacral masses or nodes, external or internal, may be seen early and biopsied.

Complications of percutaneous biopsy are relatively few and usually minor. Large series report up to 3% complications,[4, 10, 11] including pneumothorax, fever, pancreatitis, and needle tract seeding. The last is extremely rare.[20]

INTERVENTIONAL RADIOLOGY IN THE BILIARY TRACT

A host of useful diagnostic and therapeutic interventional radiology techniques exist for biliary tract and gallbladder diseases. Rarely does a patient need to be operated on without preoperative knowledge of the site, extension and cause of disease. Similarly, a bevy of preoperative and postoperative therapeutic maneuvers (percutaneous biliary drainage, percutaneous stone dissolution, balloon dilatation of strictures, percutaneous cholecystostomy, basket stone removal) provide a vast armamentarium to assist the patient and the referring physician.

Evaluation of Jaundice

For relatively rapid and inexpensive screening to differentiate "medical" from obstructive jaundice, ultrasound is generally the procedure of choice. The current accuracy of ultrasound is over 90%,[21–26] and recent advances in real-time sector scanners have increased the likelihood of suggesting a diagnosis.[27] However, ultrasound is limited in determination of the site and etiology of jaundice in up to two thirds of cases.[23, 28] This is due to duodenal and hepatic flexure gas, which obscures the middle and distal common bile duct. CT may be helpful in further evaluation for site and etiology and for biopsy guidance.[29, 39] Current practice often follows a sequence of ultrasound demonstration of dilated ducts, then percutaneous transhepatic cholangiogram (PTC) to establish the site and etiology of obstruction. PTC is accurate in over 90% of cases to predict site and etiology.[28, 31]

A few pitfalls in the above schema must be borne in mind. Specifically, obstruction may occur without dilatation, or, conversely, dilatation may occur without obstruction.[32–34] In both situations, ultrasound does not provide all necessary information. In the former category, partially obstructing stone disease, sclerosing cholangitis, and tumor infiltration or cirrhosis in the liver (limiting ductal distention) may present problems. Sonographic evaluation of the bile ducts after fatty meal administration may help to uncover occult obstruction.[35]

Percutaneous Transhepatic Cholangiography

Current refinements in technique have improved the quality and reduced the risk of PTC. Use of only 23- or 22-gauge needles, limited injection of contrast media, use of gravity in the upright and left lateral positions to fill the common bile duct, knowledge of segmental liver anatomy, peripheral needle passes, preprocedure routine use of antibiotics, and monitoring of vital signs all have helped make PTC more reliable and a relatively safer procedure than early studies indicated. A recent large series of 450 PTCs showed successful opacification of the ducts in over 95% with dilated ducts, nearly 75% with nondilated ducts, and with 5% complications.[36] PTC is

performed either by standard fluoroscopic guidance or with ultrasound in selected cases (pregnancy, children, selective left hepatic duct obstruction).[38]

Specific entities which may be diagnosed by PTC include extra- and intrahepatic bile duct carcinoma, liver metastases, periportal adenopathy, gallbladder or pancreatic carcinoma (Fig 4–7), lymphoma, ampullary tumor, benign stricture, stones, hemobilia, and sclerosing cholangitis. Although appearances frequently are diagnostic, associated biopsy may be necessary in equivocal cases or for further treatment planning.

Percutaneous Manometry and Perfusion for Biliary Pressure

Determination of biliary pressure via manometry or by perfusion challenge may be performed either at PTC, percutaneous biliary drainage, or via T tubes.[32, 39] Pressure determination is helpful in specific, and frequently the most difficult, biliary problems. These clinical situations include differentiating dilatation without obstruction from dilatation due to a subtle stricture or papillary dysfunction (Fig 4–8), uncovering obstruction without dilatation, as a predictor of potential bile leak after PTC (and the need for drainage), to determine adequacy of percutaneous biliary drainage, and to assess the efficacy and response of percutaneous balloon dilatation of strictures. Normal biliary pressure is considered up to 15–18 cm of saline; most obstructions are in the 20–30 cm saline range. Pressures at PTC over 40 cm of saline are most likely to have associated bile leak; immediate decompression is suggested in these cases.

Percutaneous Biliary Drainage

Percutaneous biliary drainage has a host of indications, some lifesaving, some cost-saving, some as a final palliative

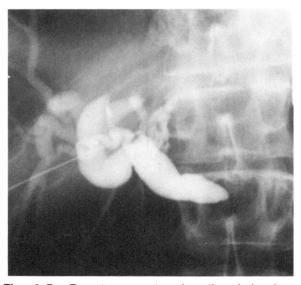

Fig 4–7.—Percutaneous transhepatic cholangiogram demonstrates site and likely etiology of biliary obstruction. 22-gauge needle PTC shows complete obstruction of the common bile duct in the suprapancreatic region. The blunt appearance of the duct region is characteristic of pancreatic carcinoma.

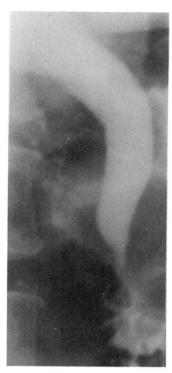

Fig 4–8.—Value of manometry at PTC to aid clinical decision making. This 44-year-old woman had a dilated bile duct but no definite lesion seen on this lateral view of the PTC. Contrast medium flowed freely into the duodenum, and the intrahepatic ducts were normal size. However, the resting pressure was 28 cm of saline (normal, to 18 cm saline), suggesting outflow obstruction. Presumptive diagnosis: ampullary dysfunction. Surgical sphincterotomy was performed with relief of preoperative symptoms.

resort, and some controversial.[40–42] Perhaps it is most valuable in overwhelming cholangitis and biliary sepsis due to obstruction (Fig 4–9).[43] Insertion of a drainage catheter may be (or lead to) definitive therapy, or it may permit general anesthesia and formal operation at a later, more optimal date. With benign disease such as calculus obstruction in the elderly or in a patient with severe cardiac or pulmonary disease, percutaneous biliary drainage may be lifesaving. Percutaneous biliary drainage is valuable in drainage of high benign lesions—e.g., after biliary-enteric bypass with a jejunal loop anastomosis which has strictured. Percutaneous stricture dilatation with a balloon catheter follows drainage. Percutaneous biliary drainage may serve as a primary route for stone removal after tract dilatation as well.

With malignant disease, percutaneous biliary drainage serves numerous functions and may avoid operation at appropriate times.[44] For unresectable disease (usually determined by CT), percutaneous biliary drainage permits definitive bypass, which may then be converted to an endoprosthesis (Fig 4–10). The latter may clog, but in patients who will succumb to their disease within months, a humane ending occurs. Percutaneous biliary drainage will relieve symptoms (pruritus, anorexia) in most patients and will uniformly decrease alkaline phosphatase and bilirubin preoperatively. Whether this is

beneficial preoperatively remains debatable.[45] Standardized controlled trials with operation and endoscopic cannulation remain to be evaluated.

Percutaneous Stone Removal

A variety of percutaneous techniques exist for bile duct or gallbladder stone removal. The steerable catheter is most frequently utilized for removal of postoperative retained calculi.[46] This technique is effective in 95% of patients, with a 3%–5% complication rate.[47]

Through the steerable catheter, baskets are placed in the tract. These engage the stone and either remove it retrograde, pass it antegrade into the intestine, or fragment and crush the stone. Fragments smaller than 0.5 cm generally will pass spontaneously. Stones may be removed from the intrahepatic or extrahepatic bile ducts by these techniques (Fig 4–11).

The surgeon's role in basket stone removal is crucial, since the type of tract created may determine the eventual outcome of the percutaneous procedure. Thus, anterior, small tracts are fraught with problems, cause unreasonable radiation exposure to the radiologist's hands, and have a higher rate of failure. Tracts should be lateral, with large-bore catheters (14–16 F), and should mature over six weeks. Although the procedure may be performed prior to six weeks, patient comfort and ease of manipulations are compromised.

In *de novo* stone cases, particularly where general anesthesia and operation are not considered optimal, percutaneous biliary drainage may serve as the main conduit for stone removal. A tract will form which can be dilated to 14 F. Management (basket removal, dissolution, stricture dilatation) may then progress as with basket stone removal.

An entity being seen in the United States with increasing frequency because of immigration is Oriental cholangiohepatitis.[48, 49] This occurs in patients from the Far East and is the commonest type of biliary disease in that environment. The disease is characterized by casts and stones—often enormous—filling the intrahepatic and extrahepatic bile ducts, strictures, and recurrent symptoms of cholangitis and pain. Inverventional radiologic techniques, along with a biliary enteric operative drainage, are extremely helpful in this complex medical problem (Fig 4–12).[49]

Percutaneous Stone Dissolution

Although the prospect is theoretically encouraging, the optimal solvent is not yet available in clinical practice. Monooctanoin is the major chemical in use today and is active against some cholesterol stones.[50, 51] This theory has been successful in over half of patients. The drug has acceptable and non-life-threatening complications. It is infused through a T tube, percutaneous biliary drainage catheter, or cholecystostomy tube. The patient is hospitalized and monitored frequently (liver function tests, infusion pressures, temperature). Complications of monooctanoin are cholangitis, nausea, diarrhea, and liver function abnormalities. Solvent infusion is reserved for cases where percutaneous removal is unsuccessful.

Percutaneous Stricture Dilatation

Derived from dilatation of arterial stenoses, balloon dilatation of biliary stenoses is a new and promising technique. Ac-

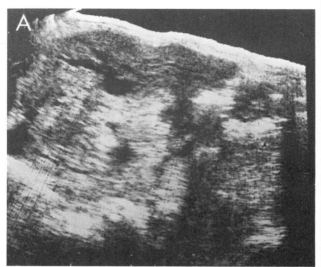

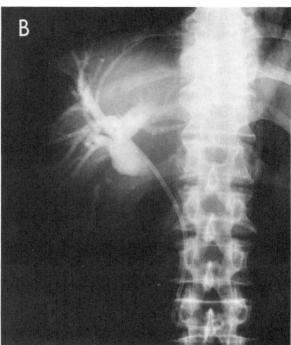

Fig 4–9.—Percutaneous biliary drainage to treat acute cholangitis: This 54-year-old man had chills, fever, elevated WBCs, and jaundice. **A,** ultrasound demonstrated dilated bile ducts in the intrahepatic system and dilatation of the proximal common hepatic duct. **B,** after diagnostic PTC, percutaneous biliary drainage yielded purulent material in the bile ducts. Six hours after PBD the patient defervesced. Final diagnosis: gallbladder carcinoma with secondary cholangitis.

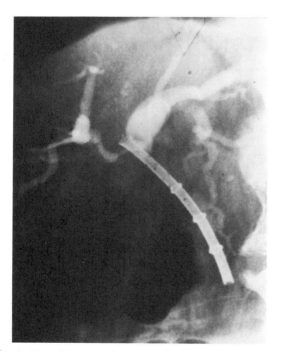

Fig 4–10.—Biliary endoprosthesis: This 72-year-old man had metastatic carcinoma to the portahepatis with contiguous invasion of the liver. PBD was performed initially, followed by insertion of a completely indwelling endoprosthesis.

cess to the biliary tract usually is made via percutaneous biliary drainage, but may be through T-tube tracts as well. A balloon catheter is inserted over a guide wire and inflated, often multiple times and in multiple sessions, depending on individual circumstances. Predilatation and postdilatation pressures are taken to help objectify morphological appearance (Fig 4–13).[32]

While strictures can be dilated physically,[52] several unanswered questions remain: (1) how many times and how long should balloons be inflated (pressures help to determine this)?, (2) should dilated strictures be stented as well, and if so, for how long?, and (3) will strictures recur?

To date, we have followed up patients for up to three years who have done well; a few have had stricture recurrence. Currently, several patients with sclerosing cholangitis who had been operated on previously are being maintained with long-term catheterization and antibiotic therapy with balloon dilatation of strictures.

Percutaneous Cholecystostomy

Percutaneous cholecystostomy is another relatively new interventional radiology procedure in the biliary tract with a host of potential applications. Percutaneous cholecystostomy has been used for: (1) relief of acute cholecystitis and empyema, (2) biliary drainage for low common bile duct lesions, (3) stone removal, (4) stone dissolution, and (5) stricture dilatation (Fig 4–14).[53–55]

Puncture may be performed under fluoroscopy with an opacified gallbladder, with palpation alone, or with CT or ul-

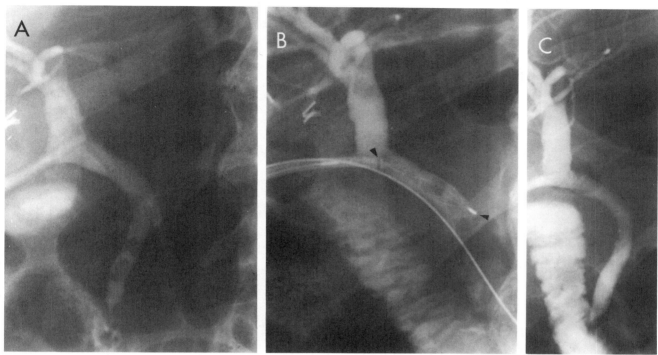

Fig 4–11.—A–C, percutaneous removal of retained biliary stones. This 52-year-old man had several stones in the distal common bile duct which could not be removed easily at operation. **A,** contrast through a 14 F T tube demonstrates retained stones. **B,** after six weeks of tract matura- tion, a steerable catheter is placed into the bile duct. A basket *(arrowheads)* placed through the tract has engaged the lucent stones. (Note safety guide wire which is in the duodenum through the tract.) **C,** the bile ducts are free of stones after the procedure.

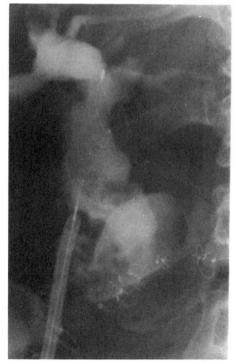

Fig 4–12.—Percutaneous basket removal of stones in Oriental cholangiohepatitis (OCH). Surgical T tube was placed in this 42-year-old woman with recurrent cholangitis and abdominal pain. Note multiple lucencies in the extremely dilated common bile duct. Several intrahepatic bile ducts are blunted, consistent with OCH. Through the T-tube tract, a steerable catheter and large basket were placed for removal of the stones.

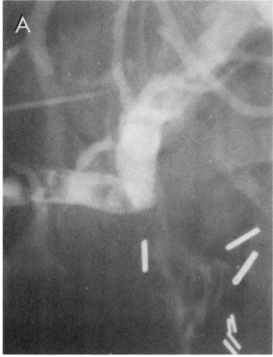
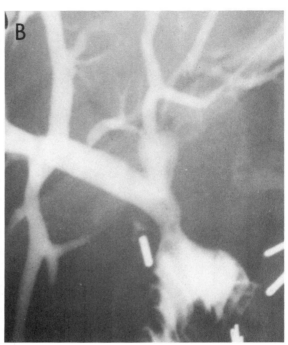

Fig 4–13.—Percutaneous balloon dilatation of biliary stricture: This woman had several previous operations and had a jejunal loop brought up to the right and left hepatic duct confluence. Recurrent cholangitis heralded **A,** anasto- motic stricture and stone formation in the ducts. **B,** after di- latation with an 8mm balloon, the anastomosis is patent. The patient has done well for the ensuing 1½ years.

trasound guidance. Our preference is combined real-time ul- trasound and fluoroscopy. Catheter entrance usually is trans- hepatic, but with extremely distended gallbladders may be directly into the fundus.

Complications have included significant vagal reactions, leakage, and cholangitis.[53, 55] Recently, large cholangioscopes

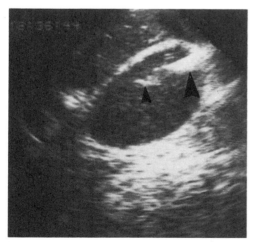

Fig 4–14.—Percutaneous cholecystostomy under ultra- sound guidance. This postoperative cardiac patient devel- oped signs of cholecystitis while in the intensive care unit. A fine needle *(small arrowhead)* and an 8.3 F catheter *(large arrowhead)* were placed in the distended gallbladder for drainage and decompression.

have been placed via these tracts for many of the above- mentioned procedures.

MANAGEMENT OF FLUIDS AND ABSCESSES

Ultrasound and CT Detection

Cross-sectional imaging revolutionized the detection of ab- scesses and fluids. Numerous studies in the 1970s showed sensitivity and specificity rates far surpassing other radio- graphic techniques. Detection rates are over 90%.[56–58] The admonition by Altemeier et al.[59] that survival with abscesses would not be modified significantly until delay in diagnosis was reduced has been partially improved by these new tech- niques.

Ultrasound is accurate for detection of fluid collections, particularly in the liver, pelvis, and superficially. Ultrasound is limited by structures which overlie the collection and impede sound transmission. Bandages, ostomies, drains, bones, and bowel gas are impediments to sound. Real-time continuous monitoring during the ultrasound examination has further added to sonographic reliability. However, ultrasound is not the optimal study in certain postoperative patients or when abscesses are intertwined within bowel.

CT is at least as accurate as sonography in fluid detection and specificity and frequently more so. CT is not impeded by the overlying structures that curtail the use of ultrasound. In approximately one third of cases, CT is able to detect gas within a collection, which adds specificity to abscess diagnosis.[60] However, CT does have limitations, such as ionizing radiation, which ultrasound does not; it is more expensive and less flexible (e.g., portable ultrasound may be used in the surgical intensive care unit).

In summary, ultrasound and CT generally are the modalities of choice for abscess and fluid detection. Ultrasound is preferred in the right upper quadrant, superficially, and in the pelvis, with the bladder filled to displace unwanted bowel loops. Ultrasound may demonstrate abscesses in other locations as well. However, a negative sonographic study does not exclude an abscess in the left upper quadrant or in the lower quadrants. In these areas and in complicated postoperative situations, CT is preferable (Fig 4–17).[61]

Radionuclide studies occasionally may be useful. We employ indium-111-labeled WBCs when an abscess is suspected, but no clinical or laboratory aids point to a particular area. Chronologically, use of gallium-67 preceded indium-111-labeled WBCs, but gallium has many more technical and interpretive problems than indium-labeled WBCs.

Diagnostic Aspiration

Diagnostic aspiration of fluid collections is accurate and necessary in most cases, offering information beyond simple imaging. While ultrasound and CT detect collections quite well, they are not always specific with respect to the contents within the collection.

Technique for diagnostic aspiration involves guidance of a 22-gauge needle into the fluid collection. The site of the collection is determined in two planes (static ultrasound and CT) or by continuous visualization of the needle (real-time ultrasound) (Fig 4–15). Depth is then calculated. Fluoroscopy occasionally is used, usually after ultrasound or CT marking; however, regional relationships of adjacent structures, including bowel, are not as accurately depicted, and hence fluoroscopy is not as safe a guidance system. In collections which are

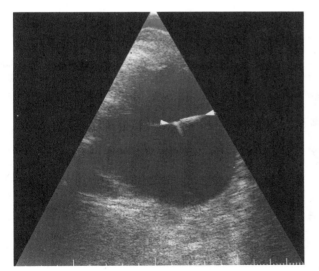

Fig 4–15.—Diagnostic percutaneous needle aspiration of a fluid collection. Under real-time sonographic monitoring, this 22-gauge needle *(arrowheads)* was passed into the rounded, postoperative fluid collection. It proved to be a noninfected lymphocele.

too viscous to extract diagnostic fluid from, a 22-gauge needle 20- or 18-gauge needles are utilized.

Once a fluid sample is aspirated, it is sent for the following evaluation: Gram stain, culture (aerobic and anaerobic), cells, amylase, and protein (optional).[62] Magnetic resonance assay of fluids is currently being evaluated as well.[63]

Diagnostic aspiration is the most commonly performed interventional radiology technique and is quite straightforward and safe. Certain pitfalls do exist. Care must be taken to avoid puncturing overlying bowel for two reasons—to avoid contaminating a sterile collection and to avoid confusion on Gram stain interpretation. Though rare, significant complications can occur even with fine needles—bleeding, pneumothorax, fever. When performed meticulously, these techniques are diagnostic and nontraumatic, even with small amounts of fluids. The information may significantly influence patient management in terms of correct antibiotic therapy, indication to operate or not, and percutaneous drainage.

Catheter Drainage of Abscesses and Fluids

Percutaneous abscess drainage (PAD) has been hailed as "one of the greatest surgical advances in the decade."[64] Utilizing ultrasound and CT for guidance, and fluoroscopy in some cases, success rates of 86%–91% have been reported. Complications have been described in 5%–15%.[65–67] Despite PAD's not being curative in some cases, significant benefit may accrue by temporizing and improving the condition of critically ill patients.[68] Temporizing PAD may then permit the patient to undergo general anesthesia and major surgery.

The technique of PAD involves initial diagnostic aspiration and planning of a safe entry into the abscess. The diagnostic needle defines the route for the catheter and insures that bowel, other viscera, and vital vessels will not be traversed. The catheter is inserted by direct trocar or guide wire exchange technique (Fig 4–16). The catheter is optimally seated, the contents evacuated, and the cavity is irrigated extensively after decompression. Catheters remain one to three weeks, depending on the complexity of abscess (e.g., one week for unilocular pyogenic liver abscess; three weeks for multiloculated pancreatic abscesses). Catheters are removed by gradual withdrawal, similar to a surgical drain, permitting healing by secondary intention.[65, 66, 69]

Previously only superficial, unilocular abscesses were drained percutaneously. Owing to accumulated experience and improved techniques and materials (multiple and large-hole catheters, sump systems, irrigation, enzymes), almost all patients with abscesses are candidates for PAD.[65, 66, 70–72] Thus, multiloculated abscesses, those with associated fistulas, and multiple abscesses are all drained (Fig 4–17). Expectation may be to debulk the abscess and to improve the patient's condition rather than to cure every case. In the overall picture, even temporizing percutaneous drainage may be extraordinarily beneficial and lifesaving.[68]

Abscesses not suitable for PAD are those in which a safe route cannot be established or there are innumerable microabscesses; *Echinococcus* may be another contraindication, although this has recently been debated.[73] CT guidance for complicated abscesses has improved the technique and reduced problems; the superior resolution of CT permits clear

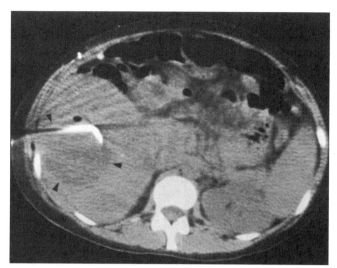

Fig 4–16.—Percutaneous abscess drainage. This 51-year-old man was septic due to a large liver abscess *(arrowheads)*. A 12 F sump catheter was placed percutaneously into the abscess cavity. After evacuation of contents and irrigation, the patient defervesced. The catheter was gradually advanced, and removed on the seventh postprocedure day.

visualization of adjacent structures that could be injured.[65–67] CT also demonstrates residual pus after the first catheter has been placed; all locules may be drained subsequently by placing more than one catheter into the nondrained purulent pockets.

Abscesses in the liver, pancreas, subphrenic subhepatic spaces, pelvis, amebic, splenic, renal, and enteric abscesses (those associated with Crohn's disease, diverticulitis, and appendicitis) have all been drained percutaneously.[74–77] In appropriate clinical situations, noninfected collections may be drained by catheters, or needle aspirated—pancreatic pseudocyst, hematoma, seroma, bile collection, lymphocele, uri-

noma.[62, 66, 78–81] When these collections are extremely viscous or associated with fistulas, drainage may be more difficult, although still potentially curable in some cases. Specifically designed catheters are used, depending on the collection (Fig 4–18).[71, 82]

ANGIOGRAPHY

The role of diagnostic angiography has changed significantly during the past ten years. Although angiography is highly accurate in diagnosing neoplasms of the liver and the pancreas, as well as in detecting traumatic changes of the spleen and the liver, it has been widely replaced by ultrasonography and CT for these common indications. Modern cross-sectional imaging modalities achieve results similar to those of angiography, but are noninvasive or significantly less invasive. Furthermore, these methods may serve to guide fine-needle biopsies, thereby leading to definitive tissue diagnoses. We will discuss some current indications for diagnostic angiography and focus on its therapeutic aspects.

Diagnostic Angiography

Diagnostic angiography is indicated in selected cases where noninvasive imaging modalities result in equivocal or controversial study results. For instance, angiography is usually diagnostic if ultrasound, CT, or scintigraphy have failed to differentiate a cavernous hemangioma of the liver from a focal neoplasm.[83] Arteriography or transhepatic catheterization of the portal vein and selective venous sampling should be considered for preoperative localization of functional endocrine tumors of the pancreas if ultrasound or CT are unsuccessful.[84]

Angiography has been the traditional method to assess local resectability of malignant tumors. Refined CT techniques such as rapid sequence scanning after single or multiple bolus injections may be equal to angiography in assessing resectability.[85, 86] However, angiography can hardly be substituted by alternative methods when a preoperative "vascular road map" is required by the surgeon (Figs 4–19, A and B).

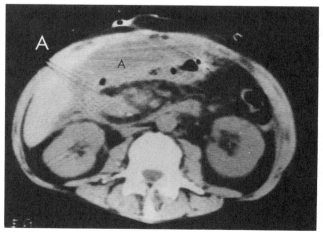

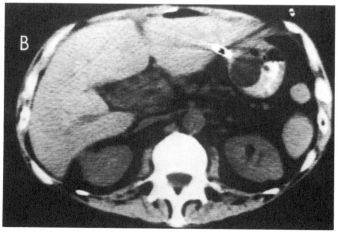

Fig 4–17.—Percutaneous drainage in a 44-year-old man who had pancreatitis complicated by a pancreatic abscess. Surgical drainage provided some improvement; however, one week later, spiking fevers recurred. **A,** undrained collection was noted by CT in the subhepatic space medially (*A* = abscess). **B,** after insertion of a 12 F sump catheter, contents were evacuated, and the postdrainage CT revealed almost complete evacuation of the abscess.

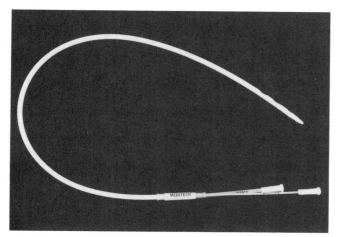

Fig 4–18.—Standard catheter for percutaneous abscess drainage. These 12 and 14 F double-lumen sump catheters are efficient for drainage of viscous and purulent collections. Irrigation is performed through the larger "drain" lumen. Organized hematomas and pancreatic phlegmons are not amenable to drainage/debridement through these catheters.

Real-time sonography (combined with Doppler scanning) and dynamic CT are capable of detecting abnormalities of large abdominal vessels such as varices secondary to portal hypertension, thrombosis or cavernous transformation of the portal vein, or large arterial aneurysms. Another promising new tool for noninvasive imaging of vascular and hemodynamic abnormalities is magnetic nuclear resonance (MNR) imaging. These methods may serve as screening modalities,

but angiography is likely to remain the gold standard for imaging vascular disorders. It is the best method to demonstrate small, disseminated aneurysms in polyarteritis nodosa or to confirm veno-occlusive changes in Budd-Chiari syndrome. Wedged hepatic venography is a simple and effective method to differentiate presinusoidal from postsinusoidal portal hypertension.[87] Arteriography is an essential and underused method to optimize management of patients with suspected acute mesenteric ischemia. Boley et al.[88] have demonstrated that treatment of this disorder based on early angiographic diagnosis may reduce the mortality from 80% to 45%.

Angiography is the method of choice to localize the site of GI bleeding and to define its cause. This will be further discussed under "Therapeutic Angiography."

Therapeutic Angiography

Angiography is frequently utilized for the diagnosis and treatment of GI bleeding. Approximately 75% of patients stop bleeding with conservative therapy.[89] However, it is important to diagnose the site and etiology of bleeding, since the hemorrhage may be recurrent and life-threatening. If the site of bleeding is suspected to be in the upper GI tract, endoscopy may identify esophageal varices, erosive gastritis, gastric or duodenal ulcers, or a Mallory-Weiss tear as the source of bleeding. If endoscopy fails to localize the cause of bleeding due to impaired visualization, angiography often is indicated. Angiographic detection of the bleeding site requires at least 0.5 ml/minute of bleeding. Hence, angiography is best performed when there is evidence of active bleeding. Proper timing of the angiographic procedure is facilitated by close monitoring of the output from a nasogastric tube. A celiac

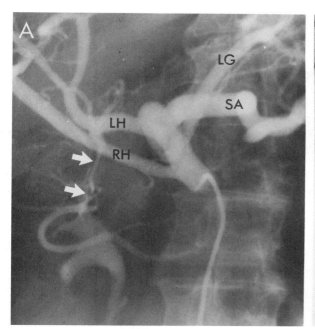

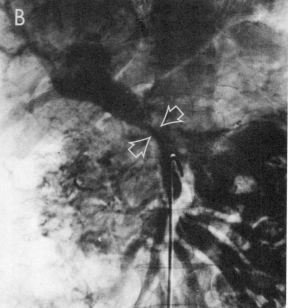

Fig 4–19.—Unresectable carcinoma of the pancreatic head. **A,** celiac arteriography demonstrates localized encasement of the gastroduodenal artery *(arrows)* typical for pancreatic cancer. Note the anatomical variant with separate origin of the left and the right hepatic arteries *(LH, RH)* from the celiac axis. These vessels as well as the splenic artery *(SA)* and the left gastric artery *(LG)* are normal. **B,** venous phase of superior mesenteric artery injection (subtraction technique). Encasement of the superior mesenteric vein *(arrows)* suggests unresectability. A tissue diagnosis of adenocarcinoma of the pancreatic head had been obtained prior to the angiogram by CT-guided fine-needle biopsy.

artery injection usually is performed, followed by selective left gastric artery or gastroduodenal artery catheterizations. If these are negative, a selective injection of the left phrenic artery should be performed; this may reveal bleeding at the esophagogastric junction.

If the bleeding site has been successfully localized, angiographic treatment by intra-arterial infusion of a vasoconstrictor such as vasopressin can be initiated. If bleeding cannot be controlled by vasopressin, embolization may be considered (Figs 4–20, A and B). Gelfoam particles or steel coils are two of several materials which have proved effective.

Massive lower GI bleed usually requires arteriography as the initial diagnostic modality. The majority of bleeding sites are located in the ascending colon, which is not readily accessible to endoscopy. Injections of the superior mesenteric artery supplemented by selective catheterization of its peripheral branches may reveal bleeding from a diverticulum of the ascending colon or from angiodysplasia of the ascending colon or ileum[90] (Fig 4–21, A and B). Intestinal tumors or inflammatory disorders such as Crohn's disease, ulcerative colitis, or ischemic colitis are less frequent causes of massive lower GI bleeding.

Diverticular bleeding can be controlled by selective intra-arterial injection of vasopressin in up to 96% of cases.[91] Due to the likelihood of rebleeding, elective surgery is often indicated in patients with diverticular bleeding, especially in patients with angiodysplasia. If a superior mesenteric arteriogram does not reveal the bleeding site, the inferior mesenteric artery is studied. Treatment with vasopressin or embolic materials often controls the bleeding but may result

in severe ischemic complications. On the other hand, this is an acceptable alternative to surgery in high-risk, elderly patients who have lower GI bleeding.

Scintigraphy is an excellent method to guide proper timing and technique of angiography in patients with low-grade or intermittent hemorrhage. Technetium Tc 99m sulfur colloid scintigraphy is more sensitive than angiography but requires active bleeding at a rate of 0.1 ml/minute to result in a positive study.[89] ^{99m}Tc-labeled RBC studies are significantly more sensitive.[92] However, they may be misleading with regard to the bleeding site unless scans are obtained at frequent, one- or two-hour, intervals.

Patients with portal hypertension and bleeding from gastroesophageal varices are candidates for transhepatic embolization. If massive hematemesis cannot be controlled medically or endoscopically, embolization of the varices and of the left gastric vein may be performed. These angiographic methods usually do not obviate surgical decompression of the portal venous system. However, bleeding is controlled by embolization in 71% of patients; thus, emergency surgery may be avoided.[93] A definitive elective surgical procedure can then be performed with less risk. Transhepatic portography with selective catheterization of the major tributaries of the splanchnic venous system, combined with cinefluorography and manometry is an excellent method to demonstrate the anatomy and hemodynamics of portal hypertension. Such information is particularly valuable when a selective distal splenorenal shunt is considered rather than a portocaval shunt.[93, 94]

Embolic therapy is an effective method to control arterial

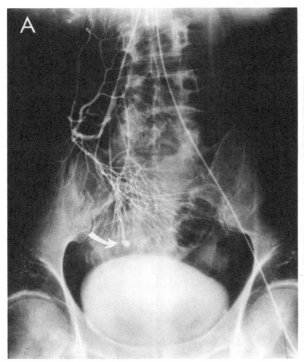

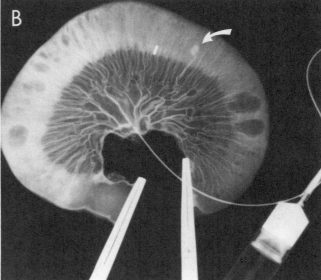

Fig 4–20.—Upper GI bleeding. **A,** contrast extravasation *(arrow)* from branches of the gastroduodenal artery in a patient with duodenal ulcer. **B,** the bleeding was controlled after selective injection of small Gelfoam particles and placement of a steel coil *(arrow)* in the gastroduodenal artery.

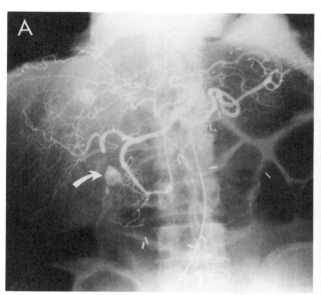
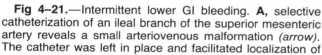
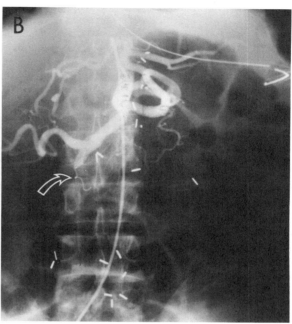

Fig 4–21.—Intermittent lower GI bleeding. **A,** selective catheterization of an ileal branch of the superior mesenteric artery reveals a small arteriovenous malformation *(arrow).* The catheter was left in place and facilitated localization of the lesion during surgery. **B,** angiography of the resected specimen confirms successful removal of the arteriovenous malformation *(arrow).*

capillary bleeding and bleeding from esophageal varices. It has been applied to treatment of malignant hepatic tumors as well. The concept of treatment of liver tumors by hepatic artery occlusion or by selective infusion of chemotherapeutic agents into the hepatic artery is based on the dual blood supply of the liver. Malignant tumors of the liver receive 90%–95% of their blood supply from the hepatic artery, while normal liver parenchyma receives 75% of its blood supply and 50% of its oxygen from the portal vein.[95] Occlusion of the hepatic artery is performed with minimal risk if portal vein patency has been demonstrated. In the series of Yamada et al.,[96] 75% of patients with unresectable hepatoma benefited from hepatic artery embolization. These patients had partial remission, with tumor reduction to at least half of the original size. Their one-year survival rate of 44% compared favorably with a 28% one-year survival after surgical tumor removal. In patients who are symptomatic from metastases of active endocrine tumors such as carcinoid, successful palliation may be achieved by hepatic artery occlusion. Patients with liver metastases from colorectal carcinoma may benefit from hepatic dearterialization if they have minimal tumor burden morphologically, if their liver function is less than twice normal, or if they are asymptomatic.[97] This form of treatment is not without potentially serious complications. In the series of Wallace et al.,[95] the 30-day mortality was 7% in 100 patients. Three of these deaths were related to the procedure. Prior to performing hepatic artery embolization, selective intra-arterial infusion of antitumor agents may be considered. The rationale for intra-arterial chemotherapy is that a higher drug concentration in the liver can be achieved than that by IV drug administration.[93] Systemic toxicity is lower because of significant drug uptake by the liver during first passage.

Transcatheter embolization of the splenic artery is an alternative to surgical splenectomy. The indications are the same for both procedures. The incidence of splenic abscess formation after embolization can be reduced by premedication with antibiotics, strict adherence to aseptic technique, and performing partial embolization.[98]

Transluminal angioplasty with balloon catheters has been performed successfully in a small group of patients with stenosis of the superior or inferior mesenteric artery[99] and in patients with closed mesocaval shunts.[100] In selected patients with acute mesenteric emboli who are at high risk for surgery and who do not have signs of peritonitis, intra-arterial thrombolysis may be attempted.[101]

NEWER TECHNIQUES IN INTERVENTIONAL RADIOLOGY

Percutaneous Pancreatic Ductography

Percutaneous pancreatic ductography is a relatively new technique that permits diagnostic evaluation of the main pancreatic duct and its branches.[102, 103] The procedure is performed under ultrasound or CT guidance. It may be used as a primary diagnostic test or after technical problems with ERCP. Pancreatic duct drainage is another potential application.[104]

With ultrasound guidance, real-time monitoring may be used. This permits the needle to be visualized and redirected if necessary as it enters the pancreatic duct.[102, 103] Fluid from the duct may be sampled for cytology and culture. Logistically, a portable ultrasound machine is used in a fluoroscopy suite to allow contrast opacification of the ducts after needle puncture.

When CT guidance is used, percutaneous pancreatic ductography has often been performed with simultaneous biopsy of the pancreas.[105] Similar to biopsy localization by CT, the needle is inserted into the duct. A drawback to percutaneous pancreatic ductography under CT control is that the patient must be transferred to fluoroscopy for standard filming after contrast injection.

Diagnostic information is gained from percutaneous pancreatic ductography regarding morphological differentiation of pancreatitis from carcinoma. Cytologic and bacteriologic evaluation is obtained from the aspirated pancreatic ductal fluid. We have also used percutaneous pancreatic ductography to help ascertain whether pancreatic pseudocysts are communicating to the pancreatic duct; this helps determine management (therapeutic needle aspiration vs. catheter drainage) and predict outcome.

To date, significant complications of percutaneous pancreatic ductography have not been reported. We have observed a slight rise in amylase in a few patients, but they were asymptomatic.

Percutaneous Gastrostomy

Percutaneous gastrostomy is created for feeding or decompression.[106–109] When used for feeding, tubes are placed into the stomach or the small bowel, depending on preference for the site of alimentation. Fluoroscopic and sonographic guidance are used; endoscopy is not required for radiologically controlled percutaneous gastrostomy.

The technique initially involves location of the appropriate site for puncture. Ultrasound is used to identify the left lobe of the liver, which occasionally overlies the stomach; the distances to the anterior and posterior wall of the insufflated stomach are determined by ultrasound as well. The transverse colon is identified fluoroscopically; contrast is infused rectally if the position of the transverse colon is uncertain. Inflation of the stomach is done with a contrast-water mixture, an intragastric balloon attached to a nasogastric tube, or with air. Puncture is made by direct trocar catheters or by guide wire exchange (Fig 4–22). The catheter size used is 8–14 F.

In most reports the stomach was not pulled up to the anterior abdominal wall with balloons attached to the gastrostomy catheters. To date, leakage has not been a problem. Other complications have occurred: dislodgment, minor oozing, and cutaneous inflammation. Success rates for the procedure are reported in the vast majority of cases.[106–109] Final catheter position is determined by contrast injection at fluoroscopy.

Celiac Ganglion Block

CT guidance for celiac ganglion block has been used due to the difficulties encountered by "blind" puncture and lack of prior success (probably due to inaccurate localization). The procedure is indicated for intractable or severe pain due to chronic pancreatitis, pancreatic cancer, or metastatic disease.

The procedure is performed in the supine or prone position under CT guidance. Needles are placed into the area of the celiac ganglion, anterior to the aorta and between the celiac

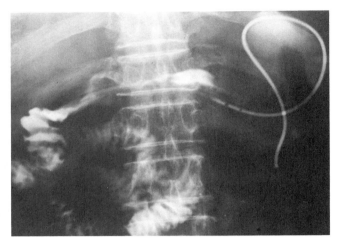

Fig 4–22.—This 64-year-old woman with a prior stroke underwent percutaneous gastrostomy. The catheter was placed directly through the abdominal wall and the tip of the catheter in the prepyloric region. Contrast material was injected to confirm appropriate position and to verify no leakage of fluid. Feedings were begun on the third postprocedure day.

and superior mesenteric arteries. In the prone position, generally two needles are used, and an angled approach to avoid the pleura is utilized. In the supine position, one needle may suffice, although overlying structures (stomach, small bowel) may need to be traversed (Fig 4–23).

Test injections with lidocaine (Xylocaine®) are used to assess the adequacy of needle position. If the patient reports "no" pain or significant improvement, contrast medium is injected to be certain there is bilateral diffusion so that all areas of the ganglia will be ablated. Once localization is correctly

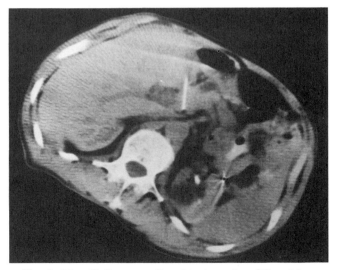

Fig 4–23.—Celiac ganglion block under CT guidance. This 72-year-old man had unrelenting pain from pancreatic carcinoma. A 22-gauge needle was inserted into the celiac plexus at the lateral aspect of the celiac artery. After confirmation of correct positioning, ethanol was injected to ablate the celiac ganglion. CT guidance ensures correct positioning of the needle, making success likely.

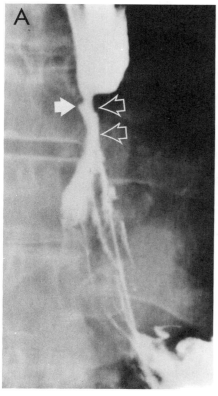

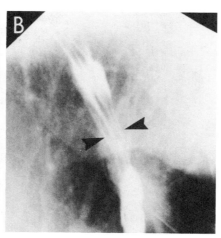

Fig 4–24.—Balloon dilatation of a benign esophageal stricture. **A,** barium swallow shows a 15-mm-long and 4-mm-wide stricture of the distal esophagus *(open arrows)* associated with a peptic ulcer *(full arrow)*. This patient would be at increased risk for perforation with bougienage. **B,** successful balloon dilatation was performed without complications, and the diameter of the stenotic segment measured 15 mm.

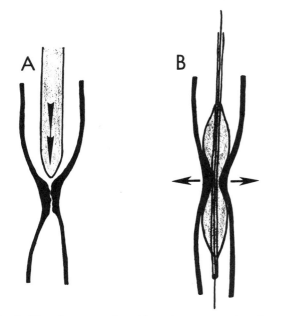

Fig 4–25.—**A,** conventional bougienage exerts a longitudinal shearing force ("snowplow" effect).[112] **B,** a tight stenosis can safely be traversed with guide wire-catheter technique. Balloon inflation exerts a radial force, with lower risk of perforation.

ascertained, ethanol is injected. Success rates are reported in 50%–100%, with a few minor complications.[109]

Balloon Catheter Dilatation of Gastrointestinal Strictures

The use of balloon catheters in the vascular system is standard practice. This method is also applicable to the percutaneous treatment of biliary, urinary, and GI strictures, which are most commonly located in the esophagus. Conventional bougienage of esophageal strictures is a well established method. Patterson et al.[111] achieved a success rate of 84% among 154 patients. This technique allows periodic self-bougienage, performed by the patient at home. However, with luminal diameters of less than 12 ml, the use of standard mercury-weighted bougies may be ineffective, and furthermore, may cause perforation.[112] The dilating force of conventional bougienage is created by a longitudinal shearing force, with the inherent risk of perforation or complete disruption of the esophagus. The rate of serious complications ranges from 0.5% to 9%.[113]

Patients with tight strictures, with tortuosity of the esophagus contiguous to the lesion, and ulcerations associated with stricture formation carry a high risk of perforation. Balloon catheter dilatation is therefore an attractive alternative (Figs 4–24, A and B). Guide wires and catheters can be safely advanced through high-grade, curved stenoses under fluoroscopic guidance. Inflation of the balloon exerts a radial rather than a shearing force (see Figs 4–25, A and B). Balloons of a diameter to 20 ml are available, and success rates from 71% to 90% have been achieved. More than one dilatation is required in 19%–25% of cases.[112–114] Ambulatory bougienage using the standard Maloney-Hurst method can be applied with less risk, once a tight stenosis has been dilated with balloon technique.

Successful balloon catheter dilatation has also been performed in a small number of patients with anastomotic strictures after surgical gastroenterostomy[113] and in children with colonic strictures after intestinal ischemia.[115]

ACKNOWLEDGMENTS

Our appreciation to Misses Deborah Lynn and Shirley Vitas for their untiring effort in preparing the manuscript.

REFERENCES

1. Meyers M.A.: *Dynamic Radiology of the Abdomen: Normal and Pathologic Anatomy*, ed. 2. New York, Springer-Verlag, 1982.
2. Whalen J.P.: *Radiology of the Abdomen*. Philadelphia, Lea & Febiger, 1976.
3. Haaga J.R.: New techniques for CT-guided biopsies. *A.J.R.* 133:633–641, 1979.
4. Ferrucci J.T. Jr., Wittenberg J., Mueller P.R., et al.: Diagnosis of abdominal malignancy by radiologic fine-needle aspiration biopsy. *A.J.R.* 134:323–330, 1980.
5. Isler R.J., Ferrucci J.T. Jr., Wittenberg J., et al.: Tissue core biopsy of abdominal tumors with a 22 gauge cutting needle. *A.J.R.* 136:725–728, 1981.
6. vanSonnenberg E., Mueller P.R.: Ultrasound, computerized body tomography and fluoroscopic guided percutaneous abdominal biopsy. *Appl. Radiol.* 10:121–123, 1981.
7. Nosher J.L., Plafker J.: Fine needle aspiration of the liver with ultrasound guidance. *Radiology* 136:177–180, 1980.
8. Rosenblatt R., Kutcher R., Moussouris H.F., et al.: Sonographically guided fine-needle aspiration of liver lesions. *J.A.M.A.* 248(13):1639–1641, 1982.
9. Torp-Pedersen S., Gronvall S., Holm H.H.: Ultrasonically guided fine-needle aspiration biopsy of gastrointestinal mass lesions. *J. Ultrasound Med.* 3:65–68, 1984.
10. Harter L.P., Moss A.A., Goldberg H.I., et al.: CT-guided fine-needle aspirations for diagnosis of benign and malignant disease. *A.J.R.* 140:363–367, 1983.
11. Pagani J.J.: Biopsy of focal hepatic lesions: Comparison of 18 and 22 gauge needles. *Radiology* 147:673–675, 1983.
12. vanSonnenberg E., Lin A.S., Deutsch A.L., et al.: Percutaneous biopsy of difficult mediastinal, hilar and pulmonary lesions by CT-guidance and a modified coaxial technique. *Radiology* 148:300–302, 1983.
13. Lee T.K.: The value of imprint cytology in tumor diagnosis. *Acta Cytol.* 169–171, 1981.
14. Lieberman R.P., Hafez G.R., Crummy A.B.: Histology from aspiration biopsy: Turner needle experience. *A.J.R.* 138:561–564, 1982.
15. Andriole J.G., Haaga J.R., Adams R.B., et al.: Biopsy needle characteristics assessed in the laboratory. *Radiology* 148:659–662, 1983.
16. Haaga J.R., LiPuma J.P., Bryan P.J., et al.: Clinical comparison of small- and large-caliber cutting needles for biopsy. *Radiology* 146:665–667, 1983.
17. vanSonnenberg E., Lin A.S., Casola G., et al.: Removable hub needle system for coaxial biopsy of small and difficult lesion. *Radiology* 152:226, 1984.
18. Berkman W.A., Chowdhury L., Brown N.L., et al.: Value of electron microscopy in cytologic diagnosis of fine-needle biopsy. *A.J.R.* 140:1253–1258, 1983.
19. vanSonnenberg E., Wittenberg J., Ferrucci J.T. Jr., et al.: Triangulation method for percutaneous needle guidance: The angled approach to upper abdominal masses. *A.J.R.* 137:757–761, 1981.
20. Ferrucci J.T. Jr., Wittenberg J., Margolies M.N., et al.: Malignant seeding of the tract after thin-needle aspiration biopsy. *Radiology* 130:345–346, 1979.
21. Cooperberg P.L.: High-resolution real-time ultrasound in the evaluation of the normal and obstructed biliary tract. *Radiology* 129:477–480, 1978.
22. Haubek A., Pedersen J.H., Burcharth F., et al.: Dynamic sonography in the evaluation of jaundice. *A.J.R.* 136:1071–1074, 1981.
23. Koenigsberg M., Wiener S.N., Walzer A.: The accuracy of sonography in the differential diagnosis of obstructive jaundice: A comparison with cholangiography. *Radiology* 133:157–165, 1979.
24. Malini S., Sabel J.: Ultrasonography in obstructive jaundice. *Radiology* 123:429–433, 1977.
25. Behan M., Kazam E.: Sonography of the common bile duct: Value of the right anterior oblique view. *A.J.R.* 130:701–709, 1978.
26. Nieman H.L., Mintzer R.A.: Accuracy of biliary duct ultrasound: Comparison with cholangiography. *A.J.R.* 129:979–982, 1977.
27. Laing F.C., Jeffrey R.B., Jr.: Choledocholithiasis and cystic duct obstruction: Difficult ultrasonographic diagnosis. *Radiology* 146:475–479, 1983.
28. Honickman S.P., Mueller P.R., Wittenberg J., et al.: Ultrasound in obstructive jaundice: Prospective evaluation of site and cause. *Radiology* 147:511–515, 1983.
29. Baron R.L., Stanley R.J., Lee J.K.T., et al.: Computed tomographic features of biliary obstruction. *A.J.R.* 140:1173–1178, 1983.
30. Jeffrey R.B., Federle M.P., Laing F.C., et al.: Computed tomography of choledocholithiasis. *A.J.R.* 140:1179–1183, 1983.
31. Vas W., Salem S.: Accuracy of sonography and transhepatic cholangiography in obstructive jaundice. *J. Can. Assoc. Radiol.* 32:111–113, June 1981.
32. vanSonnenberg E., Ferrucci J.T. Jr., Neff C.C., et al.: Percutaneous recordings and applications of biliary pressure: Manometric and perfusion studies at transhepatic cholangiography and percutaneous biliary drainage. *Radiology* 148:41–50, 1983.
33. Zimmon D.S., Ferrara T.P., Clemett A.R.: Radiology of papilla of Vater stenosis. *Gastrointest. Radiol.* 3:343–348, 1978.
34. Muhletaler C.A., Gerlock A.J., Fleischer A.C., et al.: Diagnosis of obstructive jaundice with nondilated bile ducts. *A.J.R.* 134:1149–1152, 1980.
35. Simeone J.F., Mueller P.R., Ferrucci J.T. Jr., et al.: Sonography of the bile ducts after fatty meal. *Radiology* 143:211–215, 1982.
36. Mueller P.R., Harbin W.P., Ferrucci J.T. Jr., et al.: Fine needle transhepatic cholangiography: Reflections after 450 cases. *A.J.R.* 136:85–90, 1981.
37. Mueller P.R., vanSonnenberg E., Simeone J.F.: Fine needle transhepatic cholangiography. *Ann. Intern. Med.* 97:567–572, 1982.
38. Nakamoto S., vanSonnenberg E.: Cholangiocarcinoma in pregnancy: The contributions of ultrasound guided interventional techniques. *J. Ultrasound Med.* In press.
39. Beinart C., Sniderman K.W., Tamura S., et al.: Biliary pressure measurement: An aid in the management of patients on internal biliary drainage. *Invest. Radiol.* 17(4):356–361, 1982.
40. Mueller P.R., Ferrucci J.T. Jr., vanSonnenberg E., et al.: Obstruction of the left hepatic duct: Diagnosis and treatment by selective fine needle cholangiography and percutaneous biliary drainage. *Radiology* 145:297–302, 1982.
41. Carrasco C.H., Zornoza J., Bechtel W.J.: Malignant biliary obstruction: Complications of percutaneous biliary drainage. *Radiology* 152:343–346, 1984.
42. Gobien R.P., Stanley J.H., Soucek C.D., et al.: Routine preoperative biliary drainage: Effect and management of obstructive jaundice. *Radiology* 152:353–356, 1984.
43. Kadir S., Baassiri A., Barth K.H., et al.: Percutaneous biliary drainage in the management of biliary sepsis. *A.J.R.* 138:25–29, 1982.
44. Ferrucci J.T., Jr., Mueller P.R., vanSonnenberg E., et al.: Percutaneous biliary drainage, in Ferrucci J.T. Jr., Wittenberg J. (eds.): *Interventional Radiology of the Abdomen*. Baltimore, Williams & Wilkins Co., pp. 53–110, 1981.

45. Bonnel D., Ferrucci J.T. Jr., Mueller P.R., et al.: Surgical and radiological decompression in malignant biliary obstruction: A retrospective study using multivariate risk factor analysis. *Radiology* 152:347–351, 1984.
46. vanSonnenberg E., Neff C.C., Simeone J.F.: Percutaneous basket removal of retained biliary stones. *Appl. Radiol.* 10:35–38, 1981.
47. Burhenne H.J.: Percutaneous extraction of retained biliary tract stones: 661 patients. *A.J.R.* 134:888–898, 1980.
48. Ralls P.W., Colletti P.M., Quinn M.F., et al.: Sonography in recurrent oriental pyogenic cholangitis. *A.J.R.* 136:1010–1012, 1981.
49. vanSonnenberg E., Casola G., Nakamoto S.K., et al.: Radiologic contributions to the diagnosis and interventional management in oriental cholangiohepatitis. In press.
50. Thistle J.L., Carlson G.L., LaRusso N.F., et al.: Effective dissolution of biliary duct stones by intraductal infusion of monooctanoin (abstract). *Gastroenterology* 74:1103, 1978.
51. Mack E.A., Saito C., Goldfarb S., et al.: A new agent for gallstone dissolution: Experimental and clinical evaluation. *Surg. Forum* 29:438–439, 1978.
52. Salomonowitz E., Castaneda-Zuniga W.R., Lund G., et al.: Balloon dilatation of benign biliary strictures. *Radiology* 151:613–616, 1984.
53. Shaver R.W., Hawkins I.F. Jr., Soong J.: Percutaneous cholecystostomy. *A.J.R.* 138:1133–1136, 1982.
54. Teplick S.K., Wolferth C.C. Jr., Hayes M.F. Jr., et al.: Percutaneous cholecystostomy in obstructive jaundice. *Gastrointest. Radiol.* 7:259–261, 1982.
55. vanSonnenberg E., Wing V.W., Pollard J.W., Casola G.: Life-threatening vagal reactions associated with percutaneous cholecystostomy. *Radiology* 151:377–380, 1984.
56. Wolverson M.K., Jagannadharao B., Sundaram M., et al.: CT as a primary diagnostic method in evaluating intraabdominal abscess. *A.J.R.* 133:1089–1095, 1979.
57. Koehler P.R., Moss A.A.: Diagnosis of intra-abdominal and pelvic abscesses by computerized tomography. *J.A.M.A.* 244(1):49–52, 1980.
58. Taylor K.J.W., DeGraff C., Wasson J.F., et al.: Accuracy of grey scale ultrasound diagnosis of abdominal and pelvic abscess in 220 patients. *Lancet* 1:83–84, 1978.
59. Altemeier W.A., Culbertson W.R., Pullen W.D., et al.: Intraabdominal abscesses. *Am. J. Surg.* 125:70–79, 1973.
60. Callen P.W.: Computed tomographic evaluation of abdominal and pelvic abscesses. *Radiology* 131:171–175, 1979.
61. vanSonnenberg E., Ferrucci J.T. Jr., Wittenberg J., et al.: Comparative utility of ultrasound and computed body tomography in suspected abdominal abscesses. Presented at the Radiological Society of North America Meeting, Dallas, November 1980.
62. vanSonnenberg E., Ferrucci J.T. Jr., Mueller P.R., et al.: Percutaneous drainage of abscesses and fluid collections: Technique, results and applications. *Radiology* 142:1–10, 1982.
63. Brown J.J., vanSonnenberg E., Strich G., et al.: Magnetic resonance of percutaneously obtained normal and abnormal body fluids. *Radiology* 154:727, 1985.
64. Welch C.E., Malt R.A.: Abdominal surgery (three parts). *N. Engl. J. Med.* 308:753–760, 1983.
65. Gerzof S.G., Robbins A.H., Johnson W.C., et al.: Percutaneous catheter drainage of abdominal abscesses: A five-year experience. *N. Engl. J. Med.* 305:653–657, 1981.
66. vanSonnenberg D., Mueller P.R., Ferrucci J.T. Jr.: Percutaneous drainage of 250 abdominal abscesses and fluid collections: Part I. results, failures, and complications. *Radiology* 151:337–341, 1984.
67. Haaga J.R., Weinstein A.J.: CT-Guided percutaneous aspiration and drainage of abscesses. *A.J.R.* 135:1187–1194, 1980.
68. vanSonnenberg E., Wing V.W., Casola G., et al.: Temporizing effect of percutaneous drainage of complicated abscesses in critically ill patients. *A.J.R.* 142:821–826, 1984.
69. Mueller P.R., vanSonnenberg E., Ferrucci J.T. Jr.: Percutaneous drainage of 250 abdominal abscesses and fluid collections. *Radiology* 151(2):343–347, 1984.

70. Van Waes P.F.G.M., Feldberg M.A.M., Mali W.P., et al.: Management of loculated abscesses that are difficult to drain: A new approach. *Radiology* 147:7–63, 1983.
71. vanSonnenberg E., Mueller P.R., Ferrucci J.T. Jr., et al.: Sump catheter for percutaneous abscess and fluid drainage by trocar or seldinger technique. *A.J.R.* 139:613–614, 1982.
72. Bernardino M.E., Berkman W.A., Plemmons M., et al.: Percutaneous drainage of multiseptated hepatic abscess. *J. Comput. Assist. Tomogr.* 8(1)38:41, 1984.
73. Mueller P.R., Dawson S.L., Ferrucci J.T. Jr., et al.: Percutaneous drainage of hepatic echinococcal cyst. Presented at The Society of Gastrointestinal Radiologists' 14th Annual Meeting and Postgraduate Course, Napa Valley, Calif. Sept. 29–Oct. 3, 1984.
74. Greco R.S., Kamath C., Nosher J.L.: Percutaneous drainage of peridiverticular abscess followed by primary sigmoidectomy. *Dis. Colon Rectum* 25:53–55, 1982.
75. Cronan J.J., Amis E.S. Jr., Dorfman G.S.: Percutaneous drainage of renal abscesses. *A.J.R.* 142:351–354, 1984.
76. Crass J.R.: Liver abscess as a complication of regional enteritis: Interventional considerations. *Am. J. Gastroenterol.* 78(11):747–749, 1983.
77. vanSonnenberg E., Mueller P.R., Schiffman H.R., et al.: Percutaneous catheter drainage of intrahepatic amebic abcesses: Indications and results. *Radiology* In press.
78. vanSonnenberg E., Wittich G.R., Casola G., et al.: Interventional radiology in complicated pancreatic inflammatory disease: Diagnostic and therapeutic results and benefits. *Radiology* In press.
79. Karlson K.B., Martin E.C., Fankuchen E.I., et al.: Percutaneous drainage of pancreatic pseudocysts and abscesses. *Radiology* 142:619–624, 1982.
80. Mueller P.R., Ferrucci J.T. Jr., Simeone J.F., et al.: Detection and drainage of bilomas: Special considerations. *A.J.R.* 140:715–720, 1983.
81. Bhatt G.M., Jason R.S., Delany H.M., et al.: Hepatic hematoma: Percutaneous drainage. *A.J.R.* 135:1287–1288, 1980.
82. Sacks B.A., Vine H.S., Bartek S., et al.: Postoperative abscess drainage in patients with established sinus tracks or drains. *Radiology* 142:537–538, 1982.
83. Freeny P.C., Vimont T.R., Barnett D.C.: Cavernous hemangioma of the liver: Ultrasonography, arteriography, and computed tomography. *Radiology* 132:143–148, 1979.
84. Krudy A.G., Doppman J.L., Jensen R.T., et al.: Localization of islet cell tumors by dynamic CT: Comparison with plain CT, arteriography, sonography, and venous sampling. *A.J.R.* 143:585–589, 1984.
85. LaBerge J.M., Laing F.C., Federle M.P., et al.: Hepatocellular carcinoma: Assessment of resectability by computed tomography and ultrasound. *Radiology* 152:485–490, 1984.
86. Jafri S.Z.H., Aisen A.M., Glazer G.M., et al.: Comparison of CT and angiography in assessing resectability of pancreatic carcinoma. *A.J.R.* 142:525–529, 1984.
87. Heeney D.J., Bookstein J.J., Bell R.H., et al.: Correlation of hepatic and portal wedged venography and manometry with histology in alcoholic cirrhosis and periportal fibrosis. *Radiology* 142:591–597, 1982.
88. Boley S.J., Brandt L.J., Veith F.J.: Ischemic disorders of the intestines. *Curr. Probl. Surg.* 15:1–85, 1978.
89. Baum S.: Angiography and the gastrointestinal bleeder. *Radiology* 143:569–572, 1982.
90. Baum S., Athanasoulis C.A., Waltman A.C., et al.: Angiodysplasia of the right colon: A cause of gastrointestinal bleeding. *A.J.R.* 129:789–794, 1977.
91. Baum S., Athanasoulis C.A., Waltman A.C.: Angiographic diagnosis and control of large-bowel bleeding. *Dis. Colon Rectum* 17:447–453, 1974.
92. Gupta S., Luna E., Kingsley S., et al.: Detection of gastrointestinal bleeding by radionuclide scintigraphy. *Am. J. Gastroenterol.* 79:26–31, 1984.
93. Widrich W.C., Sequeira S.R.: Interventional radiology of the liver and related structures. *Radiol. Clin. North Am.* 18:297–314, 1980.

94. Wittich G., Czembirek H., Appel W., et al.: Angiography in distal spleno-renal shunts. *Radiologe* 20:528–533, 1980.

95. Wallace S., Chuang V.P.: The radiologic diagnosis and management of hepatic metastases. *Radiologe* 22:56–64, 1982.

96. Yamada R., Sato M., Kawabata M., et al.: Hepatic artery embolization in 120 patients with unresectable hepatoma. *Radiology* 148:397–401, 1983.

97. Barone R.M., Byfield J.E., Goldfarb P.B., et al.: Intra-arterial chemotherapy using an implantable infusion pump and liver irradiation for the treatment of hepatic metastases. *Cancer* 50:850–862, 1982.

98. Mozes M.F., Spigos D.G., Pollak R., et al.: Partial splenic embolization, an alternative to splenectomy—Results of a prospective, randomized study. *Surgery* 96:694–700, 1984.

99. Castaneda-Zuniga W.R., Gomes A., Ween C., et al.: Transluminal angioplasty in the management of abdominal angina. *R.O.F.O.* 137:330–332, 1982.

100. Cope C.: Balloon dilatation of closed mesocaval shunts. *A.J.R.* 135:989–993, 1980.

101. Flickinger E.G., Johnsrude I.S., Ogburn N.L., et al.: Local streptokinase infusion for superior mesenteric artery thromboembolism. *A.J.R.* 140:771–772, 1983.

102. Ohto M., Karasawa E., Tsuchiya Y., et al.: Ultrasonically guided percutaneous contrast medium injection and aspiration biopsy using a real-time puncture transducer. *Radiology* 136:171–176, 1980.

103. Makuuchi M., Bandai Y., Ito T., et al.: Ultrasonically guided percutaneous transhepatic cholangiography and percutaneous pancreatography. *Radiology* 134:767–770, 1980.

104. Gobien R.P., Stanley J.H., Anderson M.C., et al.: Percutaneous drainage of pancreatic duct for treating acute pancreatitis. *A.J.R.* 141:795, 1983.

105. vanSonnenberg E., Casola G., Tanenbaum L.B.: CT-Guided percutaneous pancreatic ductography: Results, uses and problems. Presented at the Radiological Society of North America Meeting, Chicago, November 1983.

106. Wills J.S., Ogelsby J.T.: Percutaneous gastrostomy. *Radiology* 149:449–453, 1983.

107. Ho C.S.: Percutaneous gastrostomy for jejunal feeding. *Radiology* 149:595–596, 1983.

108. vanSonnenberg E., Cubberley D.A., Brown L.K., et al.: Percutaneous gastrostomy: Use of intragastric balloon support. *Radiology* 152:531–532, 1984.

109. vanSonnenberg E., Brown L.K., Tanenbaum L.B., et al.: Percutaneous gastrostomy and gastroenterostomy (parts I and II). *A.J.R.* In press.

110. Haaga J.R., Kori S.H., Eastwood D.W., et al.: Improved technique for CT-guided celiac ganglia block. *A.J.R.* 142:1201–1204, 1984.

111. Patterson D.J., Graham D.Y., Smith J.L., et al.: Natural history of benign esophageal stricture treated by dilatation. *Gastroenterology* 85:346–350, 1983.

112. Dawson S.L., Mueller P.R., Ferrucci J.T. Jr., et al.: Balloon catheter dilatation of severe esophageal strictures. *Radiology* 153:631–635, 1984.

113. Götberg S., Afzelius L.E., Hedenbro J., et al.: Balloon catheter dilatation of strictures in the upper digestive tract. *Radiologe* 22:479–483, 1982.

114. Starck E., Paolucci V., Herzer M., et al.: Esophageal stenosis: Treatment with balloon catheters. *Radiology* 153:637–640, 1984.

115. Ball W.S. Jr., Seigel R.S., Goldthorn J.F., et al.: Colonic strictures in infants following intestinal ischemia: treatment by balloon catheter dilatation. *Radiology* 149:469–472, 1983.

5

The Role and Effects of Parenteral and Enteral Nutrition in Digestive Diseases

HERBERT R. FREUND, M.D.
ROBERT H. BOWER, M.D.
JOSEF E. FISCHER, M.D.

INTRODUCTION AND HISTORY OF PARENTERAL NUTRITION

It is now accepted that starvation, malnutrition, or both, and the inability of patients to be nourished adequately during severe illness, injury, major trauma, or sepsis have far-reaching effects on the immunologic system and host defense against infection, wound healing, and respiratory and cardiac function. With persistence of starvation and sepsis, multiple organ system failure results. The goals of nutritional support are the maintenance of lean body mass and other vital functions important for recovery of the severely ill patient.

When the history of medicine in the 20th century is written, nutritional support will rank high among advances in medicine, particularly in surgery. Although the field of nutritional support and parenteral nutrition in this country is but 15 years old, it has become one of the more important therapeutic weapons.

The first recorded account of "parenteral nutrition" is that of Sir Christopher Wren, who in 1656 injected wine and ale into a vein of a dog; the dog became intoxicated. Caspar Scotus (1664) performed a similar experiment, while a year later Lower successfully transfused a dog. In 1667 Lower and King, and Denys transfused sheep or lamb blood into a human. The first account of fat embolism is that of William Courten (1710–12), who infused olive oil into a dog, with a dismal outcome. Similar attempts, but via the subcutaneous route, were successfully undertaken by Mentzel and Perco (1869) in both dog and man. Hodder (1873) successfully injected milk into two patients, while Biedle and Krause (1886) were the first to introduce glucose as an IV nutrient.

The beginning of this century saw Friedrich (1904) administer a combination of peptone solution, fat, glucose, and salt, to become the first investigator to carry out complete parenteral nutrition. In 1913 Henriques and Andersen were able to induce nitrogen equilibrium in a goat by infusing amino acids produced by enzymatic hydrolysis. Sansum and Wilder (1915) advocated the use of large amounts of glucose as caloric supply. In the 1940s and '50s Rose published his classic work on the essentiality of certain amino acids, which was followed by Elman infusing a casein hydrolysate fortified by tryptophan and cystine into dogs and patients. Another major landmark in the development of surgical metabolism and nutrition arose from the extensive studies by Sir David Cuthbertson during the 1930s characterizing the metabolic response to injury.

Following Rose's work with essential amino acids, Wretlind developed the technique of dialysis to obtain a casein hydrolysate containing mostly amino acids and some low molecular peptides for improved efficacy and fewer allergic reactions. Wretlind and Schuberth also pioneered nonprotein caloric sources. Apparently, one of the very first attempts to use IV fat emulsions in man was made in 1920 by Yamakawa. In 1944 Helfrick and Abelson successfully fed a 5-month-old child by vein using a combination of water, saline, olive oil in lecithin, carbohydrate, and amino acids. Later attempts to use fat as a caloric source included the use of coconut, olive, peanut, and cottonseed oil emulsions. It was finally Wretlind and Schuberth (1961) who succeeded in producing and testing a safe and nontoxic soybean oil and egg-yolk phospholipid emulsion (Intralipid), which has been widely used for over 20 years.

While in Europe a fat emulsion was developed, the Department of Surgery and its research laboratory at the University of Pennsylvania continued working on the hypertonic glucose-protein hydrolysate concept. In 1949 Rhoads and co-workers infused hypertonic glucose and protein hydrolysate into dogs for 4–20 weeks. Subsequently, it was shown that puppies fed entirely by IV for 72–255 days gained more weight and matched their litter-mate enterally fed controls in skeletal growth, development, and activity. It remained for Dudrick and associates[1] to combine their many years of research with the technical description of the subclavian venipuncture by Aubiniac, to begin the modern era of total parenteral nutrition (TPN). Although only 15 years old, TPN has been widely accepted and has made excellent progress. Indications have been refined, crystalline amino acids introduced, techniques and protocols improved, nutritional requirements defined, nutritional assessment attempted, and definition of nutritional needs in specific disease states undertaken.

PROTEIN METABOLISM AND REQUIREMENTS

Of the three major foodstuffs—protein, carbohydrate, and fat—protein is most important, since it is the effector of all vital organic function, whether mechanical, enzymatic, or immunologic.

The balance between protein synthesis and degradation is critical for normal homeostasis. Synthesis of protein is a highly complex, energy-requiring process, whereas breakdown of protein yields only one fourth of the energy-rich phosphate invested in its synthesis. In a 70-kg man there is between 10 and 11 kg of protein, largely contained as muscle but also as viscera. With a daily protein turnover of 250–300 gm, the gut is responsible for the largest component: approximately 90 gm/day of ingested protein and 70 gm of protein from desquamated gut cells and enzymes secreted into the gut. After digestion, almost all of these amino acids are absorbed, with the exception of approximately 1 gm of nitrogen excreted in the stool. Muscle breakdown accounts for another 50–70 gm of amino acids, most of which are resynthesized provided enough energy is present. Twenty grams of plasma protein, 8 gm of hemoglobin, 20 gm of white cells, and a few grams of skin compose the remainder of total body synthesis.

Protein turnover does not remain constant; it decreases with age. Turnover in a neonate is 25 gm/kg/day and decreases to 7 gm/kg/day by one year of age. Protein turnover in adults approximates 3 gm of protein/kg/day, greater in males than in females. Thus, the rate of turnover decreases with age, but as percentage of lean body mass per body weight increases, total turnover for the organism remains the same.

The nature of calories is also important to the regulation of protein turnover. Carbohydrate increases muscle protein synthesis, presumably under the influence of insulin, while fat increases both muscle and hepatic protein synthesis. In addition, carbohydrate depresses hepatic albumin synthesis compared with an optimal combination of fat and carbohydrate.

True protein requirement can be measured using the assumption that during a protein-free diet, the minimal nitrogen excretion observed represents true protein requirements. Thus, with a calorically adequate, protein-free diet, 37 mg of nitrogen/kg is excreted into the urine, 12 mg of nitrogen/kg is lost in the feces, integumentary losses account for another 5 mg/kg, and evaporation to 2–3 mg/kg, making a total of 56–57 mg/kg of nitrogen or, in terms of whole protein, 0.34 gm/kg/day. With various corrections, coefficients of variation and allowances for low biologic value protein, the average normal requirement is 0.8 gm of protein/kg or between 56 and 60 gm protein/day; injury, trauma, or sepsis increases protein requirements. In infants, between 40% and 50% of the protein intake should be administered as essential amino acids, whereas baseline adult requirements include only about 20% as essential amino acids. The percentage of essential amino acids should be increased with injury or depletion. As parenteral nutrition is claimed (but certainly not proved) to be less effective than the gut, and the liver is bypassed during parenteral nutrition, a safe figure for patients receiving parenteral nutrition is 250 mg N/kg or 1.7 gm protein/kg/day of crystalline amino acids.

CALORIE:NITROGEN RATIO

The energy required for protein synthesis has been estimated as a calorie:nitrogen ratio of 100–150:1 (i.e., 100–150 nonprotein calories are required per 1 gm of nitrogen) in relatively average patients.[2] The calorie:nitrogen ratio presumably changes in various disease states. In sepsis higher intakes of nitrogen and smaller intakes of nonprotein calories are probably useful, while in uremia a calorie:nitrogen ratio of between 300–400:1 has been advocated, although we do not subscribe to this figure.

ENERGY REQUIREMENTS AND CALORIC SOURCES

The body can utilize three sources of energy: protein, fat, and carbohydrate. Amino acids contribute approximately 15% of normal energy expenditure, 6%–7% from oxidation of branched-chain amino acids oxidized directly to high-energy phosphate, and the remaining 8%–9% derived from gluconeogenesis. The remaining 85% of normal energy expenditure is obtained from carbohydrate or fat. As most of the body's energy stores exist as fat, and as hepatic and muscle glycogen are almost totally expended after a 24-hour fast, approximately 70%–75% of the resting metabolic expenditure will be the result of fat utilization, either via direct oxidation or via ketone body production and utilization.

The ability to measure respiratory quotient (R.Q.) makes it clinically feasible to determine which fuel is being consumed. An R.Q. of 1 or greater indicates pure carbohydrate utilization, and, on a theoretical basis, with continuing lipogenesis the R.Q. can reach as high as 9, although rates greater than 1 are rarely seen clinically. Alternatively, an R.Q. of 0.7 indicates primary reliance on fat as a fuel, while an R.Q. of less than 0.7 indicates ketogenesis.

Indirect calorimetry also enables determination of caloric requirements in the clinical setting. Whereas ten and even five years ago it was common for patients to receive 3,500–4,000 calories/day, now mean caloric supplementation is closer to 2,000–2,500 calories/day. In the absence of direct measurements, the Harris-Benedict equation may be a useful guide:

$$\text{BEE} = \begin{array}{l} 66.5 + 13.7\,\text{W} + 5.0\,\text{H} - 6.8\,\text{A} \; [\text{male}] \\ 65.5 + 9.6\,\text{W} + 1.7\,\text{H} - 4.7\,\text{A} \; [\text{female}] \end{array}$$

where W = weight in kg, H = height in cm, and A = age in years.

In the absence of severe sepsis, trauma, or major burn, 30–35 kcal/kg of body weight/day is probably adequate, mostly as carbohydrate, and 25%–35% of nonprotein calories as fat.

Carbohydrates

Over the past 10–15 years, glucose has been the preferred carbohydrate source for parenteral nutrition, with other possibilities including fructose, sorbitol, xylitol, and glycerol. Administration of about 1,800 calories as glucose in the resting fasting state will minimize protein breakdown, particularly after adaptation to starvation (Fig 5–1). In addition to this protein-sparing quality, glucose is the preferred fuel for red cells,

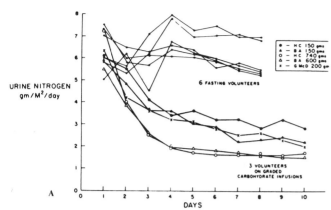

Fig 5–1.—Nitrogen-sparing effect of carbohydrate. Above are shown nitrogen excretion rates in starvation. The curves below demonstrate the remarkable decline in urinary nitrogen excretion when carbohydrate is given intravenously in the doses shown. With 600 to 740 gm/day (2,400 to 3,000 calories), a lower limit or "nitrogen floor" is achieved, at about 1.5 gm/sqm/day. (From Moore F.D., Brennan M.F., in *ACS Manual of Surgical Nutrition,* 1975, p. 205. Used by permission.)

white cells, and to a certain degree the CNS. Similarly, wound repair requires glucose. The theoretical limit to the use of glucose has been estimated at 0.4–1.2 gm/min in the normal adult, depending on age and disease. In practice, most nondiabetic adults will tolerate 0.8–1.0 gm glucose/min, or a total of 4.5–5.0 L of 25% dextrose/day, although whether it is utilized effectively is another matter. More recent data suggest that oxidation of glucose is limited to 2,000 calories, or 500 gm; the remainder is utilized for lipogenesis.

There are also deleterious effects to glucose, particularly when given in excess, such as hyperglycemia and its consequences, accumulation of body fat and fatty liver. Blood glucose levels in excess of 300–350 mg/dl adversely affect neutrophil function.

Other carbohydrate sources have not been commonly utilized in the United States. Fructose, proposed as a preferred carbohydrate source under circumstances of glucose intolerance, may cause fatal lactic acidosis. Furthermore, fructose requires expenditure of high-energy phosphate through the pentose-monophosphate shunt for its utilization, and 80% of the administered fructose is finally metabolized in the form of glucose.

The polyalcohols xylitol and sorbitol also undergo transformation to glucose. Xylitol is hepatotoxic and has caused several deaths in the Australian experience. Despite this, xylitol and sorbitol are used in Europe and are being reexamined as substrates under special circumstances.

Glycerol is another potential source of glucose. It has the advantages that it may be sterilized in solution with amino acids without undergoing the caramelization reaction and that its osmolality is low. These properties of glycerol have been recently utilized in a new commercial solution (Procalamine®), which is administered peripherally, does not require pharmacy mixing, and thus saves expensive pharmacy costs. This solution is used as an intermediate solution (not for seriously ill patients) with relatively low

cost, but its efficacy and place in the armamentarium remain to be identified. Glycerol in large doses may cause renal failure in experimental animals, and caution is therefore necessary.

Fat

In normal individuals in resting starvation, caloric expenditure is largely in terms of fat and ketone bodies. Fat constitutes the largest caloric store of the body, the equivalent of approximately 60,000 kcal in the normal person. Lipolysis is encouraged by steroids, catechols, and glucagon, and is extremely sensitive to inhibition by insulin. The omission of fat in the initial stages of parenteral nutrition in the United States was due partially to the lack of a safe fat emulsion. Initially, administration of fat was to prevent essential fatty acid deficiency by giving 4%–6% of daily caloric supply as fat. Now the pendulum has swung to encourage the utilization of fat both as a major caloric source and as a source of essential fatty acids. All seem to agree that under normal circumstances or in patients with only moderate stress, fat and carbohydrate are indistinguishable with respect to nitrogen conservation and balance,[3] 25% of nonprotein calories as fat seeming optimal for hepatic protein synthesis.[4] If all nonprotein calories are given as carbohydrate, amino acids are preferentially diverted to muscle protein synthesis under the influence of insulin.

One remaining area of controversy is the use of fat in severe stress and sepsis. It is not clear at which point in severe stress and/or sepsis fat oxidation and/or utilization becomes impaired. All seem to agree that fat clearance remains relatively normal until comparatively late in sepsis, but fat oxidation is impaired somewhat earlier. We thus believe that the degree of stress will determine the use of fat and that in the severely stressed patient, especially one with sepsis, reliance should be placed primarily on glucose and amino acids, mainly branched-chain amino acids.

In our normal practice, excluding severely septic patients, we administer 25% of the nonprotein calories as a fat emulsion, limited to 2 gm of fat emulsion/kg in adults and 4 gm/kg in neonates and infants. In patients with severe sepsis, it is necessary either to measure R.Q. or to monitor continually the lipemia to make certain that administered fat is adequately both cleared and oxidized. The accumulation of fat within the plasma indicates lack of utilization.

NUTRITIONAL ASSESSMENT

Nutritional assessment is an attempt to evaluate body nutritional composition to predict the risk for illness or the necessary therapy, generally surgery, chemotherapy, and/or radiation. The current status of nutritional assessment, however, is disappointing. Although the ability to predict statistical risk in severely malnourished populations in Third World countries has been well established, we cannot yet predict risk accurately in a U.S. hospital setting. Moreover, except for retrospective statistical analyses, one cannot accurately predict outcome in a given patient.

Theoretically, one should measure lean body mass, specifically as it affects important functions, such as muscular, respiratory, and cardiac work. However, in the surgical patient, hepatic, renal, immunologic, and host defense functions are also of utmost importance.

A brief review of current clinical and laboratory nutritional assessment follows.

LEAN BODY MASS.—Accumulation of lean body mass is the principal objective of nutritional support, so determination of lean body mass would be the most appropriate means of nutritional assessment. Such determinations, which are complicated and usually available only on a research basis, include the following.

A. Displacement, in which the various body components are estimated by immersion in a tank with displacement of water volume.

B. Exchange of labeled ions, by which total body water (tritated water), lean body mass (^{42}K), and extracellular water (^{22}Na) can be determined. A ratio of exchangeable sodium to exchangeable potassium of greater than 1.22 has been suggested by Shizgal[5] as indicating increased extracellular water and decreased body mass accompanying malnutrition.

C. Neutron activation analysis: This sophisticated and expensive apparatus bombards the body with activated neutrons to measure total body nitrogen. Other ions may be determined as well.

D. Total body counters: These can measure spontaneous decay of naturally occurring ions, such as K_{40}, which reflects lean body mass. However, these measurements are not suitable for patients who are severely ill, as they must remain stationary within the counter for prolonged periods.

E. Nuclear magnetic resonance (NMR): The advent of NMR may enable accurate measurement of body composition and lean body mass in many centers. Little data are currently available.

F. With the recent developments in gas chromatography-mass spectrometry, the use of heavy isotopes to determine protein turnover and flux is becoming more widespread. Here, too, methodology is complex and the equipment expensive.

HISTORY AND PHYSICAL EXAMINATION.—A history of weight loss (10% or more), weakness, anorexia, or a disease process that interferes with intake, such as esophageal carcinoma, should alert the examiner to the possibility of malnutrition. This can be verified on physical examination by muscle wasting; loss of thenar eminence; loose, flabby skin owing to loss of body fat; and the edema of hypoproteinemia. Anthropometric measurement, which enjoyed a brief and very disappointing flurry of utilization, adds little useful information, even if measurements are done accurately.[6]

NITROGEN BALANCE.—In the clinical setting, nitrogen balance is generally determined by measuring urinary urea or total nitrogen excretion and any GI losses. Since most patients receiving TPN are not eating, stool nitrogen can usually be disregarded. Measuring urea nitrogen excretion is within the capacity of any hospital laboratory, but the urinary collection must be accurate, which can be monitored by the simultaneous measurement of urinary creatinine. If one measures total urinary urea nitrogen excretion, 2–3 gm of nitrogen should be added for insensible and non-urea losses. A better alternative is to measure total urinary nitrogen excretion, in which case a small amount of nitrogen, about 1 gm, should be added for insensible losses.

NITROGEN BREAKDOWN AND TURNOVER.—These events, particularly concerning lean body mass, can be estimated by urinary excretion of 3-methylhistidine (3-MH). It is now clear that urinary excretion of 3-MH, a methylated derivative of histidine which is not reutilized for nitrogen synthesis,[6] measures not merely breakdown but probably turnover as well. It is also likely that 3-MH measures not only muscle lean body mass but also a relatively small, rapidly turning-over protein pool derived from the gut. Most authorities now believe that while 3-MH will measure lean body mass, it cannot be taken as a measurement of skeletal muscle turnover.[7]

OTHER MEASUREMENTS.—Indirect calorimetry, now more widely available with bedside metabolic carts, is increasingly utilized to measure energy balance, which may be as important as nitrogen balance in determining equilibrium.

The parameters commonly used today are generally disappointing. Consecutive patients studied prospectively in equally large numbers failed to reveal a group at risk. Other investigators have convincingly demonstrated that accurate clinical observations by experienced observers not particularly skilled in "nutritional assessment" provide the same accuracy as a series of extensive and complex tests. More recent studies which emphasize hepatic synthesis of short-turnover proteins and neutrophil function may prove to be more successful in nutritional assessment of patients.

GENERAL INDICATIONS FOR NUTRITIONAL SUPPORT

Because accurate prediction of risk in a given patient is impossible, indications for parenteral nutrition should depend on the following criteria:

1. The premorbid state (healthy or otherwise), especially the nutritional status;
2. Age of the patient;
3. Duration of starvation;
4. Degree of the insult;
5. The likelihood of resuming normal intake within a finite period (Fig 5–2).

Based on these general guidelines, each practitioner must choose his own criteria on the basis of available evidence in a given patient. In general, patients up to 60 years old can tolerate a 12–14-day period of fast, beyond which continuous starvation is deleterious. This is not to say that such patients should be allowed to starve for 12–14 days, merely that this can perhaps be tolerated. In a septuagenarian 7–8 days is the limit, and probably only 5–6 days in a patient of 80 years or older. Obviously, in a critically ill patient with little likelihood of return of oral intake, nutritional supplementation should be undertaken almost immediately.

ROUTES OF ADMINISTRATION

Two routes are possible—the enteral route, utilizing either the stomach or small intestine as an entry point, and the parenteral route. The enteral route is generally regarded as more physiologic; the liver is not bypassed and hepatic ability to take up, process, and store the various nutrients for later re-

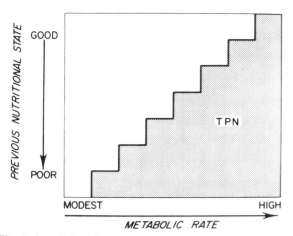

Fig 5–2.—A helpful scheme for deciding whether or not nutritional support is required in a given patient, taking into account previous nutritional state and the degree of injury presented. Under these circumstances a graded response to the need for parenteral nutrition is apparent. (From Fischer J.E.: *Curr. Probl. Surg.* 16 (No. 9):490, September 1980. Used by permission. After Winters and Dudrick.)

lease on appropriate stimuli is intact. Furthermore, there is some evidence that additional work, such as increased cardiac output, is required when the gut is bypassed. With parenteral nutrition, gut blood flow increases about 15%–20%, especially when certain amino acids are administered, presumably to allow the gut to process those nutrients which it usually metabolizes, such as transamination.

It is often claimed that enteral nutrition is safer and more efficacious than the parenteral route, but recent studies carried out in our unit have failed to confirm this view. Enteral nutrition is not more efficacious than parenteral nutrition either in experimental animals or in patients, comparing needle catheter jejunostomy and hyperalimentation.[8] However, it is a common observation in severely catabolic patients receiving TPN that plasma albumin levels will not return to normal until oral intake is resumed. Nor is it true that enteral nutrition is safer, since aspiration is an ever-present danger, and gut motility may change suddenly, for example, with sepsis. One death from aspiration is equivalent to the mortality of a well-run parenteral nutrition program of two or three years. Despite the ever-present hazard of catheter sepsis, the sepsis rate in a well-run parenteral nutrition program should not exceed 2%–4%, and there should be little mortality from the program itself.

PRINCIPLES AND PRACTICE OF ENTERAL NUTRITION

The stomach is the principal defense against an osmotic load. Following bolus administration of hyperosmotic fluid, gastric motility decreases, and gastric secretion dilutes the gastric contents until they are iso-osmotic, at which point transfer across the pylorus accelerates. The small bowel is less able to dilute osmotic loads directly presented. Furthermore, gastric acid secretion, which prevents bacterial contamination of the GI tract, may be neutralized by constant infusion into

the stomach and thus enable bacterial overgrowth in the GI tract.

The small bowel is the principal area for nutrient absorption. As suggested by Silk,[9] dipeptides are the preferred configuration for protein absorption, not, as commonly supposed, single amino acids. Under normal circumstances, with normal gut function, this is unimportant, since protein is completely absorbed in the first 120 cm of jejunum. With short or diseased bowel, there may be a decided advantage to diets in the dipeptide form. Carbohydrate is also absorbed high in the jejunum, with simple sugars preferred. Complex sugars, such as disaccharides, require enzymatic cleavage. A common difficulty with seriously ill patients is acquired lactase deficiency, which corrects itself on recovery. However, in the early post-injury recovery phase, lactose-containing products may cause diarrhea. Fat is the most difficult nutrient to absorb, dependent on proper release and mixing of bile and pancreatic enzymes. Following gastrectomy or pancreatic resection, such relationships are disturbed. Calcium, iron, and other metals tend to be absorbed in the duodenum. Consequently, duodenal bypass (as in following Billroth II gastrectomy) may result in long-term deficiencies.

In addition to its absorptive capacity, the gut serves numerous other functions. The gut may be the most important endocrine organ in the body, since at least 22 putative gut hormones (peptides) have been described, and immunohistochemical examinations have revealed an equally complex series of endocrine-like cells (the amine-precursor uptake decarboxylation, or APUD, series). The gut also performs important immunologic functions, producing large amounts of globulins.

Since hyperosmolar solutions are better tolerated by stomach than by intestine, enteral feeding is best given by the smallest possible nasogastric tube. A 10 French silastic catheter is perfectly adequate for most enteral diets, whereas an 8 French tube can be utilized for some of the more dilute diets. Infusion should be constant, with the bolus technique reserved for special situations. To prevent reflux and aspiration, patients should be kept upright at 30°, and, in general, tube feedings should be stopped at night when only skeleton nursing shifts are present. Gastric and/or intestinal motility may change rapidly with the onset of sepsis; with continued feeding, aspiration may result. From the standpoint of safety, but not physiology, it is safer to give diets into the small intestine, either by passing a tube through a gastrostomy into the duodenum, nasally into the duodenum under fluoroscopy, or by needle catheter jejunostomy, which we find very useful following operations on the esophagus, stomach, or pancreas.[10]

For gastric feeding, osmolality and then volume are gradually increased. In general, we begin with solutions diluted to iso-osmotic strength. If administration is into the small bowel, volume is increased first and then osmolality. Some patients may not tolerate small-bowel administration of greater than 500–600 milliosmols (mOsm).

An abundance of enteral products is available, varying in the quality and quantity of protein, carbohydrate, fat, vitamins, and minerals. For patients with normal gut function, a sterilized hydrolysate (a more accurate version of blenderized meal) is usually well tolerated, inexpensive, and contains all that is required. Patients so treated include those who simply cannot eat but whose GI tract is functional, such as the elderly, patients with carcinoma of the head and neck, or patients with neurologic disease. Additionally, the products have various degrees of complexity and predigestion, ranging from oligopeptides to individual amino acids. The caloric supply varies, ranging from dextrose to complex starches with or without fats. One may also utilize a series of modular diets in which the protein, fat, and carbohydrate components can be individually mixed and modified to suit the needs of specific disease states.

Much has been made of the advantages and disadvantages of elemental diets over hydrolysates. With reasonably normal gut function, there appears to be no advantage. Peptide formulas, as opposed to amino acid solutions, are less osmotically active and more palatable. Elemental diets, however, are more easily administered through needle catheter jejunostomies or 8 French catheters and still find a place (as will be subsequently discussed) in the treatment of inflammatory bowel diseases, GI fistulas, and perhaps the short-bowel syndrome.

In addition to the technical problems of administration, such as malposition or obstruction of the catheter, perforation owing to a rigid tube or introducer, and aspiration owing to changes in gastric motility or overloading, the most common complications of enteral feedings are the result of solute overload. Inappropriately rapid administration of hyperosmolar solutions will result in diarrhea, dehydration, electrolyte imbalance, or hyperglycemia (with glucose-containing solutions), as well as loss of potassium, magnesium, and other ions lost in diarrhea. Hyperosmolar, nonketotic coma can complicate both enteral feedings and parenteral nutrition. If nutritional solutions are not properly refrigerated or allowed to hang unprotected for prolonged periods, bacterial overgrowth may occur.

All of these complications can be avoided. Aspiration, as stated earlier, can be avoided by maintaining the head-upright position of 30°, the judicious advancing of enteral diets, and the checking of residual, particularly in the presence of fever. Hyperosmolarity and dehydration can be prevented by gradually increasing ingested osmolar load, using Kaopectate and opiates to prevent excessive diarrhea, and by the addition of free water to each diet.

Enteral feeding is much less expensive than parenteral nutrition, in some institutions in the United States costing as little as $6–$12/day by utilizing the cheaper hydrolysates, as compared with up to $200/day for TPN. However, enteral nutrition is often not possible in patients who are sicker and whose situation is complicated by intra-abdominal sepsis, and it is then necessary to use a parenteral approach.

THE PARENTERAL ROUTE

The two most important components of central parenteral nutrition are the route of administration and the solution infused. The basic ingredients of the TPN solution are:

1. The protein component is usually a mixture of single amino acids of synthetic origin, largely produced by "intelligent bacteria" cultures. While hydrolysates are available, they are used very little, as there is much protein wastage, since hydrolysis is incomplete (only 55% of the protein is hydro-

lyzed to amino acids). A further advantage of the synthetic amino acid solutions is the ability to tailor solutions for different disease states (such as hepatic and renal disease, and perhaps high branched-chain solutions for patients with sepsis).

2. In the United States, the caloric supply is predominantly carbohydrate, usually hypertonic dextrose. A few solutions, especially those intended for peripheral use, utilize fructose and/or glycerol.

3. Fat emulsions, used for caloric supply, consist of 10% or 20% soy or safflower oil emulsions, usually emulsified and stabilized with egg phosphatide and lecithin.

4. To the amino acid-glucose mixture, adequate amounts of electrolytes, minerals, water- and fat-soluble vitamins, and trace elements are added.

The Peripheral Route

Most urban centers in North America utilize a central venous approach, particularly for patients who will require parenteral nutrition for 2–3 weeks or longer. Many, however, prefer the peripheral route because of its relative safety and the ability to practice it without the help of a well-trained pharmacy and TPN team. In institutions in which the risk of central line complications and sepsis is significant because of the lack of a protocol as well as a nutritional support team to enforce that protocol, peripheral hyperalimentation or, as some call it, the "lipid system," may prove effective. In this system, caloric needs are largely satisfied by the use of fat emulsions combined with 3%–4% amino acids and 5% dextrose.

Most institutions utilize a "Y" tube with 10% or 20% lipid emulsion to meet the caloric requirements in patients who are not severly ill or septic. It is our experience that the lipid system uses up peripheral arm veins very quickly by causing phlebitis and sclerosis. Thus, after one or two weeks, the necessity for utilizing a central line becomes obvious. Moreover, the lipid system uses fat as the almost exclusive caloric source and is very often unable to supply the full nutritional support needed.

This technique cannot and should not be utilized in circumstances of high caloric demands, which it cannot fulfill. Furthermore, fat is expensive, and it is not yet clear that fat can be adequately utilized in severe sepsis. The advantages, on the other hand, are the avoidance of the central line and the attendant complications of placement (about 4%–6% in most institutions) and the ever-present possibility of sepsis, especially Candida sepsis.

The practice of hypocaloric peripheral parenteral nutrition is, to our mind, unacceptable, being both expensive and inappropriate. However, it is used in some institutions for short periods, until full-strength enteral nutrition can be resumed or until the patient clearly requires TPN.

Central Approach

Central hyperalimentation (total parenteral nutrition) utilizes a catheter terminating in a central vein, usually the superior vena cava, although recent data suggest that with appropriate care the inferior vena cava may be utilized as well. For short-term parenteral nutrition, polyvinyl chloride- or Teflon-coated catheters are most commonly used. Silastic catheters are less reactive and probably associated with a lower incidence of thrombosis, but are more difficult to use. Because of the easy and safe percutaneous placement of indwelling "permanent" (Broviac® or Hickman®) catheters, these are now being placed early in patients in whom the need of a central indwelling line for prolonged periods (weeks or months) is obvious. It is likely that the incidence of infection is lower with these catheters because of the barrier provided by the subcutaneous tunnel.

The infusate usually consists of 3%–5% crystalline amino acids, 20%–44% glucose, electrolytes, minerals, vitamins, and trace elements, all premixed in the pharmacy under a laminar flow hood. Recently, fat emulsions have been added into the mixture with no ill effects, although most units will administer IV lipid through a terminal accessory tube distal to the final filter. The rate of infusion is determined by the patients' nutritional requirements, glucose tolerance, renal function, liver function, and ability to excrete large volumes of fluid.

Safe and successful TPN requires an organization made up of physicians, nurses, dieticians, and pharmacists enforcing a strict protocol. In our own institution, such an organization increased the efficacy and safety of TPN and decreased the TPN-related sepsis rate from 22% to 2%–3%, the current figure.

INFLAMMATORY BOWEL DISEASES
Granulomatous Inflammatory Bowel Disease (GIBD)

Since its first description by Crohn and colleagues,[11] the spectrum of GIBD has changed from a localized lesion of the ileum to a panenteric disease reported to occur anywhere from the mouth to the anus. Clinical manifestations, pathology, and diagnosis are extensively discussed elsewhere in this book. The present discussion will be limited to the controversial role of nutritional support, mainly TPN, in the management and therapy of GIBD.

The majority of patients (65%–75%) with GIBD coming to the attention of the surgeon suffer some degree of malnutrition, the result of many factors: catabolism secondary to an ongoing active and/or chronic inflammatory process and drugs, such as steroids, which are used for its treatment; ulceration and inflammation in the involved bowel resulting in increased protein loss; diarrhea with massive losses of nutrients through malabsorption, which is further augmented by repeated bowel resection with resultant short bowel; and inadequate dietary intake. Adequate nutritional support in patients with GIBD thus seems paramount in view of this commonly occurring malnutrition.

The rationale for the use of TPN in GIBD is to: (1) replete nutritional deficits; (2) allow complete bowel rest for repair and healing of diseased bowel; (3) provide, if surgery is required, perioperative nutritional support in an attempt to minimize complication, morbidity, and mortality rates.

The objective of TPN in the primary treatment of GIBD is to place the patient on complete bowel rest while offering aggressive nutritional support to reverse nutritional depletion and enable healing of the bowel. Bowel rest presumably decreases the mechanical, hormonal, and chemical activities of the gut, enabling healing and regeneration. Studies in animals are supportive of this concept, demonstrating fewer intestinal myoelectric action potentials, decreased gastric, intestinal, and pancreatic fluid and enzyme secretion, and mucosal atrophy during bowel rest induced by TPN.[12] However, studies on humans offer conflicting results. Understandably, bowel rest must be accompanied by nutritional support; otherwise nutritional depletion, so common in inflammatory bowel disease, will progress, making any healing process impossible. Protein-calorie malnutrition not only inhibits healing of diseased bowel, wounds, and fistulas, but may also contribute to deranged immunologic competence, and increase the tendency for infection and sepsis, perhaps operative morbidity and mortality, and specific organ derangements (renal, cardiac, hepatic, and pulmonary failure), the preservation of all of which is crucial for the recovery of the depleted patient suffering a severe acute exacerbation of GIBD.

Until TPN was introduced in the late 1960s, adequate nutrition with coincident bowel rest were impossible. However, although more than a dozen years have passed, the role of TPN in the management of GIBD is still unsettled (Table 5–1). Fischer et al.[13] reported a 67% remission rate and nutritional repletion. Only four of eight patients reported by Vogel et al.[14] remained in complete clinical remission for 4–36 months of follow-up, although only one of nine patients required surgery. Dudrick et al.[15] reported clinical remission in 54% of 52 patients with inflammatory bowel disease. Greenberg et al.[16] achieved clinical remission in 77% of 43 patients with an acute inflammatory process, subacute obstruction, or extensive disease. After a two-year follow-up, 91% remained in clinical remission. Driscoll and Rosenberg,[17] after treating 16 patients in whom previous medical management had failed, reported nutritional and symptomatic improvement in all, with a 75% continued remission rate. However, only 25% remained in complete remission after 20–48 months. Forty-two percent remained in partial remission after 10–38 months, their disease controlled by medication, and 33% required surgery after 1–16 months. Fazio et al.[18] obtained a 65.2% remission rate in patients with inflammatory bowel disease (mostly Crohn's disease) in whom TPN was planned and used as primary therapy. An additional 13 patients for whom TPN was planned as an adjunct to seemingly inevitable surgery enjoyed remission and avoided surgery, bringing the overall remission rate to 77.1%. In a later publication from the same center, results seem less favorable. After a follow-up of 27 months, only four of 19 patients avoided surgery, while 14 were eventually treated surgically. The mean interval between the course of TPN and operation was ten months.[19] Dean et al.[20] treated 16 patients with TPN for inflammatory bowel disease, of whom seven avoided surgery. In a prospective study, Elson et al.[21] achieved immediate positive response to TPN in 65% of 20 patients. Of the 13 responders, five were subjected to surgery 1–6 months after the course of TPN.

In another series of 115 patients with GIBD treated by TPN for a variety of indications, remission or improvement occurred in only 41%.[22] Two of 31 patients, responding favorably, improved initially and had recurrence after 17 and 35 months, respectively. In the Mullen et al.[23] group of 50 patients with GIBD, 62% had surgery during their course of

TABLE 5–1.—RESULTS OF TPN AND BOWEL REST IN PATIENTS WITH GIBD

STUDY		NO. OF PATIENTS	DURATION OF TPN (Days)	NUTRITIONAL RESPONSE (%)	HOSPITAL REMISSION (%)	LATE REMISSION (%)
Fischer et al.	(1973)[13]				67	
Vogel et al.	(1974)[14]	14	9–50	78	100	50
Eisenberg et al.	(1974)[6]	46	5–46			
Reilly et al.	(1976)[26]	23	29–36	74	61	
Fazio et al.	(1976)[18]	67	20		77	
Greenberg et al.	(1976)[16]	43	25		77	67
Dudrick et al.	(1976)[15]	52			54	
Dean et al.	(1976)[20]	16			43	
Harford et al.	(1978)[19]					21
Mullen et al.	(1978)[23]	50	26–37		38	
Driscoll and Rosenberg	(1978)[17]	16		100	75	50
Elson et al.	(1980)[21]	20	36	100	65	25
Dickinson et al.	(1980)[27]	9	18–24		66	16
Bos and Weterman	(1980)[22]	115	41		41	
Holm	(1981)[77]	6	60–98		86	86
Shiloni and Freund	(1983)[25]	19	21–150	100	56	37.5
Muller et al.	(1983)[24]	30	84		83	43

TPN. Muller et al.,[24] in a prospective study of 30 cases of complicated GIBD hyperalimented for about 12 weeks, found a response rate of 83%. However, the recurrence rate was 60% after two years and 85% after four years.

In our own more recent group of 19 patients representing failures of medical therapy, 56.2% responded well to TPN and avoided surgery, at least temporarily. Forty-two percent had had previous bowel resection, while 84.2% had received steroids. Of our group of nine responders to TPN, two were operated on for recurrence within three and 15 months, respectively. A 13-year-old girl was operated on two years after TPN in an attempt to correct growth retardation, reducing the long-term success rate to 37.5%. The other six patients remained well, although some still require drug therapy. Of the ten patients operated on, one suffered an early acute exacerbation of his disease, necessitating resumption of steroid therapy, while two were hospitalized for incomplete bowel obstruction.[25]

Taken together, despite the lack of a prospective randomized trial, several statements can be made:

1. Bowel rest and nutritional support, in the form of TPN, can induce remission in 60%–75% of patients with inflammatory bowel disease.

2. The most favorable group are those with Crohn's disease confined to the small bowel.

3. Colonic disease has a less favorable prognosis.

4. Recurrence ranges from 50%–75%, with a mean recurrence of 10–11 months.

5. Recurrence may be decreased by maintaining patients on small doses of steroids (5–10 mg prednisone/day).

The goal of nutritional support and repletion is clearly attainable; almost all patients gain weight, feel better, and experience a rise in albumin, transferrin, and hemoglobin levels. This positive nutritional response to TPN is supported by most authors. Similarly, those patients requiring operation do exceptionally well, with a benign and brief postoperative course, although evidence that this is directly attributable to nutritional support is lacking.

Since GIBD is a chronic, recurrent disease, every effort should be made to avoid operation, reserving surgery for complications such as fistulas, perforation, or fibrous strictures. In our own series, as in many other nonrandomized studies, TPN combined with bowel rest served as an effective primary modality of treatment in 56% of 16 patients. Unfortunately, the response is unpredictable, and even more unpredictable is the longevity of remission.

In summary, despite the lack of prospective double-blind studies, one can make a strong case for TPN in the treatment of GIBD, either as primary therapy or to prepare the usually depleted GIBD patient for surgical intervention. The development of safe and effective home TPN introduces a completely new dimension to the treatment of severe GIBD (and will be subsequently discussed in that section).

ENTERAL NUTRITION.—The chemically-defined, low-residue, elemental formulas, containing amino acids or a mixture of di- and tri-peptides, require minimum digestive capacity. They are completely absorbed in the upper intestine, decrease intestinal secretion and gut flora in animals, and reduce stool frequency. In a few studies in which elemental diets were used in a fashion similar to TPN in GIBD, patients achieved nutritional rehabilitation and, in many cases, clinical remission. Unfortunately, most of these reports were retrospective, small, or even anecdotal, and applied to patient groups with a combination of various unrelated indications. In some patients, simultaneous courses of TPN were administered, making any objective evaluation impossible. It is our belief that in the medically failed, severely ill GIBD patient, when prolonged bowel rest is suggested as the last resort, this rest should be complete and be supported by TPN. Elemental diets may be utilized in the interim periods between bowel rest with TPN and return to regular diet, although in our experience a low-fat diet is equally efficacious. Some home patients will tolerate long-term intake of elemental diets, either in addition to TPN or food or as sole nutritional support, although long-term compliance is unusual. In the short-bowel syndrome elemental diets may be less well-tolerated than food because of their osmotic load, provoking rather than minimizing diarrhea.

Inflammatory bowel disease in the pediatric patient.—Gastrointestinal problems requiring nutritional support in the pediatric age group will be discussed separately, but one specific aspect of GIBD in children is worth special emphasis; namely, growth retardation. Delayed growth and sexual maturation occur in at least 20%–30% of children with GIBD. When adequate nutrition is provided by either TPN or the continuous or intermittent administration of elemental diets, most children will gain weight, achieve positive nitrogen balance, and establish linear growth. An increasing number of children are being treated with TPN to encourage stable or accelerated growth. In our opinion, growth retardation in a child with GIBD is a valid indication for hospital-based TPN, which often results in a six-month growth spurt, or even for home TPN.

Ulcerative Colitis

Even less information is available on the role of TPN in the treatment of acute ulcerative colitis. Reilly et al.[26] found remission to occur in only one of 11 patients, while favorable nutritional response occurred in only 54%. Fazio et al.[18] reported a 36% hospital remission rate and a 21% long-term remission rate. Elson et al.[21] reported good nutritional response in 90% of his ulcerative colitis patients, but only 40% immediate and 30% long-term remissions. In the prospective controlled trial of TPN in acute ulcerative colitis by Dickinson et al.,[27] 46% avoided surgery. Mullen et al.[23] showed a similar hospital remission rate of 38%. Similar remission rates are also reported in a small number of studies utilizing elemental diets. In general, ulcerative colitis is less likely than GIBD to respond to bowel rest and TPN. However, in young people and patients experiencing their first acute attacks and in whom no surgical emergency exists, a trial of bowel rest, TPN, sulfasalazine (Azulfidine®), and/or steroids should be initiated in an effort to induce remission. In patients who do not experience complete remission, the combination of bowel rest and TPN provides adequate nutritional repletion if they subsequently are to undergo major surgery. Furthermore, it enables converting an emergency operation into an elective one, which is of particular importance with the recent introduction of Soave-like pull-through procedures, which should always be performed on the quiescent and well-healed bowel.[28] In Martin and Fischer's[29] extensive experience with the Soave procedure, preoperative TPN and IV antibiotics resulted in a quiescent rectal segment, which aids the mucosal stripping. This careful preoperative preparation contributes to their excellent results.

RADIATION ENTEROPATHY

Radiation therapy, commonly used in the treatment of abdominal and especially pelvic malignancies, may result in severe damage to the GI tract. The acute form of radiation enteropathy is more common, usually self-limiting, and largely reversible. Patients suffer nausea, vomiting, abdominal cramps, and watery (sometimes bloody) diarrhea. These symptoms usually occur during or immediately following the therapeutic course of irradiation and can make it difficult or even impossible to complete the planned course of therapy. In most patients, however, symptoms of acute radiation enteropathy abate shortly after the completion of therapy with repopulation of the intestinal crypt cells. Adjuvant nutritional support, in the form of a lactose-free concentrated enteral formula, low in fat and milk protein, may carry these patients over this difficult period until adequate oral intake without severe diarrhea is possible. Some reports favor the use of gluten-free diets in acute radiation enteropathy. In severe cases complete bowel rest and TPN are necessary. Total parenteral nutrition should be accompanied by symptomatic therapy, including antispasmodic and anticholinergic drugs as well as opiates, to relieve pain, cramps, and diarrhea. Cholestyramine®, a nonabsorbable ion exchange resin which binds bile salts, and buffered acetylsalicylate to minimize the number and amount of bowel movements can be used with variable success.

The chronic or late-onset form of radiation enteropathy, estimated to occur in 0.5%–15% of patients, appears months or years after the injury. Typically, however, initial signs and symptoms occur within 6–18 months of treatment completion and is directly related to the radiation dose, various dose-rate-time parameters; volume of intestine irradiated, and predisposing factors such as hypertension, diabetes, previous chemotherapy, and intra-abdominal and pelvic adhesions that fix the bowel, resulting in an increased dose to a given segment. It appears that a radiation-induced vasculitis with major damage to endothelial and connective tissue accounts for most pathologic and clinical manifestations. These include fibrosis with complete or partial bowel obstruction, devitalized intestine with perforation, hemorrhage, and abscess or fistula formation. Colicky abdominal pain is the most common symptom and may be associated with bloody diarrhea, tenesmus, steatorrhea, and weight loss. Steatorrhea is usually not severe, although bacterial overgrowth owing to stricture formation and partial obstruction may aggravate malabsorption. Progressive intestinal obstruction is very common in late-onset radiation enteropathy, while acute perforations and enteroenteral or enterocutaneous fistulas are less frequent. The rectum, colon, and small bowel are involved in order of decreased frequency, and multiple areas are frequently involved. Small-bowel injuries account for 30%–50% of all severe late radiation injuries of the bowel; small-bowel obstruction is the most common. However, these chronic small-bowel obstructions are very commonly associated with severe injuries to other parts of the small or large bowel or to the urinary system.

Medical management of mild to moderate malabsorption includes the use of antispasmodic and anticholinergic drugs; low residue, gluten-free diets; cholestyramine; and even steroids. However, severe late radiation enteropathy is usually refractory to medical management, and, if untreated by nutritional support, patients can deteriorate to extreme malnutrition and debility. Some patients are mistakenly believed to have recurrent cancer and relegated to institutions for the terminally ill, when all they require for complete rehabilitation is treatment for severe radiation enteropathy and nutritional support. Once it can be established that recurrent cancer is not present (the CT scanner has made this easier), an aggressive approach to this relatively small but very sick group of patients is warranted. Prolonged periods of TPN, including home hyperalimentation, combined with resection and/or bypass of involved bowel will salvage most of these patients who otherwise, cured of their malignant disease, would be permanently incapacitated by the sequelae of antineoplastic therapy.

Once recognized, these patients are admitted to the hospital for total parenteral nutrition. Being severely depleted, they usually require prolonged periods of TPN with adequate amounts of protein and calories (i.e., 250 mg N/kg/day and 30–35 cal/kg). One should carefully increase the protein and calories administered, as severe liver function derangements during TPN are more common in very depleted patients, particularly when repletion occurs too quickly. TPN and complete bowel rest, in addition to nutritional repletion, also relieve abdominal complaints. It may take as long as 3–6 weeks to achieve complete repletion in such a patient and to prepare him for surgery or sometimes only 10–14 days. Meanwhile, the patient is extensively investigated to gain maximum preoperative information. At surgery, stenosed or very inflamed areas of affected bowel are resected or bypassed, establishing continuity of the GI tract and eliminating the major disease sites. Surgery should be as conservative as possible, as the process may be progressive and is diffuse, impairing the healing properties of the bowel. However, obstruction-free continuity may be restored. This exploration also firmly establishes the absence of residual or recurrent tumor. A gastrostomy should be placed. Following surgery, TPN is continued for at least 10–14 days while food is withheld. Only when healing of all anastomoses is certain should food be slowly introduced while TPN is continued. Patients often do not tolerate clear liquids to start; thus, starting on a soft diet is preferable. Codeine, calcium, and Kaopectate may help reduce the amount and number of bowel movements. When the patient is able safely to take in 1,500–2,000 calories and 60 gm of protein by mouth, TPN is discontinued. While elemental or chemically defined diets are sometimes useful, in patients with short-bowel syndrome they usually provoke more diarrhea than does food.

Most patients will be able to resume a near-normal lifestyle given an adequate investment in the form of combined aggressive nutritional support and surgery. However, some patients will never be able to use their gut adequately, particularly those with diffuse, multiple small-bowel strictures and chronic intestinal obstruction. For those patients, home TPN is essential (discussed subsequently under Home TPN). Permanent home TPN should be reserved for and applied only as a last resort to patients with *no evidence* of residual or recurrent tumor.

GASTROINTESTINAL-CUTANEOUS FISTULAS

Most fistulas are iatrogenic and follow operations for neoplastic disease, intestinal obstruction, inflammatory bowel disease, or trauma. Nonoperative fistulas usually complicate inflammatory bowel diseases, irradiation, and/or malignancy.

Fistula management has evolved significantly over the past 20 years. In their classic paper in 1960, Edmunds et al.[30] called attention to the serious nature and high mortality of such fistulas, owing to the relationship they described among infection, malnutrition, fistula output, and mortality. They advocated earlier surgical intervention in all high-output fistulas, recommending total resection of the fistula with end-to-end anastomosis or complete bypass of the fistula when resection was impossible. With early restoration of bowel continuity, malnutrition and its attendant complications were less likely to develop. The overall mortality in their series was 44%. Many similar reports demonstrate the gravity of this condition, with overall mortalities ranging from 20%–62%.

In 1964 Chapman et al.[31] emphasized that one key to successful management was to maintain adequate nutritional support from the very beginning. They stressed the vital role of nutrition and reported an increased fistula closure rate and a decreased mortality rate (14%) in those patients treated with an excess of 1,600 calories/day using a combination of peripherally administered protein hydrolysates and tube feedings. They also emphasized that supportive and surgical treatment go hand in hand; the two are not mutually exclusive. Their indications for operative closure of the fistula included the presence of distal intestinal obstruction, continued massive loss of fluid from the fistula despite control of infection and an adequate nutritional regimen, and persistence of the fistula even without high losses over a prolonged period. In a follow-up report in 1971, Sheldon and co-workers[32] documented the success of this treatment regimen, noting that most patients could be offered adequate nutrition by standard methods such as tube and enterostomy feedings. At the time of this latter report, TPN was a new technique just gaining acceptance.

With the widespread use of parenteral nutrition in the 1970s, many reports initially proclaimed TPN as a revolutionary modality in the treatment of gastrointestinal fistulas (GIF) with markedly decreased mortality (Table 5–2). However, the real impact of TPN on spontaneous fistula closure, timing and indications for surgery, and the change in mortality rate have not been totally established. When trying to evaluate the beneficial effects and efficacy of TPN in the treatment of GIF, four aspects should be discussed: (1) spontaneous fistula closure rate; (2) efficacy of nutritional support; (3) preparation for corrective surgery; and (4) mortality. The early reports of TPN treatment of GIF claimed a high rate of spontaneous fistula closure and a significantly lower mortality, in the range of 5%–20%.

However, two large longitudinal studies of 186 patients[33] and 404 patients,[34] covering 10 and 30 years' experience, respectively, in two large institutions placed TPN in the treatment of gastrointestinal-cutaneous fistulas in its proper perspective. They emphasized that its impact must be separated from other advances in the management of the surgical patient, such as fluid and electrolyte therapy, improved respiratory therapy, acid-base balance, antibiotics, monitoring, and intensive care. In their study of 186 patients treated over a ten-year period, Reber et al.[33] divided the group in 1971. They found that in the pre-TPN era, 35% of patients with gastrointestinal fistulas were treated nonoperatively and 65% operatively, compared to 49% and 51%, respectively, in the TPN era. Despite these differences, the results were similar,

TABLE 5–2.—RESULTS OF TPN AND PRE-TPN STUDIES IN PATIENTS WITH
GASTROINTESTINAL FISTULAS

STUDY	NO. OF PATIENTS	SPONTANEOUS CLOSURE, (%)	SURGICAL CLOSURE, (%)	TOTAL CLOSURE, (%)	MORTALITY, EXCLUDING CANCER, (%)
Edmunds et al. (1960)[30]	157				44
Chapman et al. (1964)[31]	56		>1,000–2,000 cal:89		16.6
			<1,000 cal/day: 37		57.8
Sheldon et al. (1971)[32]	51				12
Roback and Nicoloff (1972)[78]	55				30
MacFadyen et al. (1972)[79]	62	70.5	21.8		6.5
Aguirre et al. (1974)[80]	38	28	50		21
Himal et al. (1974)[81]	25	56	36	92	8
Freund et al. (1976)[82]	18	60	13	73	27
Deitel (1976)[83]	86	81	8	89	1965–69 40
					1969–75 9.3
Graham (1977)[84]	39	89.7	2.5		7.7
Reber et al. (1978)[85]	186	31.7	47.3	79	11.0
Thomas and Rosalion (1978)[86]	73				
No TPN	38			35	60
With TPN	35			65	23
Blackett and Hill (1978)[87]	25	60	12	72	12
Coutsoftides and Fazio (1979)[88]	174	9	61.5		22.4
Soeters et al. (1979)[34]	404				
1946–59	157				44
1960–70	119	10	68	78.2	15.1
1970–75	128	31	51.5	79	21.1
Silberman et al. (1980)[89]	35			51	29
Thomas (1981)[90]	40			71	26
Sitges-Serra et al. (1982)[91]	75	71.2	13.8	85	21.3
Zera et al. (1983)[92]	50	22.0	52	72	22
Allardyce (1983)[93]	52	36.5	30.7	67.2	23

with nonoperative treatment being successful in 71%–76%, operative treatment successful in 83%–84%, and a mortality rate of 10%–13%. Of the 43 patients whose fistulas closed without surgery, 91% did so within one month after sepsis was controlled, sepsis being the major determinant of fistula nonclosure. When sepsis was controlled within one month, spontaneous closure rate was 48% compared with only 6% when sepsis was never adequately brought under control, with an 85% mortality rate (Table 5–3).

The shift in the cause of mortality from electrolyte imbalance and malnutrition to sepsis was even more obvious in the Massachusetts General Hospital collective series of 404 patients over 30 years.[34] In the first study period (1946–59), 157 patients were treated. The most significant complications were fluid and electrolyte imbalance, malnutrition and sepsis, resulting in an overall mortality rate of 43.3%. During 1960–70, 119 patients were treated; 68% were successfully closed surgically and 10% closed spontaneously. Again, the major

TABLE 5–3.—SURVIVAL AND CLOSURE RATES OF GASTROINTESTINAL FISTULAS

STUDY (No. of Patients)	SURVIVAL, %	CLOSURE RATE, % Total	CLOSURE RATE, % Spontaneous
Reber et al. (186)[85]			
1968–71	78	79	26
1972–77	78	78	35
Soeters et al. (404)[34]			
1946–59	56	—	—
1960–70	84.1	78.2	10
1970–75	78.9	62.2	31

determinants of mortality were electrolyte imbalance, malnutrition, and sepsis, resulting in a mortality rate of only 15.1% (see Table 5–2). Sepsis in this group correlated well with malnutrition and mortality, and was inversely related to fistula closure rate. In the third period of this study (1970–75), 128 patients with fistulas were treated, 73 with TPN. A large number of patients had controlled or uncontrolled infection, leading to a mortality rate of 19%. Closure of fistula was successfully achieved operatively in 68% and spontaneously in 32%.

Comparing these three periods, it becomes obvious that mortality and closure rates improved dramatically during the last two periods (see Table 5–2). However, the decrease in mortality had already been achieved in the pre-TPN era, leading to the conclusion that the improvement in management and results of treating GIF cannot be attributed solely or perhaps at all to the introduction and widespread use of TPN, but rather to improved care. Whereas in the first period electrolyte imbalance contributed heavily to mortality, uncontrolled infection and sepsis were the main causes of death in the two later periods. Uncontrolled sepsis was the one major determinant of mortality in the 1970–75 period, TPN being unable to alleviate this problem. TPN alleviated malnutrition in the third period, reducing it from 87% to 51%, the residual malnutrition in this group secondary only to uncontrolled sepsis. When sepsis is controlled or no sepsis is present, TPN will result in improved nutritional status, healing of wounds, and eventually, in some cases, closure of fistulas. If spontaneous closure does not occur, surgery in a well-nourished patient will likely result in a low-mortality operative closure of fistulas.

A systematic approach combining diagnostic, supportive, and operative procedures is essential in the management of fistulas (Table 5–4). The first step is stabilization: the bowel is put to rest by stopping oral intake and placing decompressive tubes (e.g., nasogastric and long GI tubes). Recognition and restoration of fluid, electrolyte, and acid-base balance must be achieved. Blood volume must be restored with crystalloid, colloid, and blood transfusions. Any obvious abscess collections associated with the fistula must be promptly drained. Total parenteral nutrition should be instituted as early as possible and carried to the maximum, taking into consideration the patient's nutritional needs, resting energy expenditure, activity of disease, GI losses, and presence of infection. Care of the skin surrounding the fistula is instituted by sump drainage of the fistula and the application of various protective substances. Antibiotics should be reserved for specific instances when sepsis cannot be controlled by other means and then, if possible, only after adequate cultures and sensitivity studies have been obtained. Some authors advocate the use of cimetidine, somatostatin, or aprotinin (Trasylol®) to reduce the GI losses, while others recycle fistula fluid losses back into the GI tract. A high percentage of patients have sepsis at the time they develop the fistula or when transferred from another hospital. Early surgical drainage of intra-abdominal abscess(es) is a very critical part of management, and a continuous, unrelenting search for new abscesses is necessary during the entire treatment period.

Once blood volume has been restored, abscesses drained, parenteral nutrition begun, sump drainage instituted, skin protected, and, if necessary, proper antibiotics selected, fairly rapid improvement should occur. The next step in management is the investigation and definition of the fistula. A collaborative effort should be made involving the responsible surgeon and radiologist. Contrast medium administered through the fistula is most efficient in delineation of anatomy, including intrinsic bowel disease, location and number of fistulas, the length and course of fistula tract, associated abscess cavities, and the presence of distal obstruction. Full-scale contrast investigations of the GI tract, such as barium enema or upper GI series with small-bowel follow-through, are sometimes necessary, but not in most patients in our experience. Chest films, excretory urograms, ultrasonography, and CT scans may be indicated in certain patients.

With the patient stabilized and ambulating and the nature and anatomy of the fistula thoroughly delineated, it is possible adequately to nourish the patient and to allow a trial of bowel rest and TPN. As long as the patient is improving metabolically, it is reasonable to pursue conservative therapy with the aid of adequate nutrition in the hope that the fistula will close. With control of sepsis and restoration of nutrition, about 50% of external cutaneous fistulas will close spontaneously over a period of 3–6 weeks, particularly postoperative fistulas. Even if spontaneous closure does not occur, a period of 3–6 weeks is often invaluable in improving the patient's condition prior to operation, allowing subsidence of intraperitoneal inflammation and restoration of a positive nitrogen balance, lean body mass, immunologic competence, and healing capacity. Fistulas associated with Crohn's disease, irradiated bowel, cancer, foreign body, the presence of a large abscess cavity, distal obstruction, extensive disruption of GI continuity, and a short fistula tract with a mature fistula (i.e., an enterostomy) are unlikely to heal spontaneously and are usually indications for corrective surgery once the sepsis, metabolism, and nutritional status are improved.

In general, TPN is of value in enabling simple, effective, and safe nutritional support and management. This allows the surgeon to delay operative intervention while sustaining the patient and hoping for spontaneous closure of fistulas, which will be the case in about 50% of patients whose radiologic criteria indicate that closure is possible within 3–6 weeks of TPN. If the fistula does not close spontaneously, the patient is nutritionally and metabolically prepared more safely to undergo definitive surgical resection.

It has been consistently demonstrated that the best operation is excision of the segment of bowel from which the fistula arises and end-to-end anastomosis, although total bypass of the fistula may be useful in situations where excision is judged to be too hazardous, such as for lateral duodenal fistulas (Fig 5–3). Direct suture closure of the fistula without resection is usually followed by breakdown. Several reports have advocated Roux-en-Y bypass or serosal patching of fistulas in specific difficult cases; we have had little experience with such approaches, but it seems that if the fistula can be sufficiently mobilized for Roux-en-Y, it should be resected.

Nutritional management and continued support as outlined in the stabilization phase must be maintained during the final stage, until the fistula is solidly healed. Only then should parenteral nutrition be tapered, after oral intake of 1,500 calories has been achieved.

ELEMENTAL DIETS.—Two basic forms of chemically defined diets are commercially available for nutritional support. Initially it was assumed that diets containing crystalline amino acids were better because they were more readily absorbed.

TABLE 5–4.—PHASES IN THE MANAGEMENT OF A GASTROINTESTINAL-CUTANEOUS FISTULA

Stabilization
  Restoration of fluid, electrolyte, and acid-base balance
  Drain obvious abscesses
  Total parenteral nutrition
  Skin care surrounding fistula(s)
  Antibiotics only if indicated
Investigation
  Fistulogram
  BaE and/or UGIS-SBFT* (only if indicated)
  Excretory urograms
  Ultrasonography
  Computerized tomography
Decision
  Is operation indicated?
    Nature and behavior of drainage
    Nature of fistula
      Radiographic criteria
      Cancer
      Radiation
      Inflammatory bowel disease
    Nature of abdominal wall
Definitive therapy
  Spontaneous closure
  Operative correction
    Resection and end-to-end anastomosis vs. other choices
Healing phase
  *BaE, barium enema; UGIS-SBFT, upper gastrointestinal series with small bowel follow-through.

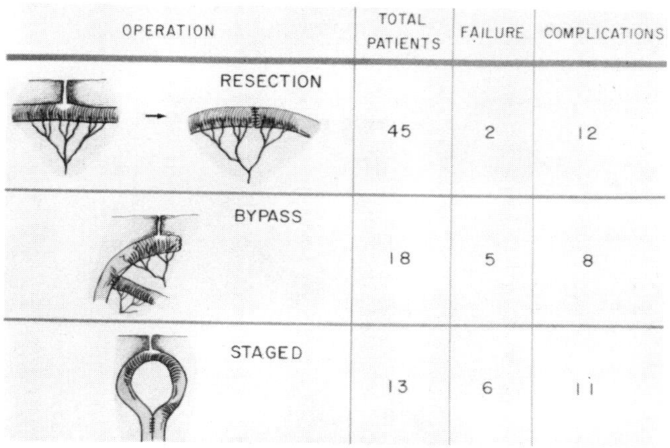

OPERATION		TOTAL PATIENTS	FAILURE	COMPLICATIONS
	RESECTION	45	2	12
	BYPASS	18	5	8
	STAGED	13	6	11

Fig 5–3.—Complication and failure rate of surgery for gastrointestinal fistulas. Note the high complication rate and failure of bypass or staged surgical procedure as opposed to resection and primary anastomoses.

However, increasing evidence indicates that diets based on dipeptides are more readily absorbed, although not necessarily more effective. Experimental animal and clinical data point toward a reduction in gastric, pancreatic, and GI secretion during use of elemental diets.[35] Furthermore, myoelectric studies have indicated that chemically defined diets provide relative mechanical rest to the gut. However, both gut secretion and mechanical activity are significantly more inhibited by TPN.

A few studies, usually with small numbers of patients, show drainage with elemental diet feeding and spontaneous closure in approximately 50% of patients with fistulas.[36] Although experimentally and clinically not as effective as TPN, the use of elemental or chemically defined diets is appealing due to low cost compared with TPN. It is our practice to use elemental diets in the treatment of GIF in only selected cases, principally in low-output distal or colonic fistulas or in proximal GIF, when elemental diets can be introduced by a variety of means into the gut distal to the fistula (esophagus, esophagogastric, anastomotic, gastric, and pancreaticobiliary fistulas).

THE SHORT-BOWEL SYNDROME

Absorption of nutrients from the gut is dependent on the number of villi and the number of cells per villus as well as the degree of cell maturity. Patients who have undergone massive small-bowel resection as a result of mesenteric vascular insufficiency, volvulus, or internal hernia, and patients who have had repeated small-bowel resections as a result of obstruction, fistulas, or inflammatory bowel disease may be left with an insufficient absorptive surface to maintain normal nutrition. Dietary protein, carbohydrate, and fat are lost in the stool, as are fat-soluble vitamins, some of the water-soluble vitamins, folate, B_{12}, bile salts, and iron. Unabsorbed food may result in secretory diarrhea with further loss of nutrients as well as fluid and electrolyte imbalance.

Nutritional support of the patient with short-bowel syndrome should initially be by the parenteral route. Rapid adaptation begins soon after resection, provided there is ade-

quate nutritional support to sustain it. Exposure of the bowel lumen to nutrients appears to have a stimulatory effect on adaptation. Therefore, enteral nutrition must be administered gradually and concomitant with parenteral nutrition. The ideal diet is rapidly absorbed with a minimum of small bowel and provides maximal trophic stimulation to increase small-bowel hypertrophy and hyperplasia. We know little about which nutrients are most effective in providing stimulation for regrowth.

The degree of malabsorption and fluid and electrolyte loss will vary with the underlying disease process, length and location of bowel resected, the presence of an ileocecal valve, and the residual length of colon. Since the degree of malabsorption is variable, and since no consensus has been achieved in regard to the best diet for the short-bowel syndrome, dietary therapy often proceeds with a systematic trial-and-error approach.

In general, patients with a moderate amount of small bowel (more than 60–80 cm) will ultimately tolerate a regular diet without developing nutritional deficiencies. For patients with some small bowel left, but less than about 80 cm, a slow and progressive feeding schedule should be carried out while simultaneously maintaining adequate nutritional state with TPN. Despite the traditional view that low-fat diets are preferable, recent studies found no differences between high-fat and high-carbohydrate diets in patients with 50% bowel resections. Other studies even claimed that high-fat diets were more efficient. In patients who require specialized diets, peptide or whole-protein formulas are generally tolerated better than elemental ones. Absorption of protein occurs for the most part as dipeptides, with hydrolysis to amino acids occurring intracellularly or, at the very least, at the brush borders. Continuous or intermittently continuous infusions of nutrients are tolerated better than bolus feeding.

Although oral diets of varying composition are necessary for stimulation of gut adaptation, parenteral nutrition may be necessary for months to years before adequate absorptive surface is present for maintenance of nutritional integrity. Such an approach is possible outside the hospital setting through the technique of home parenteral nutrition.

HOME PARENTERAL NUTRITION

Even more recent than the widespread use of parenteral nutrition in the clinical setting is the use of parenteral nutrition in ambulatory patients living independently away from the hospital. The concept of an "artificial gut" appeared in the literature as early as 1970. Infusion of nutrient solutions containing hypertonic dextrose required angioaccess with high flow rates to dilute rapidly the hyperosmolar infusate. Arteriovenous shunts and fistulas, similar to those used for renal dialysis, were employed initially, although the high incidence of thrombosis prompted the search for alternative routes of access. Long, silicone rubber right atrial catheters tunneled beneath the skin have been available since 1973. Evolution of catheters and of electronic infusion devices has enabled infusion schedules to be carried out safely and intermittently overnight while the patient sleeps, and permit rehabilitation of many patients with debilitating GI disease from a variety of causes.

Selection of patients for home parenteral nutrition (HPN) is dependent on disease state, physical factors, psychosocial factors, and prognosis. Pathologic conditions which may be treated by HPN include short-bowel syndrome resulting from mesenteric vascular thrombosis, volvulus, internal hernia, or multiple resections; Crohn's disease; intestinal insufficiency; GI motor disturbances; certain low-output fistulas; and malignancy (Table 5–5). The last indication is controversial. In general, patients with malignancy are candidates for HPN as supportive therapy only while chemotherapy or radiation therapy render them unable to eat, or for nutritional support in patients who are free of tumor but who have inadequate absorption as a result of antineoplastic therapy, but never, in our opinion, for terminal support in the cancer patient.

Patients must have adequate intelligence to learn procedures involving sterile technique, catheter care, and basic problem solving. Manual dexterity and vision must be sufficient to manipulate the catheter connections safely. Despite willingness of family members to assist the patient, therapy is most successful when patients are trained to be self-reliant and independent. Commitment to the success of HPN is critical. In this regard, patients who have been chronically debilitated by GI disease and become rehabilitated may fare better than those who have been previously healthy and later suffer an intra-abdominal catastrophe.

Placement of the central venous catheter and training in techniques of HPN take place in the hospital, usually during the convalescent phase of the primary illness. The Broviac® and Hickman® right atrial catheters perform well for HPN and are easily inserted in most adults. Catheter insertion may be performed via internal jugular, common facial, cephalic, axillary veins or their branches, or the saphenous vein. Sites of access should be carefully planned, since therapy may be complicated by thrombosis, and many patients will require catheters for years.

Catheters may be introduced percutaneously under fluoroscopic guidance or by cutdown. Our preference is for cutdown in the axilla with catheter insertion via a pectoral branch of the axillary vein (Fig 5–4). Such an approach allows catheter introduction without ligation of major veins and minimizes endothelial injury to major veins. Additional advantages include the ability to introduce subsequent catheters into neighboring veins using the same wound and a cosmetically acceptable scar.

The catheter exit site is marked preoperatively on the up-

TABLE 5–5.—INDICATIONS FOR HOME PARENTERAL NUTRITION

Short-bowel syndrome
   Mesenteric vascular event
   Multiple or extensive bowel resections (malrotation and volvulus, internal hernia, Crohn's disease)
Gastrointestinal motor disturbances
   Chronic pseudo-obstruction
   Scleroderma
Radiation enteritis
Crohn's disease
Mesenteric insufficiency
Recurrent multiple intra-abdominal adhesions
Malignancy (rarely and must be concomitant with antineoplastic therapy)

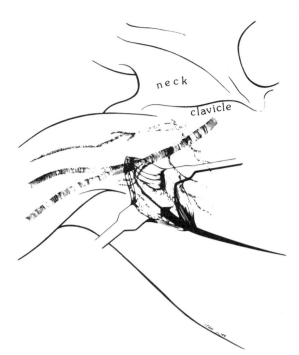

Fig 5–4.—Approach for insertion of Hickman catheter into pectoral branch of right axillary vein.

per abdomen after the patient has worn a sample catheter dressing to determine optimal placement (Fig 5–5). Abdominal placement allows convenient catheter care and manipulation under direct vision by the patient.

Education of the patient begins with the first infusion. Procedures are written in detail for each patient. An initial period of observation is followed by the patient's performing procedures under supervision of the nurses of the nutritional support service. Time required to instruct patients is generally 30–40 hours, following which procedures are performed independently.

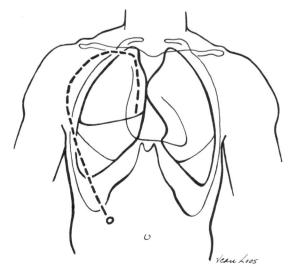

Fig 5–5.—Hickman catheter in place, with tip in right atrium and exit site over right upper quadrant of the abdomen.

Infusate consists of a 4.25% amino acid/23% dextrose solution, with appropriate electrolytes, multivitamins, and trace elements mixed in a single container. In patients who ingest a portion of their nutrients orally, essential fatty acid deficiency occurs infrequently. Patients who have inadequate oral intake and/or absorption of fat receive IV lipid emulsion 2–3 times weekly as a source of essential fatty acids. A typical 2,000-kcal infusion of 2,000 ml would be administered over 12 hours nocturnally. Following infusion, the catheter is flushed with heparinized saline solution and capped, enabling the patient to engage in an active and productive life during the day. An occlusive dressing is maintained at the catheter insertion site at all times. Strict sterile technique, including mask, is employed for all procedures. Solutions are delivered premixed to patients at least weekly.

Technical, septic, and metabolic complications are essentially those of inpatient parenteral nutrition. Migration of the catheter tip may cause thrombosis of great veins by the hypertonic solution; the catheter is placed again. Clotting of the catheter can be managed in most instances with thrombolytic agents. Broken external segments of catheters can be repaired with a kit supplied by the manufacturer. Patients maintain a diary of temperature, urine sugar, amount of infusion, daily weight, oral intake, and untoward reactions.

Initially monitoring is done weekly. Visits are lengthened to once every two months after patients become stable. In addition to monitoring blood chemistries, patient care techniques are reviewed and reinforced.

In selected patients with good prognosis, HPN provides excellent rehabilitation and return to a nearly normal life-style despite major GI dysfunction.

GASTROINTESTINAL MALIGNANCY

Nutritional impairment may develop in patients with cancer as a result of the systemic effects of cancer, the local effects of the tumor, and secondary to therapy. Among the systemic effects are anorexia, most common in patients with GI tumors but present even in patients with a miniscule tumor burden, changes in taste, an unexplained catabolic drive, increased energy requirements, and many other conditions. Local effects are most commonly caused by mechanical encroachment or obstruction. Of particular importance and significance are nutritional problems arising as a result of the treatment of cancer by surgery, irradiation, or chemotherapy. Thus, most patients with cancer will lose weight during the course of their disease, forming a large pool of candidates for nutritional support at some stage of their disease and treatment. Unfortunately, the present role of nutritional support in the cancer patient is not yet well defined and the controversy as to its efficacy ongoing.

Two basic questions must be answered concerning nutritional support in cancer patients:

1. Can feeding benefit the host without stimulating tumor growth?

2. Does nutritional support improve the outcome of cancer therapy?

The working hypothesis is that nutritional support during cancer therapy may improve host nutritional status, resulting in improved immunologic status and resistance to both tumor and infection, and thus permitting complication-free therapy, including uneventful surgical procedures, irradiation and chemotherapy.

The use of nutritional support in the cancer patient undergoing surgery is similar to its use in the depleted general surgical patient, presumably resulting in correction of protein-calorie malnutrition, which in turn will induce weight gain, nitrogen balance, increased total body protein turnover, restoration of visceral proteins, and a decreased operative and postoperative morbidity rate. Results of several studies support the working hypothesis. A comparison of patients with cancer of the larnyx undergoing surgery and irradiation showed more complications occurring in control than in parenterally nourished patients.[37] Patients with esophageal cancer receiving TPN of other forms of nutritional support exhibited better maintenance of body weight and nitrogen balance and far fewer postoperative complications.[38] Preoperative TPN in gastric cancer patients resulted in significantly less weight loss, reduced infection rate, and reduced mortality compared to matched nutritionally unsupported patients.[39] In patients with GI cancer, both weight loss and wound healing improved as a result of nutritional support, as did complications of cancer surgery, which are often successfully treated by TPN.[40] However, in numerous other studies, little difference has been found in complication rates, improved survivals, and increased duration of remission following TPN in cancer patients (Table 5–6); some have questioned the efficacy of this treatment modality.[41]

Additional studies have addressed the issue of whether survival following chemotherapy and/or radiotherapy is improved with adjuvant parenteral nutrition in cancer patients. Despite early suggestive data, not a single current study has supported the concept that cancer patients undergoing chemotherapy and/or radiotherapy demonstrate improved survival following parenteral nutrition. In many studies of different patient groups and treatment modalities, there has been little, if any, difference in outcome with respect to complications, improved survival, or prolonged duration of remission following TPN of cancer patients. In two recent studies in patients with disseminated colon cancer[42] and in patients with a mixed group of sarcomas,[43] a trend toward an increased number of early deaths or a decreased duration of remission was reported in the TPN groups (see Table 5–6). Although not statistically significant, this raises the question of increased tumor growth during nutritional support. While previous experimental studies have suggested such a possibility,[44] most animal studies concluded that the rate of tumor growth is at best the same as the host's carcass, although close examination of the data reveals this as borderline.[45] However, one recent study in untreated tumor-bearing rats demonstrated that with the administration of excessively high caloric and protein intake, tumor growth was enhanced out of proportion to the growth of the host carcass.[46] On the other hand, animal studies in which nutritional support was combined with chemotherapy were more equivocal, the authors claiming improved host nutritional status and maximal tumor inhibition.[47]

At present, TPN as a treatment modality in cancer presumably allows antineoplastic therapy to be administered to malnourished patients who otherwise might not have been ac-

TABLE 5–6.—STUDIES OF THE EFFECTS OF TP NUTRITION ON PATIENTS WITH CANCER UNDERGOING SURGERY, IRRADIATION, OR CHEMOTHERAPY

STUDY	NO. OF PATIENTS	TYPE OF TUMOR	TYPE OF THERAPY	NUTRITIONAL EFFECTS PN	NUTRITIONAL EFFECTS CONTROL	RESPONSE TO THERAPY, % PN	RESPONSE TO THERAPY, % CONTROL	COMPLICATIONS OF THERAPY, % PN	COMPLICATIONS OF THERAPY, % CONTROL	SURVIVAL, % PN	SURVIVAL, % CONTROL	COMMENTS
Holter and Fischer (1977)[40]	56	GI cancer	Surgery	Decreased weight loss and increased albumin level with PN*			Same	13	19	93.4	92.4	Lower major complication rate with PN
Moghissi et al. (1977)[94]	15	Esophageal cancer	Surgery	Better N balance with PN			Same	0	20	NA*	NA	Lower rate of wound infection with PN
Issell et al. (1978)[95]	26	Squamous cell lung cancer	Chemotherapy	Improved weight gain and arm circumference with PN		31	7	15	77	NA	NA	Less myelosuppression, less toxic effect of chemotherapy with PN
Heatley et al. (1979)[96]	74	Esophageal/gastric cancer	Surgery	Same			Same	35	83	15	22	Significant reduction in postoperative wound infection
Simms et al. (1980)[97]	30	Esophageal/gastric cancer	Surgery	Improved N balance and albumin level with PN			Same	NA	NA	10	10	
Lanzotti et al. (1980)[98]	56	Non-oat cell lung cancer	Chemotherapy	NA	NA	10	23	NA	NA	MEDIAN 11 wk	MEDIAN 12 wk	
Sako et al. (1981)[37]	69	Head and neck cancer	Surgery	Weight gain and better N balance with PN			Same	50	56	NA	NA	Significantly better long-term survival curve for PN
Valdivieso et al. (1981)[99]	49	Small cell bronchogenic cancer	Chemotherapy	Weight gain with PN		85	59	NA	NA	Survival advantage for PN		PN did not ameliorate hematologic, GI, or infectious morbidity
Thompson et al. (1981)[100]	41	GI cancer	Surgery	Improved weight gain with PN			Same	17	11	100	100	
Popp et al. (1981)[101]	36 42	Diffuse lymphoma	Chemotherapy	Marked weight gain with PN; lean body mass, anthropometry albumin, transferrin, and total lymphocytes similar for both groups				11% Subclavian vein thrombosis		69	66	No difference in drug tolerance or total drug dose between control and TPN
Nixon et al. (1981)[42]	45	Metastatic colon cancer	Chemotherapy	Weight gain with PN; no other differences		15	12			79 Days	308 Days	
Serrou et al. (1981)[102]	19	Anaplastic lung cancer	Chemotherapy	Same		83	80	Same		84	80	
Samuels et al. (1981)[103]	30	Metastatic testicular cancer	Chemotherapy	Less weight loss with PN		63	79	Increased incidence of noncatheter infections with PN		75	79	
Lim et al. (1981)[38]	24	Esophageal cancer	Surgery	Better weight gain and N balance with PN				6 Complications	12 Complications	90	80	Preoperative TPN and gastrostomy feeding compared
Muller et al. (1982)[39]	125	GI cancer	Surgery	Improved weight gain, visceral proteins and immunologic status with PN				17	32	96	81	
Shamberger et al. (1983)[104]	27	Sarcomas	Chemotherapy					42	33			Similar granulocyte and platelet recovery following chemotherapy-induced myelosuppression
Shamberger et al. (1984)[43]	32	Sarcomas	Chemotherapy	Improved N balance with PN, but similar visceral proteins		71	86			Long-term survival rate similar		Shorter remissions for PN

*PN = Parenteral nutrition; NA = information not available.

ceptable candidates for intensive oncologic therapy because of the increased risk. Furthermore, malnourished patients who are successfully repleted nutritionally may show a better response to therapy than those patients who are and stay malnourished. However, this does not mean that TPN can affect or alter the course of a rapidly progressing malignancy or improve the response to a poor or inadequate oncological treatment modality. Because the danger of early or vigorous recurrences of a malignant process as a result of excessive nutritional supplementation is very real, it is our practice to limit nutritional support to those patients who are feeble as a result of cancer cachexia and may have difficulty withstanding a major surgical procedure or aggressive oncological treatment.[41] Even then, nutritional support should be limited in duration and should not exceed basic energy expenditure and nitrogen requirements. Indiscriminate feeding of all cancer patients, except those at risk of increased morbidity or even mortality because of profound wasting, should be abandoned until more well-controlled trials with many more patients are available.

PANCREATITIS

Pancreatitis is a disease of varying presentation and severity. In its more severe forms, it may cause profound physiologic derangements of the cardiovascular, pulmonary, renal, and GI systems. Dysfunction of the GI tract may manifest itself as exocrine pancreatic insufficiency with malabsorption, paralytic ileus, or both. When alcoholism is the cause of pancreatitis, chronic malnutrition is often present. Nutritional reserves are taxed still further if acute operative intervention becomes necessary or there are late complications. Thus, nutritional support is critical in this group of malnourished, hypercatabolic patients who are subject to repeated stresses and prolonged GI dysfunction with little nutritional reserve.

Historically, the overall mortality from acute pancreatitis has been reported to be 20%–48%. In assessing the impact of nutritional support in the treatment of patients with acute pancreatitis, one must take into account the advances in critical care, including ventilatory and hemodynamic monitoring and support, which have attended the same period.

The goals of traditional management include metabolic support of the patient and bowel rest. Nasogastric suction and pharmacologic agents have been used to decrease gastric acid, thereby decreasing its stimulation of pancreatic secretion. Parenteral nutrition is employed as part of the metabolic support of the patient, although the effect of parenteral nutrition on the rate of complications and outcome remains unclear.

Goodgame and Fischer[48] reported a series of patients with acute pancreatitis who were treated with amino acid-hypertonic dextrose parenteral nutrition. Overall mortality in this group was 20%. Parenteral nutrition seemed to have little effect on early mortality. The supportive value of parenteral nutrition was demonstrated by equivalent survival between the group of patients whose disease resolved in fewer than 30 days and the group of patients who were unable to eat for up to six months. Parenteral nutrition was complicated by a higher incidence of central venous catheter-related sepsis, especially during the first week, than in the general patient population. Nevertheless, it appears that parenteral nutrition is reasonably safe and is useful as supportive therapy in these

severely ill patients with GI dysfunction, although a direct benefit of parenteral nutrition on the course of the disease has not been identified.

The proposed mechanism by which nutritional support reduces pancreatic exocrine secretion is not well established. Intravenous hypertonic dextrose has been suggested as the component of parenteral nutrition which is responsible for reduction of protein secretion and total volume of pancreatic secretion, presumably due to increased serum osmolality. Conflicting evidence exists regarding the role of the amino acid infusion. Studies on animals have demonstrated both an increased and a decreased exocrine secretory response, although minor, to parenteral infusion of amino acids. Other studies on humans have shown little effect of amino acids. Comparison of peripheral vein parenteral nutrition to central vein parenteral nutrition in patients with pancreatic ascites showed a decrease in secretion with the latter but not the former, lending suggestive evidence that the hypertonic dextrose, more than the amino acid infusion, was responsible.

The use of IV lipid emulsions in patients with pancreatitis has likewise been controversial. Although initial observations in animals and humans indicated increased pancreatic secretion in response to IV lipid emulsion, subsequent studies have shown no stimulation of exocrine secretion or influence on amylase or pancreatic histology. Studies on humans with pancreatitis have shown no exacerbation of the disease as a result of infusion of lipid, although one of the authors (J. E. F.) is aware of a fatality in a patient with pancreatitis secondary to hyperlipidemia in whom a fatal attack may have been provoked by infusion of a 20% lipid emulsion. Recent observations by Bivins et al.[49] in a patient with pure pancreatic fistula confirmed no increase in pancreatic secretion with parenteral nutrition containing fat, but increases in both volume and protein content in response to enteral protein and fat.

The role of elemental diets and enteral nutrition in patients with pancreatitis is as yet undefined. In theory, these diets provide nutrition without stimulating the pancreas. In general, studies have demonstrated a decreased volume of pancreatic secretion in response to gastric administration of elemental diets compared to orally ingested food. Further reduction in secretion has been achieved by administration of nutrients into the small bowel. Secretion of pancreatic enzymes appears to be affected more by the content of protein and fat than by the route of administration of nutrients. Uncontrolled studies of elemental diets in patients with pancreatitis have reported tolerance without exacerbation of the disease.

In the absence of controlled randomized trials, it is difficult to evaluate the role of nutritional support in the treatment of the patient with acute pancreatitis. Our preference is for early institution of parenteral nutrition with continuation of therapy until resolution of symptoms, signs, and biochemical abnormalities is achieved. A randomized prospective trial is in progress to evaluate this approach. The intolerance and mechanical problems associated with elemental diets in these patients have made them of limited usefulness in our experience.

LIVER DISEASES

Hepatic insufficiency is a common consequence of critical illness as well as a result of chronic liver disease. Since the liver has an extensive ability to regenerate, therapy is aimed at metabolically supporting the patient until regeneration has occurred. Numerous factors have been proposed to exert a trophic influence on hepatic regeneration, including growth hormone, triiodothyronine, adrenal corticosteroids, an "ileal factor," insulin, glucagon, and nutrition.[50] Of these, certainly nutrition is the most easily manipulated in the clinical setting. The provision of adequate protein and calories is essential for the maintenance of homeostasis and the reversal of catabolism to prevent further deterioration of hepatic function as well as to provide substrate for hepatic protein synthesis and regeneration. Unfortunately, the administration of adequate protein to patients with hepatic insufficiency often results in encephalopathy. The challenge remains to administer adequate nutritional support to these catabolic patients to prevent protein breakdown and to promote hepatic regeneration while preventing encephalopathy.

Appropriate nutritional support of the patient with hepatic insufficiency requires an understanding of the nature and causes of encephalopathy. Hepatic encephalopathy may manifest itself with a variety of presentations, from coma or psychosis to subtle errors in judgment or changes in day/night rhythm. Classic teaching attributes these disorders to ammonia, which is liberated by gut bacteria and exerts its effect as a CNS toxin. The variety of presentations of encephalopathy as well as the lack of correlation of blood ammonia levels with the severity of encephalopathy had led to extensive research into alternative explanations for the cause of encephalopathy; most authorities now accept that ammonia is not the sole cause of encephalopathy.

The neurotransmitter amino acid hypothesis of hepatic encephalopathy states that under conditions of hepatic dysfunction, an imbalance in plasma amino acids occurs which leads to alterations in brain neurotransmitters, resulting in metabolic encephalopathy.[51] The inadequate production of conventional energy sources by the failing liver results in utilization of the branched-chain amino acids (BCAA) valine, leucine, and isoleucine by skeletal muscle and fat for energy, lipogenesis, and gluconeogenesis. Simultaneously, the aromatic amino acids escape inactivation by the failing liver and accumulate in plasma. This reduction in the concentration of BCAA and increased concentration of aromatic amino acids in the plasma lead to accumulation of aromatic amino acids within the brain and resultant derangements of neurotransmission.

The patient with cirrhosis has threshold derangements of neurotransmission which "sensitize" the brain to stress. Clinical events such as catabolism, sepsis, starvation, GI hemorrhage, or overdiuresis may further derange the amino acid pattern by increasing the aromatic amino acids, decreasing the BCAA, or both. Thus, any superimposed stress may result in hepatic encephalopathy.

Standard therapy of hepatic encephalopathy should include the maintenance of adequate oxygenation and careful regulation of fluid and electrolytes. Urinary sodium excretion is a helpful guide to sodium replacement. Gastrointestinal hemorrhage should be controlled and the gut purged of blood. Nonabsorbable antibiotics such as neomycin, kanamycin, or paromomycin are administered in initial doses of 6–8 gm/day followed by maintenance doses of 1–4 gm/day. In addition to

decreasing ammonia absorption by suppressing urease-producing organisms in the gut, they may also allow selective malabsorption of the aromatic amino acids. Lactulose, a nonabsorbable synthetic disaccharide, is administered in dosages of 60–160 gm/day. It is hydrolyzed by bacteria to produce an acidic diarrhea which purges the gut. In addition, the lowered pH may decrease the absorption of ammonia or the aromatic amino acids.

Administration of protein in modest amounts is an essential feature of therapy. Complete restriction of protein may precipitate encephalopathy due to accumulation of aromatic amino acids liberated during muscle breakdown. In the surgical setting, 50%–60% of patients with preexisting liver disease, even with grade I encephalopathy, will tolerate up to 60–80 gm of a standard amino acid mixture as parenteral nutrition with hypertonic dextrose as a caloric source and a modicum of fat to prevent essential fatty acid deficiency. In this way, nitrogen equilibrium is achieved without a specialized amino acid solution. Patients who present with grave II–IV encephalopathy or who deteriorate on the above regimen become candidates for a specialized nutritional support solution.[52, 53]

Specialized nutritional support is aimed at restoration of a normal plasma amino acid pattern through administration of an amino acid solution with increased concentrations of BCAA and decreased concentrations of aromatic amino acids. Such a liver disease–specific amino acid solution, known experimentally as F080,[52, 53] is now available commercially as Hepatamine®. It contains 35% of its amino acids as BCAA in comparison to standard commercial amino acid mixtures containing 14%–25% BCAA. Phenylalanine and methionine are present in decreased concentrations, while concentrations of arginine and alanine are increased.

Theoretical benefits of BCAA infusion in patients with liver disease include:

1. Although they normally provide only 6%–7% of the total energy requirements, under circumstances of decreased energy production and stress, the BCAA may constitute up to 30% of total energy needs.

2. Under conditions of stress, the BCAA may serve to regulate the flux of amino acids across the myocyte membrane.

3. Individual BCAA may increase protein synthesis. Leucine appears to be the most important regulator in man.

4. Hepatic protein synthesis is increased by administration of all BCAA with an energy source.

5. BCAA administration results in decreased plasma concentrations of aromatic amino acids by decreasing proteolysis and stimulating protein synthesis.

6. At the blood-brain barrier, the BCAA compete with the neutral amino acids (of which the aromatic amino acids are a subgroup) for transport into the brain.

7. In experimental animals following total hepatectomy, infusion of BCAA has been demonstrated to increase synthesis of norepinephrine in certain areas of the brain.

8. On a theoretical basis, the BCAA may improve peripheral catecholamine synthesis.

9. BCAA increase the rate of ammonia metabolism by muscle.

Numerous anecdotal series utilizing BCAA-enriched solutions in the treatment of encephalopathic patients who are intolerant of standard amino acid solutions have been reported since 1975. From these reports, it appears that in cirrhotic patients who experience encephalopathy as the result of intercurrent illness, infusion of 80 gm of protein equivalent as a 35% BCAA-enriched solution is associated with awakening from encephalopathy and nitrogen equilibrium.[54-56] In many patients who were intolerant of standard amino acid mixtures, up to 125 gm of BCAA-enriched solutions daily was well tolerated.[54] Patients with fulminant hepatitis who exhibit diffuse hyperaminoacidemia with normal concentrations of the BCAA require hemodialysis or polyacrylonitrile membrane perfusion as well as specialized nutritional support[53] to normalize their plasma amino acid pattern.[57, 58] Despite these encouraging reports, only randomized prospective trials can demonstrate the efficacy of BCAA therapy in a clinical syndrome as variable as hepatic encephalopathy.

Several properly done randomized prospective trials have recently been reported which compare BCAA therapy to a standard form of therapy (Table 5–7).[59-65] Those studies which utilized hypertonic dextrose as a caloric source[59-63] differ in outcome from those which used lipid as the major source of calories,[64, 65] suggesting that beneficial effects of the BCAA are dependent, among others, upon caloric substrate.[66]

An Italian multicenter trial reported by Rossi-Fanelli et al.[62] comparing a 100% BCAA-hypertonic dextrose solution to isocaloric dextrose and lactulose showed no statistically significant difference between groups, but a trend which clearly favored the group receiving BCAA. Response rate appeared better in the BCAA group despite the fact that entry criteria suggested they were a sicker group of patients (see Table 5–7).

Fiaccadori et al.[60] reported three treatment groups: one received lactulose, one received a BCAA-enriched balanced amino acid formulation with hypertonic dextrose, and a third group received both. Resolution of encephalopathy was significantly better in those groups receiving BCAA. In addition, survival was improved in the groups which received BCAA over that of the group which received lactulose (see Table 5–7).

Similar results were reported in a U.S. multicenter trial which compared Hepatamine and hypertonic dextrose to isocaloric dextrose and oral neomycin in a prospective double-blind randomized trial.[59] Global assessment and resolution of encephalopathy were significantly better in the BCAA group as measured both clinically and electroencephalographically.

Also improved was the nitrogen balance in the BCAA group. Of note was the increased survival in the group which received nutritional support (see Table 5–7).

Both Brazilian[61] and Danish studies[63] which compared Hepatamine® and hypertonic dextrose with isocaloric dextrose and oral neomycin failed to demonstrate improved wake-up rate or survival. Time required for resolution of encephalopathy in the Brazilian study appeared less in the BCAA group,[61] while the Danish trial[63] suggested resolution at twice the rate in the group receiving BCAA (see Table 5–7).

The two trials which have failed to demonstrate a benefit for the BCAA[64, 65] have in common the use of fat as a major caloric source. Michel et al.[64] utilized 70% of calories as fat and failed to find a difference in rate of resolution of encephalopathy. A multicenter French and Swedish trial reported by Wahren et al., which used fat for 50% of calories, similarly failed to confirm efficacy of the BCAA[65] (see Table 5–7). In addition, the overwhelming amount of leucine utilized may have created plasma amino acid imbalance and depressed concentrations of valine and isoleucine below levels which could sustain protein synthesis. The marked difference in results between the latter two studies and those which used hypertonic dextrose suggests that the use of the appropriate caloric source is paramount. Whether the difference is on the basis of higher levels of plasma-free tryptophan and CSF tryptophan in the lipid trial[67] or better utilization of BCAA with hypertonic dextrose is unclear at present.[66]

In summary, randomized prospective trials have demonstrated that in patients with hepatic encephalopathy, BCAA-enriched solutions are at least as efficacious as standard therapy in resolution of encephalopathy when administered with hypertonic dextrose as a caloric source. Efficacy has not been demonstrated in trials which have used fat as a major source of calories.

Following hepatitis or portasystemic shunting, patients may occasionally manifest stable hepatic insufficiency and chronic encephalopathy. Despite standard therapy, their encephalopathy may limit daily dietary protein to 20 gm or less. Such patients may be nutritionally supplemented with an elemental diet supplemented with 35% BCAA, available commercially as HepaticAid®. Up to 36 gm daily may be administered to supplement a 30-gm protein oral diet to promote positive nitrogen balance without encephalopathy.[68] Patients who are unable to tolerate the large glucose load contained in Hepat-

TABLE 5–7.—Results of Prospective, Randomized, Controlled Trials of Branched-chain Amino Acids in the Treatment of Hepatic Encephalopathy*

STUDY	YEAR	NO. OF PATIENTS/ CENTERS	WAKE-UP RATE, %		TIME INTERVAL TO REACH GR 0–1/0		MORTALITY, %	
			C	S	C	S	C	S
Rossi-Fanelli[62]	(1982)	34/4	47	70	31.5 hr	27.6 hr	29	23
Fiaccadori[60]	(1982)	48/1	62	94	NA	NA	62†	94†
Michel[64]	(1982)	30/1	33	33	NA	NA	20	33
Wahren[65]	(1983)	50/5	48	56	NA	NA	20	40
Cerra[59]	(1983)	22/1	25	56	NA	NA	25†	0
Gluud[63]	(1983)	20/4	60	70	4 Days	2 Days	10	20
U.S. Multicenter[59]	(1983)	75/8	17	53	Never	5–6 Days	55†	17
Strauss[61]	(1983)	30/2	67	93	71 hr	33 hr	13	13

*C = Control; S = study; NA = information not available.
†$P < 0.05$.

amine may be given up to 24 gm of BCAA in equimolar concentrations to supplement a 40–50-gm protein diet. As with IV BCAA therapy, administration of oral BCAA supplements has been shown in randomized prospective trials to be of benefit in promoting positive nitrogen balance while preventing or ameliorating encephalopathy.[69]

INTRA-ABDOMINAL SEPSIS

Intra-abdominal infection is common, may be life-threatening, and remains the most common cause of death in diseases commonly encountered by the general surgeon. In most cases intra-abdominal sepsis is secondary to an acute inflammatory, localized process, such as acute appendicitis or acute cholecystitis, which usually resolves with appropriate surgical treatment, and occasionally, when appropriate treatment is delayed, becomes complicated. However, at times an acute catastrophic or lethal event, causing abdominal and eventually systemic sepsis, occurs (gangrenous or perforated viscera, leaking intestinal anastomoses, or postoperative abscess) and will not resolve by surgical treatment alone, since these processes trigger a whole spectrum of hemodynamic and metabolic events which must be dealt with appropriately before they lead to multiple-system organ failure and death. Predisposing factors in intra-abdominal sepsis are advanced age, protein-calorie malnutrition, associated diseases such as hypertension and diabetes, and derangements of the immune mechanism secondary to coincident medication such as steroids.

The following discussion will deal primarily with the metabolic derangements resulting from intra-abdominal sepsis and the nutritional therapeutic modalities available for dealing with them. The metabolic response to sepsis is characterized by increased proteolysis, flow of amino acids from periphery to the liver to be used for hepatic protein synthesis and gluconeogenesis, use of BCAA as a peripheral fuel source (Fig 5–6), negative nitrogen balance, and weight loss. Absence of adequate intake with increased catabolism may contribute to respiratory insufficiency, immunoincompetence with increased susceptibility to infection and sepsis, derangements of wound healing, and multiple organ failure. Thus, aggressive nutritional and metabolic support should be added early as part of the complex multidisciplinary management of patients with severe sepsis or injury.

In recent years the metabolic alterations in the highly stressed and/or septic patient have become better understood, leading to extensive investigations of a specifically designed amino acid formulation for patients with sepsis. In addition, caloric requirements, appropriate calorie:nitrogen ratio and the relationship between glucose and fat are now better understood. The hypothesis that patients with significant metabolic stress and/or sepsis might benefit from amino acid formulations adapted to meet the altered metabolic requirements was a logical development from formulations developed for patients in liver failure and hepatic encephalopathy. The plasma amino acid profile of patients with hepatic failure reflects alterations in the ability of the patient to utilize classic energy sources; i.e., glucose intolerance and, presumably, although difficult to establish, diminished ability to utilize fatty acids and diminished ability of the failing liver to

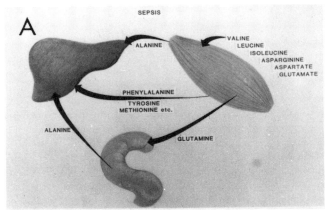

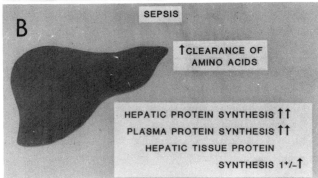

Fig 5–6.—A, metabolic derangements during sepsis: amino acid fluxes across the liver, muscle, and gut. **B,** hepatic protein synthesis during sepsis.

manufacture ketone bodies. Thus, BCAA are utilized by the skeletal muscle and fat tissue for energy and for lipogenesis. Simultaneously, there is a decreased splanchnic clearance of aromatic amino acids due to liver function derangements; the aromatic and sulfur-containing amino acids accumulate in the circulation. Manipulating this deranged plasma amino acid pattern by the administration of amino acid formulations low in aromatic and sulfur-containing amino acids and high in BCAA resulted in wake-up from septic encephalopathy, improved nitrogen balance, and even improved survival in animals and patients with liver failure.[54]

The plasma amino acid pattern of septic patients shows significant similarities to patients with hepatic failure, not surprising in view of the hepatic dysfunction which occurs relatively early in sepsis. High levels of aromatic (phenylalanine and tyrosine) and sulfur-containing amino acids (methionine, cysteine, and taurine), and low-normal levels of BCAA are seen (Fig 5–7). The increase in sulfur-containing amino acids, particularly cysteine and methionine, is more prominent in septic patients than in patients with liver disease alone. Proline is increased and arginine reduced. This amino acid pattern reflects the "peripheral energy deficit" of sepsis, resulting in increased proteolysis and the utilization of BCAA for energy and gluconeogenesis, coupled with a certain and variable degree of hepatic dysfunction. Despite this early liver dysfunction, the liver continues to synthesize and to deliver acute phase proteins, at least early on, and surviving patients with sepsis had higher plasma BCAA and alanine levels and

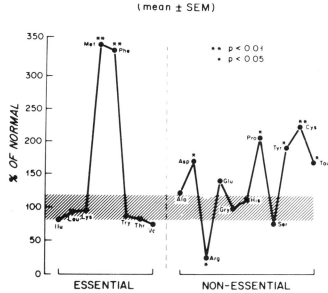

Fig 5–7.—Amino acid pattern in 15 septic patients, demonstrating a significant increase in the aromatic and sulfur-containing amino acids in the presence of the normal branched-chain amino acids. Arginine is decreased. This pattern was initially obtained in a group of 15 septic patients and was subsequently confirmed in a much larger group and by others as well. (From Freund H.R., Ryan J.A., Fischer J.E.: *Ann. Surg.* 188:423, 1978. Used by permission.)

lower aromatic and sulfur-containing amino acid levels than patients who died.[70] Discriminant analysis using plasma concentrations of alanine, cysteine, methionine, isoleucine, arginine, tyrosine, and phenylalanine correctly predicted outcome in 79% of survivors and 91% of nonsurvivors. In a preliminary study, the infusion of a liver-adapted amino acid formulation to septic patients resulted in normalization of the deranged plasma amino acid pattern and reversal of septic encephalopathy.[70, 71]

Following extensive experiments with BCAA-enriched formulations in an injured rat model, the following conclusions were reached. Administration of BCAA alone or as part of a BCAA-enriched nutritional formulation: (1) normalized the deranged plasma amino acids of injury and sepsis[72]; (2) improved nitrogen conservation[72]; and (3) increased both muscle and liver protein synthesis.[72]

Based on nitrogen balance data, plasma albumin levels, and plasma amino acid patterns, the use of a balanced amino acid solution containing adequate amounts of essential, nonessential, and 45% BCAA was advocated as the most appropriate formulation in the highly catabolic injury state.[72] Initial clinical studies were undertaken in patients undergoing elective moderate-to-severe surgical procedures. The BCAA-enriched formulations administered proved to be safe and nitrogen sparing. Recent studies in highly-stressed, severely catabolic septic patients demonstrated BCAA-enriched solutions to be superior to standard solutions.

Compared with standard amino acid solutions, infusion of BCAA-enriched amino acid formulations in severely stressed

and/or septic patients exhibited improved nitrogen conservation, a normalized plasma amino acid pattern, a rise in the absolute lymphocyte count, reversal of anergy, and an increase in transferrin, retinol-binding protein, prealbumin, and albumin levels. No difference in 3-methylhistidine excretion was demonstrated.[73]

Quantitatively, protein requirements are elevated above the usually recommended 1–1.5 gm/kg/day. Faced with an extreme demand for caloric substrate in the presence of glucose intolerance, impaired ketogenesis, and less than optimal fat utilization, the body increases peripheral catabolism with a flow of amino acids from the periphery to the liver. Amino acids are required not only for energy but also for the synthesis of acute-phase proteins, wound healing, and other lifesaving functions of the injured organism. The recommended dose of exogenous protein during this phase ranges from 1.5–3.0 gm/kg/day in hypermetabolic patients, almost half as BCAA. Concomitant with the increase in protein intake, the nonprotein intake should be modified in the presence of glucose resistance. High glucose calorie:nitrogen ratios are associated with complications such as hyperglycemia, hyperosmolarity, increased O_2 consumption, and excess CO_2 production and accumulation, perhaps contributing even to pulmonary insufficiency and certainly to increased cardiopulmonary work. The combination of a high-protein intake and reduced fractional glucose requirement will dictate a reduction in the calorie:nitrogen ratio to approximately 80:1 to 120:1. With a reduction of glucose, the requirement for fat as an energy source increases, reflected by the respiratory quotient of 0.8 during early sepsis, when fat utilization and ketogenesis are substantial. Eventually, however, with the progression of sepsis, lipid metabolism becomes deranged with elevated serum triglycerides, a result of overproduction and reduced clearance. Thus, in late sepsis only the BCAA may be efficiently utilized as energy sources, as utilization of both glucose and fat are impaired.

Our current concept of nutritional support of the severely catabolic and septic patient should include high-protein intake, generally 2.0 gm/kg/day, but perhaps up to 3.0 gm/kg/day, about 45%–50% of it in the form of BCAA, and a calorie:nitrogen ratio of about 100:1, with 65% of the nonprotein calories administered as glucose and 35% as fat. This specific form of nutritional support should be administered in addition to hemodynamic support, monitoring, appropriate antibiotics, respiratory care, and surgical treatment of intraabdominal sepsis.

ABDOMINAL TRAUMA

Trauma remains a major source of injury and a leading cause of death. Recovery from trauma requires prompt diagnosis of site and extent of injury, appropriate operative intervention, and intensive metabolic support to prevent the life-threatening complications of sepsis and multisystem organ failure. Although most victims of trauma are young, previously healthy, and well nourished, the altered metabolism of the postinjury state, as well as extensive damage to the GI tract, may necessitate nutritional supplementation as an important part of overall support.

Metabolic derangements which occur following trauma may

be similar to those described above for sepsis, although onset, duration, and severity may differ, and there are likely nuances in metabolic responses as yet unknown. Following injury there is increased protein breakdown, release of amino acids for hepatic synthesis of acute-phase reactants, and increased use of the BCAA as a fuel source. In trauma both synthesis and breakdown of protein increase, with the relatively larger increase of breakdown resulting in negative nitrogen balance. The hormonal response includes increased levels of catecholamines, adrenal corticosteroids, and glucagon. Elevated levels of insulin suppress fat mobilization, although skeletal muscle becomes glucose-resistant despite high plasma insulin, leading to hyperglycemia. In the presence of inadequate energy production from fat and glucose, the deficit is made up by increased muscle protein breakdown.

Immediate priorities in the management of the trauma victim include maintenance of hemodynamic stability by fluid and blood resuscitation, adequate ventilatory support, and repair of injuries. Often, resuscitation with fluids and pressors precludes nutritional support in the first 24–48 hours following injury. In the absence of severe multisystem injury or extensive damage to the GI tract, the patient's nutritional reserves may be adequate to withstand four or five days without oral intake, although we believe that nutritional supplementation should begin as soon as patients are stabilized.

In those patients with extensive injury to the GI tract, multisystem trauma, or previous malnutrition, or who are unable to eat for more than seven days, or who are likely to require further operative procedures, nutritional support should be instituted early. The type of nutritional support and route of delivery will be dictated by the condition of the GI tract, clinical condition, and severity of injury.

Gastrointestinal tract injury and paralytic ileus associated with severe stress often necessitate long periods of parenteral nutritional support following abdominal trauma. A classic example would be the patient with multiple pelvic fractures and retroperitoneal hematomas in whom a paralytic ileus can last for many weeks. Modification of amino acid composition and substrate may be necessary. Protein requirements are elevated in the posttraumatic state to 1.5–3.0 gm/kg/day from the usual recommendations of 1.3–1.7 gm/kg/day. Studies which have compared standard amino acid formulations to those of varying concentrations of BCAA in a population of highly stressed, injured and septic patients have shown an apparent advantage for a balanced solution containing 45% BCAA. The BCAA are provided in increased amounts both for energy and for increased protein synthesis. Use of the high-BCAA solutions appears to have been associated with increased nitrogen conservation and increased synthesis of rapid turnover proteins.

Altered substrate metabolism requires modification of the energy source as well. Greater understanding of energy requirements following injury has led to changes in amounts and sources of energy administered. Insulin-resistant hyperglycemia limits the amount of glucose infused. Infusion of glucose in excess of requirements may result in hyperosmolar nonketotic dehydration, increased oxygen consumption, increased carbon dioxide production, and fatty liver. Problems associated with excessive glucose infusion may also be pre-

vented by substitution of lipid emulsion for a portion of total calories. Although lipid emulsions have been used to provide up to 60% of total calories in nonstressed individuals, use in trauma patients should generally be limited to 25%–35% of calories. Clearance of fat is generally good at this level of administration, but triglyceride levels should be carefully monitored with any changes in the patient's condition. Optimal calculation of caloric requirements is obtained from measurements of oxygen consumption and carbon dioxide production. In the absence of such measurements, approximately 35 kcal/kg/day may be administered, 65% as glucose and 35% as lipid emulsion. The increased protein requirements and relatively decreased energy requirements decrease the calorie:nitrogen ratio from the conventional 150–160:1 to 100–120:1.

When possible, enteral nutrition may be used alone or in combination with parenteral nutrition. A frequent consequence of trauma, especially to the abdomen, is paralytic ileus. Studies of various segments of the GI tract have demonstrated that although the stomach and colon are susceptible to paralytic ileus for 24–72 hours, return of small-bowel motility generally occurs within hours. Such findings have generated interest in early use of small-bowel feeding. Needle catheter jejunostomy is an increasingly used technique of postoperative feeding in patients who have undergone abdominal operations.[74, 75] Placement of the catheter requires only an additional ten minutes of operating time and is associated with a low incidence of early and late complications. Placement of such a catheter should be considered in all patients with extensive intra-abdominal injury, especially to esophagus, stomach, duodenum, pancreas, or biliary tree. Jejunal feeding may also be accomplished by placement of a small-bore nasoenteric tube under fluoroscopic guidance.

At present, enteral formulations with modified amino acid configuration and lower calorie:nitrogen ratios have become commercially available. Although GI tolerance has been improved, diarrhea and distention remain frequent problems. In general, five to seven days may be required to achieve adequate protein and calorie intake without significant intolerance. During the initial period of nutritional support and in patients who require frequent operative procedures, a combination of enteral and parenteral nutrition will allow adequate provision of protein and calories when enteral administration is insufficient.

NUTRITIONAL SUPPORT FOR PEDIATRIC GASTROINTESTINAL SURGICAL DISEASES

Nutritional support of the pediatric patient presents a unique problem. In addition to the problems encountered in the adult patient, we are faced with the necessity of normal growth requirements, growth and maturation of developing organ systems, and prevention of deficiency states—all in the presence of limited endogenous nutrient stores. What follows is a brief discussion of the more common surgical indications for nutritional support in the pediatric surgical age group.

Congenital Gastrointestinal Anomalies

The mortality of infants with congenital GI anomalies has decreased in recent years from 75% to less than 10%, and parenteral nutrition is thought of as being largely responsible for this marked decrease in mortality. These anomalies include intestinal atresias at various levels of the GI tract, tracheoesophageal fistulas, congenital diaphragmatic hernia, gut malrotation-volvulus-short gut, meconium ileus, Hirschsprung's disease, omphalocoele, and gastroschisis, the last being the most obvious example of the decisive role of TPN in the pediatric surgical patient. Gastroschisis, although primarily an abdominal wall defect, results in a prolonged adynamic ileus owing to the prolonged intrauterine exposure of the gut to chemical irritation and peritonitis. Following successful surgical correction, these infants frequently died of inanition secondary to prolonged ileus, often lasting up to six weeks. Presently, these patients are placed on TPN immediately following surgery and supported for as long as necessary, until bowel function is regained.

Necrotizing Entercolitis (NEC)

NEC is a serious disease of the newborn characterized by necrosis of portions of the GI tract and previously carrying a mortality of about 50%. It has been associated with low birth weight or low gestational age babies sustaining perinatal stress such as asphyxia or hypothermia.

One of the initial steps in the management of NEC is the discontinuation of oral intake, making TPN mandatory treatment. Even when symptoms abate, it is customary to wait at least another week before resumption of oral intake. In babies undergoing bowel resection for necrosis or late stricture, TPN is required perioperatively, including at times the treatment of late short-bowel syndrome resulting from resection. Recent studies have implicated enteral overfeeding as contributing to NEC and suggested withholding enteral feeding in infants susceptible to NEC, using TPN for the first 2–3 weeks of life. This is controversial and has not been generally adopted.

Inflammatory Bowel Disease (IBD)

Both ulcerative colitis and Crohns' disease can and do occur early in life, even in infancy. Symptoms of IBD begin before the age of 20 years in about 15% of patients with ulcerative colitis and up to 30% of those with Crohn's disease. Presentation, clinical features, signs, symptoms, laboratory, endoscopic, and radiologic studies are similar to those of the adult patient (discussed earlier in this chapter). Growth failure, however, is specific to the pediatric patient with IBD. Impaired linear growth and delayed sexual maturation occurs in 15%–30% of children afflicted with Crohn's disease before puberty. Growth retardation may occasionally be the presenting symptom and is unrelated to the severity of the disease. Growth retardation may be aggravated by steroid treatment or by repeated or extensive bowel resections.

With the improvement in long-term TPN techniques, vascular accesses and the reduction in TPN-associated complications, severe cases of Crohns' disease-associated growth failures are logical candidates for long-term, generally home TPN. Home TPN proved to be safe and effective, with remission induced, nutritional status improved (with weight gain), normalization of serum albumin, increase in height, and marked improvement in well-being and quality of life.

Since growth failure was corrected in many of these children despite continuation of some disease activity, it was suggested that growth failure in Crohn's disease is most likely the result of chronic malnutrition. The direct effect of TPN on the bowel itself and the disease activity is only marginal when considering growth failure. Thus, some authors advocate the use of continuous enteral alimentation with elemental diets in children with Crohn's disease and growth failure. Under this treatment regimen, complete remission of symptoms, improved nutritional status, and significant height and weight gains were reported. Pediatric patients with severe, unresponsive Crohn's disease, particularly those with growth retardation, will benefit from home TPN, if only to reduce stunting and promote a growth spurt.

SUMMARY

Parenteral nutrition in digestive disease has become an increasingly important part of the therapeutic armamentarium. Many of the diseases discussed in this chapter form the classic indications for nutritional support. The availability of specially designed formulations, such as those for patients with hepatic failure, have increased the opportunities for more appropriate support in these patients.

REFERENCES

1. Dudrick S.J., Wilmore D.W., Vars H.M., et al.: Long-term total parenteral nutrition with growth, development, and positive nitrogen balance. *Surgery* 64:134, 1968.
2. Peters C., Fischer J.E.: Studies on calorie to nitrogen ratio for total parenteral nutrition. *Surg. Gynecol. Obstet.* 151:1, 1980.
3. Jeejeebhoy K.N., Marliss E.B.: Energy supply in total parenteral nutrition, in Fischer J.E. (ed.): *Surgical Nutrition.* Boston, Little, Brown & Co., 1983, pp. 645–662.
4. Buzby G.P., Mullen J.L., Matthews D.C., et al.: Prognostic nutritional index in gastrointestinal surgery. *Am. J. Surg.* 139:160, 1980.
5. Shizgal H.M.: Body composition, in Fischer J.E. (ed.): *Surgical Nutrition.* Boston, Little, Brown & Co., 1983, pp. 1–17.
6. Jeejeebhoy K.N., Baker J.P., Wolman S.L., et al.: Critical evaluation of the role of clinical assessment and body composition studies in patients with malnutrition and after total parenteral nutrition. *Am. J. Clin. Nutr.* 35:1117, 1982.
7. Young V.R., Munro H.N.: N^t-methylhistidine (3-methylhistidine) and muscle protein turnover: An overview. *Fed. Proc.* 37:2291, 1978.
8. Muggia-Sullam M., Bower R.H., Murphy, R.F., et al.: Postoperative enteral versus parenteral nutritional support in gastrointestinal surgery: A matched prospective study. *Am. J. Surg.* 149:106, 1985.
9. Silk D.B.A.: Intestinal absorption of nutrients, in Fischer J.E. (ed.): *Surgical Nutrition.* Boston, Little, Brown & Co., 1983, pp. 19–64.
10. Hoover H.C., Ryan J.A., Anderson E.J., et al.: Nutritional benefits of immediate postoperative jejunal feeding of an elemental diet. *Am. J. Surg.* 139:153, 1980.
11. Crohn B.B., Ginzburg L., Oppenheimer G.D.: Regional ileitis. *J.A.M.A.* 99:1323, 1932.
12. Copeland E.M., Dudrick S.J.: Intravenous hyperalimentation in inflammatory bowel disease, pancreatitis, and cancer. *Surg. Ann.* 12:83, 1980.
13. Fischer J.E., Foster G.S., Abel R.M., et al.: Hyperalimentation as primary therapy for inflammatory bowel disease. *Am. J. Surg.* 125:165, 1973.
14. Vogel C.M., Corwin T.R., Baue A.E.: Intravenous hyperalimentation in the treatment of inflammatory diseases of the bowel. *Arch. Surg.* 108:460, 1974.
15. Dudrick S.J., MacFadyen B.V., Daly J.M.: Management of inflammatory bowel disease with parenteral hyperalimentation, in Clearfield H.R., Dinoso V.P. (eds.): *Gastrointestinal Emergencies.* New York, Grune & Stratton, 1976, pp. 193–199.

16. Greenberg G.R., Haber G.B., Jeejeebhoy K.N.: Total parenteral nutrition and bowel rest in the management of Crohn's disease (abstract). *Gut* 17:828, 1976.

17. Driscoll R.H., Rosenberg I.H.: Total parenteral nutrition in inflammatory bowel disease. *Med. Clin. North Am.* 62:185, 1978.

18. Fazio V.W., Kodner I., Jagelman D.G., et al.: Inflammatory disease of the bowel: Nutrition as primary or adjunctive treatment. (Symposium) *Dis. Colon Rectum* 19:574, 1976.

19. Harford F.J., Fazio V.W.: Total parenteral nutrition as primary therapy for inflammatory disease of the bowel. *Dis. Colon Rectum* 21:555, 1978.

20. Dean R.F., Campos M.M., Barrett B.: Hyperalimentation in the management of chronic inflammatory intestinal disease. *Dis. Colon Rectum* 19:601, 1976.

21. Elson C.O., Layden T.J., Nemchausky B.A., et al.: An evaluation of TPN in the management of inflammatory bowel disease. *Dig. Dis. Sci.* 25:42, 1980.

22. Bos L.P., Weterman I.T.: TPN in Crohn's disease. *World J. Surg.* 4:163, 1980.

23. Mullen J.L., Hargrove W.C., Dudrick S.J., et al.: Ten years' experience with intravenous hyperalimentation and inflammatory bowel disease. *Ann. Surg.* 187:523, 1978.

24. Muller J.M., Keller H.W., Erasmi H., et al.: Total parenteral nutrition as the sole therapy in Crohn's disease: A prospective study. *Br. J. Surg.* 70:40, 1983.

25. Shiloni E., Freund H.R.: Total parenteral nutrition in Crohn's disease: Is it primary or supportive mode of therapy? *Dis. Colon Rectum* 26:275, 1983.

26. Reilly J., Ryan J.A., Strole W., et al.: Hyperalimentation in inflammatory bowel disease. *Am. J. Surg.* 131:192, 1976.

27. Dickinson R.J., Ashton M.G., Axon A.T.E., et al.: Controlled trial of intravenous hyperalimentation and total bowel rest as an adjunct to the routine therapy of acute colitis. *Gastroenterology* 79:1199, 1980.

28. Martin L.W., LeCoultre C., Schubert W.K.: Total colectomy and mucosal proctectomy with preservation of continence in ulcerative colitis. *Ann. Surg.* 186:477, 1977.

29. Martin L.W., Fischer J.E.: Preservation of anorectal continence following total colectomy. *Ann. Surg.* 196:700, 1982.

30. Edmunds L.H., Williams G.M., Welch C.E.: External fistulas arising from the gastrointestinal tract. *Ann. Surg.* 152:445, 1960.

31. Chapman R., Foran R., Dunphy J.E.: Management of intestinal fistulas. *Am. J. Surg.* 108:157, 1964.

32. Sheldon G.F., Gardiner B.N., Way L.W., et al.: Management of gastrointestinal fistulas. *Surg. Gynecol. Obstet.* 113:490, 1971.

33. Reber H.A., Roberts C., Way L.W., et al.: Management of external gastrointestinal fistulas. *Ann. Surg.* 188:460, 1978.

34. Soeters P.B., Ebeid A.M., Fischer J.E.: Review of 404 patients with gastrointestinal fistulas: Impact of parenteral nutrition. *Ann. Surg.* 190:189, 1979.

35. Rombeau J.L., Caldwell M.D.: *Enteral and Tube Feeding.* Philadelphia, W.B. Saunders Co., 1984.

36. Voitk A.J., Echave A.J., Brown R.A., et al.: Elemental diet in the treatment of fistulas of the alimentary tract. *Surg. Gynecol. Obstet.* 137:68, 1973.

37. Sako K., Lore J.M., Kaufman S., et al.: Parenteral hyperalimentation in surgical patients with head and neck cancer: A randomized study. *J. Surg. Oncol.* 16:391, 1981.

38. Lim S.T.K., Choa R.G., Lam K.H., et al.: Total parenteral nutrition versus gastrostomy in the preoperative preparation of patients with carcinoma of the oesophagus. *Br. J. Surg.* 68:69, 1981.

39. Muller J.M., Dienst C., Brenner V., et al.: Preoperative parenteral feeding in patients with gastrointestinal carcinoma. *Lancet* 1:68, 1982.

40. Holter A., Fischer J.E.: The effects of perioperative hyperalimentation on complications in patients with carcinoma and weight loss. *J. Surg. Res.* 23D:31, 1977.

41. Fischer J.E.: Adjuvant parenteral nutrition in the patient with cancer (editorial). *Surgery* 96:578, 1984.

42. Nixon D.W., Moffitt S., Lawson D.H., et al.: Total parenteral nutrition as an adjunct to chemotherapy of metastatic colorectal cancer. *Cancer Treat. Rep.* 65(suppl. 5):121, 1981.

43. Shamberger R.C., Brennan M.F., Goodgame J.T. Jr., et al.: A prospective randomized study of adjuvant parenteral nutrition in the treatment of sarcomas: Results of metabolic and survival studies. *Surgery* 96:1, 1984.

44. Steiger E., Oram-Smith J., Miller E., et al.: Effects of nutrition on tumor growth and tolerance to chemotherapy. *J. Surg. Res.* 18:455, 1975.

45. Ota D.M., Copeland E.M. III, Strobel H.W. Jr., et al.: The effect of protein nutrition on host and tumor metabolism. *J. Surg. Res.* 22:181, 1977.

46. Popp M.B., Wagner S.C., Brito O.J.: Host and tumor responses to increasing levels of intravenous nutritional support. *Surgery* 94:300, 1983.

47. Daly J.M., Reynolds H.M., Rowlands B.J., et al.: Tumor growth in experimental animals: Nutritional manipulation and chemotherapeutic response in the rat. *Ann. Surg.* 191:316, 1980.

48. Goodgame J.T., Fischer J.E.: Parenteral nutrition in the treatment of acute pancreatitis: Effect on complications and mortality. *Ann. Surg.* 186:651, 1977.

49. Bivins B.A., Bell R.M., Rapp R.P., et al.: Pancreatic exocrine response to parenteral nutrition. *J.P.E.N.* 8(1):34, 1984.

50. Nachbauer C.A., Fischer J.E.: The failing liver. *Surg. Clin. North Am.* 61:221, 1981.

51. Fischer J.E., Baldessarini R.J.: False neurotransmitters and hepatic failure. *Lancet* 2:75, 1971.

52. Fischer J.E., Funovics J.M., Aguirre A., et al.: The role of plasma amino acids in hepatic encephalopathy. *Surgery* 78:276, 1975.

53. Fischer J.E., Rosen H.M., Ebeid A.M., et al.: The effect of normalization of plasma amino acids on hepatic encephalopathy in man. *Surgery* 80:77, 1976.

54. Freund H.R., Dienstag J., Lehrich F., et al.: Infusion of BCAA solution in patients with hepatic encephalopathy. *Ann. Surg.* 196:209, 1982.

55. Okada A., Kamata S., Kim C.W., et al.: Treatment of hepatic encephalopathy with BCAA-rich amino acid mixtures, in Walser M., Williamson R. (eds.): *Metabolism and Clinical Implications of Branched Chain Amino and Ketoacids.* New York, Elsevier North Holland, 1981, pp. 447–452.

56. Capocaccia L., Calcaterra V., Cangiano C., et al.: Therapeutic effect of branched chain amino acids in hepatic encephalopathy: A preliminary study, in Orloff M.J., Stippa S., Ziparo V. (eds.): *Medical and Surgical Problems of Portal Hypertension.* New York, London, Academic Press, 1979, pp. 239–249.

57. Rosen H.M., Yoshimura N., Hodgman J.M., et al.: Plasma amino acid patterns in hepatic encephalopathy of differing etiology. *Gastroenterology* 72:483, 1977.

58. Record C.O., Bruxton B., Chase R.A., et al.: Plasma and brain amino acids in fulminant hepatic failure and their relationship to hepatic encephalopathy. *Eur. J. Clin. Invest.* 6:387, 1976.

59. Cerra F.B., Cheung N.K., Fischer J.E.: A multicenter trial of branched chain enriched amino acid infusion (FO80) in hepatic encephalopathy (HE). *Hepatology* 2:699 (abstract), 1982; Disease specific amino acid infusion (FO80) in hepatic encephalopathy: a prospective, randomized, double-blind, controlled trial. *J.P.E.N.* (in press), 1985.

60. Fiaccadori F., Ghinelli F., Pedretti G., et al.: Branched chain amino acid enriched solutions in the treatment of hepatic encephalopathy: A controlled trial, in Capocaccia L., Fischer J.E., Rossi-Fanelli F. (eds.): *Hepatic Encephalopathy in Chronic Liver Failure.* New York, Plenum Press, 1984, pp. 323–334.

61. Strauss E., Santos W.R., DaSilva E.C., et al.: A randomized controlled clinical trial for the evaluation of the efficacy of an enriched branched chain amino acid solution compared to neomycin in hepatic encephalopathy (abstract). *Hepatology* 3(5):862, 1983.

62. Rossi-Fanelli F., Riggio O., Cangiano C., et al.: Branched chain amino acids vs. lactulose in the treatment of hepatic coma: A controlled study. *Dig. Dis. Sci.* 27:929, 1982.

63. Gluud C., Dejgaard A., Hardt F., et al., and the Copenhagen Coma Group: Preliminary treatment results with balanced amino acid infusion to patients with hepatic encephalopathy. *Scand. J. Gastroenterol.* 18(suppl. 86):19, 1983.

64. Michel H., Pomier-Layrargues G., Duhamel O., et al.: Intravenous infusion of ordinary and modified amino acid solutions in the management of hepatic encephalopathy (controlled study, 30 patients) (abstract). *Gastroenterology* 79(5):1038, 1980.

65. Wahren J.J., Denis J., Desurmont P., et al.: Is intravenous administration of branched chain amino acids effective in the treatment of hepatic encephalopathy? A multicenter study. *Hepatology* 3:475, 1983.

66. Gelfand R.A., Hendler R.G., Sherwin R.S.: Dietary carbohydrate and metabolism of ingested protein. *Lancet* 1:65, 1979.

67. Cangiano C., Cascino A., Del Signore S., et al.: Cerebro-spinal fluid amino acid pattern in hepatic encephalopathy, in Capocaccia L., Fischer J.E., Rossi-Fanelli F. (eds.): *Hepatic Encephalopathy in Chronic Liver Failure.* New York, Plenum Press, 1984, pp. 87–94.

68. Freund H., Yoshimura N., Fischer J.E.: Chronic hepatic encephalopathy: Long-term therapy with a branched chain amino acid-enriched elemental diet. *J.A.M.A.* 242:347, 1979.

69. Horst D., Grace N.D., Conn H.O., et al.: Comparison of dietary protein with an oral, branched chain-enriched amino acid supplement in chronic portal-systemic encephalopathy: a randomized controlled trial. *Hepatology* 4:279, 1984.

70. Freund H.R., Ryan J.A., Fischer J.E.: Amino acid derangements in patients with sepsis: treatment with branched chain amino acid rich infusions. *Ann. Surg.* 188:423, 1978.

71. Freund H.R., Atamian S., Holroyde J., et al.: Plasma amino acids as predictors of the severity and outcome of sepsis. *Ann. Surg.* 190:571, 1979.

72. Freund H.R., Gimmon Z., Fischer J.E.: Nitrogen sparing effects and mechanisms of branched chain amino acids, in Kleinberger G., Deutsch E. (eds.): *New Aspects of Clinical Nutrition.* Basel, S. Karger-Verlag, 1983, pp. 346–360.

73. Bower R.H., Muggia-Sullam M., Vallgren S., et al.: Branched chain amino acid-enriched solutions in the septic patient: a randomized, prospective trial. *Ann. Surg.* In press.

74. Delaney H.M., Carnevale N.J., Garvey J.W., et al.: Postoperative nutritional support using needle catheter jejunostomy. *Ann. Surg.* 186:165, 1977.

75. Ryan J.A. Jr.: Jejunal feeding, in Fischer J.E. (ed.): *Surgical Nutrition.* Boston, Little, Brown & Co., 1983, pp. 757–777.

76. Eisenberg H.W., Turnbull R.B., Weakley F.L.: Hyperalimentation as preparation for surgery in transmural colitis (Crohn's disease). *Dis. Colon Rectum* 17:469, 1974.

77. Holm I.: Benefits of total parenteral nutrition in the treatment of Crohn's disease and ulcerative colitis. *Acta Chir. Scand.* 147:271, 1981.

78. Roback S.A., Nicoloff D.M.: High output enterocutaneous fistulae of the small bowel. *Am. J. Surg.* 123:317, 1972.

79. MacFadyen B.V., Dudrick S.J.: Management of gastrointestinal fistulae with parenteral hyperalimentation. *Surgery* 74:100, 1973.

80. Aguirre A., Fischer J.E., Welch C.E.: The role of surgery and hyperalimentation in therapy of gastrointestinal-cutaneous fistulae. *Ann. Surg.* 180:393, 1974.

81. Himal H.S., Allard J.R., Nadeau J.E., et al.: The importance of adequate nutrition in closure of small intestinal fistulas. *Br. J. Surg.* 61:724, 1974.

82. Freund H., Anner C., Saltz N.J.: Management of gastrointestinal fistulas with total parenteral nutrition. *Int. Surg.* 61:273, 1976.

83. Deitel M.D.: Nutritional management of external gastrointestinal fistulas. *Can. J. Surg.* 19:505, 1976.

84. Graham J.A.: Conservative treatment of gastrointestinal fistulas. *Surg. Gynecol. & Obstet.* 144:512, 1977.

85. Reber M.A., Roberts C., Way L., et al.: Management of external gastrointestinal fistulas. *Ann. Surg.* 188:460, 1978.

86. Thomas R.J.S., Rosalion A.: The use of parenteral nutrition in the management of external gastrointestinal tract fistulae. *Aust. N. Z. J. Surg.* 48:535, 1978.

87. Blackett R.L., Hill G.L.: Postoperative external small bowel fistulas: a study of a consecutive series of patients treated with intravenous hyperalimentation. *Br. J. Surg.* 65:775, 1978.

88. Coutsoftides T., Fazio V.W.: Small intestine cutaneous fistulas. *Surg. Gynecol. Obstet.* 149:333, 1979.

89. Silberman H., Granson M., Fong G., et al.: Management of external gastrointestinal fistulas with glucose and lipids. *Surg. Gynecol. Obstet.* 150:856, 1980.

90. Thomas R.J.S.: The response of patients with fistulas of the gastrointestinal tract to parenteral nutrition. *Surg. Gynecol. Obstet.* 153:77, 1981.

91. Sitges-Serra A., Jaurrieta E., Sitges-Creus A.: Management of postoperative enterocutaneous fistulas: the roles of parenteral nutrition and surgery. *Br. J. Surg.* 69:147, 1982.

92. Zera R.T., Bubrick M.P., Sternquist J.C., et al.: Enterocutaneous fistulas: effects of total parenteral nutrition and surgery. *Dis. Colon Rect.* 26:109, 1983.

93. Allardyce D.B.: Management of small bowel fistulas. *Am. J. Surg.* 145:593, 1983.

94. Moghissi K., Hornshaw J., Teasdale P.R., et al.: Parenteral nutrition in carcinoma of the oesophagus treated by surgery: nitrogen balance and clinical studies. *Br. J. Surg.* 64:125, 1977.

95. Issell B.F., Valdivieso M., Zaren H.A., et al.: Protection against chemotherapy toxicity by IV hyperalimentation. *Cancer Treat. Rep.* 62:1139, 1978.

96. Heatley R.V., Williams R.H.P., Lewis M.H.: Preoperative intravenous feeding: a controlled trial. *Postgrad. Med. J.* 55:541, 1979.

97. Simms J.M., Oliver E., Smith J.A.R.: A study of total parenteral nutrition (TPN) in major gastric and esophageal resection for neoplasia. *J.P.E.N.* 4:422 (abstract), 1980.

98. Lanzotti V., Copeland E., Bhuchar V., et al.: A randomized trial of total parenteral nutrition (TPN) with chemotherapy for non-oat cell lung cancer (NOCLC). *Proc. Am. Assoc. Cancer Res. Am. Soc. Clin. Oncol.* 21:377, 1980.

99. Valdivieso M., Bodey G.P., Benjamin R.S., et al.: Role of intravenous hyperalimentation as an adjunct to intensive chemotherapy for small cell bronchogenic carcinoma. *Cancer Treat. Rep.* 65(suppl. 5):145, 1981.

100. Thompson B.R., Julian T.B., Stremple J.F.: Perioperative total parenteral nutrition in patients with gastrointestinal cancer. *J. Surg. Res.* 30:497, 1981.

101. Popp M.B., Fisher R.I., Wesley R., et al.: A prospective study of adjuvant parenteral nutrition in the treatment of advanced diffuse lymphoma: influence on survival. *Surgery* 90:195, 1981.

102. Serrou B., Cupissol D., Plagne R., et al.: Parenteral intravenous nutrition (PIVN) as an adjunct to chemotherapy in small cell anaplastic lung carcinoma. *Cancer Treat. Rep.* 65(suppl. 5):151, 1981.

103. Samuels M.L., Selig D.E., Ogden S., et al.: IV hyperalimentation and chemotherapy for state III testicular cancer: a randomized study. *Cancer Treat. Rep.* 65:615, 1981.

104. Shamberger R.C., Pizzo P.A., Goodgame J.R., et al.: The effect of total parenteral nutrition on chemotherapy-induced myelosuppression: a randomized study. *Am. J. Med.* 74:40, 1983.

6

Intra-Abdominal Infections

DAVID H. AHRENHOLZ, M.D.
RICHARD L. SIMMONS, M.D.

FOR SEVERAL thousand years, untreated peritonitis has been recognized as a rapidly fatal disease. Even with remarkable advances in antibiotics; surgical techniques; diagnostic imaging procedures; and physiologic, metabolic, and nutritional support, the mortality has remained 20%–30%.[1-4] Recent experimental and clinical studies of intra-abdominal infections have suggested new methods for the surgical management of this problem.

ANATOMY OF THE PERITONEAL CAVITY

A single layer of mesothelial cells resting on a basement membrane covers the intra-abdominal viscera and is reflected onto the anterior and lateral abdominal walls as the parietal peritoneum. Usually the two peritoneal surfaces are in contact with one another and lubricated by less than 50 ml of isotonic peritoneal fluid.[5] Thus, the normal volume of the peritoneal cavity is small, but the anterior abdominal wall is not rigid, and this potential space can readily expand to accommodate several liters of fluid. Because small molecules readily equilibrate across the entire peritoneal membrane, peritoneal dialysis has become an effective treatment of renal failure.[6] Larger protein molecules cross the surface only in the presence of inflammation.

The peritoneal fluid normally contains fewer than 300 cells/ml, which are almost all mononuclear.[5] Inflammation and/or infection rapidly increases the volume of fluid and produces cell counts of more than 3,000 cells/ml with a high percentage of neutrophils.[7]

Von Recklinghausen[8] first described in 1863 the modified lymphatics, which remove particulate material from the peritoneal cavity. These lymphatics are found only along the undersurface of the diaphragm. Stomas connect the peritoneal cavity with the lymphatic lacunae and permit the escape of fluid and particles as large as 10 or 20 μ.[9] As the diaphragm relaxes, a negative pressure is generated beneath the diaphragms. The relaxed, upward-stretched diaphragm opens the stomas, and fluid enters the lymphatics. Diaphragmatic muscle contractions pump the lymphatic fluid cephalad, aided by one-way valves within the retrosternal lymphatics.[10] Early in the 20th century this work was discredited, until Allen and Weatherford[9] in 1959 conclusively demonstrated the presence and function of these modified lymphatics.[11]

Thus, the mechanics of respiration produce an upward circulation of peritoneal fluid. In 1900, Fowler[12] treated nine patients with peritonitis by placing them in a semi-upright position to minimize the absorption of toxins from the peritoneal cavity. As a secondary benefit respiratory efficiency was probably improved in patients with abdominal splinting and distention. All nine of his patients survived and the "semi-Fowler's position" became popular as part of the standard treatment for peritonitis. Recently, Last and associates[13] demonstrated that positive-pressure ventilation impairs bacterial clearance from the peritoneal cavity of animals, probably by impairing diaphragmatic lymphatic flow.

Surgeons have long advocated the "semi-Fowler's position" to minimize subphrenic infections vs. pelvic infections which can be drained transrectally. However, the removal of fluid from the diaphragmatic surface results in an upward circulation of peritoneal fluid. Autio[14] has shown that contrast material injected into the abdominal cavity flows cephalad along the lateral pericolic space to the diaphragm as well as into the pelvis in patients in the supine position. This allows bacteria to spread to the areas where abscesses are most frequently encountered including the subphrenic spaces, the subhepatic space, the lateral pericolic spaces, and the pelvis.[15]

The omentum seems to have two principal functions.[16] It can absorb into the circulation fluid and particulate material up to 10 μ in size. Larger material is trapped and remains in situ. The highly mobile omentum readily attaches itself by means of inflammatory exudate to any site of inflammation and frequently seals a perforated viscus or walls off an abscess cavity. This effect may be mediated in part by a recently described lipid angiogenic factor in omentum.[17]

Mesothelial cells which line the peritoneum are readily sloughed after almost any minor trauma including abrasion, drying, or prolonged exposure to saline. After brief insults healing is usually complete within a week as round cells from the peritoneal cavity adhere to the damaged surface and differentiate into mesothelial cells.[18] Ultrastructural studies by Janik and associates[19] suggest these mesothelial cells have a unique surface structure which lubricates viscera on their peritoneal surfaces.

Bacterial contamination or other trauma triggers an acute inflammatory process as injured cells, including mast cells, release their vasoactive granular contents.[20] A rapid transudation of fibrinogen-rich fluid into the peritoneal cavity is the result of increased local vascular permeability. Thromboplastin from damaged tissues converts prothrombin to thrombin, which splits fibrinogen to fibrin monomers; these monomers polymerize within the peritoneal cavity. The intraperitoneal polymerization of fibrin has multiple functions, including the ability to remove bacteria from fluid suspensions during polymerization.[21] The mechanically trapped bacteria are not systemically absorbed and bacteremia is delayed or prevented. Fibrin can also seal a perforated viscus, especially in the presence of omentum. Fibrin is readily lysed by fibrinolytic enzymes within the peritoneal cavity, but inflammation inactivates these enzyme systems so that fibrin deposits persist until fibroblasts invade to produce permanent adhesions.[22]

Bacteria trapped within fibrin deposits can have adverse effects as well. The trapped bacteria are relatively isolated from the phagocytic neutrophils, macrophages, and monocytes which have been attracted by the chemotactic factors released by bacteria growth.[21] As neutrophils accumulate around the fibrin deposit, they release their granular contents. These neutrophil enzymes are very caustic and are capable of digesting healthy tissue as well as bacteria. Further local inflammation leads to walling off of the infection and an abscess results.

The uninjured peritoneal cavity contains few phagocytic cells, but trauma or bacterial contamination produces a dramatic cellular response. Within a few hours large numbers of neutrophils arrive, followed later by monocytes and macrophages. These phagocytes are attracted by a variety of chemotactic factors including products of the complement cascade (C3a, C5a) and the products of bacterial metabolism. Neutrophils are capable of ingesting and killing large numbers of bacteria, but apparently never return to the systemic circulation. Thus, they remain and ultimately release their cellular contents, which are capable of digesting normal tissue as well as bacteria. The high levels of neutrophil elastase and collagenase found by Ohlsson[23] in the peritoneal fluid of patients with peritonitis suggest that these enzymes may augment the inflammatory response.

Normally the α-globulins of the blood, especially α_1-antitrypsin, neutralize the enzymes released from dead and dying neutrophils. But in large extravascular spaces such as the peritoneal cavity, little α_1-antitrypsin is available to neutralize these caustic enzymes. The cycle becomes self-sustaining as incoming neutrophils devour bacteria and then contribute to the local inflammatory process if the phagocytic cells cannot rapidly eradicate the bacterial inoculum. Experimentally, fibrin clots with entrapped bacteria lead to abscesses because the organisms remain protected within the clot while stimulating the continual influx of neutrophils.[21, 24] Effective therapy is necessary to interrupt this cycle and prevent persistent infection.

ETIOLOGY AND PATHOGENESIS OF PERITONITIS

Contamination of the peritoneal cavity can occur from a variety of sources, including penetrating external trauma or hematogenous seeding from distant sites. Most commonly, however, the bacteria arise from disruptions of the GI tract.

Thus, the bacteria which normally occur in the GI tract are those which most frequently produce peritonitis.

The human body can be visualized as enclosing a hollow GI tract which connects with the environment at the mouth and the anus. Although the human gut is sterile at birth, colonization of the mouth and ultimately of the entire GI tract occurs very soon after birth. The human mouth contains very large numbers of both anaerobic and aerobic bacteria which have adapted to the continual flow of saliva and the abrasion of chewing and swallowing food.[25] The oral streptococci are very resistant to abrasion and adhere specifically to the oral mucosa. Anaerobes reside in gingival pits along the gum line; bacteria commonly found here include anaerobic streptococci, *Bacteroides*, *Veillonella*, spirochetes, and *Candida*. Usually, swallowed bacteria are killed in the stomach, which has a pH of 1.5–2 between meals, but when food is present, the pH rises and bacteria rather easily reach the duodenum.[26] Achlorhydria from any cause increases the bacterial counts within the stomach.[27]

Lactobacilli are more common in the proximal small intestine because of their tolerance of acidic environments. Bacterial counts are low, however, because of the rapid transit times in jejunum and proximal ileum. In the distal ileum there is a transition to the fecal flora characteristic of the large bowel. The organisms which predominate include the gram-negative rods of the Enterobacteriaceae, the fecal streptococci, and the anaerobes, including streptococci, *Bacteroides*, and clostridia.

Not all bacteria found in the colon are pathogenic.[28] Many abundant colonic species such as eubacteria and bifidobacteria rarely establish infection in humans. The most common aerobic pathogen in the colon and distal ileum is *Escherichia coli*. Other gram-negative facultative organisms usually present include the *Klebsiella*, *Enterobacter*, *Proteus*, and *Pseudomonas* species. Group D, β-hemolytic, gram-positive, facultative organisms, known collectively as the enterococci, are the most common gram-positive aerobic organisms.[29] Approximately $10^8–10^9$ *E. coli* are characteristically present per gram of stool; in contrast, usually $10^{10.5}$ or 10^{11} anaerobic bacteria per gram of stool. Of these, *Bacteroides fragilis* is not the most common anaerobe, but it is the most common pathogenic anaerobic organism.[28] Present in lesser numbers are other anaerobic pathogens, including clostridia, peptostreptococci, peptococci, fusobacteria, and veillonellae.

Experimentally it is very difficult to produce intra-abdominal infection with pure cultures of a single bacterial species. The defenses of the peritoneal cavity are so efficient that, even though inflammation occurs, the bacteria are rarely able to persist, and the animal either dies rapidly of massive bacteremia or survives without residual intra-abdominal infection. However, in the presence of other substances, including hemoglobin, gastric mucin, bile, urine, or sterilized feces, bacteria may proliferate to produce a mortality higher than that seen with bacteria alone.[3] The term "adjuvant substances" has been applied to those materials which increase the lethality of an intraperitoneal bacterial inoculum. A variety of mechanisms has been suggested, including a direct stimulation of bacterial growth, induction of virulence factors within the bacteria, or blockade of the defense mechanisms of the peritoneal cavity.

Under normal conditions, bacteria appear in the bloodstream within minutes after peritoneal injection. It is possible that some adjuvants adhere to the bacteria, increasing their physical size and decreasing their removal via the diaphragmatic lymphatics. These adjuvants can also interfere with bacterial killing by neutrophils. Particulate materials, such as sterile feces or barium, cannot be engulfed by neutrophils, which degranulate and die in the attempt.

Many agents, such as the acidic gastric contents after peptic ulcer perforation, are irritating and cause an exudate of peritoneal fluid. Bacteria suspended in fluid are protected from phagocytosis because neutrophils require a surface for efficient phagocytosis.[30, 31] Since isotonic fluid is absorbed at a fixed rate by the lymphatic vessels, fewer suspended bacteria are removed per unit of time. The bacteria, thus protected from in situ killing mechanisms and lymphatic clearance, can proliferate. If bacteria are opsonized, either by antibody or complement, phagocytosis of bacteria in suspension can still occur.[31] Patients with ascites from cirrhosis or acute peritonitis have peritoneal fluid depleted in opsonins and bacteria are relatively protected.[1] More specifically, if C3b of the complement cascade does not attach to bacteria, it can actually protect bacteria from the intraperitoneal defenses.[32]

Certain combinations of bacteria interact synergistically to produce a more virulent intra-abdominal infection.[33] Meleney et al.[34] in 1932 showed that the combination of E. coli with an anaerobe caused an increased lethality when injected into the peritoneal cavity of animals. More recently, Onderdonk and co-workers[35] implanted gelatin capsules containing sterile stool, nutrient broth, and barium sulfate into the peritoneal cavity of rats. They recorded the effects of various combinations of bacteria when added to the capsules. If a single organism was added, abscesses and mortality were rare. Even combinations of only aerobes or only anaerobes produced few complications. However, the combination of an aerobe such as E. coli or the enterococcus and an anaerobe such as Bacteroides or Fusobacterium consistently produced abscesses. More recent work has indicated that the capsule of B. fragilis inhibits neutrophil phagocytosis of many bacteria.[36] Aerobic organisms probably promote the growth of anaerobes by consuming the oxygen locally and allowing anaerobic proliferation. A variety of other synergistic mechanisms have been proposed.[33]

The bacteria recovered from a given patient with peritonitis are determined by the source of the bacteria, presence of perioperative antibiotics, and the duration of intraperitoneal contamination. Many anaerobes and nonpathogens disappear within a few minutes or hours after perforation of the colon.[37] If an operation is delayed, fewer bacterial species, but more virulent organisms, will be isolated intraoperatively. If the stomach or upper GI tract is the source of contamination, rarely is more than one organism isolated.[38] These findings have important implications in the treatment of peritonitis (see below).

LOCAL EFFECTS OF PERITONITIS

The early effects seen in acute peritonitis are the result of the local inflammatory process of the peritoneal cavity. There is an acute increase in vascular permeability to both fluids and protein. Fluid containing many serum proteins such as fibrinogen enters the free peritoneal cavity. There is a rapid accumulation of neutrophils, followed within 24 hours by monocytes and macrophages. Although bacteria do not cross the general peritoneal surface, even in severe inflammation, there is an increased permeability to absorption of bacterial products and toxins which exert systemic effects.

Irritation of the peritoneal surface also causes edema of the bowel wall. A general adynamic ileus is characteristic of acute peritoneal contamination after a transient hypermobility. Associated with ileus is accumulation of fluid within the bowel lumen which, combined with the other losses from the intravascular space, produces a systemic hypovolemia. The patient, experiencing pain, unconsciously swallows air, which accumulates rapidly in the small bowel and is visible radiographically as air-fluid levels. Nausea, anorexia, and vomiting are frequent symptoms.

SYSTEMIC EFFECTS OF PERITONITIS

The marked systemic effects seen in general peritonitis are mediated by a variety of factors. With acute generalized inflammation of the peritoneal cavity, there is a rapid translocation of fluid from the intravascular space, resulting in an acute systemic hypovolemia. Uncomplicated hypovolemia produces a decreased cardiac output, an increased total peripheral resistance, and ultimately systemic hypotension, if untreated.[39] As a result of decreased systemic perfusion and oxygen delivery, anaerobic metabolism occurs in the peripheral muscle beds, with a resultant lactic acidosis and a fall in systemic pH. Acidosis has adverse effects on myocardial contractibility, further decreasing tissue perfusion. These effects are reversible to a greater or lesser degree by fluid resuscitation. Superimposed on this hypovolemia are the effects of other factors including bacterial products and endotoxin, systemic acidosis, complement activation, and other inflammatory mediators.[40, 41]

Sepsis without hypovolemia is usually caused by a localized rather than a generalized peritonitis. These patients have an increased cardiac output with a decreased total peripheral resistance, an effect possibly caused by endotoxin, the lipopolysaccharide component of gram-negative bacterial cell walls. When endotoxin is infused by IV in experimental animals, there is marked dilatation of the venous bed with local extravasation of fluid.[42] But endotoxin produces markedly different effects in different animal species. For example, in dogs there is an early splanchnic pooling of blood with an acute fall in cardiac output and blood pressure. In primates, there is transient vasoconstriction and then peripheral vasodilatation, with an early rise of cardiac output followed by a slow decline.

It is probable that the clinical manifestations of peritonitis are mediated not only by endotoxin but also by absorption of live bacteria, bacterial exotoxins, and products of inflammation including neutrophil products, activated complement, fibrin monomers, and bacterial debris. Therefore, no experimental infusion of purified bacterial products or even live bacteria can be expected to mimic exactly the human condition, even in primates.[41]

Two distinct septic states can be identified in humans. MacLean and associates[43] found that patients who are normovolemic before the onset of sepsis develop a hyperdynamic circulatory pattern characterized by hypotension, high cardiac output, normal or somewhat increased blood volume, normal or somewhat high venous pressure, and low total peripheral systemic resistance. There is usually a decreased oxygen utilization, thought previously to be caused by arteriovenous shunting but more likely to be due to a primary cellular defect in oxygen utilization.

In their study, patients who were hypovolemic before onset of septic shock developed hypotension, low cardiac output, high peripheral resistance, and a low central venous pressure. Early respiratory alkalosis progressed to metabolic acidosis if inadequately treated. Vincent et al.[39] studied 31 patients with generalized peritonitis who presented with systemic hypotension. Those patients who were truly hypovolemic responded to fluid resuscitation and had a better prognosis than those patients who were normovolemic and were unable to increase their cardiac output in response to increased cardiac filling pressures. Experimentally, acute infusion of endotoxin has no effect on cardiac function, but over six hours there is a gradual impairment of right ventricular function. Such an effect has never been conclusively demonstrated in humans. Nevertheless, Siegel et al.[40] identified a small subset of patients with sepsis and myocardial depression in spite of relatively large blood volumes apparently caused by direct myocardial contractile depression. This is very close to the state found in patients with primary cardiogenic shock. More commonly, however, septic patients demonstrate an extreme hyperdynamic state with a very low total peripheral resistance and very high cardiac outputs. These patients produce an extreme amount of flow-related work.

A progressive decrease in respiratory function is present in human sepsis.[44] Hyperventilation and disorientation may be the earliest signs of sepsis. Endotoxin and other mediators cause a loss of vascular and capillary integrity with leakage of fluid into the interstitial pulmonary space. Oxygenation across the pulmonary vascular bed falls, and systemic hypoxia ultimately results, further contributing to the lactic acidosis found with poor tissue perfusion. The increased fluid in the lung also decreases its elasticity (compliance) and leads to pulmonary hypertension.

Ultimately, protein-rich fluid accumulates within the alveolar spaces and progressive subsegmental and segmental collapse may ensue, manifested on a chest x-ray as diffuse fluffy infiltrates. Pulmonary A-Vo$_2$ differences show ventilation-perfusion defects within the lung tissue and a further fall in oxygenation across the pulmonary vascular bed.[45] This adult respiratory distress syndrome, characteristic of severe systemic sepsis, may be aggravated by fluid resuscitation with colloid. Further loss of compliance, pulmonary hypertension, and severe systemic hypoxemia require ventilatory support.[46]

Complement activation may specifically accentuate the pulmonary dysfunction by increasing the severity of the endothelial leak, or increase the shunting by causing leukocyte and platelet aggregation and obstruction of pulmonary vascular flow. This effect has been documented in patients undergoing dialysis when complement is activated by flow across the dialysis bed.[47] Saba and associates[48] found increased lung lymph flow in septic sheep which was significantly reduced in ani-

mals treated with fibronectin. The significance of fibronectin levels is discussed subsequently.

Kirton and associates[49] induced repeated episodes of peritonitis with *E. coli* and *B. fragilis* in rats. Serial examinations of lung specimens revealed a progressive fibrosis of the alveolar walls and ducts indicating sepsis may produce permanent long-term changes in pulmonary beds. Lanser and Saba[50] have attributed this to a neutrophil-mediated lung localization of bacteria in sepsis.

In the kidneys, hypovolemia and hypotension initially decrease the glomerular filtration rate (GFR), which may proceed to acute tubular necrosis. More commonly, there is an opening of cortical-medullary shunts within the renal parenchyma.[44] Decreased perfusion of the cortex and glomeruli results in an acute fall in urine output. Adequate fluid resuscitation with resumption of urine flow is a goal of the treatment of sepsis.

Increased attention has been focused on the endocrine effects of sepsis. Initially there is a large production of epinephrine and norepinephrine and a marked increase in cortisol release during the first two or three days. Systemic hyponatremia often results from aldosterone and antidiuretic hormone release due to hypovolemia.

Bessie et al.[51] have tried to mimic the hypermetabolic response to trauma by infusion of cortisol, glucagon, and epinephrine in normal human volunteers. Their data suggest that many of the metabolic responses of the hypermetabolic state following injury may be mediated by changes in the levels of these hormones.

Patients with major septic stress exhibit a hypermetabolic state with marked protein catabolism. There is a decreased ability to utilize glucose stores and a gradual shift to peripheral utilization of ketone bodies and free fatty acids as a primary energy source.[52] Many patients show decreased peripheral oxygen utilization, possibly because of a generalized cellular metabolic dysfunction. In hypovolemic states with peripheral hypoperfusion, the oxygen delivery is inadequate to meet oxygen demands, and there is a shift to anaerobic metabolism. In addition, there is a marked metabolic acidosis as lactate accumulates. In the hypotensive patient, reflex vasoconstriction further decreases the tissue perfusion of muscle, gut, and skin to preserve perfusion of the brain and heart. Local acidosis causes vasodilation of tissue, an antagonistic effect.

After an initial mobilization of glycogen stores within the liver, other tissues become the source of further energy.[40] Lipolysis can lead to production of ketone bodies but these are relatively inefficiently used. Protein catabolism is an early hallmark of sepsis, leading to rapid muscle wasting as muscle proteins are used as a source of glucose and blood protein production. It appears that interleukin I, a protein produced by leukocytes, is the mediator of this breakdown.[53] One of the major goals of therapy in patients with peritonitis is to meet the metabolic energy demands and minimize protein catabolism.

The immunologic system is also compromised in patients with sepsis. Experimental work in our laboratory indicates that neutrophils readily lose their ability to respond to chemotactic stimuli when exposed to circulating complement products such as C5a and C3a.[54] These "deactivated" cells in vitro are unable efficiently to phagocytose and kill bacteria.

Cutaneous anergy has also been documented in many patients with systemic sepsis. Whether this is a factor which predisposes to the infection or a complication of the infectious process is unclear.[55] In vitro tests of neutrophil and lymphocyte function also show depressed activity in patients with sepsis in parallel with this anergy.[56]

Serum fibronectin (cold insoluble globulin) in the bloodstream functions to promote the clearance of particulate matter and immune complexes by the Kupffer cells in the liver. Patients with prolonged sepsis show marked falls in serum fibronectin levels, and preliminary data indicate that these patients have a decreased survival compared to controls.[57] Low fibronectin levels have also been associated with onset of multiple-organ failure. Early studies with fibronectin replacement therapy have been encouraging.[58]

CLINICAL MANIFESTATIONS

Clinical manifestations of peritoneal irritation are determined by a variety of factors. The innervation of the bowel wall is via the splanchnic nerves, and pain sensation, produced principally by dilatation of the bowel, is diffuse and crampy. In contrast, the inner surface of the anterior abdominal wall is innervated by the somatic nerves which produce marked, well-localized pain in response to irritation. Thus, the signs of rebound tenderness and guarding, which are characteristic of generalized peritonitis, are found principally with irritation of the anterior muscle wall. More localized processes, especially between visceral surfaces, produce a nonspecific, dull, aching pain which is difficult to localize. Major texts have been written describing the differential diagnosis of acute intra-abdominal pathologic conditions.[59]

Nevertheless, in patients with acute intra-abdominal infection, abdominal pain and tenderness are characteristic. A progressive increase in symptoms with nausea and anorexia is most common. Ultimately, localized tenderness, rebound, and guarding are associated with irritation of the anterior abdominal wall. Fever and leukocytosis are usually present in proportion to the degree of intra-abdominal contamination; localized processes tend to produce less marked symptoms. Multiple conditions can modify the presentation of patients with intra-abdominal sepsis. Patients taking steroids or other immunosuppressive agents, those receiving chemotherapy, or those with chronic malignancy or starvation tend to have a less marked response to intra-abdominal contamination. Postoperative patients who have continuing or recurrent sepsis initally have minimal physical findings. For this reason, the diagnosis of occult intraperitoneal infection usually requires radiographic techniques.

When the diagnosis of peritonitis has been made, fluid resuscitation is mandatory. In the modern era, the vast majority of intra-abdominal infections are treated by urgent surgery to repair any breaks in the continuity of the GI tract and to remove bacteria and those contaminating materials that foster bacterial growth. Preparation for surgery, however, involves restoration of the circulating fluid volume, cardiac output, and peripheral perfusion, usually with Ringer's lactate.[60] Young patients manifest adequate rehydration by prompt resumption of adequate urine flow. Elderly patients, including those with histories of congestive heart failure or other cardiac disease, are more accurately managed by monitoring of central venous or pulmonary artery wedge pressures. Cardiac output, total peripheral venous resistance, and oxygen consumption measurements are sensitive indicators of adequate fluid resuscitation.

EMPIRIC ANTIBIOTIC THERAPY

Since the mid-20th century, antibiotics have become the cornerstone of treatment for virtually all infections. Experimental studies have shown that after tissue contamination, there is a brief period of several hours during which antibiotics are especially effective in preventing established infections.[30] This "grace period" has been estimated as approximately four to six hours. Additional studies on prophylactic use of antibiotics indicate that effective tissue levels of antibiotics must be present as early as possible after contamination for maximal benefit.[37] All patients should have systemic broad-spectrum antibiotics instituted before surgery. Patients with suspected primary peritonitis (i.e., those not requiring surgical intervention) should have immediate paracentesis followed by institution of antibiotic therapy based on the Gram stain results.[1] Anaerobes can be detected very rapidly by gasliquid chromatography of ascitic fluid.[61]

The choice of antibiotics for intra-abdominal sepsis remains difficult. Factors such as cost of therapy, spectrum of efficacy, and risk of complications must be weighed. In patients with acute contamination the virulence of the inoculum is determined by the site of perforation, the presence of adjuvant substances, and whether this contamination resulted from a previously localized infection.

For example, in patients with peptic perforation of the duodenum, the bacterial counts are relatively low, and no organisms are cultured at the time of surgery in about two thirds of patients.[38] A cephalosporin is usually adequate systemic therapy in this disease. Patients with traumatic perforation of the colon, however, have contamination with an inoculum containing a multitude of gram-positive and gram-negative organisms, many of which are pathogens. A broad-spectrum cephalosporin (e.g., cefoxitin) effective against aerobes and anaerobes is probably adequate in uncomplicated cases with early surgical intervention, if delayed primary wound closure is used.

Patients who have secondary perforation of inflammatory conditions within the GI tract present a greater challenge. These patients have sudden release of a virulent inoculum consisting of multiple aerobic and anaerobic bacterial pathogens, dead and dying neutrophils, and bacterial cell products. Because the organisms are more virulent, the infection is more difficult to eradicate, and a combination of antibiotics is probably more appropriate than a single agent. The most difficult infections are those where diagnosis has been delayed or where infection has recurred despite antibiotic therapy. Antibiotic choices for these patients cannot be based on cultures obtained intraoperatively, because multiple pathogens are found and unnecessary, dangerous delays in therapy would occur. For these reasons empirical therapy based on knowledge of the common pathogens is required.

There has been little argument that gram-negative facultative organisms of the group Enterobacteriaceae are the organisms routinely isolated after perforation of the distal GI tract.[3] These organisms are sensitive to some of the newer cephalosporins but the gold standard has been an aminoglycoside such as gentamicin, tobramycin, or amikacin. These agents bind irreversibly to the bacterial ribosome and are bactericidal rather than bacteriostatic. However, aminoglycosides have no effect against anaerobic organisms and have a relatively high incidence of renal and ototoxicity. Careful monitoring of aminoglycoside levels has resulted in more adequate treatment, since many patients require higher than expected amounts of the antibiotic to achieve appropriate tissue levels.[62] The renal and ototoxicity problems have also been reduced, but not eliminated, by monitoring serum levels.

It is becoming increasingly clear that antibiotics effective against anaerobic organisms should be instituted in all cases of small- and large-bowel perforations.[63] Work several years ago by Stone et al.[37] indicated that the numbers of anaerobes isolated from the contaminated abdominal cavity decreased markedly with time during an operation. They suggested that if aerobic organisms were eliminated, the anaerobes would be unable to grow. This may be true in patients with acute traumatic perforations which are treated early, but it is not true in most patients.

More commonly, a local inflammatory process such as appendicitis or diverticulitis has allowed anaerobic growth in a localized area of necrotic tissue. Anaerobes can persist, even if an operation is carried out. Since aminoglycosides have no effect against pathogenic anaerobes, we routinely use either clindamycin or metronidazole preoperatively in patients with diseases of the distal half of the GI tract.

Each agent has advantages and disadvantages. Clindamycin appears to be a bacteriostatic rather than a bactericidal agent which has had a high degree of clinical success in treating anaerobic infections. Anaerobes exposed to clindamycin are more readily phagocytosed by neutrophils.[64] Adequate doses, at least 600 mg, four times a day for adults, are necessary. Antibiotic-associated colitis caused by Clostridium difficile has been its major drawback.[65]

Metronidazole has a much more narrow spectrum and is effective only against anaerobes, but it is bactericidal and rarely causes clostridial enterocolitis. Experimental work indicates a remarkable ability to penetrate abscess cavities.[66] Also unique are its irreversible binding to bacteria and its ability to kill bacteria which are undergoing little or no growth.[67] Debate continues over its mutagenicity.[68]

The combination of an aminoglycoside with either clindamycin or metronidazole effectively treats most intraperitoneal infections.[69] But the enterococcus is not susceptible to these antibiotics and may break through as a pathogen.[29, 70] Since Onderdonk and co-workers[35] found that the enterococcus is a synergistic organism comparable to E. coli in producing intra-abdominal sepsis, we have most commonly added ampicillin, 1 gm every six hours in adults, until cultures of the abdominal fluid are available. We then alter the antibiotic therapy to specifically treat the organisms isolated.

Recently, a great deal of interest has been shown in the use of single antibiotic agents to treat intra-abdominal sepsis. The second- and third-generation cephalosporins have little or no renal and ototoxicity and in clinical trials have been effective

in intra-abdominal sepsis.[70–75] Most of the reported trials have found no significant difference between third-generation cephalosporins and gentamycin-clindamycin. However, serious defects exist in almost all clinical antibiotic trials, as reviewed by Solomkin and associates.[76] This review should be read by every clinician before evaluating the results of antibiotic treatment for peritonitis. A major problem remains—that standard treatment is so effective that small improvements in therapy can only be demonstrated by treating hundreds of patients in each treatment group. It is probable that differences in efficacy of antibiotic combinations will only be demonstrated in animal models where human pathogens are implanted in the peritoneal cavity.[77]

Only a few disadvantages with cephalosporins are evident. Some agents such as moxalactam have been associated with a high incidence of postoperative bleeding which is only partially reversible with parenteral vitamin K.[78] More significant, however, is the ability of many pathogenic organisms to elaborate cephalosporinase enzymes which confer bacterial resistance.[79] Exogenously secreted cephalosporinases may inactivate locally all the administered antibiotic and thus protect all organisms in the pathogenic inoculum. Many cephalosporinases are carried on bacterial plasmids which are exchanged freely by gram-negative bacteria. Rapid spread of cephalosporin resistance has been reported. This has tempered our enthusiasm for such agents.

Chloramphenicol is the other single agent which has been used for generalized intra-abdominal sepsis, but treatment failures have been reported.[80] The complications of generalized myelosuppression and rare, but usually lethal, aplastic anemia have significantly reduced its popularity. At this time it is not a first-line drug in the treatment of intra-abdominal sepsis.

Candida peritonitis is usually found in patients on antibiotics or after gastric perforation. Low-dose amphotericin-B has been effective treatment in such patients.[81] It has not been determined that treatment should be instituted when candida are isolated as part of a mixed flora in acute peritonitis.

OPERATIVE TREATMENT

After adequate fluid resuscitation and institution of systemic antibiotics, the patient must be explored surgically without delay. Except in cases of clearcut appendicitis or cholecystitis, we most commonly use a vertical midline approach because of its ease of opening and closure and ready access to the entire abdominal cavity. Upon opening the peritoneum, a specimen of fluid is aspirated for gram staining and aerobic and anaerobic cultures. These results will be used subsequently to determine the appropriateness of extended antibiotic therapy.

The abdomen is rapidly explored and any continuing contamination from a perforated viscus is controlled with sutures or atraumatic clamps. The entire abdomen is then lavaged repeatedly with antibiotic saline solution. A description of the specific surgical intervention for each possible intra-abdominal condition is beyond the scope of this discussion. However, continuity of the GI tract is reestablished except that primary colonic anastomoses are avoided in the face of extensive or neglected infection, advanced age, or multisystem organ failure.

A number of controversial methods of operative management deserve discussion. Surgeons have used intraoperative saline lavage routinely to remove the visible contamination found at operation.[82] Often antibiotics have been added to the final lavage and clinical and experimental data suggest that this reduces the incidence of infectious complications.[83, 84] Significant decrease in morbidity and mortality has not been demonstrated using antibiotic lavage in animals treated with systemic antibiotics, suggesting the additional benefit is small.[85, 86]

Topical antibiotics clearly reduce the incidence of wound infection.[87] However, since β-lactam antibiotics require a prolonged time of contact with bacteria, we feel that immediate and repeated use of antibiotic lavage throughout the procedure is appropriate. It has been our practice not to use the agents which have been given systemically, especially aminoglycosides, since these have been associated with postoperative depression of respiration when neuromuscular-blocking agents have been used intraoperatively. Our preference has been to use a first-generation cephalosporin diluted in 1 gm/L of saline and used liberally throughout the operation. At this concentration (1,000 μcg/ml) the cephalosporins are effective against even resistant organisms, since these concentrations cannot be achieved by systemic administration. Antibiotics are rapidly absorbed across inflamed peritoneal surfaces, so they are reapplied frequently during an operation. Inexpensive cephalosporins with prolonged half-lives have been our preference.

Multiple experimental and clinical reports have appeared regarding the use of intra-abdominal lavage with antiseptic solutions such as povidone-iodine,[88] noxythiolin,[89] and taurolin.[90] Povidone-iodine (PVP-I) is cheap, readily available, and assumed to be relatively safe. It is bactericidal on contact with virtually all bacteria except clostridial spores. Ideally, the operating surgeon can immediately reduce the local bacterial contamination in the operative field by antiseptic lavage. However, experimental work indicates that even dilute PVP-I solutions permanently inactivate neutrophil chemotactic functions, and higher concentrations kill not only bacteria but also neutrophils and mesothelial cells.[91] The resulting chemical burn of the peritoneal cavity produces an exudation of intra-abdominal fluid which impedes the clearance of bacteria. Unlike antibiotics, PVP-I has a very brief duration of action and is rapidly inactivated by interaction with tissue. Bacteria can grow readily in the presence of inactivated PVP-I solutions. Since antibiotics have a prolonged postoperative beneficial effect without damaging human cells, we feel they are always preferred over antiseptics within the peritoneal cavity.

A variety of antibiotics for intra-abdominal lavage have been proposed.[3] Many, however, including bacitracin, polymyxin, and the aminoglycosides have significant systemic toxicity if they are absorbed across the peritoneal membrane. In contrast, the cephalosporins are relatively safe in patients who are not allergic to penicillins. We prefer to use a bimodal attack, treating free intra-abdominal bacteria with topical antibiotics and bacteria deep within tissue with systemic antibiotics.

Some patients continue to have a consistently high mortality with conventional therapy. These include patients with ascites, alcoholic liver disease, immunosuppression, and cancer chemotherapy. In such patients, prolonged postoperative intra-abdominal lavage using crystalloids or antibiotic solutions have been proposed.[92, 93] Washington and associates[94] were able to reduce their intra-abdominal abscess rate from 16% to 0% in patients treated for two days with continuous intraperitoneal antibiotic lavage. Lavage is a demanding task for the nursing staff and is frequently complicated by poor drainage of the abdominal cavity after infusion of antibiotic solutions. This results in abdominal distention, pain, and elevation of the diaphragms with relatively poor ventilation. However, when the catheters function, the system can also be used for postoperative dialysis in patients with renal failure. This is especially important, since patients with systemic sepsis demonstrate hemodynamic instability on hemodialysis.

The major problem with postoperative lavage is that the inflamed peritoneal surfaces seal off the catheters and form relatively narrow tracts between the inflow and outflow catheters.[95] Prolonged drainage is thus almost impossible to maintain. An alternative to maintaining continuous postoperative drainage of the peritoneal cavity is the placement of porous Marlex or Vicryl mesh with a running monofilament suture around the edges of the abdominal wound. This has multiple potential advantages.[96] The patient can be placed prone to allow continuous postural drainage. On the ward a small incision can be made in the mesh and loculations broken up by a gloved finger with minimal discomfort to the patient. In the most critically ill patients this procedure allows serial reexploration of the abdominal cavity using general anesthesia without the cumbersome task of repeated wound closure and its risk of necrotizing fasciitis. The patient may be placed in a Hubbard tank to facilitate irrigation and removal of infected contents.[97] After the sepsis is controlled, the Marlex may be removed and wound closure attempted, or it may be left in situ until granulation tissue forms which can be skin grafted. This is equally effective in patients who have lost portions of the abdominal wall from necrotizing fasciitis. One must remember, however, that Marlex, when left in place, has significant long-term complications of fistula formation or mesh extrusion.[98–100] Jenkins and associates[101] suggest that Vicryl may be better material for closure of abdominal wall defects. Open packing of the abdomen has also been used,[102–104] but reports of fistula formation are discouraging.[105]

Radical peritoneal debridement has been proposed as a method to reduce the incidence and severity of recurrent intra-abdominal sepsis. Experimental data indicate that small fibrin deposits even containing very high bacterial counts are well tolerated, but that large deposits result in abscess formation.[20] Although some clinical studies have been encouraging, Polk and Fry[106] found radical peritoneal debridement was not effective in minimizing postoperative infectious complications.[107] We try to remove all obviously necrotic tissue including large fibrin deposits, but do not expend extra time debriding fibrinous wisps. Bleeding must be avoided.

Intra-abdominal drains are contraindicated except where abscess walls cannot be adequately debrided (e.g., appendiceal abscess) or fistula formation is expected (e.g., pancreatic or biliary trauma).[108] Drains do not evacuate the general peritoneal cavity in diffuse peritonitis but may serve as outlet tracts for localized virulent collections or leaking enteric secretions that would otherwise spread throughout the peritoneal cavity. Drains near anastomoses increase the incidence of anastomotic failure.

The abdominal wound is routinely closed with running or interrupted nonabsorbable monofilament sutures which have a high resistance to infections.[109–111] Mattress sutures are rarely used but may be placed and tied over buttresses separated from the wound margin. The skin is not closed in contaminated abdominal operations but a 2–0 or 3–0 running monofilament suture is placed loosely in the wound, which is then packed with dry gauze. On the fourth or fifth postoperative day the gauze is removed, and the running suture is pulled up and tied. This minimizes the risk of deep wound infection and allows delayed primary wound closure. The suture is usually removed after two additional weeks.

As an alternative, suction catheters may be placed in the subcutaneous wound, which is then closed.[112] Antibiotic solution is instilled intermittently for two days, after which catheters are removed. The catheters are able to remove the fluid accumulations, and topical antibiotics suppress bacterial proliferation. Staples minimize infectious complications in contaminated wounds.[113]

Surprisingly, recent studies have shown that irrigation of contaminated wounds with dilute povidone-iodine reduces the wound infection rate in patients treated with systemic antibiotics.[114–116] We expect that a similar effect can be achieved by irrigation of the contaminated wound with topical antibiotics.

LOCALIZED PERITONITIS AND INTRA-ABDOMINAL ABSCESSES

Unfortunately, the distinctions and definitions applied to infections of the abdominal cavity have been rather arbitrarily defined. For our purposes, generalized peritonitis is bacterial contamination and growth within the preformed peritoneal space. From this large surface bacterial products and toxins are absorbed and bacterial invasion may occur. Abscesses, however, imply a process contained by either a normal anatomical boundary, such as within the mesocolon in diverticulitis, or by adherence of the serosal surfaces of visera or omentum. An abscess may occur when bacteria invade tissue and cause suppuration or when they proliferate in a localized portion of the preformed peritoneal cavity. A phlegmon, on the other hand, implies a generalized bacterial cellulitis within living tissue, especially the mesentaries or retroperitoneal structures. Surgical therapy is of little benefit and the process may proceed to complete resolution or the production of single or multiple abscesses. Little is known about the pathophysiology of cellulitis, but abscesses have received the attention of surgeons for centuries.

An abscess is essentially a collection of fluid containing necrotic debris, leukocytes, and bacteria. Sterile abscesses are possible in the presence of sufficient local tissue necrosis.[1] Unlike generalized peritonitis, abscesses are the result of subacute or chronic inflammation because the accumulation of leukocytes and fluid and the necrosis of tissue requires time. For example, if bacteria become isolated in a portion of the

peritoneal cavity after generalized peritonitis, adherent adjacent viscera and fibrin deposits can loculate fluid within which bacteria can grow. Neutrophils aggregate, and this cavity becomes purulent with increasing local inflammation. Further fibrin deposits occur and fibroblasts invade this matrix, protecting the surrounding tissue from spillage.

Alternatively, an inflammatory process may occur within the wall of the intra-abdominal organ. In this case, tissue necrosis and surrounding cellulitis develop as bacteria invade subjacent structures. The contents of the abscess become hypertonic with enzymatic digestion of the tissue and ultimately rupture in the peritoneal space. If the local defenses are effective this produces a walled-off abscess; if not, free peritonitis results.

The walling-off process retards bacterial escape and resulting tissue invasion, septicemia, or infection of a preformed space. It also decreases the access of bacteria to oxygen and glucose. Thus, bacteria within an abscess are metabolically inactive with very retarded growth rates.[118] Chronic abscesses have thick fibrin deposits forming a barrier to penetrating phagocytes and systemic antibiotics. However, bacteriostatic antibiotics are unable to eradicate bacteria which already have minimal growth rates.[119] Many bactericidal antibiotics disrupt the growth of bacterial cell walls. In an iso-osmotic environment these defective bacteria rupture and die. In the hypertonic abscess, however, they are able to persist and grow as vegetative forms with defective cell walls. When the antibiotic concentration falls, the dividing bacteria can begin to produce normal cell walls.

Thus, the inflammatory process produces barriers which inhibit bacterial spread but also delays or prevents eradication of the bacteria even with the help of antibiotics. The surgical principle that abscesses must be drained appears valid.

An exhaustive discussion of the sites where abdominal sepsis can occur is probably not necessary. Common sites remain the right and left subphrenic spaces, the right subhepatic space, the lesser sac, the right and left pericolic-spaces, the pelvis.[15] Abscesses between adjacent viscera also occur. Infections of the kidney, pancreas, duodenum, and colon can cause intramesenteric or retroperitoneal abscesses.

The incidence of intra-abdominal abscesses is decreasing. In the past, perforated appendicitis was the most common cause of intra-abdominal abscess,[120] but colonic diverticulitis is increasing as earlier treatment of appendicitis decreases this complication.[121] With advances in overall care of trauma patients, the incidence of abscesses is increasing, as severely injured patients survive longer than previously.[122–124]

Not surprisingly, contiguous or nearby organs most frequently give rise to abscesses in a given location. With the decreasing incidence of perforated appendicitis, left subphrenic abscesses are now more common than right.[125] These are usually associated with trauma or operations on the pancreas, spleen, stomach, and duodenum. Incidental splenectomy during operations on the stomach or bowel has an especially high risk for left subphrenic abscess.[126] It is apparent that subphrenic abscess is becoming more common in the elderly population.[127]

DIAGNOSIS OF INTRA-ABDOMINAL ABSCESS

Unlike diffuse generalized peritonitis which produces marked, diffuse abdominal pain, intra-abdominal abscesses rarely cause such marked symptoms. Contributing factors include walling off by bowel or omentum which has visceral rather than somatic innervation, and the subacute or chronic time course compared to generalized peritonitis. However, localizing abdominal pain, ileus, and even a palpable mass generally become apparent with time in patients without previous trauma or operation. Intraloop retroperitoneal pelvic and subphrenic abscesses are more difficult to palpate and produce fewer symptoms.[117, 128] Ileus, diarrhea, or tenesmus may be the earliest findings in these patients.

Patients who develop intra-abdominal sepsis in the postoperative period have even fewer signs or symptoms. The abdominal findings are frequently masked by perioperative analgesics, incisional pain, or perhaps even decreased sensitivity of the peritoneal innervation. Often an unexplained fever, leukocytosis, and persistent ileus are the only signs of developing or persisting infection. With minimal objective findings it is difficult for any surgeon to admit that his patient may require reoperation. Only changes in the abdominal findings on serial examinations which document failure of the patient to improve will lead to early, appropriate intervention.

A variety of signs and symptoms occur in patients with subphrenic abscesses.[125, 127–135] Typically fever and tachycardia are more prominent than abdominal pain, which may be difficult to differentiate from postoperative incisional pain.[130] Occasionally patients will have abdominal guarding or distention and ileus. Hiccups, tachypnea, cough, and jaundice are also associated with subphrenic abscess.[133] If patients have not received antibiotics, pain ultimately develops over the anterior costal margin or posterior 12th rib.[128] If antibiotics have been given, abdominal tenderness, fever, and leukocytosis are less frequent, and the abscesses probably are smaller.[132] Patients who have a prolonged ileus or develop nausea and vomiting after initial return of bowel function have an increased risk of intra-abdominal abscesses. Nonspecific chest signs include pleural effusions, decreased breath sounds, and elevation of the diaphragm on one side.[134]

The diagnosis of pelvic abscesses is especially difficult unless a vaginal or rectal examination is carried out. Patients with a tubo-ovarian abscess or pelvic inflammatory disease often have symptoms similar to appendicitis, with low abdominal tenderness, fever, leukocytosis, and ileus. Pelvic examination may reveal a palpable pelvic mass or marked pain when the cervix is moved. Development of a pelvic abscess after laparotomy is usually associated with relatively mild findings.[115]

A variety of diagnostic criteria have been suggested in evaluating the possibility of postoperative intra-abdominal infection. In the absence of antibiotics, the most consistent finding is an elevated WBC count with increased precursor cells. However, the total count may be below 10,000/cu mm if the patient has received antibiotics. Lennard et al.[136] studied 65 patients treated for intra-abdominal sepsis with antibiotics and recorded the WBC count on the day that antibiotics were discontinued. Fifty-one patients were afebrile, and of these, seven of 21 who had persistent leukocytosis developed intra-abdominal infections. None of the 30 patients with normal WBC counts developed abscesses. They suggest that a normal WBC count at the conclusion of antibiotic treatment predicts a minimal risk for recurrent intra-abdominal sepsis.

Freischlag and Busuttil[131] have evaluated the significance of fever in postoperative patients. Of 71 patients with postoperative fever, only 19, or 27%, had an infection as the cause. None had intra-abdominal sepsis, and five had wound infections. Other causes included pulmonary sepsis, urinary tract sepsis, IV catheter-associated sepsis, and meningitis. Epididymitis, prostatitis, parotitis, and sinusitis may also cause unexplained postoperative fever and leukocytosis.[138] Leukocytosis and fever per se are not specific indicators of intra-abdominal infection. Coon[139] found only one of 38 patients undergoing laparotomy for fever of undetermined origin to have an abscess. Malignancy was the most frequent diagnosis.

Martin and associates[140] monitored the gastric pH in patients after surgical treatment of intra-abdominal sepsis. Patients were given standard regimens of antacids or cimetidine. In those patients who failed to maintain a pH above 4, 20 of 28 patients were septic vs. 8 of 49 patients with easily corrected hyperacidity. However, of these patients, 19 of 28 had bacterial pneumonia, and only eight had wound infection or abscess as an etiology. Stothert and associates,[141] however, were unable to identify septic patients by their response to either antacids or cimetidine.

Ing and co-workers[142] studied 125 bacteremic episodes over a two-month period in 83 surgical patients. Of these, more than one species of bacterium was isolated by blood culture in 32 episodes. Twenty-four of the 32 episodes were related to intra-abdominal pathology. It is of interest that enterococci and *E. coli* were especially common in multiple-organism sepsis.

Postoperative *Bacteroides* bacteremia also suggests recurrent intra-abdominal sepsis, according to data presented by Fry et al.[143] In their series of 98 patients with *Bacteroides* bacteremia over a 28-month period, 46 patients had intra-abdominal sepsis and an additional 31 had a surgically treatable focus of infection. Bryan and associates[144] found one third of 142 patients with *Bacteroides* bacteremia in four community hospitals had intra-abdominal sepsis.

Schentag and associates[145] have measured C-reactive protein in 97 patients treated for intra-abdominal sepsis. Nearly all patients had a sharp rise in C-reactive protein level after surgery, but by day 8 those successfully treated had levels below 5 mg/dl vs. 10 mg/dl for those with persistent or recurrent intra-abdominal sepsis. Aasen and associates[146] found that of 18 surgical patients with septicemia, all nine nonsurvivors had low plasma prekallikrein levels. Reduced plasma kallikrein inhibition appeared in those patients who developed fatal septic shock.

All of these factors lead to a high index of suspicion, especially in postoperative patients. But postoperative infections cause continuing diagnostic difficulties.[147] Routinely, surgeons attempt to confirm the diagnosis by radiographic means. The presence of intra-abdominal air is an obvious indication for exploratory laparotomy, except in postoperative patients where intra-abdominal air may persist for several days. However, a reticulated pattern or an air-fluid level outside the bowel may demonstrate a septic process dramatically. More often air-fluid levels are seen within the small bowel as a result of localized ileus. Chest findings, including pleural effusion or pulmonary infiltrate, with elevation of the diaphragm suggest a subphrenic abscess,[134] but subhepatic abscesses have minimal radiologic findings. Occasionally contrast material instilled into the GI tract may show compression of the stomach or bowel or even extravasation from an anastomotic dehiscence.

Of the available specific diagnostic modalities, gray-scale ultrasonography is safe because of its absence of radiation dosage.[148] It can be performed rapidly but is dependent on the skill of the operator to adequately localize collections of fluid. Intact skin is required over the area to be visualized; air in the GI tract or bone will degrade the image obtained. The major problem, however, is its failure to reassure the surgeon that a septic focus has not been missed.

Although high-resolution CT is associated with some radiation exposure, it has become the diagnostic test of choice in patients with suspected intra-abdominal abscesses.[149] A negative study is highly reliable except for interloop abscesses. The technique cannot always differentiate between a sterile or a contaminated fluid collection. Combined with diagnostic percutaneous fine-needle aspiration, however, the diagnostic accuracy is very high indeed.

Gallium-67 and indium-111 scans are only occasionally used in our institution. In theory, these agents will localize to areas of inflammation, but the test has an overall accuracy below that of CT scanning.[150, 151]

Recently, Richardson and associates[152] have used diagnostic peritoneal lavage in 138 patients with suspected peritonitis. In 65 of 77 patients with more than 500 leukocytes/cu mm, peritonitis was found at laparotomy. In eight of 77 cases, other causes of leukocytosis were found. But four of 61 patients with a negative lavage also had peritonitis. We have not found it helpful in patients with occult diverticulitis, for example, and blind peritoneal lavage can be dangerous in distention with abscess. Percutaneous, CT-guided diagnostic aspiration has replaced peritoneal lavage in the usual postoperative situation.

TREATMENT OF INTRA-ABDOMINAL INFECTIONS

Drainage of an infected collection of fluid combined with appropriate systemic antibiotics remains the treatment of choice. However, concepts in the drainage of intra-abdominal fluid have changed radically in the past few years. The principle remains, however, that a patient with suspected intra-abdominal sepsis is best treated by early drainage, without wasting time in a prolonged attempt to localize precisely the site of infection.

As surgery became a rigorous discipline in the early part of this century, extraserous drainage of intra-abdominal abscesses was adopted as the norm.[153] Contamination of otherwise uninfected sites was a dreaded complication, to be avoided at all costs. However, with the advent of antibiotics, adequate fluid resuscitation, and other modern treatment modalities, contamination of otherwise uninfected sites has become less dangerous. The risk of distant abscess is minimal,

provided perioperative antibiotics and intra-abdominal lavage are adequate. Transabdominal exploration of the entire peritoneal cavity has the advantages of allowing fibrin debridement, complete mobilization of the bowel to minimize adhesions, and thorough exploration to minimize the risk of missed synchronous abscesses, which occur in up to 23% of patients.[135] Until recently, this had become the standard of therapy against which other modalities are compared.[154-156]

As high-resolution CT scanning has become available, wide experience has been gained in visualizing intra-abdominal collections of fluid. Many of these sites can be aspirated by percutaneous needle puncture and fluid obtained for gram stain and culture, with selection of appropriate antibiotics. Currently, catheters are routinely placed in these intra-abdominal fluid collections.[155-160] This technique is successful only if the fluid is in continuity with the abdominal wall and is not applicable for intraloop abscesses, where the risk of bowel perforation is high. Nevertheless, the technique avoids the risk and pain of a general anesthetic and surgical exploration, much to the relief of most surgeons. We expect that with increasing experience, this technique will become standard in the treatment of intra-abdominal infections.

We have recently identified subsets of patients in whom CT-directed catheter drainage of intra-abdominal abscesses is unsuccessful.[159] Patients with a phlegmon rather than a localized fluid collection do not respond to either surgery or catheter drainage. Peripancreatic phlegmons and infected organized hematomas fall in this group.[160] Patients with enteric fistulas also are better treated by operative exploration to control the source of leak. Fungal infections or abscesses within infected tumor are also relative contraindications to catheter drainage. Associated complications include significant bleeding or inadvertent puncture of the GI tract.

The antibiotic choice in treatment of intra-abdominal abscesses is best determined by aspiration and culture of the purulent material. The most frequent aerobic organisms recovered are *E. coli*, other facultative Enterobacteriaceae, and enterococci. The most common anaerobes are *B. fragilis*, other *Bacteroides* spp., anaerobic cocci, and occasionally, clostridia. We expect that instillation of antibiotics into the abscess cavity may also be of benefit in the treatment of intra-abdominal abscesses. Experience with this treatment is very limited at this time.

A guiding principle remains that if the septic focus can be surgically excised, i.e., acute diverticulitis, the overall prognosis is markedly improved over other treatments. Unfortunately, grave infections such as phlegmons in the pancreatic area are usually unresectable.

PROGNOSIS

The prognosis for patients with intra-peritoneal sepsis remains guarded with reported mortalities of 20%–50%.[4, 147, 161-167] The degree of contamination (generalized peritonitis vs. localized abscess) is an important factor. There is also a variety of host factors which determine the immunocompetence of the patient, including the presence of associated injuries, duration of contamination, presence of intra-abdominal inflammatory conditions, and other chronic illnesses. In general, appendicitis, because of its frequent presentation as a highly symptomatic, localized inflammation before perforation, is treated earlier and has a lower mortality than other causes of peritonitis.[168] Perforated duodenal ulcer has a relatively nonvirulent inoculum and also has an excellent prognosis—sometimes even without operative treatment.[169] In contrast, gastric ulcer perforations often produce a significant bacterial contamination, since high acid production is less characteristic of this disease process. In general, the virulence of the inoculum and the mortality increase with progressively more distal perforations. Some subsets of patients, especially those who are elderly, receiving immunosuppressive agents, or with renal failure, have an especially high mortality.[1]

Stephen and Lowenthal[167] studied 68 patients with diffuse peritonitis, 33 of whom died. Fatalities were higher in older patients, those with fecal peritonitis or anastomotic leak, and those with a delay of more than 24 hours before the diagnosis of peritonitis was made. Twenty-seven of 29 patients with multiple-organ failure (discussed below) died of persistent sepsis. The two survivors underwent operative control of persistent sepsis.

The group of patients which presents with hypotension has a high mortality. Vincent and co-workers[39] reviewed 24 patients with generalized peritonitis and hypotension. Eleven of the 24 had uncorrectable shock and died. Seven of the remaining 11 died as a result of uncontrolled sepsis. Adverse factors included shock exceeding 24 hours, older age group, normal initial blood volume with little response to fluid resuscitation, and elevated blood lactate levels eight hours after institution of fluid resuscitation.

Dellinger and co-workers[4] reviewed 187 patients from five intensive care units with documented intra-abdominal infection. The mortality was 24%, and only 48% of patients were cured with one operation and one course of antibiotics. Patients with appendicitis had a good prognosis and perforated duodenal ulcer patients were excluded. Multivariate analysis showed that a poor acute physiology score (a measure of physiologic response to sepsis), advanced age, shock, malnutrition, and diffuse peritonitis all adversely affected survival.

So many factors contribute to the mortality and morbidity in peritonitis that it is difficult to categorize patients into groups of equivalent severity. This complicates the evaluation of efficacy for various operative and antibiotic therapies in the treatment of generalized peritonitis. However, the data of Dellinger and co-workers provide a preliminary basis for stratification in clinical trials of the treatment of intra-abdominal sepsis.

Baue in 1975[170] described a clinical syndrome of sequential multiple-system organ failure leading to death. In subsequent years it has become clear that the most common cause of multiple-system organ failure in surgical patients is uncontrolled sepsis.[171–173] Increasingly, the development of progressive remote organ failure has been recognized as an indication for surgical reexploration after other common sites of sepsis are ruled out.[161, 171, 173] The pathophysiology of multiple-organ failure is complex and beyond the scope of this chapter.[172, 174, 175] The mediators of this failure are poorly understood.[175] Aggressive treatment of residual sepsis offers the best chance for survival.[147, 162, 171, 173]

The majority of patients who succumb after intra-abdominal

infection have uncontrolled sepsis at death. This may be the result of inadequate or inappropriate antibiotics, incomplete drainage, or unsuspected focus of infection within the peritoneal cavity or elsewhere. As experience grows with broader-spectrum antibiotics and more sophisticated and sensitive diagnostic modalities, intra-abdominal infections will be treated earlier and more completely, further reducing the mortality of this condition.

REFERENCES

1. Ahrenholz D.H., Simmons R.L.: Peritonitis and other intraabdominal infections, in Simmons R.L., Howard R.J. (eds.): *Surgical Infectious Diseases.* New York, Appleton-Century-Crofts, 1982.
2. Steinberg B.: *Infections of the Peritoneum.* New York, Paul B. Hoeber, 1944.
3. Hau T., Ahrenholz D.H., Simmons, R.L.: Secondary bacterial peritonitis: The biologic basis of treatment. *Curr. Probl. Surg.* 16:1, 1979.
4. Dellinger E.P., Wertz M.J., Meakins J.L., et al.: Multicenter trial of a surgical infection stratification (SIS) system for intraabdominal infection. *Surgery* In press.
5. Bercovici B., Michel J., Miller J., et al.: Antimicrobial activity of human peritoneal fluid. *Surg. Gynecol. Obstet.* 141:885, 1975.
6. Henderson L.W., Nolph K.D.: Altered permeability of the peritoneal membrane after using hypertonic peritoneal dialysis fluid. *J. Clin. Invest.* 48:992, 1969.
7. Golden G.T., Shaw A.: Primary peritonitis. *Surg. Gynecol. Obstet.* 135:513, 1972.
8. von Recklinghausen F.T.: Zur Fettresorption. *Arch. Pathol. Anat. Physiol.* 26:172, 1863.
9. Allen L., Weatherford T.: Role of fenestrated basement membrane in lymphatic absorption from the peritoneal cavity. *Am. J. Physiol.* 197:551, 1959.
10. Higgins G.M., Beaver M.G., Lemon W.S.: Phrenic neurectomy and peritoneal absorption. *Am. J. Anat.* 45:137, 1930.
11. Yoffey J.M., Courtice F.C.: *Lymphatics, Lymph and Lymphoid Tissue.* Cambridge, Mass., Howard Press, 1956.
12. Fowler G.R.: Diffuse septic peritonitis, with special reference to a new method of treatment, namely, the elevated head and trunk posture, to facilitate drainage into the pelvis: With a report of nine consecutive cases of recovery. *Med. Rec.* 57:617, 1900.
13. Last M., Kurtz L., Stein T.A., et al.: Effect of PEEP on the rate of thoracic duct lymph flow and clearance of bacteria from the peritoneal cavity. *Am. J. Surg.* 145:126, 1983.
14. Autio V.: The spread of intraperitoneal infection. *Acta Chir. Scand.* [Suppl.] 321:1, 1964.
15. Altemeier W.A., Culbertson W.R., Fullen W.D., et al.: Intraabdominal abscesses. *Am. J. Surg.* 125:70, 1973.
16. Shipley P.G., Cunningham R.S.: Studies on the absorption from serous cavities: I. The omentum as a factor in absorption from the peritoneal cavity. *Am. J. Physiol.* 40:75, 1916.
17. Goldsmith H.S., Griffith A.L., Kupferman A., et al.: Lipid angiogenic factor from omentum. *J.A.M.A.* 252:2034, 1984.
18. Watters W.B., Buck R.C.: Scanning electron microscopy of mesothelial regeneration in the rat. *Lab. Invest.* 26:604, 1972.
19. Janik J.S., Apkarian R., Nagarah H.S., et al.: An ultrastructural study of enteric serosa after surgical management. *Surg. Gynecol. Obstet.* 154:491, 1982.
20. Opie E.L.: Inflammation in serous cavities: Definition and measurement. *Arch. Pathol.* 78:1, 1964.
21. Ahrenholz D.H., Simmons R.L.: Fibrin in peritonitis: I. Beneficial and adverse effects of fibrin in experimental *E. coli* peritonitis. *Surgery* 88:41, 1980.
22. Hau T., Payne W.P., Simmons R.L.: Fibrinolytic activity of the peritoneum during experimental peritonitis. *Surg. Gynecol. Obstet.* 148:415, 1979.
23. Ohlsson K.: Collagenase and elastase released during peritonitis

are complexed by plasma protease inhibitors. *Surgery* 79:652, 1976.

24. Dunn D.L., Rotstein O.D., Simmons R.L.: Fibrin in peritonitis: IV. Synergistic intraperitoneal infection caused by *E. coli* and *B. fragilis* within fibrin clots. *Arch. Surg.* 119:139, 1984.

25. Rosebury T.: *Microorganisms Indigenous to Man.* New York, McGraw-Hill Book Co., 1962.

26. Drasar B.S., Hill M.J. (eds.): *Human Intestinal Flora.* London, Academic Press, 1974.

27. Long J., DeSantis S., State D., et al.: The effect of antisecretagogues on gastric microflora. *Arch. Surg.* 118:1413, 1983.

28. Balows A., DeHann R.H., Dowell V.R., et al. (eds.): *Anaerobic Bacteria: Role in Disease.* Springfield, Ill. Charles C Thomas Publisher, 1974.

29. Dougherty S.H.: Role of enterococcus in intraabdominal sepsis. *Am. J. Surg.* 148:308, 1984.

30. Miles A.A., Miles E.M., Burke J.: The value and the duration of defense reactions of the skin to the primary lodgement of bacteria. *Br. J. Exp. Pathol.* 38:79, 1957.

31. Ahrenholz D.H.: Effect of intraperitoneal fluid on mortality of *Escherichia coli* peritonitis. *Surg. Forum* 30:272, 1979.

32. Ogle C.K., Ogle J.D., Alexander J.W.: Inhibition of bacterial clearance in the guinea pig by fluid-phase C3b. *Arch. Surg.* 119:57, 1984.

33. Ahrenholz D.H., Simmons R.L.: Mixed and synergistic infections, in Simmons R.L., Howard, R.J. (eds.): *Surgical Infectious Diseases.* New York, Appleton-Century-Crofts, 1982.

34. Meleney F., Olpp J., Harvey H., et al.: Peritonitis: II. Synergism of bacteria commonly found in peritoneal exudates. *Arch. Surg.* 25:709, 1932.

35. Onderdonk A., Bartlett J., Louie T., et al.: Microbial synergy in experimental intraabdominal abscesses. *Infect. Immun.* 13:22, 1976.

36. Onderdonk A.B., Kasper D.L., Cisneros R.L., et al.: The capsular polysaccharide of *Bacteroides fragilis* as a virulence factor. *J. Infect. Dis.* 136:82, 1978.

37. Stone H.H., Kolb L.D., Geheber, C.E.: Incidence and significance of intraperitoneal anaerobic bacteria. *Ann. Surg.* 181:705, 1975.

38. Boey J., Wong J., Ong G.B.: Bacteria and septic complications in patients with perforated duodenal ulcers. *Am. J. Surg.* 143:635, 1982.

39. Vincent J., Weil M.H., Puri V., et al.: Circulatory shock associated with purulent peritonitis. *Am. J. Surg.* 142:262, 1981.

40. Siegel J.H., Cerra F.B., Coleman B., et al.: Physiological and metabolic correlations in human sepsis. *Surgery* 86:163, 1979.

41. Parker M.M., Parrillo J.E.: Septic shock: Hemodynamics and pathogenesis. *J.A.M.A.* 250:3324, 1983.

42. Hinshaw L.B.: Overview of endotoxin shock, in Crowley R.A., Trump B.F. (eds.): *Pathophysiology of Shock, Anoxia, and Ischemia.* Baltimore, Williams & Wilkins, 1982, pp. 254–270.

43. MacLean L.D., Mulligan W.G., McLean A.P.H., et al.: Patterns of septic shock in man—a detailed study of 56 patients. *Ann. Surg.* 166:543, 1967.

44. Condon R.E.: Peritonitis and intraabdominal abscesses, in Schwartz S.I. (ed.): *Principles of Surgery,* ed. 3. New York, McGraw-Hill Book Co., 1979.

45. Clowes G.H.A. Jr., Hirsch E., Williams L., et al.: Septic lung and shock lung in man. *Ann. Surg.* 181:681, 1975.

46. Lava J., Rice C.L., Moss G.S., et al.: Pulmonary dysfunction in sepsis: Is pulmonary edema the culprit? *J. Trauma* 22:280, 1982.

47. Craddock P.R., Fehr J., Brigham K.L., et al.: Complement and leukocyte-mediated pulmonary dysfunction in hemodialysis. *N. Engl. J. Med.* 296:769, 1977.

48. Saba T.M., Niehaus G.D., Scovill W.A., et al.: Lung vascular permeability after reversal of fibronectin deficiency in septic sheep. *Ann. Surg.* 198:654, 1983.

49. Kirton O.C., Jones R., Zapol W.M., et al.: The development of a model of subacute lung injury after intra-abdominal infection. *Surgery* 96:384, 1984.

50. Lanser M.E., Saba T.M.: Neutrophil-mediated lung localization

of bacteria: A mechanism for pulmonary injury. *Surgery* 90:473, 1981.

51. Bessey P.Q., Watters J.M., Aoki T.T., et al.: Combined hormonal infusion simulates the metabolic response to injury. *Ann. Surg.* 200:264, 1984.

52. Visner M.S., Cerra F.B., Anderson R.W.: Hemodynamic and metabolic responses to sepsis, in Simmons R.L., Howard R.J. (eds.): *Surgical Infectious Diseases.* New York, Appleton-Century-Crofts, 1982.

53. Baracos V., Rodemann H.P., Dinarello C.A., et al.: Stimulation of muscle protein degradation and prostaglandin E_2 release by leukocytic pyrogen (Interleukin-1). *N. Engl. J. Med.* 308:553, 1983.

54. Solomkin J.S., Jenkins M.K., Nelson R.D., et al.: Neutrophil dysfunction in sepsis: II. Evidence for the role of complement activation products in cellular deactivation. *Surgery* 90:319, 1981.

55. Bohnen J.M., Christou N.V., Chiasson L., et al.: Anergy secondary to sepsis in rats. *Arch. Surg.* 119:117, 1984.

56. Buffone W., Meakins J.L., Christou N.V.: Neutrophil function in surgical patients. *Arch. Surg.* 119:39, 1984.

57. Richards W.O., Scovill W.A., Shin B.: Opsonic fibronectin deficiency in patients with intra-abdominal infection. *Surgery* 94:210, 1983.

58. Scovill W.A., Saba T.M., Blumenstock F.A., et al.: Opsonic alpha-2-surface binding glycoprotein therapy during sepsis. *Ann. Surg.* 188:529, 1978.

59. Cope Z. (ed.): *The Early Diagnosis of the Acute Abdomen.* London, Oxford University Press, 1957.

60. Lucas C.E., Weaver D., Higgins R.F., et al.: Effects of albumin versus non-albumin resuscitation on plasma volume and renal excretory function. *J. Trauma* 18:564, 1978.

61. Spiegel C.A., Malangoni M.A., Condon R.E.: Gas-liquid chromatography for rapid diagnosis of intra-abdominal infection. *Arch. Surg.* 119:28, 1984.

62. Zaske D.E., Cipolle R.J., Rotschafer J.C., et al.: Gentamicin pharmacokinetics in 1,640 patients: Method for control of serum concentrations. *Antimicrob. Agents Chemother.* 21:407, 1982.

63. Nichols R.L., Smith J.W., Fossedal E.M., et al.: Efficacy of parenteral antibiotics in the treatment of experimentally induced intraabdominal sepsis. *Rev. Infect. Dis.* 1:302, 1979.

64. Gemmell C.G., Peterson P.K., Schmeling D., et al.: Antibiotic-induced modification of *Bacteroides fragilis* and its susceptibility to phagocytosis by human polymorphonuclear leukocytes. *Eur. J. Clin. Microbiol.* 2:327, 1983.

65. Dowell V.R. Jr.: Antibiotic-associated colitis. *Hosp. Pract.* 14:75, 1979.

66. Joiner K., Lowe B., Dzink J., et al.: Comparative efficacy of 10 antimicrobial agents in experimental infections with *Bacteroides fragilis. J. Infect. Dis.* 145:561, 1982.

67. Ralph E.D., Kirby W.M.M.: Unique bactericidal action of metronidazole against *Bacteroides fragilis* and *Clostridium perfringens. Antimicrob. Agents Chemother.* 8:409, 1975.

68. Beard C.M., Noller K.L., O'Fallon W.M., et al.: Lack of evidence for cancer due to use of metronidazole. *N. Engl. J. Med.* 301:519, 1979.

69. Smith J.A., Skidmore A.G., Forward A.D., et al.: Prospective, randomized, double-blind comparison of metronidazole and tobramycin with clindamycin and tobramycin in the treatment of intra-abdominal sepsis. *Ann. Surg.* 192:213, 1980.

70. Horvitz R.A., Von Graevenitz A.: A clinical study of the role of enterococci as sole agents of wound and tissue infection. *Yale J. Biol. Med.* 50:391, 1977.

71. Berne T.V., Yellin A.W., Appleman M.D., et al.: Antibiotic management of surgically treated gangrenous or perforated appendicitis: Comparison of gentamicin and clindamycin versus cefamandole versus cefoperazone. *Am. J. Surg.* 144:8, 1982.

72. Stone H.H., Geheber C.E., Kolb L.D., et al.: Clinical comparison of cefotaxime versus the combination of gentamicin plus clindamycin in the treatment of peritonitis and similar polymicrobial soft-tissue surgical sepsis. *Clin. Ther.* 4(suppl. A):67, 1981.

73. Schentag J.J., Wels P.B., Reitberg D.P., et al.: A randomized

clinical trial of moxalactam alone versus tobramycin plus clindamycin in abdominal sepsis. *Ann. Surg.* 198:35, 1983.

74. Stone H.H., Strom P.R., Fabian T.C., et al.: Third-generation cephalosporins for polymicrobial surgical sepsis. *Arch. Surg.* 118:193, 1983.

75. Harding G.K.M., Buckwold F.J., Ronald A.R., et al.: Prospective, randomized comparative study of clindamycin, chloramphenicol and ticarcillin, each in combination with gentamicin, in therapy for intra-abdominal and female genital tract sepsis. *J. Infect. Dis.* 142:384, 1980.

76. Solomkin J.S., Meakins J.L. Jr., Allo M.D., et al.: Antibiotic trials in intra-abdominal infections: A critical evaluation of study design and outcome reporting. *Ann. Surg.* 200:29, 1984.

77. Louie T.J., Onderdonk A.B., Gorbach S.L., et al.: Therapy for experimental intraabdominal sepsis: Comparison of four cephalosporins with clindamycin plus gentamicin. *J. Infect. Dis.* 135:518, 1977.

78. Joehl R.J., Rasbach D.A., Ballard J.O., et al.: Moxalactam: Evaluation of clinical bleeding in patients with abdominal infection. *Arch. Surg.* 118:1259, 1983.

79. Neu H.C.: Mechanisms of bacterial resistance to antimicrobial agents, with particular reference to cefotaxime and other B-lactam compounds. *Rev. Infect. Dis.* 4(suppl.):S288, 1982.

80. Thadepalli H., Gorbach S.L., Bartlett J.G.: Apparent failure of chloramphenicol in the treatment of anaerobic infections. *Obstet. Gynecol. Surg.* 33:334, 1978.

81. Solomkin J.S., Flohr A.B., Quie P.G., et al.: The role of *Candida* in intraperitoneal infections. *Surgery* 88:524, 1980.

82. Rosato E.F., Oram-Smith J.C., Mullis W.F., et al.: Peritoneal lavage treatment in experimental peritonitis. *Ann. Surg.* 175:384, 1972.

83. Rambo W.M.: Irrigation of the peritoneal cavity with cephalothin. *Am. J. Surg.* 123:192, 1972.

84. Smith E.B.: Adjuvant therapy of generalized peritonitis with intraperitoneally administered cephalothin. *Surg. Gynecol. Obstet.* 136:441, 1973.

85. Hau T., Nishikawa R., Phuangsab A.: Irrigation of the peritoneal cavity and local antibiotics in the treatment of peritonitis. *Surg. Gynecol. Obstet.* 156:25, 1983.

86. Lally K.P., Trettin J.C., Torma M.J.: Adjunctive antibiotic lavage in experimental peritonitis. *Surg. Gynecol. Obstet.* 156:605, 1983.

87. Halasz N.A.: Wound infection and topical antibiotics. *Arch. Surg.* 112:1240, 1977.

88. Sindelar W.F., Mason G.R.: Intraperitoneal irrigation with povidone-iodine solution for the prevention of intra-abdominal abscesses in the bacterially contaminated abdomen. *Surg. Gynecol. Obstet.* 148:409, 1979.

89. Pickard R.G.: Treatment of peritonitis with pre- and postoperative irrigation of the peritoneal cavity with noxythiolin solution. *Br. J. Surg.* 59:642, 1972.

90. Browne M.K., MacKenzie M., Doyle P.J.: A controlled trial of taurolin in established bacterial peritonitis. *Surg. Gynecol. Obstet.* 146:721, 1978.

91. Ahrenholz D.H., Simmons, R.L.: Povidone-iodine in peritonitis: I. Adverse effects of local instillation in experimental *E. coli* peritonitis. *J. Surg. Res.* 26:458, 1979.

92. DeVincenti F.C., Cohn I. Jr.: Prolonged administration of intraperitoneal kanamycin in the treatment of peritonitis. *Am. Surg.* 37:177, 1971.

93. Bushan C., Mital V.K., Elhence I.P.: Continuous postoperative peritoneal lavage in diffuse peritonitis using balanced saline antibiotic solution. *Int. Surg.* 60:526, 1975.

94. Washington B.C., Villalba M.R., Lauter C.B., et al.: Cefamandole-erythromycin-heparin peritoneal irrigation: An adjunct to the surgical treatment of diffuse bacterial peritonitis. *Surgery* 94:576, 1983.

95. Silenas R., O'Keefe P., Gelbart S., et al.: Mechanical effectiveness of closed peritoneal irrigation in peritonitis. *Am. J. Surg.* 145:371, 1983.

96. Wouters D.B., Krom R.A.F., Slooff M.J.H., et al.: The use of Marlex mesh in patients with generalized peritonitis and multiple organ system failure. *Surg. Gynecol. Obstet.* 156:609, 1983.

97. Lally K.P., Torma M.J.: The Hubbard tank as an adjunct to drainage in overwhelming intra-abdominal sepsis. *Arch. Surg.* 118:989, 1983.

98. Kendrick J.H., Casali R.E., Lang N.P., et al.: The complicated septic abdominal wound. *Arch. Surg.* 117:464, 1982.

99. Stone H.H., Fabian T.C., Turkleson M.L., et al.: Management of acute full-thickness losses of the abdominal wall. *Ann. Surg.* 193:612, 1981.

100. Voyles C.R., Richardson J.D., Bland K.I., et al.: Emergency abdominal wall reconstruction with polypropylene mesh. *Ann. Surg.* 194:219, 1981.

101. Jenkins S.D., Klamer T.W., Parteka J.J., et al.: A comparison of prosthetic materials used to repair abdominal wall defects. *Surgery* 94:392, 1983.

102. Steinberg D.: On leaving the peritoneal cavity open in acute generalized suppurative peritonitis. *Am. J. Surg.* 137:216, 1979.

103. Duff J.H., Moffat J.: Abdominal sepsis managed by leaving abdomen open. *Surgery* 90:774, 1981.

104. Maetani S., Tove T.: Open peritoneal drainage as effective treatment of advanced peritonitis. *Surgery* 90:804, 1981.

105. Richardson J.D., Polk H.C. Jr.: Newer adjunctive treatments for peritonitis. *Surgery* 90:917, 1981.

106. Polk H.C., Fry D.E.: Radical peritoneal debridement for established peritonitis: The results of a prospective randomized clinical trial. *Ann. Surg.* 192:350, 1980.

107. Hudspeth A.S.: Radical surgical debridement in the treatment of advanced generalized bacterial peritonitis. *Arch. Surg.* 110:1233, 1975.

108. Haller J.A. Jr., Shaker I.J., Danahoo J.S., et al.: Peritoneal drainage versus non-drainage for generalized peritonitis from ruptured appendicitis in children: A prospective study. *Ann. Surg.* 177:595, 1973.

109. Chu C., Williams D.F.: Effects of physical configuration and chemical structure of suture materials on bacterial adhesion. *Am. J. Surg.* 147:197, 1984.

110. Sharp W.V., Belden T.A., King P.H., et al.: Suture resistance to infection. *Surgery* 91:61, 1982.

111. Bucknall T.E., Ellis H.: Abdominal wound closure—a comparison of monofilament nylon and polyglycolic acid. *Surgery* 89:672, 1981.

112. McIlrath D.C., van Heerden J.A., Edis A.J., et al.: Closure of abdominal incisions with subcutaneous catheters. *Surgery* 80:411, 1976.

113. Stillman R.M., Marino C.A., Seligman S.J.: Skin staples in potentially contaminated wounds. *Arch. Surg.* 119:821, 1984.

114. Galland R.B., Heine K.J., Trachtenberg L.S., et al.: Reduction of surgical wound infection rates in contaminated wounds treated with antiseptics combined with systemic antibiotics: An experimental study. *Surgery* 91:329, 1982.

115. Sherlock D.J., Ward A., Holl-Allen R.T.J.: Combined preoperative antibiotic therapy and intraoperative topical povidone-iodine. *Arch. Surg.* 119:909, 1984.

116. Zamora J.L.: Povidone-iodine and wound infection. *Surgery* 93:121, 1984.

117. Hau T., Haaga J.R., Aeder M.I.: Pathophysiology, diagnosis, and treatment of abdominal abscesses. *Curr. Probl. Surg.* 21(7):1, 1984.

118. Simmons R.L. (ed.): *Topics in Intraabdominal Surgical Infection.* Norwalk, Conn., Appleton-Century-Crofts, 1982.

119. Condon R.E., Gorbach S.L. (eds.): *Surgical Infections: Selective Antibiotic Therapy.* Baltimore, Williams & Wilkins, 1981.

120. Stafford E.S., Sprong D.H. Jr.: The mortality from acute appendicitis in the Johns Hopkins Hospital. *J.A.M.A.* 115:1242, 1940.

121. Berne C.J., Pattison A.C.: Diverticulitis of the colon. *Calif. West Med.* 52:225, 1940.

122. Serrano A., Dahl E.P., Rubin R.H., et al.: Eclectic drainage of subphrenic abscesses. *Arch. Surg.* 119:942, 1984.

123. Gibson D.M., Feliciano D.V., Mattox K.L., et al.: Intraabdominal abscess after penetrating abdominal trauma. *Am. J. Surg.* 142:699, 1981.

124. Dellinger E.P., Oreskovich M.R., Wertz M.J., et al.: Risk of

infection following laparotomy for penetrating abdominal injury. *Arch. Surg.* 119:20, 1984.

125. Wang S.M.S., Wilson S.E.: Subphrenic abscess: The new epidemiology. *Arch. Surg.* 112:934, 1977.

126. Klaue P., Eckert P., Kern E.: Incidental splenectomy: Early and late postoperative complications. *Am. J. Surg.* 138:296, 1979.

127. Halliday P.: The surgical management of subphrenic abscess: An historical study. *Aust. N.Z. J. Surg.* 45:235, 1975.

128. DeCosse J.J., Pulin T.L., Fox P.S., et al.: Subphrenic abscess. *Surg. Gynecol. Obstet.* 138:841, 1974.

129. Doberneck R.C., Mittelman J.: Reappraisal of the problems of intra-abdominal abscess. *Surg. Gynecol. Obstet.* 154:875, 1982.

130. Bonfils-Roberts E.A., Barone J.E., Nealon T.F. Jr.: Treatment of subphrenic abscess. *Surg. Clin. North Am.* 55:1361, 1975.

131. Halliday P., Loewenthal J.: Subphrenic abscess. *Aust. N.Z. J. Surg.* 33:260, 1964.

132. Carter R., Brewer L.A. III: Subphrenic abscess: A thoracoabdominal clinical complex. *Am. J. Surg.* 108:165, 1964.

133. Sherman N.J., Davis J.R., Jesseph J.E.: Subphrenic abscess: A continuing hazard. *Am. J. Surg.* 117:117, 1969.

134. Boyd D.P.: The intrathoracic complications of subphrenic abscess. *J. Thorac. Cardiovasc. Surg.* 38:771, 1959.

135. Halasz N.A.: Subphrenic abscess: Myths and facts. *J.A.M.A.* 214:724, 1970.

136. Lennard E.S., Dellinger E.P., Wertz M.J., et al.: Implications of leukocytosis and fever at conclusion of antibiotic therapy for intra-abdominal sepsis. *Ann. Surg.* 195:19, 1982.

137. Freischlag J., Busuttil R.W.: The value of postoperative fever evaluation. *Surgery* 94:358, 1983.

138. O'Reilly M.J., Reddick E.J., Black W., et al.: Sepsis from sinusitis in nasotracheally intubated patients. *Am. J. Surg.* 147:601, 1984.

139. Coon W.W.: Diagnostic celiotomy for fever of undetermined origin. *Surg. Gynecol. Obstet.* 157:467, 1983.

140. Martin L.F., Max M.H., Polk H.C. Jr.: Failure of gastric pH control by antacids or cimetidine in the critically ill: A valid sign of sepsis. *Surgery* 88:59, 1980.

141. Stothert J.C. Jr., Simonowitz D.A., Dellinger E.P., et al.: Randomized prospective evaluation of cimetidine and antacid control of gastric pH in the critically ill. *Ann. Surg.* 192:169, 1980.

142. Ing A.F.M., McLean A.P.H., Meakins J.L.: Multiple-organism bacteremia in the surgical intensive care unit: A sign of intraperitoneal sepsis. *Surgery* 90:779, 1981.

143. Fry D.E., Garrison R.M., and Polk, H.C., Jr.: Clinical implications in *Bacteroides* bacteremia. *Surg. Gynecol. Obstet.* 149:189, 1979.

144. Bryan C.S., Reynolds K.L., Kirkhart B., et al.: *Bacteroides* bacteremia: Analysis of 142 episodes from one metropolitan area. *Arch. Surg.* 119:894, 1984.

145. Schentag J.J., O'Keeffe D., Marmion M., et al.: C-reactive protein as an indicator of infection relapse in patients with abdominal sepsis. *Arch. Surg.* 119:300, 1984.

146. Aasen A.O., Smith-Erichsen N., Amundsen E.: Plasma kallikrein-kinin system in septicemia. *Arch. Surg.* 118:343, 1983.

147. Harbrecht P.J., Garrison R.N., Fry D.E.: Early urgent relaparotomy. *Arch. Surg.* 119:369, 1984.

148. Taylor K.J.W., Wassan J.F.M., Graff C.D., et al.: Accuracy of grey-scale ultra-sound diagnosis of abdominal and pelvic abscesses in 220 patients. *Lancet* 1:83, 1978.

149. Daffner R.H., Halber M.D., Morgan C.L., et al.: Computed tomography in the diagnosis of intra-abdominal abscesses. *Ann. Surg.* 189:29, 1979.

150. Ascher N.L., Ahrenholz D.H., Simmons R.L., et al.: Indium-111 autologous tagged leukocytes in the diagnosis of intraperitoneal sepsis. *Arch. Surg.* 114:386, 1979.

151. Sugerman H.J., Tatum J.L., Hirsch J.I., et al.: Gamma scintigraphic localization of platelets labeled with indium 111 in a focus of infection. *Arch. Surg.* 118:185, 1983.

152. Richardson J.D., Flint L.M., Polk H.C. Jr.: Peritoneal lavage: A useful diagnostic adjunct for peritonitis. *Surgery* 94:826, 1983.

153. Ochsner A.: Reappraisal: The value of extraserous drainage in subphrenic abscesses. *Surgery* 43:319, 1958.

154. Glick P.L., Pellegrini C.A., Stein S., et al.: Abdominal abscess. *Arch. Surg.* 118:646, 1983.

155. Johnson W.C., Gerzof S.G., Robbins A.H., et al.: Treatment of abdominal abscesses: Comparative evaluation of operative drainage versus percutaneous catheter drainage guided by computed tomography or ultrasound. *Ann. Surg.* 194:510, 1981.

156. Glass C.A., Cohn I. Jr.: Drainage of intraabdominal abscesses: A comparison of surgical and computerized tomography guided catheter drainage. *Am. J. Surg.* 147:315, 1984.

157. Gerzof S.G.: Surgical and computerized tomography guided drainage for intraabdominal abscess. *Am. J. Surg.* 147:426, 1984.

158. Aeder M.I., Wellman J.L., Haaga J.R., et al.: Role of surgical and percutaneous drainage in the treatment of abdominal abscesses. *Arch. Surg.* 118:273, 1983.

159. Pruett T.L., Rotstein O.D., Crass J., et al.: Percutaneous aspiration and drainage for suspected abdominal infection. *Surgery* 96:731, 1984.

160. Gerzof S.H., Johnson W.C., Robbins A.H., et al.: Percutaneous drainage of infected pancreatic pseudocysts. *Arch. Surg.* 119:888, 1984.

161. Sinanan M., Maier R.V., Carrico C.J.: Laparotomy for intra-abdominal sepsis in patients in an intensive care unit. *Arch. Surg.* 119:652, 1984.

162. Hinsdale J.G., Jaffe B.M.: Re-operation for intra-abdominal sepsis: Indications and results in modern critical care setting. *Ann. Surg.* 199:31, 1984.

163. Bohnen J., Boulanger M., Meakins J.L., et al.: Prognosis in generalized peritonitis. *Arch. Surg.* 118:285, 1983.

164. Fry D.E., Garrison R.N., Heitsch R.C., et al.: Determinants of death in patients with intraabdominal abscess. *Surgery* 88:517, 1980.

165. Pine R.W., Wertz M.J., Lennard E.S., et al.: Determinants of organ malfunction or death in patients with intra-abdominal abscess. *Arch. Surg.* 118:242, 1983.

166. Dawson J.L.: A study of some factors affecting the mortality rate in diffuse peritonitis. *Gut* 4:368, 1963.

167. Stephen M., Loewenthal J.: Generalized infective peritonitis. *Surg. Gynecol. Obstet.* 147:231, 1978.

168. Bradley E.L., Isaacs J.: Appendiceal abscess revisited. *Arch. Surg.* 113:130, 1978.

169. Donovan A.J., Vinson T.L., Maulsby G.O., et al. Selective treatment of duodenal ulcer with perforation. *Ann. Surg.* 189:627, 1979.

170. Baue A.E.: Multiple, progressive, or sequential systems failure: A syndome of the 1970s. *Arch. Surg.* 110:779, 1975.

171. Fry D.E., Pearlstein L., Fulton R.L., et al.: Multiple system organ failure: The role of uncontrolled infection. *Arch. Surg.* 115:136, 1980.

172. Cerra F.B., Border J.R., McMenamy R.H., et al.: Multiple systems organ failure, in Crowley R.A., Trump B.F. (eds.): *Pathophysiology of Shock, Anoxia, and Ischemia.* Baltimore, Williams & Wilkins, 1982, pp. 254–270.

173. Ferraris V.A.: Exploratory laparotomy for potential abdominal sepsis in patients with multiple-organ failure. *Arch. Surg.* 118:1130, 1983.

174. Bartlett R.H., Dechert R.E., Mault J.R., et al.: Measurement of metabolism in multiple organ failure. *Surgery* 92:771, 1982.

175. Ozawa K., Aoyama H., Yasuda K., et al.: Metabolic abnormalities associated with postoperative organ failure. *Arch. Surg.* 118:1245, 1983.

7

Surgical Treatment of Pediatric Digestive Disease

JOHN R. LILLY, M.D.
GERALD M. HAASE, M.D.
FRITZ M. KARRER, M.D.

IN THIS CHAPTER, we would like to cover the entire field of pediatric surgical digestive disease; however, space constraints prohibit an in-depth analysis of all topics. Emphasis is placed on those lesions that either are unique to children or have manifestations significantly different from those of their adult counterparts. Diseases that occur in both age groups with similar manifestations, e.g., peptic ulcer disease, cholelithiasis, achalasia, are mentioned briefly or only in passing.

The majority of gastroenterologic diseases in the infant are congenital; intestinal atresia, Meckel's diverticulum, and malrotation are examples. In addition, several afflictions (of uncertain pathogenesis) are seen almost exclusively in the child. Therefore, lesions such as hypertrophic pyloric stenosis, intussusception, necrotizing enterocolitis, and biliary atresia are covered in some depth. On the other hand, GI cancer and colonic diverticulitis are rare in children and not discussed in this chapter.

Finally, we advance our surgical bias for diseases which may begin in childhood and continue into adulthood. Since the aim is to achieve a result which will be complication-free for 70 years, performing a more definitive, albeit radical, procedure is often elected. For example, rather than recommend ileostomy for the adolescent with ulcerative colitis, we prefer whenever feasible to perform an ileorectal pull-through operation, despite the significant early postoperative complications of the latter procedure. Although technically more demanding, we believe that a choledochal cyst should be completely resected rather than simply drained, because of the remote complications of cholangitis, anastomotic stricture, and malignancy. Esophageal varices are preferably treated by endosclerosis rather than risk the development of hepatic encephalopathy and liver impairment consequent to a portosystemic shunt operation. In brief, when surgical therapy is chosen in the child, the lifetime implications are taken into account.

This work was supported in part by a grant (RR-69) from the General Clinical Research Centers Program of the Division of Research Resources, National Institutes of Health.

The chapter is divided by organ systems, beginning with the liver and bile ducts and concluding with the anus.

THE LIVER AND BILE DUCTS

In infants and children, the major surgical lesions of the liver and bile ducts are: (1) biliary atresia; (2) choledochal cyst; (3) perforation of the extrahepatic bile ducts; and (4) cholecystitis and cholelithiasis.

Biliary Atresia

Biliary atresia is a condition in which the extrahepatic bile ducts are not patent. The disease has been arbitrarily divided into a "correctable" type, in which the proximal extrahepatic bile ducts are patent and the distal ducts occluded, and a "noncorrectable" type, where the proximal extrahepatic ducts are occluded.[1] The sclerotic process in biliary atresia is panductular, afflicting the intrahepatic biliary tree as well as the extrahepatic system. Ten to fifteen percent of patients with biliary atresia have associated anomalies[2]; e.g., absent inferior vena cava, preduodenal portal vein, intestinal malrotation and polysplenia, suggesting that the developmental insult in biliary atresia may occur early in embryonic life.

Jaundice in the first months of life may be on a mechanical, obstructive basis or on a hepatic parenchymal basis (Table 7–1). Serologic, radioisotopic, and ultrasonographic investigations will differentiate most cases of surgical obstruction from parenchymal jaundice, but in a small group of patients operative cholangiography is necessary. Cholangiography is done via the gallbladder and should demonstrate continuity of the biliary tree between liver and duodenum. If biliary continuity cannot be demonstrated or the gallbladder contains "white bile," full exploration of the extrahepatic biliary tree should be undertaken.

For correctable biliary atresia, a Roux-en-Y intestinal anastomosis to the proximal patent bile duct is recommended. Operation is not curative, and most infants have some degree of residual liver damage.

The great majority of patients with biliary atresia have non-

TABLE 7–1.—JAUNDICE IN INFANCY

SURGICAL	MEDICAL
Biliary atresia	Infectious
Choledochal cyst	Viral (cytomegalovirus,
Perforation of the bile ducts	herpes, rubella)
Biliary hypoplasia (Alagille's	Others (*Listeria,*
syndrome)*	toxoplasmosis,
Inspissated bile syndrome	syphilis)
Choledocholithiasis	Metabolic (α_1-antitrypsin,
	cystic fibrosis,
	galactosemia)
	Neonatal hepatitis
	Hemolytic disease
	Sepsis
	Hyperalimentation

*Anatomical defect, not surgically correctable.

patent bile ducts at the liver hilus, noncorrectable biliary atresia. About 15% of this group have residual patency of the distal biliary tree, i.e., gallbladder, cystic duct, and common bile duct.[3] In either case, bile flow from the liver is impossible without surgical intervention.

In the standard operation, hepatic portoenterostomy, the extrahepatic bile ducts are removed and bile drainage established by anastomosis of an intestinal conduit to the transected duct at the liver hilus. Operative success depends on the presence of microscopic biliary structures at the liver hilus and is inversely proportional to the age of the patient. The diminutive biliary structures drain bile into the approximated intestinal conduit and, in time, an autoanastomosis between the intestinal and ductal epithelial elements occurs. Most methods of biliary reconstruction temporarily exteriorize the conduit to help control postoperative cholangitis (Fig 7–1).

In the presence of a still patent gallbladder, cystic duct, and distal common duct, these extant natural structures are used for biliary reconstruction rather than an intestinal conduit. The common hepatic duct is resected, and the gallbladder is opened and anastomosed to the transected duct at the liver hilus. This procedure almost completely eliminates the risk of postoperative cholangitis.

Most surgeons report successful bile drainage in about half of the infants operated upon under 4 months old and success may approach 80% in infants less than 10 weeks old. Of the 185 patients treated by Kasai's hepatic portoenterostomy operation since 1973 in Denver and Washington, D.C./New York City, 90 are alive for at least one year and as long as ten years after operation. Twenty-three of these 90 survivors are alive at five or more years from operation (R.P.A. Altman and J.R. Lilly, personal communication, 1985).

Choledochal Cyst

Popular classification of choledochal cyst is in three types.[4] Type 2 (diverticulum of the common bile duct) and type 3 (intraduodenal duct cyst) are extremely rare and will not be discussed here. The classic features of type 1 choledochal cyst are cystic dilation of the common bile duct, partial obstruction of the terminal common bile duct, and normal liver paren-

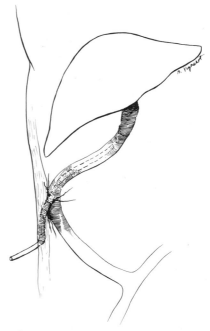

Fig 7–1.—Catheter decompression of bilioenteric conduit after a Kasai et al.[3] hepatic portoenterostomy operation for biliary atresia. For the first three to six months after operation, the conduit is exteriorized as a double-barreled enterostomy. Subsequently, the stomas are resected and direct continuity with the GI tract reestablished. Catheter decompression as shown is employed for an additional three months to facilitate management of cholangitis.

chyma. Microscopically, the cyst wall is almost exclusively composed of fibrous connective tissue, and the mucosal lining is ulcerated or absent.

The classic triad of abdominal pain, jaundice, and abdominal mass occurs in only one third of patients, primarily in older children. The most common presenting symptom in most children is mild, intermittent jaundice, often overlooked for months to years. Additional early manifestations include cholangitis and pancreatitis. Ultrasonography is the best initial investigational method.

Total excision of the cyst and mucosa-to-mucosa anastomosis by Roux-en-Y choledochojejunostomy is the treatment of choice. Anastomotic drainage of the cyst into the duodenum or jejunum has a high incidence of late anastomotic stricture, recurrent cholangitis, and the risk of cyst malignancy. Cyst excision is easier and safer by approaching the cyst from its inside and leaving a rim of the posterior wall behind (overlying the hepatic artery and portal vein).[5] If the diagnosis is made early and biliary obstruction corrected, reversal of minor degrees of hepatic damage is anticipated.

Choledochal cyst may also present in the first months of life. In this age the presenting symptom is almost always obstructive jaundice, since complete biliary obstruction is usually present. The infant, therefore, enters into the diagnostic mix of infantile jaundice, the work-up of which is described under the section on biliary atresia. Surgical treatment is identical to that outlined for choledochal cyst in the older child, i.e., complete operative resection and biliary reconstruction by choledochoenterostomy (Roux-en-Y).[6]

Idiopathic Perforation of the Extrahepatic Bile Ducts

The malformation is rare. Afflicted infants present in the first 3 to 9 months of life with jaundice, ascites, and occasionally fever. The location of the ductal perforation is invariably at the union of the common bile and cystic ducts, suggesting a congenital weakness in this area. At operation, sterile bilious ascites and a bile-filled pseudocyst are usually found.[7] The operative cholangiogram (via the gallbladder) is sometimes misleading in that phantoms may be seen in the distal common duct, e.g., stenosis or calculi. In most cases this merely represents bilious sludge, which resolves spontaneously. The lesion is self-limited and seals several weeks after operation. Therefore, treatment is simple drainage of the area of perforation.[8] Residual hepatobiliary disease is rare.

Gallbladder Disease

CHOLECYSTITIS AND CHOLELITHIASIS.—Gallstone disease in children is commonly believed to be predominantly due to hemolytic anemia, e.g., spherocytosis, sickle cell disease, thalassemia. In reality, the majority of cases, about 80%,[9] are nonhemolytic. The pathogenesis is obscure in most patients with nonhemolytic gallstone disease. Congenital malformations are occasionally incriminated.[10] Symptoms are often vague or are absent altogether. Except in adolescents, fatty food intolerance is unusual. Parenthetically, for reasons that are still unclear, gallbladder disease is becoming more common in adolescents. Because of the ill-defined symptomatology, diagnosis is often delayed or mistaken as appendicitis. In contrast to adults, the majority of gallbladder calculi are radiopaque.[11] Surgical treatment is as described in chapter 19.

ACUTE HYDROPS.—Acute distention of the gallbladder occurs infrequently in children and usually is secondary to a systemic infectious disease. Most patients do not require operation unless gangrene supervenes.

ACALCULOUS CHOLECYSTITIS.—Acute inflammation of the gallbladder in children may occur during a severe intercurrent illness. The attack is characterized by pain and tenderness in the upper right abdomen, fever, and leukocytosis. Cholecystectomy should be done.

PORTAL HYPERTENSION

Portal hypertension in most children is due to extrahepatic obstruction of portal flow. Thrombosis of the portal vein may be secondary to perinatal omphalitis, umbilical catheterization, or intra-abdominal sepsis. The portal vein and often its tributaries undergo a cavernomatous transformation. Intrahepatic obstruction is a less frequent cause of portal hypertension. Cirrhosis as an end stage of chronic, active viral hepatitis or mononucleosis and, recently, of biliary atresia that has been alleviated but not cured account for most cases of intrahepatic obstruction of portal flow.

For reasons that have never been clearly stated, esophageal variceal hemorrhage in many children with portal hypertension appears to be of limited duration; i.e., the frequency and severity of hemorrhagic episodes decrease after adolescence. For many children, therefore, surgical measures which permanently eradicate esophageal varices may be unnecessary and, in fact, those which do so by reduction in hepatic portal flow are probably actually harmful.[12]

Most conventional surgical temporizing procedures for variceal hemorrhage are of such limited benefit as to be basically ineffective. Splenectomy and direct variceal ligation are examples. Portosystemic shunt operations (portocaval, mesocaval, splenorenal) have been the standard treatment for variceal hemorrhage in children. Technically, the relatively small caliber of vessels predisposes to shunt thrombosis. On the other hand, the penalties for a successful shunt may be hepatic encephalopathy and impairment of hepatic function.[12] The distal splenorenal shunt theoretically should preserve hepatopedal flow and thus prevent the complications of encephalopathy and the portoprival state. Unfortunately, the surgical division of the portal circuit into two separate compartments by this technique is, from a child's standpoint, of relatively short duration. Eventually the high-pressure "hepatic compartment" decompresses itself into the low-pressure "splenic compartment" in effect, transforming itself into a standard portosystemic shunt.

Because of these overt and latent shunt complications, for the past five years we have treated all children with esophageal variceal hemorrhage by endosclerosis (Fig 7–2).[13] Our approach has been to do serial injections until all varices are eradicated. Subsequently, esophagoscopy is done periodically to determine recurrence and for endosclerosis, if new varices are developing. Recurrent hemorrhage has not been encountered in the follow-up for as long as 6½ years.

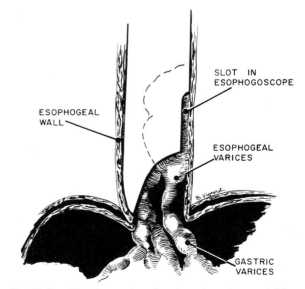

Fig 7–2.—Esophageal endosclerosis using a rigid, specially slotted esophagoscope. A distal esophageal varix is "trapped" in the slot and directly injected with sodium morrhuate. Retrograde thrombosis of incontinuity gastric varices often occurs.

THE PANCREAS

Pancreatitis

Acute pancreatitis in childhood is unusual. Afflicted children are usually diagnosed as having acute appendicitis. Pancreatitis may occur from blunt trauma or after a febrile illness associated with vomiting and secondary dehydration. Also, steroid therapy, renal disease, and familial aminoacidemia and hyperlipidemia predispose to pancreatitis.[14] Biliary tract disease, on the other hand, is an unusual cause of pancreatitis in children except, as alluded to earlier, in some cases of choledochal cyst. Pancreatitis induced by mumps is usually quite rare and mild. Surgical intervention is done for complications; e.g., resection of necrotic tissue, drainage of a pancreatic abscess or pseudocyst. The indications for operation and types of surgical procedures employed are the same as those described for adults detailed elsewhere in this book.

Pancreatic Cysts

Pancreatic cysts may be classified as: (1) congenital, (2) retention, (3) neoplastic, and (4) pseudocysts.[15]

CONGENITAL CYSTS.—Congenital cysts are usually unilocular, lined with epithelium, most common in the body and tail, and seldom give rise to symptoms, unless there is extrinsic pressure on neighboring organs. Surgical treatment is total excision (with distal pancreatectomy) or internal drainage for cysts located in the head of the pancreas.

RETENTION CYSTS.—Retention cysts of the pancreas are a result of ductal obstruction. They contain pancreatic enzymes. Treatment is excision or Roux-en-Y jejunostomy, again depending on location.

NEOPLASTIC CYSTS.—Papillary neoplastic cysts are premalignant and rare in children.

PSEUDOCYSTS.—In children, the majority of pancreatic pseudocysts are caused by trauma. A pseudocyst is composed of inflammatory tissue, has no epithelial lining and often communicates with the pancreatic duct system. Its usual location is in the lesser sac. Symptoms are epigastric pain and anorexia. A mass is usually palpable. Ultrasonography is diagnostic, and CT may aid further in localization.

Treatment is cystogastrostomy in most cases. If not strategically located (adherent to the stomach), Roux-en-Y cystojejunostomy or excision may be done. Often in traumatic pancreatitis, small pseudocysts may be followed (to disappearance).

Pancreatic Neoplasms

Malignant tumors of the pancreas in infants and children are usually carcinoma and extremely rare.[16]

Nesidioblastosis

Nesidioblastosis is primarily a condition of infancy (the first six months of life) and is one of the prime causes of hypoglycemia in the neonate. There is inappropriate insulin secretion. The diagnosis is based on the histologic appearance of a diffuse scattering of β cells among ductile and acinar tissues.

The hypoglycemic manifestations are multiple including frank seizures, lethargy, and twitching. Some patients are asymptomatic until an intercurrent infection or some other event prevents oral intake. Diagnosis is suggested by insulin levels greater than 10 μU/ml when the blood glucose is lower than 50 mg/dl. Fasting insulin levels are frequently greater than 20 μU/ml. Absolute blood glucose levels are not correlated with symptoms, however.

Prolonged medical treatment (diazoxide or somatostatin) may control the hyperinsulinemia. Failure to maintain blood glucose levels at normal levels results in mental retardation, a not infrequent consequence of conservative obstinacy. As stated by Welch:[15]

The numerous reports of poor outcome in hypoglycemia of infancy unresponsive to medical management, the poor ability to detect hyperinsulinism and rule out other endocrine dysfunction and the rapidly growing evidence of specific histopathology in hyperinsulin states in infancy, especially nesidioblastosis, suggest that surgical exploration and partial pancreatectomy should be performed early in these children rather than as a last resort.

Preparation for operation includes maintaining blood glucose levels above 50 mg/dl; parenteral glucose may need to be given at 0.5 gm/kg/hour. Most patients are cured by an operation in which 85%–90% of the pancreas is removed.[17] The risk of diabetes mellitus is relatively small. The spleen is preserved at operation.

Islet Cell Adenoma

Islet cell adenoma occurs uncommonly in children; only about 50 cases have been reported. Selective arteriography may identify the tumor.[18] If found in the body or tail of the pancreas, excision of the tumor is feasible; if not, a subtotal (85%–90%) resection of the gland is done.

MESENTERIC CYSTS

Mesenteric cysts are derived from lymphatic spaces associated with embryonic lymph sacs. Most cysts are asymptomatic until their progressive increase in size encroaches on the adjacent bowel lumen, causing partial intestinal obstruction. Some patients may present with a freely mobile abdominal mass. Occasionally, their weight may precipitate a volvulus and a surgical emergency. Ultrasound is diagnostic. In some cases mesenteric cysts may be excised from the mesentery without damage to the intestinal blood supply. Resection of the cyst with the corresponding mesentery and intestine is generally safer.

ESOPHAGUS

Esophageal Atresia

Esophageal atresia (EA) occurs once in 5,000 live births. One half of the patients have one or more associated cardiac, genitourinary, skeletal, anorectal or other GI anomalies. The lesion is classified anatomically: EA with distal tracheoesophageal fistula (TEF), 84%; isolated EA, 10%; isolated TEF, 5%; and EA with proximal or double TEF, 1%.[19]

Infants show excess drooling and regurgitate when fed. Respiratory symptoms such as cough, dyspnea, and cyanosis may be prominent when a TEF is present. The diagnosis is suggested by the inability to pass a catheter into the stomach or confirmed by demonstrating the proximal pouch or fistula with small amounts of contrast medium. An x-ray shows the level of the catheter in the esophagus, the status of the lungs and the presence or absence of intestinal gas (isolated EA is likely in the latter case). Endoscopy is helpful in detecting the isolated TEF.

Risk factors for therapy are summarized by the Waterston et al.[20] classification: group A—weight over 2,500 gm with no other anomalies; group B—weight 1,800 to 2,500 gm with no other anomalies; group C—weight under 1,800 gm or presence of a major associated anomaly. Patients with pulmonary disease are placed into the next greater risk category. Table 7–2 outlines the trends in survival from several series.[20–25]

Infants in group A undergo immediate retropleural division of the TEF with primary esophageal anastomosis. A preliminary gastrostomy tube placement is beneficial when repair is delayed because of the patient's size or pulmonary status. High-risk neonates (group C) are candidates for staged management with gastrostomy tube placement and division of the TEF performed in one or two procedures. Esophageal repair awaits delineation of major associated anomalies and appropriate treatment to maximize patient survival.

The long esophageal gap, common in isolated EA, is the most challenging technical problem in surgical management. Introduction of the circumferential esophagomyotomy by Livaditis[26] has allowed primary anastomosis in cases in which this otherwise would have been impossible. Combining bougienage and myotomy to elongate the esophagus is also effective, but ballooning at the myotomy site can cause dysphagia or respiratory obstruction.[27] Esophageal replacement with gastric tube or colon interposition is a reasonable alternative if primary esophageal repair cannot be accomplished.

Complications of definitive surgery include anastomotic leak (12%), stricture requiring dilation (25%), and recurrent TEF.[28] Dysphagia and chronic respiratory disease secondary to esophageal dysfunction has been documented by manometry. Peristaltic wave incoordination, gastroesophageal reflux, and abnormal peak and resting pressures in the lower esophagus are noted. Dramatic postprandial episodes of cyanosis, bradycardia, apnea, and "dying spells" are thought to be due to tracheomalacia and compression. Aortopexy is often required.[29]

TABLE 7–2.—SURVIVAL IN PATIENTS WITH ESOPHAGEAL ATRESIA BY WATERSTON'S RISK CATEGORIES

AUTHOR	YEAR	NO. OF PATIENTS	GROUP A, %	GROUP B, %	GROUP C, %	TOTAL SURVIVAL, %
Waterston et al.[20] (categorized patients only)	1962	113	95	68	6	60
Cozzi and Wilkinson[21]	1967	93	94	68	18	57
	1975	60	95	72	37	67
German et al.[22]	1976	102	100	96	43	82
Randolph et al.[23]	1977	56	86	84	62	82
Strodel et al.[24] (last decade only)	1979	77	97	95	59	86
Touloukian[25]	1981	38	100	83	50	87

Achalasia

Achalasia is a motility disorder of the esophagus with only about 5% of cases described in childhood.[30] It is characterized by absent or diminished peristalsis in the body of the esophagus and failure of relaxation of the lower esophageal sphincter with an elevated resting pressure. Loss of vagal innervation to the esophagus is thought to be the primary etiologic factor. Most young patients present with regurgitation, failure to thrive, or pulmonary symptoms such as chronic cough, recurrent pneumonia, or aspiration.

The diagnosis is made on barium esophagram. The esophagus is dilated, patulous, aperistaltic, and ends in a narrow "parrot's beak" (Fig 7–3). Manometry confirms the absence of a propagated wave and incoordinated spasm in response to parasympathomimetic stimulation. The lower esophageal sphincter has a resting pressure in the 40–50 mm Hg range and does not relax.[31] Radionuclide scintigraphy can also detect the abnormalities.[32] Esophagoscopy rules out mechanical obstruction.

Anticholinergics, β-adrenergics, long-acting nitrates, and glucagon may enhance esophageal emptying and reduce sphincter pressure, but their efficacy is unproved. Dilation with bougienage is only transiently effective. Although often requiring several procedures, pneumatic or hydrostatic dilation is successful in approximately 80% of adults and may

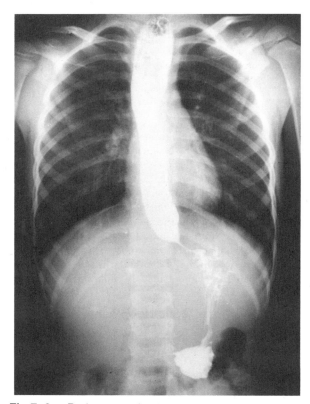

Fig 7–3.—Barium completely retained in dilated, patulous esophagus with the narrow "parrot's beak" at the esophagogastric junction, a configuration seen in advanced achalasia.

have a place in the initial treatment of children.[33] The Heller esophagomyotomy has about a 90% success rate in pediatric patients.[34, 35] Gastroesophageal reflux (25%) and esophagitis can occur after the Heller operation, so concomitant reconstruction of the hiatus or an antireflux procedure should be considered.

Cricopharyngeal achalasia is associated with congenital CNS abnormalities (70%) and manifests symptoms in the first few months of life.[36] The defect is in the parasympathetic innervation with failure of relaxation of the cricopharyngeus muscle in response to presentation of food or saliva. Affected infants feed poorly, with choking and coughing, and may demonstrate nasal reflux, regurgitation, and pulmonary aspiration.

A barium esophagram is often diagnostic (Fig 7–4). Manometry shows that the muscle may not relax at all or may contract discordantly. Endoscopy will rule out vocal cord abnormalities and mechanical esophageal obstruction.

Upright positioning of the infant and intermittent gavage feedings can be effective treatment if there is no associated progressive CNS disease. Dilation of the "sphincter area" is generally ineffective in older children, although improvement in infants with dilation is reported.[37] Cricopharyngeal myotomy generally results in relief of symptoms in otherwise

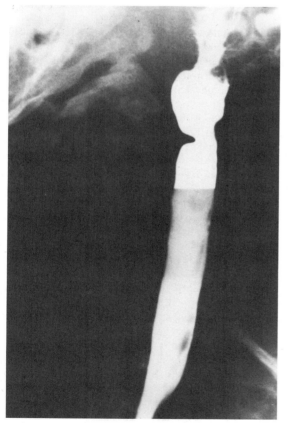

Fig 7–4.—Fixed posterior indentation at level of cricopharyngeus muscle on upper esophagus. This persistent spastic defect in the barium column appears to be cricopharyngeal achalasia.

normal patients.[36, 38] Severely affected children who have failed other maneuvers should be considered for gastrostomy tube feedings.

Gastroesophageal Reflux

Stomach contents reflux into the esophagus because of high intragastric pressure, lower esophageal sphincter incompetence, and distal esophageal dysfunction. By several weeks of age, the sphincter pressure increases and neurologic control over the swallowing, and esophageal relaxation mechanisms occur.[39] Delayed maturation of this neuromuscular function is responsible for clinical gastroesophageal reflux (GER), often termed chalasia in infancy. Ten percent of symptomatic children have associated CNS disorders and mental retardation. Young patients demonstrate vomiting, dysphagia, and failure to thrive. Hematemesis and anemia secondary to esophagitis are common in older children. GER also causes aspiration pneumonitis, asthma, nocturnal cough, apneic episodes, and perhaps the sudden infant death syndrome.[40]

Several studies may be used to detect reflux but these must be correlated with clinical symptoms. GER or stricture formation can be seen on the upper GI series, and radionuclide esophageal scintigraphy is accurate in demonstrating reflux and pulmonary aspiration.[41] Esophageal manometry may show reduced lower esophageal sphincter pressure. Esophagoscopy with biopsy can detect inflammatory changes of esophagitis. The most sensitive indicator of clinically significant GER is continuous esophageal pH monitoring.[42] Reflux episodes during sleep or more than two hours after meals correlate with the presence of pulmonary symptoms. Also, a prolonged esophageal clearance time, the time for pH to return to baseline level, suggests pathologic GER.[43]

Many infants with GER will be symptom-free at 18 months of age without treatment. Initial medical therapy consists of head-up positioning and frequent, small-volume, thickened feedings. Pharmacologic manipulation includes the use of antacids, cimetidine, metoclopramide, and bethanecol. Only the last has produced significant manometric, pH, and clinical improvement in childhood.[44]

Surgery is reserved for those patients who have esophagitis, esophageal stricture, life-threatening or recurrent pulmonary complications, or failure to respond to an adequate medical regimen.[45] All antireflux procedures have been employed successfully in children, but the Nissen fundoplication, perhaps because of its technical simplicity, is currently the most frequently performed operation. Control of reflux and improvement in patients with failure to thrive and esophagitis can generally be expected, but only about 75% of those with pulmonary symptoms get better.[46] Concomitant temporary gastrostomy tube placement is recommended, because the gas bloat syndrome is particularly distressing in the pediatric age group. The tube is also placed in neurologically damaged patients where feeding difficulties may be prominent.

Foreign Bodies of the Gastrointestinal Tract

Fortunately, most foreign bodies pass through the GI tract without mishap. Those that do not become lodged at sites of physiologic sphincters or at sites of acute angulation or GI abnormalities; e.g., cricopharyngeus, cardioesophageal junction, pylorus, C-loop, ligament of Treitz, distal ileum, rectosigmoid, prior anastomoses, or congenital stenoses.

Esophageal foreign bodies often are heralded by choking, dysphagia, fever, or cough. Gastrointestinal foreign bodies may present with signs of perforation, obstruction, or bleeding. The diagnosis is usually made by plain roentgenograms of the abdomen or chest, since many foreign bodies are radiopaque. Radiolucent objects require contrast studies.

Foreign bodies that lodge in the esophagus require removal. Blunt objects (coins, toys, marbles, buttons) may occasionally be removed by an experienced radiologist with a Foley catheter, but if the foreign body is sharp (open safety pins, needles, tacks, glass), esophagoscopy should always be performed.[47] Neglected esophageal foreign bodies have a propensity to ulcerate and perforate, with resultant mediastinitis or erosion into the great vessels. Regarding the latter, foreign bodies producing hemorrhage should never be removed endoscopically but by thoracotomy because of the likelihood of a vascular fistula.

Nonoperative management is successful in 90%–95% of objects reaching the stomach.[48] The indications for intervention via endoscopic extraction or operative removal are dependant on the nature of the foreign body. Round, blunt objects may be observed safely for several weeks; however, sharp, pointed or long, thin objects raise more concern, and if they become stationary, suggesting impending perforation, removal is indicated. A special group of foreign bodies requiring more aggressive management are "button" batteries. These may leak mercury, lead, or alkali and should be removed immediately if not progressing or fragmenting.[49] Foreign-body perforations rarely present with generalized peritonitis or free air because of the slow penetration of the bowel wall resulting in fistulas, hemorrhage, or, more commonly, a localized abscess. Operative therapy consists of drainage of the abscess and removal of the foreign body via a longitudinal enterotomy with transverse closure to avoid stenosis.

Bezoars, usually in the stomach, consist of hair (trichobezoar), vegetable matter (phytobezoar), milk curd (lactobezoars), or concretions of shellac, varnish, or medication. Most patients present with GI obstruction and require operative removal.

STOMACH AND DUODENUM

Volvulus of the Stomach

Gastric volvulus is an unusual condition in children which occurs when the ligamentous attachments to the stomach are loose or absent.[50, 51] Rotation may be organoaxial (longitudinal) or mesenteroaxial (transverse). The lesion can be associated with diaphragmatic defects,[52] abnormalities of mesenteric fixation, and intestinal rotation in infants, and with peptic ulcer disease, carcinoma, and trauma in adults.

The acute form of volvulus leads to sudden pain and an urge but inability to vomit. A nasogastric tube cannot be passed. Uncorrected torsion results in obstruction, strangulation, and shock. The chronic form can be asymptomatic or cause dyspepsia, distention, and weight loss. In acute lesions, an upright film will show a double fluid level in the left upper abdomen. An upper GI series may disclose an inverted stomach in chronic cases.

Prompt exploratory laparotomy and derotation of the volvulus is indicated. Any gangrenous portion of stomach is resected with primary closure. A gastropexy or temporary gastrostomy tube placement may aid in fixation. If there is an associated hiatal or foramen of Bochdalek hernia, the abdominal approach is still preferred, and the diaphragmatic defect is closed from below. There are reports of correction of chronic volvulus with a flexible endoscope, but there were recurrences, and adequate long-term follow-up is not available.

Peptic Ulcer Disease

Ulcers of the stomach and duodenum occur infrequently in the pediatric population. Peptic ulcers are categorized as primary or secondary. Secondary or stress ulcers are associated with some underlying cause; e.g., burns or trauma. Primary ulcers occur in the absence of precipitating factors.

The incidence of primary ulcers increases with age, males being affected more frequently than females. A familial history is present in 30%–40%.[53] The majority are located in the duodenum. Infants and toddlers present with perforation, recurrent vomiting, failure to thrive, or GI hemorrhage. Older children and adolescents usually present with abdominal pain not different from that seen in adults. A contrast study of the upper GI tract misses approximately 25% of peptic ulcers. Therefore, flexible endoscopy should be undertaken if the diagnosis is suspected.

Treatment of perforation is immediate laparotomy. Neonates may require urgent peritoneal aspiration to relieve the pneumoperitoneum that prevents diaphragmatic excursion. At operation, most perforations can be closed primarily. Rarely, with large or multiple perforations, partial gastric resection is required. Many children presenting with upper GI hemorrhage can be managed nonoperatively with blood replacement and iced saline lavage. Hypothermia must be avoided in infants. Arteriographic embolization is reserved for patients at excessive operative risk. A transfusion requirement equal to the blood volume in infants (80 ml/kg), or one half the blood volume in older children, is an indication for operative intervention. After transfixing the bleeding site, a truncal vagotomy and pyloroplasty is preferred. In selected cases with diffuse gastric hemorrhage, antrectomy is appropriate and may not result in severe growth disturbance as previously believed. Other operative indications include obstruction and intractability.

Stress ulcers arise in all age groups. Precipitating lesions include shock, hypoxia, prematurity, sepsis, CNS lesions (Cushing's ulcer), burns (Curling's ulcer), neoplasms, and trauma.[54] The ulcers are nearly equally distributed between gastric and duodenal sites. In neonates, perforation is not unusual. Older children more commonly present with hemorrhage. Treatment should be directed at prevention with antacids and possibly cimetidine. The diagnosis is most reliably confirmed by flexible endoscopy.

Prepyloric Obstruction

Pyloric atresia, antral webs, and prepyloric diaphragms account for fewer than 1% of all intestinal obstructions in the newborn.[55] With complete obstruction, forceful nonbilious vomiting becomes evident soon after birth. Partial luminal blockage can be asymptomatic or cause chronic abdominal pain, weight loss, and emesis. Associated anomalies include other GI obstructions, cardiovascular disease, and a specific autosomal recessive syndrome consisting of pyloric atresia, epidermolysis bullosa, and aplasia cutis congenita.[56]

The barium upper GI series is performed as soon as the diagnosis is suspected and shows a band-like defect in the prepyloric area at right angles to the gastric wall, often with a visible central aperture.[57] Flexible endoscopy can be used to make the diagnosis or to confirm the x-ray findings in equivocal cases. Although dietary manipulation and endoscopic resection of antral membranes have been attempted, patients are best managed by operation.[58] The distal stomach and duodenum are fully mobilized, and intraluminal inspection of the defect is mandatory. Pyloric atresia requires resection and gastroduodenostomy. Webs and diaphragms are excised and other distal obstructions must be excluded. The gastric outlet may be enlarged by a pyloroplasty, and adjunctive gastrostomy tube placement is often used in younger patients.

Hypertrophic Pyloric Stenosis

Hypertrophic pyloric stenosis results from overgrowth of the pyloric smooth muscle causing progressive gastric outlet obstruction. The cause remains obscure, although there is a familial predilection.

The average age of onset is three to five weeks, with a male predominance (4:1), often the first-born. The typical presentation begins with nonbilious, occasionally "coffee ground" vomiting, with progression to persistent projectile emesis after every meal. The diagnosis is made by visible gastric peristalsis and a palpable pyloric tumor, or "olive." About 10%–15% of patients require barium meal confirmation. Recently, ultrasonography has been shown to be highly accurate in diagnosis[59] and may replace barium studies (Fig 7–5).

The characteristic dehydration and hypochloremic alkalosis, resulting from losses of gastric secretions, must be corrected preoperatively. This is achieved by administration of normal saline with added potassium 20 mEq/L. Treatment is by Fredet-Ramstedt pyloromyotomy. Mucosal perforation during the muscle splitting can almost always be avoided, but if it occurs, the perforation and muscle are closed, and the remyotomy done 90° from the original. Postoperatively, some vomiting is not unusual. Incomplete pyloromyotomy is rare, but if suspected, an interval of 14 days prior to reoperation is suggested since many resolve spontaneously. Pyloromyotomy carries such low mortality (<1%) that attempts at medical management are unjustified.[60]

Congenital Duodenal Obstruction

Congenital duodenal obstruction is common and either intrinsic or extrinsic (Table 7–3).[61] The former are usually postampullary and consist of atresia, stenosis, web, and the rare intraluminal diverticulum. Extrinsic causes are due to intestinal malrotation, anular pancreas, duplications, and vascular compression. Complete obstruction, i.e., duodenal atresia, presents in the neonate with bilious vomiting. Partially ob-

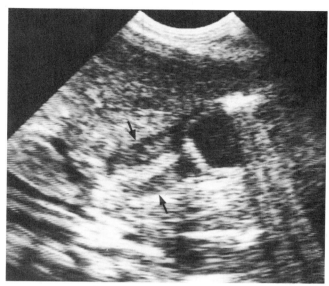

Fig 7–5.—Hypertrophic pylorus as seen by ultrasonography. The diameter of the pylorus *(arrows)* exceeding 1.5 cm confirms the diagnosis.

structing intrinsic lesions cause abdominal pain, distention, and weight loss.

Intrinsic defects are due to failure of vacuolation of the "solid" duodenum and are associated with Down's syndrome (30%), congenital heart disease (20%), esophageal atresia (15%), and urologic and vertebral anomalies.[62, 63] Most adult cases demonstrate long-standing, nonspecific symptoms caused by webs and stenosis, often secondary to peptic ulcer disease or chronic pancreatitis.[64] Anular pancreas is due to persistence of its ventral anlage in the anterior position while rotating around the duodenum and may be associated with an intrinsic lesion. In childhood, anular pancreas may be a source of recurrent abdominal pain,[65] and in adults with peptic ulcer disease, pancreatitis, biliary tract obstruction, and pancreatic carcinoma.

In duodenal atresia, the upright abdominal film will show a "double bubble" without distal air. Partial obstruction ex-

TABLE 7–3.—TYPES OF DUODENAL OBSTRUCTION

	FREQUENCY, %	COMMON PRESENTATION AGE	TREATMENT
Intrinsic			
Atresia	25	Newborn	Bypass*
Stenosis	10	Infancy Adult	Duodenoplasty
Web	20	Infancy Adult	Excise web Duodenoplasty
Extrinsic			
Malrotation	35	Newborn	Ladd's procedure
Anular pancreas	10	Newborn	Bypass
Duplication	<5	Childhood	Excise
Vascular compression	<5	All	Marsupialization

*Bypass: Duodenoduodenostomy or retrocolic duodenojejunostomy.

hibits the same picture, but there is distal intestinal gas (Fig 7–6). In this case, barium studies are indicated immediately to rule out malrotation because of the risk of midgut volvulus. Both the upper GI series and barium enema can detect anomalous rotation, and the procedure of choice is left to the discretion of the surgeon and radiologist. Studies such as CAT scan, ERCP, and angiography have also been used to diagnose anular pancreas.[66]

Except for malrotation, duodenal obstruction lends itself to an elective operation. In patients with atresia, anular pancreas and preduodenal portal vein, a bypass such as a duodenoduodenostomy or retrocolic duodenojejunostomy is necessary. Webs and membrane can be excised and the channel widened by duodenoplasty. A dilated proximal duodenum is often reduced in size by serosal plication or a tapering (V-excision) duodenoplasty. Afferent and blind loop syndromes can occur after bypass, causing stasis, malabsorption, and long-term stooling abnormalities.

SMALL INTESTINE, COLON, AND RECTUM

Malrotation

Normal rotation of the gut occurs in three stages: (1) the intestine is in the umbilical sac; (2) the midgut enters the abdomen with counterclockwise rotation of the duodenojejunal and cecocolic loops; and (3) the cecum descends into the right lower abdomen and is fixed to the posterior abdominal wall. Malrotation is present when the intestine fails to follow this pattern. The lesion occurs with volvulus of the midgut half the time and is also associated with abdominal wall defects, diaphragmatic hernia, and congenital heart disease.[67]

In the newborn, volvulus causes rapid vascular compromise and intestinal infarction with a 10%–15% mortality. In the older child, partial obstruction may cause pain, vomiting, and diarrhea. Malrotation with intermittent volvulus can also be a source of chronic abdominal pain and acute intestinal obstruction in older patients (Fig 7–7).[68, 69] After a partial duodenal

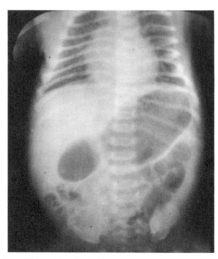

Fig 7–6.—"Double bubble" with distal intestinal gas. There is a partial duodenal obstruction. An immediate contrast study is indicated to rule out malrotation (with potential volvulus).

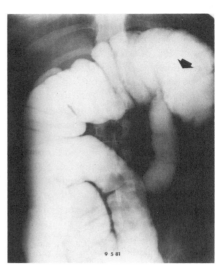

Fig 7–7.—Barium enema in a patient after many episodes of partial bowel obstruction. There is nonfixation of the colon, and the cecum (arrow) is in the left upper quadrant.

obstruction is suggested by plain abdominal films, an immediate contrast study is indicated to detect the rotational abnormality.

The upper GI series outlines a "beak sign" at the obstructed duodenum, and the barium enema shows the colonic malrotation.

Prompt operation is mandatory. The bowel is eviscerated, and if a midgut volvulus is present, the volvulus is reduced by counterclockwise rotation. Only frankly gangrenous bowel is resected. All peritoneal adhesions are divided, especially the Ladd's bands from the cecum and right colon crossing over the duodenum to the posterior parietes. The base of the mesentery is widened to separate the duodenojejunal and cecocolic loops. The duodenum is straightened down the right side of the abdomen, while the colon is moved to the left. An appendectomy is performed. No intestinal fixation is indicated.

Intestinal Duplications

One half of alimentary tract duplications occur in the small bowel, 20% in the thorax, and the remainder are either gastroduodenal or colonic. The diagnosis is made in early childhood in 85% of cases, yet some patients are asymptomatic until adult life.[70] Cystic duplications usually do not communicate with the adjacent intestinal lumen, whereas tubular lesions usually do. The latter often contains ectopic mucosa and may be associated with peptic ulceration, or perforation, and may, therefore, be detected by technetium scan. Intraluminal duplications are generally found in the ileocecal region and cause obstruction often by intussusception. The diagnosis is made in early childhood in 85% of cases; some patients are asymptomatic until adult life.[23] Duplications may be associated with cancer.

Thoracic duplications result from herniation of endoderm through the embryonic notochord, and thus vertebral defects are common.[71] Patients have symptoms of obstruction with cough, stridor or dysphagia, and recurrent pneumonia. Ectopic gastric mucosa may cause peptic ulceration with pain, bleeding, and perforation. The chest x-ray will show a posterior mediastinal mass, and barium swallow may demonstrate esophageal compression.[72] Operative resection of the thoracic duplication may be complicated if there is a common wall with the esophagus. In this case only, the cyst mucosa should be removed with the duplication.

Intestinal duplications present as an abdominal mass or with symptoms of obstruction or peptic ulceration. An extrinsic mass effect may be identified on the stomach or duodenum by upper GI series or on the colon by barium enema. Gastric lesions are resected and duodenal cysts may be excised, marsupialized into the normal duodenal lumen, or drained by a Roux-en-Y cyst enterostomy. Localized spherical lesions of the intestine are resected. Duplications of the hindgut, especially the tubular total colonic type, are complicated by genitourinary anomalies. They are discovered because of bleeding, obstruction, or the presence of an abdominal or rectal mass. Long tubular lesions are treated by creating a distal fenestration to drain the end into the normal bowel lumen.

Intestinal Atresia

Jejunoileal and colonic atresias are caused by an in utero mesenteric vascular accident. Colonic lesions make up fewer than 10% of cases and may be associated with abdominal wall defects.[73] Proximal lesions in the newborn are indicated by bilious vomiting, while abdominal distention and failure to pass meconium are signs of distal lesions.

Jejunoileal atresia can be: (1) a membrane or cord-like obstruction, 85% survival; (2) a single atresia with discontinuity of the bowel and mesentery, 66% survival; (3) multiple atresias (shortgut), 29% survival; (4) the "apple peel" anomaly (shortgut), 57% survival.[74] In type 4 lesions, the superior mesenteric artery is lost, and the ileocolic or right colic artery supplies the distal small bowel, which wraps itself around the vessel like an "apple peel".[75] Abdominal films delineate an obstructive bowel gas pattern. Barium enema shows the unused microcolon in jejunoileal lesions and "cut-off" of the contrast column in colonic atresia.

The dilated proximal intestine functions poorly, and 4 to 10 cm is resected. Tapering enteroplasty or serosal plication may be done to further reduce the bowel size and enhance functional motility.[76, 77] Primary end-to-end or end-to-oblique anastomosis in jejunoileal atresia is the treatment of choice. Colonic atresia forms a closed loop obstruction if there is a competent ileocecal valve. Resection with exteriorization of the bowel is preferred, although primary anastomosis is reasonable in proximal colonic lesions.[78]

Meconium Disease

Meconium diseases encompass meconium ileus, meconium plug syndrome, and meconium peritonitis. Meconium ileus is associated with cystic fibrosis (> 95%), and the neonate presents with distal small-bowel obstruction.[79] In the usual simple form, viscous meconium obstructs the terminal ileum. In complicated cases, a vascular accident has caused associated ileal atresia or perforation, resulting in meconium peritonitis. In this case sterile meconium causes a nonbacterial, chemical inflammation of the peritoneum. Early in utero perforation

may seal with or without atresia formation. Late perforation results in meconium ascites.

The meconium plug syndrome is a distal colonic obturator obstruction. Twenty-five percent of the patients have cystic fibrosis and ten percent have Hirschsprung's disease.[80] Barium enema will either demonstrate the unused microcolon and distal ileal obstruction or outline the meconium plug. In meconium peritonitis 95% of patients will show intestinal obstruction and calcification of the parietes on plain films, and 20% will already have pneumoperitoneum.[81]

The meconium plug is evacuated by Gastrografin enema. If a normal stooling pattern does not ensue, Hirschsprung's disease must be ruled out. Simple meconium ileus can be successfully treated in many patients by Gastrografin enema. If unsuccessful, operative ileotomy with meconium evacuation is needed. The bowel is usually exteriorized by a Mikulicz or Bishop-Koop ileostomy. In complicated meconium ileus and meconium peritonitis, resection and primary anastomosis or stoma diversion is performed depending on the operative circumstances.

Meckel's Diverticulum

Meckel's diverticulum represents a remnant of the omphalomesenteric duct. Failure of obliteration of this duct can result in enteroumbilical fistula, umbilical mucosal remnant, or, most commonly, Meckel's diverticulum. These diverticula are located on the antimesenteric border of the ileum, proximal to the ileocecal valve. They are present in nearly 2% of the population and occur twice as frequently in males. Heterotopic tissue (gastric, pancreatic, duodenal, or colonic) is present in over 50% of symptomatic diverticuli, whereas ectopic tissue is found in only 5% of diverticuli removed incidentally. The majority are asymptomatic, but 4% present with complications—hemorrhage, obstruction, or inflammation—most before the age of 2.[82]

Hemorrhage, the most common presentation, is usually painless and may range from massive to occult. Nearly all cases are the result of ectopic gastric mucosa within the diverticulum, with subsequent erosion/ulceration of the adjacent ileal mucosa.

Obstruction occurs by two mechanisms: (1) intussusception with the diverticulum as the lead point; and (2) congenital bands with torsion or internal herniation. The latter can present catastrophically resulting from closed loop obstruction with strangulation, necrosis, and perforation if not diagnosed and treated early.

Acute Meckel's diverticulitis, sometimes complicated by perforation, can mimic acute appendicitis. The usual etiology is impaction of the diverticulum by fecolith or luminal stricture secondary to peptic ulceration.

The diagnosis of Meckel's diverticulum is difficult and dependent on clinical suspicion. Technetium 99mTc pertechnetate scan may be useful in delineating those diverticuli containing ectopic gastric mucosa.[83] The sensitivity may be improved by administration of cimetidine before the examination.[84] Contrast studies, enteroclysis, or barium enema with ileal reflux rarely demonstrate diverticuli.

Surgical therapy of Meckel's diverticuli should begin with preoperative stabilization by administration of IV fluids, blood, or antibiotics as needed. In the majority, simple diverticulectomy via wedge excision and transverse closure is all that is required. Some cases of intussusception, volvulus, or perforation may require small-bowel resection with end-to-end anastomosis. Incidental removal remains controversial, but should probably be done only when there is palpable ectopic mucosa or associated bands.

Intussusception

Intussusception is a frequent cause of intestinal obstruction during the first two years of life. In infants, the etiology may be hypertrophied lymphoid elements in the bowel wall that are drawn into the bowel lumen. The seasonal peaks (midsummer and midwinter) implicate a viral etiology. In older children, an identifiable lead point is more common; e.g., Meckel's diverticulum, polyps, tumors, intramural hematoma, or duplication.[85]

Symptoms begin with intermittent colicky abdominal pain and vomiting, followed by bloody mucoid, "current jelly" stools. A sausage-shaped mass is often palpable in the right upper quadrant, and there may be absence of bowel in the right lower quadrant (Dance's sign).

Management with barium enema is not only diagnostic but also therapeutic in many cases. Strict guidelines must be followed to avoid perforation.[86] In the presence of peritonitis or profound shock, no attempt at barium enema should be made. Intravenous rehydration should be under way and a nasogastric tube passed prior to any attempt at hydrostatic reduction. The barium is run in under fluoroscopic control. The level is never placed higher than 100 cm above the table. If no progress is made for five minutes, the patient is allowed to evacuate and the enema restarted. The reduction is considered incomplete unless small-bowel reflux is seen. Prompt laparotomy is indicated if barium enema reduction fails. At operation, manual reduction is accomplished by pressure at the distal end, not by proximal traction. Rarely, if operative reduction is not possible, the involved bowel is resected with primary anastomosis. With perforation and peritonitis, enterostomy and mucous fistula are preferable.

Necrotizing Enterocolitis

Necrotizing enterocolitis (NEC) has become the most frequent neonatal surgical emergency; 2,000–4,000 cases are reported annually. The etiology is probably related to stress, reduced mesenteric blood flow, hypoxia, hyperosmolar feedings, infectious agents, and/or altered immunity of the gut.[87] Most infants are premature or of low birth weight.

The disease usually begins within the first week of life and presents with signs of GI dysfunction or systemic manifestations (Table 7–4). Physical findings include abdominal disten-

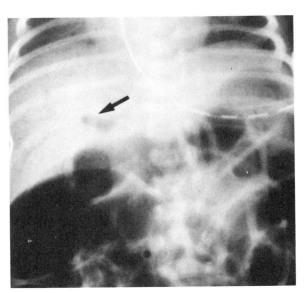

Fig 7–8.—Radiograph of a one-week-old infant demonstrating hepatic portal vein gas *(arrow).*

tion, tenderness, peritonitis, mass, or erythema and edema of the abdominal wall. The hallmark of NEC is the identification of pneumatosis intestinalis (streaks or bubbles of gas parallel to the bowel lumen) on abdominal radiographs: the ileum and right colon are most commonly involved. Other radiographic signs include nonspecific intestinal distention, pneumoperitoneum, and portal vein gas (Fig 7–8).

In the absence of perforation, treatment is by bowel rest and treatment of sepsis. An oral-gastric tube is placed on gravity drainage. Intravenous fluids are administered to replace third space losses and correct acid-base derangements. Parenteral antibiotics are administered, usually ampicillin and an aminoglycoside, with adjustments based on culture results. Frequent reassessment is required, since clinical deterioration can occur quite rapidly. Abdominal radiographs and serologic studies are obtained every six hours.

Surgical intervention is indicated for free perforation or intestinal gangrene. Paracentesis has been used to identify the latter. Aspirates of peritoneal fluid are examined for the presence of bacteria, indicative of gangrene.[88] Relative operative indications include: clinical deterioration based on worsening physical findings, thrombocytopenia, progressive metabolic acidosis, persistent gas collections indicating partial or complete obstruction, mass, localized abscess, or late stricture formation.

The basic principles at operation are resection of obviously perforated or gangrenous bowel (questionably viable bowel is spared to avoid short gut syndrome) and exteriorization of the divided ends. Primary anastomoses in this setting have been done with success in highly selected cases. A second-look operation within 48 hours allows reassessment in cases where viability of the gut is in question. In some neonates considered to be at excessive operative risk, a Penrose drain may be placed intraperitoneally through a stab wound in the right lower abdomen.[89] Infants should be at a relatively normal weight before intestinal continuity is restored. Prior to ostomy closure, contrast radiography of the distal gut is man-

TABLE 7–4.—FREQUENCY OF CLINICAL SIGNS IN INFANTS WITH NEC

SYMPTOM	INCIDENCE, %
Abdominal distention	90
Lethargy	84
Gastric retention or vomiting	85
Temperature instability	81
Apneic spells	66
Hematochezia (gross or occult)	60

datory to rule out secondary strictures. Patients requiring surgical intervention have about a 50% survival.

Appendicitis

Appendicitis is the most common condition requiring intra-abdominal surgery in the pediatric age group. The presentation, findings, and management in children and adolescents differ little from the adult and are well described elsewhere. Appendicitis in infancy, however, warrants separate consideration owing to the atypical nature of the signs and symptoms and the special management required.

The incidence of appendicitis in the first two years of life is less than 2% of all childhood cases.[9] The most frequent symptoms are vomiting and fever, often accompanied by irritability, lethargy, or anorexia. Unfortunately, these symptoms are nonspecific and are often seen with common nonsurgical illnesses. The physical findings are abdominal distention and tenderness, localized or diffuse. Sometimes an abdominal mass, spasm, or rigidity of the abdominal wall is present, as well as a rectal mass. Leukocytosis is present in over 50%, and nearly all patients will have a left shift on the differential smear.[91] An ileus pattern, free intraperitoneal fluid, soft tissue mass, right scoliosis, thickened lateral abdominal wall, or appendicolith may be seen on abdominal x-rays.

Prior to operation, the infant's intravascular volume must be restored. Intravenous antibiotic therapy is begun. A transverse right lower quadrant incision is used, and the appendix removed. Drains are placed in the presence of a perforation or abscess. Complications in infants are more frequent, including prolonged ileus, wound infection, and abscess formation. The mortality has improved but still exceeds that of older children or adults.

Inflammatory Bowel Disease

About 15% of patients with ulcerative colitis or Crohn's disease develop symptoms before age 20; 2% before age 10. The relative frequency of each is nearly equal in children.

The presentation may be insidious, with a long prodrome of extraintestinal symptoms including weight loss, arthritis or arthralgia, growth failure, retardation of sexual development, cutaneous manifestations, and hepatic disease. Ulcerative colitis typically is manifested by gradually worsening diarrhea, rectal bleeding and tenesmus, or, rarely, toxic megacolon. Crohn's disease also may present with progressively worsening diarrhea, infrequently bloody, or with chronic, colicky abdominal pain, symptoms mimicking appendicitis, or anorectal lesions (fistula, abscess, or fissures).

Certain differences between the adult and the pediatric disease bear emphasis. Ulcerative colitis in children commonly affects the entire colon, and the colonic disease frequently is more severe than is the rectal involvement. In Crohn's disease, colonic involvement is more common than in adults.

The acute indications for operative intervention include perforation, unremitting hemorrhage, toxic megacolon, and severe fulminant disease. More often the indications are due to chronic disabilities, intractability with retardation of growth and sexual development being the most common. The risk of neoplastic change is increased in both diseases, but markedly so for ulcerative colitis (3% in the first ten years after the onset of symptoms and increasing to 20% each decade there-

after).[92] Recent application of a rectal mucosectomy with total colectomy and pull-through ileoanal anastomosis for ulcerative colitis has had overall good results (Fig 7–9).[93] The avoidance of a permanent ileostomy is seen as a distinct advantage in children.

The majority of patients with Crohn's disease will eventually require operative intervention. Resection of the diseased bowel with end-to-end anastomosis is preferred. One third of the reported carcinomas in Crohn's disease develop in bypassed segments.

Polyps

Juvenile polyps are the most common pediatric intestinal tumors, comprising 90% of all childhood polyps.[94] The majority are confined to the rectum and sigmoid colon, usually as a single polyp, but they are occasionally multiple[3–22] and only rarely numerous. The cause is unknown, but mechanical, inflammatory, and allergic factors have been implicated. The polyps are usually pedunculated, round, smooth, and may reach 2–3 cm. Histologically, they consist of numerous mucin-filled cysts, lined by columnar epithelium. They have no malignant potential.[95]

They most commonly present between 2 and 8 years of age with rectal bleeding. The bleeding is intermittent and generally bright red on the surface or mixed throughout the stool. Presentation with prolapse of the polyp through the anus is not unusual. Rectal examination will identify many cases of juvenile polyps. Proctosigmoidoscopy affords direct visualization and excisional biopsy. Barium enema may identify the unusual polyp beyond the research of the proctosigmoidoscope. Once the diagnosis has been confirmed histologically, the treatment should be very conservative. The natural history of juvenile polyps is self-limited and many infarct or autoamputate. There is a rapid decline in the incidence in adolescence.

The remaining 10% of polyps seen in childhood are either adenomatous polyps or part of one of the polyposis syndromes

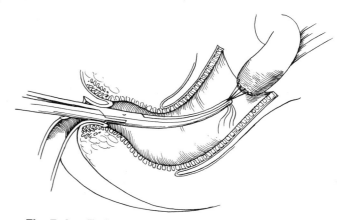

Fig 7–9.—Endorectal pull-through for ulcerative colitis. The rectal mucosal-submucosal tube is everted and the terminal ileum brought down through the muscular cuff. (From Coran A.G., Sarahan T.M., Dent T.L., et al.: The endorectal pull-through for the management of ulcerative colitis in children and adults. *Ann. Surg.* 197:99, 1983. Used by permission.)

TABLE 7–5.—POLYPOSIS SYNDROMES

	JUVENILE POLYPOSIS	PEUTZ-JEGHERS SYNDROME	FAMILIAL POLYPOSIS	GARDNER'S SYNDROME	TURCOT SYNDROME	CRONKHITE-CANADA SYNDROME	LYMPHOID POLYPOSIS
Anatomical involvement	Mainly colon, occasionally entire GI tract	Entire GI tract, esp. small bowel	Colon	Colon mainly, occasionally stomach, duodenum	Colon	Entire GI tract, mainly stomach, colon	Colon, rectum
Pathology	Retention or juvenile polyps	Hamartoma	Adenoma	Adenoma	Adenoma	Retention or juvenile polyps	Large lymphoid follicle, usually sessile
Onset of symptoms	Infancy, childhood	Childhood, adolescence	Childhood, adolescence	Adult	Childhood to young adult	Adult	Childhood
Inheritance	Familial in many	Autosomal dominant	Autosomal dominant	Automosal dominant	Autosomal recessive	None	None
Extraintestinal manifestations	Occasional heart lesions, malrotation, hydrocephalus, porphyria, hypertelorism, protein-losing enteropathy	Mucocutaneous pigmentation, exostoses, ovarian cysts or tumors	None	Sebaceous cysts desmoids, osteomas, mesenteric fibromas, lipomas, exostoses, dentigerous cysts, odontomas	CNS tumors (ependymoma, glioblastoma, medulloblastoma)	Hyperpigmentation Alopecia Nail atrophy	None
Malignant potential	None	Low	High (colorectal)	High (colorectal or duodenal)	Probable	Multiple carcinomata	None

(Table 7–5).[96, 97] These are discussed in detail in other sections of this book.

Hirschsprung's Disease

Arrest of the caudal migration of neuroblasts in the embryonic alimentary canal results in congenital aganglionic megacolon. While the involved segment may extend proximally for any distance, in 70% of patients the disease begins at the sigmoid colon. Absence of ganglion cells causes bowel spasm, producing partial functional obstruction. Presentation in Hirschsprung's disease may be as: (1) vomiting, distention, and no passage of meconium in the newborn; (2) delayed passage of meconium and chronic obstipation; (3) mild initial obstipation followed by sudden enterocolitis; (4) acute intestinal obstruction; or (5) chronic obstipation, poor nutritional status, and chronic illness.

Hirschsprung's disease must be differentiated from functional obstruction and the meconium diseases described earlier. Barium enema is 85% accurate if a transition zone, irregular bowel contractions, and prolonged barium retention are seen.[98] Anorectal manometry is accurate for diagnosis except in stressed neonates and children with fecal impaction. Its greatest value is to exclude Hirschsprung's disease. Rectal biopsy shows absence of ganglion cells and the presence of excess nerve fibers, which establishes the diagnosis. Full-thickness biopsy techniques under general anesthesia are no longer necessary. Punch biopsy with Hartmann forceps or suction biopsies provide adequate tissue for examination. Acetylcholinesterase is readily found in aganglionic bowel and detecting its activity facilitates the histologic interpretation of superficial specimens. Combined manometry and acetylcholinesterase staining is very effective in diagnosing Hirschsprung's disease (Tables 7–6 and 7–7).[99]

Intestinal decompression should be carried out as soon as the diagnosis is made. Rectal tube placement and normal saline irrigation have been used but may be inadequate. A diverting colostomy is preferable, placed in the ganglionic bowel just proximal to the transition zone. Definitive surgical treatment is performed after the patient weighs about 20 lb. or is about 9 months old.

One of three operations is currently popular. In the Swenson procedure, the aganglionic bowel is resected, a posterior sphincterotomy performed, and the pulled-through normal colon anastomosed to the rectum. In Duhamel's operation, the aganglionic intestine is resected down to the peritoneal reflection and the rectum is closed. The proximal normal bowel is brought through a retrorectal tunnel, and the anterior wall of the colon and posterior wall of the retained rectum are anastomosed by surgical staples. Soave's endorectal pull-through involves removal of the distal bowel mucosa by submucosal dissection to the anus and passage of the normal colon through the remaining rectosigmoid muscular tube with anastomosis at the anal verge.

Complication rates vary widely but all procedures are prone to anastomotic leak (average 5%), stricture (average 6%), and pelvic sepsis (average 3%). There is also long-term risk for enterocolitis, impotence, ejaculatory failure, and fecal incontinence.[100–102]

Imperforate Anus

Anorectal malformations are initiated early in gestation while the urinary, genital, and rectal tracts open into a common cloaca. The mesodermal urorectal septum moves craniocaudally to perforate the cloacal membrane and form an

TABLE 7–6.—ANORECTAL MANOMETRY IN DIAGNOSIS OF HIRSCHSPRUNG'S DISEASE

RESULTS*	PATIENTS WITH AGANGLIONOSIS	NORMAL SUBJECTS
Normal	1	93
Abnormal	17	11†

*Accuracy, 90%.
†All false positive results were obtained in premature newborns or in children with severe fecal impaction.

TABLE 7–7.—ACETYLCHOLINESTERASE
STAINING IN DIAGNOSIS OF
HIRSCHSPRUNG'S DISEASE

RESULTS*	PATIENTS WITH AGANGLIONOSIS	NORMAL SUBJECTS
Positive	9	0
Negative	1	15

*Accuracy, 96%.

open urogenital sinus and rectum. Infralevator lesions consist of anal stenosis (5%), anal membrane (5%), and anal agenesis (40%).[103] Three fourths of the last have fistulas, commonly to the perineum or vulva. The major supralevator defect is rectal agenesis (50%), two thirds of which have fistulas, commonly to the urethra or vagina.

The diagnosis is made by visual examination. The urine is checked for the presence of meconium. Genitourinary anomalies, esophageal atresia, and congenital heart disease may be anticipated. The Wangensteen-Rice "invertogram" may demonstrate the level of the distal bowel and distance from the anal skin.[104] Swallowed air will move to the terminal gut by about 12 hours of age. Thus, a lateral film taken after this time with the buttocks elevated straight up may allow measurement of the distance between the gas-filled distal blind rectal pouch and the perineal surface. However, the patient's crying and straining as well as the presence of trapped meconium in the terminal bowel decreases the accuracy of this technique.

Infralevator lesions with a visable fistula or those ending within 1–2 cm of the anal skin can be repaired by direct perineal operation. Ninety percent continence can be expected. All high lesions require a preliminary diverting colostomy (which protects the definite pull-through six to 12 months later). Abdominal perineal, sacrococcygeal, and combined operations have been described to place the rectum through the puborectalis sling and the external sphincter. Fifty to seventy-five percent continence is achieved. Recently, Pena and deVries[105] used a midline vertical incision from the navicular fossa to the site of the neoanus to better expose and mobilize the rectum. This posterior saggital anorectoplasty allows bowel tapering, reconstruction of the striated muscle complex, and circumferential suture of the pull-through to the layers of the external sphincter. No long-term follow-up is available, but preliminary experience suggests that the incidence of mucosal prolapse is reduced and continence is improved.

REFERENCES

1. Gross R.E.: *The Surgery of Infancy and Childhood.* Philadelphia, W.B. Saunders Co., 1954.
2. Lilly J.R., Chandra R.: Surgical hazards of co-existing anomalies in biliary atresia. *Surg. Gynecol. Obstet.* 139:49, 1974.
3. Kasai M., Kimura S., Asakura Y., et al.: Surgical treatment of biliary atresia. *J. Pediatr. Surg.* 3:665, 1968.
4. Alonso-Lej F., Rever W.B., Pessagno D.J.: Congenital choledochal cyst with a report of 2 and an analysis of 94 cases. *Int. Abstr. Surg.* 108:1, 1959.
5. Lilly J.R.: Surgical treatment of choledochal cysts. *Surg. Gynecol. Obstet.* 149:36, 1979.
6. Kasai M., Asakura Y., Taira Y.: Surgical treatment of choledochal cyst. *Ann. Surg.* 182:844, 1970.
7. Prevot J., Babut J.M.: Spontaneous perforations of the biliary tract in infancy. *Prog. Pediatr. Surg.* 3:187, 1971.
8. Lilly J.E., Weintraub W.H., Altman R.P.: Spontaneous perforation of the extrahepatic bile ducts and bile peritonitis in infancy. *Surgery* 75:664, 1974.
9. Harned R.K., Babbitt D.P.: Cholelithiasis in children. *Radiology* 117:391, 1975.
10. Natar G.: Gall bladder disease in childhood. *Aust. Paediatr. J.* 8:147, 1972.
11. Zwart W.A.J., Megens J.G.N.: Cholelithiasis and cholecystitis in children. *Arch. Chir. Neerl.* 27:187, 1975.
12. Starzl T.E., Halgrimson C.G., Francavilla F.R., et al.: The origin, hormonal nature, and action of hepatotrophic substances in portal venous blood. *Surg. Gynecol. Obstet.* 137:179, 1973.
13. Stellin G.P., and Lilly J.R.: Esophageal endosclerosis in children, *Surgery.* In press.
14. Comfort M.W., Steinberg A.G.: Pedigree of a family with hereditary chronic relapsing pancreatitis. *Gastroenterology* 21:54, 1952.
15. Welch K.J.: The pancreas and spleen, in Ravitch M.M., Welch K.J., Benson C.D., et al. (eds.): *Pediatric Surgery.* Chicago, Year Book Medical Publishers, 1979, pp. 857–877.
16. Grosfeld J.L., Clatworthy H.W., Hamoudi A.B.: Pancreatic malignancy in childhood. *Arch. Surg.* 101:370, 1970.
17. Harken A.H., Filler R.M., AvRuskin T.W., et al.: The role of "total" pancreatectomy in the treatment of unremitting hypoglycemia of infancy. *J. Pediatr. Surg.* 6:284, 1971.
18. Kirkland J., Ben-Menachem Y., Akhtar M., et al.: Islet cell tumor in a neonate: Diagnosis by selective angiography and histological findings. *Pediatrics* 61:790, 1978.
19. Mollitt D.L., Golladay E.S.: Management of the newborn with gastrointestinal anomalies and tracheoesophageal fistula. *Am. J. Surg.* 146:792, 1983.
20. Waterston D.J., Carter R.E., Aberdeen E.: Oesophageal atresia: Tracheoesophageal fistula: A study of survival in 218 infants. *Lancet* 1:819, 1962.
21. Cozzi F., Wilkinson A.W.: Mortality in esophageal atresia. *J. R. Coll. Surg. Edinb.* 20:236, 1975.
22. German J.C., Mahour G.H., Woolley M.M.: Esophageal atresia and associated anomalies. *J. Pediatr. Surg.* 11:299, 1976.
23. Randolph J.G., Altman R.P., Anderson K.D.: Selective surgical management based upon clinical status in infants with esophageal atresia. *J. Thorac. Cardiovasc. Surg.* 74:335, 1977.
24. Strodel W.E., Coran A.G., Kirsh M.M., et al.: Esophageal atresia: A 41-year experience. *Arch. Surg.* 114:523, 1979.
25. Touloukian R.J.: Long-term results following repair of esophageal atresia by end-to-side anastomosis and ligation of the tracheoesophageal fistula. *J. Pediatr. Surg.* 16:983, 1981.
26. Livaditis A.: Esophageal atresia: A method of overbridging large segmental gaps. *Z. Kinderchir.* 13:293, 1973.
27. Otte J.B., Gianello P., Wese F.X., et al.: Diverticulum formation after circular myotomy for esophageal atresia. *J. Pediatr. Surg.* 19:68, 1984.
28. Holder T.M., Ashcraft K.W.: Developments in the care of patients with esophageal atresia and tracheoesophageal fistula. *Surg. Clin. North Am.* 61:1051, 1981.
29. Schwartz M.Z., Filler R.M.: Tracheal compression as a cause of apnea following repair of tracheoesophageal fistula: Treatment by aortopexy. *J. Pediatr. Surg.* 15:842, 1980.
30. Azizkhan R.G., Tapper D., Eraklis A.: Achalasia in childhood: A 20-year experience. *J. Pediatr. Surg.* 15:452, 1980.
31. Cohen S.: Motor disorders of the esophagus. *N. Engl. J. Med.* 301:184, 1979.
32. Rozen P., Gelford M., Zaltzman S., et al.: Dynamic, diagnostic and pharmacological radionuclide studies of the esophagus in achalasia. *Radiology* 144:587, 1982.
33. Boyle J.T., Cohen S., Watkins J.B.: Successful treatment of achalasia in childhood by pneumatic dilatation. *J. Pediatr.* 99:35, 1981.
34. Payne W.S., King R.M.: Treatment of achalasia of the esophagus. *Surg. Clin. North Am.* 63:963, 1983.

35. Starinsky R., Berlovitz I., Mares A.J., et al.: Infantile achalasia. *Pediatr. Radiol.* 14:113, 1984.

36. Reichert T.J., Bluestone C.D., Stool S.E., et al.: Congenital cricopharyngeal achalasia. *Ann. Otol. Rhinol. Laryngol.* 86:603, 1977.

37. Lernau O.Z., Sherzer E., Mogle P., et al.: Congenital cricopharyngeal achalasia treatment by dilatations. *J. Pediatr. Surg.* 19:202, 1984.

38. Orringer M.B.: Extended cervical esophagomyotomy for cricopharyngeal dysfunction. *J. Thorac. Cardiovasc. Surg.* 80:669, 1980.

39. Weissbluth M.: Gastroesophageal reflux: A review. *Clin. Pediatr.* 20:7, 1981.

40. Euler A.R., Byrne W.J., Ament M.E., et al.: Recurrent pulmonary disease in children: A complication of gastroesophageal reflux. *Pediatrics* 63:47, 1979.

41. Jona J.Z., Sty J.R., Glicklich M.: Simplified radioisotope technique for assessing gastroesophageal reflux in children. *J. Pediatr. Surg.* 16:114, 1981.

42. Sondheimer J.M.: Continuous monitoring of distal esophageal pH: A diagnostic test for gastroesophageal reflux in infants. *J. Pediatr.* 96:804, 1980.

43. Koch A., Gass R.: Continuous 20–24 hr. esophageal pH-monitoring in infancy. *J. Pediatr.* 16:109, 1981.

44. Euler A.R.: Use of bethanechol for the treatment of gastroesophageal reflux. *J. Pediatr.* 96:321, 1980.

45. Leape L.L., Ramenofsky M.L.: Surgical treatment of gastroesophageal reflux in children: Results of Nissen's fundoplication in 100 children. *Am. J. Dis. Child.* 134:935, 1980.

46. Johnson D.G., Jolley S.G.: Gastroesophageal reflux in infants and children: Recognition and treatment. *Surg. Clin. North Am.* 61:1101, 1981.

47. O'Neill J.A., Holcomb G.W., Noblett W.W.: Management of tracheobronchial and esophageal foreign bodies in childhood. *J. Pediatr. Surg.* 18:475, 1983.

48. Pellerin D., Fortier-Beaulieu M., Gueguen J.: The fate of swallowed foreign bodies: Experience of 1250 instances of sub diaphragmatic foreign bodies in children. *Prog. Pediatr. Radiol.* 2:286, 1979.

49. Temple D.M., McNeese M.C.: Hazards of battery ingestion. *Pediatrics* 71:100, 1983.

50. Carter R., Brewer L.A., Hinshaw D.B.: Acute gastric volvulus. *Am. J. Surg.* 140:99, 1980.

51. Smith R.J.: Volvulus of the stomach. *J. Natl. Med. Assoc.* 75:393, 1983.

52. Starshak R.J., Sty J.R.: Diaphragmatic defects with gastric volvulus in the neonate. *Wis. Med. J.* 82:28, 1983.

53. Kumar D., Spitz L.: Peptic ulceration in children. *Surg. Gynecol. Obstet.* 159:63, 1984.

54. Tolia V., Dubois R.S.: Peptic ulcer disease in children and adolescents. *Clin. Pediatr.* 22:665, 1983.

55. Andrews E.C., Stem J.M.: Pyloric atresia. *South. Med. J.* 75(9):1122, 1982.

56. Cowton A.L., Beattie T.J., Gibson A.A., et al.: Case report: Epidermolysis bullosa in association with aplasia curtis congenita and pyloric atresia. *Acta Paediatr. Scand.* 71:155, 1982.

57. Clements J.L. Jr., Jinkins J.R., Torres W.E., et al.: Antral mucosal diaphragms in adults. *A.J.R.* 133:1105, 1979.

58. Bell M.J., Ternberg J.L., Keating J.P., et al.: Prepyloric gastric antral web: A puzzling epidemic. *J. Pediatr. Surg.* 13:307, 1978.

59. Khamapirad T., Athey P.A.: Ultrasound diagnosis of hypertrophic pyloric stenosis. *J. Pediatr.* 102:23, 1983.

60. Spicer R.D.: Infantile hypertrophic pyloric stenosis: A review. *Br. J. Surg.* 69:128, 1982.

61. Salonen I.S.: Congenital duodenal obstruction—a review of the literature and a clinical study of 66 patients, including a histopathological study of annular pancreas and a follow-up study of 36 survivors. *Acta Paediatr. Scand.* [Suppl.] 272, 1978.

62. Atwell J.D., Klidjian A.M.: Vertebral anomalies and duodenal atresia. *J. Pediatr. Surg.* 17:237, 1982.

63. Wesley J.R., Mahour G.H.: Congenital intrinsic duodenal obstruction: A twenty-five year review. *Surgery* 82:143, 1983.

64. Killebrew L.H., Kukora J.S.: Adult duodenal webs—a difficult diagnosis. *Arch. Surg.* 118:875, 1983.

65. Liebman W.M.: Recurrent abdominal pain: Apparent association with annular pancreas. *Am. J. Gastroenterol.* 71(5):522, 1979.

66. Inamoto K., Ishikawa Y., Itoh N.: CT demonstration of annular pancreas: Case report. *Gastrointest. Radiol.* 8:143, 1983.

67. Stewart D.R., Colodny A.L., Daggett W.C.: Malrotation of the bowel in infants and children: A 15 year review. *Surgery* 79:716, 1976.

68. Janik J.S., Ein S.H.: Normal intestinal rotation with non-fixation: A cause of chronic abdominal pain. *J. Pediatr. Surg.* 14(6):670, 1979.

69. Rao P.L., Katariya R.N., Rao P.G., et al.: Malrotation of midgut causing intestinal obstruction in adults. *J. Assoc. Physicians India* 7:493, 1977.

70. Bower R.J., Sieber, W.K., Kiesewetter W.B.: Alimentary tract duplications in children. *Ann. Surg.* 188(5):669, 1978.

71. Steinhagen R.M., Pertsemlidis D., Feld H.J.: Spontaneous perforation of intestinal duplications. *Mt. Sinai J. Med. (N.Y.)* 49:406, 1982.

72. Tschappeler H., Smith W.B.: Duplications of the intestinal tract: Clinical and radiological features. *Ann. Radiol.* 20:133, 1977.

73. Powell R.W., Raffensperger J.G.: Congenital colonic atresia. *J. Pediatr. Surg.* 17(2):166, 1982.

74. Martin L.W., Zerella J.T.: Jejunoileal atresia: A proposed classification. *J. Pediatr. Surg.* 11:399, 1976.

75. Haller J.A. Jr., Tepas J.J., Pickard L.R., et al.: Intestinal atresia: Current concepts of pathogenesis, pathophysiology, and operative management. *Am. Surg.* 49:385, 1983.

76. Weber T.R., Vane D.W., Grosfeld J.L.: Tapering enteroplasty in infants with bowel atresia and short gut. *Arch. Surg.* 117:684, 1982.

77. deLorimier A.A., Harrison M.R.: Intestinal plication in the treatment of atresia. *J. Pediatr. Surg.* 18:734, 1983.

78. Schiller M., Aviad I., Freund H.: Congenital colonic atresia and stenosis. *Am. J. Surg.* 138:721, 1979.

79. Mabogunje O.A., Wang C.-I., Mahour G.H.: Improved survival of neonates with meconium ileus. *Arch. Surg.* 117:37, 1982.

80. Olsen M.M., Luck S.R., Lloyd-Still J., et al.: The spectrum of meconium disease in infancy. *J. Pediatr. Surg.* 17(5):479, 1982.

81. Pan E.Y., Chen L.Y., Yang J.Z., et al.: Radiographic diagnosis of meconium peritonitis: A report of 200 cases including six fetal cases. *Pediatr. Radiol.* 13:199, 1983.

82. Williams S.: Management of Meckel's diverticulum. *Br. J. Surg.* 68:477, 1981.

83. Sfakianakis G.N., Haase G.M.: Abdominal scintigraphy for ectopic gastric mucosa: A retrospective analysis of 143 studies. *A.J.R.* 138:7, 1982.

84. Baum S.: Pertechnetate imaging following cimetidine administration in Meckel's diverticulum of the ileum. *Am. J. Gastroenterol.* 76:464, 1981.

85. Eklof O.A., Johanson L., Lohr G.: Childhood intussusception: Hydrostatic reducibility and incidence of lead points in different age groups. *Pediatr. Radiol.* 10:83, 1980.

86. Ravitch M.M.: Intussusception, in Ravitch M.M., Welch K.J., Benson C.D., et al. (eds.): *Pediatric Surgery.* Chicago, Year Book Medical Publishers, 1979, pp. 989–1003.

87. Kliegman R.M., Fanaroff A.A.: Necrotizing enterocolitis. *N. Engl. J. Med.* 310:1093, 1984.

88. Kosloske A.M., Lilly J.R.: Paracentesis and lavage for diagnosis of intestinal gangrene in neonatal necrotizing enterocolitis. *J. Pediatr. Surg.* 13:315, 1978.

89. Janik J.S., Ein S.H.: Peritoneal drainage under local anesthesia for necrotizing enterocolitis (NEC) perforation: A second look. *J. Pediatr. Surg.* 15:565, 1980.

90. Bartlett R.H., Eraklis A.J., Wilkinson R.H.: Appendicitis in infancy. *Surg. Gynecol. Obstet.* 130:99, 1970.

91. Grosfeld J.L., Weinberger M., Clatworthy H.W.: Acute appendicitis in the first two years of life. *J. Pediatr. Surg.* 8:285, 1973.

92. Devroede G.J., Taylor W.F., Sauer W.G., et al.: Cancer risk

and life expectancy of children with ulcerative colitis. *N. Engl. J. Med.* 285:17, 1971.

93. Coran A.G., Sarahan T.M., Dent T.L., et al.: The endorectal pull-through for the management of ulcerative colitis in children and adults. *Ann. Surg.* 197:99, 1983.

94. Holgersen L.E., Miller R.E., Zintel H.A.: Juvenile polyps of the colon. *Surgery* 69:288, 1971.

95. Chang J.H., Lilly J.R., Sautulli T.V.: Alimentary tract neoplasms, in Rudolph A.M., Hoffman J.I. (eds.): *Pediatrics.* Norwalk, Conn.: Appleton-Century-Crofts, 1982, pp. 992–993.

96. Schwabe, A.D., Lewin, K.J.: Gastrointestinal polyposis syndromes. *Viewpoints Dig. Dis.* 12:1, 1980.

97. Jagelman D.G.: Familial polyposis. *Surg. Clin. North Am.* 63:117, 1983.

98. Rosenfield N.S., Ablow R.C., Markowitz R.I., et al.: Hirschsprung disease: Accuracy of the barium enema examination. *Radiology* 150:393, 1984.

99. Morikawa Y., Donahoe P.K., Hendren W.H.: Manometry and histochemistry in the diagnosis of Hirschsprung's disease. *Pediatrics* 63:865, 1979.

100. Swenson O., Sherman J.O., Fisher J.H., et al.: The treatment and postoperative complications of congenital megacolon: A 25 year follow-up. *Ann. Surg.* 182:266, 1975.

101. Soper R.T., Miller F.E.: Modification of Duhamel procedure: Elimination of rectal pouch and colorectal septum. *J. Pediatr. Surg.* 3:376, 1968.

102. Klotz D.H. Jr., Velcek F.T., Kottmeier P.H.: Reappraisal of the endorectal pull-through operation for Hirschsprung's disease. *J. Pediatr. Surg.* 8:595, 1973.

103. Santulli T.V., Schullinger J.N., Kiesewetter W.B., et al.: Imperforate anus: A survey from the members of the surgical section of the American Academy of Pediatrics. *J. Pediatr. Surg.* 6:484, 1971.

104. Wangensteen O.H., Rice C.O.: Imperforate anus. *Ann. Surg.* 92:77, 1930.

105. deVries P.A.: Complication of surgery for congenital anomalies of the anorectum, in deVries P.A., Shapiro S.R. (eds.): *Complications of Pediatric Surgery.* New York, John Wiley & Sons, 1982, pp. 233–262.

PART II

Esophageal Disorders

8

Motor Disturbances of the Esophagus

W. Spencer Payne, M.D.
Takuo Murakami, M.D.
Victor F. Trastek, M.D.

Motor disturbances of the esophagus and its sphincters encompass a wide range of clinically recognized conditions. At one time it appeared that all esophageal motility problems could be clearly classified under the headings "achalasia," "diffuse spasm," and "scleroderma of the esophagus." In achalasia, as classically defined, the patient has a nonrelaxing, often hypertensive, lower esophageal sphincter (LES), and the body of the esophagus is amotile, which leads to the triad of esophageal obstruction, retention, and regurgitation. Diffuse spasm is characterized by episodic, spontaneous, high-amplitude, painful contractions throughout the smooth muscle portion of the esophagus, including the LES. On the other hand, scleroderma of the esophagus is defined as a hypomotility disorder, with absence of contractions in the body of the esophagus and a hypotensive or absent high-pressure zone (HPZ) in the region of the LES. This leads to severe gastroesophageal reflux and its complications. As knowledge of esophageal function in health and disease increased, it was recognized that some of these conditions are less clearly delineated than initially anticipated and that there are transitions and overlapping relationships among these manometrically defined conditions.

Furthermore, it has been more clearly appreciated that there is a wider spectrum of motor disorders with both primary and secondary manifestations. Zenker's diverticulum has come to be appreciated as a secondary manifestation of upper esophageal sphincter (UES) dysfunction. Cricopharyngeal dysfunction can occur without diverticulum and is more clearly recognized under the broad term "cricopharyngeal dysphagia." Similarly, symptomatic pulsion diverticula of the lower esophagus have been recognized as secondary manifestations of distal esophageal obstruction due especially to achalasia or diffuse spasm. Transitions between diffuse spasm and achalasia are recognized under the term "vigorous achalasia." Gastroesophageal imcompetence is a motor failure of the LES mechanism, irrespective of the presence or absence of esophageal hiatal hernia, with both hypotensive LES and inappropriately relaxing LES being implicated.

The clear definition of motor disorders entirely on the basis of laboratory investigation remains difficult in many circumstances. The achalasia motility pattern may be seen secondary to neoplasms of the cardia. Overly vigorous destruction of the LES in achalasia, by either forceful dilatation or surgery, can produce the laboratory manometric picture of scleroderma. Diffuse spasm on occasion has been seen to evolve into classic achalasia, with vigorous achalasia having features of both. Severe reflux esophagitis may present with a scleroderma motility pattern only to revert to normal with the restoration of competence. In other cases, the scleroderma motility pattern may be a first manifestation of systemic sclerosis and the motor abnormality not reversible by restoration of competence. Similarly, diffuse spasm may present as a motor manifestation of reflux esophagitis. In a few achalasia patients, return of peristalsis has been observed after relief of distal esophageal sphincteric obstruction, raising questions regarding additional subgroups in that condition. Diffuse spasm appears to be less well-defined with various hypermotility subgroups being recognized under the descriptive headings of "hypertensive lower esophageal sphincter," "hypercontracting lower esophageal sphincter," and "segmental esophageal spasm."

Finally, a vague wastebasket laboratory term, "nonspecific esophageal motility disorder," has evolved to cover those conditions not clearly classifiable under the usual headings. Increasingly, matters of esophageal and esophageal sphincteric dysfunctions are being linked with organic or motility dysfunctions of the more distal alimentary tract as well as to various systemic and neurologic conditions. Table 8–1 attempts to provide a comprehensive overview of this complex problem.

It should be apparent that objective laboratory investigation of esophageal motor activity is still the best available means of defining esophageal motor disturbances, but, as with any laboratory test, the results must be considered in context with the individual patient's clinical problems and other function studies and findings.

DYNAMICS OF SWALLOWING AND THEIR INVESTIGATION

Deglutition, or swallowing, begins in the mouth and terminates at the esophagogastric junction. Thus, oral, pharyngeal, and esophageal phases of swallowing are recognized which involve muscles innervated by cranial nerves V, VII, IX, X and XII. Swallowing is generally considered as being a

TABLE 8–1.—ESOPHAGEAL MOTILITY DISTURBANCES*

UES (either isolated cricopharyngeal or more diffuse oropharyngeal
   dysphagia)
   Central nervous system disease
      Cerebrovascular accident with pseudobulbar palsy
      Parkinson's disease
      Bulbar poliomyelitis
      Multiple sclerosis
      Amyotrophic lateral sclerosis
   Muscular disease
      Muscular dystrophy (myotonic, oculopharyngeal)
      Inflammatory (dermatomyositis, polymyositis)
      Metabolic myopathy (thyrotoxicosis, hypothyroidism)
      Myasthenia gravis
   Miscellaneous
      Radical oropharyngeal surgery
      Hypertensive UES
      Poorly relaxing UES
      Premature contraction of the UES (pharyngoesophageal
         diverticulum)
Body of esophagus and LES
   Achalasia
   Vigorous achalasia
   Diffuse spasm of the esophagus
   Hypertensive LES
   Hypercontracting LES
   Nutcracker esophagus
   Hypotensive LES
   Inappropriately relaxing LES
   Scleroderma of the esophagus
Miscellaneous
   Dermatomyositis
   Myasthenia gravis
   Muscular dystrophy
   Cerebrovascular accident
   Parkinson's disease
   Amyotrophic lateral sclerosis
   Diabetic neuropathy
   Alcoholic neuropathy
   Presbyesophagus

*UES = upper esophageal sphincter; LES = lower esophageal
sphincter.

voluntarily initiated act associated with the ingestion of food-stuff, but under resting conditions, normal individuals swallow subconsciously, or involuntarily, at a frequency ranging from 4 to 40 times per hour. Whether initiated voluntarily or unconsciously, swallowing is a complex, automated act required to conduct nutrients and saliva from the mouth to the GI tract for digestion and absorption.

During the pharyngeal phase, this conduit function is especially complicated by special requirements imposed by the sharing of space with and proximity to upper airways. Specifically required and provided are mechanisms to prevent laryngotracheal contamination and nasal regurgitation during swallowing. Thus, in addition to a propulsive mechanism to aid transit, respiration must be coordinated with swallowing, and both laryngeal and nasal airways must be sealed and then opened and cleared alternatingly at critical moments to prevent catastrophe.

A propulsive mechanism, assisted by gravity, involves sequential peristaltic muscular contractions beginning in the mouth and extending to the pharynx, hypopharynx, and length of the esophagus. Propulsion is associated with time-appropriate relaxation of the UES and LES. The whole se-

quence, occupying a little over one second, is precisely programmed in the "swallowing center" of the brain stem and is facilitated by sensory and proprioceptive neural inputs.

Salivary secretions, more than 1 L/day, provide the stimuli for unconscious swallowing, lubrication of mucosal surfaces, dilution, pH control, enzymatic activity, and, along with peristalsis, a clearing action on the conduit itself.

The need for both the UES and LES brings into focus a mechanism that not only protects airways from retrograde flow but also protects sensitive esophageal mucosa from the corrosive effects of refluxed gastroduodenal secretions. The resting tone of each of these sphincters is reflexly augmented by distention of the segment of alimentary tract immediately distal to it. Through this adaptive mechanism, both gastroesophageal and esophagopharyngeal reflux are minimized. The time of contact of esophageal mucosa with refluxed or ingested corrosive material is significantly reduced by the clearing, dilution, and neutralization provided by primary and secondary peristalsis and saliva.

It should be apparent from this preliminary discussion of the mechanisms of swallowing that not all problems of deglutition are confined to the esophagus and its sphincters. Indeed, it is incumbent on anyone investigating swallowing difficulties in a given patient to define clearly the integrity of oral and pharyngeal phases of swallowing before attributing the difficulties entirely to esophageal malfunction. Such investigation should include careful history taking and also visual observation of the patient during the simple act of swallowing solids and liquids. Video or cine fluoroscopy during the ingestion of radiopaque liquids and solids provides a unique opportunity to observe each of the phases of swallowing with stop-frame or slow-motion sequencing. The latter is not commonly required, but it can provide an added dimension of time sequence of events, especially of the oral and pharyngeal phases of swallowing; these findings often correlate well with manometric events in the body of the esophagus and sphincteric areas. Esophageal motility study by manometry, however, has been the most reliable, objective means of defining esophageal motility problems and dysfunction of its sphincters.

Although many of the motor disturbances of the esophagus and its sphincters occasionally were suspected with remarkable clarity and insight in previous centuries, modern manometric investigation can be traced to the balloon kymographic studies by Kronecker and Meltzer in 1883.[1] Subsequent early technical modifications and clinical correlations are notably associated with the names Ingelfinger, Kramer, Code, and Olsen.

Current modern clinical manometric testing utilizes three or four pressure-detecting units (fine water-filled and perfused polyvinyl chloride tubes attached to strain-gauge manometers) with lateral openings positioned at 5-cm intervals in the esophagus for simultaneous recording of pressure events. With the recording device operating at constant speed, time is recorded on the horizontal axis and simultaneous pressure events are recorded on the vertical axis. At the Mayo Clinic we use a terminal balloon-covered transducer in addition to the perfused tubes for nonquantitative higher sensitivity in studies of sphincter function (Fig 8–1). Measurements are made with the esophagus at rest and after swal-

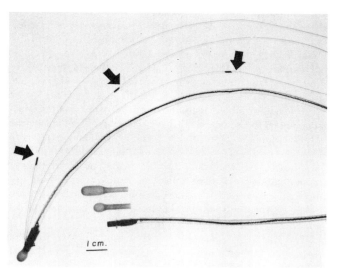

Fig 8–1.—Balloon-covered differential transformer and cluster of three polyvinyl chloride tubes used in measurement of esophageal and sphincteric pressures. Each tube has side opening *(arrows)* 5 cm from opening in next tube, is infused with water at rate of 1.4 ml/min by individual pump, and is attached to pressure-sensitive recording device. At Mayo Clinic, balloon-covered pressure transducer is routinely included at the end as highly sensitive additional means of studying sphincter function. (From Code C.F., Kelley M.L. Jr., Schlegel J.F., et al.: Detection of hiatal hernia during esophageal motility tests. *Gastroenterology* 43:521, 1962. By permission of the American Gastroenterological Association.)

lowing. Resting pressures are measured while the units are being withdrawn in stepwise fashion from the stomach up the esophagus to record especially the length and pressure of the sphincteric high-pressure zones (Fig 8–2).

Fluoroscopic observations of the esophagus with contrast medium often give results closely paralleling the manometric events during swallowing, but the latter method provides a convenient, objective, quantitative record of pressure events and their timing at multiple sites simultaneously for careful and leisurely analysis. Often, manometry provides supplementary information about the esophagus not provided by radiography and vice versa. In addition, endoscopy and various other specific esophageal function tests provide additional insight into mechanisms of dysfunction. These include standard and 24-hour acid (pH) reflux tests, galvanometric potential difference (PD) used to identify the squamous-columnar epithelial junction, acid-clearing, acid perfusion, esophageal and gastric emptying studies, and pharmacologic esophageal responses. These are covered in more detail in the chapter devoted to gastroesophageal reflux but will be alluded to in subsequent sections of this chapter.

MOTOR DISTURBANCES OF UES

Dysfunctions of the UES are being recognized with increasing frequency, although their manometric definition is not always needed clinically or always well defined objectively. Little is actually known about the cause of UES dys-

function in many patients, but the symptoms may be progressive and incapacitating from even minimal dysfunction.

Normal UES

The high-pressure zone (HPZ) of the UES corresponds closely to the anatomical cricopharyngeal muscle, although manometrically it exceeds the anatomical length of this muscle by several centimeters. This may be due to the fact that lower pharyngeal constrictor fibers and upper esophageal circular musculature contribute fibers to sphincter function. When studied at rest with low-perfusion (1.6 ml/min), open-tip, fine, polyvinyl chloride pressure-detection catheters, the UES is definable as a 30- to 90-mm Hg HPZ, 2.5–4.5 cm long, at approximately the C5 or C6 level. Anatomically, the cricopharyngeal sphincter site is considered to be the narrowest point of the entire alimentary tract. Unlike most sphincters, the UES has a radial pressure profile that is more oval in contour, with higher pressures being recorded in the anteroposterior (AP) axis than in the lateral. This occurs in part because of the nonanular nature of the cricopharyngeal muscle which is seen as a bowstring across the posterior aspect of the pharyngoesophageal juncture with musculature absent over the cricoid plate anteriorly. Upon the initiation of deglu-

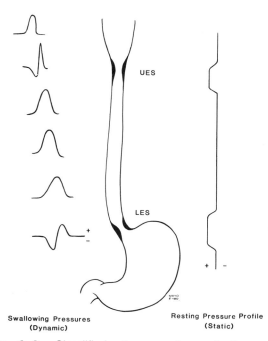

Fig 8–2.—Simplified diagram demonstrating normal physiologic manometric pressures in pharynx, UES, and LES. *Right,* static or resting high-pressure zones of LES and UES are defined as pressure-sensing catheter is withdrawn from stomach below to pharynx above. *Left,* normal sequential swallowing pressure events from pharynx downward. Note that these dynamic events are peristaltic, with both upper and lower sphincters showing relaxation prior to contraction and return to resting tone. (From Payne W.S., Ellis F.H. Jr.: Esophagus and diaphragmatic hernias, in Schwartz S.I., Shires G.T., Spencer F.C., et al. (eds.): *Principles of Surgery,* ed. 4. New York, McGraw-Hill Book Co., 1984, pp. 1063-1112. Used by permission.)

tition, the UES relaxes to a baseline of nearly atmospheric pressure and remains thus throughout the sequential pharyngeal contractions, permitting unobstructed passage of the ingested bolus into the esophagus. After completion of pharyngeal motor activity, the UES contracts vigorously and then returns to resting tone.

Abnormal UES

Various sphincter abnormalities have been defined either manometrically or radiographically. Care should be taken in interpreting radiographic findings alone because they do not always correlate with manometric findings or clinical symptoms. For example, the persistence of a radiographic indentation of the cricopharyngeal muscle has been interpreted by some as evidence of a nonrelaxing sphincter, dubbed "achalasia of the cricopharyngeus." Such radiographic sphincteric prominence is usual and is characteristic of Zenker's pharyngoesophageal diverticulum, but careful and repeated manometric observations in that condition show that quantitatively the sphincter relaxes and contracts in an entirely normal fashion. The problem is not that of a manometrically definable failure to relax but is a premature contraction of the UES while the pharynx is still contracting. Indeed, the problem is even more complicated in Zenker's diverticulum because only about 60% of swallows show the characteristic incoordination. Furthermore, the radiographic definition of a prominent cricopharyngeal muscle indentation may be seen in apparently normal persons who have no manometric abnormality, diverticulum, or symptoms.

Oropharyngeal and Cricopharyngeal Dysphagia

UES dysfunction may occur either as an isolated problem (cricopharyngeal dysphagia) or in combination with varying degrees of oral and pharyngeal dysfunction (oropharyngeal dysphagia). Cricopharyngeal myotomy has been used in the empirical management of both of these conditions, often without distinction. The results have been quite variable. In the Mayo Clinic experience, patients with isolated cricopharyngeal dysfunction without diverticulum have responded better to myotomy than those with the more diffuse oropharyngeal dysfunctions. Almost all of those with associated diverticulum have responded well to myotomy.

Various specific UES dysfunctions without diverticulum that are potentially amenable to cricopharyngeal myotomy have been defined manometrically. These include hypertensive, premature-contracting, incomplete, or nonrelaxing UESs. In other patients who gain significant benefit from myotomy, no specific sphincter disturbance can be identified manometrically, although the pharynx may be seen to contract feebly or the cricopharyngeal muscle may be prominent on radiography or endoscopy.

CLINICAL FEATURES.—Irrespective of specific mechanism, clinically these patients, cricopharyngeal and oral pharyngeal dysphagic, present with difficulty with the initial phases of swallowing. Prominent features are "food sticking in the throat," regurgitation, salivation, respiratory aspiration, and weight loss. Many of these patients have definable systemic or neurologic conditions. Because the results of medical therapy for most of these disorders have been disappointing,

cricopharyngeal myotomy has been suggested as an alternative. The procedure is relatively safe and occasionally effective, and so it is often a tempting alternative. Too often, it is undertaken with unrealistic expectations.

Patients undergoing extensive head and neck surgery (laryngeal release procedures for tracheal reconstruction or laryngectomy patients, etc.) often benefit from cricopharyngeal myotomy, but these patients often recover spontaneously with time. Duranceau et al.[2] have described excellent results with myotomy in 70% of 15 patients with oculopharyngeal muscular dystrophy. This is a rare, genetically transmitted (autosomal dominant) condition seen, mainly in North America in members of a French-Canadian family. Henderson[3] defined a group of patients with cricopharyngeal dysphagia secondary to isolated, recurrent laryngeal nerve paralysis and reported excellent results with myotomy. Orringer[4] reported quite satisfactory results with cricopharyngeal myotomy when swallowing dysfunction could be clearly localized to the cricopharyngeal muscle.

Despite these and other enthusiastic reports, one should apply cricopharyngeal myotomy cautiously and preferably in patients with clearly defined manometric changes and dysfunction isolated to the UES. At the Mayo Clinic only four of the 14 patients with oropharyngeal or cricopharyngeal dysphagia without diverticulum benefited from myotomy. Although the results were excellent in these four, the remaining ten experienced no detectable improvement.

TECHNIQUE OF CRICOPHARYNGEAL MYOTOMY.—There have been some minor variations in the actual techniques of cricopharyngeal myotomy reported by various authors. All use a cervical incision for exposure. Payne, Belsey, and Ellis use a posterior midline vertical extramucosal myotomy, 3–4 cm long, extending from the lower border of the inferior pharyngeal constrictors through the cricopharyngeal muscle and caudally well onto the esophagus. Divided musculature is allowed to retract, permitting mucosa to pout through the muscular defect. Duranceau et al.[2] perform essentially the same myotomy but raise a flap of muscularis off the mucosa and either excise this pedicle or tack it to adjacent tissue, exposing a large area of mucosa. However, Orringer[4] extends the myotomy cephalad 3–4 cm onto the hypopharynx as well as 3–4 cm distally onto the esophagus. It is not known whether differences in reported results are related to these technical aspects or to patient selection.

While one may wish to give patients the benefit of the doubt by performing cricopharyngeal myotomy with the hope of improving or restoring swallowing, the procedure apparently is not without risk of sudden death from aspiration in patients with manifest gastroesophageal reflux.[5] With this single exception, myotomy poses few risks for the patient.[6–16]

Pharyngoesophageal (Zenker's) Diverticulum

A pharyngoesophageal diverticulum is a pouch of herniated pharyngeal mucosa that protrudes through a muscular defect in the posterior pharyngeal wall just above the cricopharyngeal muscle. Dysfunction of the UES has been implicated in its genesis, but definable CNS disease is very rare and, with appropriate surgical treatment, the prognosis is excellent. Although the condition was recognized as a distinct clinical entity over 200 years ago by the English surgeon Ludlow,[17] it was not until 1874 that the German pathologist Zenker appreciated the pulsion nature of this diverticulum, and his name became synonymous with the condition.

The pharyngoesophageal diverticulum is clearly an acquired condition seen almost exclusively in adults; the incidence increases with age. The diverticulum seems to develop as a consequence of an increased intraluminal pressure caused by functional obstruction at the level of the cricopharyngeal muscle. This, in combination with a congenitally weak area in the musculature of the lower pharyngeal constrictors just above the cricopharyngeal muscle, is thought to be the reason for its development and constant location. The nature of the functional obstruction during swallowing has been defined as frequent premature contraction of the UES during pharyngeal contraction in patients with diverticula of all sizes.[18] Although such uncoordinated events could provide a reasonable explanation for the development of the diverticulum, even this mechanism has been challenged.[19]

Irrespective of the precise mechanism, once a diverticulum is established in this area it progresses in size, in frequency, and in severity of symptoms and complications. Not only does the sac increase in diameter, but it also tends to elongate and descend between the esophagus and the vertebral column (Fig 8–3, A–C). Eventually the sac becomes huge, occupying the posterosuperior mediastinum and displacing the esophagus anteriorly. Such an advanced diverticulum will be seen to fill preferentially—esophageal filling occurs as a spillover phenomenon after the sac is distended and filled. Filling defects from retained food are commonly seen on contrast radiography, and a prominent cricopharyngeal muscle is usually evident just below the neck of the sac. Radiographic examination of the esophagus is otherwise negative, except for an unusually high incidence of associated asymptomatic esophageal hiatal hernia.

CLINICAL FEATURES.—A pharyngoesophageal diverticulum produces cervical obstruction to swallowing, diverticular retention of food, and spontaneous regurgitation of fresh, bland, undigested food and saliva. Swallowing is characteristically noisy, and the breath smells foul. Eating and drinking may be interrupted by episodes of regurgitation—with or without coughing or choking if respiratory aspiration occurs. On occasion, especially in very elderly persons and debilitated patients, respiratory complications such as hoarseness, asthma, pneumonitis, and lung abscess are the only signs. When treatment is neglected, serious nutritional depletion and suppurative lung disease may occur. Squamous cell carcinoma is known to develop in long-standing pharyngoesophageal diverticula, but this complication fortunately is infrequent.

Findings at physical examination usually are unremarkable unless a large diverticulum can be palpated as a soft, doughy cervical mass. The diagnosis of pharyngoesophageal diverticulum is usually suspected on the basis of history alone, but confirmation requires demonstration of the sac by contrast radiography. Manometry has little place in the usual diagnostic work-up of these patients. Endoscopic examination is hazardous if such a diverticulum is present. Unless an attendant malignant growth or other esophageal condition is suspected from a previous roentgenographic study, esophagoscopy usually is not indicated. When esophagoscopy is required, however, safety may be enhanced by carrying out the procedure over a previously swallowed thread as a guide. Diverticular perforation is the chief risk of any esophageal intubative procedure. Both the rigid and the flexible esophagoscopes have been implicated, and so has the simple attempt to pass a nasogastric tube.

SURGICAL TREATMENT.—At the Mayo Clinic, we have long favored a one-stage transcervical diverticulectomy for the

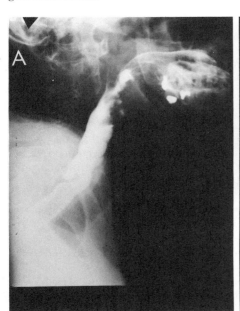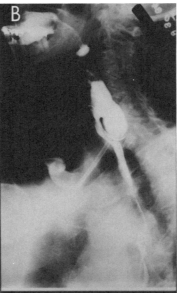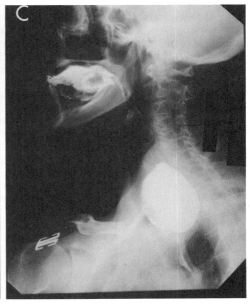

Fig 8–3.—Various sizes of pharyngoesophageal diverticula (lateral radiographic views). **A,** small. **B,** moderate. **C,** large. (From Payne W.S.: Esophageal diverticula, in Shields T.W. (ed.): *General Thoracic Surgery,* ed. 2. Philadelphia, Lea & Febiger, 1983, pp. 859–872. Used by permission.)

management of moderate to large diverticula. During the past decade, cricopharyngeal myotomy has been added to diverticulectomy (Fig 8–4), and myotomy alone (Fig 8–5) has been used for extremely small, early diverticula.[20]

Others have used other approaches. Sutherland[21] and Ellis and associates[18] performed myotomy alone for diverticula of all sizes, whereas Belsey[22] favored diverticulopexy with myotomy. Dohlman and Mattsson,[23] Holinger and Schild,[24] and van Overbeek[25] reported experience with multistage peroral endoscopic diathermic procedures in which the common sep-

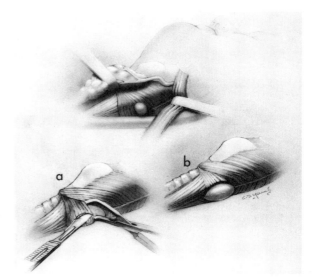

Fig 8–5.—Technique of cricopharyngeal myotomy. Myotomy alone is used for treatment of small pharyngoesophageal diverticula. Surgical exposure of retropharyngeal space is gained through oblique left cervical incision oriented along anterior border of sternomastoid muscle (not shown). *Top,* retraction of sternomastoid and carotid sheath laterally and of thyroid, pharynx, and larynx medially provides necessary exposure of diverticulum, which is located at cervical level where the omohyoid muscle crosses surgical field. (Note that the omohyoid muscle in upper center of drawing has been retracted cephalad to show diverticulum.) After connective tissue is dissected off mucosal sac to identify defect in posterior pharyngeal wall *(a),* a right-angle forceps is used to develop dissection plane inferiorly between muscularis and mucosa. Posterior midline extramucosal myotomy is effected with scalpel from neck of small sac inferiorly for 3 cm. With retraction of ends of cut muscle *(b),* almond-shaped, diffuse bulge of mucosa through myotomy is seen. Small Penrose drain is brought from region of myotomy and retropharyngeal space through lower end of cervical wound to outside, and platysma and skin are closed in layers around drain. (From Payne W.S.: Esophageal diverticula, in Shields T.W. (ed.): *General Thoracic Surgery,* ed. 2. Philadelphia, Lea & Febiger, 1983, pp. 859–872. Used by permission.)

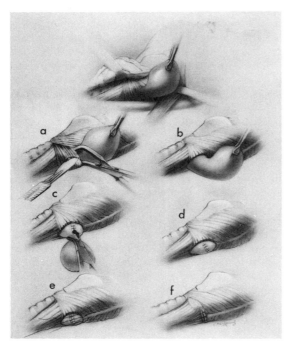

Fig 8–4.—One-stage pharyngoesophageal diverticulectomy with myotomy. This procedure is used to manage medium- and large-sized diverticula. *Top,* medium-sized diverticulum is exposed through left cervical incision (see legend for Fig 8–5). Note that omohyoid is retracted cephalad, diverticulum is dissected out to its neck, and apex of diverticulum is held cephalad. Right-angle forceps *(a)* is used to develop dissection plane between muscularis and mucosa just below neck of sac in preparation for extramucosal myotomy with scalpel. After 3-cm vertical myotomy is completed *(b),* neck of mucosal sac appears to have widened. With 28 F catheter in esophagus *(c),* curved clamp is placed across neck of diverticulum at right angle to long axis of esophagus at point of planned amputation. With cut-and-sew technique, sac is amputated stepwise and closed with fine vascular silk (5–0), placed so that knots are within esophageal lumen. Alternatively, a stapling device can be used. Diverticulectomy and closure are completed *(d).* Absorbable vertical sutures are placed in edges of muscular defect after myotomy and diverticulectomy *(e).* This completed transverse closure *(f)* provides muscular layer closure over mucosal suture line, which further minimizes leakage without restitution of cricopharyngeal muscle. Drainage and closure are effected. (From Payne W.S.: Esophageal diverticula, in Shields T.W. (ed.): *General Thoracic Surgery,* ed. 2. Philadelphia, Lea & Febiger, 1983, pp. 859–872. Used by permission.)

tum between the diverticulum and the esophagus is divided. Our approach, we believe, provides a safer and more definitive solution to the pharyngoesophageal diverticulum problem, and we continue to recommend its use.

TECHNIQUE OF ONE-STAGE PHARYNGOESOPHAGEAL DIVERTICULECTOMY WITH CRICOPHARYNGEAL MYOTOMY.—The patient is placed in the supine position on the operating table (see Fig 8–4). While the patient is awake, tracheal intubation is accomplished with topical pharyngeal anesthesia to prevent aspiration. General anesthesia is promptly induced once the airway is sealed by the inflation of a cuffed endotracheal tube. Esophageal intubation is avoided until later in the procedure. After preparation of the skin and draping of the neck into the operative field, a 5-cm left oblique cervical skin incision is made along the anterior border of the left sternomastoid muscle. This incision extends from a point two fingerbreadths above the clavicle to the level of the hyoid bone. The sternomastoid muscle is retracted laterally, and the strap muscles and omohyoid muscle are identified. By blunt and sharp dissection, the retropharyngeal space is entered just cephalad to the omohyoid muscle. This latter landmark is at the approximate level of the diverticular neck. Goiter retractors are inserted to retract the carotid sheath and its contents laterally and the pharynx and larynx to the right. The cervical vertebral bodies make up the floor of the space entered; the pharynx and esophagus are in front. A band retractor placed over the omohyoid to retract it caudally exposes the entire diverticulum unless it is huge and extends into the mediastinum. In either event, the diverticulum is grasped with an Allis forceps and by blunt dissection is elevated and separated from the esophagus. Eventually, the apex of the diverticulum is grasped and brought cephalad.

At this point in the procedure, it is desirable and safe for the anesthesiologist to insert an esophageal stethoscope (28 F catheter) down the esophagus. The surgeon can help move this tube past the diverticulum into the upper esophagus. The tube itself provides a palpable identifying landmark for the pharynx and esophagus. Later in the procedure, at diverticulectomy, its presence prevents excessive loss of lumen when traction is applied to the diverticulum for amputation.

Once the diverticulum is completely mobilized and held at a right angle to the long axis of the esophagus, its neck is dissected out at the point where the mucosal sac protrudes through the muscular defect of the pharynx just above the cricopharyngeal muscle. Often, a coat of attenuated muscle and connective tissue 3–4 mm thick covers the mucosal sac. When this circumferential dissection of the diverticular neck is complete, the defect in the pharyngeal musculature is apparent.

A posterior vertical cricopharyngeal myotomy is now performed. This is effected by use of a right-angle forceps to develop an extramucosal dissection plane just inferior to the neck of the diverticulum, between muscularis and mucosa. The transverse fibers of the cricopharyngeal muscle are divided vertically for a distance of 3–4 mm. A TA 30 stapling device is then applied to the neck of the diverticulum at a right angle to the long axis of the esophagus. With the esophageal stethoscope in place, traction on the diverticulum draws the sac into the jaws of the stapling device, which is tightened onto the neck before the staples are delivered. The protruding sac is amputated with a scalpel. After the stapler is removed, the transverse closure retracts and contours onto the esophageal catheter-stethoscope. The mucosal closure is covered with musculature by vertically placed extramucosal sutures. The result is a transverse closure of the defect. Two small Penrose drains are brought from the retropharyngeal space to the outside through the lower end of the cervical wound, which is otherwise closed. The esophageal tube is removed at the end of the procedure.

TECHNIQUE OF CRICOPHARYNGEAL MYOTOMY.—After the preparation for anesthesia, draping, and surgical incision described for diverticulectomy are done, the retropharyngeal space is entered just above the level of the omohyoid muscle (see Fig 8–5). The small sac, 3–10 mm in diameter, is apparent just above the transverse fibers of the cricopharyngeal muscle. A right-angle forceps is used to develop an extramucosal dissection plane between esophageal mucosa and muscularis just inferior to this small mucosal sac. A vertical incision is made just inferior to the diverticulum for 3–4 cm. A cabochon-like bulge of mucosa occurs as the muscle fibers retract after division. No attempt is made to close the muscularis over the mucosa. The wound is drained and closed in the same way as that with diverticulectomy.

POSTOPERATIVE CARE.—The morning after the operation, the patient is examined radiographically with oral ingestion of diatrizoate meglumine and diatrizoate sodium solution (Gastrografin). If there is no sign that the mucosal closure is leaking, a liquid diet is begun, and rapid progress is made to a general diet in the next 72 hours. Wound drains are shortened and removed on postoperative days 3 and 4, and the patient is dismissed from the hospital on day 5. Full normal activities are resumed as comfort permits.

Although leakage from the esophageal repair is rare, studies should be carried out and a plan of management outlined. If there is evidence of mucosal leak on radiographic study, or if signs of excessive wound drainage develop, drains are left in place and the patient is fed nothing by mouth for 7–10 days. If repeated radiographic studies still show leakage, a parenteral alimentation line is inserted to restore a positive nitrogen balance within the next week. By that time, with a well-established drainage tract, it usually is possible to begin oral feedings. Eventually, the drains can be removed with the expectation of spontaneous closure of the fistula.

In the unusual patient who is severely depleted nutritionally or has pulmonary sepsis, parenteral alimentation is begun 1–2 days before operation. Efforts should be made to restore normal fluid and electrolyte balance and hemoglobin concentration and to improve oxygen transport and cardiorespiratory function. Bronchoscopic toilet and massive antibiotic therapy are indicated for those with pulmonary sepsis and copious secretions. Early surgical intervention is desirable, and parenteral nutrition should be continued until uncomplicated oral ingestion is possible. In these severely depleted patients, parenteral feedings rarely need to be continued for more than 7–10 days. We have never found it necessary or desirable to use feeding gastrostomy or nasogastric tube feeding. Thin barium suspension is used in lieu of diatrizoate meglumine or diatrizoate sodium solution for radiographic study because it is a safer medium if accidentally aspirated by a patient with preexisting pulmonary complications.

RESULTS.—During the 35-year period 1944–78, 888 patients were treated at the Mayo Clinic by means of a one-stage pharyngoesophageal diverticulectomy.[26–28] Thirty-five patients had cricopharyngeal myotomy in addition to diverticulectomy.[27] The results are shown in Tables 8–2 and 8–3. The late results of myotomy with diverticulectomy were nearly identical to those of diverticulectomy alone. During the latter decade of this experience, nine additional patients were treated by cricopharyngeal myotomy alone for small diverticula.[27] Seven of them had excellent results, but two had diverticular progression and recurrent symptoms, justifying subsequent diverticulectomy.

TABLE 8–2.—RESULTS IN 888 PATIENTS UNDERGOING ONE-STAGE PHARYNGOESOPHAGEAL DIVERTICULECTOMY AT THE MAYO CLINIC, JAN. 1, 1944, THROUGH DEC. 31, 1978

RESULT	PATIENTS	
	No.	%
Morbidity		
Vocal cord paralysis	28	3.2
Wound infection	27	3.0
With fistula	16	1.8
Mortality	11	1.2
Recurrence	32	3.6

From Payne W.S., Reynolds R.R.[27] By permission of Surgical Rounds Publishing Corporation.

TABLE 8–3.—LATE RESULTS (5–14 YEARS) AFTER ONE-STAGE PHARYNGOESOPHAGEAL DIVERTICULECTOMY*

RESULT	NO.	%	
Excellent	135	82	93
Good	18	11	
Fair	5	3	
Poor	6	4	
Total	164	100	

*Definitions: excellent and good, highly satisfactory; fair, improved but symptomatic; poor, recurrence established. These results are identical to the results in 888 patients followed up for 1–20 years. (From Payne W.S., Reynolds R.R.[27] By permission of Surgical Rounds Publishing Corporation.)

One-stage pharyngoesophageal diverticulectomy with or without myotomy is a highly effective, relatively safe procedure that provides long-term control in more than 93% of patients. There is little deterioration of the good results with the passage of time (see Table 8–3).[26, 27] Although it is difficult to justify myotomy as an adjunct to diverticulectomy on the basis of the present data, we are encouraged that no leaks occurred when the procedure was performed as described and that, when there was anatomical recurrence, the symptoms often were less severe. Obviously, myotomy adds little time and no morbidity to diverticulectomy. Continued use of the combination seems warranted.

Cricopharyngeal myotomy alone for small diverticula has been less rewarding. In our small series, only 78% of the patients had complete and permanent control of symptoms. Both patients with symptoms at late follow-up had diverticular recurrence and progression in diverticular size. Although recurrences were resolvable by diverticulectomy, it was disappointing that the initial effort had failed. Nevertheless, knowing that this is the only currently available method of managing this symptomatic problem, we continue to suggest myotomy alone for the small diverticulum.

Although diverticular recurrences are uncommon after properly performed first surgical procedures, we have had considerable experience with reoperation for persistent and recurrent pharyngoesophageal diverticula after many different kinds of procedures.

In a recent analysis and comparison of the results of primary operations and reoperations for diverticulum,[28] it was found that almost all the morbidity and mortality previously reported by us for this operation was seen among 31 patients undergoing reoperation (Table 8–4). It was clear that, although recurrent diverticulum is uncommon after one-stage diverticulectomy with or without myotomy, it poses a major technical challenge, irrespective of the type of previous operation performed. Happily, late results of reoperation were highly satisfactory.

MOTOR DISORDERS OF BODY OF ESOPHAGUS AND LES

Achalasia of the Esophagus

Thomas Willis[29] is credited with the first description of this condition. His report in 1674 not only provided a clear description of the clinical syndrome but also suggested an accurate pathophysiologic mechanism, described a method of treatment using forceful dilatation, and reported a 15-year follow-up of sustained good results from that treatment. This extraordinary report was lost from the mainstream of medicine for nearly 300 years,[30] leaving the problem for others to rediscover.

Achalasia is a specific motility disturbance of the esophagus characterized by an absence of peristalsis in the body of the esophagus and a nonrelaxing, often hypertensive, LES. It affects males and females of all ages, from childhood through adult life to old age. It has been shown to be related to a loss of vagal innervation to the body of the esophagus and the LES. Neural degeneration from the vagal motor nucleus in the brainstem to the myenteric plexus in the esophageal wall has been documented. No specific cause for the neural degeneration has been defined. Although *Trypanosoma cruzi* may produce a picture identical to that of achalasia, it is improbable that Chagas' disease is responsible for the cases of achalasia seen throughout the world outside the endemic areas of South America.

TABLE 8–4.—COMPARISON OF RESULTS OF PRIMARY OPERATIONS AND OF REOPERATIONS FOR PHARYNGOESOPHAGEAL DIVERTICULUM IN 356 PATIENTS

RESULTS	PRIMARY OPERATIONS (n = 325)		REOPERATIONS (n = 31)	
	No.	%	No.	%
Morbidity				
Vocal cord paralysis	5	1.5	6	19.4
Wound infection	3	0.9	10	32.2
With fistula	2	0.6	6	19.4
Mortality	3	0.9	1	3.2
Recurrence	10	3.1	2	6.4
Functional result	277*	. . .	29†	. . .
Excellent-good	258	93	28	97
Fair-poor	19	7	1	3

*Among the 325 patients, 25 were lost to follow-up and there were 20 late deaths and 3 operative deaths.
†Based on number of survivors. One patient having reoperation died late of an unrelated cause. (From Huang B.S., Payne W.S., Cameron A.J.[28] By permission of Little, Brown & Co.)

CLINICAL FEATURES.—The clinical features of achalasia are distal esophageal obstruction with esophageal retention and spontaneous, effortless regurgitation of bland, undigested, fresh food and saliva. The major complications of the condition are nutritional depletion and suppurative lung disease (Table 8–5). The suppurative lung disease is secondary to accidental respiratory aspiration of regurgitated esophageal contents. Initially, dysphagia is episodic and unrelated to the mechanical properties of the material ingested. At times, entire meals may be ingested with little or no distress; then, inexplicably, symptoms worsen to the extent that all or portions of a meal fail to pass. The frequency and duration of dysphagia imperceptibly increase and are interspersed with irregular and unpredictable episodes of apparent remission.

Patients with achalasia not only experience respiratory and nutritional problems but also have an increased incidence of esophagitis and cancer. Approximately one third of the patients with achalasia have subjective heartburn and a few have objective esophagitis, but this is not due to gastroesophageal reflux. Such changes in the untreated patient are caused by chronic esophageal retention and stasis secondary to achalasia. The cause for the increased incidence of cancer of the esophagus and cardia in patients who have achalasia is not known, although cancer tends to occur in patients who have long-standing (more than 20 years in duration) untreated achalasia. Such cancers are distributed throughout the length of the esophagus and have no specific anatomical predilection. Because of the long-standing preexisting esophageal symptoms of achalasia, most of these cancers are undiagnosed until quite advanced.

The diagnosis of achalasia usually can be suspected from the clinical symptoms alone, but esophageal radiography, manometry, and endoscopy are required for complete evaluation. There appears to be some vague correlation between the degree of esophageal dilatation and tortuosity seen on the x-ray film (Fig 8–6) and the duration or severity of obstructive esophageal symptoms; for example, esophageal retention and regur-

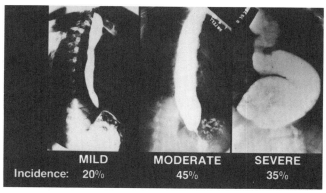

MILD   MODERATE   SEVERE
Incidence: 20%   45%   35%

Fig 8–6.—Radiographic findings in patients undergoing treatment for achalasia of esophagus. Note that 20% of patients had minimal or no increase in esophageal caliber, 45% showed moderate dilatation and tortuosity, and 35% showed severe or advanced dilatation and tortuosity. (From Payne W.S.: Disorders of oesophageal motility, in Dyde J.A., Smith R.E. (eds.): *The Present State of Thoracic Surgery: The Fifth Coventry Conference.* London, Pitman Medical, 1981, pp. 137–158. Used by permission.)

gitation are more bothersome in patients with more advanced radiographic stages. In our experience, only one third of patients have classic megaesophagus, and in many of these the symptoms are of relatively short duration and indistinguishable from those in patients with less significant radiographic changes. Thus, we regard radiographic stages as interesting but noncritical descriptive features of a patient's condition. Incidentally, radiographic features are unlikely to improve significantly after successful treatment of achalasia.

Manometric study of esophageal motility with the use of perfused catheters is the most reliable and sensitive method of diagnosing achalasia. Classically, esophageal contractions are small, repetitive, simultaneous, and nonperistaltic. Eighty-seven percent of our patients have this finding, whereas 13% have the manometric features of vigorous achalasia.[31] The resting pressure tone of the LES in all patients with achalasia is often above normal, and the sphincter fails to relax normally with swallowing. This latter feature is essential for establishing the diagnosis of achalasia. Endoscopy should always be performed at diagnosis to rule out other esophageal and gastroduodenal conditions; for instance, in rare cases, the x-ray and manometric findings of classic achalasia actually are manifestations of cancer of the esophagogastric junction.

TREATMENT.—The goal of treatment in patients with achalasia is to relieve symptoms of obstruction by weakening the LES and thereby improving the emptying of the esophagus. There is no medical or surgical cure for this disease, and all current efforts at treatment should be considered palliative. Regardless of the type of current therapy used, peristalsis and LES function are not restored. Treatment consists of either forceful pneumatic dilatation or surgical esophagomyotomy.[32]

FORCEFUL DILATATION.—Pneumatic dilatation (Fig 8–7) is performed by passing an inflatable bag over a previously swallowed thread to straddle the gastroesophageal junction

TABLE 8–5.—COMPLICATIONS
OF ACHALASIA*

Obstruction to swallowing
  Malnutrition
  Dehydration
  Delayed growth and development
Regurgitation
  Respiratory aspiration
Esophageal retention
  Subjective heartburn
  Stasis esophagitis
Neurosis
  Solitary dining
  Valsalva's maneuver
  Drinking of copious liquids
  Coughing and choking
  Regurgitation
  Sleep deprivation
Late development of carcinoma of esophagus

*(From Payne W.S.: Disorders of oesophageal motility, in Dyde J.A., Smith R.E. (eds.): *The Present State of Thoracic Surgery: The Fifth Coventry Conference.* London, Pitman Medical, 1981, pp. 137–158. By permission.)

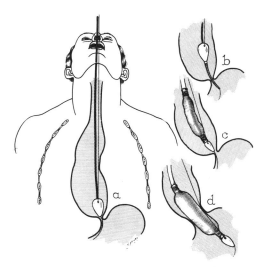

Fig 8–7.—Method of performing dilatations: *a,* olive-tipped (41 F) bougie being passed to stomach; *b,* sound (50 or 60 F) guided by flexible wire spiral is passed into stomach; *c,* hydrostatic dilator is passed to cardia and distended within cardia *(d).* (From Olsen A.M., Harrington S.W., Moersch H.J., et al.: The treatment of cardiospasm: Analysis of a twelve-year experience. *J. Thorac. Cardiovasc. Surg.* 22:164, 1951. Used by permission of the C.V. Mosby Company.)

and then inflating it. Proper positioning of the bag at the cardia and in the region of the LES is determined either by fluoroscopy or by inference after the preliminary passage of a bougie. The recent modification of fixing the dilating balloon to a fiberoptic scope has permitted retroflexed viewing of the balloon during dilation. After proper positioning, balloon inflation is carefully performed with pressures of 549–670 cm H_2O (hydrostatic dilatation) or 150–200 mm Hg (pneumatic dilatation). With either method, the pressure is sustained for several seconds before the procedure is terminated. The patient is allowed to resume a normal diet after the procedure.

ESOPHAGOMYOTOMY.—The current technique of esophagomyotomy is identical to that used at the Mayo Clinic since 1949 (Fig 8–8,A and B).[33, 34] The procedure consists of a left transthoracic longitudinal esophagomyotomy that begins at the esophagogastric junction and extends 7–10 cm proximally to the level of the left inferior pulmonary vein. Care is taken to avoid undue traction on the esophagus and dissection around the esophageal hiatus, which might lead to the development of hiatal hernia. Approximately 50% of the circumference of the esophageal mucosal tube is free of overlying muscularis to allow the mucosa to pout through the site of the myotomy. Care is taken to avoid injury to vagal fibers and to avoid extending the myotomy onto the stomach. If an anatomical sliding esophageal hiatal hernia is present, it is repaired. The esophagus is returned to its mediastinal bed, and the mediastinal pleura is reapproximated. The lung is reexpanded, a nasogastric tube and a chest tube are inserted, and the chest is closed. On the morning after operation, the nasogastric tube and chest tube are removed, and normal diet is resumed.

If a defect is created in the esophageal mucosa at the time of myotomy, it is repaired with interrupted 5–0 silk sutures in the mucosal layer only. In such circumstances, radiographic examination is performed the morning after operation before the nasogastric tube and chest tube are removed and before the normal diet is resumed. If there is good esophageal emptying and no leakage is apparent, the normal postoperative routine is followed. However, if there is a delayed esophageal emptying or leakage, parenteral alimentation is begun and is continued for at least ten days or until complete sealing is apparent radiographically. By following this routine, we have avoided significant clinical morbidity in those patients in whom mucosal tear has occurred.

RESULTS.—During the 27-year period 1949 through 1975, 899 patients underwent treatment for achalasia of the esoph-

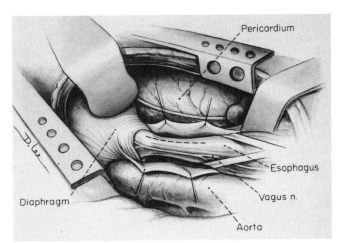

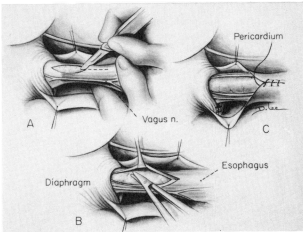

Fig 8–8.—**Upper,** transthoracic exposure of distal esophagus for esophagomyotomy. Note that left lung has been retracted cephalad, and the mediastinal pleura has been opened. This procedure exposes the distal esophagus, which has been encircled by a soft rubber drain. **Lower,** technique of esophagomyotomy. *A,* beginning the incision. *B,* dissection of the mucosa from the muscularis. *C,* restoration of esophagogastric junction to intra-abdominal position with sutures to narrow esophageal hiatus, if necessary. (From Ellis F.H. Jr., Olsen A.M.: Achalasia of the esophagus. *Major Probl. Clin. Surg.* 9:1, 1969. Used by permission.)

agus at the Mayo Clinic: 468 by transthoracic esophagomyotomy and 431 by one or more forceful hydrostatic or pneumatic dilatations (Fig 8–9).[35]

EARLY RESULTS.—The early complications of treatment are compared in Table 8–6. Except for transient, rare episodes of cardiac arrhythmia or retention of tracheobronchial secretions, the early postoperative course of patients undergoing esophagomyotomy was usually benign. In five patients, however, a definable esophageal leak developed; three of them required additional surgical intervention for management. The single death among the 468 patients treated by esophagomyotomy was unrelated to the operation. In fact, malignant hyperthermia developed in this patient while anesthesia was being induced, and so the operation was not actually performed. Nevertheless, the outcome is counted as a surgical death.

Among the 431 patients managed by forceful dilatation, most had minimal morbidity after treatment. Nineteen patients experienced esophageal perforation, and 10 of these required surgical management; all 19 survived. The two early postdilatation deaths were due to acute myocardial infarction and were not directly attributable to the dilatation.

LATE RESULTS.—Table 8–7 compares the late follow-up results on 767 patients at 1–18 years after treatment. The criteria for assessing results of treatment were identical in the two treatment groups.[36] The late results of esophagomyotomy were significantly better than those for forceful dilatation (P < 0.001): 85% of those treated surgically had "excellent" or "good" results on late follow-up compared with only 65% of those treated by dilatation. Among those patients treated by dilatation, most underwent the treatment once, 16% required two treatments, and 2% required three or more.

The late results of surgical treatment were analyzed by pa-

TABLE 8–6.—EARLY COMPLICATIONS OF TREATMENT OF ACHALASIA

	DILATATION (n = 431)	ESOPHAGOMYOTOMY (n = 468)
Deaths	2*	1*
Esophageal leak†	19(10)	5(3)

*Deaths not related to procedure.
†Numbers in parentheses are operations required to control leakage.
(Data from Okike N., et al.[35])

TABLE 8–7.—LATE RESULTS OF TREATMENT OF ACHALASIA

	DILATATION (n = 431)		ESOPHAGOMYOTOMY (n = 468)	
Result, %*				
Excellent	28	65†	50	85†
Good	37		35	
Fair	16		9	
Poor	19		6	
Follow-up, yr	1–18		1–17	
Patients followed				
No.	311		456	
Percent	72		97	
Ages of patients at operation, yr	1–85		4–81	

*Criteria, from Payne and King,[36] were as follows: excellent = asymptomatic, gained weight, returned to normal activities; good = significant improvement, occasional dysphagia, no regurgitation; fair = definite improvement, occasional dysphagia with regurgitation; poor = worsening of achalasia or no improvement.
†Significantly different, P < 0.001.
(From Okike N., Payne W.S., Neufeld D.M., et al.[35] By permission of Little, Brown Co.)

tient's age and sex, duration of symptoms, degree of esophageal dilatation, presence or absence of hiatal hernia, or presence of classic or vigorous achalasia on manometric study, and one of these factors appeared to be important in determining the outcome. Even previous forceful dilatation did not affect results, provided it had not been performed more than once or twice before operation. Multiple forceful dilatations occasionally resulted in fusion and fibrous obliteration of the tissue plane between the mucosa and the muscularis and made effective myotomy technically difficult or, at times, impossible to perform. Results were uniformly poor under such circumstances.

DISCUSSION.—From our experience it is evident that esophagomyotomy is more effective and safer than forceful dilatation and provides a longer-lasting favorable result. "Fair" or "poor" results occurred twice as often among patients undergoing dilatation as among those treated by myotomy. Failure to relieve the obstructing LES is more often the defined cause for these residual symptoms. Gastroesophageal reflux and its complications are rare (2.5%) after a properly performed esophagomyotomy. The chief cause for such reflux complications can clearly be defined as overzealous extension of the esophageal myotomy onto the stomach. Those intent on performing esophagogastric myotomy have uniformly reported a higher incidence of postoperative reflux

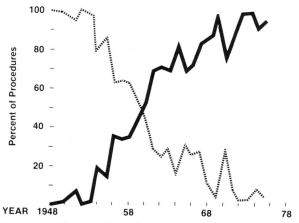

Fig 8–9.—Observed trends in management of achalasia of the esophagus in 899 patients seen at the Mayo Clinic from 1949 through 1975. Percentage distribution of the two forms of treatment by year is shown. Note shift in emphasis toward esophagomyotomy *(solid curve)* and away from forceful hydrostatic or pneumatic dilatation *(dotted curve)* since 1949. (From Okike N., Payne W.S., Neufeld D.M., et al.: Esophagomyotomy versus forceful dilatation for achalasia of the esophagus: Results in 899 patients. *Ann. Thorac. Surg.* 28:119, 1979. Used by permission of Little, Brown & Co.)

problems. Similarly, those in the past who adhered to the classic Heller procedure[37] or to the procedures that totally destroy or bypass the LES, such as the pyloroplasty-like procedures of the cardia described respectively by Heyerovsky, Grondahl, and Wendel, have had disastrously high incidences of reflux problems.[38]

In recent years there has been renewed interest in performing incompetence-producing esophagogastric myotomy by one of the standard antireflux procedures to restore competence.[39] We recognize the necessity for hiatal hernia repair in the rare achalasia patient with preexisting hiatal hernia,[35] but results have not been significantly different from those observed when esophagomyotomy alone is done in the absence of hiatal hernia. Furthermore, it has been our observation among achalasia patients undergoing reoperation[40] that the addition of antireflux procedures to esophagogastric myotomy can be associated with unpredictable obstruction of the esophagus or, at other times, failure to produce competence, especially when the esophagus has become greatly dilated, hypertrophied, and tortuous.

For the present at least, we see the routine addition of an antireflux procedure to the modified Heller procedure described as being an unnecessary complication and a potential source of complicating consequences.

Over the past decade one of us (W.S.P.) has attempted to investigate the possibility of improving the results of esophagomyotomy by insuring more complete destruction of the suprahiatal portion of the LES.[41] On the basis of the previous observations by Olsen et al.[42] (Fig 8–10), a technique for intraoperative esophageal manometry has been used, first to document the effect of myotomy and subsequently as a guide

to the extent of distal myotomy extension. Early postoperative results have been excellent, but sufficient time has not elapsed to determine whether this approach will improve late results. A similar approach has been reported recently by Hill et al.[43]

A discussion of achalasia of the esophagus would not be complete without some reference to some of the newer calcium antagonists that are known to decrease the contraction of smooth muscle.[44] Our rather limited clinical experience with such agents at times has been impressive, but the side effects of the medication and the chronicity of treatment detract from its use.

Reoperations for achalasia have received little notice in the literature since our 1971 report.[45] We have continued to use remyotomy in those patients in whom a previous myotomy has healed. In a more recent review of that subject,[46] we were discouraged that, with further experience and additional follow-up, only 60% of the patients had "good" or "excellent" late results. These results were not enhanced by adding antireflux procedures. It was significant, however, that remyotomy could be effected with minimal morbidity and no mortality.

Management alternatives beyond myotomy for reoperations for achalasia are legion. These include, in our experience, long and short colon interpositions, esophagogastrostomy combined with gastric antrectomy with long-limb Roux-en-Y gastric drainage procedure, total thoracic blunt esophagectomy without thoracotomy, and the Ivor-Lewis type esophagogastric resection and reconstruction with thoracotomy. Each of these procedures carries considerably more risk than does myotomy alone, and each has specific early and late complications. Each is also capable of producing excellent results. Not enough time has elapsed and not enough cases have accrued to permit a final judgment as to which procedure is most desirable. It should be apparent, however, that reoperation should be required infrequently if the initial myotomy is properly performed.

It becomes mandatory to reoperate, however, when a patient's clinical course becomes complicated by respiratory aspiration or nutritional depletion. Short of these serious complications, there is another 5%–10% of myotomized patients who, although improved, have varying degrees of imperfection in their clinical results that they would like to eliminate. The decision to reoperate on this mildly symptomatic but not threatened subgroup should be undertaken with caution. Some have sufficient interference with daily function and comfort that reoperation is reasonable. Others have misconceptions regarding the significance of residual symptoms rather than being incapacitated by them. Always it should be kept in mind that none of the techniques for the management of achalasia is curative in the sense of restoring the motor activity to the esophagus or its lower sphincter. All have as their goal the palliation of the symptoms of achalasia and the prevention of serious complications.

Diffuse Spasm of the Esophagus and Allied Hypermotility Disturbances

CLINICAL FEATURES.—Diffuse spasm of the esophagus is less clearly defined than achalasia. The dominant and most consistent clinical feature is pain. Characteristically, this pain

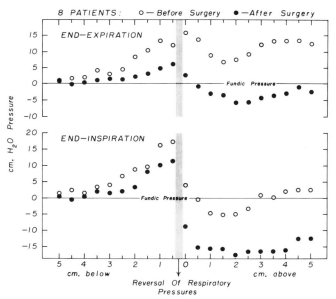

Fig 8–10.—Mean resting pressures at gastroesophageal junction in eight patients before *(open circles)* and after *(solid circles)* esophagomyotomy. Note reduction in pressure after operation with partial retention of subhiatal segment. (From Olsen A.M., Schlegel J.F., Creamer B., et al.: Esophageal motility in achalasia (cardiospasm) after treatment. *J. Thorac. Cardiovasc. Surg.* 34:615, 1957. Used by permission of the C.V. Mosby Co.)

is spontaneous, retrosternal, and crushing, identical to that of myocardial infarction, with radiation into the neck, jaw, or ear and not infrequently down the ulnar aspect of one or both upper extremities. Because there often are no accompanying esophageal symptoms and distress often occurs spontaneously, these patients frequently have been managed as if they had acute myocardial ischemia, even with coronary arteriography, before other diagnostic possibilities are entertained. In other patients, the pain is more clearly induced during swallowing, with extremely cold or carbonated liquids being provocative. In still others, the pain is more clearly associated with esophageal dysfunction; esophageal obstruction, retention, and regurgitation are common in this subgroup.

Contrast radiograms are normal at the time of examination in nearly half of patients; the classic findings of "curling," "corkscrew," "rosary," or "pseudodiverticulosis" of the esophagus are seen with varying intensity in the remainder. Epiphrenic pulsion diverticulum, with or without other classic radiographic signs of diffuse spasm, is seen in less than 5% of patients.

Manometric studies usually identify the hypermotility nature of the problem, whether the patient is symptomatic or not at the time of study (Fig 8–11). Swallowing studies show that orderly sequential peristaltic contractions are lost in the lower half to two thirds of the thoracic esophagus and are replaced by simultaneous, repetitive, prolonged contractions of high amplitude. Similar spontaneous contractions of this type are seen in resting studies as well as during swallowing and are almost always confined to the smooth muscle portion of the esophagus. The incidences of associated hiatal hernia or gastroesophageal reflux problems reported have varied depending both on the method of study and the authors' conviction that patients with manifest reflux belong in this or a separate category of secondary motility disturbances.

Results of psychometric examinations of patients with diffuse spasm of the esophagus are frequently abnormal.[47] It is not entirely clear whether this is a cause or an effect of the disease. There is no question that, in some individuals, episodes of severe distress are precipitated by emotional tension, an association well recognized by patients and physicians.

Various associated hypermotility disturbances are recognized manometrically although they are usually indistinguishable clinically from pure diffuse spasm in their subjective manifestations. It has been noted that 60% of patients with the manometric features of diffuse spasm have an entirely normal LES mechanism during both rest and swallowing. Such cases may be considered to be a type of segmental esophageal spasm. Leonardi et al.[48] have reported excellent results after sphincter-saving esophagomyotomy in a high proportion of these patients (Fig 8–12). Other variations include both the hypertensive esophageal sphincter and the hypercontracting LES. Either of these has been seen alone or in combination with diffuse spasm of the entire lower esophagus. These latter two types of sphincter abnormalities have required myotomy of the sphincteric area for management.

Another variant of esophageal hypermotility disturbance is the so-called nutcracker esophagus. Although these patients have sequential peristaltic esophageal motility, the contractions are of high amplitude with prolonged duration. The condition can be associated with both pain and esophageal dysfunction.

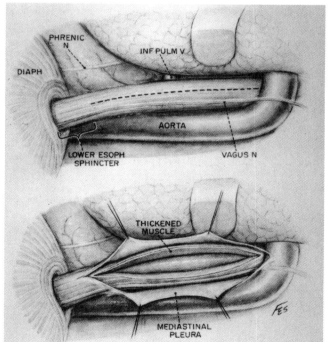

Fig 8–12.—Lower esophageal sphincter-sparing extended esophagomyotomy, as suggested by group at Lahey Clinic, for selected patients with segmental diffuse spasm of the esophagus in whom LES was normal and not involved as determined by preoperative manometry. In their experience, exclusion of the LES from myotomy afforded satisfactory antireflux protection without an ancillary antireflux procedure. (From Leonardi H.K., Shea J.A., Crozier R.E., et al.: Diffuse spasm of the esophagus: Clinical, manometric, and surgical considerations. *J. Thorac. Cardiovasc. Surg.* 74:736, 1977. Used by permission of C.V. Mosby Co.)

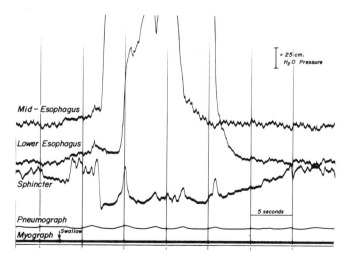

Fig 8–11.—Diffuse spasm: motility in esophagus and sphincter. Note giant repetitive contractions. Sphincter relaxes normally. Although usually absent, peristalsis is present in this case. (From Ellis F.H. Jr., Code C.F., Olsen A.M.: Long esophagomyotomy for diffuse spasm of the esophagus and hypertensive gastroesophageal sphincter. *Surgery* 48:155, 1960. Used by permission of the C.V. Mosby Co.)

TREATMENT.—Many patients with hypermotility disturbances of the esophagus have such mild and intermittent distress that diagnosis alone provides sufficient reassurance that no further treatment is required. Others will require intermittent treatment with nitroglycerin, long-acting nitrates, calcium-blocking agents, or periodic bougienage to control symptoms.[49–51] Few patients present with continuous, severe symptoms. Long-term medical management in this latter group often is ineffectual or is abandoned because of annoying side effects of medication or lack of response. A few patients are seriously disabled by their severe but non–life-threatening symptoms and often seek surgical treatment.

Long esophagomyotomy has been the standard surgical approach, but how long, in which direction, and whether to carry out rouine antireflux procedures remain as controversial as individual enthusiasm about results of such surgery (Figs 8–12 and 8–13).[3, 48, 52, 53]

At the Mayo Clinic, our enthusiasm for the surgical management of patients with diffuse spasm and allied hypermotility disturbances is considerably less than that reported by others.[3, 48, 52, 53] Although the initial response to long myotomy with or without antireflex measures usually is quite satisfactory, there is serious deterioration in quality of results with the passage of time. Indeed, we have seen patients with persistent good results after treatment inexplicably revert to preoperative status or worse at 3–5 years postoperatively. This is in sharp contrast to the achalasia patient: once "good" or "excellent" results are attained after myotomy, they are usually sustained for many decades.

Secondary operations may become necessary and are usually required to manage patients with sustained and persistent severe disability after myotomy. Esophagectomy has been the most reliable approach, with either stomach or colon used in reconstruction.

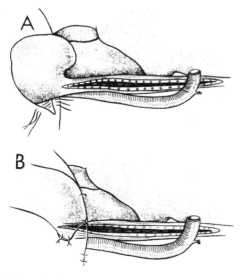

Fig 8–13.—A, drawing illustrating extent of myotomy to apex of chest and including HPZ. **B,** reflux control is achieved with a modified Nissen fundoplication in which the completion fundoplication is reduced to less than 0.5 cm in total length. (From Henderson R.D.: Diffuse esophageal spasm. *Surg. Clin. North Am.* 63:951, August 1983. Used by permission.)

It should be recognized that many patients with hypermotility disturbances carry a heavy emotional burden, and transference—in terms of incisional distress or emotional intolerance to imperfection in function or comfort at any level—is poorly managed. Because of the highly subjective nature of disability in many, selection of patients for operation should be undertaken with caution. Those with combined motility and x-ray findings generally respond better than do those with just manometric findings. Interestingly, those cases with associated epiphrenic diverticulum have had the best results, while those with manifest reflux problems are least satisfactory in our experience.

Epiphrenic Diverticulum of the Thoracic Esophagus

Pulsion diverticula of the thoracic esophagus tend to occur in the lower smooth muscle portion of the thoracic esophagus. Because of a predilection for the 10 cm above the diaphragm, the term "epiphrenic diverticula" is commonly used to differentiate these from "traction diverticula," which tend to occur at the carinal level, and "pharyngoesophageal diverticula," which occur in the neck.

Epiphrenic diverticula are relatively common, with an incidence relative to pharyngoesophageal diverticula of 1:5. The condition is clearly acquired in most instances, although a few have been reported associated with bronchopulmonary foregut malformation with various heterotopic epithelial linings. Such cases are undoubtedly congenital. A few have been reported in association with mediastinal granuloma or leiomyoma, and the term "pulsion traction diverticula" has evolved to describe these circumstances, whether fully justified or not.

Although epiphrenic diverticulum was first described by Deguise in 1804, little was known regarding the significance of this problem until relatively recently. Clairmont, who performed the first extirpation of this type of diverticula in 1927, used an extrapleural approach. A transpleural approach was first reported by Barrett[54] in 1933.

Functional and organic mechanical esophageal obstructions were probably first appreciated in the genesis of these diverticula by Vinson[55] at the Mayo Clinic in 1934. This feature was subsequently emphasized by Harrington[56] in 1939, Goodman and Parnes[57] in 1952, Habein et al.[58] in 1956, Effler et al.[59] in 1959, Cross et al.[60] in 1961, Allen and Clagett[61] in 1965, and by Debas et al.[62] in 1980. Unfortunately, almost all of our information regarding these diverticula relates to symptomatic patients. Most patients seen with epiphrenic diverticula are either asymptomatic or have had such mild symptoms at diagnosis that neither extensive investigation nor therapy is warranted. This is unfortunate from the viewpoint of complete understanding of the genesis of all diverticula in this region.

The inference is that at least the symptomatic epiphrenic diverticulum develops as a mucosal protrusion through some weak point in the esophageal musculature as a consequence of increased intraluminal pressure caused by either distal esophageal obstruction or a motor disorder. In a recent report from the Mayo Clinic by Debas et al.,[62] 65 patients with symptomatic epiphrenic diverticulum were reviewed in whom radiographic, endoscopic, and manometric studies were performed. Fifty patients (77%) had manometric evidence of abnormal esophageal motility: 21 had diffuse spasm, 13 had hiatal hernia, and 5 of the 13 had distal, high-grade, reflux-induced, esophageal stenosis. Only 8 of the 65 patients had no definable organic or functional abnormality to explain the development of diverticulum or its symptoms.

CLINICAL FEATURES.—Most patients with epiphrenic diverticula either have been asymptomatic or have such mild symptoms at diagnosis that extensive investigation and therapy are not warranted. In others, the symptoms seem to be compatible with a diverticulum. However, at times the symptoms have been difficult to differentiate from those of associated mechanical and functional conditions. Dysphagia, esophageal retention, and regurgitation are frequent and characteristic of diverticulum, but symptoms of associated diaphragmatic hernia, esophagitis, stricture, diffuse spasm, or achalasia may dominate. Secondary symptoms of respiratory aspiration are seen but are less frequent than in patients with pharyngoesophageal diverticulum. Primary carcinoma has been noted occasionally with epiphrenic diverticulum, as reported by Allen and Clagett,[61] as have rare benign neoplasms, particularly leiomyoma and lipoma.

Radiographic examination of the esophagus is the most reliable means of determining the presence of a pulsion diverticulum of the thoracic esophagus (Fig 8–14). Endoscopic examination and studies of esophageal motility are essential in evaluating patients and defining the nature and severity of associated conditions. Esophagoscopy also may be required not only for diagnosing the condition but also for removing retained debris from the sac before operation in patients with severe retention and regurgitation.

TREATMENT AND RESULTS.—Treatment is surgical and is indicated chiefly in patients with symptoms, particularly when the symptoms are progressive or incapacitating. Simple medical measures often provide good temporary control in mildly symptomatic patients. Diverticulectomy should be considered when an operation is planned for the management of associated esophageal conditions, even when symptoms cannot be definitely attributed to the diverticulum. Surgical treatment also should be considered for any diverticulum that is progressively enlarging or has already attained considerable size, irrespective of symptoms.

The technique currently used at the Mayo Clinic is a transthoracic diverticulectomy, usually with a long extramucosal esophagomyotomy (Fig 8–15). The frequently associated slid-

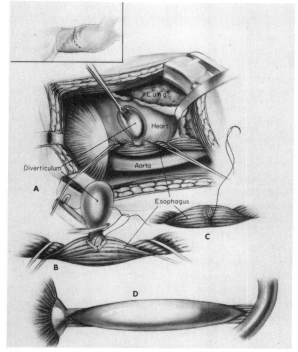

Fig 8–15.—Surgical management of pulsion diverticulum of the lower portion of the esophagus. *Inset,* placement of left posterolateral thoracotomy incision. *A,* exposure of diverticulum obtained when the chest is entered through bed of left eighth rib. Note that the esophagus has been delivered from its mediastinal bed, tapes have been passed around esophagus, and esophagus has been rotated to bring diverticulum into view. Neck of mucosal diverticulum has been dissected to allow identification of the defect in the esophageal muscular wall. *B,* cut-and-sew technique of diverticulectomy. Note that amputation and closure are effected in a transverse axis. Mucosal sutures are tied with knots within the esophageal lumen. *C,* closure of esophageal musculature over mucosal suture line. *D,* site of diverticular incision has been rotated back to right and is not visible. A long esophagomyotomy, extending from esophagogastric junction to aortic arch, has been performed. Musculature of esophagus has been freed from approximately 50% of circumference of esophageal mucosal tube to allow mucosa to bulge through muscular incision. Frequently associated sliding esophageal hiatal hernia is shown; when present, it should be repaired at this operation. (From Payne W.S.: Diverticula of the esophagus, in Payne W.S., Olsen A.M. (eds.): *The Esophagus.* Philadelphia, Lea & Febiger, 1974, pp. 207-223. Used by permission.)

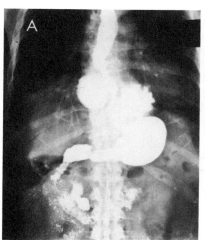
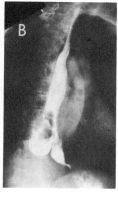

Fig 8–14.—Radiographs of esophagus and stomach showing epiphrenic diverticula. **A,** large, right-sided epiphrenic diverticulum, large combined sliding and paraesophageal hiatal hernia, and diffuse spasm of the esophagus. **B,** large epiphrenic diverticulum with filling defect that proved to be carcinoma arising in the diverticulum.

ing esophageal hiatal hernia is repaired at the same operation. One of the nonobstructive antireflux procedures is advised. Any associated esophageal obstructive condition must be corrected at or before operation, not only to prevent suture line leak and diverticulum recurrence but also to relieve the symptoms from the associated condition. No operative mortality has occurred, and long-term results of 18 patients treated in this manner have been good. In our total experience with 55 patients who underwent surgical treatment for epiphrenic diverticulum, two deaths have occurred. One death happened with induction of anesthesia; there was regurgitation and massive respiratory aspiration before the operation was performed. The other death occurred after operation, as a consequence of suture line leak and empyema. Four patients in the series had late recurrent epiphrenic diverticula.

Although the failure to utilize esophagomyotomy in conjunction with diverticulectomy may be equated with recurrence or suture line complication and postoperative death, these sequelae are not inevitable results of this omission. One may infer from the data, however, only that every effort should be made to correct associated esophageal conditions to minimize postoperative complications and symptoms. My colleagues and I have found that it is particularly valuable, in the postoperative management of these patients, to do early radiographic examination of the esophagus using an absorbable contrast medium—e.g., Gastrografin. This examination permits a final assessment of the suture line at the diverticulectomy site and evaluation of the esophagogastric lumen. When leak or obstruction is encountered, parenteral hyperalimentation is continued for three weeks before restudy and resumption of oral diet. Patients are generally asymptomatic after operation if associated esophageal conditions have been adequately dealt with at operation.

REFERENCES

1. Kronecker H., Meltzer S.: Der Schluckmechanismus, seine Erregung und seine Hemmung. *Arch. Anat. Physiol. (Physiol. Abteil.)* Suppl. 1883, pp. 328–360.
2. Duranceau A.C., Beauchamp G., Jamieson G.G., et al.: Oropharyngeal dysphagia and oculopharyngeal muscular dystrophy. *Surg. Clin. North Am.* 63:825, August 1983.
3. Henderson R.D.: *Motor Disorders of the Esophagus.* Baltimore, Williams & Wilkins, 1976.
4. Orringer M.B.: Extended cervical esophagomyotomy for cricopharyngeal dysfunction. *J. Thorac. Cardiovasc. Surg.* 80:669, 1980.
5. Hurwitz A.L., Duranceau A.: Upper-esophageal sphincter dysfunction: Pathogenesis and treatment. *Am. J. Dig. Dis.* 23:275, 1978.
6. Black R.J.: Cricopharyngeal myotomy. *J. Otolaryngol.* 10:145, 1981.
7. Duranceau A., Forand M.D., Fauteux J.P.: Surgery in oculopharyngeal muscular dystrophy. *Am. J. Surg.* 139:33, 1980.
8. Ellis F.H. Jr.: Upper esophageal sphincter in health and disease. *Surg. Clin. North Am.* 51:553, June 1971.
9. Ellis F.H. Jr., Crozier R.E.: Cervical esophageal dysphagia: Indications for results of cricopharyngeal myotomy. *Ann. Surg.* 194:279, 1981.
10. Fischer, R.A., Ellison G.W., Thayer W.R., et al.: Esophageal motility in neuromuscular disorders. *Ann. Intern. Med.* 63:229, 1965.
11. Palmer E.D.: Progress in gastroenterology: Disorders of the cricopharyngeus muscle; a review. *Gastroenterology* 71:510, 1976.
12. Paterson D.R.: A clinical type of dysphagia. *J. Laryngol. Otol.* 34:289, 1919.
13. Smith A.W.M., Mulder D.W., Code C.F.: Esophageal motility in amyotrophic lateral sclerosis. *Proc. Staff Meet. Mayo Clin.* 32:438, 1957.
14. Watson W.C., Sullivan S.N.: Hypertonicity of the cricopharyngeal sphincter: A cause of globus sensation. *Lancet* 2:1417, 1974.
15. Winans C.S.: The pharyngoesophageal closure mechanism: A manometric study. *Gastroenterology* 63:768, 1972.
16. Zaino C., Jacobson H.G., Lepow H., et al.: *The Pharyngoesophageal Sphincter.* Springfield, Ill.: Charles C Thomas, Publisher, 1970.
17. Ludlow A.: A case of obstructed deglutition, from a preternatural dilatation of, and bag formed in the pharynx. *Med. Observations Inquiries* (ed. 2) 3:85, 1769.
18. Ellis F.H. Jr., Schlegel J.F., Lynch V.P., et al.: Cricopharyngeal myotomy for pharyngo-esophageal diverticulum. *Ann. Surg.* 170:340, 1969.
19. Knuff T.E., Benjamin S.B., Castell D.O.: Pharyngoesophageal (Zenker's) diverticulum: A reappraisal. *Gastroenterology* 82:734, 1982.
20. Payne W.S.: Diverticula of the esophagus, in Payne W.S., Olsen A.M. (eds.): *The Esophagus.* Philadelphia, Lea & Febiger, 1974, pp. 207–223.
21. Sutherland H.D.: Cricopharyngeal achalasia. *J. Thorac. Cardiovasc. Surg.* 43:114, 1962.
22. Belsey R.: Functional disease of the esophagus. *J. Thorac. Cardiovasc. Surg.* 52:164, 1966.
23. Dohlman G., Mattsson O.: The endoscopic operation for hypopharyngeal diverticula: A roentgencinematographic study. *Arch. Otolaryngol.* 71:744, 1960.
24. Holinger P.H., Schild J.A.: The Zenker's (hypopharyngeal) diverticulum. *Ann. Otol. Rhinol. Laryngol.* 78:679, 1969.
25. Van Overbeek J.J.M.: *The Hypopharyngeal Diverticulum: Endoscopic Treatment and Manometry.* Assen, Netherlands, Van Gorcum, 1977.
26. Welsh G.F., Payne W.S.: The present status of one-stage pharyngo-esophageal diverticulectomy. *Surg. Clin. North Am.* 53:953, August 1973.
27. Payne W.S., Reynolds R.R.: Surgical treatment of pharyngoesophageal diverticulum (Zenker's diverticulum). *Surg. Rounds* 5:18, June 1982.
28. Huang B.-S., Payne W.S., Cameron A.J.: Surgical management for recurrent pharyngoesophageal (Zenker's) diverticulum. *Ann. Thorac. Surg.* 37:189, 1984.
29. Willis T.: *Pharmaceutice Rationalis Sive Diatriba de Medicamentorum Operationibus in Humano Corpore.* London, Hagae-Comitis, 1674.
30. Major R.H.: *Classic Descriptions of Disease: With Biographical Sketches of the Authors,* ed. 3. Springfield, Ill., Charles C Thomas, Publisher, 1945, p. 628.
31. Sanderson D.R., Ellis F.H. Jr., Schlegel J.F., et al.: Syndrome of vigorous achalasia: Clinical and physiologic observations. *Dis. Chest* 52:508, 1967.
32. Bortolotti M., Labò G.: Clinical and manometric effects of nifedipine in patients with esophageal achalasia. *Gastroenterology* 80:39, 1981.
33. Ellis F.H. Jr., Olsen A.M.: Achalasia of the esophagus. *Major Probl. Clin. Surg.* 9:1, 1969.
34. Payne W.S., Olsen A.M.: *The Esophagus.* Philadelphia, Lea & Febiger, 1974.
35. Okike N., Payne W.S., Neufeld D.M., et al.: Esophagomyotomy versus forceful dilation for achalasia of the esophagus: Results in 899 patients. *Ann. Thorac. Surg.* 28:119, 1979.
36. Payne W.S., King R.M.: Treatment of achalasia of the esophagus. *Surg. Clin. North Am.* 63:963, August 1983.
37. Heller E.: Extramuköse Cardioplastik beim chronischen Cardiospasmus mit Dilation des Oesophagus. *Med. Chir.* 27:141, 1913.
38. Riply H.R., Olsen A.M., Kirklin J.: Esophagitis after esophagogastric anastomosis. *Surgery* 32:1, 1952.
39. Jamieson G.G., Duranceau A.C.: Esophageal myotomy and gastroesophageal reflux. *Surg. Clin. North Am.* 63:877, August 1983.

40. Payne W.S.: Unpublished data, 1984.
41. Payne W.S., Ferguson T.B. (Conferee): Esophagomyotomy for achalasia of the esophagus. *Cardiothoracic Techniques* (Presented by Smith Kline & French Laboratories). New Scotland, New York, Learning Technology, 1984.
42. Olsen A.M., Schlegel J.F., Creamer B., et al: Esophageal motility in achalasia (cardiospasm) after treatment. *J. Thorac. Cardiovasc. Surg.* 34:615, 1957.
43. Hill L.D., Asplund C.M., Roberts P.N.: Intraoperative manometry: Adjunct to surgery for esophageal motility disorders. *Am. J. Surg.* 147:171, 1984.
44. Becker B.S., Burakoff R.: The effect of verapamil on the lower esophageal sphincter pressure in normal subjects and in achalasia. *Am. J. Gastroenterol.* 78:773, 1983.
45. Patrick D.L., Payne W.S., Olsen A.M., et al.: Reoperation for achalasia of the esophagus. *Arch. Surg.* 103:122, 1971.
46. Payne W.S., Neufeld D.M.: Unpublished data, 1984.
47. Clouse R.E., Lustman P.J.: Psychiatric illness and contraction abnormalities of the esophagus. *N. Engl. J. Med.* 309:1337, 1983.
48. Swamy N.: Esophageal spasm: Clinical and manometric response to nitroglycerin and long acting nitrites. *Gastroenterology* 72:23, 1977.
49. Richter J.E., Sinar D.R., Cordova C.M., et al.: Verapamil—a potent inhibitor of esophageal contractions in the baboon. *Gastroenterology* 82:882, 1982.
50. Mellow M.H.: Effect of isosorbide and hydralazine in painful primary esophageal motility disorders. *Gastroenterology* 83:364, 1982.
51. Ellis F.H. Jr., Code C.F., Olsen A.M.: Long esophagomyotomy for diffuse spasm of the esophagus and hypertensive gastroesophageal sphincter. *Surgery* 48:155, 1960.
52. Leonardi H.K., Shea J.A., Crozier R.E., et al.: Diffuse spasm of the esophagus: Clinical, manometric, and surgical considerations. *J. Thorac. Cardiovasc. Surg.* 74:736, 1977.
53. Henderson R.D.: Diffuse esophageal spasm. *Surg. Clin. North Am.* 63:951, August 1983.
54. Barrett N.R.: Diverticula of thoracic oesophagus: Report of a case in which the diverticulum was successfully resected. *Lancet* 1:1009, 1933.
55. Vinson P.P.: Diverticula of the thoracic portion of the esophagus: Report of forty-two cases. *Arch. Otolaryngol.* 19:508, 1934.
56. Harrington S.W.: Pulsion diverticula of the hypopharynx: A review of forty-one cases in which operation was performed and a report of two cases. *Surg. Gynecol. Obstet.* 69:364, 1939.
57. Goodman H.I., Parnes I.H.: Epiphrenic diverticula of the esophagus. *J. Thorac. Cardiovasc. Surg.* 23:145, 1952.
58. Habein H.C. Jr., Kirklin J.W., Clagett O.T., et al.: Surgical treatment of lower esophageal pulsion diverticula. *Arch. Surg.* 72:1018, 1956.
59. Effler D.B., Barr D., Groves L.K.: Epiphrenic diverticulum of the esophagus: Surgical treatment. *Arch. Surg.* 79:459, 1959.
60. Cross F.S., Johnson G.F., Gerein A.N.: Esophageal diverticula: Associated neuromuscular changes in the esophagus. *Arch. Surg.* 83:525, 1961.
61. Allen T.H., Clagett O.T.: Changing concepts in the surgical treatment of pulsion diverticula of the lower esophagus. *J. Thorac. Cardiovasc. Surg.* 50:455, 1965.
62. Debas H.T., Payne W.S., Cameron A.J., et al.: Physiopathology of lower esophageal diverticulum and its implications for treatment. *Surg. Gynecol. Obstet.* 151:593, 1980.

9

Gastroesophageal Reflux Disease

TOM R. DEMEESTER, M.D.

INTRODUCTION

Foregut symptoms are among the most common complaints encountered by physicians. This statement is substantiated by data obtained by the Freedom of Information Act on the sales of antacid products (Table 9–1), and the report that cimetidine sales have surpassed Valium as number one in the marketplace. The degree to which gastroesophageal reflux is the cause of these symptoms is difficult to evaluate, because the disease has such a variety of presentations that there is no one symptomatic complex that can be used to indicate its presence. Further, many individuals consider the sensation of typical heartburn to be normal and do not seek medical attention.

Palmer[1] in his classic article reviewed 196 symptomatic patients assumed to have incompetence of the cardioesophageal junction because of the presence of a hiatus hernia. Only 15% of the patients complained of the classic syndrome of epigastric or substernal burning pain, exaggerated by recumbency. An additional 19% complained of epigastric or substernal burning pain without relationship to position but aggravated by meals. Thus, only one third of the patients had symptoms that would suggest the presence of gastroesophageal reflux. The magnitude of the problem is further increased by the observation that gastroesophageal reflux can cause chest pain that masquerades as heart disease or pulmonary symptoms that masquerade as respiratory disease, both of which do not suggest an esophageal etiology.[2, 3]

The basic pathophysiologic abnormality of gastroesophageal reflux disease is an excessive reflux of gastric juice into the esophagus. In the past this was inferred by the presence of a hiatal hernia, later by endoscopic esophagitis, and more recently, by a hypotensive lower esophageal sphincter pressure. Although these findings can occur with gastroesophageal reflux, their presence or absence cannot be equated with the presence or absence of the disease. Until esophageal exposure to gastric juice could be quantitated by prolonged monitoring of esophageal pH, documentation of the disease was difficult. Consequently, the information obtained from 24-hour esophageal pH monitoring provided an opportunity to conceptualize the pathophysiology of a complicated disease process. It stimulated a rational, stepwise approach to determining the cause of abnormal esophageal exposure to gastric juice and the design of specific therapy for correcting the abnormality.

TABLE 9–1.—MARKETING SURVEY OBTAINED THROUGH FREEDOM OF INFORMATION ACT

ANTACID SALES, 1979*	IN WHOLE DOLLARS
Liquid	153,000,000
Tablet	146,000,000
Effervescent	62,000,000
Total	361,000,000

*1974–79 = 9.3% Annual increase in sales.

PHYSIOLOGIC REFLUX IN ASYMPTOMATIC HUMAN SUBJECTS

Healthy individuals have occasional episodes of gastroesophageal reflux. Prolonged pH monitoring of the distal esophagus has shown that asymptomatic subjects with normal manometric measurements of length, position, and pressure of the distal esophageal sphincter have physiologic reflux episodes that account for a normal level of esophageal exposure to gastric juice. These physiologic reflux episodes rarely occur during sleep but are common during and after eating. They are responsible for a total esophageal acid exposure time equal to 2% of the time spent in the upright position and 0.3% of the time spent in the supine position. When a physiologic episode occurs, normal subjects rapidly clear the acid gastric juice from the esophagus regardless of their position. A single reflux episode rarely causes a drop in esophageal pH below 4 for longer than nine minutes, and over a 24-hour period, no more than three reflux episodes last longer than five minutes.[4, 5] To this normal esophageal acid exposure, individuals suspected of having gastroesophageal reflux disease must be compared.

The observation that the cardia is significantly more competent in normal subjects during sleep in the supine position than while up and about in the upright posture seems paradoxical. Why should it be easier for gastric juice to flow upward, against gravity, into the esophagus rather than spilling into the esophagus when the subject is supine? There are several explanations for this. First, in the upright position there is a 12 mm Hg pressure gradient between the resting, positive intra-abdominal pressure measured in the stomach and the most negative intrathoracic pressure measured in the esophagus at midthoracic level.[6] This gradient favors the flow of gastric juice up into the thoracic esophagus when upright. The gradient diminishes in the supine position.[7] Second, reflux episodes can occur in healthy volunteers on swallowing due to the relaxation of the lower esophageal sphincter.[8, 9] These reflux episodes occur because of a "failed" peristaltic sequence; i.e., during an "unguarded moment" when the relaxed sphincter is not protected by an oncoming peristaltic wave.[8] The average swallowing frequency is 72 swallows per hour for normal subjects while awake and in the upright position, and only seven per hour while asleep and in the supine position.[10, 11] Consequently, there are fewer opportunities for reflux to occur secondary to swallowing while supine. Third, the lower esophageal sphincter pressure in normal subjects is significantly higher in the supine position than in the upright position.[12] This is due to the apposition of the hydrostatic pressure of the abdomen to the abdominal portion of the sphincter when supine. In the upright position, the abdominal pressure surrounding the sphincter is negative compared to atmospheric pressure, and, as expected, the abdominal pressure gradually increases the more caudally it is measured (Table 9–2). This pressure gradient tends to move the gastric contents toward the cardia and encourages the occurrence of reflux into the esophagus when the individual is upright. In contrast, in the supine position the gastroesophageal pressure gradient diminishes, and the abdominal hydrostatic pressure under the diaphragm increases, causing an increase in sphincter pressure and a more competent cardia.

PATHOPHYSIOLOGY OF GASTROESOPHAGEAL REFLUX DISEASE

The pathophysiologic abnormalities in patients with gastroesophageal reflux disease are: (1) abnormal esophageal exposure to gastric juice, and (2) an increased sensitivity of the esophagus to gastric juice. The latter gives rise to a variety of symptoms, of which heartburn and regurgitation are most common. A sensitive esophagus may not always be present or may occur as an isolated abnormality unassociated with an increased esophageal exposure to gastric juice. Therefore, the absence of classic symptoms in a patient cannot be used to exclude the presence of pathologic reflux, nor does the experience of symptoms definitely indicate the existence of pathologic reflux (Fig 9–1).

In approximately 50% of patients with increased esophageal exposure to gastric juice, mucosal inflammation, scarring, and metaplasia occur as a complication.[12] Usually, but not always,

TABLE 9–2.—INTRA-ABDOMINAL PRESSURE, CM H₂O

| | UNDER DIAPHRAGM | | IN LOWER PART OF ABDOMEN |
POSITION OF ANIMAL	On Inspiration	On Expiration	
Supine	3.0	3.5	5.5
Erect	−3.5	−3.0	10.0
Head down	11.0	16.0	0.5
Head up (45°)	−2.5	−2.0	8.0
Head down (45°)	6.0	5.5	2.0
Supine (second reading)	3.0	3.5	5.5

Courtesy of Lam C.R.: Intra-abdominal pressure: A critical review and an experimental study. *Arch Surg.* 39:1006, 1939. Copyright 1939, American Medical Association.

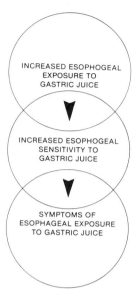

Fig 9–1.—Pathophysiologic sequence of gastroesophageal reflux disease.

the development of these sequelae is preceded by symptoms from a sensitive esophagus. Consequently, the monitoring of symptoms cannot be depended on to reflect the severity of the disease. This requires esophagoscopy, but the visual confirmation of the presence of such complications is not a dependable indicator of reflux disease. There are other causes of esophagitis and stricture besides reflux, such as caustic drugs, *Candida (Monilia)* infection, and repetitive vomiting. Similarly, a normal endoscopic examination does not exclude reflux disease, but only the complications of the disease. Consequently, the diagnosis of the disease requires measuring the exposure of the esophagus to gastric juice.[12]

Etiology of Increased Esophageal Acid Exposure

The causes of increased esophageal acid exposure in patients with gastroesophageal reflux disease are now known to be four. The first is a mechanically incompetent gastroesophageal junction. The introduction of esophageal manometry demonstrated that the distal esophageal sphincter pressure in patients with symptoms of gastroesophageal reflux, as a group, was lower than that measured in normal subjects.[13] This finding focused attention on the sphincter pressure as the mechanism by which competency of the cardia was maintained. Various factors were suggested to explain the decrease in sphincter pressure, including neural, humeral, sphincter location, and myogenic influences. A neural excitatory mechanism for the maintenance of basal sphincter pressure was questioned, since truncal vagotomy has no effect on sphincter pressure.[14] Similarly, a pharmacologic mechanism has been proposed, since doses of cholinergic agents can cause an increase in the sphincter pressure, and anticholinergics reduce it, but the relevance of these observations to explain a low sphincter pressure has not been shown.[15] The influence of many hormones on the distal esophageal sphincter has been investigated, but the effects noted are associated with pharmacologic doses and probably do not represent the true physiologic situation.[15] The position of the distal esophageal sphincter, either in the abdomen or in the chest, does not seem to be a major factor in the genesis of the pressure, since it can be measured when the chest and abdomen are surgically opened and the distal esophagus is held freely in the surgeon's hand.[16] The explanation for a lower esophageal sphincter pressure in symptomatic individuals is most likely due to an abnormality of myogenic function. Biancini and co-workers[17] have shown that the distal esophageal sphincter's muscle response to stretch is reduced in patients with incompetent cardias. This suggested that sphincter pressure depends on the length and tension properties of the sphincter's smooth muscle. Indeed, a reduction in the pressure is associated with measured abnormalities in length-tension characteristics. Furthermore, a surgical fundoplication that restores sphincter pressure to normal also corrects the abnormal length-tension characteristics.[17]

Despite the statistical correlation between the amplitude of the lower esophageal sphincter pressure and the presence of gastroesophageal reflux on a population basis, it became evident that the magnitude of the pressure in the distal esophagus was not always related to competency of the cardia.[18] Some individuals with a low pressure had competent cardias, while others with a high pressure had incompetent cardias. It further became evident that there was a marked overlap between the lower esophageal sphincter pressure in normal control subjects and in patients with gastroesophageal reflux and that the administration of atropine, which reduces sphincter pressure, did not increase the incidence of gastroesophageal reflux in normal subjects.[19, 20]

Until the technique of prolonged esophageal pH monitoring was developed, this observation defied explanation. Data obtained from 266 patients who underwent both esophageal manometry and 24-hour esophageal pH monitoring indicated that the competency of the cardia to challenges of intra-abdominal pressure was related to two manometric measurements; namely, the amplitude of the distal esophageal sphincter pressure zone and the length of sphincter exposed to abdominal pressure. From these studies, it became evident that a patient who had an average sphincter pressure of 5 mm Hg, or an average length of less than 1 cm of sphincter exposed to abdominal pressure, had a 90% probability of having abnormal esophageal acid exposure.[21]

These findings drew attention to the intra-abdominal position of the lower esophageal high-pressure zone as an additional factor contributing to the incompetency of the cardia.

This observation was supported by the anatomical measurements of Bombeck and co-workers,[22] who showed a correlation between the level of insertion of the phrenoesophageal membrane on the esophagus and the presence of esophagitis. Patients with esophagitis statistically had a shorter portion of the sphincter exposed to the abdominal environment compared to those who did not. Even when a hiatal hernia was present, this held true. Subsequent studies have shown that in this situation, a portion of the distal esophageal sphincter is still exposed to the abdominal pressure because of the hernia sac, which acts as a conduit to transmit changes in intra-abdominal pressure around the abdominal portion of the sphincter.[23] This structural arrangement allows for extrinsic compression of that portion of the sphincter and provides protection against reflux secondary to changes in intra-abdominal pressure. The shortening of the abdominal portion of the distal esophageal sphincter, whether in a hernia sac or not, results in an incompetent cardia, because the sphincter cannot be affected extrinsically by changes in intra-abdominal pressure. Since these changes in intra-abdominal pressure cannot be countered successfully by intrinsic sphincter pressure alone, free reflux occurs.

What remained to be discerned was whether the extrinsic pressure acted directly on the intra-abdominal segment of the sphincter or through an adoptive neural reflex response intrinsic to the stomach and distal esophagus. In the former, behavior of the distal esophageal sphincter could be explained simply on extrinsic mechanical factors, whereas the latter implies the presence of complex neural reflexes, with less emphasis on the mechanical function of the cardia. To differentiate between these two possibilities, we have challenged the distal esophageal sphincter with variations in intra-abdominal and intrathoracic pressure to determine their effect on the thoracic and abdominal segments of the sphincter in patients whose reflux status was defined by standard acid reflux test and 24-hour pH monitoring of the esophagus.[24] Table 9–3 shows the changes in pressure induced by respiratory and positional maneuvers in ten such patients.

The results showed that each portion of the distal esophageal sphincter, abdominal or thoracic, was markedly affected by changes in environmental pressure, and each was affected independently. An increase in abdominal pressure caused an increase in the luminal pressure of the abdominal portion of the sphincter and stomach, while the thoracic portion of the sphincter and esophagus remained unaffected and vice versa. The varied response of different portions of the sphincter to

TABLE 9–3.—CHANGE IN PRESSURE INDUCED BY RESPIRATORY AND POSITIONAL MANEUVERS IN TEN PATIENTS*

MANEUVER	THORACIC ESOPHAGUS	DISTAL ESOPHAGEAL SPHINCTER (DES)		GASTRIC FUNDUS
		Thoracic part (DES-T)	Abdominal part (DES-A)	
Valsalva	30.2 (±3.6)	24.9 (±4.6)‡	30.7 (±2.3)‡	36.4 (±1.3)
Leg raising	0.38 (±0.1)	3.7 (±3.5)†	16.3 (±2.8)	17.2 (±3.3)
Muller	>−22 mm Hg	14.9 (±3.8)	16.1 (±4.7)	7.3 (±1.9)

Note: All measurements differ significantly from resting pressure (P < .05) except those marked †.

*Adapted from Pellegrini C.A., et al.[24]

‡Comparison between thoracic and abdominal portions of DES are all significant (P < .05) except those marked ‡.

environmental pressure at the same time strongly indicates that the distal esophageal sphincter reflects changes in environmental pressure by simple extrinsic mechanical compression rather than complicated neural reflex, and that the intraluminal pressure measured in the sphincter results from both applied extrinsic environmental pressure plus the intrinsic myogenic tone. Consequently, only that portion of intragastric pressure due to gastric muscle tone must be exceeded by the muscle of the distal esophageal sphincter to prevent reflux, so long as both the abdominal portion of the sphincter and the stomach are able to respond similarly to environmental pressure changes. This study further suggested that at least 1 cm of the lower esophageal sphincter must be exposed to the positive pressure of the abdomen for this aspect of the antireflux mechanism to function adequately. Lesser amounts place the cardia at a mechanical disadvantage, and reflux is likely to occur when there is an increase in intra-abdominal pressure secondary to straining or changing body position.

To understand the relationship between the amplitude of the distal esophageal sphincter pressure and the length of sphincter exposed to abdominal pressure, an in vitro model was developed that enabled us to study the function of these two components individually and together.[21] This model showed that the competency of the cardia to challenges of intra-abdominal pressure was primarily the function of the length of the distal esophageal sphincter exposed to the positive pressure environment of the abdomen. If the intrinsic sphincter pressure was negligible—i.e., less than 6 mm Hg— greater than 4 cm of abdominal sphincter was necessary to achieve competence. The shorter the length of sphincter exposed to the abdominal pressure environment, the greater the intrinsic pressure of the sphincter had to be to maintain competency. The model further demonstrated, as the earlier clinical study suggested, that under ideal conditions a minimum length of 1 cm of sphincter was required to protect against challenges of increases in intra-abdominal pressure. The reason for this was that the mechanical advantage was lost with less than 1 cm of abdominal sphincter, and as a consequence the amplitude of intrinsic sphincter pressure necessary to achieve competency became infinite.

The predictions of the in vitro model were evaluated in a clinical study done in patients with abnormal esophageal exposure to gastric juice who had esophageal manometry and simultaneous 24-hour monitoring of their esophageal pH and intra-abdominal pressure.[25] Figure 9–2 shows that when normal mechanical components are present, the cardia is more resistant to intra-abdominal pressure challenges than when they are absent.

Table 9–4 shows the results of clinical experience that support the findings of both the in vitro model and clinical study.[26] Three hundred ninety-one consecutive patients with symptoms suggestive of gastroesophageal reflux had both esophageal manometry and 24-hour esophageal pH monitoring. The table was constructed by stratifying the patients as to the length of sphincter exposed to the positive pressure environment of the abdomen and the amplitude of its intrinsic pressure. The competency of the cardia was evaluated using 24-hour esophageal pH monitoring to measure the amount of esophageal acid exposure. Acid exposure was considered abnormal when it exceeded 2 SD above the mean of normal subjects. The results showed that a high incidence of incom-

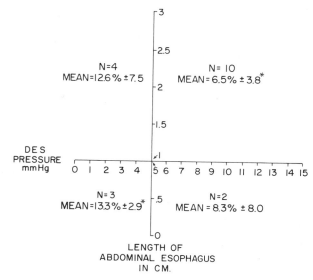

Fig 9–2.—Relationship between distal esophageal pressure (DES) and length of abdominal esophagus in preventing reflux from intra-abdominal pressure (IAP) challenges. Patients with a mechanically defective cardia *(left lower quadrant)* were statistically less able to protect against challenges of IAP than those with normal mechanical components *(right upper quadrant)*. (From DeMeester T.R., in van Heukelem H.A., Gooszen H.G., Terpstra J.L., Belsey R.H.: *Pathological Gastro-oesophageal Reflux.* Amsterdam, Zuid-Nederlandse Uitgevers Maatschappij BV, 1982, p. 26. Used by permission.)

petency of the cardia occurred when either the intrinsic sphincter pressure was 5 mm Hg or below, or a length of sphincter exposed to abdominal pressure was less than 1 cm.

A secondary observation from the data in Table 9–4 is that a sphincter pressure below 5 mm Hg can occur when an adequate length of sphincter is exposed to abdominal pressure, and a normal amplitude of pressure (15–20 mm Hg) can occur when a sphincter length of less than 1 cm is exposed to ab-

TABLE 9–4.—INCIDENCE OF ABNORMAL GASTROESOPHAGEAL REFLUX STRATIFIED FOR LENGTH AND PRESSURE OF DISTAL ESOPHAGEAL SPHINCTER (DES)*

PRESSURE OF DES, mm Hg	LENGTH OF DES BELOW RESPIRATORY INVERSION POINT, cm		
	0–1	1–2	2
0–5	92%	88%	87.5%
	34/37	22/25	7/8
> 5–10	90%	58%	68%
	19/21	29/50	17/25
>10–15	86%	77%	76%
	14/16	34/44	26/34
>15–20	67%	60%	71%
	4/6	15/25	20/28
>20	90%	40%	19%
	9/10	10/25	7/37

Note: No./No. = Number of patients with a positive 24-hour pH score over the total number of patients monitored in each cell (total number, 391; total number of refluxers, 267). Results of analysis of variance incorporating Tukey's test for nonadditivity; determinants of competence: pressure $F_{(4,7)} = 4.885$ ($P<0.05$); length $F_{(2,7)} = 5.203$ ($P<0.005$); interaction $F_{(1,7)} = 7.027$ ($P<0.05$).
*Adapted from O'Sullivan G. C., et al.[26]

dominal pressure. This observation supports the concept that the intrinsic sphincter pressure is not caused by the positive pressure of the abdomen acting extrinsically on the intra-abdominal segment, but rather is due to an intrinsic myogenic property as discussed previously.

In an additional clinical study, the two components responsible for incompetency of the cardia; i.e., the distal esophageal sphincter pressure and the length of it exposed to the positive pressure environment of the abdomen, were measured in 20 normal subjects and 126 previously untreated patients with gastroesophageal reflux.[27] On 24-hour esophageal pH monitoring, all of the normal control subjects were shown to have competent cardias, whereas the patients' were incompetent. The results were again plotted on the grid with the horizontal bar representing the length of sphincter exposed to abdominal pressure and the vertical bar representing the amplitude of the intrinsic sphincter pressure. Poor mechanical components, i.e., a sphincter pressure less than 5 mm Hg or an abdominal length less than 1 cm, were seen in 31% of the patients with reflux and none of the normal subjects. Excellent mechanical components—i.e., a sphincter pressure greater than 15 mm Hg and an abdominal length greater than 3 cm—were seen in only 10 percent of the normal subjects and none of the patients with reflux. On the other hand, 69% of the patients with reflux had mechanical components of their cardia similar to 90% of the normal subjects. This finding suggested that factors other than sphincter pressure and the length of sphincter exposed to the positive pressure environment of the abdomen were important in the antireflux mechanisms. This began to focus attention on a *second* cause for abnormal esophageal exposure to gastric juice; i.e., gastric function. Could abnormal esophageal exposure to gastric juice result from overwhelming a mechanically normal cardia by increases in intragastric pressure independent from rises in intra-abdominal pressure?

We made use of an in vitro model similar to the one described before to analyze the relationship between intragastric pressure and distal esophageal sphincter pressure.[28] The results of the study showed that a ratio of at least one between the pressure of a distal esophageal sphincter with an overall length of five cm; i.e., the length of both the abdominal and thoracic portions, and gastric pressure was necessary for the cardia to protect against rises in intragastric pressure independent from intra-abdominal pressure. The model also showed that the shorter the overall length of sphincter became, the greater the pressure ratio required for competency. For example, if the overall length of the lower esophageal sphincter was 4 cm, a ratio between sphincter pressure and gastric pressure of 1.5 was necessary to maintain competence of the cardia, whereas a sphincter with an overall length of 2 cm required a ratio of 3 for competency. According to the model, the pressure necessary to give competency to a sphincter with an overall length of 2 cm against independent rises in gastric pressure was 25–30 mm Hg. This is well above the sphincter pressure measured in our normal control subjects with a normal overall sphincter length of 4 cm. Consequently, most individuals with an overall length of 2 cm would be expected to have incompetent cardias when studied by 24-hour esophageal pH monitoring. This hypothesis was tested in the clinic in 191 patients with a mechanically defec-

tive cardia and foregut symptoms. Sixty-six of the patients had a resting overall sphincter length of 2 cm or less, and this was associated with an abnormal esophageal acid exposure on 24-hour pH monitoring in 74.2%. The finding of a resting overall sphincter length 2 cm or less can occur as an isolated abnormality, in association with a sphincter pressure of 5 mm Hg or less, and/or an abdominal sphincter length of 1 cm or less.

The short sphincter syndrome is in reality a third measurable mechanical deficiency of the sphincter, not a gastric cause for reflux of gastric juice into the esophagus. There are, however, a number of gastric abnormalities that can cause reflux of gastric contents through a mechanically normal cardia. For example, transient rises in intragastric pressure, independent from an increase in intra-abdominal pressure, can occur from increased gastric contractions in response to a gastric outlet obstruction from an anatomical lesion or pyloric and duodenal motor abnormalities, or the loss of active relaxation of the stomach secondary to a previous vagotomy. Occasionally, these increases in gastric pressure can exceed the ability of a normal cardia to remain competent.

Abnormally slow gastric emptying secondary to gastric atony from advanced diabetes, diffuse neuromuscular disorders, or idiopathic gastroparesis that follows a viral infection increases the probability of regurgitating gastric juice into the esophagus through a mechanically normal cardia, simply because the gastric reservoir remains full for a longer period and accentuates physiologic reflux.[29] When the cardia is mechanically incompetent, delayed gastric emptying potentiates the abnormality by increasing the severity of reflux with incremental increases in retained gastric volume. This has been shown experimentally in patients with symptomatic gastroesophageal reflux disease; i.e., reflux as measured by pH monitoring increased from 20% in the basal state to 100% following gastric loading with 300 ml of 1/10N hydrochloric acid. It appears that the volume of gastric contents available for reflux dictates not only the probability of reflux occurring, but also the volume of material refluxed.[30] Of a similar nature is the observation that patients who have increased gastric acid secretion also have increased esophageal acid exposure. This is probably due to both increased gastric volume and the high acidity of that volume.[31]

Excessive gastric distention without increases in gastric pressure can decrease the overall length of the distal esophageal sphincter, similar to the decrease in the length of the neck of a balloon as it is inflated. This results in an incompetent cardia and increased esophageal acid exposure by the mechanism similar to the short sphincter syndrome previously discussed. The cause of gastric distention is usually a voluntary process that occurs during awake hours and is secondary to aerophagia or gluttony.[5] These individuals have increased esophageal acid exposure from repetitive belching or excessive postprandial reflux and are termed "upright refluxers." As mentioned previously, the upright body position results in a gradation of intra-abdominal pressures exerted over the stomach and the abdominal portion of the distal esophageal sphincter. This gradation of extrinsic pressure can affect the relationship between the intragastric pressure and the lower esophageal sphincter pressure, resulting in a ratio between the two that is inadequate for competency while in the upright position. This is particularly so when gastric distention has caused a shortening of the overall sphincter length. Thus, any gastric condition that predisposes toward reflux is more likely to result in reflux when the patient is in the upright position.

Increased esophageal exposure to gastric juice, secondary to a gastric disorder, is a commonly unrecognized facet of gastroesophageal reflux disease. Clinical studies have indicated that upward to 40% of patients with gastroesophageal reflux have a disturbance of upper GI motility that is manifested by delayed gastric emptying.[32] This delay is most pronounced in patients who have endoscopic esophagitis.[33] This suggests that transmural esophagitis could involve the vagi fibers in direct contact with the esophageal muscle and produce a vagoparesis, resulting in delayed gastric emptying. In this situation, the delayed gastric emptying would be a consequence rather than the cause of gastroesophageal reflux disease. On the other hand, delayed gastric emptying could result from a primary stomach or duodenal motility abnormality. The latter would not only reduce gastric emptying but also cause an inefficient flow of duodenal contents in the aboral direction. Consequently, bile could regurgitate into the stomach and change the composition and pH of the gastric juice refluxing into the esophagus. The bile regurgitation could also explain the observed correlation between chronic gastritis and the symptoms of heartburn.[34]

Dodds and associates[35] suggested transient spontaneous relaxation of the distal esophageal sphincter as a *third* cause for increased esophageal exposure to gastric juice. In this situation, the sphincter relaxes spontaneously, unrelated to swallowing, with a drop in pressure to gastric baseline, allowing reflux of gastric contents to occur. The cause of the spontaneous relaxation is unknown. To diagnose this condition requires continuous pressure monitoring of the sphincter and esophageal body over a 24-hour period, with simultaneous pH monitoring.[36] Episodes of spontaneous relaxation are unlikely to be recorded during a short motility study. According to the Dodds group, patients with normal mean distal esophageal sphincter pressure refluxed mainly by transient sphincter relaxation, whereas those with low resting sphincter pressure had a high frequency of reflux unrelated to sphincter relaxation. The latter group probably represented patients with a mechanically incompetent cardia. Thus the Dodds mechanism of reflux is the most likely explanation for patients who have increased esophageal exposure to gastric juice in the presence of normal manometric measurement of their sphincter on standard motility studies and no evidence of gastric dysfunction. In these patients an antireflux procedure, which incorporates a fundic wrap, can provide effective therapy by preventing the sphincter pressure from dropping below gastric pressure during a transient spontaneous relaxation episode.

A *fourth* factor that can cause increased esophageal exposure to gastric juice is inefficient esophageal clearance of refluxed material. This can result in an abnormal esophageal exposure to gastric juice in individuals who have a mechanically competent distal esophageal sphincter and normal gastric function by ineffectual clearing of physiologic reflux episodes.[27] This situation, however, is relatively rare, and ineffectual clearance is more apt to be seen in association with a mechanically incompetent cardia, where it augments the

esophageal exposure to gastric juice by prolonging the duration of each reflux episode.

Four factors important in esophageal clearance are gravity, esophageal motor activity, salivation, and the presence of a hiatal hernia.[5, 23, 37, 38] The upright position enhances esophageal emptying compared to the supine position and explains the occurrence of severe reflux disease in patients who are nocturnal refluxers.[39] Normally, the esophagus is adequately cleared by a peristaltic pressure wave after a pharyngeal swallow; i.e., a primary peristalsis; or after local esophageal distention; i.e., a secondary peristalsis. The former is initiated voluntarily and is the major esophageal motor activity that clears the esophagus of reflux material in normal subjects. Secondary peristalsis can be initiated by a bolus of refluxed material or a sudden drop in intraesophageal pH, and has a contributing role in clearing the esophagus, particularly in patients with gastroesophageal reflux disease.[40] The esophageal contractions initiated can be a normal peristaltic pattern or a nonspecific abnormal motility pattern consisting of broadbased, powerful, and synchronous contractions.[41] When a motility abnormality is induced, it rarely causes dysphagia, but reduces the efficiency of esophageal clearance, encourages the regurgitation of refluxed material into the pharynx, and predisposes the patient to aspiration.[3]

Salivation contributes to esophageal clearance by neutralizing the minute amount of acid that is left following a peristaltic wave.[42] Esophageal clearance time is increased significantly when saliva is removed by suction and conversely decreased when salivation is stimulated by oral lozenges. Thus, esophageal acid clearance normally occurs as a two-step process and is aided by gravity when in the upright position. First, virtually all of the acid volume that is refluxed is emptied from the esophagus by one or two peristaltic sequences, leaving a minimal residual amount that sustains a low pH. Second, the residual acid is neutralized by the swallowed saliva. The effectiveness of saliva in neutralizing the residual acid may contribute to a habit of repetitive pharyngeal swallowing and gum chewing in patients who reflux. This can result in excessive aerophagia and a cyclic process of gastric distention and further gastroesophageal reflux.

The presence of a hiatal hernia can cause an esophageal propulsion defect and inadequate esophageal acid clearance.[23] Recent studies have shown that the presence of a hernia is unrelated to the competency of the cardia but does contribute to a longer esophageal transit time. The decrease in transit time is not due to a manometric motility disorder but is secondary to the hiatal hernia, which significantly interferes with the mechanical ability of esophageal contractions in the distal third of the esophagus to clear refluxed gastric contents. Reduction of the hernia and anchoring the esophagus in the abdomen effectively improve the mechanics and as a consequence esophageal acid clearance.

In this regard, patients with a mechanically defective cardia and a large hiatal hernia have a severely compromised antireflux mechanism. They lack an adequate overall sphincter length and pressure to protect against independent rises in intragastric pressure, an adequate length of intra-abdominal sphincter to protect against the challenge of intra-abdominal pressure, and an effective clearance mechanism to evacuate refluxed gastric juice back into the stomach. In addition, the possibility of developing a reflux-induced motility abnormality can add to the clearance abnormality and predispose the patient to propel the refluxed gastric juice into the pharynx, with the potential hazards of aspiration.

In some patients a hiatal hernia not only interferes with esophageal clearance but also restricts the passage of a swallow bolus by what Edwards has termed abnormal hiatal flow.[43] If the diaphragmatic hiatus forms a narrow slit, there can be an accumulation of swallowed material within the hernia above the diaphragm, resulting in delayed propulsion of food into the stomach and the symptoms of dysphagia. When the herniated portion of the stomach contracts, the resistance of flow through the diaphragmatic hiatus may be sufficient so that the intragastric pressure within the hernia overcomes the sphincter pressure and the contents regurgitate into the esophagus. As expected, these patients do not complain of heartburn but of regurgitation and dysphagia.

Patterns of Esophageal Gastric Juice Exposure

Patients with gastroesophageal reflux disease do not appear to be a homogeneous population with regard to their reflux patterns.[5] When compared to asymptomatic normal subjects, some patients have excessive upright acid exposure while awake, but a normal supine acid exposure at night while asleep. They are called "upright refluxers," named for the period during which they are abnormal. Other patients have excessive supine acid exposure at night while asleep, but normal amounts of reflux when upright. They are called "supine refluxers." A third group had excessive acid exposure in both postures and were called "combined," or "bipositional," refluxers.

A retrospective comparison of the results of surgical antireflux procedures on patients with upright reflux compared to those with supine reflux suggested that each had different mechanisms of reflux. Patients who had excessive upright acid exposure (upright and bipositional refluxers) had an increased incidence of gas bloat syndrome after surgery as opposed to supine refluxers.[5] We have observed that the upright refluxers are habitual air swallowers and repetitive belchers, with each belch causing a reflux episode. The bipositional refluxers have a mechanically deficient cardia, and the resulting reflux stimulates multiple dry pharyngeal swallows to clear the reflux acid from the esophagus, i.e., a secondary form of aerophagia. Each pharyngeal swallow pumps 1 to 2 cc of air into the stomach.[44] This leads to a cyclic process of excessive gastric distention, belching, and recurrent reflux. An antireflux procedure does not correct the basic abnormality in upright refluxers and results in a severe persistent postoperative gas bloat syndrome. Bipositional refluxers, on the other hand, eventually lose the swallowing habit and become free of the gas bloat problem.

Supine refluxers have excessive supine acid exposure of a different etiology. In normal subjects, swallowing during sleep occurs with arousal and occasionally triggers reflux episodes, whereas reflux episodes do not occur during stable sleep, and abdominal contractions do not cause reflux episodes.[8] Patients with supine reflux have several reflux episodes during sleep; some are due to a mechanically defective cardia,[25] and others, with a mechanically normal cardia, are due to cyclic periods of lower esophageal sphinc-

ter relaxation that last 5–30 seconds.[35] Studies have shown that these patients do rouse more quickly than normal subjects when acid is infused into their esophagus but have difficulty in initiating esophageal contractions to clear the refluxed material. Normal subjects, although less likely to be aroused, do respond with more esophageal swallows than refluxers, and the lower the drop in esophageal pH, the more peristaltic activity generated. The esophageal peristaltic waves initiated are not primary, but secondary; i.e., without a pharyngeal component; consequently, gastric distention is not a problem.[44] Therefore, patients who are supine refluxers not only are less able to clear reflux episodes that occur during sleep, but are more easily roused when they occur, which interferes with their sleep pattern. It is believed that combined, or bipositional, refluxers are patients who initially started with supine reflux but, as the severity of the clearance increased, began to show abnormal esophageal exposure to gastric juice during the day, despite the benefit of gravity on esophageal clearance.

Esophageal Exposure to Gastric Juice and the Development of Esophagitis

Chronic irritation of the esophageal mucosa by noxious gastric juice has been implicated as the cause of increased loss of epithelial cells, reflected by the closer approximation of the papillar to the mucosal surface and basal zone hyperplasia in epithelial biopsies in patients who have gastroesophageal reflux disease.[45] This hypothesis has been supported by objective data that quantitatively correlated esophageal mucosa exposure to acid gastric juice with 24-hour pH monitoring to the epithelial papillary length and the thickness of the basal zone hyperplasia in esophageal mucosal biopsies.[46] Patients with a positive 24-hour pH record had a significantly greater mean percentage of papillary extension (representing a loss of surface epithelial cells) than those with a normal test, and a regression analysis showed a significant direct correlation between the percent of papillary length and the degree of distal esophageal acid exposure. This reactive epithelial change was reversible in that it significantly decreased in five patients during the early postoperative period, after antireflux surgery had returned the distal esophageal acid exposure to normal.

The relationship between esophageal acid exposure time and the epithelial reaction is also demonstrated by studies on the pattern of reflux in patients with gastroesophageal reflux disease; i.e., upright, supine, or bipositional refluxers. When categorized, the mean papillary extension was found to exceed 60% of the width of the epithelium (representing epithelial cell loss) only in the supine and bipositional refluxers; i.e., acid exposure that resulted from few reflux episodes but of long duration. In contrast, the mean papillary length was found to be normal in those patients who had only upright reflux; i.e., acid exposure that resulted from frequent reflux episodes of short duration. Of importance is that although the total duration of the upright reflux episodes significantly exceeded the total duration of recumbent reflux episodes, the upright acid exposure was less damaging to the esophageal mucosa because of rapid clearance. Thus, esophageal acid clearance time is more important in determining the epithelial reaction than the total magnitude of esophageal acid exposure. The concept appears to be that acid exposure of low frequency but long duration is more deleterious to the mucosa than that of high frequency but short duration.

A similar effect is observed when the patterns of reflux are related to the incidence and severity of endoscopic esophagitis.[5] Isolated supine acid exposure is associated with a high incidence of a severe form of esophagitis, while isolated upright reflux is associated with a low incidence of a mild form of esophagitis. These studies also suggested that bipositional refluxers, who had the highest incidence and most severe grades of endoscopic esophagitis, represent a severe form of gastroesophageal reflux disease that probably started as only supine reflux. Thus, supine reflux appears to be the most critical factor in the development of esophagitis as a complication of gastroesophageal reflux disease.

There is considerable discussion over what the offensive ingredient is in the refluxed gastric juice that produces esophagitis, and components from both gastric and duodenal secretions have been implicated. Quincke[47] in 1879 first drew the correlation between esophagitis and the digestive action of acid gastric juice. The concept of injury to the esophageal mucosa by gastric juice was further developed by Hamperl, who introduced the term "peptic esophagitis."[48] Subsequent to this, several studies were designed to identify the offensive agent in the gastric juice. These consisted of infusion experiments in which the substance under question was dripped continuously into the esophagus of an anesthetized animal, or experiments in which the lower esophageal sphincter was destroyed so that the reflux of gastric juice could occur. In the latter type of study, it was difficult to determine the exact composition of refluxed juice, and this led to surgical experiments in which the esophagus was exposed to intestinal juices in such a manner that their composition could be controlled. The results of these studies seem to show that a combination of acid and pepsin has a damaging effect on the esophageal mucosa of the species tested. However, in all of the experiments, a prolonged continuous exposure of the esophageal mucosa to the substance studied was necessary to produce a deleterious effect, and rarely are these exposure times found on esophageal pH monitoring in patients with esophagitis. In the most severely affected patients, the esophageal pH is below 4 in only 20%–30% of the 24-hour period, and this exposure is not continuous but broken up into several episodes. It must be recognized, however, that the low pH in the distal esophagus on 24-hour pH monitoring reflects only the exposure of the esophagus to acid gastric juice. There may be periods when alkaline gastric juice is refluxed into a monitored esophagus, and the reflux episode goes undetected because of its high alkaline pH.

The occurrence of esophagitis in patients with achlorhydria or after total gastrectomy is a well-established clinical observation.[49, 50] In these circumstances, the offensive agents can only be in the duodenal juice. This clinical observation has suggested that the noxious agent in the duodenal juice may also be the active ingredient in patients with a normal secreting stomach.[51, 52] In support of this, several authors have demonstrated concomitant increases in duodenal gastric reflux in patients with symptomatic gastroesophageal reflux disease,[53–56] and 24-hour esophageal pH monitoring has shown that episodes of alkaline reflux are mixed with acid reflux in patients with esophagitis.[57] If this is the case, the duodenal juice that is to reach the esophagus must pass through the stomach, an environment that is deleterious to most duodenal enzymes.

The potential injurious ingredient of duodenal juice is bile, pancreatic, or duodenal in origin. Bile salts are considered to be the corrosive component of bile, and their presence in the esophagus has been correlated with symptomatic heartburn.[58] The corrosive components of pancreatic juice are activated enzymes such as trypsin, lipase, and carboxypeptidase, all of which have been shown to produce epithelial changes when incubated with strips of esophageal mucosa.[59] These proteolytic enzymes are generally thought to be rapidly inactivated in the stomach. Experiments have demonstrated that the inactivation of trypsin by pepsin takes place at a pH below 3.5.[60] In the absence of pepsin, trypsin is stable in acid solution and present in an active form.[61] Furthermore, active trypsin has been demonstrated in the stomach at pH values between 3.5 and 7 as long as 90 minutes after a test meal.[62]

The conclusion of these experimental studies seems to show that components from bile, pancreatic juice, and gastric juice can produce esophageal damage under given conditions. In this regard, the elegant experiments of Kivilaakso et al.[63] showed that in the presence of hydrogen ions, pepsin, and conjugated bile salts were the substances responsible for mucosal damage; however, in the absence of hydrogen ions, trypsin and deconjugated bile salts were the crucial factors.

In summary, the development of esophagitis requires exposure of the esophageal mucosa to harmful elements in the gastric juice, whether of gastric or duodenal origin. The exposure of the esophageal mucosa to gastric content can be measured by the use of the hydrogen ion as a tag, even though the hydrogen ion may not be responsible for the injury. The composition of the gastric juice consists of both gastric secretions and duodenal secretions that are regurgitated back into the stomach. The latter has been shown to be increased in patients with symptoms of reflux esophagitis, and is thought to be caused by pyloric dysfunction resulting from a duodenal motility disorder.[34] This may explain why delayed gastric emptying is seen in patients with reflux esophagitis as compared to those who reflux and do not have esophagitis.[33] Twenty-four-hour esophageal pH monitoring studies have shown that in patients with severe esophagitis the esophageal pH is above 4, and in the range of 5 to 6 approximately 80% of the time. This is the pH at which trypsin is most active and pepsin least active. The demonstration of the prolonged presence of stable and partially active trypsin in the stomach after a test meal with a pH between 3.5 and 7 explains how trypsin could get into the esophagus without being deactivated.[62] In support of this, active trypsin has been demonstrated in the stomach of patients with symptoms of esophagitis, and there was a significant relationship between a high level of active trypsin in the stomach and the finding of ulcerative esophagitis.[64] Thus, a reasonable conclusion is that in man it appears that in the environment of strong gastric acidity, activated pepsin causes esophagitis, and in the presence of weak gastric acidity, activated trypsin is responsible for its development.

Increased Esophageal Sensitivity to Gastric Juice

There are two primary symptoms resulting from esophageal dysfunction, dysphagia and chest pain. Heartburn is considered part of the latter and is a form of chest pain that is typically esophageal in origin. Because we evaluate patients more frequently than normal subjects, physicians become programmed into thinking that the experience of heartburn indicates that acid has contacted the esophageal mucosa. This may not be true. Rather, the studies of Jones[65] showed that the symptom of heartburn can arise from a variety of esophageal stimuli that are unrelated to the presence of regurgitated gastric acid in the esophagus. He recorded the sensation experienced by subjects during the distention of a balloon at different levels in the esophagus (Table 9–5). The majority of the subjects felt a sensation of choking or fullness in the upper portion of the esophagus, and a small percentage reported a burning sensation. As the point of stimulation descended, there was a diminishing sensation of choking or fullness and more one of burning. Over one half of the subjects examined felt definite burning the moment the balloon was distended in the region of the cardia. Of interest was that in a few instances, in addition to the sensation of burning, subjects felt as if something hot or sour was being carried up toward the mouth when a balloon was inflated near the cardia. Such findings explain why heartburn can be experienced by patients who are achlorhydric and that heartburn can occur from causes other than irritation of the lower esophagus by regurgitation of gastric acid.

In additional studies, Jones placed a nasogastric tube just above the cardia in eight normal subjects and made repeated observations on the effects of introducing various amounts of warm water, cold water, 0.1N sodium hydroxide, 0.1N hydrochloric acid, and gastric juice into the esophagus. From this simple experiment, several observations are noteworthy. First, there was a wide variation in the amount of fluid that could be introduced into the esophagus before heartburn or any other sensation was experienced. Discomfort of one sort or another, usually burning, was produced with as little as 5 ml or as much as 35 ml of fluid. The speed with which the fluid was introduced was also an important factor. When it was allowed to run in slowly, frequently no sensation was produced. On the other hand, the rapid introduction of 10–15 ml of fluid with a syringe produced almost an instantaneous sense of discomfort or pain. It was further noted that the more frequent the injections of fluid were made, the more easily discomfort was produced and the longer it persisted. Table 9–6 gives the findings in these normal subjects related to the infusion of different fluids. Of note is that when warm water was introduced, five of eight subjects noted a cool sensation, and three had a feeling of heartburn. When ice water was injected, all eight subjects had a distinct sensation of heartburn. The introduction of 0.1N hydrochloric

TABLE 9–6.—SENSATION NOTED IN EIGHT NORMAL SUBJECTS FOLLOWING INFUSION OF THE LOWER ESOPHAGUS WITH VARIOUS FLUIDS (N = 8)*

FLUID EMPLOYED	SUBJECTS EXPERIENCING COLD	SUBJECTS EXPERIENCING "HEARTBURN"
Cold water	0/8	8/8
Warm water	5/8	3/8
n/10 HCl	1/6	5/6
n/10 NaOH	1/7	6/7
Gastric juice	1/3	2/3

*Adapted from Jones C.M.: *Digestive Tract Pain.* New York, Macmillan Co., 1938.

acid produced a sensation of coolness in one subject, and in five subjects caused a definite burning feeling, which was described as heartburn. In six of seven subjects, 0.1N sodium hydroxide had the same effects but to a greater degree. Three subjects had their own gastric contents introduced in the lower end of the esophagus, and in two of these, heartburn was produced. In the third, only a sensation of coolness.

From a clinical point of view, these studies indicate that the experience of heartburn by a normal subject is more dependent on the speed of distending the esophagus and the repetition of the event than the chemical composition of the fluid in the lower esophagus. Consequently, in patients who complain of heartburn, chemical neutralization cannot be expected to bring universal relief of the discomfort. Although the presence of acid within the esophagus is central to the pathophysiology of gastroesophageal reflux, the symptoms that it elicits can be variable. The development of an acid-sensitive esophagus appears to be largely dependent on the volume of each reflux episode and the rapidity with which the episodes occur.

The mechanism by which acid provokes pain has been a matter of controversy. Some investigators suggested that the pain associated with reflux was due to acid-induced muscle spasms.[41] Others believed that induced motility changes were not an integral part of the pain mechanism.[66] The work of Atkinson and Bennett[67] suggests that the presence of acid in the esophagus has two independent effects: (1) to produce pain and (2) to increase nonpropulsive muscular activity, and the motor changes are not an essential part of the pain mechanism. The latter is based on the observation that: (1) pain and nonperistaltic contractions may each occur in the absence of the other, and (2) when both pain and a change in motility occur together, sodium bicarbonate infusion will relieve the

TABLE 9–5.—PREDOMINATE SYMPTOM EXPERIENCED WITH BALLOON DISTENTION OF THE ESOPHAGUS*

SIGN	UPPER ESOPHAGUS	MID ESOPHAGUS	LOWER ESOPHAGUS
Choking or fullness	62% (18/29)	20% (5/25)	10% (3/29)
Heartburn	14% (4/29)	44% (11/25)	59% (17/29)†
Chest pain	10% (3/29)	8% (2/25)	10% (3/29)
Uncomfortable	14% (4/29)	20% (7/25)	21% (6/29)

*Adapted from Jones C.M.: *Digestive Tract Pain.* New York, Macmillan Co., 1938.
†Seven patients also complained of chest pain.

pain without affecting the motility, and propantheline will abolish motility without relieving the pain.

THE EVOLUTION OF SURGICAL THERAPY FOR GASTROESOPHAGEAL REFLUX DISEASE AND THE CRITERIA FOR SUCCESS

The development of surgical therapy for the treatment of gastroesophageal reflux disease has paralleled our gradual understanding of esophageal physiology. In many situations, clinical experience with various antireflux operations contributed to this understanding. Gastroesophageal reflux disease was not recognized as a significant clinical problem until the mid-1930s and was not identified as a precipitating cause for esophagitis until after World War II.[68]

An important advance in the treatment of a hiatal hernia occurred when it was recognized that the symptoms associated with a hernia were actually caused by gastroesophageal reflux. This led to the conclusion that the hernia itself must be the cause of the reflux. It therefore seemed reasonable to attempt to correct reflux by surgically reducing the hernia with simple closure of the crura. The result of this first surgical effort was an unacceptably high failure rate.[69] For a long period, the failures did not become evident because of inadequate diagnostic tools. Only rigid endoscopy was available for evaluating esophagitis. Radiologic methods for the detection of reflux were inaccurate. Esophageal motility was just being introduced into clinical practice, and pH testing was not widely used or standardized. This experience, along with increased understanding of esophageal physiology, encouraged surgeons to improve the function of the cardia rather than simply reducing the hernia. The Allison repair, introduced in 1951, represented the first efforts in this direction.[70] He emphasized the need to place the gastroesophageal junction in its normal intra-abdominal position to improve its function. Although the repair was associated with a high incidence of recurrence, Allison has received the credit for initiating the modern day concepts of antireflux surgery. The experience with the Allison repair demonstrated that relief from the symptoms of reflux occurred in those patients whose gastroesophageal junction remained in the intra-abdominal position. Consequently, surgeons were stimulated to develop procedures designed to place and anchor the lower esophagus more effectively in the intra-abdominal position. Initially, these operations consisted of various forms of gastropexy in which an intra-abdominal esophagus was achieved by pulling the stomach down in the abdomen, whether it was herniated or not, and attaching it to the anterior abdominal wall or to any posterior peritoneal structure that seemed strong enough to maintain it there. The design of the gastropexy operation placed the stomach and esophagus on a great deal of continual tension due to normal respiratory and swallowing movements. Consequently, there was a dislodgment of the gastropexies with the return of reflux symptoms.[71–73] The most popular of these operations was the Hill procedure, which anchors the gastroesophageal junction posteriorly to the median arcuate ligament.[74]

With the exception of the Hill procedure, these operations did not stand the test of time and were gradually abandoned as more durable methods were sought to achieve an intra-abdominal esophagus. One of these was the Belsey Mark IV repair[75] and another the Nissen fundoplication.[76] Both procedures incorporate a portion of the distal esophagus into the stomach to ensure that it will be affected by changes in intra-abdominal pressure transmitted by the gastric conduit. The Belsey Mark IV procedure is, in essence, a partial fundoplication, or a 280° gastric wrap around the distal esophagus, while the Nissen is a complete fundoplication, or a 360° gastric fundic wrap. According to Bombeck,[77] the Nissen has become the more popular of the two operations, and variations of the operation are now used by the majority of surgeons worldwide for the treatment of reflux. Hill has added a degree of fundoplication to his operation that improved the results of the procedure to nearly the same as those of the Nissen.

It became obvious in the 1970s that the Nissen fundoplication was not without hazards. If the fundoplication is too long or wrapped too tightly, dysphagia results, which can be permanent. Experience with the operation has shown that the complete fundoplication functions as a very effective one-way valve, preventing reflux of any sort. This precludes physiologic belching and vomiting, both of which can become unacceptable side effects of the operation. Consequently, abdominal surgeons began to introduce a variety of incomplete fundoplications to avoid these problems.[78, 79] A partial fundoplication is usually constructed by covering either the anterior or the posterior wall of the distal esophagus with the stomach. This necessitates suturing the fundus of the stomach to the esophagus as the primary and most important portion of the procedure. This suture line is subject to a great deal of stress, and, as a consequence, has a limited durability. Although the partial fundoplication operations are successful in preventing reflux and permitting physiologic belching when they remain intact, they disrupt with a distressing frequency. The most durable of the partial fundoplication procedures is the Belsey Mark IV operation.[80] In this procedure the attachment of the esophagus to the stomach is more extensive than that advocated for the other partial fundoplications, and the procedure is performed transthoracically, so that the esophagus can be adequately mobilized to construct the repair without undue tension. The main drawback of the Belsey procedure is that, with its universal application by surgeons with varied skills, the antireflux protection achieved is not as dependable as that of a complete Nissen fundoplication. This is because the Belsey procedure is difficult to teach and to communicate and has less margin for error. In experienced hands, the success of the Belsey operation appears similar to that of the Nissen.

With wider application of the Nissen procedure, it became evident that a successful Nissen fundoplication is not simply a matter of wrapping the stomach around the lower esophagus and sewing it in place. Rather, a good deal of judgment and experience is required to determine how tight to make the fundoplication, how long, where it should start, and what portion of the stomach should be used. Consequently, Nissen fundoplications have contributed to a number of severe postoperative complications.[81] Some can be attributed to surgical technique, but the majority probably occurred from inaccurate selection of patients for operation.

Aware of the complications associated with the Nissen fundoplication, and desiring a procedure which can be performed by a less experienced surgeon, Angelchik and Cohen[82] designed a silicone prosthetic collar which can be easily placed around the abdominal esophagus as an antireflux device. The collar is made of material that resembles the silicone breast implant. On this basis, the silicone antireflux prosthesis was approved for human implantation without adequate clinical or animal investigation. It is now evident that this was an unfortunate mistake which has resulted in a loss of confidence regarding the use of an implantable device as a surgical solution to the problem of gastroesophageal reflux. This, coupled with the natural reluctance of surgeons to implant a prosthetic device adjacent to bowel and the increasing acceptance of the Nissen fundoplication, gave rise to the attitude that the use of a prosthetic device was an unnecessary risk. Despite this, there have been increasing reports of its safety and effectiveness in the control of reflux.[83, 84]

The introduction of the Angelchik prosthesis has been plagued with difficulties not uncommon to prosthetic devices.[85] In an early version of the prosthesis, the tabs which were used to tie the device in place had a tendency to become detached. Several became dislodged into the peritoneal cavity and produced symptoms, depending on where they came to rest. The tie tabs were changed to a continuous strip of silastic-impregnated Dacron. This completely encircles the outside of the prosthesis so that detachment is not possible; the only way that it can become dislodged is for the tabs to break.

A second problem has been the inappropriate use of the prosthetic device in the presence of an esophageal or high gastric suture line. This has led to the dramatic complication of erosion of the prosthesis into the GI tract, with subsequent passage of the device in the feces or its retrieval endoscopically. This complication, however, has been reported in fewer than 1% of the reported implantations. A bizarre complication occurs from puncturing the prosthesis by improper instrumentation during its implantation, with leakage of the silastic filling into either the mediastinum or abdomen. Sepsis around the prosthesis has not been a problem, although the device should never be employed in the presence of preexisting sepses or in patients whose esophagus or stomach has been severely traumatized or perforated during the dissection. Incidental implantation of the device for a hiatal hernia discovered at the time of another abdominal procedure is especially to be condemned.

The principal difficulty with the prosthesis has been that transit postoperative dysphagia occurs in 30% of the patients following implantation. In about 2% of all implants, persistence of dysphagia has necessitated the removal of the device.

The main dangers associated with the use of the Angelchik prosthesis are its ease of implantation and the potential long-term deleterious effects of an implantable material. The ease of implanting the device has tempted surgeons with little experience in other antireflux procedures to use it for lesser indications than proved gastroesophageal reflux. The second danger is the unknown consequences of having an implantable material around the cardia for a period of 10–20 years. Although this appears to be minimal, there have been sufficient long-term problems with silastic breast implants to suggest that similar problems might occur with the prosthesis. On the other hand, the Angelchik prosthesis may be an ac-

ceptable alternative to the Nissen fundoplication, when one considers the difficulties in standardizing the technique of the latter, due to the number of surgeons attempting to perform the procedure without specific training, and the lack of sufficient patient volume in training programs to teach proper technique.[86]

A discussion on the evolution of surgical treatment for gastroesophageal reflux might be interpreted to encourage broader use of medical treatment for this entity. It should be remembered, however, that medical treatment of gastroesophageal reflux is directed toward changing the pH of the reflux material and decreasing the incidence and duration of reflux episodes by postural and dietetic therapy. Changing the pH alters the symptoms of reflux to less heartburn and more regurgitation; avoiding certain positions reduces the number of reflux episodes; and assuming the upright position improves esophageal clearance. Despite these benefits, the cardia remains incompetent. Thus, the monitoring of medical therapy is necessary, since patients who continue to reflux without the symptoms of heartburn may develop a chronic cough from repetitive occult aspiration or dysphagia from persistent and progressive esophagitis. The end stage of reflux which responds symptomatically to medical therapy can be development of Barrett's esophagus with its recognized premalignant potential. In contrast, an antireflux procedure provides immediate correction of an incompetent cardia after one short surgical procedure. Long-term studies indicate that this correction will last well over 12 years, remove the life-style restraints of medical management, and relieve the expense necessary to provide for and monitor effective drug therapy.

To be competitive, it is necessary that surgical therapy achieve its goals without complications. To accomplish this, it is paramount that the surgeon understands the physiology of the cardia, learns how its function can be improved by surgical reconstruction, knows the benefits of the various procedures (Table 9–7), and has obtained training to perform the operations. Antireflux surgery is different from the extirpation of a diseased organ whose function is of no concern, since it will be destroyed with its removal. Rather, antireflux surgery is designed to improve the function of an organ that will remain in the patient and provide complete and permanent relief of all symptoms and complications of gastroesophageal reflux secondary to an incompetent cardia. Ideally, the reconstructed cardia should permit the patient to swallow normally, belch to relieve gaseous distention, or vomit when necessary. The end result should restore the patient to normal life, with no further need for medical, postural, or dietary therapy. As antireflux operations achieve these goals with greater safety and dependability, indications for the operation will increase.

The persistence of nausea, heartburn, regurgitation, dysphagia, chest pain, or epigastric pain after an antireflux procedure represents a clinically poor result due to either an incorrect initial diagnosis or technical failure. The problem with using symptoms as an indicator of success is that often a patient who has undergone surgery will not readily admit to the presence of postoperative symptoms. Gauging operative success by only the lack of postoperative symptoms is inadequate. Similarly, the report of a normal barium swallow is not a dependable criterion of success, since the symptoms of re-

TABLE 9–7.—COMPARISON OF CURRENT ANTIREFLUX PROCEDURES

OPERATION	CONCEPTUALITY	EASE OF INSTRUCTION	EFFECTIVENESS OF THE VALVE	OUTFLOW RESISTANCE	TOLERATION OF TENSION	BEST USE
Hill posterior gastropexy	Complex	Difficult	Dependent on intraoperative manometrics	Dependent on degree of imbrication of cardia	Best	Previous gastric resection
Belsey partial fundoplication	Simple	Most difficult	Effective valve—usually able to belch	Lowest resistance	Poor	Poor esophageal pump
Nissen fundoplication	Simple	Average	Most effective valve—unable to belch	Highest resistance Long and tight wrap can cause permanent dysphagia	Fair	Standard antireflux procedure
Angelchik prosthesis	Poorly understood	Easiest	Appears effective	Average pseudocapsule can cause permanent dysphagia	Fair	Undetermined

flux or its complications may be present in a patient who has no radiologic evidence of a hiatal hernia or regurgitation of barium from the stomach into the esophagus. Rather, the success of a procedure depends on achieving the combination of: (1) relief from symptoms, (2) objective evidence on 24-hour esophageal pH monitoring that reflux has been reduced to physiologic levels, and (3) evidence on esophageal manometry that the mechanical defect of the cardia has been corrected.

THE DEFINITION AND RECOGNITION OF A MECHANICALLY INCOMPETENT CARDIA

In man, the antireflux mechanism consists of a valvular cardia and the propulsive pump-like function of the body of the esophagus. Failure of one of these components can usually be compensated for by the other. Failure of both components inevitably leads to abnormal esophageal exposure to gastric juice.[27]

Mechanical failure of the valvular component of the antireflux mechanism is diagnosed by measuring inadequate mechanical characteristics of the sphincter on manometry. Based on our experience correlating esophageal manometry with 24-hour esophageal pH monitoring in both control subjects and patients, we have defined a mechanically incompetent cardia as having (1) an average sphincter pressure of 5 mm Hg or less, (2) an average length of sphincter exposed to the positive pressure environment of the abdomen of 1 cm or less, and/or (3) a sphincter with an average overall resting length of 2 cm or less.[21, 25, 26] These values are 2 SD below the mean measurement in normal control subjects and are associated with an 85%–90% incidence of increased esophageal acid exposure on 24-hour esophageal pH monitoring.

The key factor in the competency of the cardia is the distal esophageal sphincter pressure, but the efficiency of the pressure can be nullified by an inadequate abdominal length or an abnormally short overall resting length of the sphincter. Patients with a low sphincter pressure or those with a normal pressure but a short abdominal length are unable to protect against reflux caused by fluctuations of intra-abdominal pressure that occur with daily activities and changes in body position. Patients with a low sphincter pressure or those with a normal pressure but a short overall length are unable to pro-

tect against reflux caused by independent increases in gastric pressure over intra-abdominal pressure. In this situation, reflux can occur whenever an increase in gastric pressure exceeds the sphincter pressure that is necessary to provide competency for the overall length of sphincter present. Conversely, reflux of gastric contents can occur whenever gastric distention results in shortening of the overall length of the sphincter, like the shortening of the neck of a balloon on inflation, to the point where the sphincter length drops below that which is necessary for the sphincter pressure present to maintain competency. Thus, persons who have a short overall sphincter length on a resting esophageal motility study are at a disadvantage in protecting against reflux caused by normal gastric pressure and dilatation. On the other hand, in those who have a normal overall sphincter length on a resting esophageal motility study, it is possible for primary gastric pathology to cause gastric dilatation, shortening of the sphincter length, and reflux of gastric contents through a sphincter which, when the stomach is decompressed, has normal mechanical parameters. The first situation is a form of a mechanically incompetent cardia and can be corrected by an antireflux procedure. The second situation may require gastric surgery to correct.

The patient who has, on a resting motility study, a deficiency of one, two, or all three of the components of a competent valve—sphincter pressure, abdominal length and overall length—has a mechanically defective cardia as a basis for experiencing the symptoms and complications associated with the regurgitation of gastric contents into the esophagus. Such patients are less apt to receive benefits from medical therapy because their problem is a mechanical deficiency. They have a pathophysiologic defect that a surgical antireflux procedure is designed to correct.

Failures of the esophageal pump component of the antireflux mechanism often occur with a mechanical deficiency of the valvular component. This is usually caused by a reflux-induced or primary motility disorder, the presence of a hiatal hernia, or a myogenic abnormality. Each of these abnormalities produces inefficiency in the propulsive pumping action of the body of the esophagus, and potentiates the effects of a mechanically defective valve. Studies have indicated that surgery can improve the efficiency of the esophageal pump by reducing the hiatal hernia, but is not effective in improving the other causes of pump failure, with the exception of a reflux-induced motility disorder.[23] The latter, however, is often difficult to differentiate from a primary motility disorder.

Habitual pharyngeal swallowing is an effort to compensate for a mechanically defective valve of the antireflux mechanism and can result in pumping an excessive amount of air into the stomach. This leads to gastric dilatation and repetitive belching with further reflux of gastric contents into the esophagus. Surgical correction of the defective valvular component will usually remove the need for the excessive swallowing and alleviate the symptoms of gastric distention. Other causes for habitual swallowing resulting in excessive air intake, gastric dilatation, and reflux are attempts to compensate for a decreased saliva production and the loss of secondary peristalis. A surgical antireflux procedure has no benefit in these situations and may potentiate the gastric dilatation causing a gas bloat syndrome.

PATIENT SELECTION AND INDICATIONS FOR ANTIREFLUX SURGERY

Prior to any rational therapy for gastroesophageal reflux, a precise diagnosis as to the cause for abnormal acid exposure of the esophagus is necessary. An antireflux procedure should be considered only for those patients with a mechanically incompetent cardia. If the cardia is manometrically normal, the patient should be evaluated for gastric or esophageal causes for abnormal esophageal acid exposure. If neither is found, the increased acid exposure is probably due to transient spontaneous relaxation of the sphincter. These patients usually can be managed by medical therapy, but in severe cases an antireflux procedure can be very beneficial. The clinical indications to proceed with an antireflux operation in patients with a mechanically incompetent cardia are the presence of a complication of reflux; namely, persistent endoscopic esophagitis, esophageal stricture, Barrett's columnar line esophagus, or radiographic evidence of repetitive aspiration pneumonia.

As discussed previously, the development of esophagitis as a complication of gastroesophageal reflux appears to be related to the composition of the refluxed material and the pattern in which it is exposed to the esophageal mucosa.[5, 64] Thus, it is possible to have a mechanically incompetent cardia and not develop esophagitis. This occurs in about 50% of symptomatic patients.[12] In our experience, patients with esophagitis and a mechanically incompetent cardia commonly receive little long-term benefit from medical therapy and will usually require a surgical antireflux procedure to correct the condition. If severe endoscopic esophagitis is present, surgery should be performed rather quickly, since strictures can develop during medical therapy.[87] If 24-hour esophageal pH monitoring is normal in a patient with unequivocal endoscopic esophagitis, the possibilities of alkaline, drug-induced, or retention esophagitis should be considered.

A benign esophageal stricture secondary to reflux esophagitis in a patient with a mechanically incompetent cardia represents a failure of medical management and is an indication for surgical therapy.[88] Prior to surgery a malignant etiology of the stricture should be excluded. This can be difficult, and the roentgenographic barium swallow can be misleading. To make this differentiation, several biopsies and brushings from within the lumen of the stricture should be obtained. Occasionally, rigid endoscopy may be required to get an adequate biopsy. When a malignant etiology has been excluded, the stricture is progressively dilated up to a 60 F bougie prior to surgery. When fully dilated, esophageal manometry and 24-hour pH monitoring are performed. Manometry is used to determine the adequacy of peristalsis in the distal esophagus and the ability of the distal esophageal sphincter to relax on deglutition. If the stricture is so severe that normal function cannot be restored, caution should be exercised in performing an antireflux procedure and serious consideration given to a colon interposition. If 24-hour esophageal pH monitoring is normal, the cardia is either competent, indicating that the stricture is probably secondary to drug ingestion and dilation may be all that is needed, or pure alkaline reflux is present.

Barrett's esophagus is a columnar-lined esophagus acquired as a complication of persistent reflux esophagitis. It is almost always associated with a severe mechanical defect of the cardia.[89] A patient with a Barrett's esophagus is at risk of developing a stricture, hemorrhage from esophageal ulcer, and adenocarcinoma. It is established that control of reflux by an antireflux procedure can avert the complications of bleeding ulceration and stricture and probably protect against the development of adenocarcinoma by causing a reduction in the degree of pleomorphism and anaplasia.[90] The presence of a Barrett's esophagus is an indication for multiple mucosal biopsy. If severe mucosal dysplasia or carcinoma in situ is found, an esophageal resection should be done. If these changes are not found, an antireflux procedure should be performed.

Patients with roentgenographic evidence of previous recurrent pneumonias and a history of episodes of nocturnal choking, waking up with gastric contents in the mouth or soilage of the bed pillow may be suffering from repetitive pulmonary aspiration secondary to gastroesophageal reflux. The chest roentgenogram often shows a large hiatal hernia and signs of pleural thickening, bronchiectasis, and pulmonary fibrosis. In such patients 24-hour pH monitoring should be done to confirm the presence of increased esophageal acid exposure. If present, esophageal manometry should be performed; if a mechanical defect of the cardia is found, an antireflux procedure is indicated. Usually, these patients have a nonspecific motility abnormality of the esophageal body which tends to propel the refluxed material toward the pharynx.[3] Other esophageal disorders that can cause repetitive aspiration are achalasia, a hiatal hernia with a competent sphincter but a narrow diaphragmatic hiatus (to be discussed subsequently), and a pharyngeal or esophageal diverticulum.

The indication for antireflux surgery in a patient with a mechanically incompetent cardia and the absence of complications of reflux is the patient's unwillingness to put up with the chronic symptoms of heartburn or regurgitation that persist despite the best medical therapy. In this situation, it is important to demonstrate objectively the presence of abnormal reflux with 24-hour pH monitoring. If reflux is objectively shown but the complications of reflux are not present, the patient should receive medical therapy. If the symptoms persist over four to six months, an antireflux repair should be done. If there are normal mechanical components of the cardia, a gastric or esophageal cause for the increase in esophageal acid exposure should be sought. If the 24-hour esophageal pH monitoring test is normal, a cause for the symptoms other than reflux should be investigated.

Chronic atypical symptoms of reflux that can indicate the need for operative therapy in a patient with a mechanically incompetent cardia are chest pain from a reflux-induced esophageal irritation or spasm and pulmonary symptoms such as chronic cough, hoarseness or wheezing.[91] Generally, these atypical symptoms overshadow any gastroesophageal complaints and focus the physician's attention on the heart or lungs. Chest pain indistinguishable from coronary artery disease can be caused by reflux. These patients are usually thought to have coronary artery disease but have normal coronary arteries on arteriography or have had a previous coronary artery bypass procedure without relief of their chest pain. The tip-off that the pulmonary symptoms may be related to reflux is the history of recurrent pneumonias, the presence of chronic interstitial pulmonary fibrosis on the chest x-ray, adult onset of asthma, or a chronic cough that eludes all efforts to uncover its etiology.

The relationship of the cardiac or pulmonary symptoms to reflux can be clarified with 24-hour esophageal pH monitoring by correlating the timing of the onset of the symptom with a reflux episode. If the symptom occurs during or immediately after a reflux episode and the patient has a mechanically defective cardia but no complication of reflux, medical therapy should be tried. This consists of reducing the number of reflux episodes by elevating the head of the bed and prescribing cimetidine to alkalinize the pH of the refluxed gastric juice.[39] Urecholine can be added to increase esophageal clearance of the refluxed material.[39] If this therapy fails, an antireflux procedure can be helpful in controlling or abolishing the symptoms. If normal mechanical components of the cardia are found, a gastric or esophageal cause for the increase in esophageal acid exposure should be sought. If the 24-hour pH monitoring test is normal, the presence of a motility disorder in the body of the esophagus should be investigated. Attempts to induce esophageal spasm and precipitate an episode of chest pain may be helpful.[92]

A third indication for an antireflux procedure is dysphagia, regurgitation, or chest pain on eating. These symptoms are usually related to the presence of a large paraesophageal hernia, intrathoracic stomach, or a small hiatal hernia with a Schatzki ring or a narrow diaphragmatic hiatus.[93] These conditions are easily identified with an upper GI roentgenographic barium examination done by a knowledgeable radiologist. Heartburn can be associated with a paraesophageal hernia but is uncommon in the latter two conditions. It is absent in patients with an intrathoracic stomach because saliva pools within the stomach and neutralizes the gastric acid. A patient with a small, sliding hiatal hernia and a Schatzki ring or narrow diaphragmatic hiatus can have dysphagia and chest pain during eating due to the Schatzki ring or distention and contraction of that portion of the stomach above the narrow diaphragmatic opening. Occasionally, the contents in the herniated portion of the stomach can be regurgitated into the esophagus and, in some patients, up into the pharynx. These patients have little or no heartburn, since only swallowed food is regurgitated. Between meals, the cardia may be competent, and reflux of gastric contents does not occur. A cine- or

video-esophagogram using thick barium or a barium-coated hamburger can be helpful in identifying this problem. The surgical repair of these abnormalities includes an antireflux procedure because of an associated incompetency of the cardia initially or the potential of destroying the competency of the cardia during the repair of the hernia. In a patient in whom only a Schatzki ring is identified as the cause of dysphagia, dilatation with a 60 F dilator is usually effective therapy without operation.

In addition to these general indications for antireflux surgery, there are specific clinical situations in which an antireflux procedure is indicated. In children with incompetent cardias, the complications of reflux are esophagitis, recurrent pneumonia, anemia, and failure to thrive. Esophagitis is rapidly progressive in this age group, and a stricture may develop in a matter of weeks, even while the child is undergoing an acceptable form of medical therapy. Consequently, once the complication of esophagitis has been confirmed in a child with documented reflux, the need for a surgical antireflux procedure becomes urgent. In infants, failure to thrive, anemia, and aspiration pneumonia may be the only evidence that reflux is present. Once gastroesophageal reflux is objectively established by 24-hour esophageal pH monitoring, surgical correction should be performed.

The presence of gastroesophageal reflux in association with scleroderma or after balloon dilatation for achalasia is an indication for early surgical therapy, since reflux in the presence of a severe motility disorder progresses rapidly to esophagitis with stricture formation. The Belsey Mark IV procedure should be done in this situation because its low outflow resistance makes it particularly suitable to an esophageal body that has poor peristaltic activity.[88, 94]

The presence of a mechanically defective cardia after vagotomy and gastric resection or pyloroplasty can allow reflux of gastric and pancreaticobiliary secretions into the esophagus. This problem is usually manifested by symptoms of pulmonary aspiration. Endoscopic esophagitis can occur but is usually absent. Medical therapy designed to control both acid and alkaline reflux usually fails, and a bile-diverting procedure, without reconstruction of the cardia, is of little benefit in preventing the symptoms of aspiration. The proper surgical therapy is an antireflux operation, with the addition of a bile-diverting procedure if symptomatic alkaline gastritis is present.[95]

Prior to proceeding with a surgical antireflux repair, there are two things a surgeon should do. First, he should specifically query the patient for complaints of epigastric pain, nausea, vomiting, and loss of appetite. In the past, we accepted these symptoms as part of the reflux syndrome, but now realize that they can be due to bile reflux gastritis which occurs independently or in association with gastroesophageal reflux. As mentioned above, the problem is usually seen in patients who have had previous upper GI surgery, although this is not absolutely necessary.[96] In such patients, the correction of only the incompetent cardia will result in a disgruntled individual who continues to complain of nausea and epigastric pain on eating. In these patients, 24-hour pH monitoring of the stomach for the percent of time the pH is below 3 is being evaluated as a method of documenting the duodenogastric reflux.[97, 98] The diagnosis can also be documented with a ^{99m}Tc-

HIDA scan if excessive reflux of bile from the duodenum into the stomach can be demonstrated.[96] If surgery is necessary to control gastroesophageal reflux and if severe duodeno-gastric reflux is present, consideration should also be given to performing a bile diversion procedure. When diagnosed after an antireflux repair, the administration of sucralfate may relieve the persistent complaint of nausea and epigastric pain. Second, the surgeon should evaluate the propulsive force of the body of the esophagus to determine if there is sufficient power to propel a bolus of food through a newly reconstructed valve. This can be done by esophageal manometry or, better, using radioisotopic studies of esophageal transit time.

SURGICAL PRINCIPLES FOR THE RECONSTRUCTION OF THE ANTIREFLUX MECHANISM

As emphasized, it is necessary for the surgeon to understand the physiology of the foregut when performing an antireflux procedure. Regardless of the type of antireflux repair used, five principles must be kept in mind when surgically constructing a competent and permanent antireflux mechanism.

First, the operation should maintain or restore the overall length of the distal esophageal sphincter to at least 3 cm and its pressure to a level two times resting gastric pressure (12–20 mm Hg). As previously discussed, mechanical incompetency of the cardia can result from either a reduction in the distal esophageal sphincter pressure or its overall length. The probability of gastroesophageal reflux secondary to increases in intragastric pressure, independent of intra-abdominal pressure, is 77% for a cardia with an overall sphincter length of less than 2 cm. The ratio of resting gastric to sphincter pres-

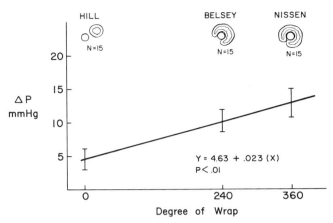

$$Y = 4.63 + .023\,(X)$$
$$P < .01$$

Fig 9–4.—The relationship between the augmentation of sphincter pressure over preoperative pressure (ΔP) and the degree of gastric fundic wrap.

sure of at least 3 is necessary to make a sphincter of this length competent; i.e., 18–30 mm Hg (Fig 9–3). This magnitude of sphincter pressure is rarely achieved by an antireflux procedure. Therefore, the overall sphincter length must be corrected to restore competency. If the preoperative sphincter pressure is abnormally low, then it, as well as the sphincter length, if also abnormally short, must be increased by the operation. Preoperative and postoperative esophageal manometry measurements have shown that the overall sphincter length and the resting sphincter pressure can be surgically augmented over preoperative values, and that the change in the latter is a function of the extent of the gastric wrap around the distal esophagus (Fig 9–4).

Second, the operation should place an adequate length of the distal esophageal sphincter in the positive pressure environment of the abdomen by a method that ensures its response to changes in intra-abdominal pressure. As previously discussed, the degree of competency provided by a segment of intra-abdominal sphincter to challenges in intra-abdominal pressure in the absence of intrinsic sphincter tone is a function of its length (Fig 9–5). Its efficiency is augmented by the presence of intrinsic sphincter pressure in that the greater the pressure, the shorter the abdominal length required to maintain competency. To function mechanically, however, a minimum of 1 cm of abdominal sphincter must be present. The probability of gastroesophageal reflux secondary to challenges of intra-abdominal pressure is 90% if the length of sphincter exposed to the abdomen is less than 1 cm, irrespective of its resting pressure. Since the abdominal sphincter length rarely exceeds 2 cm, a minimum intrinsic pressure of at least 5 mm Hg is required for competency. The permanent restoration of 1.5–2 cm of abdominal esophagus in a patient with a sphincter pressure greater than 10 mm Hg will maintain the competency of the cardia over various challenges of intra-abdominal pressure. Figure 9–6 shows that all three of the popular antireflux procedures increased the length of sphincter exposed to abdominal pressure by an average of 1 cm. However, this did not consistently occur, and in some patients the operation actually resulted in a reduction of the length of abdominal sphincter. If the operation results in less than 1 cm

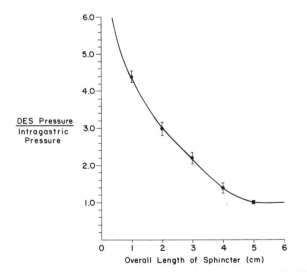

Fig 9–3.—The relationship of the ratio of sphincter (DES) pressure/intragastric pressure and overall length of sphincter to competency of the cardia. *Plotted line* represents the pressure ratio necessary to maintain competence for a given overall sphincter length. As the sphincter length shortens, a greater ratio is required for competency. For example, a sphincter length of 2 cm requires a ratio of 3, whereas a sphincter length of 4 cm requires a ratio of 1.5.

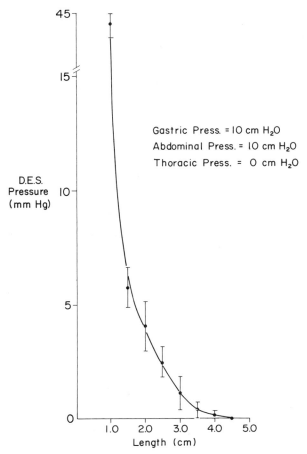

Gastric Press. = 10 cm H_2O
Abdominal Press. = 10 cm H_2O
Thoracic Press. = 0 cm H_2O

D.E.S. Pressure (mm Hg)

Length (cm)

Fig 9–5.—The relationship of sphincter (DES) pressure and length of sphincter exposed to the positive pressure environment of the abdomen to competency of the cardia. *Plotted line* represents the pressure necessary for a given length to obtain competence. Patients with 1.5–2 cm of abdominal sphincter require at least 5–7 mm Hg of sphincter pressure to remain competent. If abdominal length is less than 1 cm, competency is difficult to achieve irrespective of the level of sphincter pressure.

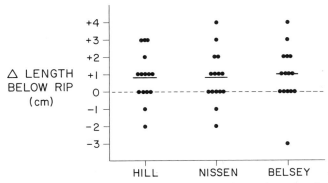

Δ LENGTH BELOW RIP (cm)

HILL   NISSEN   BELSEY

Fig 9–6.—The change over preoperative values in abdominal sphincter length expected after the three major antireflux procedures. On the average, all the procedures increase the length by 1 cm. However, it is possible for the procedure actually to decrease the length.

of sphincter exposed to abdominal pressure, incompetency of the cardia to challenges of intra-abdominal pressure results, regardless of the amount that the sphincter pressure was increased by the procedure.

Increasing the length of sphincter exposed to abdominal pressure will improve competency of the cardia only if it can be acted on by challenges of intra-abdominal pressure. Thus, the creation of a conduit that will ensure the transmission of intra-abdominal pressure changes around the abdominal portion of the sphincter is a necessary aspect of the surgical repair. The fundoplication in the Nissen and Belsey repairs serves this purpose (Fig 9–7). In the absence of a fundic wrap, as in the original Hill procedure, the development of periesophageal adhesions can prevent the transmission of intra-abdominal pressure to the abdominal esophagus. This will allow for postural-induced pressure changes in the abdominal cavity to be transmitted unequally to the stomach and the abdominal portion of the sphincter and result in a reflux episode.

Third, the operation should ensure that the reconstructed cardia relaxes on deglutition. To facilitate normal swallowing after an operative repair, the distal esophageal sphincter must be able to relax. On deglutition, a vagally mediated relaxation of the distal esophageal sphincter and fundus of the stomach occurs. The relaxation lasts for approximately ten seconds and is followed by rapid recovery to its former tonicity. To ensure relaxation of the cardia, only the fundus of the stomach should be used, since it is known to relax in concert with the sphincter.[99] It is paramount that the innervation of the cardia be protected, since inadvertent vagal damage during dissection of the thoracic esophagus may result in failure of relaxation.

Fourth, the operation should not increase the resistance of the reconstructed cardia to a level that exceeds the peristaltic power of the body of the esophagus. The resistance of a reconstructed cardia depends on the degree, length, and diameter of the gastric fundic wrap and on the variation in intra-abdominal pressure (Fig 9–8). A 360° gastric wrap should be no longer than 2 cm and large enough to allow a 60 F bougie to pass into the stomach with ease. This will ensure that the relaxed cardia will have an adequate lumen size and minimal changes in resistance with variation in intra-abdominal pressure. This is not necessary when constructing a partial wrap. The choice between a total 360° or a partial 240° gastric wrap is influenced by the strength of the peristaltic contractions in the body of the esophagus. The esophagi that have normal motility and strong peristaltic contractions do well with a 360° fundoplication. When peristalsis is absent, severely disor-

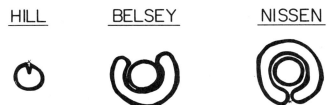

HILL   BELSEY   NISSEN

Fig 9–7.—Schematic cross section of the cardia after the three major repairs. The Belsey and Nissen repair creates a conduit that ensures the transmission of intra-abdominal pressure changes around the abdominal portion of the sphincter.

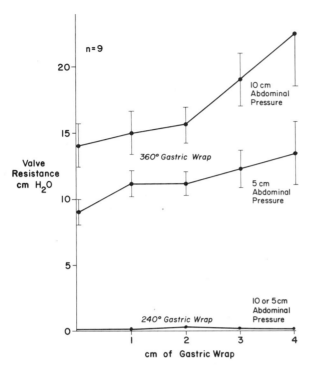

Fig 9–8.—The hydrostatic pressure necessary to overcome the resistance of a 360° or 240° gastric fundic wrap of various lengths constructed over a 60 F bougie in the absence of intrinsic tone at different levels of abdominal pressure.

dered, or of low magnitude (below 20 mm Hg), the Belsey two thirds partial fundoplication is the procedure of choice.

Fifth, the operation should ensure that the repair will remain within the abdomen by not placing the reconstructed cardia under undue tension and approximate the crura of the diaphragm above the fundoplication, if used. Failure to do so results in the operative conversion of a sliding hiatal hernia into a paraesophageal hernia, with all the complications associated with that condition.[100]

TECHNIQUE OF THE NISSEN FUNDOPLICATION

Through ten years of personal experience, I have come to settle on the following operative technique for the transabdominal and transthoracic Nissen fundoplication. Several of my patients have submitted themselves voluntarily to postoperative studies consisting of esophageal manometry, 24-hour esophageal pH monitoring, and a thorough questioning about their esophageal symptoms. Comparison of the postoperative to preoperative studies and to similar studies obtained from normal volunteers has helped me to evaluate objectively what I have accomplished by the surgical repair. I selected the Nissen operation because it initially gave the best early results in a randomized study of the three available operations.[101] I have continued to follow up these and subsequent patients who have had the Nissen operation and made modifications in the operative technique only when the results of the postoperative studies indicated that I was not achieving

the stated goals. The current technique represents only minor refinement over the method initially published by Nissen[76] and, if performed as I have described, will give excellent results to surgeons endowed with average skill.

The Nissen fundoplication, as initially described, consists of wrapping the fundus of the stomach 360° around the lower esophagus for a distance of 4–5 cm. I have modified the originally described procedure only by limiting the length of the wrap to 1.5 cm. When done transthoracically, the fundic wrap lies primarily over the anterior and lateral surfaces of the esophagus with the sutures posterior. When done transabdominally, the fundic wrap lies primarily over the posterior, left lateral, and anterior surfaces of the esophagus, with the sutures on the right anterolateral surface, in line with the insertion of the gastrohepatic ligament along the lesser curve of the stomach. The modifications I have made arose out of my experience in redoing previously failed Nissen operations. These patients made up a sizable portion of my referral practice, so I took a special interest in determining why the procedures failed. In some patients who complained of recurrent heartburn and regurgitation traces of a previously performed fundoplication were completely absent. It was my impression that this was due to the breakage or pulling out of the fundic sutures and indicated the need to use stronger sutures placed in a more durable manner. Other patients had marked dysphagia. In some, a 60 F dilator could be passed into the stomach with ease and in others only with force. In the former patients the fundic wrap was too tight; in the latter, too long. From these clinical observations, along with observations made from a model of the cardia, it became evident that the gastric wrap should be only 1.5–2 cm long and held in place with permanently reinforced sutures. A technique was developed which used one permanent 2–0 Prolene horizontal mattress suture reinforced with four 1.5 × 0.5-cm Teflon pledgets placed in a manner described subsequently. It is important that Teflon pledgets are cut to exact size. This keeps the wrap a standard length and gives reproducible results. With experience, the technique has matured into that described below, and if followed exactly, will give the surgeon gratification and the patient dramatic relief of symptoms coupled with a return to the joy of eating.

The Transabdominal Approach

The transabdominal Nissen fundoplication is performed through an upper midline abdominal incision extending from the lower end of the sternum laterally around the xiphoid process and down to the umbilicus. Paramount in performing the procedure is to have excellent exposure of the esophageal hiatus. We have constructed a specialized upper abdominal retractor for this purpose by welding a Weinberg retractor to a Balfour handle. This retractor is placed under the liver down to the esophageal hiatus. The patient is placed in a reverse Trendelenburg position, and the retractor is lifted cephalad in a 45° angle and secured to an overhead bar attached to the table (Fig 9–9). This elevates the anterior chest wall and lifts the liver out of the way, providing excellent exposure to the area of the esophageal hiatus. Without this exposure, careful dissection of the hiatus is difficult, time consuming, and dangerous. A Balfour retractor is used to open the incision laterally, and the exposure obtained with the

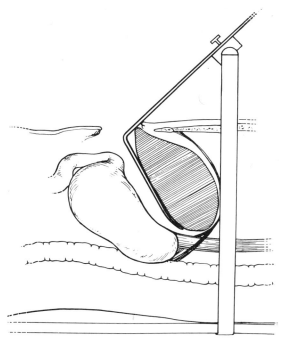

Fig 9–9.—Position of a modified Weinberg retractor to provide exposure of the esophageal hiatus.

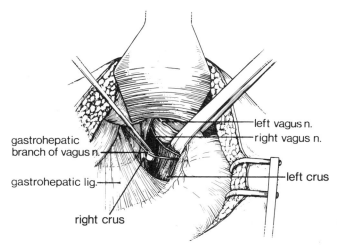

gastrohepatic branch of vagus n.

gastrohepatic lig.

right crus

left vagus n.

right vagus n.

left crus

Fig 9–10.—Completed hiatal dissection done through the transabdominal approach showing the vagal nerves, position of the rubber drain around the esophagus, and the right and left crus.

combination of the two retractors makes the operation a pleasure to perform.

The first step is to dissect out the esophageal hiatus by dividing the gastrohepatic ligament in the area where it is thin and usually transparent. Care should be taken not to damage the hepatic branch of the anterior vagus nerve. The temptation to divide this nerve should be resisted, even though it appears initially that it will compromise the exposure. The portion of the gastrohepatic ligament cephalad to the nerve should be palpated between the thumb and index finger prior to its division to prevent inadvertent injury to an aberrant left hepatic artery coming directly from the celiac axis. If a large artery is identified, it should be spared and the operation performed by working around the isolated artery. The cephalad portion of the gastrohepatic ligament is divided and the incision carried superiorly over the anterior surface of the esophagus, dividing the reflection of the parietal peritoneum from the diaphragm onto the esophagus and stomach, where it forms the visceral peritoneum. This incision should not be made on the diaphragm, as this will engender bleeding from the phrenic veins, but within the esophageal hiatus, taking care not to damage the anterior vagal trunk. The incision is continued down the left lateral surface of the esophagus until the left crus of the esophageal hiatus is identified.

The loose areolar tissue over the superior surface of the esophagus is removed. The esophagus is dissected circumferentially within the posterior mediastinum using blunt finger dissection over the anterior surface of the aorta encircling both the vagal trunks and the esophagus. When a large hiatal hernia is present, it is helpful to perform this finger dissection high within the posterior mediastinum. This will allow for an easier dissection around the esophagus and aids in reducing the hiatal hernia. When encircled, the right or posterior va-

gus is identified and a soft rubber drain is passed around the esophagus, excluding the posterior vagal trunk. While retracting on the rubber drain, the loose fibroareolar tissue within the hiatus is divided to identify clearly the right and left crus. The decussation of the right and left crus over the anterior surface of the aorta represents the inferior extent of the dissection (Fig 9–10).

The second step of the procedure is to mobilize the fundus of the stomach by dividing the short gastric vessels. This is started at the point where the greater curvature veins drain superiorly toward the spleen, rather than inferiorly toward the right gastroepiploic vein. This is approximately at the junction of the proximal third of the greater curvature and the distal two thirds (Fig 9–11). It should be remembered that

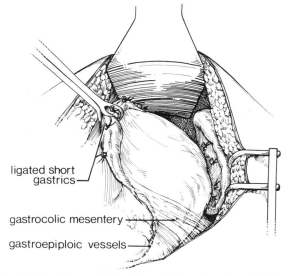

ligated short gastrics

gastrocolic mesentery

gastroepiploic vessels

Fig 9–11.—The mobilized gastric fundus after division of the short gastric vessels. Some of these vessels can take a retroperitoneal course, tethering the fundus of the stomach posteriorly.

the gastric epiploic mesentery "V"s out along the greater curvature to both the anterior and posterior surface of the stomach. In each of these mesentery leaves are branches of the short gastric vessels. It is helpful to divide the vessels in the anterior leaf of the mesentery first and then those in the posterior leaf. This avoids crimping of the gastric wall when both leaves are taken together with bulk ties. Occasionally at the most superior aspect of the greater curvature, the short gastric vessels take a retroperitoneal course, tethering the fundus of the stomach to the posterior abdominal wall.[102] One can appreciate how these vessels, if not divided, force the surgeon to construct the fundoplication with a portion of the body of the stomach rather than the fundus. Excellent exposure is required to free a tethered gastric fundus; and if the retractor described is used, the dissection is not difficult.

The third stage of the operation is to close the esophageal hiatus. The esophagus is retracted to the left with a specially designed esophageal retractor, and the right and left crura are approximated with interrupted 0 silk sutures. The closure is started inferiorly, where the crura decussate over the aorta. The sutures are placed at 1 cm intervals, advancing the esophageal body anteriorly as the hiatus is closed. Usually six sutures are required to complete the closure (Fig 9–12). Care is taken not to place the uppermost sutures on the right side in the fascia of the diaphragm, as this will result in a constriction of the hiatus and dysphagia. All sutures should be placed within the muscle of the crura and tied with a tension that causes tissue approximation without strangulation. When complete, the hiatus should freely admit a fingertip adjacent to the esophagus. It is better to err in making the hiatal closure too loose rather than too tight. The purpose of the crural closure is only to maintain the repair within the abdomen.

The fourth step of the operation is to construct the fundic wrap. A 60 F bougie is passed by the anesthesiologist into the stomach to display the gastroesophageal junction. The pad of areolar tissue which lies on the anterior surface of the gastroesophageal junction is removed to allow proper identification of the junction and encourage the fusion of the fundic wrap to the esophagus. Care should be taken to avoid injury of the anterior vagus nerve while removing the fat pad. The bleeding that occurs during removal can be controlled by placing a lap pad on the esophagus and squeezing it around the bougie for a few moments. Any remaining bleeding points can be ligated or cauterized. To attempt to clamp and tie all the

small vessels while removing the fat pad is both time consuming and potentially damaging to the anterior vagus. Failure to control the bleeding can result in a postoperative hematoma within the fundic wrap and dysphagia.

The freed posterior wall of the fundus is pulled between the right vagal trunk and the posterior wall of the esophagus containing the 60 F bougie. The anterior wall of the fundus is pulled across the anterior wall of the esophagus. This results in wrapping the distal esophagus with the stomach by enveloping it within the fundus. The needles at both ends of a 2.0 Prolene suture are passed through a 1.5×0.5-cm Teflon pledget 1 cm apart and then through the left lip of the fundic wrap, again 1 cm apart. Both ends of the suture are passed through a second pledget sandwiching the lip of the stomach between the two pledgets. One of the limbs of the suture is then passed through the anterior wall of the esophagus at the gastroesophageal junction, incorporating the tissue down to, but not through, the muscularis mucosa. The second limb is similarly passed through the anterior wall of the esophagus 1 cm cephalad to the first stitch. Both ends of the suture are passed through a third Teflon pledget, again 1 cm apart, and then through the right lateral lip of the fundic wrap. Both ends of the suture are then passed through the fourth and final Teflon pledget. The completed horizontal mattress stitch, or U-stitch, sandwiches the stomach between the first and second pledget, the esophagus between the second and third pledget, and the stomach again between the third and fourth pledget (Fig 9–13).

A single tie is then placed in the suture approximating the two lips of the fundic wrap around the esophagus containing the 60 F bougie. The ability for Prolene suture to slide through tissue without sawing allows for this test approximation of the fundic wrap without causing tissue damage or hematoma formation. When drawn together, the fundic wrap

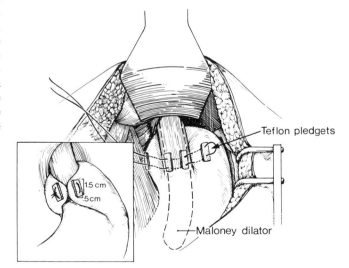

Fig 9–13.—Construction of the fundoplication by the transabdominal approach illustrating the placement of the horizontal mattress stitch and the positions of the pledgets. The wrap is formed over a 60 F bougie with enough space left over to allow the passage of an index finger through the wrap adjacent to the bougie. *Inset,* the completed fundoplication.

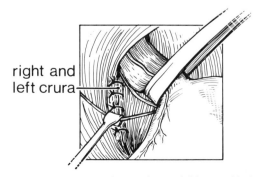

Fig 9–12.—The closed esophageal hiatus. Notice that the esophageal body has been displaced anteriorly by the approximation of the right and left crura.

should be large enough to accept the insertion of the surgeon's index finger alongside the esophagus containing the 60 F bougie. If the surgeon is unable to insert his finger or feels tight bands over his finger, the wrap is too tight, and the left end of the horizontal U-stitch must be replaced more laterally and inferiorly on the anterior wall of the fundus. This enlarges the internal diameter of the wrap. If there is excessive space, the wrap is too floppy, and the left end of the U-stitch must be replaced more medially and superiorly on the anterior wall of the fundus. This reduces the internal diameter of the wrap. When the wrap is proper size, the bougie is removed and the limbs of the U-stitch are tied securely (see Fig 9–13).

Since only one U-stitch suture is used to hold the wrap, it is important that it is made of permanent material and that the Teflon pledgets are used to reinforce its purchase on the tissue. The use of Teflon pledgets has not resulted in the development of postoperative infection or wall erosion. This is probably due to the compression of one pledget against the other, excluding the lumen of the esophagus and stomach (Fig 9–14). The placement of the fundic wrap between the esophagus and right vagal trunk posteriorly and passing the U-stitch through the anterior wall of the esophagus holds the fundic wrap around the gastroesophageal junction and prevents the development of a slipped Nissen.

Figure 9–14 is a transverse section of the stomach and distal esophagus at the level of the fundoplication. It illustrates the position of the four pledgets and the placement of the U-stitch. The completed fundoplication has an external length of only 1.5 cm and a circumference of slightly less than 360° wrap. Both factors reduce the resistance to the passage of food through the cardia. The illustration also shows how intragastric pressure, intra-abdominal pressure, and gastric muscle tone are applied to the distal esophageal sphincter.

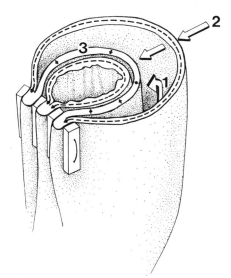

Fig 9–14.—Schematic cross section of a Nissen fundoplication done with 1.5 × 0.5-cm pledgets illustrating how the pledgets compress the stomach and esophagus together and how intragastric *(1)*, intra-abdominal pressure *(2)*, and gastric fundic muscle tone *(3)* are transmitted to the sphincter.

The Transthoracic Approach

The indications for performing an antireflux procedure by transthoracic approach are: (1) The patient who has had a previous hiatal hernia repair. With a transthoracic approach, a peripheral circumferential incision in the diaphragm can be made for simultaneous exposure of the upper abdomen, allowing safe dissection of the previous repair from both the abdominal and thoracic sides of the diaphragm. (2) The patient who requires a concomitant esophageal myotomy for achalasia or diffuse spasm. (3) The patient who has an esophageal stricture. In this situation, the thoracic approach is preferred to obtain maximum mobilization of the esophagus and place the repair without tension below the diaphragm. (4) The patient with a sliding hiatal hernia that does not drop below the diaphragm during a roentgenographic barium study in the upright position. This can indicate esophageal shortening and, again, a thoracic approach is preferred for maximum mobilization of the esophagus. (5) The patient who has associated pulmonary pathology. In this situation, the nature of the pulmonary pathology can be evaluated and the proper pulmonary surgery in addition to the antireflux repair can be performed. (6) The obese patient. In this situation, the abdominal procedure is difficult because of poor exposure, whereas the thoracic approach gives better exposure and allows a more precise repair.

The hiatus is approached transthoracically through a left posterior lateral thoracotomy incision in the sixth intercostal space; i.e., over the upper border of the seventh rib. For patients who have a failed antireflux repair and are undergoing a second procedure, I prefer to use the seventh intercostal space; i.e., above the superior border of the eighth rib. This allows better exposure of the abdomen through the diaphragm incision. When necessary, the diaphragm is incised circumferentially 2–3 cm from the chest wall for a distance of approximately 10–15 cm. An adequate fringe of diaphragm must be preserved along the chest wall to allow for reapproximation of the muscle. This diaphragm incision also provides excellent exposure of the left upper abdomen for a concomitant surgical procedure on the stomach or performing a left colon interposition following resection of the distal esophagus. If further abdominal exposure is necessary, the thoracic incision can be extended across the costal margin and bridge of the diaphragm and diagonally across the rectus muscle to the abdominal midline. The operation is made easier if the anesthetic is delivered through a double-lumen endotracheal tube and the left lung is selectively deflated.

The first step in the operation is to mobilize the esophagus from the level of the diaphragm to the aortic arch. Care is taken not to injure the vagal nerves. There are two arteries which arise from the proximal descending thoracic aorta and pass over the left lateral surface of the esophagus to the left main stem bronchus. They are the left superior and inferior bronchial arteries. These are ligated individually and represent the cephalad extension of the esophageal mobilization. In addition to these arteries there are two or three esophageal arteries coming directly from the distal descending thoracic aorta to the lower third of the esophagus. They are also ligated and divided. One need not worry about ischemic necrosis of the esophagus with this degree of dissection. In our experience (Belsey, DeMeester, Skinner), this has not occurred in over 1,000 antireflux procedures in which the esophagus has been so mobilized. There is sufficient blood supply through the intrinsic arterial plexus of the esophagus, fed by the inferior thyroid artery in the neck and branches of the right brachial artery in the thorax, to maintain the integrity and prevent ischemic necrosis of the muscle. This degree of mobilization is absolutely necessary to place the reconstructed cardia into the abdomen without undue tension. Failure to mobilize the esophagus adequately is one of the major causes for subsequent breakdown of a transthoracic repair and return of symptoms.

The second step of the operation is freeing the cardia from the diaphragm and is the most difficult portion of the transthoracic procedure. To accomplish this, it is not necessary to make an incision through the central tendon of the diaphragm or to enlarge the hiatus by dividing the crura. With experience, this portion of the operation can be completed through the hiatus. The dissection is started by gaining access into the abdominal cavity through the phrenoesophageal membrane. It can be difficult to find the right tissue plane, since the properitoneal fat tends to protrude through the incision once the superior leaf of the membrane has been divided. Persistence and close dissection to the wall of the stomach, away from the gastric vessels, will eventually be rewarded with entry into the free peritoneal space. Entry into the abdominal cavity is easier when a hiatal hernia is present.

The proper stance of the surgeon at the operating table will aid him in the dissection of the hiatus. He should stand adjacent to the patient, facing the head of the table. The left index and middle fingers are placed through the diaphragmatic hiatus into the abdominal cavity with the palm of the hand facing the patient's feet. The surgeon's line of vision is down and backward under his left axilla. With judicial use of the left thumb, index, and middle fingers, the surgeon is able to spread the hiatal tissues and guide the dissection done with scissors controlled by his right hand. In this position, the left hand is also used to retract the esophagus and protect the vagal trunks. Although the description of this stance sounds somewhat awkward, its use greatly facilitates the most difficult part of the operation. In fact, the stance is quite natural and would be assumed eventually by any surgeon who, on numerous occasions, has experienced the struggle of freeing the cardia from the hiatus through a transthoracic approach.

When all the attachments between the cardia and diaphragmatic hiatus are divided, the fundus and part of the body of the stomach are drawn up through the hiatus into the chest. Sometimes this requires dividing the cephalad portion of the dorsal mesentery of the stomach, just anterior to the aorta, through the hiatus. Care should be taken not to injure the left gastric artery or vagal trunks during this maneuver. This portion of the operation is completed by excising the vascular fat pad that lies on the anterior lateral surface of the cardia in a manner similar to that described for the abdominal approach (Fig 9–15).

The third step of the procedure is the placement of the crura sutures used to close the hiatus. The mobilized esophagus and cardia are retracted anteriorly to expose the right

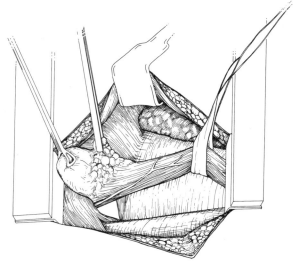

Fig 9–15.—A transthoracic antireflux procedure through a left posterolateral thoracotomy showing complete mobilization of the esophagus and freeing of the cardia from the diaphragmatic hiatus. The fundus of the stomach is drawn through the hiatus into the chest with a Babcock clamp. The forceps is on the vascular fat pad at the cardioesophageal junction.

and left crura (Fig 9–16). Usually there is a decussation of muscle fibers from the right crus around the aorta, but occasionally the aorta lies free within the enlarged hiatus. In either situation, the first crural stitch is placed as close as possible to the aorta, taking a generous bite of crural muscle.

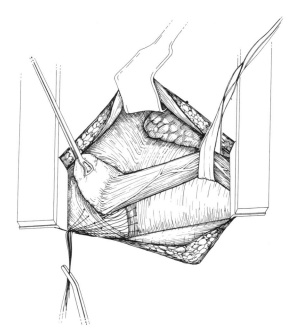

Fig 9–16.—A transthoracic antireflux procedure showing the vascular fat pad removed and anterior retraction of the esophagus with placement of the crural sutures for closure of the hiatus posteriorly.

Traction on this first suture and on a Babcock clamp attached to the anterior border of the hiatus elevates the right crus toward the surgeon and facilitates the placement of subsequent crural stitches. Occasionally it is necessary to mobilize the pericardium off the diaphragm for better exposure of the fascia and muscle of the right crus. The subsequent crural sutures should incorporate the fascia from the periphery of the central tendon that blends with the muscle fibers of the right crus. On the left, the stitches are placed through the muscle fibers of the crus and the firmly adherent overlying pleura. Approximately six sutures, placed 1 cm apart, are necessary to approximate the crura adequately and to reduce the size of the hiatus. If it is thought that more sutures are needed, they should be placed at this time, since it is easier to remove those not needed than to place additional stitches after completion of the repair. To insert the most anterior crural stitch, it is often necessary to push the esophagus posteriorly against the previously placed sutures and pass a stitch through the right crus, anterior to the esophagus, then bring it posterior to the esophagus and through the left crus. The crural sutures are not tied until the reconstruction of the cardia is complete.

The fourth step of the operation is to construct the fundoplication. The fundus of the stomach is brought up into the chest through the hiatus. The wrapping of the fundus around the distal esophagus is performed in a manner similar to that described for the abdominal approach, except that the fundus is anterolateral instead of posterolateral and the hold suture posterior instead of anterior. As in the abdominal approach, the distal esophagus is invaginated into the stomach by pulling the walls of the fundus around posteriorly (Fig 9–17). The technique used to secure the wrap is similar to that described in the transabdominal approach. The needles of a double armed 2.0 Prolene suture are passed through a 1.5 × 0.5-cm

Teflon pledget 1 cm apart and then through the right lateral lip of the fundic wrap, again 1 cm apart. This is the inferior lip of the wrap as seen by the surgeon when operating through a left lateral thoracotomy incision. Both ends of the suture are passed through a second Teflon pledget, sandwiching the lip of the stomach between the two pledgets. A 60 F bougie is passed by the anesthesiologist into the stomach for accurate sizing of the wrap and proper identification of a posterior border of the gastroesophageal junction (Fig 9–18). One of the limbs of the stitch is then passed through the posterior wall of the esophagus at the level of the gastroesophageal junction, incorporating tissue down to, but not through, the muscularis mucosa. The second limb is similarly passed through the posterior wall of the esophagus 1 cm cephalad to the first stitch. Both ends of the suture are passed through a third Teflon pledget, again 1 cm apart, and then through the left lateral lip of the fundic wrap. This is the superior lip of the wrap as seen by the surgeon when operating through a left lateral thoracotomy incision. Both ends of the suture are then passed through the fourth and final Teflon pledget (Fig 9–19). A single tie is used initially to approximate the two lips of the fundoplication around the esophagus containing the 60 F bougie. Again, as with the abdominal repair, the wrap, when drawn together, should be large enough to accept the insertion of the surgeon's index finger between the stomach and the esophagus containing the 60 F dilator (Fig 9–20). If unable to do so, or if the wrap is too loose, the size of the wrap must be adjusted as discussed in the abdominal approach. If the size of the wrap is correct, the suture is tied sandwiching the stomach and esophagus together (Fig 9–21).

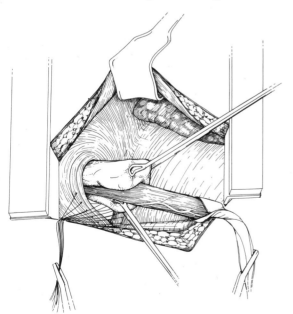

Fig 9–17.—Construction of a Nissen 360° gastric fundic wrap showing the fundus of the stomach brought up through the hiatus anterior to the esophagus.

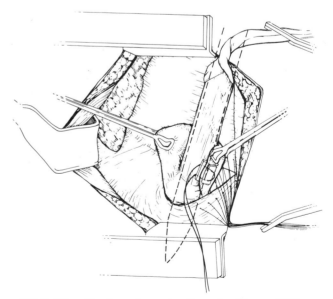

Fig 9–18.—Continued construction of a Nissen 360° gastric wrap showing placement of the U-stitch with the Teflon pledgets in the right lateral lip of the fundic wrap. The esophagus and stomach have been rotated to the right for easier placement of this suture. When the suture has been placed, a 60 F bougie is passed into the stomach to allow accurate sizing of the wrap and to allow identification of the posterior border of the gastroesophageal junction.

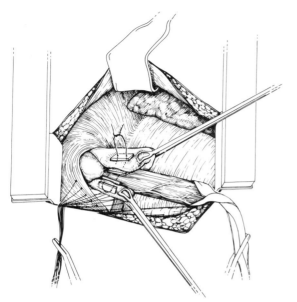

Fig 9–19.—Continued construction of a Nissen 360° gastric fundic wrap showing the position of the U-stitch and the four Teflon pledgets. Again, the stomach and esophagus have been rotated to the right for easier placement of the U-stitch.

When complete, the fundoplication is placed into the abdomen by compressing the fundic ball with the hand and manually maneuvering it through the hiatus. Resistance to placing the repair into the abdomen can result from the shoelace obstruction of the previously placed crural sutures. Opening the crural sutures, like loosening the laces of a shoe,

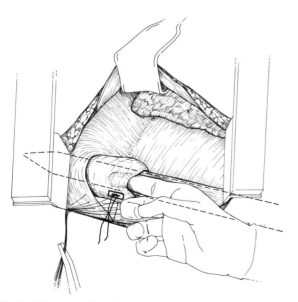

Fig 9–20.—Continued construction of a Nissen 360° gastric fundic wrap. The size of the diameter of the wrap is tested by insertion of the tip of the surgeon's index finger between the gastric wrap and the esophagus containing the 60 F dilator. The stomach and esophagus have rotated back to their normal positions with the U-stitch located posteriorly.

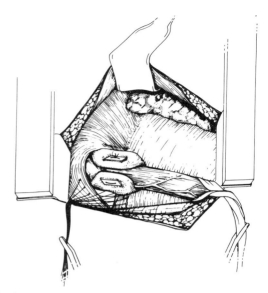

Fig 9–21.—Continued construction of a Nissen 360° gastric fundic wrap. The U-stitch is tied over 1.5 × 0.5-cm Teflon pledgets. Again, the stomach and esophagus have been rotated to the right to demonstrate the U-stitch.

relieves the obstruction and aids in placing the reconstructed cardia into the abdomen. Once in the abdomen, the fundoplication should remain there, and a gentle up-and-down motion on the diaphragm should not encourage it to emerge back through the esophageal hiatus into the chest. If the repair remains in the abdomen unaided, the previously placed crural sutures are tied (Fig 9–22).

If the fundoplication tends to ride up through the hiatus, tension on the repair is too great, usually due to inadequate mobilization of the esophagus. If there has been complete mobilization and the fundoplication still tends to ride up through the hiatus, the branches of the left vagus nerve to the left pulmonary plexus can be divided in an effort to re-

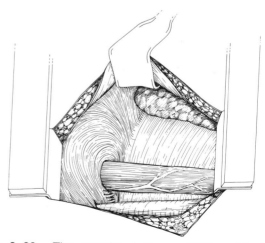

Fig 9–22.—The completed Nissen 360° gastric fundic wrap. The reconstructed cardia in the abdomen and the right and left crura have been approximated by tying the previously placed sutures.

duce the tension and allow for easier placement of the reconstructed cardia in the abdomen. If, after this maneuver, the tendency to ride up through the hiatus persists, a Collis gastroplasty or a resection of the cardia using a short left colon interposition to reestablish GI continuity is done. This becomes a serious consideration in only two out of every 100 uncomplicated repairs.

When performing the repair, it is important that the vagus nerves are protected and not injured. This will ensure the relaxation of the gastric fundic wrap in concert with the distal esophageal sphincter on deglutition. At the completion of the procedure, a nasal gastric tube should be able to be passed, without guidance from the surgeon, directly into the stomach to ensure that there has been no angulation of the distal esophagus. A chest tube for drainage of the pleural cavity is properly placed and the chest incision closed.

TECHNIQUE OF BELSEY MARK IV REPAIR

The techniques of the Belsey Mark IV and the transthoracic Nissen operations are the same, differing only in the construction of the gastric fundoplication. To perform the Belsey Mark IV reconstruction, the esophagus and cardia are mobilized, and the fundus of the stomach is brought up through the hiatus as described for the transthoracic Nissen procedure. In contrast to the Nissen, the Belsey Mark IV procedure is a partial fundoplication of the stomach around the anterior two thirds of the lower 3–4 cm of the esophagus. The partial wrap is held in place by two rows of three horizontal mattress sutures placed equidistantly between the seromuscular layers of the stomach and the muscular layers of the esophagus. Number 00 silk sutures are used, and each suture obtains a firm grip of the esophageal muscle fibers by passing down to, but not through, the muscularis mucosae. The first row of sutures is placed 1.5 cm above the cardia and is tied only tightly enough to obtain tissue apposition without disrupting the muscle fibers of the esophagus. It is important to remember that the hiatus is approached surgically from the left lateral position. To construct the fundoplication over the anterolateral two thirds of the esophagus, it is necessary that the far right suture be placed in the right lateral wall of the esophagus. This is out of the surgeon's view and requires rotating the esophagus before placement of the suture (Fig 9–23). A common mistake is placing this suture too far anteriorly, resulting in an anterolateral fundoplication displaced to the left. This is a less effective gastric wrap and can result in an incompetent cardia.

A second row of sutures is placed 1.5–2.0 cm above the first row, using the position of the previously placed first row of sutures as a guide (Fig 9–24). Once again the sutures in the second row are tied carefully to achieve tissue apposition without strangulation. The tails of these sutures are not cut, but are separately rethreaded on a large thin Ferguson needle and passed 0.5 cm apart from each other through the diaphragm from the abdominal to the thoracic surface, 1.0–1.5 cm from the edge of the hiatus. The diaphragmatic sutures are placed at the 4, 8, and 12 o'clock positions on a clock face, oriented with the 6 o'clock position on the posterior margin of the hiatus between the right and left crus just anterior to the aorta (Fig 9–25). It is important to place the right lateral,

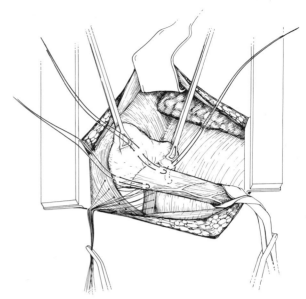

Fig 9–23.—Construction of a Belsey 240° gastric fundic wrap showing placement of the first row of sutures 1.5 cm above the gastroesophageal junction. Particular attention must be given to placement of the right lateral suture.

or 4 o'clock suture, correctly to avoid the common error of putting this stitch too far anteriorly, in the 1 or 2 o'clock position, and ending with an anterolateral fundoplication displaced to the left. These sutures must be carefully placed to avoid injury to the abdominal structures. Belsey has popularized the spoon retractor to aid in their placement. I use the Army-Navy right-angle retractor with the long right-angle limb placed through the hiatus. The needle is guided along

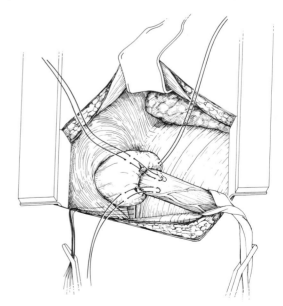

Fig 9–24.—Continued construction of the Belsey 240° gastric fundic wrap showing placement of the second row of sutures 1.5–2.0 cm above the previously tied sutures of the first row.

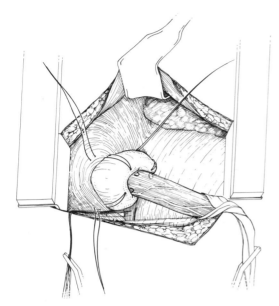

Fig 9–25.—Continued construction of the Belsey 240° gastric fundic wrap showing placement of the tails of the previously tied second row of sutures through the diaphragm, 0.5 cm apart and 1.0–1.5 cm from the edge of the hiatus. Note the placement of the sutures at the 4, 8, and 12 o'clock positions on an imaginary clock face oriented with the 6 o'clock position posterior in the hiatus between the right and left crura just anterior to the aorta.

the inner surface of the retractor limb before passing it through the diaphragm.

The reconstructed cardia is passed through the hiatus and placed in the abdomen. It is not dragged down into the abdomen by pulling on the diaphragmatic sutures, but rather placed into the abdomen by compressing the fundic ball with the hand and manually maneuvering it through the hiatus as described for the transthoracic Nissen procedure. Once in the

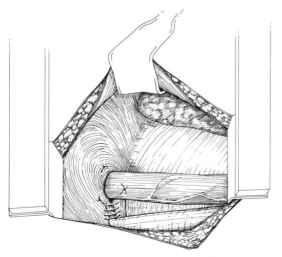

Fig 9–26.—The completed Belsey 240° gastric fundic wrap showing the right and left crura approximated by tying the previously placed sutures. The position of the tied holding sutures is also shown.

abdomen, the cardia should remain there without tension on the holding sutures. As with the transthoracic Nissen repair, a gentle up-and-down motion on the diaphragm should not allow the repair to emerge back through the esophageal hiatus. If it does, the tension on the repair is too great, and the problem is managed as described previously for the transthoracic Nissen procedure. If the repair remains in the abdomen unaided, the previously placed crural sutures are tied. The holding sutures are then tied, approximating the knot against the previously tied knot so as to avoid any redundancy in the suture between the repair and the diaphragm (Fig 9–26). An additional safety factor of the double-knot technique is that if one of the tails of the holding sutures breaks while it is being tied, it is not necessary to take the repair down, pull the stomach back up into the chest, and insert a new suture. Simple anchoring of the single remaining tail to the diaphragm is sufficient to hold the cardia in position. This technique also prevents tying the sutures too tight and causing necrosis of the incorporated tissue.

POSTOPERATIVE MANAGEMENT

After either the abdominal or thoracic repair, the patient is kept on nasogastric suction for approximately five days to prevent distention of the stomach during the healing period. Gastric distention prior to complete healing can cause a breakdown of the repair. A barium swallow is obtained on the seventh postoperative day to demonstrate the unobstructed passage of barium into the stomach prior to starting a solid oral diet. Initially, a slight dysphagia may be experienced by the patient, but this will disappear as the traumatic edema resolves. Dysphagia may occasionally persist for a longer period due to an intramural hematoma at the site of the fundoplication. If present, the hematoma will usually be absorbed within four to six weeks, and the dysphagia will subside. One of the immediate benefits of an antireflux procedure is that from the time the patient recovers from anesthesia, he notes and enjoys relief from heartburn and regurgitation. Before discharge, the patient should be counseled that until the habit of air swallowing is broken, he may experience increased flatus and gastric distention due to trapping of the air in the stomach.

Our patients are readmitted one year after the operation for a critical symptomatic evaluation, upper GI contrast study, esophageal manometry, and 24-hour esophageal pH monitoring. These studies ensure us that we have accomplished the goals of: (1) correcting the patient's symptoms without contributing to dysphagia; (2) establishing a mechanically competent cardia by increasing the distal esophageal sphincter pressure without interfering with its ability to relax, increasing the overall length of the sphincter if inadequate preoperatively, and increasing the length of the sphincter exposure to the positive pressure environment of the abdomen; and (3) the cessation of gastroesophageal reflux documented by 24-hour esophageal pH monitoring.

REFERENCES

1. Palmer E.D.: Hiatus hernia in the adult: Clinical manifestations. *Am. J. Dig. Dis.* 3:45–58, 1958.
2. DeMeester T.R., O'Sullivan G.C., Bermudez G., et al.: Esoph-

ageal function in patients with angina type chest pain and normal coronary angiograms. *Ann Surg.* 196:488–498, 1982.

3. Pellegrini C.A., DeMeester T.R., Johnson L.F., et al.: Gastroesophageal reflux and pulmonary aspiration: Incidence, functional abnormality, and results of surgical therapy. *Surgery* 86:110–119, 1979.

4. Johnson L.F., DeMeester T.R.: Twenty-four hour pH monitoring of the distal esophagus: A quantitative measure of gastroesophageal reflux. *Am. J. Gastroenterol.* 62:325–332, 1974.

5. DeMeester T.R., Johnson L.F., Guy J.J., et al.: Patterns of gastroesophageal reflux in health and disease. *Ann. Surg.* 184:459–470, 1976.

6. Johnson L.F., Lin T.C., Hong S.K.: Gastroesophageal dynamics during immersion in water to the neck. *J. Appl. Physiol.* 38:449–454, 1975.

7. Banchero N., Schwartz P.E., Wood E.H.: Intraesophageal pressure gradient in man. *J. Appl. Physiol.* 22:1066–1074, 1967.

8. Dent J., Dodds W.J., Friedman R.H., et al.: Mechanism of gastroesophageal reflux in recumbent asymptomatic human subjects. *J. Clin. Invest.* 65:256–267, 1980.

9. Leon C.S.C., Flanagan J.B. Jr., Moorrees C.F.A.: The frequency of deglutition in man. *Arch. Oral. Biol.* 10:83–96, 1965.

10. Orr W.C., Robinson M.G., Johnson L.F.: Acid clearing during sleep in patients with esophagitis and controls. *Dig. Dis. Sci.* 26:423–427, 1981.

11. Babka J.C., Hagar G.W., Castell D.O.: The effect of body position on lower esophageal sphincter pressure. *Am. J. Dig. Dis.* 18:441–442, 1973.

12. DeMeester T.R., Wang C.I., Wernly J.A., et al.: Technique, indications and clinical use of 24-hour esophageal pH monitoring. *J. Thorac. Cardiovasc. Surg.* 79:656–667, 1980.

13. Haddad J.K.: Relation of gastroesophageal reflux to yield sphincter pressures. *Gastroenterology* 58:175–184, 1970.

14. Mann C.V., Hardcastle J.D.: The effect of vagotomy of the human gastroesophageal sphincter. *Gut* 9:688–695, 1968.

15. Castell D.O.: The lower esophageal sphincter: Physiologic and clinical aspects. *Ann. Intern. Med.* 83:390–401, 1975.

16. DeMeester T.R.: What is the role of intraoperative manometry? *Ann. Thorac. Surg.* 30:1–4, 1980.

17. Biancani P., Zabinsky M.P., Behar J.: Pressure, tension, and force of closure of the human lower esophageal sphincter and esophagus. *J. Clin. Invest.* 56:476–483, 1975.

18. Thurer R.L., DeMeester T.R., Johnson L.F.: The distal esophageal sphincter and its relationship to gastroesophageal reflux. *J. Surg. Res.* 16:418–423, 1974.

19. DeMeester T.R., Johnson L.F.: The evaluation of objective measurements of gastroesophageal reflux and their contribution to patient management. *Surg. Clin. North Am.* 56:39–53, 1976.

20. Skinner D.B., Camp T.R. Jr.: Relation of esophageal reflux to lower esophageal sphincter pressures decreased by atropine. *Gastroenterology* 54:543–551, 1968.

21. DeMeester T.R., Wernly J.A., Bryant G.H., et al.: Clinical and in vitro analysis of gastroesophageal competence: A study of the principles of antireflux surgery. *Am. J. Surg.* 137:39–46, 1979.

22. Bombeck C.T., Dillard D.H., Nyhus L.M.: Muscular anatomy of the gastroesophageal junction and role of phreno-esophageal ligament: Autopsy study of sphincter mechanism. *Ann. Surg.* 164:643–654, 1966.

23. DeMeester T.R., Lafontaine E., Joelsson B.E., et al.: The relationship of a hiatal hernia to the function of the body of the esophagus and the gastroesophageal junction. *J. Thorac. Cardiovasc. Surg.* 82:547–558, 1981.

24. Pellegrini C.A., DeMeester T.R., Skinner D.B.: Response of the distal esophageal sphincter to respiratory and positional maneuvers in humans. *Surg. Forum* 27:380–382, 1976.

25. Wernly J.A., DeMeester T.R., Bryant G.H., et al.: Intra-abdominal pressure and manometric data of the distal esophageal sphincter. *Arch. Surg.* 115:534–539, 1980.

26. O'Sullivan G.C., DeMeester T.R., Joelsson B.E., et al.: The interaction of the lower esophageal sphincter pressure and length of sphincter in the abdomen as determinants of gastroesophageal competence. *Am. J. Surg.* 143:40–47, 1982.

27. Joelsson B.E., DeMeester T.R., Skinner D.B., et al.: The role

of the esophageal body in the antireflux mechanism. *Surgery* 92:417–424, 1982.

28. DeMeester T.R.: Experimental and clinical evidence for mechanical factors in the competency of the cardia, in Van Heukelem H.A., Gooszen H.G., Terpstra J.B., et al. (eds.): *Pathological Gastroesophageal Reflux.* Amsterdam, Zuid Nederlandse Uitgevers Maatschappij BV, 1982, pp. 17–34.

29. Malagelada J.R.: Physiologic basis and clinical significance of gastric emptying disorders. *Dig. Dis. Sci.* 24:657–661, 1979.

30. Ahtaridis G., Snape W.J., Cohen S.: Lower esophageal sphincter pressure as an index of gastroesophageal acid reflux. *Dig. Dis. Sci.* 26:993–998, 1981.

31. Boesby S.: Relationship between gastroesophageal acid reflux, basal gastroesophageal sphincter pressure and gastric acid secretion. *Scand. J. Gastroenterol.* 12:547–551, 1977.

32. McCallum R.W., Berkowitz D.M., Lerner E.: Gastric emptying in patients with gastroesophageal reflux. *Gastroenterology* 80:285–291, 1981.

33. Little A.G., DeMeester T.R., Kirchner P.T., et al.: Pathogenesis of esophagitis in patients with gastroesophageal reflux. *Surgery* 88:101–107, 1980.

34. Kaye M.D., Showalter J.P.: Pyloric incompetence in patients with symptomatic gastroesophageal reflux. *J. Lab. Clin. Med.* 83:198–206, 1974.

35. Dodds W.J., Dent J., Hogan W.J., et al.: Mechanisms of gastroesophageal reflux in patients with reflux esophagitis. *N. Engl. J. Med.* 307:1547–1552, 1982.

36. Dent J.: A new technique for continuous sphincter pressure measurements. *Gastroenterology* 71:263–267, 1976.

37. Helm J.F., Riedel D.R., Dodds W.J., et al.: Determinants of esophageal acid clearance in normal subjects. *Gastroenterology* 85:607–612, 1983.

38. Helm J.F., Dodds W.J., Hogan W.J., et al.: Acid neutralizing capacity of human saliva. *Gastroenterology* 83:69–74, 1982.

39. Johnson L.F., DeMeester T.R.: Evaluation of elevation of the head of the bed, Bethanechol, and antacid foam tablets on gastroesophageal reflux. *Dig. Dis. Sci.* 26:673–680, 1981.

40. Madsen T., Wallin L., Boesby S., et al.: Oesophageal peristalsis in normal subjects: Influence of pH and volume during imitated gastroesophageal reflux. *Scand. J. Gastroenterol.* 18:13–18, 1983.

41. Siegel C.I., Hendrix T.R.: Esophageal motor abnormalities induced by acid perfusion in patients with heartburn. *J. Clin. Invest.* 42:686–695, 1963.

42. Helm J.F., Dodds W.J., Pelc L.R., et al.: Effect of esophageal emptying and saliva on clearance of acid from the esophagus. *N. Engl. J. Med.* 310:284–288, 1984.

43. Edwards D.A.W.: Radiological examination and quantitation of reflux in the hiatal hernia—reflux syndrome, in Van Heukelem H.A., Gooszen H.G., Terpstra J.B., et al. (eds.): *Pathological Gastroesophageal Reflux.* Amsterdam, Zuid Nederlandse Uitgevers Maatschappij BV, 1982, pp. 47–53.

44. Maddock W.G., Bell J.L., Tremaine M.J.: Gastrointestinal gas. *Ann Surg.* 130:512–521, 1949.

45. Ismail-Beigi F., Pope C.E.: Distribution of histological changes of gastroesophageal reflux in the distal esophagus of man. *Gastroenterology* 66:1109–1113, 1975.

46. Johnson L.F., DeMeester T.R., Haggitt R.C.: Esophageal epithelial response to gastroesophageal reflux: A quantitative study. *Am. J. Dig. Dis.* 23:498–509, 1978.

47. Quincke H.: Ulcus oesophagi ex digestione. *Deutsch. Arch. Klin. Med.* 24:72–78, 1879.

48. Hamperl H.: Peptic esophagitis (Peptische oesophagitis). *Verh. Dtsch. Ges. Pathol.* 27:208, 1934.

49. Palmer E.D.: Subacute erosive ("peptic") esophagitis associated with achlorhydria. *N. Engl. J. Med.* 262:927–929, 1960.

50. Helsingen N.: Oesophagitis following total gastrectomy. *Acta Chir. Scand.* [Suppl.] 273:5–21, 1961.

51. Gillison E.W., de Castro V.A.M., Nyhus L.M., et al.: The significance of bile in reflux esophagitis. *Surg. Gynecol. Obstet.* 134:419–424, 1972.

52. Rovati V., Bastagli A., Foschi D.: Duodenoesophageal reflux in sliding hiatus hernia. *Chir. Gastroenterol.* 9(2):183–187, 1975.

53. Donovan I.A., Harding L.K., Keighley M.R.B., et. al.: Abnormalities of gastric emptying and pyloric reflux in uncomplicated hiatus hernia. *Br. J. Surg.* 64:847–848, 1977.

54. Stol D.W., Murphy G.M., Collis J.L.: Duodeno-gastric reflux and acid secretion in patients with symptomatic hiatal hernia. *Scand. J. Gastroenterol.* 9:97–101, 1974.

55. Crumplin M.K.H., Stol D.W., Murphy G.M., et al.: The pattern of bile salt reflux and acid secretion in sliding hiatal hernia. *Br. J. Surg.* 61:611–616, 1974.

56. Clemencon G.: Nocturnal intragastric pH measurements. *Scand. J. Gastroenterol.* 7:293–298, 1972.

57. Pellegrini C.A., DeMeester T.R., Wernly J.A., et al.: Alkaline gastroesophageal reflux. *Am. J. Surg.* 135:117–184, 1978.

58. Gillison E.W., Nyhus L.M.: Bile reflux, gastric secretion and heartburn (abstract). *Br. J. Surg.* 58:864, 1971.

59. Bateson M.C., Hopwood D., Milne G., et al.: Oesophageal epithelial ultrastructure after incubation with gastro-intestinal fluids and their components. *J. Pathol.* 133:33–58, 1981.

60. Heizer W.D., Cleveland C.R., Iber F.L.: Gastric inactivation of pancreatic supplements. *Johns Hopkins Med. J.* 116:261–270, 1965.

61. Northrop J.H., Kunitz M., Herriott R.M.: *Crystalline Enzymes,* ed. 2. New York, Columbia University Press, 1948.

62. Wenger J., Trowbridge C.G.: Bile and trypsin in the stomach following a test meal. *South Med. J.* 64:1063–1064, 1971.

63. Kivilaakso E., Fromm D., Silen W.: Effect of bile salts and related compounds on isolated esophageal mucosa. *Surgery* 87:280–285, 1980.

64. Kranendonk S.E.: Reflux oesophagitis: An experimental study in rats. Thesis, Rotterdam, Erasmus University, 1980.

65. Jones C.: *Digestive Tract Pain.* New York, Macmillan, 1938.

66. Tuttle S.G., Rufin F., Bettarello A.: The physiology of heartburn. *Ann. Intern. Med.* 55:292–300, 1961.

67. Atkinson M., Bennett J.R.: Relationship between motor changes and pain during esophageal acid perfusion. *Am. J. Dig. Dis.* 13:346–350, 1968.

68. Allison P.R.: Peptic ulcer of the esophagus. *J. Thorac. Surg.* 15:308–317, 1946.

69. Richter J.E., Castell D.O.: Gastroesophageal reflux: Pathogenesis, diagnosis and therapy. *Ann. Intern. Med.* 97:93–103, 1982.

70. Allison P.R.: Reflux esophagitis, sliding hiatus hernia and the anatomy of repair. *Surg. Gynecol. Obstet.* 92:419–431, 1951.

71. Boerema I.: Gastropexia anterior geniculata for sliding hiatus hernia and cardiospasm. *J. Int. Coll. Surg.* 29:533–541, 1958.

72. Nissen R.: Gastropexy as the lone procedure in the surgical repair of hiatus hernia. *Am. J. Surg.* 92:389–392, 1956.

73. Ziperman H.H., Mathewson C. Jr., Starck R.G., et al.: Hiatal hernia repair by interperitoneal gastric fixation. *Surg. Gynecol. Obstet.* 116:608–612, 1963.

74. Hill L.D., Tobias J.A.: An effective operation for hiatal hernia: An eight year appraisal. *Ann. Surg.* 166:681–692, 1967.

75. Skinner D.B., Belsey R.H.R.: Surgical management of esophageal reflux with hiatus hernia: Long-term results with 1,030 cases. *J. Thorac. Cardiovasc. Surg.* 53:33–54, 1967.

76. Nissen R.: Gastropexy and 'fundoplication' in surgical treatment of hiatus hernia. *Am. J. Dig. Dis.* 6:954–961, 1961.

77. Bombeck C.T.: The choice of operations for gastro-oesophageal reflux, in Watson A., Celestin L.R. (ed.): *Disorders of the Oesophagus.* London, Pitman Publishing, 1984, pp. 112–128.

78. Donahue P.E., Bombeck C.T.: The modified Nissen fundoplication—reflux prevention without gas bloat. *Chir. Gastroenterol. (Surg. Gastroenterol.)* 11:15–21, 1977.

79. Behar J., Biancani P., Spiro H., et al.: Effect of an anterior fundoplication on lower esophageal sphincter competence. *Gastroenterology* 67:209–215, 1974.

80. Baue A.E., Belsey R.H.R.: The treatment of sliding hiatus hernia and reflux esophagitis by the Mark IV technique. *Surgery* 62:396–406, 1967.

81. Negre J.B.: Hiatus hernia: Post-fundoplication symptoms: Do they restrict the success of Nissen fundoplication? *Ann. Surg.* 198:698–700, 1983.

82. Angelchik J.P., Cohen R.: A new surgical procedure for the treatment of gastroesophageal reflux and hiatal hernia. *Surg. Gynecol. Obstet.* 148:246–248, 1979.

83. Starling J.R., Reichelderfer M.D., Pellett J.R., et al.: Treatment of symptomatic gastroesophageal reflux using the Angelchik prosthesis. *Ann. Surg.* 195:686–691, 1982.

84. Kozarek R.A., Phelps J.E., Grobe J.L., et al.: Assessment of a prosthetic device for the correction of esophagel reflux. *Gastroenterology* 82:1106, 1982.

85. Angelchik J.P., Cohen R., Kravetz R.E.: A ten year appraisal of the antireflux prosthesis. *Am. J. Gastroenterol.* 78:671, 1983.

86. Gear M.W.L., Gillison E.W., Dowling B.L.: Randomized prospective trial of the Angelchik antireflux prosthesis. *Br. J. Surg.* 71:681–683, 1984.

87. Behar J., Sheahan G.G., Biancani P.: Medical and surgical management of reflux esophagitis. *N. Engl. J. Med.* 293(6):263–268, 1975.

88. DeMeester T.R.: Management of benign esophageal strictures, in Stipa S., Belsey R.H.R., Moraldi A. (eds.): *Medical and Surgical Problems of the Esophagus.* New York, Academic Press, 1981, Serona Symposia 43:173–176.

89. Iascone C., DeMeester T.R., Little A.G., et al.: Barrett's esophagus: Functional assessment, proposed pathogenesis and surgical therapy. *Arch. Surg.* 118(5):543–549, 1983.

90. Skinner D.B., Walther B.C., Ridell R.I., et al.: Barrett's esophagus: Comparison of benign and malignant cases. *Ann. Surg.* 198:554, 1983.

91. DeMeester T.R., Iascone C., Courtney J.V., et al.: Prospective evaluation of patients with chronic respiratory symptoms for the presence of occult esophageal disease. *J. Thorac. Cardiovasc. Surg.,* in press.

92. Benjamin S.B., Richter J.E., Cardova C.M., et al.: Prospective manometric evaluation with pharmacologic provocation of patients with suspected esophageal motility dysfunction. *Gastroenterology* 84:393–401, 1983.

93. Walther B.S., Courtney J.V., DeMeester T.R., et al.: The effect of paraesophageal hernia on sphincter function and its implication on surgical therapy. *J. Surg.* 147:111–116, 1984.

94. Orringer M.B., Dabich L., Zarafonetis C.J.D., et al.: Gastroesophageal reflux in esophageal scleroderma: Diagnosis and implications. *Ann. Thorac. Surg.* 22:120, 1976.

95. O'Sullivan G.C., DeMeester T.R., Smith R.B.., et al.: Twenty-four hour pH monitoring of esophageal function: Its use in evaluation in symptomatic patients after truncal vagotomy and gastric resection or drainage. *Arch. Surg.* 116:581–590, 1981.

96. Tolin R.D., Malmud L.S., Stelzer F., et al.: Enterogastric reflux in normal subjects and patients with Billroth II gastroenterostomy: Measurement of enterogastric reflux. *Gastroenterology* 77:1027–1033, 1979.

97. Little A.G., DeMeester T.R., Skinner D.B.: Combined gastric and esophageal 24-hour pH monitoring in patients with gastroesophageal reflux. *Surg. Forum* 30:351–353, 1979.

98. Little A.G., Martinez E.L., DeMeester T.R., et al.: Duodenogastric reflux and reflux esophagitis. *Surgery* 96(2):447–454, 1984.

99. Lind J.F., Duthie H.L., Schlegal, J.F., et al.: Motility of the gastric fundus. *Am. J. Physiol.* 201:197–202, 1961.

100. Richardson J.D., Larson G.M., Polk H.C.: Intrathoracic fundoplication for shortened esophagus: Treacherous solution to a challenging problem. *Am. J. Surg.* 143:29–35, 1982.

101. DeMeester T.R., Johnson L.F., Kent A.H.: Evaluation of current operations for the prevention of gastroesophageal reflux. *Ann. Surg.* 180:511–525, 1974.

102. Wald H., Polk H.C.: Anatomical variations in hiatal and upper gastric areas and their relationship to difficulties experienced in operations for reflux esophagitis. *Ann. Surg.* 197:389–392, 1983.

10

Surgical Treatment of Esophageal Neoplasms

DAVID B. SKINNER, M.D.

ESOPHAGEAL CARCINOMA shares with pancreatic carcinoma the reputation of being the least curable of neoplasms. In most reports, fewer than 5% of patients who present with symptomatic esophageal cancer are living five years later.[1] Yet the discovery of an occasional early case of esophageal carcinoma and the success of screening techniques in identifying presymptomatic patients with this disease demonstrate that esophageal neoplasms can be cured by surgery when detected at an early stage.[2] Determining the stage of the disease is the single most important consideration in the planning and choice of treatment and in evaluating the outcome of therapy for esophageal cancer.

Dysphagia is the common presenting symptom of esophageal cancer, but obstruction to swallowing does not occur until approximately 90% of the circumference of the esophagus is invaded.[3] Like bladder muscle, the esophagus can dilate rapidly without causing sensation, so that a small segment of normal smooth muscle permits a bolus to pass without the sensation of obstruction. When a patient develops dysphagia caused by an esophageal cancer, the tumor is already large and almost always extends more than 2 cm along the esophageal axis.[4, 5] In the TNM classification used for other organs such as breast or lung cancer, tumors of this size are at least T2 lesions and frequently are accompanied by positive lymph nodes (N2) or extension beyond the original organ (T3).

The likely advanced state of the symptomatic esophageal cancer, coupled with the inaccessible location of the esophagus in the central mediastinum adjacent to vital structures, explains why surgical resection employing the standard esophagectomy technique accomplishes removal of the visible and palpable tumor in only about one half of cases,[6, 7] and also explains the poor long-term survival rates of 10%–15% usually reported among such patients undergoing resection.[8, 9] In selecting treatment, it is important to identify the half or more of symptomatic patients who cannot benefit from surgical removal of the tumor and to strive for new therapy approaches that can improve the results for those in whom the disease is still localized although symptomatic.

The poor results of surgical treatment of esophageal cancer as practiced over the past 45 years led some to question about whether the disease should always be treated as if incurable, with the objective of therapy focused upon relief of symptoms.[10] Standing against this view are the reports of high long-term cure rates from surgical resection of tumors that do not extend through the esophageal muscle and to lymph nodes. Based on cytologic detection of presymptomatic esophageal cancer in high risk areas, Huang and his Chinese colleagues[2] reported three-year survival of 89% and five-year survival of 86% among 237 stage 1 (T1 N0 M0) operative survivors. A low operative mortality of 2.5% was achieved. Among 13 such stage 1 cases without esophageal wall penetration or lymph node metastases referred for en bloc resection, ten are long-term survivors in our series, results equivalent to the Chinese experience.[11] Such results show that esophageal carcinoma is no more lethal than other types of neoplasms if detected and treated early. Accordingly, most of the effort to improve survival should be focused upon early case detection. The variability in results achievable from treatment depends so heavily upon the stage of the disease that detailed staging information must be provided whenever results of treatment are compared or new treatments advocated.

Except in such well-known locations as portions of China, the Caspian littoral, and regions in South Africa and southwestern France, where the incidence of esophageal carcinoma is extraordinarily high, efforts at mass population screening for early cancer detection are not likely to be cost effective. Of the means available for early esophageal cancer detection, cytologic screening appears to have advantages of both accuracy and lower cost when compared to endoscopy or radiology. In North America and other low-incidence areas, certain groups of patients are known to have a higher than normal risk of esophageal carcinoma in whom periodic cytologic screening for early case detection appears warranted. Such people include those with achalasia,[12, 13] caustic strictures,[14, 15] Barrett's columnar lined esophagus,[16–19] the Plummer Vinson syndrome,[20] and alcoholics who are heavy smokers.[21, 22] Whether patients with long-standing symptomatic gastroesophageal reflux but without transformation to Barrett's esophagus should be considered in the high-risk group remains more controversial.[23]

Several techniques for esophageal cytology preparation are described.[24, 25] We prefer a simple method in which a standard gastroscopy brush with 6-mm bristles is passed through

159

a standard nasogastric tube with the end split.[11, 26] The tube is advanced to approximately 35 cm from the nostril or incisors. The brush is advanced out of the end of the tube and passed up and down several times, rotating the bristles. The tube is withdrawn 5 cm and the brushing is repeated, and then a third set of brushings is performed after withdrawal of the tube for another 5 cm. The bristles are left exposed as the apparatus is withdrawn back through the cricopharyngeus. The material accumulated is promptly smeared and quick-fixed on two glass microscope slides. Using the same techniques as in the Papanicolaou screening methods for uterine cervical carcinoma, the slides are subjected to cytologic screening, which can be done by computerized techniques to reduce cost and cytopathologist's time. Results are comparable to those achieved by brushing under direct vision in patients with known esophageal carcinoma, and a definite diagnosis of carcinoma is achieved in more than 85% of cases with known carcinoma. This method yielded the anticipated results when applied in a field trial in the Caspian littoral region of Iran just prior to the Iranian revolution. Three asymptomatic cases of esophageal cancer were detected and verified by later biopsy among 1,800 people undergoing screening in a district where the case incidence was known to be in excess of 1/1,000 adults per year. The more widespread use of cytology for early case detection offers the best promise that this dread disease can be discovered early, when surgical resection can be successful, and the survival from this type of cancer can be improved.

TREATMENT CHOICES FOR SYMPTOMATIC PATIENTS WITH LOCALIZED ESOPHAGEAL CANCER

When a symptomatic patient with esophageal carcinoma is identified, initial evaluations include preoperative staging techniques to determine whether the disease is likely to be localized to the region of the esophagus or to spread more widely. Possible palliative treatments for patients with more widespread disease are discussed later. For those with localized disease, the primary treatment considerations are radiation therapy vs. surgical resection. Neither alone gives satisfactory results to the symptomatic patient for the reasons mentioned above, so more extended or combined forms of treatment are under evaluation. As primary treatment, radiation therapy is usually reported to yield five-year survival rates in the range of 2%–10% in favorable cases;[27–29] only one report claims 20% survival at five years among selected patients.[30] This result was not duplicated by the original reporter or others in more than a decade since first claimed. Similarly, except for the rare series in which more than 20% five-year survival is reported in selected cases subjected to surgery,[31] the usual reports for survival at five years after standard or palliative esophagectomy is in the range of 10%–15%. While conventional surgery appears to have a slight advantage over radiation therapy, the mortality resulting from either treatment must also be considered. Reports of surgical mortality vary from 2% to 30%, with an average of approximately 10%, depending to some degree on the definition of mortality employed in each series. Although radiation therapy is sometimes considered less hazardous during the immediate

time of treatment, deaths do occur from hemorrhage, perforation, and sepsis during radiation therapy. Among patients referred from our clinic for radiation therapy, approximately 10% died during treatment or could not complete the prescribed therapy.[32] Such results from conventional radiation or surgical treatment have encouraged efforts to alter therapy in hopes of achieving better results.

Preoperative irradiation to obtain the benefits of both types of treatment has long attracted interest. For many years, Nakayama's group advocated brief intense preoperative irradiation employing 2,000 rad over four consecutive days, followed on the next day by surgical resection. They estimated a 10% improvement in five-year survival compared to results achieved in patients not receiving irradiation therapy. This experience has been difficult to assess, since the selection of patients for preoperative irradiation, the precise staging of the disease, and the total group of patients from whom the group chosen for irradiation have never been clearly stated. A recent report from the authors ascribed no significant benefit to preoperative irradiation.[6] In the Western world, efforts at preoperative irradiation have not resulted in improved results. A standard approach has been the use of 3,000–5,000 rad in three to five weeks, followed by surgical resection at approximately a one-month interval. Parker and associates[34] found no significant improvement in long-term survival in their large experience. Other smaller series have confirmed lack of benefit from preoperative irradiation therapy.[35–38] Currently such combined treatment is not usually recommended for patients judged suitable for primary surgical treatment. For palliation of dysphagia from unresectable carcinoma, radiation therapy still has a major role, and the value of irradiation postoperatively for patients in whom the tumor has extended to the region adjacent to but not beyond the esophagus remains under active evaluation.

Another more recent approach to combined therapy has been based on the observation that bleomycin and cis-platinum chemotherapy can reduce dramatically the size of squamous cell carcinoma of the esophagus in some cases. At present there are several experimental protocols under evaluation employing combined-drug preoperative chemotherapy, with or without preoperative irradiation therapy, followed by surgical resection in favorable cases. Similar combined-drug therapy programs are under evaluation for esophageal adenocarcinoma using programs similar to those employed for gastric cancer chemotherapy.[39–41] Dramatic reduction in the volume of tumor has been achieved in some patients, and detectable residual carcinoma has not been found in some patients undergoing subsequent surgical resection. Whether these methods will result in improved long-term cure rates remains uncertain. It is not yet clear whether use of these strong chemotherapeutic agents will cause increased surgical mortality and morbidity. Assessment of long-term results may be difficult because of alteration in the pathologic staging caused by the preoperative therapy. Careful and extensive preoperative staging followed by a randomized trial of preoperative chemotherapy compared to extensive surgical resection will be necessary to evaluate the long-term value of combined preoperative therapy protocols. As with irradiation therapy, it appears that chemotherapy does have a role to play in patients with systemic spread of esophageal carcinoma who are fit to withstand a palliative chemotherapy program. Whether postoperative chemotherapy used as a prophylactic is worthwhile is currently under investigation in patients with unfavorable pathologic staging after surgical resection.

Modest improvement in surgical results may be anticipated by employing the concept of en bloc resection for carcinoma of the esophagus. The standard esophagectomy technique attributed to Adams and Phemister,[42] Garlock,[43] and others, and evaluated thoroughly by Sweet,[3] Belsey and Hiebert,[10] Ellis et al.,[31, 44] and others is comparable to treating cancer in other organs by simple extirpation of the organ and sampling of adjacent lymph nodes. Removal of the cancer-bearing organ in continuity with its vascular and lymphatic connections is now standard practice for treating cancers in other portions of the alimentary tract and elsewhere, with modest improvement in five-year survival, in the range of 10% or more, following en bloc resection compared to a more localized procedure. For treating esophageal carcinoma, en bloc resections were not initially developed because the esophagus did not appear to have a definite mesentery and boundary, and because of the difficulty in working on the esophagus in close proximity to other vital organs. However, the esophagus distal to the aortic arch does have a mesoesophagus during embryonic life, which determines the direction of its vascular and lymphatic drainage.[45] This dorsal mesentery of the esophagus can be resected en bloc and includes removal of the azygos vein and thoracic duct drainage system, as well as dividing the bronchoesophageal arteries at the aortic wall. The esophagus also has a serosal-like relationship to adjacent organs, as the esophageal longitudinal muscle fibers arise in part from subpleural and subpericardial fibrous tissue.[46] By resecting all of these structures in continuity with the esophagus, the en bloc concept is applicable to treating esophageal cancer (Fig 10–1). The two vital structures which determine whether total clearance of the tumor from the mediastinum can be achieved are the airways and the aorta.

A technique for en bloc resection for the distal third of the esophagus and cardia was described by Logan in 1963.[47] The 16% five-year survival obtained was the best result reported to that time. However, an operative mortality of 21% dis-

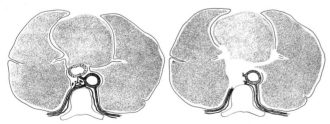

Fig 10–1.—Schematic for the concept of en bloc resection of the esophagus and posterior mediastinum. After removal of the esophagus surrounded by pericardium anteriorly, pleura laterally, and mesoesophageal tissues including azygos vein and thoracic duct and esophageal arteries posteriorly, the entire posterior mediastinum can be removed, leaving only the aorta, vertebral body, lungs, and myocardium as the margins of the resection. (From Skinner D.B.: En bloc resection for neoplasms of the esophagus and cardia. *J. Thorac. Cardiovasc. Surg.* 85:59–70, 1983. Used by permission.)

couraged widespread adoption of this approach. After developing the technical approach for an en bloc resection for middle third as well as lower third neoplasms, I have used the radical resection approach for carcinoma of the thoracic esophagus in each consecutive favorable case referred since 1969. The concept was extended to carcinoma of the cervical esophagus in 1974 by adding bilateral limited radical neck dissections to achieve clearance of the blood supply and lateral lymphatic drainage of the cervical esophagus. Favorable cases were defined as those in which the tumor identifiable preoperatively and at surgery could be completely encompassed within an envelope of normal tissue. In the following discussion of surgical therapy, this en bloc approach to extirpation of the esophagus and adjacent tissue is described in detail. The widely practiced standard operation for removing the esophagus and obvious adjacent lymph nodes is now referred to as a standard or palliative esophagectomy. The selection of the overall type of treatment and type of surgical resection planned depends heavily on correct staging. Much of this is accomplished during preoperative preparation of the patient for surgery.

PREOPERATIVE ASSESSMENT AND PREPARATION

In any patient presenting with the symptom of dysphagia or in whom a structural abnormality of the esophagus is seen on barium swallow, the diagnosis of carcinoma should be expected until ruled out by establishing a definite alternative diagnosis. This requires obtaining a tissue diagnosis from the strictured area, which should be done preoperatively and before the planned investigations are performed. Repeated endoscopy may be required. The use of a rigid, open tube esophagoscope allows dilatation and larger biopsies of the region of a stricture than possible with a flexible endoscope. On rare occasions, a tissue diagnosis cannot be obtained preoperatively, and a patient is evaluated and treated with the assumption that a carcinoma is present. This setting occurs when a stricture is difficult to dilate, the radiographic appearance suggests possible neoplasm, and no definitive tissue diagnosis for benign or malignant causes of stricture is obtained. In such instances, the preoperative assessment and operation are carried out with the assumption that carcinoma will be found in the resected specimen. Esophagectomy performed as for esophageal cancer is undertaken unless the operative findings establish an alternative diagnosis.

In addition to establishing the diagnosis of esophageal carcinoma, three further objectives are met in the preoperative assessment, including staging for the extent of the tumor, assessment of the patient's overall condition and ability to withstand major surgery, and assessment of the patient's nutritional status. Preoperative staging includes the evaluation of any symptom or abnormal physical finding which might indicate a metastasis. When the patient's history and physical examination do not point toward possible metastatic disease, the preoperative search employs a CAT scan, including the neck, chest, and upper abdomen to detect possible enlarged lymph nodes, the size and extent of the primary tumor and its possible invasion of adjacent organs, and evidence of liver or adrenal metastases. Since the esophagus normally lies contiguous to the trachea and aorta, direct contact of the tumor mass with these organs does not establish inoperability, as normal esophageal tissue may intervene. However, when the tumor shadow encompasses more than 90° of the circumference of the aorta or distorts the tracheal lumen in an irregular fashion, these findings strongly suggest direct invasion and inoperability (Fig 10–2). Enlarged lymph nodes measuring more than 1 cm are highly likely to contain metastatic tumor. The CAT finding alone of enlarged nodes does not preclude resection for cure, but directs the operative biopsies to the sites of the enlarged lymph nodes early in the procedure. The CAT scan appears at least as sensitive as a liver-spleen scan for the detection of squamous carcinoma metastatic to liver, but the density of adenocarcinoma in the liver may be sufficiently close to the density of liver tissue, so that the CAT scan can be difficult to interpret. For adenocarcinoma of the distal esophagus, a standard liver-spleen scan is obtained.

Two other scans are obtained routinely. The bone scan is used to detect unsuspected osseous metastases, which are common in esophageal carcinoma. When the bone scan is positive, bone radiographs are obtained. A positive bone scan followed by a normal bone radiograph showing no cause for the abnormal bone scan is highly suspicious of a metastatic lesion. In such instances, the bone scan is used to place a marking solution injected to guide biopsy of the abnormal area, since the bone itself may not appear remarkable at bone biopsy yet contain microscopic zones of carcinoma. The most common cause of false positive bone scans results from arthritic changes which are usually confirmed by bone radiographs and do not require biopsy. The third scan that has proved useful in patients with squamous cell carcinoma is the gallium scan, which frequently demonstrates the primary tumor and may point to regional or systemic spread not demonstrated by other techniques (Fig 10–3).

In patients harboring carcinomas of the upper or midesophagus, bronchoscopy is obtained routinely to detect direct invasion of the membranous portion of the airway. When bronchial or tracheal distortion is seen, brushings and biopsies are taken to detect microscopic evidence of an invasion as opposed to compression, which would not preclude resection.

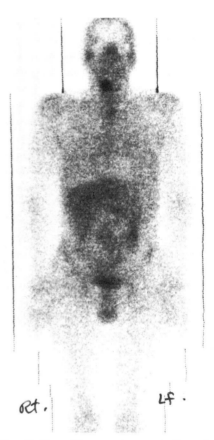

Fig 10–3.—Gallium 67 scan demonstrating slight uptake in a primary esophageal carcinoma in the upper mediastinum and a large uptake in a previously undetected retropharyngeal mass.

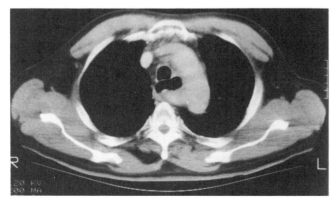

Fig 10–2.—Chest CAT scan demonstrating partial engulfment of the aorta by a large esophageal cancer. When more than one quarter of the aortic circumference is lost in the tumor shadow, the cancer is regarded as unresectable.

Palpable lymph nodes in the neck or elsewhere are biopsied. Based upon the detailed history and physical examination, CAT scan, bone, gallium, and possibly liver-spleen radioisotope scans and bronchoscopy or lymph node biopsy when indicated, a thorough preoperative assessment of the extent of the tumor is obtained.

Patients presenting with esophageal cancer are frequently elderly or suffering from other diseases, so an assessment of the patient's overall health and ability to withstand major surgery is an important part of the evaluation. Cardiovascular or respiratory diseases present special hazards. When chest pain is a symptom, the patient should undergo a full cardiological evaluation, which may necessitate stress testing and even coronary angiography to determine the presence and extent of coronary disease prior to a decision about therapy for the esophageal cancer. A normal resting ECG is not sufficient evidence of the absence of coronary disease when chest pain is a symptom. When coronary artery disease is detected, the overall prognosis of the esophageal cancer must be assessed in deciding whether coronary artery bypass grafting is indicated. This would be undertaken only in very early stage 1 cases of esophageal carcinoma. When the cancer is more advanced, surgical resection may still be carried out in the presence of known coronary artery disease, but with the understanding of a significantly increased risk of operative mortality. In patients having angina on mild exertion, a better decision is to treat the esophageal carcinoma for palliation of symptoms by radiation therapy.

Aspiration from the obstructed esophagus occurs frequently in patients with esophageal carcinoma, so careful evaluation of pulmonary function and intensive preoperative pulmonary physical therapy is important. In patients having a total vital capacity of less than 2 L, or less than 50% of the vital capacity exhaled during a forced expiratory volume in one second test, the risks for life-threatening complications following esophagectomy are usually too high to warrant surgery. Alternative means of palliation should be considered. On the other hand, patients with recent aspiration may improve significantly with pulmonary physical therapy, postural drainage, and antibiotics, so the pulmonary function assessment may be repeated later in the evaluation. The risk of esophageal carcinoma is increased in patients with heavy alcohol intake, so liver function should be carefully evaluated in such patients. The presence of portal hypertension greatly increases the risk of attempted esophagectomy and is generally a contraindication to surgery.

Age alone is not a contraindication to operation, nor is weight loss, if the other assessments of overall condition are favorable. Weight loss is a common complaint in patients admitted for evaluation of esophageal neoplasms. When weight loss is noted, nutritional therapy is started promptly and is an important part of the preoperative preparation. In patients who can swallow liquids, several cans of liquid diet supplement are added to the daily menu. If the patient is unable to swallow large amounts of liquid, or is unwilling to do so because of poor appetite, the insertion of a feeding tube beyond the obstruction may allow administration of high-caloric liquids containing appropriate mixtures of vitamins. When the esophageal obstruction is too tight, parenteral hyperalimentation is carried out through a central venous line. In addition to weight loss, measurements of nutritional status include serum albumin and serum iron-binding capacity, triceps muscle and skin thickness, and response to several skin test antigens. When two or more of these assessments for nutritional status are abnormal, nutritional supplemental therapy is started and carried out for at least 10–14 days before the patient's status is reevaluated. Since the preoperative staging and assessments of the patient's medical condition consume the better part of a week, such time spent for nutritional preparation does not lengthen the preoperative interval unduly.

In anticipation of esophageal replacement, a barium enema is obtained to be certain whether polyps or diverticulosis would make the colon a poor choice for reconstruction. Similarly, an upper GI radiograph is done to determine the suitability of the stomach as an esophageal replacement. Duodenal or gastric ulcers make this undesirable. Prior colon or stomach operations probably preclude use of that organ. Just before operation, a three-day mechanical and 12-hour antibiotic bowel preparation are performed. Systemic antibiotics are given prophylactically on call to the operating room, during the operation, and postoperatively until the risk of wound contamination is reduced—usually two to three days or until the majority of the multiple tubes and lines are removed.

EN BLOC ESOPHAGECTOMY FOR POSSIBLE CURE

When preoperative staging shows no evidence of systemic spread of the esophageal cancer, when there is no evidence of invasion of adjacent structures or enlarged lymph nodes away from the primary tumor, when the patient's overall medical condition is favorable, and when nutritional status is adequate, conditions are favorable to attempt surgical cure of an esophageal neoplasm. Under these circumstances, the preferred technique is an en bloc resection of the esophagus in continuity with its surrounding tissues for a distance 10 cm above and below the extent of the palpable growth whenever possible.[37] This procedure is performed for squamous carcinomas arising at any level in the esophagus and for adenocarcinoma arising from Barrett's epithelium or from the distal tubular esophagus, which is normally lined with columnar epithelium.

Correlation of pathologic findings in resected specimens with survival shows that extension through the muscular wall of the esophagus or spread to four or more lymph nodes is a bad prognostic sign.[11] When positive lymph nodes are encountered at the margins of the planned en bloc resection; i.e., 10 cm beyond the tumor in either direction, or when the tumor is fixed to an adjacent structure demonstrating full-thickness penetration, these operative findings predict that cure cannot be achieved by radical surgical resection. The operation is converted to a palliative or standard esophagectomy with removal of as much tumor and adjacent lymph nodes as possible, and still securing adequate margins (5–10 cm) above and below the tumor to avoid recurrent dysphagia from suture lined implantation of the cancer.

Distal Esophageal Tumors

When the proximal edge of the tumor is at least 10 cm caudal to the aortic arch as measured at esophagoscopy, the en bloc resection is performed through a left thoracotomy. This allows optimal exposure of the region of the hiatus, retroperitoneum, and proximal stomach, as well as affording exposure for the 10-cm resection of the lower posterior mediastinum. The incision is made through the sixth intercostal interspace, dividing a segment of the seventh rib posteriorly. The diaphragm is detached at its periphery from behind the sternum to the edge of the spleen. By reattaching the diaphragm at the end of the procedure, herniation through the diaphragm or phrenic nerve paralysis is avoided. The initial dissection is begun 10 cm proximal to the tumor under the arch of the aorta to determine whether positive lymph nodes at this location signal incurability (Fig 10–4). Frozen section biopsies are obtained. Next, the celiac axis region of the upper abdomen is explored and the liver carefully palpated for evidence that would make the tumor incurable. If these findings are favorable and the tumor is movable from adjacent fixed tissues, the en bloc resection is carried out.

The omentum is mobilized from the transverse colon, taking care to preserve the right gastroepiploic vessels at their origin. The splenic flexure of the colon is mobilized and retracted caudally. The omentum and spleen are freed from the retroperitoneum in the left upper quadrant, and the splenic artery and vein are ligated and divided to enter the lesser sac.

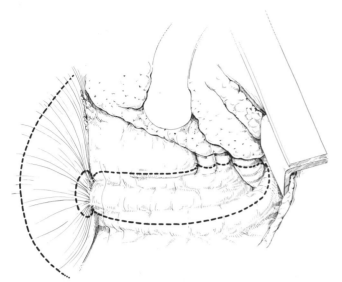

Fig 10–4.—Outline of the mediastinal incisions made through a left thoracotomy for en bloc resection of the mediastinum below the aortic arch. The abdomen is entered through a circumferential peripheral incision in the diaphragm. (From Skinner D.B.: En bloc resection for neoplasms of the esophagus and cardia. *J. Thorac. Cardiovasc. Surg.* 85:59–70, 1983. Used by permission.)

Dissection is carried along the cephalic margin of the pancreas toward the celiac axis. The left gastric artery is ligated and divided at its origin, and the coronary vein is similarly divided. The mobilized retrogastric tissues are dissected upward into the hiatus. Using electrocautery dissection, a cuff of diaphragm muscle is left attached to the cardia in the hiatus (Fig 10–5).

Through this enlarged hiatal opening, the most distal thoracic aorta and prevertebral tissues adjacent to the aortic hiatus are exposed. The thoracic duct is doubly ligated and divided through this exposure in the hiatus. The ascending lumbar veins which unite to form the azygos vein are ligated and divided in the same field.

The en bloc resection is completed on the thoracic side of the diaphragm (Fig 10–6). Pleura overlying the anterior aorta is incised, and communicating lymphatic and venous branches crossing over the aorta are divided. The dissection on the aorta is carried medially. The esophageal and bronchoesophageal vessels are divided flush with the aorta. The medial aortic dissection is carried dorsally to the vertebral body. The right intercostal arteries are ligated and divided on the vertebral bodies along with their adjacent left intercostal veins coursing to join the azygos vein. Beginning caudally, the plane on the vertebral body is developed so that the thoracic duct system and azygos vein with ligated intercostal vessels are elevated off the vertebral bodies. This dissection is carried out with ligation of all tributary lymphatic channels as well as vessels up to the previously determined 10-cm margin above the tumor. During this dissection, the esophagus remains imbedded under the left pleura laterally and with its venous and lymphatic mesentery dorsally. The posterior dissection is completed by dividing the right intercostal arteries and veins

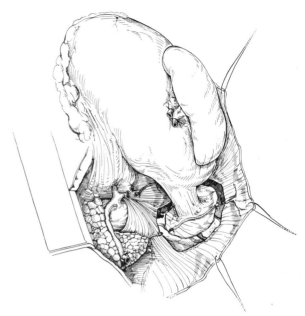

Fig 10–5.—Abdominal mobilization for en bloc resection of the distal esophagus. After division of the left gastric artery and splenic artery and vein with retroperitoneal node dissection, the stomach is elevated and the lower mediastinum is entered by incising a cuff of diaphragm around the tumor bearing esophagus. The thoracic duct and azygos vein origins are exposed through the hiatus. These structures are ligated and divided. (From Skinner D.B.: En bloc resection for neoplasms of the esophagus and cardia. *J. Thorac. Cardiovasc. Surg.* 85:59–70, 1983. Used by permission.)

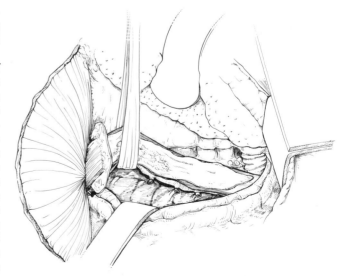

Fig 10–6.—After completion of the abdominal mobilization the en bloc resection continues medial to the aortic arch on the vertebral body. The mesoesophagus is elevated with the esophagus.

as they pass off the vertebral body into the right hemithorax, and incising the right pleura at its reflection off the vertebral body.

Anteriorly the pericardium is opened on the inferior pulmonary vein. The pericardial incision is carried cephalad to the top of the pericardial sac, and the subcarinal lymph nodes are removed with the specimen at this level. The pericardial incision is carried caudally down to the diaphragm, where it connects with the previously incised muscle of the hiatus. The right side of the pericardium is incised on the right pulmonary veins. This incision enters the right pleural cavity anterior to the right pulmonary ligament. The superior dissection of the pericardium and subcarinal lymph nodes is completed. Incision down the right side of the posterior pericardium is carried along its reflection with the right pleura. When this is completed, the right pulmonary ligament is visible, and the bronchial collateral vessels in this ligament are divided flush with the right lung to complete the entire mobilization of the subaortic posterior mediastinum.

If the tumor is a squamous cell carinoma, the remaining intrathoracic esophagus above the level of the 10 cm en bloc resection is mobilized by dissection on the wall of the esophagus under the aortic arch and upward to the level of the clavicles. By incising the pleura cephalad to the aortic arch, the lower cervical esophagus can be reached, divided, and closed temporarily with interlocking mattress sutures. A blunt dissection is carried out into the neck circumferentially around the esophagus to facilitate later mobilization of the cervical esophagus for the final anastomosis. When the cell type is an adenocarcinoma, and 10-cm margins above the tumor are obtained caudal to the aortic arch, the esophagus can be transected at this level and the anastomosis performed just below the aortic arch.

The gastric transection line is determined by measuring 10 cm from the palpable tumor along the lesser curvature and a similar distance along the greater curvature. Connecting these two points determines the transection line when the stomach is to be preserved. The resection always includes the lesser curvature lymph nodes and left gastric pedicle as well as the spleen and short gastric vessels on the greater curvature. The omentum is removed with the specimen, leaving the right gastroepiploic vessels intact along with the right gastric artery as the blood supply for the residual stomach. If the cancer is an adenocarcinoma, consideration is given to adding a total gastrectomy to the resection. Reports of Akiama and associates[48] and Castrini and Pappalardo[49] suggest that a higher survival rate is achieved when total gastrectomy is added to radical resection for adenocarcinoma at the cardia. The decision to proceed with total gastrectomy and reconstruction depends in part on the patient's condition at this stage of the operation, and also upon the availability of an adequate segment of properly prepared intestine to perform the reconstruction.

When the situation appears favorable for possible cure of the tumor after the complete en bloc resection, the patient's condition at this point is satisfactory, and the colon is suitable and prepared for interposition, reconstruction of the esophagus by an isoperistaltic colon interposition is preferred (Fig 10–7). The interposition is based on the ascending branch of

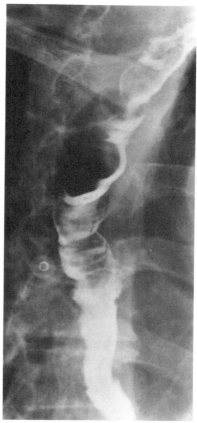

Fig 10–7.—X-ray demonstrating long segment of isoperistaltic colon anastomosed to the residual esophagus in the neck.

the left colic artery as initially described by Belsey.[50] Preference for reconstruction by colon interposition compared to esophagogastrostomy is based upon long-term follow-up of surviving patients. Approximately one third of long-term survivors after reconstruction with stomach have subsequent difficulty with esophagitis, even progressing to tight stricture of bleeding. Such long-term complications are not encountered following replacement of the esophagus with an isoperistaltic intestinal segment. However, if the patient's condition is precarious at this time in the operation, or if the colon is unsuitable for reconstruction, completion of the operation by advancement of the stomach for anastomosis to the esophagus, at either its subaortic or cervical transection point, is the most rapid and satisfactory way to complete the operation. When the anastomosis is done to the upper esophagus, the connection is carried out through a separate cervical incision after completion of the abdominal and thoracic portions of the operation. Our preference for an anastomotic technique is a 5–0 monofilament wire running anastomosis performed end-to-end between the colon and esophagus or side-to-end between the gastric pouch and esophagus (Fig 10–8). Leakage rate from this anastomosis is under 5%, and the incidence of stricture is less than 2%.[51] These results compare favorably with other anastomotic techniques, including the end-to-end stapling device.

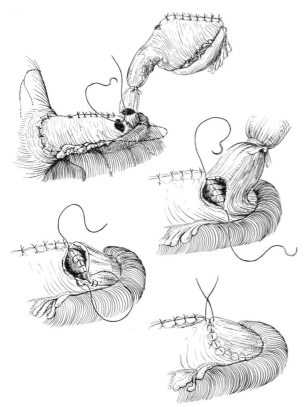

Fig 10–8.—Preferred technique for an esophagogastric anastomosis just below the aortic arch. 5-0 monofilament stainless steel wire is used. (From Nora P.F.: *Operative Surgery and Principles and Techniques,* ed. 2. Philadelphia, Lea & Febiger, 1980. Used by permission.)

Middle Third Tumors

For neoplasms arising in the middle or lower esophagus less than 10 cm distal to the aortic pulsation determined endoscopically, the operative approach for en bloc resection is through a right thoracotomy. When the tumor is 10 cm or more cephalad to the hiatus, and the patient has not had previous abdominal surgery and is not unduly obese, the entire dissection can be performed through a right thoracotomy, as described by Belsey and Hiebert,[10] with the stomach advanced through the hiatus for an esophagogastric anastomosis. When the tumor is closer to the hiatus, or abdominal conditions are unfavorable for transhiatal mobilization of the stomach, or reconstruction by colon is desired, a simultaneous midline incision is made. Two teams can work simultaneously in the thorax and abdomen to speed the dissection of the mediastinum and upper abdomen.

Initially the upper- and lower-most extents of the dissection are inspected to determine evidence of positive lymph nodes, which would preclude attempted curative resection. Similarly, the mobility of the tumor from the trachea and aorta is determined early, before the commitment is made to perform a curative resection. When conditions are favorable, the en bloc resection of the posterior mediastinum is carried out to include the esophagus 10 cm proximal and distal to the tumor enveloped in its normal surrounding tissues.

The dissection is started posteriorly on the vertebral body, ligating and dividing the right intercostal vessels to mobilize the azygos vein and thoracic duct off the vertebral bodies. This dissection is carried the full 20 cm length of the planned radical resection. By proceeding across the vertebral bodies, the aorta is exposed from the arch to the diaphragm. The intercostal vessels are again divided on the left side of the vertebral bodies, and the esophageal bronchial vessels are divided flush with the aortic wall. The dissection is carried off the aorta anteriorly to enter the left pleural cavity from the arch of the aorta down to the diaphragm. The left recurrent nerve is identified and spared unless it is close to the tumor.

Anteriorly the pleura is incised along the edge of the trachea at the superior margin of the planned resection. The plane between the membranous portion of trachea and esophagus is cleared to the level of the carina. The azygos arch is encountered, divided, and oversewn. Subcarinal lymph nodes are mobilized and bronchial arteries divided. The pericardium is entered at the right pulmonary vein, and the pericardial incision is carried down to the diaphgram at the reflection of the pleura and pericardium onto the esophagus. By reaching across through the pericardium, the left pericardial incision is made on the left pulmonary veins and a similar incision made down to the diaphragm in the left pleural cavity. The left pulmonary ligament is now divided to complete the resection of the posterior mediastinum (Fig 10–9).

For tumors less than 10 cm from the hiatus, the left gastric pedicle and retroperitoneal tissues into the hiatus are divided through the abdominal incision. A point for transection of the stomach is identified at least 10 cm from the lower edge of the tumor. For tumors of the midesophagus, there is no need to perform a major gastric resection, once the adequate 10 cm margins are achieved and left gastric lymph nodes removed. The splenectomy is optional depending upon location of the

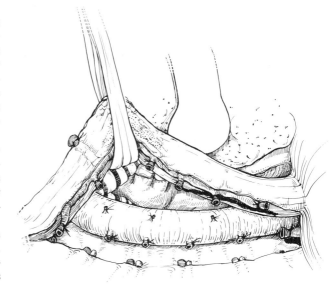

Fig 10–9.—Mobilization of the entire esophagus for en bloc resection of a middle third carcinoma. (From Skinner D.B.: En bloc resection for neoplasms of the esophagus and cardia. *J. Thorac. Cardiovasc. Surg.* 85:59–70, 1983. Used by permission.)

tumor and the possibility of operative injury to the spleen.

Based upon the visible and palpable findings of the tumor and possible enlarged lymph nodes, a decision is made as to whether the reconstruction should be done by mobilizing and advancing the entire stomach to the neck, or by preparing and advancing an isoperistaltic segment of transverse and left colon based upon the left colic artery. This decision is influenced by the condition of the colon and its preoperative preparation, by evidence of ulcer disease which might interfere with the gastric advancement, and by the patient's condition at the time, recognizing that a gastric advancement entails less surgery at this point of the operation than would a colon interposition. Whichever organ is selected is advanced through the esophagus hiatus and up the posterior mediastinum for attachment to the temporarily closed stump of the esophagus at the root of the neck. The organ used for reconstruction is attached around the margins of the hiatus to prevent herniation of other abdominal organs into the thorax. The chest and abdominal wounds are closed, and the final anastomosis is done through a separate cervical incision (Fig 10–10).

For carcinoma arising in the cervical esophagus or cricopharyngeal region, the operation is performed through a long collar incision, elevating skin flaps to expose the entire neck. Most carcinomas at this level involve the cricopharyngeal sphincter, so laryngectomy is frequently required as part of the procedure. Modified bilateral radical neck resections are performed with the laryngectomy and mobilization of the cervical esophagus. These dissections spare the internal jugular vein. Depending upon location of the tumor, one lobe of the thyroid gland with attached parathyroids can usually be preserved. If not, and if total thyroidectomy is necessary, the parathyroids are dissected free from the specimen in the operating room and reimplanted to avoid permanent hypocalcemia.

While the neck dissection is proceeding, a second team enters the abdomen through a midline incision, divides and closes the cardia, and prepares the stomach or colon segment for advancement to the neck. When the cervical dissection is completed, an esophagectomy without thoracotomy is performed by working upward on the wall of the esophagus through the hiatus and downward on the thoracic esophagus through the neck dissection. Since the lymphatic drainage of the cervical esophagus goes laterally into the tissues removed by the modified neck dissections, no efforts are made to include mediastinal lymph node dissection. The purpose of the esophagectomy is to remove potential tumor-bearing squamous epithelium, which would be inaccessible for future follow-up investigation. The mobilized stomach or colon is passed through the posterior mediastinum to the neck, where anastomosis is made to the hypopharynx. The end tracheostomy is brought out in the sternal notch, and the incisions are closed after anchoring the esophageal replacement organ to the margins of the hiatus.

Standard or Palliative Esophagectomy

This operation might be selected as dictated by the experience and judgment of the surgeon or as a purely palliative procedure when preoperative staging shows extension of the tumor beyond the region encompassed by an en bloc resection. When such extension of tumor is found before surgery, the indications for palliative resection depend upon the degree of symptomatic dysphagia experienced by the patient. The operation will not cure the cancer, so its only purpose is to relieve symptoms. A standard palliative esophagectomy may also be performed when operative findings at the time of an attempted curative resection show that the tumor cannot be cured because of invasion of adjacent structures or spread to remote lymph nodes. Although more limited in the amount of tissue removed surrounding the esophagus, the standard palliative esophagectomy should still strive for 10-cm margins above and below the tumor to eliminate the problem of a suture line recurrence and subsequent dysphagia. Recurrence of dysphagia completely defeats the purpose of palliative resection to relieve this symptom.

The operative approach can be either through the left or right thoracotomy incision, depending upon the location of the tumor. Palliative resection for carcinoma of the cardia can be performed with an upper abdominal incision, with dissection carried up into the mediastinum under direct vision by excising a margin of the hiatus around the tumor and dissecting as high in the mediastinum as possible under direct vision. A large retractor under the xiphoid and diaphragm and anchored to the table frame facilitates this exposure. In thin patients, as much as 10 cm of lower mediastinum can be exposed through the hiatus. This approach may be used for attempted curative resections of carcinomas arising in the proximal stomach or at the exact gastroesophageal junction. It is not recommended for attempted curative removal of tumors within the lower thoracic esophagus.

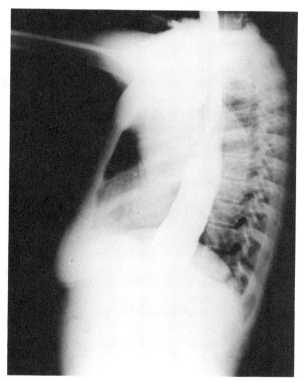

Fig 10–10.—Lateral radiograph of a barium swallow demonstrating anastomosis of the whole stomach to the pharynx in the neck.

The palliative resection removes the esophagus and any enlarged adjacent lymph nodes. The pericardium and opposite pleura are not opened intentionally, and no effort is made to remove the thoracic duct lymphatic system or azygos vein system. Much of the dissection is carried out on the muscular wall of the esophagus itself. Reconstruction is usually performed by an esophagogastric anastomosis, since the long-term outlook for the patient is not sufficiently good to warrant the additional operative maneuvers necessary to perform reconstruction by an intestinal interposition.

RESULTS

The results achieved by the en bloc resection have been analyzed in 100 consecutive patients undergoing such a radical resection between 1969 and 1983 in a personal series. These resections represented the treatment selected in approximately 40% of patients referred for treatment of esophageal cancer. An additional 33 patients underwent a palliative resection, and approximately 45% were found to have advanced incurable disease at the time of the referral or were considered unfit for resection by the patient's own choice or by the patient's medical condition. The 30-day hospital mortality for the 100 patients treated by en bloc resection has been 10%, with 4 deaths resulting from cardiovascular complications, 4 from technical complications, and 2 from respiratory disease. Nonfatal complications occurred in approximately half of the surviving patients and were frequently respiratory or cardiovascular. Two persistent lymphatic fistulas occurred, and prolonged chest tube drainage was required in approximately 10%. As determined by actuarial analysis, the three-year survival rate was 26%. Two patients died of myocardial infarction in the fourth year after radical surgery, and the five-year actuarial survival rate was 16%. Among 55 patients treated more than five years ago, the actual number surviving was 8, or 15%. The actual survival rate at four years was 19%, 24% after three years, and 32% after two years. No patient has developed recurrent disease after surviving more than three years following operation. Regional recurrence of the tumor causing dysphagia has occurred in fewer than 5%, indicating that the en bloc resection is highly effective in controlling regional disease.

Among 33 patients undergoing palliative resection, the 30-day hospital mortality has been a similar 9%. Actual survival after two years has been 7%. Among the 93 patients treated more than two years ago for palliation other than by resection, only three have lived as long as two years. Two are five-year survivors after radiotherapy.

Further evaluation of the en bloc resection depends upon correlation between detailed pathologic staging and patient survival. The prognosis is influenced independently by invasion of the tumor through the esophageal muscle wall or by the presence of lymph node metastases. When both of these negative factors have been absent, ten of 13 such patients who have survived operation lived long-term free of disease (three years or more). Among ten patients with one to five lymph nodes positive but no muscle wall penetration, six survived two years or more without evidence of disease. Among nine operative survivors with full-thickness muscle wall penetration, but without lymph node metastases, five survived two years or more free of disease. In contrast, fewer than 10% of patients with both full-thickness muscle penetration and lymph node metastases have lived as long as two years following surgery. The argument for the en bloc resection is best made by greater than 50% survival for two years or more of patients with one of the grave prognostic factors, indicating spread beyond the esophagus but still localized in the mediastinum. Those stage 1 patients with neither wall penetration nor lymph node metastases might be cured by a standard esophagectomy, but it seems unlikely that patients with early regional spread of the disease through the wall of the esophagus or into lymph nodes would be cured by a standard resection carried out on the muscle layers on the esophagus without systematic lymph node removal. Although some of these patients may develop later recurrences, a two-year or greater time free of disease is worthwile to the patient and indicates that the more extensive resection is effective in controlling regional as well as localized disease. Since the en bloc resection can be accomplished with a mortality no greater in our experience than that of a palliative resection, and no greater than the average operative mortality reported worldwide for standard esophagectomy, the advantages of the procedure in providing increased survival time for a modest number of patients and perhaps cure for a few urge the adoption of this approach.

OTHER PALLIATIVE PROCEDURES

For approximately one half of the patients presenting with symptomatic esophageal cancer, the disease is already too advanced to consider curative treatment. The role of the physician is to relieve symptoms in these patients for whom life cannot be greatly prolonged. When dysphagia is severe, and the tumor-bearing esophagus can be successfully removed, a palliative resection as described above offers the most direct, quickest, and longest-lasting means of relieving the dysphagia. However, when technical considerations such as invasion of the trachea or aorta, or the presence of widespread metastases, or medical factors contraindicate resectional therapy, other choices include radiation therapy, chemotherapy, surgical bypass procedures, and endoluminal intubation.

When dysphagia is not severe, so that the need for relief of esophageal obstruction is not urgent, radiation therapy appears to be the palliative procedure of choice for squamous cell carcinoma, and multidrug chemotherapy is selected as the first palliative maneuver for adenocarcinoma. Further discussion of the role of radiation therapy and chemotherapy has been presented previously in this chapter.

Surgical bypass operations and endoluminal intubation do not prolong the patient's life but can relieve dysphagia. A surgical bypass operation is a major procedure to carry out in a patient whose life expectancy is limited to months. Currently we reserve bypass operations for patients without systemic metastases but in whom local invasion of the tumor into the trachea or aorta precludes esophageal resection. In such patients regional radiation therapy may prolong life but raises the risk of mediastinal abscess or tracheoesophageal fistula as a complication. In such patients a substernal bypass using an isoperistaltic colon segment or the entire stomach as a bypass conduit anastomosed to the cervical esophagus can be performed prior to radiation therapy. When the colon is suitable for the interposition, we prefer this to advancing the entire stomach, since the stomach can retain its digestive function distal to the colon interposition, and the problem of draining the esophagus divided at its upper and lower end is avoided when the esophagus can be left in continuity with the stomach.

Endoluminal intubation is reserved for those patients whose life expectancy is short because of systemic metastases, but in whom near-total esophageal obstruction or tracheo-esophageal fistula makes persistent night and day cough and expectoration inevitable and, in turn, makes life unbearable. The intubation can be performed with any of several commercially available tubes. These are routinely passed over a bougie inserted through the rigid esophagoscope so that operative insertion of the tube is rarely indicated or necessary. The tubes allow ingestion of a liquid diet, but solid foods will usually not pass and should be avoided to eliminate the need for mechanical cleansing of the tube.

Occasionally a patient will be encountered with regional disease which can be treated by radiation therapy but in whom medical conditions contraindicate a bypass procedure to improve dietary intake. In such patients an extracorporeal, large-diameter esophageal tube which connects the cervical esophagus to a permanent gastrostomy can be effective.[52] In patients with regional but inoperable disease, the use of a bypass or extracorporeal tube coupled with radiation therapy to the primary tumor has achieved survival greater than 18 months in several instances, with worthwhile palliation.

SUMMARY

Current therapy for carcinoma of the esophagus does not offer high prospects of cure for many symptomatic patients. Future emphasis must be placed upon earlier case detection by cytologic screening techniques if better long-term survival rates are to be obtained. For those patients whose disease is discovered at an early stage, surgical resection offers the best chance for cure. An en bloc resection of the involved esophagus within an envelope of normal surrounding tissue is described and practiced. When extent of disease precludes curative resection, a standard or palliative esophagectomy offers the most certain, quickest, and longest-lasting relief from dysphagia. Surgical bypass, luminal intubation, radiation therapy, and chemotherapy each have a well-defined role in palliation. Future improvement in extending life for symptomatic patients may be achieved by combined forms of therapy such as those now under evaluation.

REFERENCES

1. Earlam R., Cunha-Melo J.R.: Oesophageal squamous cell carcinoma: I. A critical review of surgery. *Br. J. Surg.* 67:381, 1980.
2. Huang K.C., et al.: Diagnosis and surgical treatment of early esophageal carcinoma, in Stipa S., Belsey R.H.R., Moraldi A. (eds.): *Medical and Surgical Problems of the Esophagus.* New York, Academic Press, 1981, vol. 43, Serona Symposia, pp. 296–299.
3. Sweet R.H.: Results of radical surgical extirpation in treatment of carcinoma of the esophagus and cardia: With 5 year survival statistics. *Surg. Gynecol. Obstet.* 94:46, 1952.
4. Marshak R.H.: The roentgen findings of benign and malignant tumors of the esophagus. *J. Mt. Sinai Hosp.* 23:75, 1956.
5. Nabeya K.: Early carcinoma of the esophagus. *Stomach Intest.* (Tokyo) 5:1205, 1970.
6. Endo M., Kinoshita Y., Yamada A., et al.: Surgical treatment of thoracic esophageal cancer, including clinical evaluation of early esophageal cancer, in Pfeiffer C.J. (ed.): *Cancer of the Esophagus.* Boca Raton, Fla., CRC Press, 1982, vol. 2, pp. 57–70.
7. Gunlangsson G.H., Wychulas A.R., Roland C., et al.: Analysis of the records of 1657 patients with carcinoma of the esophagus and cardia and stomach. *Surg. Gynecol. Obstet.* 130:997, 1970.
8. Appelqvist P.: Carcinoma of the esophagus and gastric cardia: A retrospective study based on statistical and clinical material from Finland. *Acta Chir. Scand. [Suppl.]* 430, 1972.
9. Leon W., Strug L.H., Brickman I.D.: Carcinoma of the esophagus: A disaster. *Ann. Thorac. Surg.* 11:583, 1971.
10. Belsey R., Hiebert C.A.: An exclusive right thoracic approach for cancer of the middle third of the esophagus. *Ann. Thorac. Surg.* 18:1–15, 1974.
11. Skinner D.B., Dowlatshahi K.D., DeMeester T.R.: Potentially curable cancer of the esophagus. *Cancer* 50:2571–2575, 1982.
12. Just-viera J.O., Haight C.: Achalasia and carcinoma of the esophagus. *Surg. Gynecol. Obstet.* 128:1081, 1969.
13. Silber W.: Achalasia. *Lancet* 2:1287, 1965.
14. Alvarez A.F., Colbert J.G.: Lye stricture of the esophagus complicated by carcinoma. *Can. J. Surg.* 6:470, 1963.
15. Lansing P.B., Ferrante W.A., Ochsner J.L.: Carcinoma of the esophagus at the site of lye stricture. *Am. J. Surg.* 118:108, 1969.
16. Berenson M.M., Riddell R.H., Skinner D.B., et al.: Malignant transformation of esophageal columnar epithelium. *Cancer* 41:544–561, 1978.
17. Borrie J., Goldwater L.: Columnar cell-lined esophagus: Assessment of etiology and treatment. *J. Thorac. Cardiovasc. Surg.* 71:825–834, 1976.
18. Naef A.P., Savary M., Ozzell L.: Columnar-lined lower esophagus: An acquired lesion with malignant predisposition. *J. Thorac. Cardiovasc. Surg.* 70:826–835, 1975.
19. Radigan L.R., Glover J.L., Shipley F.E., et al.: Barrett's esophagus. *Arch. Surg.* 112:486–491, 1977.
20. Ahlbom H.E.: Simple achlorhydric anemia: Plummer-Vinson syndrome, and carcinoma of the mouth, pharynx, and oesophagus in women; observations in Radiumhemmet Stockholm. *Br. Med. J.* 2:331, 1936.
21. Wynder E.L., Bross I.J.: A study of etiological factors in cancer of the esophagus. *Cancer* 14:389, 1961.
22. Wynder E.L., Mabuchi K.: Etiological and environmental factors. *J.A.M.A.* 226:1546, 1973.
23. Adler R.H., Rodriguez J.: The association of hiatus hernia and gastroesophageal malignancy. *J. Thorac. Surg.* 37:553–569, 1959.
24. Li F.P., Shiang E.L.: Screening of oesophageal cancer in 62,000 Chinese. *Lancet* 2:804, 1979.
25. Berry A.V., Basking A.F., Hamilton D.G.: Cytologic screening for esophageal cancer. *Acta Cytol. (Baltimore)* 25(2):135–141, 1981.
26. Dowlatshahi K., Daneshbod A., Mobarhan S.: Early detection of cancer of the oesophagus along the Caspian Littoral. *Lancet* 1:125, 1978.
27. Earlam R., Cunha-Melo J.R.: Oesophageal squamous cell carcinoma: II. A critical review of radiotherapy. *Br. J. Surg.* 67:457, 1980.
28. VanHoutte P.: Radiotherapy of esophagus cancer: A review of 136 cases treated at the Institut Bordet. *Acta Gastroenterol. Belg.* 40:121, 1977.
29. Wara W.M., Mauch P.M., Thomas A.N., et al.: Palliation for carcinoma of the esophagus. *Radiology* 121:717, 1976.
30. Pearson J.G.: The present status and future potential of radiotherapy in the management of esophageal cancer. *Cancer* 39:882, 1977.
31. Ellis F.H. Jr., Gibb S.P., Watkins E. Jr.: Esophagogastrectomy: A safe, widely applicable, and expeditious form of palliation for patients with carcinoma of the esophagus and cardia. *Ann. Surg.* October 1983.
32. Skinner D.B.: Esophageal malignancies: Experience with 110 cases. *Surg. Clin. North Am.* 56:137–147, 1976.
33. Nakayama K., Kinoshita Y.: Surgical treatment combined with

preoperative concentrated irradiation. *J.A.M.A.* 227:175, 1974.

34. Parker E.F., Gregorie H.B.: Carcinoma of the esophagus—long-term results. *J.A.M.A.* 235:1018, 1976.

35. Anabtawi I.N., Brackney E.L., Ellison R.G.: Carcinoma of the esophagus treatment by a combination of radiation and surgery. *J. Thorac. Cardiovasc. Surg.* 48:205, 1964.

36. Goodner J.T.: Surgical and radiation treatment of cancer of thoracic esophagus. *A.J.R.* 105:523, 1969.

37. Skinner D.B.: En bloc resection for neoplasms of the esophagus and cardia. *J. Thorac. Cardiovasc. Surg.* 85:59–69, 1983.

38. Walker J.H.: Carcinoma of the esophagus: Cobalt 60 teletherapy experience and comparison with surgical results. *A.J.R.* 92:67, 1964.

39. Kelson D.P., Cvitkovic E., Bains M., et al.: Cyst-dichlorodiamine-platinum (11) and bleomycin in the treatment of esophageal carcinoma. *Cancer Treat. Rep.* 62:1041, 1978.

40. McDonald J.S., Schein P.S., Woolley P.V., et al.: 5-Fluorouracil, doxorubicin, mitomycin-C (FAM) combination chemotherapy for advanced gastric cancer. *Ann. Intern. Med.* 93:533–536, 1980.

41. Steiger Z., Franklin R., Wilson R.F., et al.: Complete eradication of squamous cell carcinoma of the esophagus with combined chemotherapy and radiotherapy. *Am. J. Surg.* 47:95, 1981.

42. Adams W.E., Phemister D.B.: Carcinoma of the lower thoracic esophagus: Report of a successful resection and esophagogastrostomy. *J. Thorac. Surg.* 7:621–632, 1938.

43. Garlock J.H.: The surgical treatment of carcinoma of the thoracic esophagus with the report of three successful cases. *Surg. Gynecol. Obstet.* 66:534, 1938.

44. Ellis F.H. Jr.: Treatment of carcinoma of the esophagus and cardia. *Mayo Clin. Proc.* 35:653, 1960.

45. Arey L.B.: *Development Anatomy: A Textbook and Laboratory Manual of Embryology*, ed. 6. Philadelphia, W.B. Saunders Co., 1954.

46. Laimer E.: Beitrag zur Anatomie des Oesophagus. *Med. Jahrbucher Jahrg. Wien.* 1883, pp. 333–338.

47. Logan A.: The surgical treatment of carcinoma of the esophagus and cardia. *J. Thorac. Cardiovasc. Surg.* 46:150–161, 1963.

48. Akiyama A.H. Personal communication, 1984.

49. Castrini G., Pappalardo G: Carcinoma of the cardia: Tactical problem. *J. Thorac. Cardiovasc. Surg.* August 82(2):190–193, 1981.

50. Belsey R.: Reconstruction of esophagus with left colon. *J. Thorac. Cardiovasc. Surg.* 49:33–55, 1965.

51. Skinner D.B.: Esophageal reconstruction. *Am. J. Surg.* 139:810–814, 1980.

52. Skinner D.B., DeMeester T.R.: Permanent extracorporeal esophagogastric tube for esophageal replacement. *Ann. Thorac. Surg.* 22:107, 1976.

11

Caustic and Traumatic Injury of the Esophagus

KENNETH W. SHARP, M.D.
JOHN L. SAWYERS, M.D.

THE INJURED esophagus remains a challenging clinical problem. Patients suffering esophageal injuries may be successfully managed by early diagnosis and treatment. Sequelae of esophageal injury that are missed, however, frequently are difficult to manage and carry substantial morbidity. Esophageal strictures and the septic complications of missed esophageal injuries are difficult surgical problems, often treated by staged surgical procedures, and result in a large number of unsatisfactory results. Since caustic injuries and penetrating trauma of the esophagus have distinctly different presentations and treatment, they will be covered independently.

CAUSTIC INJURY OF THE ESOPHAGUS

Etiology

The accidental or suicidal ingestion of corrosive substances is a medical emergency with a significant mortality and substantial morbidity. The evaluation and treatment of such ingestions has changed over the past 20 years but remains a highly controversial subject. Caustic ingestion remains the most common cause of esophageal stricture in children and ranks directly behind peptic stricture as the major cause of benign esophageal stricture in adults.

The reason for caustic ingestion varies with the age group encountered. Most ingestions in childhood are accidental, and most adult ingestions are suicidal gestures. Toddlers are led to drink caustics because the substances are stored in attractively colored and painted cans or bottles. Toddlers may drink from soda bottles that are used to store cleaning solutions left around the house.

Strong alkalis and acids head the list of agents producing esophageal injury. Strong alkalis such as lye, oven and drain cleaners, and household ammonia solutions are responsible for the majority of caustic ingestions. Acid solutions such as bleaches, battery acid, swimming pool cleansers, or concrete cleansers are responsible for a significant, but smaller, number of ingestions. Miscellaneous agents such as Clinitest tablets, tetracycline, ascorbic acid, and potassium chloride tablets have been reported to cause esophageal injury but are uncommon.

Prior to 1967, most alkalis for household use were sold as solid pellets or flakes of sodium hydroxide. Ingestion of these solid pellets was less commonly followed by swallowing of the caustic, as most children accidentally ingesting the pellets would expectorate vigorously once they burned their lips or tongue.[1] Consequently, esophageal injury and stricture were infrequent unless the pellets were swallowed. In 1967, liquid lye (as a 30% sodium hydroxide solution) was introduced as a drain cleaner, and ingestion of this product led to many serious esophageal injuries because the liquid was often swallowed accidentally rather than expectorated. Recognition of the extremely toxic nature of these solutions and of the large numbers of injured children (up to 5,000 children ingest these substances each year in the United States)[2] led to the reformulation of these products after 1970 with lower concentrations of lye.

Most drain cleaners still have potentially destructive amounts of lye. Many still have a pH of 14 and are associated with the highest incidence of ulceration and stricture.[3] Other household items containing alkalis are laundry cleaning aids and household ammonia preparations. These solutions have a lower pH and result in a lesser incidence of severe injury with ingestion.

Pathophysiology

Caustic injury of the esophagus may be due to acid or alkaline agents found in solid or liquid form. The extent of the injury is dependent on the nature of the substance (acid or alkaline), the concentration of the solution (or amount of solid), and the duration of contact with the tissue. The complications of the ingestion are related to the depth of the esophageal injury—the deeper and more severe the tissue penetration, the greater the chance of immediate perforation or longer-term stricture.

Histologically, the extent of corrosive injury has been compared to burn injuries of the skin.[4] The three pathologic stages are: first-degree—a mucosal injury characterized by hyperemia, edema, and superficial epithelial sloughing; second-degree—a transmucosal injury with exudates, loss of mucosa, and erosions through the esophageal wall; and third-degree—an injury that involves periesophageal tissues in the mediastinum, pleura, or peritoneum. Acid and alkaline solutions have different pathophysiologic mechanisms in producing the depths of injury.

Alkaline agents are well known to produce a liquefactive necrosis and a more severe injury than acid ingestions. When alkaline solutions contact the esophageal mucosa, cell death occurs rapidly, and cellular fats and proteins quickly saponify. The gelatinous mass that results is no barrier to the alkali, which penetrates deeply as contact is prolonged. As deeper tissues are penetrated, small vessels thrombose, leading to local tissue ischemia, worsening the injury.

The ingestion of solid pellets of lye leads to a slightly different type of injury from liquid alkaline solutions. Solid particles of lye that are swallowed tend to adhere spottily to mucosal surfaces and tend to stick in the pharynx and in the upper esophagus, where they do their damage. The stricture rate is generally less than with concentrated liquid lye. Accidental liquid lye ingestions are generally more serious because they are more easily swallowed than solids and are generously distributed over all surfaces of the pharynx and esophagus. Suicidal ingestions of liquid lye are often very serious owing to the ease with which large quantities of lye may be gulped down.

The effect of liquid lye ingestion has been graphically described by Kirsh and Ritter.[5] Shortly after instillation of liquid lye into an anesthetized dog's esophagus, violent regurgitation of the material occurs and is followed by cricopharyngeal spasm, "to-and-fro" peristalsis, and reverse peristalsis. This results in severe esophageal injury (and reinjury) and gastric injury in all cases. Gastric injury is frequent, and its degree is dependent on the amount of caustic reaching the stomach, the presence of food in the stomach, and whether pylorospasm occurs.

Acid injury of the esophageal and gastric mucosa causes coagulative necrosis. Acid contacting the mucosa results in superficial sloughing and the formation of a protective, coagulated eschar of desquamated epithelium, preventing further penetration of the acid into the mucosa in most cases. Acid injuries are often marked by more severe gastric injury than alkaline ingestions. This is generally thought to be due to several factors: the coagulum that forms in the esophagus and a general increased resistance of esophageal mucosa to acid compared to alkali. Gastric injury may occur more frequently with acid injury because alkaline ingestions are often neutralized by acid gastric contents. Typically, pooling of acid in the stomach results in pyloric stenosis or antral stenosis, since they are dependent areas.

Esophageal injuries resulting from the use of Clinitest tablets have been reported.[6] Clinitest tablets are used for testing urine sugar and contain copper sulfate, citric acid, sodium hydroxide, and sodium carbonate. The sodium hydroxide is used to produce a strong basic pH for reducing glucose and heat (from its heat of hydration). Children have ingested these tablets by mistaking them for candy, and the tablets cause a very localized area of injury where they stick in the esophagus. They typically lodge in the upper thoracic esophagus and have a high incidence of stricture. The stricture is typically short, dense, and resistant to dilatation; it generally requires

surgery. Other agents such as potassium chloride[7] and ascorbic acid[8] have been described as causing esophageal injury but are rare.

Presentation

The clinical features of corrosive ingestion have several items common to all injuries, whether the ingestion is the result of an accident or of a suicidal gesture. Toddlers who accidentally ingest caustics are generally rushed into the hospital shortly after the incident, when the ingestion is discovered by the parents. Occasionally, the ingestion may be silent and unknown to the parents—as often happens with Clinitest tablet ingestion. Suicidal patients often present one or two days after ingesting a caustic, with drooling or inability to swallow their saliva.

The symptoms of caustic ingestion are clearly related to the amount of caustic ingested and whether the caustic is solid or liquid. The pain and symptoms are less related to the acid or alkaline nature of the caustic than to the amount of caustic taken and whether it is solid or liquid. Solid pellets or flakes of caustic, which tend to adhere to mucous membranes, usually have symptoms referrable to oral, pharyngeal, and upper esophageal injury, and are often expectorated. Liquids tend to be gulped by toddlers or suicidal adults and have slightly less predilection for the upper digestive tract.

Burning, stinging, or searing pain in the lips, mouth, and throat are common. Retrosternal chest and back pain are nearly universal symptoms of esophageal injury, and abdominal or midback pain may be a symptom of gastric or small-bowel injury from caustic ingestion. Odynophagia and dysphagia are frequent as the initial pain lessens. Emesis is common, and hematemesis may be present. Hematemesis is most frequently noted, with gagging and retching of blood-streaked saliva, but on occasion may be frank blood. The development of exsanguinating hematemesis usually heralds a terminal event such as aortoesophageal fistula complicating esophageal necrosis five to ten days after caustic ingestion. Excessive salivation and drooling in these patients is generally not the result of parasympathetic stimulation but of the inability to swallow or the fear of swallowing.

The most alarming symptoms of caustic ingestion are those related to the upper airway. Hoarseness, stridor, and aphonia may alert the examiner to an upper airway burn with edema of the epiglottis, vocal cords, or larynx. Aspiration of the caustic may occur due to spasm of the cricopharyngeus muscle, and cough and dyspnea may be present in such a patient.

The acute symptoms of pain are generally self-limited and last one or two days. The later developing symptoms are due to the early complications of caustic ingestion and are most commonly those of early esophageal obstruction.

On physical examination, the findings range from the very subtle to the flagrantly intoxicated patient in extremis. Tachycardia is the most frequent abnormality of the vital signs, but fever is very common hours after the ingestion. Hypotension due to hypovolemia is relatively infrequent with early medical attention, but as patients present later after ingestion, it becomes quite common. Hypotension due to septic shock is quite a late feature in presentation.

Erythema and ulceration of the lips, mouth, tongue, and

pharynx occur rapidly after ingestion, and the ingestion of solids typically causes more punctate and discrete patches of erythema or ulceration than does liquid caustic ingestion. With very severe ingestion, the mouth and pharynx may be covered with a gray or black pseudomembrane of necrotic tissues. Indirect laryngoscopy may reveal edema or erythema of the epiglottis and possibly of the vocal cords in the symptomatic patient. Palpation of the neck most commonly reveals very mild tenderness but may reveal subcutaneous emphysema or crepitus if there has been disruption of the cervical or thoracic esophagus.

Examination of the chest may reveal signs of aspiration such as crackles or consolidation. Examination of the abdomen must be thorough to observe the early signs of peritonitis. Epigastric tenderness over the stomach is common, but frank signs of peritonitis are rare and generally indicate full-thickness necrosis and perforation of the stomach owing to the caustic.

Evaluation

In the modern management of caustic ingestions, endoscopy has become the "gold standard" of evaluation of the injured esophagus. It is clearly superior to symptoms, physical examination, or any radiographic technique for evaluating the esophagus. Previously, the use of esophagoscopy was highly controversial, chiefly because of the risk of perforation. Perforation of the injured esophagus with the rigid esophagoscope occurred often in the past and was the main objection to the early performance of esophagoscopy. The safety of flexible endoscopy now far exceeds that of the rigid esophagoscope.

Prior to the use of esophagoscopy, clinical evaluation of esophageal burns rested on the physical examination of the oropharynx for burns and radiographic contrast studies. The physical examination of the oropharynx as an indicator of esophageal injury is notoriously inaccurate. Depending on the population surveyed, only 20%–40% of patients with oropharyngeal burns will have identifiable esophageal injuries.[9, 10] Unfortunately, in many reports, a small number of patients have no visible or symptomatic oropharyngeal injury yet have an endoscopically unequivocal esophageal injury.[11]

The main point of controversy surrounding the endoscopic evaluation of caustic esophageal injuries centers on the proper timing of the examination. There are proponents of immediate (immediately upon presentation) endoscopy, early (one to three days after ingestion) endoscopy, and late (one to three weeks after ingestion) endoscopy. Early endoscopy is the best method to ascertain which patients with unclear histories of ingestion (questionable ingestion, uncertain amount) do indeed have esophageal injury and need prolonged hospital observation and possibly treatment. Endoscopy performed within a few hours may theoretically miss subtle injuries of the esophagus that may be manifested by erythema or edema that will develop 12 to 24 hours after injury in some patients. Most proponents of immediate or early endoscopy do not believe that endoscopy is so urgent that it need be performed in the middle of the night but at the earliest convenient time. Proponents of late endoscopy cite the increased chance of perforating an edematous injured esophagus as the reason to delay the endoscopy until the edema is resolving and fibrosis is occurring, so that the risk of perforation is lessened.

The role of rigid esophagoscopy is diminishing. The flexible endoscope, especially the newest generation of pediatric-sized endoscopes, is highly satisfactory for patient comfort, safety of insertion, and accurate visualization of the esophagus. The rigid esophagoscope has the disadvantage of requiring a general anesthetic for its use, and the risk of perforation of the esophagus is high—especially with a severely injured hypopharynx and cricopharyngeal area. The flexible endoscope is usually easily passed with topical oropharyngeal anesthesia; general anesthesia is usually only required in children. The flexible endoscope is far superior to the rigid endoscope for visualizing the stomach and duodenum, and caustic injuries of the stomach may be evaluated accurately.

Controversy remains over how far to pass the endoscope. Certainly, the safest and most prudent course is to halt the endoscope at the highest level of injury encountered.[12, 13] Unfortunately, this may leave most of the esophagus uninspected, but it has the least chance of perforating the esophagus. However, with the advent of small-diameter endoscopes and the increased desire to visualize all potential sites of injury in the esophagus and stomach, there is increasing enthusiasm for visualizing the highest point of injury and very gently passing beyond, under direct visualization.[14, 15]

The principal advantage of early endoscopy in the evaluation of caustic ingestion is its accuracy in the determination of the presence or absence of caustic injury. Second, endoscopy is the most accurate way to stage the esophageal injury—to assess the depth of the burn and the extent of the esophagus involved. Prognostically, the best information concerning the long-term prospects for an esophageal caustic injury comes from a carefully performed endoscopy. Accurate assessment of the injury allows tailoring the treatment to the degree of injury: lesser injury needs lesser treatment.

Clinical staging endoscopically is an attempt to correlate the endoscopic appearance of an injured esophagus to the histopathologic staging described earlier. The depth of injury once again determines the severity of the injury more than the nature of the caustic. A first-degree burn endoscopically is described as hyperemia and superficial epithelial desquamation of the esophageal mucosa. A second-degree burn displays superficial blisters, ulcers, hyperemia, and the presence of an exudate over the mucosa. A third-degree burn shows deeper, more extensive loss of mucosa and more exudates. Some add a fourth degree—the presence of black or gangrenous patches visible through the endoscope, indicative of full-thickness injury of the esophagus or stomach, with involvement of adjacent tissue or organs in the mediastinum or peritoneum.

There are two limitations to endoscopy in the evaluation of esophageal injury. Most commonly, it is difficult to be truly certain of the exact depth of injury; repeated endoscopy may be necessary to recheck the initial findings several days after the first endoscopy. Second, if truly severe burns are encountered in the upper esophagus, the rest of the esophagus remains unvisualized, and the extent of esophageal or gastric injury is uncertain.

The radiographic evaluation of caustic ingestion plays a secondary role to endoscopy. Plain films of the chest and abdomen should be obtained for baseline evaluation and for assessment of complications. Cervical or mediastinal air may be seen, indicating esophageal disruption. Plain films of the chest are valuable for assessing the degree of pneumonitis present if aspiration of caustic has occurred.

Contrast studies of the esophagus are particularly useful if a skilled endoscopist is not available or if the esophageal injury is so severe that only a limited endoscopy has been performed. The radiographic features of both acid and alkaline injuries have been well described.[16, 17] In evaluating the fresh esophageal injury, the use of water-soluble contrast agents is advised. They are safer if a perforation is present and extravasation of contrast occurs, and they are safer if aspirated. Early contrast studies may be misleading: the freshly burned esophagus is often atonic or in spasm, and a true picture of esophageal motility is not obtained.

Later signs (more than one or two days after injury) of esophageal injury may be seen on contrast studies. If the clinical situation suggests that there is no perforation and the patient shows no sign of aspiration, barium contrast studies may be obtained. Mucosal edema and blurring of the esophageal mucosa are frequently seen owing to the severe edema after caustic ingestion. Contrast may be seen collecting in intramural recesses due to deep linear ulcerations and intramural dissections. Barium tends to be retained in the esophageal wall long after the swallow has passed if these findings are present. Pocketing and segmentation of the contrast and air may be seen if there are local areas of spasm soon after injury.

The most clearly helpful aspect of contrast studies of the esophagus comes later (beyond two weeks) after the injury. Evaluation of early and late stricture due to caustic ingestion is very easy with barium studies. Screening of all injured patients should be performed two to three weeks after injury to evaluate the possibility of stricture, even in the minimally symptomatic or asymptomatic patient.

Complications

The complications of caustic ingestion group rather easily into early (less than six weeks) and late complications. Though stricture somewhat overlaps the two time periods, it is the late strictures that are the major source of long-term morbidity for the caustic-injured esophagus.

The early complications involve the airway, aspiration, perforation, or bleeding from the esophagus, shock, and death. Strictures may occur as early as several days after injury; but the tough, dense, fibrous strictures that are such a source of misery take many weeks to develop. The two major late complications of caustic ingestion are strictures and, rarely, carcinoma.

The truly life-threatening early emergencies in caustic ingestion are those involving the upper airway. Contact of strong corrosives with the epiglottis is frequent, and edema always follows. Severe ingestions with destruction of the hypopharynx frequently involve the larynx and vocal cords, and airway obstruction may occur within hours. Though an uncommon event in general, laryngeal edema with airway obstruction is a preventable cause of death early after caustic ingestion.

The lower airway complications of caustic ingestion are as-piration and its manifestation in the tracheobronchial tree and lung parenchyma. Though not as immediately life-threatening as airway obstruction, severe pneumonitis and respiratory distress syndrome may follow corrosive aspiration. The secondary bacterial pneumonias that occur in the damaged lung are difficult to treat for two reasons: the normal host defenses such as the cilia are destroyed by the caustic, and the widespread use of broad-spectrum antibiotics in caustic ingestion selects out resistant organisms.

Perforation of the esophagus or stomach generally occurs several days after ingestion, when the slowly progressing necrosis finally breaks through the esophagus or gastric wall. Early perforation, within hours of ingestion, is dramatic and highly lethal. Early perforation of the esophagus or stomach indicates a massive ingestion, with rapid full-thickness penetration of the gastric or esophageal wall. Free air in the neck, mediastinum, or abdomen is the most dramatic evidence of perforation; but more commonly, perforation presents as a slowly smoldering mediastinitis, with several weeks of fevers and pain developing after injury. Penetration of the caustic in the region of the carina occasionally results in fistula formation to the trachea or bronchi—again usually developing slowly after the injury rather than early and dramatically. Tracheoesophageal or bronchoesophageal fistulas may present with pneumonia and signs of constant low-grade aspiration and may be difficult to diagnose in the patient who suffered caustic aspiration during the initial injury.

Bleeding occurs frequently during the course of esophageal caustic injury. Most of the time, it is low-grade bleeding, with hematemesis being the most visible manifestation. The ulcerated raw esophagus or stomach may bleed or ooze almost constantly before healing occurs. Major life-threatening hemorrhage is very unusual and is most often due to deep ulcerations eroding into vessels supplying the esophagus or stomach.

Shock may be present in some patients soon after caustic ingestion. In the early presentation, it is usually due to hypovolemia, pain, and fright. Shock developing later in the course of caustic injury generally is the result of sepsis. Pneumonia and other opportunistic infections are common in the severely injured patient, and mediastinitis causes another significant portion of the septic complications. Mediastinitis from an unsuspected or overlooked esophageal perforation should be considered in the patient with continuing fevers and intoxication two to three weeks after caustic ingestion.

The incidence of death due to caustic ingestion is low in most series. In children the incidence is very low. Haller et al.[9] reported no deaths in a series of 285 children with esophageal injuries. Children have accidental ingestions that less commonly result in the massive, severe ingestions that suicidal adults sustain. Kirsh et al.[18] reported a 12.5% mortality in a series of 32 patients with caustic ingestion that had heavy weighting by several massive ingestions, which were truly hopeless despite heroic attempts. Most series have death rates that range from 1% to 4%.[11, 13, 19] Death is most commonly due to uncontrollable infection in most cases and only rarely due to hemorrhage.

The late complications of esophageal injury by caustics are stricture and cancer. The occurrence of stricture is directly related to the severity of the caustic injury. Liquid lye products are by far the most common cause of esophageal stricture owing to their highly alkaline nature and ease of swallowing. Acid ingestions are, in general, less common than alkaline ingestions and have a lower incidence of stricture. Bleach, detergents, and ammonia ingestion have a low rate of stricture formation (Figs 11–1 and 11–2).[20]

The true rates of stricture formation must be analyzed by grouping comparable injuries. According to clinical (endoscopic) staging, there should be a negligible incidence of stricture in a patient with a first-degree burn of the esophagus. Unfortunately, endoscopic staging is not perfectly accurate, and there will be rare patients who develop a stricture after what is apparently a first-degree burn. It appears that the mode of treatment bears little influence on the outcome of the first-degree burns. It is clear that patients with second-degree burns have a lower incidence of stricture than patients suffering third-degree burns; however, it is difficult to sort out the effects of treatment from the necessarily difficult staging differences in these patients. Most reported series tend to lump the various caustic agents and resulting strictures without regard to clinical staging; but it is probable that patients suffering from second-degree burns have an incidence of stricture between 10% and 30%, whereas patients with third-degree burns have a stricture rate of 40%–70%. As an example of the difficulty in comparing series, DiCostanzo et al.[21] recently reported a series of 27 patients with second-degree esophageal and gastric injuries with not a single stricture resulting. This seems remarkable until the patient population is analyzed, and it is seen that bleach was the most commonly ingested caustic (48%), and there were a large number of acid ingestions (22%). Both acids and bleach generally have a low incidence of esophageal stricture following their ingestion. More typical is the report of Cardona and Daly,[12] who reported a 31% incidence of stricture in steroid- and antibiotic-treated patients who were "severely burned" (third-degree equivalent). Webb et al.[19] reported five "minimal" strictures in 21 patients with second-degree burns, and all eight patients with third-degree burns developed strictures.

The risk of cancer developing in the caustic-injured esophagus remains a great fear. Its incidence is not precisely

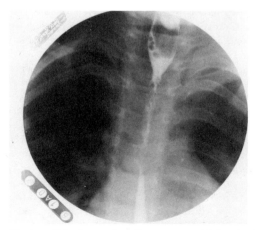

Fig 11–1.—AP view of a three-year-old boy's barium swallow demonstrating an esophageal stricture after accidental lye ingestion.

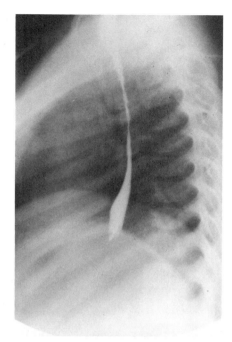

Fig 11–2.—Lateral view of the esophagus of the same three-year-old boy.

known, and the biologic aggressiveness of such a tumor is uncertain. These cancers appear insidiously in patients whose injured esophagus has required bypass or substitution (without removal of the injured esophagus), or they may occur in a functional esophagus that was injured many years earlier.

The incidence of cancer developing in a caustic-injured esophagus is unclear. There have been no large studies performed on caustic-injured patients followed for a lifetime to ascertain the true incidence. Possibly the most accurate estimate is that of Kiviranta[22] studying a Finnish population in 1952. He described nine cases of corrosion carcinoma developing in 381 known cases of corrosion injury, for an incidence of 2.4%. The obvious problem is the accurate estimation of index cases of caustic injury: it is likely there were many more caustic injuries that occurred but were not identified and entered into the denominator. Kiviranta raises the issue of latency, the long periods elapsing between injury and development of esophageal cancer. The shortest latency was 24 years and the longest 44 years. In comparing the incidence of esophageal cancer in the Finnish people as a whole as compared to a group of patients suffering lye injuries at least 24 years earlier, he found that the risk of developing esophageal cancer was at least 1,000-fold increased for lye-injured patients.[22] Another more recent report[23] gives an estimate of an 8% incidence of carcinoma developing in a caustic-injured esophagus, but again almost certainly overestimates the risk because the denominator is inadequately studied.

The latent period between caustic injury and the diagnosis of esophageal carcinoma has been reported frequently, and the agreement between reports is high. The largest reported series of caustic-related esophageal carcinomas is from Appelqvist and Salmo,[24] and the mean latent time between injury and cancer is 41 years in 63 cases of caustic-related cancer. Hopkins and Postlethwait[25] reported an average interval of 46 years in 12 patients. Most of these patients ingested lye and generally were children at the time of ingestion. The shortest interval between injury and development of cancer was nine years.

All of the reported cases of caustic-related esophageal cancer have been squamous cell cancer histologically. Their distribution in the esophagus does not parallel the usual distribution of squamous cell cancer, as it tends to have a marked predilection for the upper thoracic esophagus—generally near the carina. This is almost certainly related to the location of injury, because the majority of caustic strictures occur at or near the carina. The vast majority of cases reported have been in a functional esophagus; i.e., in a patient without symptomatic stricture during the latent period. The occurrence of carcinoma in a bypassed esophagus develops insidiously, and its incidence is as difficult to ascertain as for the nonbypassed cases.

Early Treatment

The early treatment of the patient with a caustic injury is still a highly controversial subject, especially with regard to the use of steroids. Additionally, the timing of endoscopy and the use of antibiotics, nasogastric tubes, and intraluminal stents are all debatable. The goals of early treatment are the prevention of early and late complications, especially stricture.

The management of the upper airway is undeniably the top priority in the emergency management of a patient after caustic ingestion. The control of the upper airway must be ensured in a patient with hoarseness, stridor, or aphonia. Intubation, cricothyroidotomy, or tracheostomy may be necessary and are best performed prior to total airway obstruction rather than afterward. Severe pharyngeal and epiglottic injuries are a relative contraindication to oral or nasal endotracheal intubation and suggest the need for surgical airway management.

Emetics are contraindicated in the patient with recent caustic ingestion. The stomach neutralizes all but the most massive of ingestions more safely than a physician can remove the caustic. Emetics given while the caustic is still present in the stomach would only worsen the exposure of the esophagus to the noxious agent, increase the risk of perforation from retching, and increase the chance of aspiration.

Gastric lavage with or without neutralization is usually not necessary. As mentioned previously, the stomach can quickly neutralize or dilute caustics by the normal process of gastric secretion. Neutralization is generally not only unnecessary but may be dangerous. Adding neutralizing agents to the gastric contents, which contain an unknown amount of caustic agent, runs the risk of overtitration and changing an acid injury to an alkaline one, or vice versa. The gases released by neutralization as well as the heat produced will both tend to exacerbate the injury.

The use of a nasogastric tube is not widely advocated but has several uses. Obviously, passage must be gentle to avoid perforating an injured esophagus. Once in place, it may be used to check the pH of the gastric contents. Kirsh and Ritter[5] advocate passing a nasogastric tube in patients suffering lye ingestion and aspirating the gastric contents. If the pH

is alkaline and "the alkalinity does not cease with gentle and limited irrigation, it is presumed that the stomach and esophagus are burned." At that point, abdominal exploration is carried out, with assessment of viability of the stomach and surrounding organs. If the stomach is nonviable, it is removed, and presumption of esophageal necrosis is followed by esophagectomy and cervical esophagostomy. Delayed reconstruction, six to 12 weeks later, is preferred.

A nasogastric tube may also be used for feeding the patient who cannot swallow. Cardona and Daly[12] believe that the nasogastric tube can prevent strictures by preventing adhesions between adjacent or opposing ulcerations in the esophagus and additionally serves to preserve at least a small esophageal lumen if strictures develop. Unfortunately, stricture formation is enhanced by factors that promote exuberant granulation tissue, and the irritation and trauma of an indwelling nasogastric tube in the esophagus may promote granulation and stricture; therefore, widespread support for the use of nasogastric tubes is not found.

Early endoscopy, while not a therapeutic measure in itself, is absolutely essential for the intelligent treatment of caustic ingestions. It is important to examine endoscopically all patients with a history of caustic ingestion, whatever the findings on oropharyngeal examination. At least 30% of patients with oropharyngeal burns will have no esophageal burns on esophagoscopy.[13] Conversely, it is possible to have esophageal burns without oropharyngeal injury, but this uncommon event should be excluded by endoscopy.

The most important function of early endoscopy is to stage the injury and to use staging to guide treatment. Patients with oropharyngeal burns without esophageal burns may be treated with symptomatic support and will not have the short- or long-term complications to which esophageal burns are subject. The ability to exclude esophageal injury may obviate hospital admission in many cases of suspected, but unproved or unwitnessed, ingestions. It is clear that minimal or first-degree burns of the esophagus need minimal treatment beyond supportive or symptomatic care and will not result in late strictures. Visualizing an extensive or greater-depth burn calls for more aggressive treatment and may be guided by endoscopic findings. Endoscopic findings are also the best method to predict prognosis for a given patient's injury because of its relatively accurate staging of injury.

Repeated or follow-up endoscopy is often valuable to assess the progression of healing of esophageal injury. As the acute symptoms subside, endoscopic evaluation of ulceration may reveal progression toward full-thickness ulceration in severe injuries or will easily observe ulcer healing as it progresses.

The use of steroids in the management of the caustic-injured esophagus remains highly controversial. No large prospective randomized trials have been performed, and definitive clinical results have never been obtained. Limited studies have been performed in a prospective manner. Hawkins et al.[13] were able to study 24 patients prospectively and to show a trend toward fewer strictures in steroid-treated patients as opposed to nonsteroid-treated patients, but the small number of patients studied with equal severity of burns precluded unequivocal statistical significance. By adding a group of ten patients admitted after the end of their study who were treated with steroids, they were able to demonstrate a striking difference in stricture formation in 12 patients with moderately severe or deep second-degree burns. Only one of four (25%) steroid-treated patients developed a stricture, as opposed to seven of eight (88%) developing a stricture who were not treated with steroids. Other studies[9, 12] have shown striking reductions in stricture formation with steroid treatment compared to historical controls.

Many studies question the utility of steroids. Kirsh et al.[18] and Webb et al.[19] both noted a high incidence of stricture in steroid-treated patients with third-degree burns and therefore suggest that steroids offer no benefit. Oakes et al.[26] summarized the results of 15 authors' reports on esophageal injuries and found an overall stricture rate of 16.8% in steroid-treated patients and a stricture rate of 20.1% for nonsteroid-treated patients. They concluded that steroid therapy "is of unproved efficacy in the management of *any* esophageal burn."

It is difficult to account for the different stricture rates in the many reported series. Clearly, the major problem is the uniformity of clinical staging for comparison of results. Endoscopic appearances are not totally objective; therefore, it may be that differences in endoscopists are being compared rather than injuries. It is fairly clear that minimal esophageal injuries do not require steroid treatment and equally clear that the severely injured esophagus that is transmurally destroyed over most of its length will not respond to steroid treatment.

The rationale for the use of steroids is their ability to inhibit fibroplasia and granulation tissue formation.[27] In experimental dogs, cortisone prevents lye strictures, but only if penicillin is used to control infection.[28] To prevent stricture, steroids must be used early (as soon as possible after the injury and certainly not more than 48 hours after injury) and must be used in pharmacologic doses. Standard dosage for children is 2 mg/kg of prednisone (or equivalent steroid) per day. Adult dosages have been generally 60–80 mg per day of prednisone. The duration of steroid treatment is not standardized but is at least one to three weeks, with occasional reports of several months' therapy.[12]

The potential complications of steroid therapy are frequently cited as reason against their use. Gastric and duodenal ulcers have been reported, and many authors believe that a steroid-treated esophagus is more prone to perforation but cite no incidences.[5] Predisposition to secondary infection is often cited, and most authors who advocate steroid use also advocate concomitant antibiotic use.

Current opinion of steroid use remains divided, but several generalizations may be made. First, the minimally injured esophagus with first-degree burns or small areas of second-degree burns will do well without the use of steroids. Second, the severely injured or destroyed esophagus cannot be rejuvenated with steroids. Third, the patient with extensive second-degree burns or limited amounts of third-degree burns is the patient in whom to consider steroid use. It seems likely that children may respond more favorably than adults, and steroid use in children is much less controversial.

The use of antibiotics is less controversial than the use of steroids. Most authors who advocate steroids use antibiotics, but the converse is not true. The rationale for antibiotic use is that it will decrease or eliminate the secondary infection or superinfection of damaged tissue that would tend to exacerbate the caustic injury. Antibiotics would also be helpful in treating subclinical mediastinitis or aspiration pneumonia. Generally, ampicillin is recommended for its coverage of mouth flora and some gram-negative organisms. Penicillin in combination with an aminoglycoside has also been used.

Experimentally, approaches have been made to decrease scar formation and subsequent stricture by inhibiting the cross-linking of collagen as it is synthesized. Davis et al.[29] have reduced experimental caustic stricture formation in dogs by using β-aminopropionitrile; but this compound is not approved for human use. Penicillamine is another approach, with a more acceptable drug. Gehanno and Guedon[30] reported excellent results in preventing esophageal strictures in a rat model by administering penicillamine daily via gastrostomy from the day after injury until sacrifice up to one month later. Penicillamine has not been used in human studies, however.

The nutritional support of the patient with caustic injury of the esophagus depends on the severity of the injury. As with all other therapeutic measures, more aggressive treatment is needed for the more severe injuries. Patients with minor burns of the oropharynx or esophagus will usually need IV fluids only as long as the acute pain of the ingestion persists—usually one to three days. Beyond that, they will be able to eat and drink relatively painlessly and should need little special attention to nutrition. The more severely injured patients need more aggressive support. If a patient has burns severe enough to have ulcers or areas of denuded mucosa, the effect of swallowed food passing over the ulcers or particles of food lodging in the ulcers may traumatize the esophagus, exacerbating the injury and increasing the chance of stricture. Nasogastric tubes may be used for feeding if they are placed. Gastrostomy may be helpful in the patient with the severe injury prone to stricture, and it is very helpful in children who tolerate nasogastric tubes poorly. Jejunostomy feeding is rarely necessary except in the patient with severe gastroesophageal reflux or in the patient with gastric caustic injury.

The use of parenteral nutrition has grown more popular in caustic injury management. It offers good nutritional support without the disadvantages of nasogastric tubes or surgical placement of gastrostomy. The current techniques of central venous catheterization and the use of hypertonic nutrient solutions are so safe now that indications for their use are continuing to expand. The recent report of DiCostanzo et al.[21] even ascribes a therapeutic benefit to the use of TPN for patients with esophageal caustic injuries. They describe a series of 94 patients treated without steroids or prophylactic antibiotics but with 40–50 calories per kilogram body weight of TPN until their injuries healed. The rate of stricture formation in patients with second-degree burns was *zero* and only 36% (five of 14) in the patients with third-degree burns. Analysis of the report, however, brings out the high incidence of bleach and acid ingestion in this series, and these are well known to have a low stricture rate. With severe injuries having a 36% rate of stricture formation, it is difficult to proclaim this approach superior to other therapeutic approaches.

Intraluminal stenting of the severely injured esophagus with large-bore silicone tubing has limited support.[31] This is usually only advocated for moderately severe lye injuries with high suspicion for stricture formation. Mills et al.[31] report their use of the technique in four patients with lye injuries with no stricture formation. Their technique involves endoscopy to ascertain injury, laparotomy for assessment of gastric viability, and placement of the esophageal stent via a gastrostomy. A jejunostomy tube is placed at the time and jejunostomy feedings are used to prevent gastroesophageal reflux. Steroids and antibiotics are used additionally. The stents are kept in place for three weeks, when a barium swallow is obtained; a functional esophagus without stricture was seen in all four patients. Experience with this technique is too limited for it to be widely recommended at this time. It is possible to imagine that this technique is effective for mucosal injuries, but it will not salvage an esophagus with muscular injury.

Early surgical intervention is necessary in a small number of patients with caustic ingestion. It is most commonly necessary for the patient with massive ingestion or in the patient suffering a perforation during endoscopy. If perforation happens during endoscopy, urgent surgical repair should be carried out if the esophagus is viable. If perforation during endoscopy is not noted or the patient has a later perforation of the esophagus leading to mediastinitis, esophagectomy with delayed reconstruction will usually be necessary. The patient with massive ingestion of liquid lye with necrosis of the esophagus and stomach will require emergency esophagogastrectomy. If abdominal exploration is undertaken for peritoneal signs in the patient suffering liquid lye ingestion, and the stomach is found to be necrotic, it is safe to presume that the esophagus is also necrotic and should also be removed.[18] If solid lye is ingested (or encapsulated lye, which some suicidal patients will ingest) and the stomach is found to be nonviable, it is *not* safe to assume that the esophagus is destroyed, and endoscopic evaluation of the esophagus must be carried out. If esophagogastrectomy is done within 12–24 hours following injury, it is possible in some cases without mediastinitis to perform safely esophagectomy without thoracotomy through a transcervical and transhiatal abdominal approach.[32] The patient with severe acid injury should be closely examined for small-bowel injury if gastric injury is present.

Figure 11–3 is an algorithm for the evaluation and treatment of caustic ingestion.

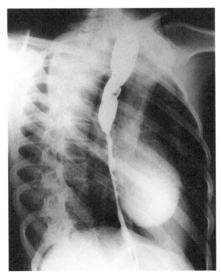

Fig 11–3.—Destroyed esophagus in a 19-year-old female who ingested lye in a suicide attempt.

Treatment of Late Complications

Stricture is such a difficult and unpleasant late complication of caustic injury that everyone agrees it is better prevented than treated. The vast array of techniques for treatment of stricture also speaks to its difficulty: if treatment were simple, there would be only a few acceptable options.

The development of a dense, fibrous stricture of the esophagus takes at least six weeks to develop. Strictures are obviously in evolution during the first several weeks after injury and may certainly be symptomatic. It is difficult in the first two to three weeks after caustic injury to determine which early strictures will be soft and easily treated by a single dilatation and which are the very tough, dense strictures that require multiple dilatation or surgical bypass. For this reason, some surgeons practice early bougienage; that is, they start early, blind esophageal dilatations in the first two or three weeks after caustic ingestions in the hope of preventing severe stricture formation. Unfortunately, this probably only submits the patient to an increased risk of perforation of the esophagus and probably traumatizes many areas of the esophagus and worsens the injury. Current opinion speaks against early dilatation in favor of delayed (more than three or four weeks) dilatation of the esophagus.

Barium contrast studies are the easiest method to evaluate stricture formation. All patients suffering caustic ingestion of any degree should undergo barium swallow two to three weeks after injury, whether symptomatic or not. The location, length, and tightness of a stricture are easily seen on barium swallow. At the early barium swallow, it is difficult to evaluate how dense the stricture is and to predict its response to treatment.

Once an esophageal stricture is located, the initial treatment should be dilatation. Many early-appearing, short-segment esophageal strictures after caustic injury will respond favorably to a single dilatation or to a few gentle serial dilatations. Several techniques are available: prograde dilatations may be done in several ways, and retrograde dilatations are useful in certain clinical settings. Prograde esophageal dilatation can be accomplished blindly with mercury-weighted dilators such as the Maloney and Hurst dilators, or dilatation can be done under direct vision through the rigid esophagoscope. Owing to the worry about perforation with blind dilatation and the need for general anesthesia for rigid esophagoscopy, many surgeons prefer to have an injured patient swallow a string early after the injury to use later to guide the use of Tucker or Eder-Puestow dilators. Retrograde dilatations are very useful for children or for adults who will not cooperate or cannot tolerate prograde dilatations. Retrograde dilatations obviously require a gastrostomy for access to the swallowed string that is used to pull the dilators through from the stomach upward. Since gastrostomies are frequently used in children with esophageal injuries (for feeding and to avoid nasogastric tubes), this is a common approach in children.

Several technical points should be discussed. The decision to begin dilatation should be made several weeks after the injury. Early dilatations are rarely indicated, and later dilatations are safer. Gentle technique is essential. The rough and forceful fracture of a soft stricture will result in further trauma and fibrosis in the area. Gently working up through several different-sized dilators is useful, but the passage of multiple dilators in one session may lead to further trauma and inflammation; therefore, sessions should be restrained to only two or three dilator passages. A final point is how long one should persist with dilatation for a refractory or recurrent stricture. Several factors point toward earlier surgical intervention and ceasing efforts at dilatation: multiple stricture, a diffusely strictured esophagus, and occurrence of complications from dilatation. When strictures have persisted beyond four to six months of dilatation, it is clear that persistence will be fruitless, and a surgical approach should be taken. Figure 11–3 shows a hopelessly destroyed distal esophagus recalcitrant to dilatation.

The operations performed for esophageal stricture following caustic injury are now solely esophageal substitutions. Early attempts at short-segment esophageal resections or Mikulicz-type esophagoplasties are followed by recurrent stricture formation in nearly all cases. The only situation in which these operations are still useful are those cases caused by extremely localized esophageal injury, such as Clinitest tablet injury in children.[6] In other caustic injuries, limited resections or plastic repairs by the Mikulicz- or Thal-type repairs fail because the esophageal fibrosis is worse than it looks on contrast swallows, and the fibrosis will recur or progress at the site of local repair.

For the same reason, even more extensive esophageal resections with intrathoracic reconstruction fail. The upper thoracic esophagus is almost always more fibrotic than appreciated on endoscopy or barium swallow, and intrathoracic esophageal anastomoses in the setting of caustic injury have a high stenosis rate. Cervical anastomosis to the esophagus is virtually always preferred for the substitution procedure.

Reconstruction is most commonly performed with the colon, followed by the stomach and then the jejunum. Antethoracic skin tubes for esophageal replacement are only of interest historically. The colon is the preferred method in most cases, because it preserves a more normal gastric food reservoir, prevents problems with gastroesophageal reflux, and has a dependable blood supply and mobility. Either the right or left colon may be used in an isoperistaltic direction, and it may be brought up to the neck either retrosternally or through the thorax. The left colon has somewhat less tendency to elongate or become saccular; but many surgeons prefer the right colon—feeling the mobility of the right colon and terminal ileum is better than the left colon. If the stomach is not damaged and colon interposition is performed, tube gastrostomy should be performed for postoperative decompression and feeding.

The stomach is probably the easiest technical substitute for the esophagus. The mobilized stomach will easily reach the cervical esophagus through either the retrosternal route or through the thorax. Pyloroplasty or pyloromyotomy should be performed in all cases to avoid emptying difficulties. Despite the concern about acid-peptic reflux, if the stomach is brought up to the neck, it has not been nearly as frequent a problem as with intrathoracic esophagogastrostomies. Some patients will have some problems with weight maintenance and eating due to decreased gastric reservoir capacity when stomach is used as an esophageal substitute. One alternative proposed has been the use of a gastric tube, such as the Heimlich or Gavriliu, to replace or bypass the esophagus. These tubes, and reversed tubes (antiperistaltic), such as the Beck, will

reach the cervical esophagus in almost all instances. One particular caveat should be kept in mind: if there is any gastric injury from the caustic injury, it is unlikely that the stomach will serve well as an esophageal substitute.

The use of the jejunum is definitely less popular than the colon or stomach. It is difficult to mobilize a segment of jejunum enough to reach the cervical esophagus and preserve a viable blood supply to the upper end. It is possible to do this in some patients primarily; but in many cases it will require microvascular techniques of revascularization of the upper end of the jejunum to the thyrocervical trunk vessels in the neck. This may be especially suitable in the patient who has previously undergone gastric resection, in whom the stomach was injured by the caustic, or in whom the colon is unsuitable for conduit use. Failed colon interpositions often require jejunal interpositions, because the stomach may not be mobile enough after previous operations.

Transhiatal, transcervical esophagectomy without thoracotomy is gaining increased use in the resection and reconstruction of the caustic-injured esophagus. It has been described in the urgent situation[32] for esophageal necrosis, in the elective treatment of stricture in adults,[33] and in children.[34] One of the favorable technical aspects of the operation is the ease with which the stomach may be brought up through the posterior mediastinum to the neck. Retrosternal colon interposition may be done for reconstruction if desired; but the colon may not pass up the posterior mediastinal route as easily as the stomach.

The special problems of the patient with severe pharyngeal or hypopharyngeal stricture should be mentioned. When esophageal substitution must be taken up to the hypopharynx, many difficulties with aspiration and relearning of the swallowing process occur. These are often the patients who have required tracheostomy early after their injury as an indication of severe high cervical injuries. When esophageal bypass must be performed above the cricopharyngeus, many patients will suffer aspiration.[35] If the cricopharyngeal muscle is stenotic along with pharyngeal constrictor injury, difficulties with swallowing postreconstruction can be expected.

The development of cancer in an injured esophagus is the most dreaded late complication of caustic ingestion. Though its incidence is low, its presence demands several questions. The most common question concerns proper treatment of the bypassed or excluded esophagus at the time of esophageal replacement. Many surgeons have regarded esophagectomy at the time of substitution as too much additional surgery in an already debilitated patient. It is difficult to balance the additional risk of esophagectomy with the incidence of late cancer development. Current opinion recommends esophagectomy at the time of esophageal substitution if it does not substantially increase the operative morbidity. This is certainly one of the attractive features of transhiatal esophagectomy without thoracotomy, since it makes a technically easy route for gastric interposition in the posterior mediastinum and does not subject the patient to the additional morbidity of a thoracotomy.

A difficult question arises with the patient whose injured esophagus does not require replacement. Most reported cases of caustic-related esophageal carcinoma occur in functional esophagi. The proper surveillance is difficult to ascertain, because most of these cancers occur so late after caustic injury, an average of 40–45 years. It seems that these patients who have had strictures dilated, or some other feature of injury that indicated moderately severe injury, should be followed up with yearly barium swallows. Periodic endoscopy could be advocated as more effective in finding cancer but probably would not be as widely accepted.

Most carcinomas developing in patients after caustic injury present exactly like a spontaneous esophageal carcinoma: dysphagia, weight loss, and, eventually, pain. The diagnostic methods—barium swallow, endoscopy, and biopsy—are the same. However, once a caustic-related carcinoma is diagnosed, there is some room for optimism. The largest series of esophageal carcinomas related to caustic injury[24, 25] find that the resectability rate is higher than that for other causes, and five-year survival is also slightly higher. The resectability rate in these two series was over 75%, and the operative survivors in one series had a 33% five-year survival. While these figures are somewhat better than for other causes of esophageal carcinomas, they still support aggressive surveillance of such patients throughout their lifetimes.

TRAUMATIC INJURIES OF THE ESOPHAGUS

Traumatic injury to the esophagus leading to perforation is a surgical emergency which is usually fatal if untreated. Perforation of the esophagus has been described as the most rapidly lethal perforation of the GI tract. Contamination of the mediastinum with corrosive fluids, food matter, and bacteria leads to cardiorespiratory embarrassment, shock, major fluid losses, and fulminating infection. However, with prompt, aggressive surgical treatment, survival can be expected in most patients.

Boerhaave's Syndrome

Boerhaave's syndrome, or spontaneous rupture of the esophagus, was described in 1724 by Hermann Boerhaave, the leading physician in Europe during the first part of the 18th century. Boerhaave was simultaneously chairman of the three departments of chemistry, botany, and medicine for many years at the University of Leyden.

Boerhaave's patient, Baron Wassenauer, Admiral of the Dutch Fleet, induced vomiting by taking emetics at the end of a very large dinner. During the violent straining while vomiting, the Baron developed an agonizing pain and sensation of something giving way in the epigastric region. He fell to the floor crying out from the intense pain. He was placed in bed but was unable to lie still and had to be supported bent over by three men. He was unable to swallow liquids. He developed a cold sweat and intense pallor with a weak pulse. His condition rapidly worsened, and he died 18½ hours later. At the autopsy performed by Boerhaave, subcutaneous emphysema was noted as well as pleural effusion, which had the smell of duck flesh, which the baron had eaten. A linear tear was present on the left side of the esophagus just above the diaphragm.

Spontaneous rupture of the esophagus was observed sporadically until the first successful operation for this condition was performed by Norman Barrett in 1947.

Pathogenesis

Two factors associated with vomiting lead to rupture of the esophagus. First, a very rapid distention of the esophagus occurs, especially in the esophageal segment immediately above the diaphragm. Second, an anatomical weakness is present in the left lateral wall of the distal esophagus. In 1952 Mackler reported that if the cardia and upper end of the esophagus of cadavers were ligated and the esophagus inflated with air, 95% of esophagi ruptured on the left lateral side just above the cardia. The spiral fibers of the internal muscular layer give way under pressure to initiate the rupture.

Vomiting leading to Boerhaave's syndrome is often associated with alcohol ingestion (Fig 11–4), but the vomiting may be induced, as in Baron Wassenauer's case, or may be associated with the vomiting of pregnancy.

The laceration in the esophagus varies from 2–20 cm long. The mucosal tear usually extends farther than that of the muscle layers. The edges of the esophageal tear become irritated by regurgitated gastric secretions and rapidly become inflamed. The resulting edema and friability make suture closure difficult in perforations not treated within 24 hours of injury. Postemetic esophageal rupture is associated with forceful extrusion of gastric juice throughout the mediastinal planes, resulting in severe mediastinitis. Added to the gastric juice losses, the pleural outpouring of fluid in response to contamination may amount to several thousand milliliters in only a few hours, leading to hypovolemic shock.

Clinical Presentation

The characteristic presentation of a patient with Boerhaave's syndrome is that of forceful vomiting followed by acute, severe pain which may be localized to the upper abdomen or retrosternal area. Later, the pain may be referred to the patient's back. Patients have difficulty staying in a recumbent position. As the condition progresses, dyspnea may develop, followed by vascular collapse.

Physical examination reveals epigastric tenderness and abdominal wall resistance, but less than that seen in patients

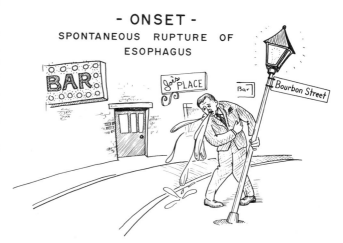

Fig 11–4.—Spontaneous rupture of esophagus may occur after forceful vomiting associated with excessive alcohol ingestion.

with a perforated peptic ulcer. Mediastinal emphysema may be found but is frequently a late sign and may not develop if the rupture proceeds through the pleura. Mediastinal air passes into the pleural space without the development of subcutaneous air.

Since spontaneous esophageal rupture is rare, physicians tend not to think of this disorder. The differential diagnosis includes pancreatitis, myocardial infarction, perforated peptic ulcer, strangulated hiatal hernia, dissecting aortic aneurysm, and spontaneous pneumothorax (Fig 11–5). While all of these conditions are associated with severe pain, they are not usually preceded by vomiting. The sequence of vomiting before pain is important in considering Boerhaave's syndrome; the other conditions give rise to pain first, followed by vomiting.

Diagnosis

A careful history may make the physician suspect esophageal perforation (Fig 11–6). The first diagnostic examination is a chest x-ray. Mediastinal widening, mediastinal or subcutaneous emphysema, and pleural effusion are the usual findings. Subcutaneous emphysema is present in about one half of patients. Hydrothorax is usually on the left but may be bilateral; pneumothorax may occur.

Aspiration of the pleural fluid to determine the amylase level may be confusing. The patient with a ruptured esophagus will swallow saliva, which enters the pleural space, giving the pleural fluid a high amylase content. Amylase isoenzyme studies will determine that the amylase is salivary in origin, not pancreatic, but such studies are not rapidly available. We have seen patients with spontaneous esophageal perforation mistakenly treated for acute pancreatitis because the "sympathetic effusion" had an elevated amylase level, thus confirming an erroneous diagnosis.

The definitive test is a Gastrografin study, which should be done immediately after the chest x-ray in patients suspected of having an esophageal perforation (Fig 11–7). If the Gastrografin esophagogram fails to show a leak, a barium esophagogram is done. Barium gives better contrast and may demon-

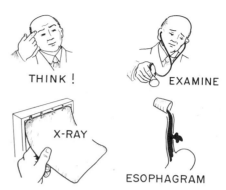

Fig 11–6.—The key to making the diagnosis of Boerhaave's syndrome is to think of the diagnosis. A gastrografin esophagogram will usually confirm the diagnosis.

strate a small leak. A prior Gastrografin study will rule out a large perforation, permitting barium to be used.

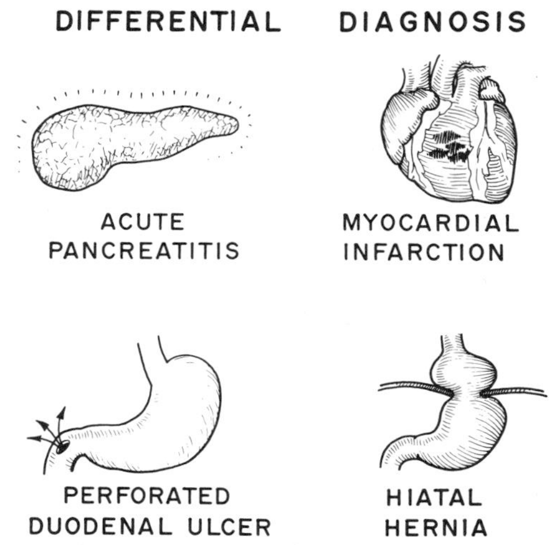

Treatment

Spontaneous perforation of the esophagus ideally is managed by prompt surgical intervention to close the site of perforation and widely drain the mediastinum. The only delay should be for emergency resuscitative measures. Antibiotic therapy to cover both gram-positive and gram-negative organisms should be started prior to operation. The interval between perforation and operative repair of the perforation influences the outcome. The mortality in our 12 patients was 25% when treatment was delayed longer than 24 hours, but no patient died when surgical treatment was initiated within 24 hours of esophageal perforation.

Operation is performed through a left posterolateral thoracotomy. After removal of necrotic and suppurative material, the site of esophageal perforation is visualized. If the esophageal wall appears viable and able to hold sutures, a primary repair is performed with nonabsorbable sutures in one or two layers. A pleural flap is raised to buttress the repair. The mediastinal pleura is incised up to the aortic arch to provide wide drainage of the mediastinum. Two chest tubes are usually inserted. A gastrostomy tube is placed for drainage of the stomach, and a jejunostomy tube for feeding. Immediately after operation, patients receive their nutritional support with parenteral hyperalimentation to reduce GI secretions. Later, enteric feedings may be given via the jejunostomy, although it is recognized that jejunostomy feedings stimulate gastric, pancreatic, biliary, and intestinal secretions.

Prognosis

Prior to Barrett's successful surgical repair in 1947, no patient was reported to have survived spontaneous esophageal perforation. Derbes in 1956 reported a series of 71 patients with Boerhaave's syndrome managed without operation. All died—60% within 24 hours and the rest by one week.

The prognosis has much improved in the past decade, with earlier recognition of the diagnosis and improved nutritional support of the patient. Symbas[36] reported a mortality of 22%

DIFFERENTIAL DIAGNOSIS

ACUTE PANCREATITIS

MYOCARDIAL INFARCTION

PERFORATED DUODENAL ULCER

HIATAL HERNIA

Fig 11–5.—Patients with spontaneous perforation of esophagus are frequently misdiagnosed when first seen by a physician.

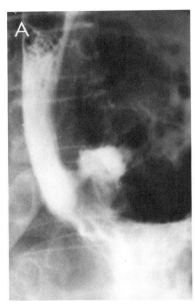
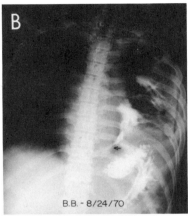
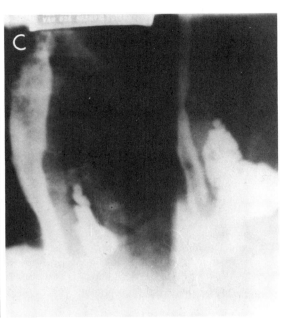

Fig 11–7.—A, gastrografin swallow in 39-year-old alcoholic showing Boerhaave's syndrome. **B,** gastrografin swallow 14 days after spontaneous rupture in a 41-year-old alcoholic. Esophageal perforation not recognized initially. **C,** gastrografin swallow showing esophageal perforation following rigid endoscopy.

and Grillo of 15%. Our mortality of 25% reported in 1975 is now under 10%, with no patient dying when operation to repair the esophageal perforation was done within 24 hours. Bradley and associates[37] from the Mayo Clinic report no deaths in patients with spontaneous rupture of the esophagus who had primary surgical repair within 24 hours. Only three of seven patients operated on after 24 hours survived. Two other patients treated conservatively, without operation, also died. Patients who come to operation after 24 hours may have an esophagus too friable for primary repair. Diversion followed by reconstruction is recommended for these patients.

Iatrogenic Perforations

Iatrogenic injuries, the most common cause of esophageal perforation, are most frequently due to endoscopy and bougienage. In 1957, Palmer reviewed 267,175 gastroscopies and reported 0.03% perforation, with a mortality of 15.5% in patients suffering an esophageal perforation. He also reviewed 40,450 rigid esophagoscopies with a 0.23% perforation and 23.2% mortality rate in patients with esophageal injury. Silvis in 1976 reviewed 211,410 fiberoptic esophagogastroscopy procedures. The perforation rate was 0.03% and the mortality for perforation was 4.3%.

The cricopharyngeal region is the site most commonly perforated by endoscopy. The lower end of the esophagus is the other area at risk.

Hydrostatic or pneumatic dilators for achalasia have been a frequent cause for iatrogenic esophageal perforation in our institution. Four of 40 patients so treated suffered esophageal perforation, while no patient sustained an esophageal leak from esophageal myotomy for achalasia.

External Trauma

Penetrating injuries of the neck or thorax from either gunshot or stab wounds may injure the esophagus. Gastrografin swallow will usually demonstrate the perforation. Blunt trauma to the neck more often injures the airway, but may avulse the esophagus from the pharynx.

The incidence of esophageal perforations continues to increase, more often from external trauma than iatrogenic injuries recently. At our hospital there was one case of esophageal perforation per 20,000 admissions during 1950–54. The incidence has risen to one case per 8,000 admissions.

Clinical Material

A review of 64 patients sustaining esophageal perforation at the Vanderbilt University Medical Center reported 10 patients with cervical esophageal perforations, 39 with thoracic esophageal perforations, and 15 with perforation in the abdominal esophagus. There were 45 males and 19 females, with an age range from 11 months to 78 years.[38] The cause of the ten cervical esophageal perforations was as follows: four perforations occurred during endoscopy and four from external trauma—three gunshot wounds and one stab wound from a sharp stick of wood. Foreign bodies (a dental prosthesis and a bone) were the cause of two perforations.

The causes of perforation of the thoracic esophagus were usually iatrogenic and followed endoscopy in 16 patients, dilatation in 6, rupture secondary to Sengstaken-Blakemore tube in two, penetration by Souttar's tube in 1, and paraesophageal surgical procedures (hiatus hernia repair 2 and vagotomy 1) in 3 patients. Spontaneous rupture occurred in five patients. Blunt trauma in two patients and a gunshot wound in one patient caused esophageal perforation. Three perforations were caused by foreign bodies.

The major cause of the abdominal esophageal perforations was paraesophageal surgery, during vagotomy in six patients and esophageal hiatus hernia repair in two patients. One patient perforated his esophagus by forcefully removing his Cantor tube. One perforation occurred during dilation, and three were from spontaneous rupture. In two patients, the perforation was thought to be secondary to an esophageal ulceration.

The signs and symptoms varied in relation to the location of the esophageal perforation. Neck pain and subcutaneous emphysema manifested by crepitus were frequent findings of cervical perforation. The most consistent symptom of thoracic perforation was chest pain, which usually occurred at the time of perforation and was frequently substernal. A significant temperature elevation was the next most frequent manifestation and usually occurred within a few hours. Upper abdominal pain, which occurred in 19 patients, often seemed to confuse the diagnosis. Crepitus was present in only eight patients; but the triad of chest pain, fever, and crepitus should establish the diagnosis of thoracic esophageal perforation. Crepitus was present in none of our 15 abdominal esophageal perforations, but upper abdominal pain and fever were frequent clinical findings.

Contrast roentgenographic studies with either a water-soluble medium or barium demonstrated a perforation in all but one of the patients who had this diagnostic examination.

The treatment of cervical esophageal perforations consisted of operation in all but one patient, who died. This patient sustained a perforation at the time of esophagogastroscopy. Antibiotic therapy was instituted at 36 hours when his neck was painful and swollen. The patient died after 96 hours of laryngeal edema and extensive cellulitis. All patients who had surgical treatment for cervical esophageal perforation survived.

Drainage is indicated treatment for all cervical esophageal perforations. Suture closure of the perforation should also be performed when technically feasible.

There were numerous treatments used for perforations of the thoracic and abdominal esophagus. The overall mortality for perforation in these sites was 35%. Thirty patients had suture closure drainage with seven deaths (23%). However, in patients who had early suture closure and drainage, there was only one death. Suture closure without drainage and drainage alone resulted in less satisfactory results than suture closure with drainage. In patients with underlying disease, such as achalasia, correction of the primary disorder should be done at the time of closure of the esophageal perforation.

The time between perforation and surgical treatment influenced the results of treatment. The mortality was more than four times as great when treatment was delayed for more than 24 hours (13% vs. 56%). Twenty-eight of the 32 patients treated within 24 hours lived, while only 10 of the 23 in whom treatment was delayed survived.

Perforation of the esophagus continues to be a challenge for physicians. The number of cases is not decreasing, even though iatrogenic perforations from instrumentation have been fewer in recent years. However, perforations from trauma, associated paraesophageal operations, and spontaneous perforation have increased.

Perforation of the esophagus should be treated surgically and treatment instituted promptly. The only delay should be for emergency resuscitative procedures. Inevitably, the availability of antibiotics induced conservative supportive measures with antibiotic therapy for small perforations. This misleading approach is still used. That some small perforations occasionally can be managed conservatively with success is not questioned; the difficulty in classifying a perforation as small, or in predicting the ultimate effects of a small perforation presents the real problem. Early suture closure when possible and drainage should be performed in all patients with esophageal perforation.

The surgeon's judgment becomes important in managing perforations of long standing. There is little advantage to placing sutures in an esophageal wall which obviously will not hold them. Adequate drainage is essential for these patients. Urschel and co-workers advocated esophageal exclusion and diversion in continuity—in addition to closure, drainage, nutritional support, and antibiotic therapy—for esophageal perforations that are diagnosed late. Their method of treatment involves placing a temporary ligature around the esophagus above the cardia to prevent gastroesophageal reflux that might interfere with healing. We have not used this procedure. Adkins advocated use of a fundic patch for treatment of later perforations in the distal esophagus. Rosoff and White favor a gastric serosal buttress. We agree with Skinner and associates[39] that resection or division should be used when primary closure of the perforation cannot be achieved. Reconstruction of the esophagus, usually by colon interposition, can be done later.

Selective nonoperative management for thoracic esophageal injuries has been advocated by Cameron and associates.[40] Eight patients with intrathoracic esophageal disruptions were treated without operation. The criteria are rigid. The esophageal disruption must be contained in the mediastinum or between the mediastinum and visceral lung pleura; the cavity must drain back into the esophagus; and the patient must have minimal symptoms with minimal signs of clinical sepsis. Patients were given broad-spectrum antibiotics and maintained on parenteral hyperalimentation until the esophagus healed. This treatment has limited application for patients with esophageal injury.

Eleven of our patients sustained esophageal perforation from paraesophageal surgical procedures, usually vagotomy. If perforation is recognized at the time of injury, immediate suture repair will usually result in healing without complications. In an extensive review of this subject, Postlethwait and associates reported 24 esophageal perforations occurring in 4,414 vagotomies, an incidence of 0.54%. Awareness of the possibility of esophageal wall perforation after a paraesophageal procedure may lead to early recognition and appropriate treatment.

When perforation occurs in an abnormal esophagus, a definitive operation for the underlying esophageal abnormality should be performed as well as closure of the perforation. Patients with achalasia who sustain an instrumental perforation are best treated by esophagocardiomyotomy in addition to early closure of the perforation. When perforation occurs in patients with carcinoma of the esophagus, immediate resection will provide a better result than closure and drainage.

REFERENCES

1. Ritter F.N., Gago O., Kirsh M.M., et al.: The rationale of emergency esophagogastrectomy in the treatment of liquid caustic burns of the esophagus and stomach. *Ann. Otol. Rhinol. Laryngol.* 80:513, 1971.
2. Leape L.L., Ashcraft K.W., Scarpelli D.G., et al.: Hazard to health—liquid lye. *N. Engl. J. Med.* 287:578, 1971.
3. Vancura E.M., Clinton J.E., Ruiz E., et al.: Toxicity of alkaline solution. *Ann. Emerg. Med.* 9:118, 1980.
4. Hollinger P.H.: Management of esophageal lesions caused by chemical burns. *Ann. Otol. Rhinol. Laryngol.* 77:819, 1968.
5. Kirsh M.M., Ritter F.: Caustic ingestion and subsequent damage to the oropharyngeal and digestive passages. *Ann. Thorac. Surg.* 21:75, 1976.
6. Burrington J.D.: Clinitest burns of the esophagus. *Ann. Thorac. Surg.* 20:400, 1975.
7. Lambert J.R., Newman A.: Ulceration and stricture of the esophagus due to oral potassium chloride (slow release tablet) therapy. *Am. J. Gastroenterol.* 73:508, 1980.
8. Walta D.C., Giddens J.D., Johnson L.F., et al.: Localized proximal esophagitis secondary to ascorbic acid ingestion and esophageal motor disorder. *Gastroenterology* 70:766, 1976.
9. Haller J.A. Jr., Andrews H.G., White J.J., et al.: Pathophysiology and management of acute corrosive burns of the esophagus: Results of treatment in 285 children. *J. Pediatr. Surg.* 6:578, 1971.
10. Gaudreault P., Parent M., McGuigan M.A., et al.: Predictability of esophageal injury from signs and symptoms: A study of caustic ingestion in 378 children. *Pediatrics* 71:767, 1983.
11. Symbas P.N., Vlasis S.E., Hatcher C.R.: Esophagitis secondary to ingestion of caustic material. *Ann. Thorac. Surg.* 36:73, 1983.
12. Cardona J.C., Daly J.F.: Current management of corrosive esophagitis. *Ann. Otol. Rhinol. Laryngol.* 80:521, 1971.
13. Hawkins D.B., Demeter M.J., Barnett T.E.: Caustic ingestion: Controversies in management. *Laryngoscope* 90:98, 1980.
14. Chung R.S.K., Den Besten L.: Fiberoptic endoscopy in treatment of corrosive injury of the stomach. *Arch. Surg.* 110:725, 1975.
15. Sugawa C., Mullins R.J., Lucas C.E., et al.: The value of early endoscopy following caustic ingestion. *Surg. Gynecol. Obstet.* 153:553, 1981.
16. Muhletaler C.A., Gerlock A.J. Jr., deSoto L., et al.: Acid corrosive esophagitis: Radiographic findings. *A.J.R.* 134:1137, 1980.
17. Martel W.: Radiologic features of esophagogastritis secondary to extremely caustic agents. *Radiology* 103:31, 1972.
18. Kirsh M.M., Peterson A., Brown J.W., et al.: Treatment of caustic injuries of the esophagus: A ten-year experience. *Ann. Surg.* 188:675, 1978.
19. Webb W.R., Koutras P., Ecker R.R., et al.: An evaluation of steroids and antibiotics in caustic burns of the esophagus. *Ann. Thorac. Surg.* 9:95, 1970.

20. Postlethwait R.W.: Chemical burns of the esophagus, in Postlethwait R.W. (ed.): *Surgery of the Esophagus.* New York, Appleton-Century-Crofts, 1979, pp. 286–317.
21. DiCostanzo J., Noirclerc M., Jonglard J., et al.: New therapeutic approach to corrosive burns of the upper gastrointestinal tract. *Gut* 21:370, 1980.
22. Kiviranta U.K.: Corrosion carcinoma of the esophagus. *Acta Otolaryngol. (Stokh.)* 42:89, 1952.
23. Ti T.K.: Oesophageal carcinoma associated with corrosive injury—Prevention and treatment by oesophageal resection. *Br. J. Surg.* 70:223, 1983.
24. Appelqvist P., Salmo M.: Lye corrosion carcinoma of the esophagus. *Cancer* 45:2655, 1980.
25. Hopkins R.A., Postlethwait R.W.: Caustic burns and carcinoma of the esophagus. *Ann. Surg.* 194:146, 1981.
26. Oakes D.D., Sherck J.P., Mark J.B.D.: Lye ingestion: Clinical patterns and therapeutic implications. *J. Thorac. Cardiovasc. Surg.* 83:194, 1982.
27. Spain D.M., Molomut N., Haber A.: The effect of cortisone on the formation of granulation tissue in mice. *Am. J. Pathol.* 26:710, 1950.
28. Rosenburg W., Kunderman P., Vroman L.: Prevention of experimental lye stricture by cortisone. *Arch. Surg.* 66:593, 1953.
29. Davis M.W., Madden J.W., Peacock E.E. Jr.: A new approach to the control of esophageal stenosis. *Ann. Surg.* 176:469, 1972.
30. Gehanno P., Guedon C.: Inhibition of experimental esophageal lye strictures by penicillamine. *Arch. Otolaryngol.* 107:145, 1981.
31. Mills L.J., Estera A.S., Platt M.R.: Avoidance of esophageal stricture following severe caustic burns by the use of an intraluminal stent. *Ann. Thorac. Surg.* 28:60, 1979.
32. Brun J.G., Celerier M., Koskas F., et al.: Blunt thorax oesophageal stripping: An emergency procedure for caustic ingestion. *Br. J. Surg.* 71:698, 1984.
33. Orringer M.B., Sloan H.: Esophagectomy without thoracotomy. *J. Thorac. Cardiovasc. Surg.* 76:643, 1978.
34. Rodgers B.M., Ryckman F.C., Talbert J.L.: Blunt transmediastinal total esophagectomy with simultaneous substernal colon interposition for esophageal caustic strictures in children. *J. Pediatr. Surg.* 16:184, 1981.
35. Berkowitz W.P., Roper C.L., Sessions D.G., et al.: Surgical management of severe lye burns of the esophagus by colon interposition. *Ann. Otol. Rhinol. Laryngol.* 84:576, 1975.
36. Symbas P.N., Hatcher C.R., Harlaftis N.: Spontaneous rupture of the esophagus. *Ann. Surg.* 187:634, 1978.
37. Bradley S.L., Pairoleo P.C., Payne W.S., et al.: Spontaneous rupture of the esophagus. *Arch. Surg.* 116:755, 1981.
38. Sawyers J.L., Lane C.E., Foster J.H., et al.: Esophageal perforation: An increasing challenge. *Ann. Thorac. Surg.* 19:233, 1975.
39. Skinner D.B., Little A.G., Demeester T.R.: Management of esophageal perforation. *Am. J. Surg.* 139:760, 1980.
40. Cameron J.L., Kieffer R.F., Hendrix T.R., et al.: Selective nonoperative management of contained intrathoracic esophageal disruptions. *Ann. Thorac. Surg.* 27:404, 1979.

PART III

Gastroduodenal Disease

12

The Pathogenesis of Acid-Peptic Disease

LAURENCE Y. CHEUNG, M.D.
STANLEY W. ASHLEY, M.D.

INTRODUCTION AND HISTORICAL PERSPECTIVE

The pathogenesis of acid-peptic disease has been the major interest of a host of investigators in a wide range of fields. Physiologists studying basic gastric processes have in part relied on the findings gleaned from pathologic models to delineate the normal mechanisms and patterns of secretion and motility. Likewise, endocrinologists, studying abnormal patterns of both gastrin production and the hormonal control of gastric secretion in peptic ulcer, have made important contributions to the relatively new field of GI endocrinology. Both surgeons and gastroenterologists, through very fundamental efforts to understand the basic pathogenesis of acid-peptic disease, have made major breakthroughs in the development of successful operative and medical therapies.

There is a long and complex history of scientific efforts in this area. Although ulcers of the stomach were first described by Galen, it was not until the 19th century that investigators began to speculate seriously about their etiology. One of the first theories was that of Gunzberg, who in 1852 attributed ulcers to an excessive acidity of gastric juice which he suggested might be the result of some disturbance in vagal control. About the same time, Virchow proposed that locally reduced blood supply might be responsible for the lesion. This theory held sway for much of the last century.

Studies by Claude Bernard and by William Beaumont, in his famous patient (Alexis St. Martin) with a gastric fistula, did much to increase our understanding of basic gastric physiology. In 1881 Heidenhain first prepared a cannulated pouch in dogs, separated from the rest of the stomach, which became an important model for the study of gastric secretion. A pupil of his, Pavlov, modified this pouch, keeping the vagus nerve intact, and used it to demonstrate the cephalic phase of gastric secretion with his famous sham feeding experiments. In 1910 Schwartz proposed his much quoted "no acid-no ulcer" dictum. About the same time, Edkins discovered a humoral factor in the gastric phase of acid secretion, gastrin. In 1941 Wangensteen, Varco, and Code took an important step toward our current understanding of peptic ulcer when they induced the lesion in dogs by injecting histamine and beeswax to prolong absorption and thus stimulation. In the mid-1940s, A. C. Ivy made one of the first major epidemiologic studies of the disease, estimating that approximately 10% of the American male population would have a peptic ulcer by age 65, a prevalence figure that has been quoted ever since. Lester Dragstedt's theories on the origin of both duodenal and gastric ulcer have had a significant impact on the direction of research in this area.[1] In 1935, based on canine experiments and a large patient experience, he hypothesized that hypersecretion of acid was the basis for duodenal ulcer and that this was in turn a consequence of vagal overactivity. Subsequently he suggested that gastric stasis with secondary hypergastrinemia was responsible for the lesion in gastric ulcer. Although his theories have largely been disproved, they dominated much of the thinking in this field until quite recently.

The past 25 years have witnessed a flurry of significant contributions in this area. Much of this work will be covered briefly, an exhaustive survey would be impossible. However, the identification of the major trends and directions in this most recent work does help to place our current concepts and understanding of acid-peptic disease in an evolutionary perspective.

Recent investigations have tended to follow one of three major approaches to examine the pathogenic basis of peptic ulcer. The most direct effort has been an attempt to identify the specific abnormalities present in patients with an ulcer diathesis. This work has included studies of secretion, motility, endocrine relationships, environmental and psychologic factors, epidemiologic data, risk factors, genetics, and disease associations. Although much of this work has been very fruitful, there have been numerous obstacles to real progress in this type of approach. Among the major problems has been the distinction between abnormalities which are actual causal factors and those that merely represent a consequence of the disease process itself. In addition, while many specific defects have been identified in acid-peptic disease, many of these are detected in only a small subpopulation of those afflicted. This has inevitably raised questions about the significance of any single finding. The relatively recent recognition of the theory of heterogeneity in peptic ulcer—the concept that ulcer is not one but a group of disorders—has done much to clarify this variety of findings.[2] The analogy has been made between our current understanding of acid-peptic disease and that of anemia before the recognition that a variety of pathophysiologic mechanisms might be responsible for the single common clinical presentation. As will be discussed, evidence for this heterogeneity continues to accumulate, and investigators are only now beginning to sort out the specifics of this variety of pathogenic entities, which all become manifest as a defect in the lining of the gastroduodenum. While doing much to explain previous inconsistencies in the findings of various studies, this recognition raises the possibility that a number of important abnormalities have been overlooked by past studies that considered all ulcer patients as a single group.

In contrast to these direct efforts to understand the etiology of acid-peptic disease, other recent researchers have approached this problem by more basic investigations of normal gastric physiology. There have been major breakthroughs in our understanding of gastric secretion, ion transport, motility, and neuroendocrine regulation. Gregory's synthesis of gastrin, the development of histamine H_2-receptor antagonists, the use of single-cell culture techniques, the clarification of regulatory mechanisms in the intestinal phase of acid-secretion, and the identification and isolation of the $H^+ - K^+$ adenosine triphosphatase (ATPase) are just a few of the many important discoveries of the past two decades. Their significance rests not only in improving our understanding of the normal gastroduodenum but also in providing a sound context for the study of physiologic derangements in peptic ulcer.

The third pattern of investigation has been an effort to determine the factors responsible for protection and repair of the stomach during injury. Under normal conditions, a balance exists between the acid-peptic secretory process and the factors defending the gastroduodenal mucosa against injury. Traditionally, most research on the pathogenesis of chronic peptic ulcer has centered on an analysis of the abnormal secretory mechanisms which might disrupt this balance. On the other hand, beginning with Code and Davenport's concept of the gastric mucosal barrier, investigators of acute mucosal lesions have focused on the mechanisms of mucosal defense. This separation between secretory abnormalities in chronic lesions and disorders of defense in acute lesions has been a useful, although perhaps somewhat artificial, distinction for a number of reasons. First, in at least some patients with chronic acid-peptic disease, particularly duodenal ulcer and definitely Zollinger-Ellison syndrome, acid-pepsin hypersecretion seems to be the critical factor. In addition, except in the case of Curling's ulcer, an acute erosion seen after burn injuries, there is little evidence that an actual increase in the quantity or corrosiveness of gastric secretion is responsible for acute injury. Rather, acute erosive gastritis usually occurs either in the context of severe injury or illness or after the exposure of the gastric mucosa to specific injurious agents, both suggesting some basic defect of mucosal defense. Several excellent animal models for the study of acute lesions have been developed and have permitted a careful analysis of the role of such factors as the gastric mucosal barrier and mucosal blood flow in protecting the gastroduodenum against acute injury. On the other hand, no really good experimental model exists for chronic ulceration, and investigators have been limited in their pathogenic studies to human patients. In this context, the detection of defensive disturbances is much more difficult than any exploration of secretory abnormalities. However, recently this distinction between an acid-peptic basis for chronic disease and a disorder in defense for acute lesions has become less clear. While the role of hypersecretion in some forms of chronic ulceration cannot be overestimated, it has become evident that in many cases, particularly in chronic gastric ulceration, a disorder in defense is responsible. The recognition that some patients with gastrinoma and marked hypersecretion do not develop ulcerations has further emphasized the importance of protective mechanisms in chronic disease. The roles of abnormalities in mucous secretion, bicarbonate formation, blood flow, epithelial renewal, and prostaglandin production are just beginning to be examined. This, more than any other area, seems to be the direction in which investigators are turning for future studies. While this subject of mucosal defense is discussed in greater detail in chapter 13 on acute lesions, an analysis of the pathogenesis of acid-peptic disease would be incomplete without some mention of this exciting topic.

ACID-PEPTIC DISEASE: GENERAL COMMENTS

In the most general sense, acid-peptic disease refers to any abnormality of the GI tract that results from the corrosive action of acid and pepsin. This includes acute lesions and chronic peptic ulcer. The esophagus, although normally protected from gastric secretions by the complex mechanisms that prevent esophageal reflux, is very susceptible to pepsin and acid digestion. Likewise, when exposed to gastric secretion following gastroenterostomy or from a Meckel's diverticulum with ectopic gastric mucosa, the lining of the more distal small intestine is by no means resistant to acid-peptic injury. This chapter will concentrate on the pathogenesis of the more common problems of duodenal and gastric ulcer.

Peptic ulcer is a chronic and recurrent disease. Usually the ulcers are less than 1 cm in diameter, sharply demarcated, and, as opposed to the superficial lesions of acute ulceration, extend down through the muscularis mucosae to the submucosa and even into the muscularis. The pathology is relatively simple—the ulcer bed is a zone of necrosis resting on granulation tissue surrounded by variable amounts of fibrosis.

Peptic ulcer is a worldwide disease which has been estimated to affect between 6% and 15% of the population of the western hemisphere at some point in their lifetime.[3] A decade ago it was estimated that it afflicted approximately 10 million people in the United States, with an estimated medical cost of more than $2 billion per year. There is considerable evidence, which will be discussed, that the incidence of at least duodenal ulcer has decreased markedly in the United States and England. This reported decline in incidence is only one part of a more profound change in almost every aspect of our knowledge and understanding of peptic ulcer disease in recent years.[4] Inevitably this evolution has had a major impact on the general surgeon. No longer is this illness a mainstay of surgical training, research, or practice. The reasons for this trend include not only these reported differences in disease prevalence but also changes in presentation, complications, and treatment. However, acid-peptic disease remains a major source of morbidity and mortality that every surgeon can expect to encounter on multiple occasions. Now, more than ever before, the choice between various treatment options depends on a firm understanding of the etiology and pathogenesis of peptic ulceration.

While our knowledge of the etiologies in acid-peptic disease has improved, the complexity of its pathogenic basis has become increasingly evident. Both duodenal and gastric ulcer are defined by an interplay of many factors. The simple pathologic process occurs within a context of hereditary, psychologic, and environmental forces, which all influence its mode of expression. In some areas our knowledge is still very rudimentary. In this chapter, after a brief discussion of relevant normal gastric physiology, it is hoped that by reviewing separately the epidemiology, heredity, risk factors, associations, and pathophysiology of this disease, a clear picture of its pathogenesis will emerge. The traditional separation between duodenal and gastric ulcer is valid not only on an anatomical basis but also on these pathogenic grounds, and will be the format for organization of this review.

NORMAL GASTRIC PHYSIOLOGY RELATED TO ACID-PEPTIC DISEASE

The stomach really performs two main functions in the initial phase of digestion.[5] Swallowed food enters and is exposed to the proteolytic action of acid and pepsin. The stomach reservoir mixes gastric secretions and food to form a more uniform consistency chyme, which it releases in small boluses, slowly, into the duodenum. Derangements in both the secretory process itself and the reservoir capacity of the stomach have been implicated in the pathogenesis of acid-peptic disease.

Acid itself is secreted directly by parietal cells in the body and fundus of the stomach through an active mechanism involving the recently characterized $H^+ - K + ATPase$ and a carbonic anhydrase. The estimated HCl concentration of parietal cell secretions is approximately 160 mM. This product is mixed with pepsinogen from chief cells and the alkaline and mucous secretions of surface epithelial cells. Acid secretory capacity correlates fairly well with the absolute number of parietal cells. The basis for control of acid secretion at the cellular level is still incompletely defined, but isolated cell studies seem to validate the three component hypotheses of interacting receptors for gastrin, histamine, and acetycholine, each of which has direct and independent effects, while their combination results in an augmentation of response.

Regulation of gastric function itself is a complex process involving intimately related neural, endocrine, and paracrine factors. The neural mechanisms involve local reflex arcs within Meissner and Auerbach's plexuses and more distant control mechanisms involving the vagus nerve. Vagal activity increases secretion by direct stimulation of parietal cells, by increasing gastrin release from the antrum, and by lowering the parietal cell threshold to circulating gastrin. Gastrin is actually a family of polypeptides, produced mainly by the antrum but also by the proximal duodenum. Two forms seem to be important—gastrin-17 (G-17), a smaller, shorter half-life molecule, which is both the major form found in antral tissue and the primary hormonal stimulus to secretion, and gastrin-34 (G-34), or "big gastrin," which is the primary circulating

form of the hormone. Histamine is present in large concentrations in mast cells of the body of the stomach and, although its importance in acid secretion has been confirmed by the efficacy of H_2-receptor antagonists, its exact role has yet to be completely defined. A number of other secretagogues including caffeine, calcium, alkaline pH, and glucagon have been identified, and although some of their effects seem to be mediated through gastrin release, their exact mechanism of action remains obscure.

Gastric secretion in response to food, the major physiologic stimulus to acid secretion, has traditionally been divided into three phases. The first, the cephalic phase, represents the response to sight, smell, and taste of food and is mediated through vagal activity which directly stimulates the parietal cells and also releases gastrin from the antrum. The second gastric phase results from both the mechanical stimulation of distention acting through vagal reflex arcs and the direct release of gastrin from the antrum by food. Intact food is not responsible for this release; in fact, it is really only the small peptide and amino acid products of protein digestion which can directly stimulate the antral G cells. Finally, food entering the duodenum initiates the third, complex, intestinal phase of acid secretion. This appears to be mediated through several pathways. Small peptides and amino acids are absorbed into the portal circulation and then act directly to stimulate parietal cell secretion. Gastrin, released from the endocrine cells of the proximal duodenum, may also have a role. In addition, some as yet unidentified hormone may be in part responsible.

Inhibition of gastric secretion is equally complex. Acid itself bathes the antral mucosa and blocks the release of gastrin. In addition, the products of gastric secretion act through a variety of neural and hormonal mechanisms. Hyperglycemia and fatty acids, monoglycerides, and hypertonic solutions in the duodenum all seem to inhibit the secretory mechanisms. Secretin, cholecystokinin, somatostatin, gastric inhibitory peptide, urogastrone, and vasoactive intestinal peptide may all serve at some level to mediate this control. The integration of this complex system is still only partially understood. Figure 12–1 illustrates some of these multiple, coexistent regulatory mechanisms.

Pepsin secretion, in most respects, is controlled by the same factors which regulate hydrochloric acid secretion. Pepsin seems to be integrally related with acid in the production of tissue damage. It is released into the stomach in an inactive form, pepsinogen, which is activated under acidic conditions. The variety of pepsinogens (PGs) have been classified by immunologic techniques as either PGI, which is found only in the corpus and PGII, which is also present in the pylorus, cardia, and duodenum. Both can be detected in plasma, while only PGI is present in urine. Blood PGI concentrations seem to correlate fairly closely with maximal acid secretory capacity.

Gastric motility is a well-coordinated function involving receptive relaxation and coordinated peristaltic contractions involving the antrum, the pylorus, and the proximal duodenum. In addition there is a propulsive and retropulsive activity in the antrum which serves to grind and mix food. Motility is regulated through a complex electrical system consisting of a

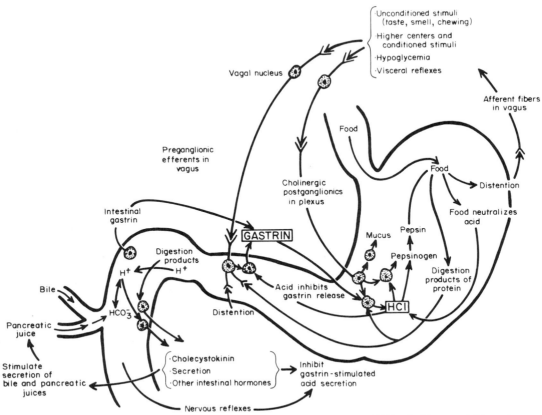

Fig 12–1.—Some of the major factors responsible for control of gastric secretion. (Reproduced with permission from Davenport H.W.: *A Digest of Digestion,* ed. 2. Copyright 1978 by Year Book Medical Publishers, Inc., Chicago.)

pacemaker in the mid-body, which establishes a baseline electrical rhythm and an electrical-response activity, consisting of spike potentials associated with muscle contraction. These in turn are controlled by cholinergic and adrenergic neural reflexes and by the GI hormones, particularly gastrin, secretin, and cholecystokinin. The pylorus remains open most of the time but appears to act as a one-directional sphincter and closes after the passage of food to prevent reflux. Derangements in these mechanisms seem to be major factors in the development of at least some forms of acid-peptic disease.

In addition to the digestive functions, several other physiologic mechanisms are important in understanding normal gastric activity. As with the rest of the GI tract, mucosal cell turnover is a major process, the surface epithelial cells being replaced every three to six days by a process under the control of trophic hormones and GI regulatory peptides such as gastrin. Gastric mucus, containing mucopolysaccharides and glycoproteins, is produced by surface epithelial cells and serves to coat and lubricate the mucosal surface. About three fourths of the population secrete AB(H) blood group substances in their mucus and are referred to as secretors as opposed to nonsecretors. Bicarbonate is another important secretory product of mucus cells. The possible role of an unstirred mucus and bicarbonate layer at the surface of the epithelia, moderating the effects of acidic luminal contents on the surface cells is just beginning to be explored.[6]

Gastric blood flow, particularly mucosal, seems to be inti-

mately related with normal gastric physiology. Increases in mucosal blood flow correlate fairly closely with increases in acid secretion, mucosal repair, and resistance to injury. Finally, the relatively impermeable gastric mucosal barrier keeps acid within the lumen, where it can perform its normal digestive functions. The barrier is provided by both the cell surfaces and the intercellular tight junctions, which are particularly resistant in the body of the stomach. That these factors may participate in mucosal protection from acid-pepsin in chronic ulcer is unproved but seems very likely. While mucous and bicarbonate production occur in the duodenum, neither the same capacity to increase mucosal blood flow nor the degree of mucosal barrier is found in the stomach. This may have some role in the proximal duodenal anatomical distribution of ulcers in association with hypersecretion. The importance of gastric mucosal injury and barrier disruption by reflux of duodenal contents or agents such as aspirin in permitting chronic gastric ulcer will be discussed.

Thus a host of normal mechanisms are responsible for the usual pattern of gastric functions. The heterogeneous group of acid-peptic diseases may be the result of disruptions in any number of these mechanisms.

PATHOGENESIS OF DUODENAL ULCER

More than 95% of duodenal ulcers occur in the first portion of the duodenum, and approximately 90% of these are located within 3 cm of the junction of the pyloric and duodenal mucosa.[7] This distribution suggests the importance of gastric acid in their pathogenesis. Only in the massive hypersecretory state of Zollinger-Ellison syndrome is it common to see ulcerations beyond the duodenal bulb. Acid hypersecretion has been the most important feature distinguishing duodenal from gastric ulcerations, and this distinction in general has survived the recent refinements in our knowledge of this disease.

As mentioned above, it is useful to separate our discussion on the basis of the types of studies which have been used to explore the pathogenic basis of duodenal ulceration. In general, researchers have approached this subject by epidemiologic studies, through a genetic approach, in terms of risk factors and disease associations, and finally, by directly examining psychologic and physiologic abnormalities.

Epidemiologic Patterns

Epidemiologic data provide a number of clues to the pathogenesis of duodenal ulcer. Trends in incidence and prevalence can help to establish a pattern of causality for the disease process itself. There are many difficulties in interpreting the data, however; investigators have used a variety of different criteria for diagnosis, and the intermittency of symptoms further complicates these studies. While approximately 10% of the population in the United States develops duodenal ulcer, only 1%–2% actually have active disease at any given time.[8]

There is a great deal of geographical variation in ulcer incidence.[9] While gastric ulcer is more frequent in the Far East, particularly Japan, duodenal ulcer is the most common entity in most of the rest of the world. In Africa, duodenal ulcer, presenting frequently with obstruction, is most common on the west coast. It is also two to four times as frequent in Scotland as England. In India, duodenal ulcer, often with pyloric obstruction, is more prevalent in the rice-eating south than in the northern regions, where wheat is the primary crop. In general the incidence of duodenal ulcer diagnosis increases with advancing age of the population, but in India it occurs in younger patients with a very high male-to-female ratio of approximately 30 to 1. In the United States the incidence of duodenal ulcer in males is double or triple that in females.

In most studies race does not appear to be an important factor. However, there is evidence that the mortality may be somewhat higher for non-whites before the age of 65. In southwestern American Indians, the frequency of duodenal ulcer is one-fortieth that in American whites, although it is difficult to attribute this solely to racial factors. Few conclusions can be drawn from the data on occupational and social factors. Studies in this area are small, but the main variation detected is the tendency for duodenal ulcer to be more frequent in the less skilled professions and the lower socioeconomic groups. A study from York in England suggested a higher incidence for urban than country dwellers, supporting the common speculation that urbanization may play a role in the pathogenesis.[3] Very little epidemiologic data exist to distinguish various patterns for chronicity and recurrence. For duodenal ulcer in this country, it does appear that periods of freedom from pain usually occur during the summer months.

Perhaps the most interesting epidemiologic data concern recent trends in the incidence of duodenal ulcer. Until the late 19th century, duodenal ulcer was so rare as to be almost unrecognized. Subsequently there was a fairly steady increase in the incidence of ulcer, until the time of A. C. Ivy's American surveys in the 1940s, which estimated a 10% prevalence figure in the United States. Recently several studies in both America and Europe have reported significant declines in the numbers of hospitalizations, complications, operations, and mortality due to duodenal ulcer.[4] A host of explanations, ranging from changes in dietary patterns to a relationship with the end of large-scale European immigrations, have been provided for this phenomenon. The suggestion that cimetidine may have played a role has been largely disproved. Evidence for these trends begins 20 years before the H_2-receptor antagonist really came into widespread use, in 1977, and there is no evidence that the drug has any long-term effects on the course of disease. Many studies have questioned whether this trend really exists. Bonnevie found little change in the incidence of duodenal ulcer in Copenhagen for the period 1963–78.[7] A recent analysis of admissions to a large health maintenance organization in California failed to demonstrate any downward trend (Fig 12–2).[10] It has been suggested that these apparent changes may be more a reflection of other factors such as a change in hospital disease classifications, an increase in patient self-medication with antacids, a greater willingness to treat ulcer patients as outpatients, and an improved diagnostic approach to peptic ulcer with the advent of more

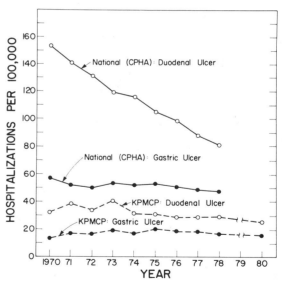

Fig 12–2.—Hospitalization discharge rates for gastric and for duodenal ulcer for the years 1970–1980. While the national data from the Commission on Professional and Hospital Activities (CPHA) suggests a marked drop in the incidence of duodenal ulcer, there was no change in rates for the Kaiser-Permanente Medical Care Program (KPMCP), a large California health maintenance organization. (Reprinted by permission of the publisher from Kurata J.H., Honda G.D., Frankl H.L.: Hospitalization and mortality rates for peptic ulcers: A comparison of a large health maintenance organization and United States data. *Gastroenterology* 83:1008, 1982. Copyright 1982 by the American Gastroenterological Association.)

widespread endoscopy. In any event, at present no firm conclusions can be drawn about the direction of these trends in the incidence of duodenal ulcer.

Epidemiologic studies do little to examine directly the pathogenesis of acid-peptic disease. However, they have generated evidence that patterns of life-style, diet, and economics may play a role in this process. Many of these studies have been limited by past uncertainty about the accuracy of diagnosis and by a failure to distinguish duodenal and gastric ulcer. It is hoped that as criteria become more standardized, epidemiologic studies will be more revealing.

Genetic Abnormalities

There is no question now that genetic factors are important in the pathogenesis of peptic ulcer. The strongest evidence for the relatively new concept of heterogeneity in peptic ulcer, perhaps the most important of the recent advances in our understanding of this disease, comes from genetic studies. Until quite recently it was thought that peptic ulcer was a single polygenic disease, the result of interactions between many different genes and environmental factors. The recent recognition of several distinct, genetically-determined subcategories of peptic ulcer has suggested instead that it is a heterogeneous group of different diseases, in some instances the result of simple Mendelian genetics, all of which present as an ulcer of the gastroduodenum.[2]

A host of studies has provided important evidence for the genetic basis of peptic ulcer.[11] Twenty to fifty percent of duodenal ulcer patients have a positive family history of duodenal ulcer in contrast to 10%–15% of controls. The increased familial risk is site specific—family members of a patient with duodenal ulcer also develop duodenal, not gastric ulcers. Even the entity of combined gastric and duodenal ulcers seems to have a separate familial aggregation. Twin studies have documented an increased concordance of duodenal ulcer in monozygotic over dizygotic twins. However, this is a less than 100% concordance, demonstrating that other factors also do have a role. Duodenal ulcers are also associated with several genetic marker traits. In contrast with other blood types, blood group O is associated with a 30% increase in incidence. Secretors of blood group antigens into the body fluids, as opposed to nonsecretors, have a 50% increase in the risk of duodenal ulcer. Several studies have suggested associations of HLA types, specifically B5 and B12, with duodenal ulcer.

The most dramatic evidence for genetic heterogeneity has come from the recognition of a number of rare genetic syndromes which all seem to include peptic ulcer as a component of the phenotype.[12] The best known is probably multiple endocrine adenoma type I, an autosomal dominant, variable penetrance disorder, characterized by parathyroid, pituitary, and, most important, pancreatic neoplasms which may be gastrinomas, producing the Zollinger-Ellison syndrome. Systemic mastocytosis, which has both dominant and recessive pedigrees, is a rare disorder characterized by histamine-producing mast cell infiltration of many tissues and a 30%–40% incidence of duodenal ulcer. An autosomal dominant disorder of tremor, nystagmus, narcolepsy, and ulcer has also been described. Amyloidosis type IV, stiff-skin syndrome (pachydermoperiostosis), and hereditary leukonychia totalis all have been associated genetically with duodenal ulcer.

Finally, a number of discrete genetic subtypes of the more common duodenal ulcer have been identified by means of both biochemical and physiologic marker abnormalities.[8] Among these is the association, in some patients, of duodenal ulcer with an elevated serum pepsinogen I. These levels are elevated in 30%–50% of duodenal ulcer patients. In a subgroup of this disease, there is an autosomal dominant pattern of inheritance for this characteristic and the risk of duodenal ulcers is increased only in hyperpepsinogenic siblings. There is another subgroup of duodenal ulcer patients for whom normopepsinogenemia is familially aggregated. In this group, only the normopepsinogenemic siblings have an increased incidence. In another subgroup of common duodenal ulcer, a familial association of the disease with a pattern of rapid gastric emptying has been demonstrated. At least in some other cases, antral G-cell hyperplasia appears to be an inherited trait underlying the development of duodenal ulcer although its specific genetic pattern has not yet been identified. It has also been suggested that childhood duodenal ulcer may have a familial basis. Fifty percent of childhood patients have a positive family history, compared with 20% of adults. In this group, there is no association between ulcer and blood group O.

In summary, genetic abnormalities have been demonstrated to be a major factor in several rare syndromes of peptic ulceration. In addition, they have become an important tool for defining subgroups in the population of common duodenal ulceration. There is little doubt that further genetic patterns will be documented in the future.

Risk Factors

Any disease as common as peptic ulcer develops a host of folklore associations which become very difficult to validate or disprove. A large number of environmental factors have been suggested as inciting agents, but very few have been definitely documented.

There is fairly definite evidence that cigarette smoking is associated with an increased incidence of duodenal ulcers.[13] Smokers seem to be about twice as likely to develop ulcers as nonsmokers, although most of the studies of this subject failed to differentiate duodenal and gastric ulcer. The mortality of ulcer is higher for smokers, although this may be more related to the secondary pulmonary disease than to the ulcer itself. Smoking also impairs the healing of ulcers. Nicotine has been demonstrated to decrease pancreatic bicarbonate secretion and increase duodenogastric reflux. It has been suggested but not proved that these may be the major basis for its effect on the disease process. On the other hand, alcohol does not appear to be a risk factor for duodenal ulcer. In man it is a very weak stimulant of acid secretion, and, although in high concentrations it may result in acute gastric mucosal injury, there is some evidence that moderate consumption may even favor ulcer healing.

There are no really solid data that diet has a role in the pathogenesis of acid-peptic disease.[9] Most patients do report that particular foods seem to exacerbate their symptoms, but it is very difficult to test the common belief that a bland diet actually improves ulcer healing. However, a few studies have implicated dietary patterns. In India, the difference between the low incidence of ulcers in the wheat-eating north and the high incidence of ulcers in the rice-eating south has been suggested to result from an increase in salivary secretion with the wheat diet.[7] Saliva does have a high concentration of epidermal growth factor, which inhibits acid secretion and stimulates epithelial renewal. One study suggested that, in college students, consuming milk was associated with a decrease and coffee and soft drinks with an increase in the later development of duodenal ulcers.[7] Caffeine itself is a rather weak stimulant of acid secretion, but coffee and soft drinks seem to be strong stimulants. However, there is no other really good evidence to implicate any of these dietary effects.

Several drugs have been incriminated in the pathogenesis of acid-peptic disease, although few studies have distinguished between duodenal and gastric ulcer.[13] Aspirin and the nonsteroidal anti-inflammatory agents have been fairly definitely implicated, although the evidence is much stronger for gastric than duodenal ulcers. Steroids, reserpine, and aminophylline have all been considered, but the evidence is still equivocal.

Disease Associations

The establishment of an association between two diseases is fraught with problems, particularly in the case of an illness as common as peptic ulcer. It requires rigorous patient and control selection criteria—and even then is plagued by the bias of hospital referral patterns and chance; the greater likelihood that a patient with one disease will have other diagnostic tests which recognize some unnoticed condition; and the sensitivity of each of the variety of diagnostic modalities that may be used to establish a diagnosis. As mentioned, duodenal ulcer has been definitely associated with a number of rare genetic conditions. In addition, it is the most characteristic feature of gastrin-producing islet cell tumors. However, most other associations are at best probable.

There does seem to be an increased incidence of peptic ulcer in patients with chronic pulmonary disease.[7] Even when the data are corrected for the predominance in the pulmonary disease group of male smokers, who would be expected to have an increase, the association persists. The mechanisms for this have not been elucidated. It is unrelated to the degree of pulmonary disease or the treatment used and, in fact, the ulcer often precedes the pulmonary problems. In addition to the more common chronic obstructive pulmonary conditions, cystic fibrosis, α_1-antitrypsin deficiency, and carcinoma of the lung all have been suggested as associations with duodenal ulcer, but firm evidence is lacking.

Cirrhosis appears to be associated with a two- to three-fold increase in the incidence of duodenal ulcer. However, the control data in most studies are inadequate, and it is difficult to draw any strong conclusions. Acid secretion is normal in cirrhotic patients, and it has been suggested that altered mucosal blood flow in the context of portal hypertension may play a role. Duodenal ulcers probably occur with increased frequency after renal transplantation, and the mortality rate is very high. Some of the concern about a relation between steroid use and ulcer has been generated in this group of patients. An association with chronic renal failure in general has been suggested, but this evidence is inconclusive. Uremia actually tends to decrease the level of acid secretion.

A host of other associations have been suggested. An increased risk of duodenal ulcer has been reported with coronary artery disease, renal stones, hyperparathyroidism, polycythemia vera, chronic pancreatitis, carcinoid syndrome, myasthenia gravis, and aortic aneurysms. The evidence for these associations is very weak.

Several other diseases may actually be associated with a decrease in ulcer incidence. Patients with achlorhydria and pernicious anemia and atrophic gastritis rarely develop peptic ulcer. There is fairly convincing evidence that hypertension can confer some protection against duodenal ulcer. Addison's disease, hypoparathyroidism, and diabetes mellitus all have been claimed to result in a decrease in incidence; firm evidence is lacking.

The association, or lack of one, in these disorders suggests some common pathophysiologic factor that is important in both disease processes. Little is yet known about these factors, but their recognition should help to enhance our understanding of the pathogenesis of both disorders.

Psychological Abnormalities

Peptic ulcer is one of the disease entities for which the psychosomatic theory of the origin for medical illness has been most strongly argued.[14] Empirical observation has repeatedly suggested that stressful life events and anxiety-producing situations affect the course of the individual patient's illness and may even be important in its genesis. However, no one has yet been able actually to document that psychodynamic factors play a role in peptic ulcer.

There is little question that emotion does affect gastric function. The observations of William Beaumont in his chronic gastric fistula patient, Alexis St. Martin, demonstrated a change in acid secretion and blood flow with emotional stimulation that has been repeatedly confirmed in more recent studies. One study in an 18-month-old child with a fistula suggested that psychodynamic states not only affect acid secretion directly but also may alter the stomach's sensitivity to other stimulation—the response to exogenous histamine was increased when this patient was interacting with others but actually fell when she was withdrawn.[7] Emotions probably do not have the same impact in all patients. In one study of the effects of hypnotically-induced emotion on acid secretion, patients with lower anxiety levels unexpectedly developed a higher acid secretion under anger conditions while those with high anxiety suppressed acid (Fig 12–3).[15]

Efforts to link psychological patterns to duodenal ulcer have attempted to characterize a personality type in whom ulcers are likely to develop. This effort has been hampered by our basic inability to define personality types in general. The common stereotype of the "ulcer personality" as an aggressive, hyperactive, overworked professional has been clearly disproved. Psychoanalytic studies of the 1930s suggested that a central feature was an excessive dependency-independency conflict. In one prospective study, a group of military recruits was selected on the basis of this type of conflict and simultaneously elevated plasma pepsinogens.[14] A significant number were found to have or to develop duodenal ulcers over the basic training periods. Others, however, have rejected this concept of a dependency conflict.

Frequent attempts have been made to correlate psychologic stress with the development of peptic ulcer. In animals,

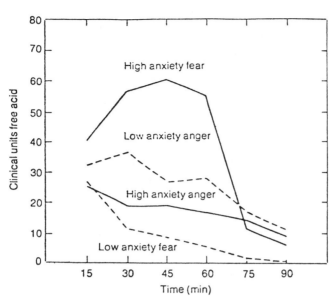

Fig 12–3.—Comparison of acid secretion in subjects with high levels of anxiety and those with low levels of anxiety when exposed to hypnotically induced fear or anger. (From Eichorn R., Trackter T.: The relationship between anxiety, hypnotically induced emotion and gastric secretion. *Gastroenterology* 29:422, 1955. Copyright 1955 by the Williams & Wilkins, Co., Baltimore.)

restraint and avoidance experiments seem to indicate a role for stress in the development of acute lesions. In human studies, however, this has been very difficult to evaluate, because for any given situation the amount of real stress experienced is in part, subjective. During the bombing of London, there was an increase in the incidence of perforated ulcers (Fig 12–4).[16] One study failed to document any increase in the incidence of peptic ulcer in air traffic controllers, who are generally considered to work in a stressful environment.[14]

In summary, the importance of psychological factors in

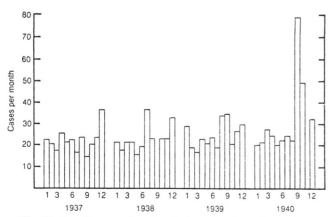

Fig 12–4.—Cases of perforated peptic ulcer charted each month from 1937 to 1940 in 16 London hospitals. The peak incidence correlates with the heaviest blitzkrieg of September and October, 1940. (From Stewart D.N., Winser D.M., De R.: Incidence of perforated ulcer. *Lancet* 1:259, 1942. Used by permission.)

duodenal ulcer remains controversial. It seems likely that, at least in some patients, a variety of psychic conflicts and stresses could upset the balance of secretion and mucosal defense in favor of peptic ulceration; however, the details of this mechanism and its proof are still lacking.

Physiologic Disturbances

A wide variety of physiologic abnormalities have been demonstrated in some but not all patients with duodenal ulcer. It is likely that, in most cases, this variation results from the heterogeneity of the disease. In general three main types of abnormality have been detected in duodenal ulcer—disturbances of acid secretion, gastric motility, and acid disposal and defense.

ABNORMALITIES OF ACID SECRETION.—Duodenal ulcer has been generally associated with hypersecretion of acid. Patients tend to secrete more acid at rest and in response to stimulation than normal controls. On the average, they have a maximal acid output of about 40 mM/hour as opposed to 20 mM/hour in controls (Fig 12–5).[17] However, there is considerable overlap, and most ulcer patients have acid outputs in the normal range. In fact, there appears to be no relationship between the degree of acid hypersecretion and the severity of the ulcer diathesis as measured by the number and magnitude of complications.

This increase in secretory capacity probably results from several different physiologic abnormalities. First, duodenal ulcer patients have an average of 1.8 billion parietal cells as compared with about one billion in normals, but again there is a great deal of overlap.[6] Parietal and chief cell numbers seem to increase together, and pepsin probably plays a role in the development of ulceration, although this has not yet been proven. Several attempts to treat ulcers with pepsin inhibitors have met with little or no success. The basis for the increase in parietal cell numbers has not yet been established, but numerous etiologies have been proposed. One suggestion is that the patients with an increase in parietal cells represent the same subset distinguished by hyperpepsinogenemia I. Thus these patients may develop the pattern of hypersecretion and hyperpepsinogenemia on the basis of simple genetic inheritance. In other cases, however, this abnormality is

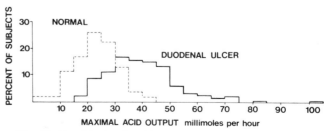

Fig 12–5.—Maximal acid response to IV infusion of histamine in normal men and men with duodenal ulcer. Median value is significantly greater in the duodenal ulcer patients, although the overlap is considerable, and about 70% of duodenal ulcer patients fall within the normal range. (From data of Kirkpatrick et al. Reproduced with permission from Grossman M.I. (ed.): *Peptic Ulcer: A Guide for the Practicing Physician.* Chicago, Year Book Medical Publishers, Inc., 1981. Copyright 1981 by the CURE Foundation.)

probably acquired. For example, in Zollinger-Ellison syndrome the increased gastrin produced by the islet cell tumor is thought to have a trophic effect, increasing parietal cell numbers. Partial pyloric obstruction in rats produces chronic antral distention, probably increasing secretory mass through the trophic effects of elevated serum gastrin.[18] Such a mechanism may have parallels in human disease. The increased histamine levels in the small group of patients with systemic mastocytosis may also stimulate an increase in cell numbers. It is also conceivable that not only are cell numbers increased but also that each individual cell may be capable of secreting more acid; this is a very difficult hypothesis to test. In some series, secretory capacity tends to increase with increasing duration of the disease. However, acid and pepsin hypersecretion return to control levels after the ulcer heals. A definite cause-and-effect relationship between this increase in secretory capacity and duodenal ulceration is by no means established.

In addition to this disorder in secretory capacity, there is also evidence of an abnormal increase in secretory stimulation both under basal conditions and after endogenous and exogenous stimuli. Not only is there an increase in basal secretion, which might only be a reflection of the increased secretory capacity, but there is also an increase in the ratio of basal secretion to total secretory capacity, suggesting some elevation in the background stimulus to acid secretion. This ratio is elevated not only in patients with Zollinger-Ellison syndrome and antral G-cell hyperplasia but also in common duodenal ulcer where serum gastrin levels are normal. Basal secretion seems to result primarily from a combination of steady-state vagal and histamine stimulation. Dragstedt's hypothesis that vagal hyperactivity is the basis for duodenal ulcer is not without basis in a subset of patients, although definite experimental evidence is lacking.[1] Some patients fail to increase acid secretion in response to sham feeding, a finding which suggests an already elevated vagal tone. Others have an increased acid response to insulin-induced hypoglycemia, a process mediated vagally, suggesting increased neural stimulation. Psychodynamic theories of pathogenesis are based on the concept of vagal mediation. The other suggestion, that an increase in basal histamine stimulation is involved, is very difficult to evaluate experimentally. There is no method to measure gastric histamine release. A decrease in the histamine content and in the activity of histamine methyltransferase in the fundic mucosa of duodenal ulcer patients has been reported but is very difficult to interpret.[12]

Duodenal ulcer patients also secrete more acid in response to meals. Some studies have documented an increase in the peak secretion, whereas others show only a more prolonged acid secretory response (Fig 12–6).[19] Duodenal ulcer patients have been variously reported to have an increase in acid responses to the cephalic, gastric, and intestinal phases of stimulation. While basal serum gastrin levels are not elevated in most patients, the rise in serum gastrin after a meal seems to be greater than in normal subjects. However, gastrin content of the antral mucosa is similar to that of controls. This postprandial hypergastrinemia has not been explained but could conceivably result from several mechanisms. In addition to an actual increase in the amount released, it could represent a decrease in gastrin metabolism and degradation. It also may

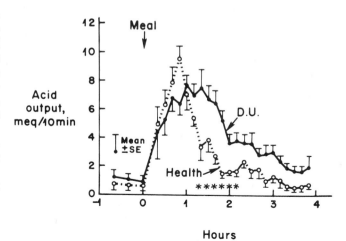

Fig 12–6.—Gastric output after meals in patients with duodenal ulcer *(DU)* and normal controls *(Health)*.* indicates a significant difference for 10-min intervals. Hourly outputs for the second, third, and fourth hours were significantly greater in DU than in normals ($P < 0.05$). There is an increased duration and total acid output in DU patients. Other studies have shown an increased peak acid output. (Reprinted by permission of the publisher from Malagelada J.R., Longstreth G.F., During T.B., et al.: Gastric secretion and emptying after normal meals in duodenal ulcer. *Gastroenterology* 73:991, 1977. Copyright 1977 by the American Gastroenterological Association.)

be a result of some defect in inhibition of gastrin secretion. Since duodenal ulcer patients tend to hypersecrete acid and since acid inhibits antral gastrin release, they would be expected to have low basal and meal-stimulated gastrin levels. Thus, even though basal gastrin levels are normal, they may be inappropriately high in relation to the increased secretory capacity. Different studies have variously shown defects in inhibition of both acid secretion and gastrin release in response to instilled acid and amino acids, although the response to fat and hypertonic glucose seems to be normal. This could represent a decrease in inhibitory peptides, disordered reflex inhibition, or a decreased sensitivity of parietal cells to inhibition. A host of as yet unidentified disorders in secretory stimulation or inhibition by gut hormones such as bombesin, cholecystokinin, gastric inhibitory polypeptide, and somatostatin are possible; evidence to date is unremarkable.

There is also evidence of an increased parietal cell sensitivity to secretagogues. Duodenal ulcer patients produce more acid in response to a wide variety of exogenously administered agents including pentagastrin, gastrin 17, histamine, and caffeine (Fig 12–7).[20] Not only is the overall response increased, but the dose of pentagastrin and G17 required to produce a half-maximal response is also much reduced. This increased sensitivity could be due to several factors, including increased mucosal levels of histamine and acetylcholine, increased parietal cell receptors for stimulants, or more efficient coupling of receptors to the secretory apparatus. At present this represents speculation.

ABNORMALITIES OF MOTILITY.—A disturbance in motility constitutes the second major category of physiologic abnormality detected in patients with duodenal ulcer. Results of

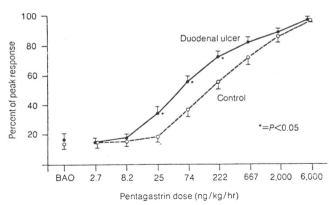

Fig 12–7.—Dose-response curve to graded doses of pentagastrin in duodenal ulcer and controls. The D50, the dose required to produce half the maximal response, is significantly lower in duodenal ulcer patients. (From Isenberg J.I., Grossman M.I., Maxwell V., et al.: Increased sensitivity to stimulation of acid secretion by pentagastrin in duodenal ulcer. *J. Clin. Invest.* 55:330, 1975. By copyright permission of The American Society for Clinical Investigation.)

many studies of gastric emptying have shown that patients with duodenal ulcer have more rapid gastric emptying of meals, particularly liquids, than controls. Normally both acid and food itself entering the duodenum slow gastric emptying. Defects in response to both these stimuli have been noted in duodenal ulcer patients.

Fluoroscopists have long noted that duodenal ulcer patients' stomachs were hypermotile during emptying of a barium meal. Attempts to characterize this abnormality have often yielded conflicting results. Some patients empty at a normal rate, while in others duodenal acidification fails to slow gastric emptying. In some it may even accelerate it (Fig 12–8).[21] There seems to be some controversy about whether nonacidic meals are also emptied more rapidly, and a difference in response between patients and controls after a fatty meal can only be detected after a delay. The etiology of this rapid emptying pattern is unclear.[11] In at least some patients, as mentioned above, there is evidence for a genetic basis for this motility abnormality. It has also been suggested that bulbar inflammation and ulceration may reduce the effectiveness of acid- or food-sensitive inhibitory mechanisms. It can only be speculated that this rapid motility overwhelms the buffering and disposal mechanisms in the duodenum.

ABNORMALITIES OF DUODENAL ACID DISPOSAL AND DEFENSE.—The third category of suggested abnormalities in duodenal ulcer, that of defects in duodenal acid disposal and defense, is probably the least understood of the three. The old theory that the jet of acid emerging from the stomach strikes the same spot on the duodenal bulb, thus determining the site of ulceration, has been dismissed. Both the tendency to secrete more acid and to empty it more rapidly from the stomach contribute to an increase in the amount of acid delivered to the duodenum in any given time (Fig 12–9).[19] This lowers the average duodenal pH in the bulb in ulcer patients under fasting conditions from approximately 4 to 3, and in the second portion of the duodenum after a meal from approximately 6 to 4.[8] Gastric acid is neutralized by pancreatic, bili-

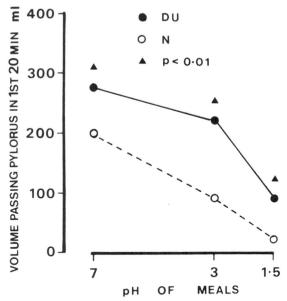

Fig 12–8.—Volume of liquid passing the pylorus during the first 20 minutes after meals at pH 7.0, 3.0, and 1.5 in duodenal ulcer patients *(DU)* and normals *(N)*. The volumes emptied by DU patients at each pH were significantly greater. (From Lam S.K., Isenberg J.I., Grossman M.I., et al.: Rapid gastric emptying in duodenal ulcer patients. *Dig. Dis. Sci.* 27:598, 1982. Used by permission.)

ary, and intestinal secretions, by the buffer capacity of food, and by hydrogen ion absorption. The suggestion from earlier studies that patients with duodenal ulcers did not produce as much bicarbonate as normals in response to an acid load has largely been disproved. Both pancreatic bicarbonate secretion in response to acidification and secretin levels during fasting

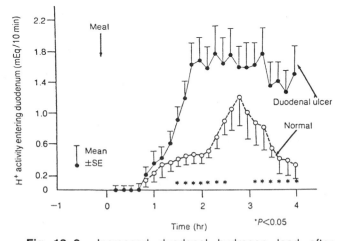

Fig 12–9.—Increased duodenal hydrogen load after meals in duodenal ulcer patients compared with normal controls. * indicates a significant difference for 10-min intervals. (Reprinted by permission of the publishers from Malagelada J.R., Longstreth G.F., During T.B., et al.: Gastric secretion and emptying after normal meals in duodenal ulcer. *Gastroenterology* 73:991, 1977. Copyright 1977 by the American Gastroenterological Association.)

and after a meal are normal in duodenal ulcer. Some studies have actually shown an increase in bicarbonate production in the response of duodenal ulcer patients to a dose of instilled acid compared with normal subjects (Fig 12–10).[22] Cigarette smoking does seem to inhibit pancreatic bicarbonate secretion, which may eventually help to explain its role as a risk factor in the development of peptic ulcer. The role of recently defined bicarbonate secretory mechanisms in the surface epithelium of the antrum and duodenum has not yet been clearly defined. As yet studies of duodenal acid absorption have not revealed any abnormality in duodenal ulcer.

Since the majority of duodenal ulcer patients have acid and pepsin secretory rates within the normal range, it seems very likely that a defect in duodenal defense exists in some of these patients. There has been a suggestion that there may be impaired motility of the proximal duodenum so that acid in the bulb is slow to be passed downward with a simultaneous reduction in the frequency of retrograde peristaltic waves, which bring alkali into the bulb from lower in the intestine.[6] Chronic duodenitis has been noted in duodenal ulcer in much the same way gastritis has been associated with gastric ulcer. It has been proposed that this chronic inflammation weakens the defenses of the mucosa. Impaired mucosal production of prostacyclin and thromboxane A_2, two factors thought to be important in cytoprotection has been reported in duodenal ulcer patients. There has also been some suggestion that mucosal blood flow may be reduced in the duodenal bulb of ulcer patients. Defects in mucous production and viscosity are possible but as yet have not been proved to be of pathophysiologic significance.

Finally, it has been suggested that in some patients the primary injury is the result of some other agent which damages the mucosa and then allows backflux of acid and pepsin, producing an ulcer. Infectious etiologies have been proposed.[7] Antibodies to herpes virus type 1 are elevated in duodenal ulcer patients, and the virus has been found in vagal ganglia. Cytomegalovirus has been isolated from the gastric mucosa of renal transplant patients. The high incidence of allergic disorders in duodenal ulcer patients and the findings of antibodies to IgA and parietal cells have been suggested as evidence for an immunologic disorder in some duodenal ulcer patients.

Summary: Pathogenesis of Duodenal Ulcer

A wide range of often unrelated abnormalities has been implicated in the pathogenesis of duodenal ulcer through epidemiologic, genetic, psychological, and physiologic studies. The synthesis of a unifying concept of the etiology of duodenal ulcer from this variety of findings is a formidable task; however, it is possible to speculate on the relative importance of some of these factors. Epidemiologic data provide some interesting observations which in general are too diverse to be conclusive. Genetic studies provide convincing evidence for an hereditary basis, at least in some subsets of patients, particularly those hypersecretors with elevated serum pepsinogen I and those with rapid gastric emptying. In addition, genetics has demonstrated the validity of heterogeneity, the concept that duodenal ulcer is not one but a group of diseases with differing pathogenic mechanisms. This finding in itself does much to explain the diversity of abnormalities. The only clear risk factor is cigarette smoking. Psychological factors probably have a role in exacerbations of the disease, but their pathogenic importance has not been clearly established. The most striking physiologic defects in duodenal ulcer involve disorders in control of acid secretion and its disposal by the duodenum. In some patients this represents an increase in secretory capacity, probably on a genetic basis. Others secrete more in what appears to be a normal physiologic response to stimulus. The roles of vagal activity and gastrin in determining this increased sensitivity are as yet undefined, but probably are of major importance in some patients. Rapid gastric emptying seems to be significant in only a small subset. Preliminary studies suggest that duodenal acid disposal and mucosal defense mechanisms are of much greater importance than has been previously recognized, and further examination of these factors may provide the basis for a more unified theory of pathogenesis.

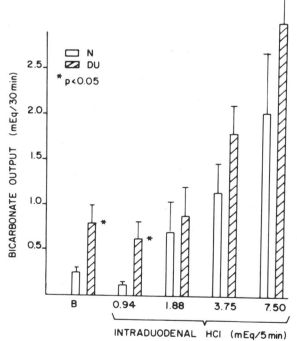

Fig 12–10.—Mean bicarbonate output before (B) and after instillation of graded doses of hydrochloric acid into the duodenum of duodenal ulcer patients vs. normal subjects. (From Isenberg J.I., Cano O.R., Bloom S.R.: Effect of graded amounts of acid instilled into the duodenum of pancreatic bicarbonate secretion and plasma secretion in duodenal ulcer and normal subjects. *Gastroenterology* 72:6, 1977.)

PATHOGENESIS OF GASTRIC ULCER

Gastric ulcers occur much less frequently than duodenal ulcers. Bonnevie's studies from Denmark suggest an incidence of three new cases for each 10,000 adult men per year as opposed to 18 new cases of duodenal ulcer.[9] In this country they are only one third to one fifth as common as duodenal ulcers although probably responsible for as many deaths. In recent years, fewer clinical studies have examined the pathogenesis of the gastric ulcer, and this is probably a reflection of this difference in incidence. Common therapeutic measures have been equally successful in healing both types of ulcer and, at least morphologically, they appear similar. Gastric and duodenal ulcer have fairly similar rates of spontaneous healing, recurrence, and complications. The two types are very difficult to differentiate symptomatically. However, in terms of their epidemiology, genetics, risk factors, associations, and physiologic abnormalities, gastric and duodenal ulcer are very different. In addition, there appears to be an increased risk of gastric carcinoma in the same patients who develop gastric ulcer which is not present in patients with duodenal ulcer.

Like duodenal ulcer, gastric ulcer is thought to represent a spectrum of different pathophysiologic entities. The pattern is less diverse but a variety of abnormalities have also been described in gastric ulcer patients. Three forms of gastric ulcer are commonly recognized. Type I lesions are primary ulcers located in the body and proximal antrum which are usually associated with hyposecretion and constitute the majority of gastric ulcers. Type II gastric ulcers, which arise secondary to duodenal ulcer with pyloric stenosis, and type III, the prepyloric gastric ulcer, are both usually associated with acid hypersecretion and assumed to share a common etiology with duodenal ulcer. Only type I ulcers will be considered here.

Epidemiologic Patterns

In the late 19th century gastric ulcer was the more frequent acid-peptic disease. Today duodenal ulcer is the more common entity and gastric ulcer is very rarely encountered in such areas as India and Africa.[3] However, there is a much higher incidence of gastric ulcer in Japan, among Indian miners in the Peruvian Andes, and in some fishing villages of northern Norway. While in the 19th century, gastric ulcer was more prevalent in higher social classes, this has shifted to the lower socioeconomic groups. Unlike duodenal ulcers, which tend to be more common in men, gastric ulcers are distributed about evenly between the sexes. The one exception is in Australia, where gastric ulcer seems to be very common among lower-class women who consume large amounts of aspirin for "tension headaches." The incidence of gastric ulcer increases with advancing age and gastric ulcer patients tend to be older than those with duodenal ulcer. It has been suggested that this may be related to the increased incidence of chronic gastritis with age.

Unlike duodenal ulcer, the overall hospitalization rates for gastric ulcer have remained relatively stable over recent years (see Fig 12–2).[10] It is not clear whether the decline in the incidence of duodenal ulcer represents a significant change, nor is it clear why gastric ulcer has not shown the same patterns. This may reflect some very different factor in their pathogenesis and response to treatment or just that gastric ulcers tend to occur more in older patients who have other reasons for entering the hospital.

In summary, several epidemiologic patterns have been recognized for gastric ulcer. Although they provide some clues, as yet these differences have not revealed the factors responsible for gastric ulceration.

Genetic Abnormalities

Compared with the extensive genetic data on duodenal ulcer, gastric ulcers are a relatively poorly studied entity. Early family studies demonstrated the familial aggregation of gastric ulcer.[23] Gastric and duodenal ulcer, as mentioned earlier, segregate independently—relatives of gastric ulcer patients tend to get gastric ulcers. In addition, twin studies have supported this separation. Blood group O is not associated with gastric ulcer. Genetic data were really the first strong evidence that gastric and duodenal ulcer are distinctly separate diseases. Chronic atrophic gastritis, usually found in association with gastric ulcer and often assumed to be a preliminary step in its development, also shows familial aggregation and probably has some genetic basis.

As yet no genetic markers for subsets of gastric ulcer patients have been identified. Thus the argument for heterogeneity within gastric ulcer has been less strong than that in duodenal ulcer, although the variation in physiologic abnormalities suggests it exists. The future identification of such markers should help to sort out the factors involved in gastric ulcer pathogenesis.

Risk Factors

Slight risk factors have been identified in gastric ulcer. None seems overriding, except perhaps aspirin ingestion.[23] Like duodenal ulcer, there is an association with cigarette smoking and a correlation between the number of cigarettes smoked and the prevalence of gastric ulcers. No definite evidence exists for a decrease in the likelihood of ulcer healing for smokers with gastric ulcer as it does for duodenal ulcer. Smoking has been shown to reduce pyloric sphincter pressure, and this may have a role in the duodenogastric reflux, which has been linked to the development of gastric ulceration. Alcohol does cause gastritis and has been implicated in the disruption of the gastric mucosal barrier in animals. However, no studies yet exist linking alcohol and chronic gastric ulcer.

Diet is often considered to be important in the pathogenesis of gastric ulceration, and one popular theory is that irritants such as spices and curries may damage the gastric mucosa. However, there is no firm evidence to support this, although undoubtedly some dietary factor will be shown to be responsible for the geographical variation in incidence. One epidemiologic study implicated coffee and soft drinks in the pathogenesis of peptic ulcer but did not separate duodenal and gastric ulcer.[3]

The only really strong risk factor is aspirin. Both in animals and man, aspirin in combination with acid produces acute gastric mucosal injury with disruption of the gastric mucosal barrier, a fall in potential difference, and gross injury.[23] Several epidemiologic studies have also demonstrated an increased frequency of chronic ulcers in patients taking large aspirin doses. There was also an increase in the incidence of chronic ulcer in patients taking three tablets of aspirin a day to reduce the risk of recurrent myocardial infarction. Similar associations between chronic ulcer and acetaminophen and the other nonsteroidal anti-inflammatory agents have been noted. It has been suggested that these agents act both through direct mucosal injury and through inhibition of prostaglandin synthesis. Prostaglandins have been shown to have multiple roles in the basic physiologic processes of the gastric mucosa. They stimulate blood flow, sodium transport, bicarbonate secretion, and cyclic AMP formation, without which the mucosa may be more susceptible to injury. While gastric ulcer patients without a history of aspirin ingestion invariably have an element of gastritis in association with their ulcer, studies of gastrectomy specimens have revealed that habitual aspirin users may develop ulcers in otherwise normal mucosa.[22]

Disease Associations

In contrast to duodenal ulcers, not many other diseases are associated with gastric ulcer. In part, this reflects the far more common occurrence of duodenal than gastric ulcer, a characteristic which in some instances suggests associations which do not really exist. Gastric ulcer has been associated with two other stomach disorders, however. First, chronic superficial and atrophic gastritis are frequently found in association with gastric ulcer. This may be limited to the area of the ulceration or be more widespread, involving both the corpus and the antrum. It is unclear whether either entity is the primary event, although the gastritis usually persists after ulcer healing, suggesting that gastric ulcer is probably the secondary process.

In contrast to duodenal ulcer, there is a strong although controversial association between gastric ulcer and gastric carcinoma. These two entities share many features. Both occur in a context of intestinal metaplasia and gastritis in the stomach. They have many epidemiologic similarities although, even in Japan, the geographical mortalities do not really seem to correlate. Gastric cancer often presents as an ulcer and even a malignant ulcer can occasionally heal with intensive medical therapy. There is no evidence that benign ulcerations eventually develop malignancy, although benign ulcers with only a small focus of malignancy have been described. The process of recurrent inflammatory injury and healing in gastric ulcer is consistent with our concepts of carcinogenesis.

Psychological Abnormalities

Psychological factors seem to have less of a role in the pathogenesis of gastric than duodenal ulcer, more an empirical observation than a proved fact. In animal experiments, stress and restraint have been used to induce acute mucosal lesions of the stomach, but their relationship to the pathogenesis of chronic ulceration is unclear.

Human studies of the relationship of psychodynamic factors to chronic gastric ulceration have not been particularly revealing. No one personality pattern has been identified in gastric ulcer patients, and studies of the role of stressful events have had conflicting findings, although some association seems valid. In one recent paper, two patients had increased acid secretion and symptomatic gastric ulcer that developed at the time of severe emotional distress.[24]

Physiologic Abnormalities

In contrast to the hypersecretion noted in duodenal ulcer patients, gastric ulcer patients secrete in a range from normal to barely detectable. Although a few patients have been reported who have no detectable acid secretion or achlorhydria, in general it is believed that at least some acid and pepsin is required for gastric ulceration. However, it is clear that the physiologic defect in gastric ulcer must include a significant disorder of mucosal defense.

It is interesting in light of our current knowledge of gastric ulceration to examine Dragstedt's theory of antral stasis, hypergastrinemia.[1] Based on extensive experimental and clinical observations, he postulated that because of pyloric stenosis or gastric atony there was a slowing of gastric emptying and a consequent distention of the antrum. This stimulated gastrin release and secondary acid hypersecretion, which resulted in ulceration. Recent evidence has largely disproved this hypothesis. Gastric ulcer patients as a rule have normal rates of emptying of solids and tend to have low rates of acid secretion, even when allowance is made for loss of acid owing to back-diffusion. Some studies have demonstrated a slowing of the gastric emptying of liquids and antral atony while ulcers are active, which returns to normal patterns after healing.[24] This suggests that the ulceration is the primary event. Gastrin levels are often elevated, but usually appropriately for the acid hyposecretion.

Current theories suggest that there are two major physiologic abnormalities in gastric ulcer—duodenogastric reflux and damaged mucosal defenses. These are very closely related.

DUODENOGASTRIC REFLUX.—Reflux of duodenal contents into the stomach is very common in gastric ulcer patients. It has been speculated that reflux into the stomach of duodenal contents and biliary and pancreatic secretions results in gastritis and eventual ulceration. Barium fluoroscopy and marker studies have in general demonstrated increased reflux in gastric ulcer patients.[9] The basis for this is not fully understood but seems to be a defect in pyloric function. Normally the pyloric sphincter has a low resting pressure that increases in response to the presence of acid, fat, amino acids, and cholecystokinin in the duodenum. Abnormally low basal pressures are found only in some patients with gastric ulcer. However, when acid or fat is infused into the duodenum, the pressure increases in gastric ulcer patients are almost always less than those of normal controls (Figs 12–11 and 12–12).[25] The pressure also increases less in response to exogenous cholecystokinin and secretin. It has been suggested that the lack of response to these hormones, when produced endogenously by acids or fat in the duodenum, is the mechanism for all of these differences. This malfunction of the pylorus presumably explains the increase in duodenogastric reflux.

Current theories suggest that the reflux somehow damages mucosal defense mechanisms, permitting ulceration by acid-pepsin. However, some normal subjects and patients with duodenal ulcers also have evidence of significant reflux, and the difference between these patients and those with gastric ulcer has not yet been determined.

DAMAGED MUCOSAL DEFENSES.—It is unclear how duodenal reflux might damage the gastric mucosa. Drainage of duodenal contents into the stomach of experimental animals can produce a chronic superficial gastritis, which is

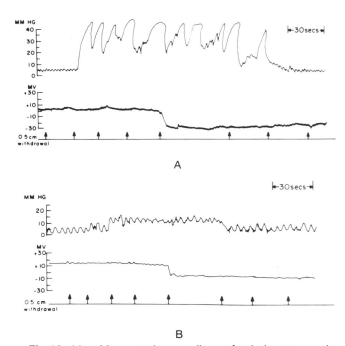

Fig 12–11.—Manometric recordings of pyloric pressure in a normal subject *(A)* and a patient with gastric ulcer *(B)* during pyloric pull-through. In the normal subject, pressure increased from its basal level of 5 mm Hg to greater than 40 mm Hg. In the gastric ulcer patient, pressure did not change significantly. Hydrochloric acid perfusion was begun 5 minutes before and continued throughout the pyloric pullthrough. (From Fisher R.S., Cohen S.: Pyloric sphincter dysfunction in patients with gastric ulcer. *N. Engl. J. Med.* 288:273, 1976. Reprinted by permission of *The New England Journal of Medicine.*)

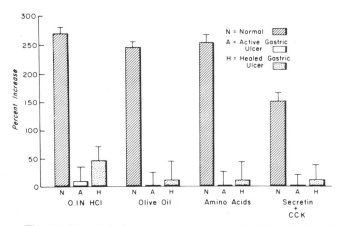

Fig 12–12.—Pyloric pressure responses to intraduodenal stimuli and exogenous hormonal administration in normals and patients with gastric ulcer before and after healing. Pyloric pressure is expressed as the percentage increase above the basal pyloric pressure. In normals hydrochloric acid, olive oil, amino acids, and IV secretin and cholecystokinin all increased pyloric pressure. In gastric ulcer all failed to produce a significant rise before and after healing of the ulcer. (From Fisher R.S., Cohen S.: Pyloric sphincter dysfunction in patients with gastric ulcer. *N. Engl. J. Med.* 288:273, 1976. Reprinted by permission of *The New England Journal of Medicine.*)

worse in the antrum.[18] However, it has not been shown to produce chronic gastric ulceration. Measurements of bile acid conjugates in the stomach suggest an increase in some gastric ulcer patients both in the fasting state and after meals. The severity of gastritis seems to correlate fairly well with a bile acid concentration. The damaging agents in duodenal contents have not been fully differentiated, but bile acids, particularly deoxycholate and taurocholate, lysolecithin, and pancreatic secretions have been postulated to have the most damaging effects. They are thought to damage the mucosa by disrupting the gastric mucosal barrier and possibly by disturbing the surface mucus, which has been suggested to form with bicarbonate an unstirred layer, protecting the mucosa from injury. Like refluxing duodenal contents, aspirin and other nonsteroidal anti-inflammatory agents also seem to damage the mucosa.

The gastric mucosal barrier, originally described by Davenport, is a conceptual explanation for the mechanism by which the gastric mucosa maintains a lumen-negative potential difference, with a high luminal acid concentration and low sodium concentration. When this barrier is disrupted the potential difference decreases, hydrogen ion refluxes into the tissue, and sodium ions enter the lumen. This barrier has been studied most extensively in relation to acute gastric mucosal lesions, the subject of the next chapter. However, this concept is also important in understanding chronic gastric injury. Both bile salts and aspirin in animal experiments can damage the mucosal barrier, producing a fall in potential and backflux of hydrogen ions. Aspirin alone produces significant gross injury; however, bile salt erosions only develop in the presence of significant luminal acid or ischemia.

Current theories on the origin of gastric ulcerations suggest that chronic reflux probably produces a low-grade disruption of the mucosal barrier. Ion transport and other metabolic processes such as ATP production may be altered. Alternatively, the refluxing detergent action of bile salts and lecithin could disrupt the glycoprotein mucous and bicarbonate layer on the epithelial surface. It has also been suggested that gastric ulcer patients might have some inherent abnormality in mucous or bicarbonate secretion. Some studies have suggested a decrease in mucous secretion with atrophic gastritis, but it is difficult to differentiate which disorder is the primary one. Another recent study has suggested that mucus in gastric ulcer patients has an increased proportion of low as opposed to high molecular weight glycoproteins.[26] However, no definite role for gastric mucus has ever been conclusively demonstrated in gastric ulcer.

Gastritis is the widely assumed intermediary step between the repeated injury of the gastric mucosal barrier by refluxing duodenal contents and gastric ulcer. Just as in acute models where aspirin can produce damage alone, so it may also produce gastric ulcer directly without this intermediary step of gastritis. This concept of gastritis prior to ulceration is generally unproved, and chronic atrophic gastritis is very common in the elderly, found in 40% of persons over age 50. Although gastritis is usually associated with gastric ulcers, it is not really known which precedes the other. Gastritis usually involves the entire antrum and sometimes even the fundus, but it may be limited to the area immediately surrounding the ulcer. It usually persists even after ulcer healing, suggesting that it is the primary defect. Gastritis seems also to be a precursor of gastric carcinoma; the reasons why one patient with gastritis will get ulcer, another cancer, and another nothing at all are totally unclear.

The extension of gastritis from antrum into the fundus explains the generally low acid secretion in gastric ulcer. This is probably further reduced by the backflux of hydrogen out of the lumen in the context of a broken gastric mucosal barrier. G cells, as mentioned above, are apparently spared by the gastritis because the fasting serum gastrin level may be slightly increased in these patients and double the normal increase after a meal. Though acid-pepsin production is low in chronic gastric ulcer, there is presumably enough to result in ulceration.

The pathologic pattern and anatomy of gastric ulceration have provided some insight into its pathogenesis. Gastric ulcers most often occur along the lesser curvature at the angularis, usually on the antral side of the junction between the acid-secreting corpus and the antrum. Several reasons for this have been suggested.[18] Near the angularis there are prominent muscle bundles underlying the mucosa which may somehow predispose this region to ulceration. With advancing age, the junction between corpus and antrum actually migrates cephalad, most rapidly on the lesser curvature. It has been suggested that ulcers develop when the junction overlies the muscle bundles. It is unclear how these bundles might predispose to ulceration. One suggestion has been that they somehow constrict the mucosal blood supply, increasing the susceptibility of the gastric mucosa to any acid-peptic injury. Mucosal ischemia has clearly been shown to have a role in acute gastric lesions; in fact, bile salts only really damage the mucosa in a setting of hemorrhagic shock. Whether changes in blood flow have a role in chronic gastric ulcer is a matter of speculation. The blood supply is different on the lesser curvature. There mucosal capillaries and submucosal arteries are actually end-vessels, arising directly from the left gastric artery. In other parts of the stomach, the mucosal vessels arise from an extensive submucosal plexus. It has been suggested that muscular contractions constrict these end-arteries and, where there are no plexuses of anastomosing vessels, produce mucosal patches of local ischemia. Several recent studies have reported at least relative focal mucosal ischemia at the site of gastric ulceration.

Summary: Pathogenesis of Gastric Ulcer

The variety of abnormalities detected in duodenal ulcer patients has not been demonstrated in patients with gastric ulceration. In fact, a relatively coherent concept of the pathogenesis of gastric ulcer is gradually emerging from the results of clinical observation and scientific inquiry. Epidemiologic studies have not been helpful except for the correlation among gastric ulcer, advancing age, and the incidence of chronic gastritis. Genetic factors are also of less importance than in duodenal lesions. Psychological factors also do not appear to be of major significance. Hypersecretion of acid is excluded categorically, since gastric ulcers occur in a normal or low secretory state. The most striking pathogenic mechanism is a decrease in gastric mucosal defense against acid-peptic epithelial injury. There is evidence that pyloric sphincter dysfunction permits duodenogastric reflux of bile salts and other endogenous agents that may, in the presence of acid, disturb mucosal function. These endogenous agents, as well as exog-

enous substances such as aspirin or nonsteroidal compounds, may weaken the resistance of the mucosa thereby disrupting the mucosal barrier and perhaps affecting mucous and bicarbonate secretion. The end result is chronic gastritis which, in combination with acid-pepsin, produces ulceration. Anatomical factors and reductions in mucosal blood flow probably have a role in determining the specific site of ulceration.

CONCLUSIONS

On the most basic level, we still have very little understanding of why patients develop peptic ulcers. We have accumulated a vast quantity of data from such disparate sources as epidemiologic studies, genetics, psychology, and physiology. Each of these disciplines has provided specific clues, but, in most cases, the underlying abnormalities are far from clear. Only in the Zollinger-Ellison syndrome, where hypersecretion and ulcer formation is unquestionably the result of elevated gastrin production by an islet cell tumor, can the basic pathophysiology be explained.

It is still very difficult to gauge the significance of any of the specific abnormalities gleaned from this variety of studies. Most functional abnormalities are found in some but not all the patients with duodenal or gastric ulcer. It is often unclear whether a given finding actually has etiologic significance or merely represents a secondary phenomenon which may only be a defensive reaction to the disease process itself.

Despite these difficulties, we have established some important distinctions which can provide a framework for our clinical understanding of these disease entities. Duodenal ulcer is firmly associated with acid hypersecretion, although rapid gastric emptying seems to have a very important role. Genetic factors also appear to be critical, and cigarette smoking probably affects the natural history of duodenal ulcer. Gastric ulcer is a disease of the elderly, marked by acid hyposecretion associated with duodenogastric reflux, gastritis, and mucosal barrier damage. Aspirin has been clearly implicated. Finally, and perhaps most importantly, the new theory of heterogeneity has provided a unifying concept which clarifies much of this confusion of data. The diversity of findings suddenly makes sense with this organization. The real significance of this, however, lies in its ultimate implications for the clinician. With this knowledge we can potentially separate these patients on the basis of their specific category of ulcer disease. Diagnostic priorities may ultimately be directed toward distinguishing specifically the type of duodenal or gastric ulcer. The real test of this theory will come when our knowledge of the pathogenesis of each subtype permits the further individualization of medical and surgical therapy.

REFERENCES

1. Dragstedt L.R.: The pathogenesis of duodenal and gastric ulcers. *Am. J. Surg.* 136:286, 1978.
2. McCarthy D.M.: Peptic ulcer heterogeneity and clinical implications (editorial). *Ann. Intern. Med.* 95:507, 1981.
3. Langman M.J.S.: Epidemiology of gastrointestinal disease, in Sircus W., Smith A.N. (eds.): *Scientific Foundations of Gastroenterology.* Philadelphia, W.B. Saunders Co., 1980, pp. 88–100.
4. Stabile B.E., Passaro E.: Duodenal ulcer: A disease in evolution. *Curr. Probl. Surg.* 21(1):1984.
5. Davenport H.W.: *A Digest of Digestion.* Chicago, Year Book Medical Publishers, Inc., ed. 2, 1978.

6. Baron J.H.: Current views on pathogenesis of peptic ulcer. *Scand. J. Gastroenterol.* 17(suppl. 80):1, 1982.

7. Soll A.H., Isenberg J.I.: Duodenal ulcer diseases, in Sleisenger M.H., Fordtran J.S. (eds.): *Gastrointestinal Disease: Pathophysiology Diagnosis Management.* Philadelphia, W.B. Saunders Co., 1983, pp. 625–672.

8. Third International Symposium on Gastroenterology, in *Peptic Ulcer Disease: An Update.* New York, Biomedical Information Corporation Publications, 1979.

9. Grossman M.I. (ed.): *Peptic Ulcer: A Guide for the Practicing Physician.* Chicago, Year Book Medical Publishers, Inc., 1981.

10. Kurata J.H., Honda G.D., Frankl H.: Hospitalization and mortality rates for peptic ulcers: A comparison of a large health maintenance organization and United States data. *Gastroenterology* 83:1008, 1982.

11. Grossman M.I. (moderator) UCLA Conference: Peptic ulcer: New therapies, new diseases. *Ann. Intern. Med.* 95:609, 1981.

12. Holtermuller K.H., Malagelada J.R. (eds.): *Advances in Ulcer Disease.* Proceedings of a Symposium on the Pathogenesis and Therapy of Ulcer Disease. Amsterdam, Excerpta Medica, 1980.

13. Carter D.C.: Aetiology of peptic ulcer, in Sircus W., Smith A.N. (eds.): *Scientific Foundations of Gastroenterology.* Philadelphia, W.B. Saunders Co., 1980, pp. 344–357.

14. Wolf S.: Peptic ulcer: Psychosomatic illness review: No. 3 in a series. *Psychosomatics* 23:1101, 1982.

15. Eichorn R., Trackter T.: The relationship between anxiety, hypnotically induced emotion and gastric secretion. *Gastroenterology* 29:422, 1955.

16. Stewart D.N., Winser D.M., De R.: Incidence of perforated peptic ulcer. *Lancet* 1:259, 1942.

17. Kirkpatrick J.R., Laurie J.H., Forrest A.P.M., et al.: The short pentagastrin test in the investigation of gastric disease. *Gut* 10:760, 1969.

18. Skillman J.J.: Pathogenesis of peptic ulcer: A selective review. *Surgery* 76:515, 1974.

19. Malagelada J.R., Longstreth G.F., During T.B., et al.: Gastric secretion and emptying after normal meals in duodenal ulcer. *Gastroenterology* 73:991, 1977.

20. Isenberg J.I., Grossman M.I., Maxwell V., et al.: Increased sensitivity to stimulation of acid secretion by pentagastrin in duodenal ulcer. *J. Clin. Invest.* 55:330, 1975.

21. Lam S.K., Isenberg J.I., Grossman M.I., et al.: Rapid gastric emptying in duodenal ulcer patients. *Dig. Dis. Sci.* 27:598, 1982.

22. Isenberg J.I., Cano O.R., Bloom S.R.: Effect of graded amounts of acid instilled into the duodenum on pancreatic bicarbonate secretion and plasma secretin in duodenal ulcer and normal subjects. *Gastroenterology* 72:6, 1977.

23. Richardson C.T.: Gastric ulcer, in Sleisenger M.H., Fordtran J.S. (eds.): *Gastrointestinal Disease: Pathophysiology Diagnosis Management.* Philadelphia, W.B. Saunders Co., 1983, pp. 672–693.

24. Peters M.N., Richardson C.T.: Stressful life events, acid hypersecretion, and ulcer disease. *Gastroenterology* 84:114, 1983.

25. Fisher R.S., Cohen S.: Pyloric sphincter dysfunction in patients with gastric ulcer. *N. Engl. J. Med.* 288:273, 1976.

26. Younan F., Pearson J., Allen A., et al.: Changes in the structure of the mucous gel on the mucosal surface of the stomach in association with peptic ulcer disease. *Gastroenterology* 82:827, 1982.

13

Stress Erosive Gastritis

THOMAS A. MILLER, M.D., F.A.C.S.

INTRODUCTION

Despite its constant exposure to high concentrations of hydrochloric acid and the potent proteolytic enzyme pepsin, the human gastric epithelium is normally not susceptible to autodigestion. Under conditions of physical stress that occur with severe injury and sepsis, however, the gastric mucosa becomes susceptible to damage by its own secretions. This form of gastric injury has been called "stress erosive gastritis." Although its incidence is unknown, evidence of gastric damage has been observed in as many as 80%–100% of critically ill patients undergoing gastroscopy.[1-3] Fortunately, only a small number of these patients develop GI bleeding or perforation, and in recent years, the incidence of stress gastritis as an important clinical problem has decreased dramatically. The explanation for this is uncertain, but may be related to the following three factors.[4, 5] First, most critically ill patients in intensive care units are routinely given vigorous antacid therapy as a preventive measure. Improved resuscitation techniques are another important development. Finally, earlier arrival at defined treatment centers allows for the management of injuries to be started more quickly than was possible a decade ago.

DEFINITION

Stress erosive gastritis* is a generic term for the multiple erosions that occur within the epithelial lining of the stomach in the clinical setting of severe injury or illness. Other terms that have been used include hemorrhagic gastritis, hemorrhagic erosive gastritis, acute peptic ulcer, acute gastroduodenal ulceration, acute mucosal lesion, stress bleeding, stress erosion, and stress ulcer. Stress ulcer is the term most commonly used to describe the gastric lesion that occurs in the acutely injured or critically ill patient. However, the term is actually a misnomer, since an erosion becomes an ulcer only after penetration of the muscularis mucosa as schematically shown in Figure 13–1. While extension through the muscularis mucosa may occur in stress erosive gastritis, it is quite uncommon. Even in this situation it can be distinguished from a true ulcer by the paucity of inflammatory cells and the

---

*Because the terms "stress ulcer" and "stress ulceration" are in such common use, they will be used interchangeably with "stress erosive gastritis" throughout this chapter.

accompanying fibrosis. Further, a true ulcer has the capability of penetrating through the entire gastric wall resulting in perforation and peritonitis. It is rare for such a circumstance to develop with stress erosive gastritis. Examples of a true ulcer and the typical lesion that is seen pathologically in stress gastritis are shown in Figures 13–2 and 13–3.

Characteristically, the gastric erosions that occur in stress erosive gastritis are acute in nature, generally multiple, shallow, and well demarcated, and they involve only the superficial layers of the gastric epithelium. They are almost always situated in the proximal stomach (the acid-secreting portion), with sparing of the antrum and duodenum. Rarely, they may involve extensive portions of the gastric epithelial lining with almost universal sloughing of the mucosa. If lesions do occur in the antrum and/or duodenum, they are rarely ever found in the absence of severe disease in the proximal stomach. The explanation for this anatomical distribution is unknown.

CLINICAL SETTING UNDERLYING ACUTE GASTRIC MUCOSAL INJURY

In virtually all patients who develop stress erosive gastritis, some form of stress has preceded the onset of the gastric lesion.[1-7] This may take the form of a traumatic injury, shock, sepsis, or some type of life-threatening illness. Occasionally, stress bleeding develops in a patient who has undergone a prolonged operation or has developed severe complications after the operation such as pulmonary, hepatic, or renal failure. The percentage of patients at risk for stress bleeding in these various clinical settings is unknown. In one large study involving trauma patients, only one patient in 64 bled from acute erosive gastritis within ten days of injury.[7] In another study involving 2,300 general surgical admissions to an intensive care unit, only 1.8% bled from stress-related gastric lesions, and of these, fewer than 20% required operation to control the hemorrhage.[8]

In addition to the acute erosive gastritis arising in the preceding clinical settings, acute gastric injury may also develop in extensively burned patients. This is often referred to as a "Curling's ulcer." In one study involving 32 adult patients who sustained severe burn injury, 86% had evidence of acute gastric mucosal injury on endoscopic evaluation.[3] Such injury was particularly common in patients with burns involving 35% or more of the body surface area. Since these lesions are

Erosion   Simple Ulcer

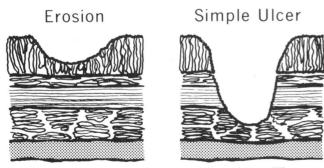

Fig 13–1.—Schematic representation of the differences between a true ulcer and the lesion seen in stress erosive gastritis.

similar morphologically and temporally to the process referred to here as stress erosive gastritis, it is our opinion that they should be classified as a variant of stress ulceration. There is a major difference, though, between the lesions that develop in the burned patient and those observed in the traumatically injured or seriously ill patient. A duodenal distribution is more commonly observed in the burn case, but the

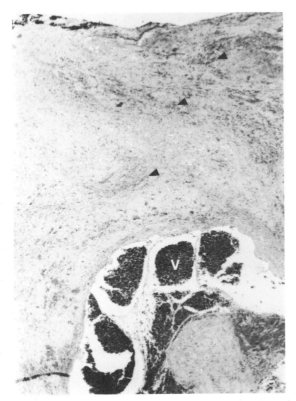

Fig 13–2.—Light micrograph of the crater of a true ulcer. The mucosa has been replaced by fibrous connective tissue infiltrated by numerous inflammatory cells *(arrowheads)*. No epithelium remains, and the ulcerative process and its accompanying scar extends into the submucosa. Note the large, partially thrombosed vessel *(V)* in the submucosa; ×25. (Courtesy of Karmen L. Schmidt, Department of Pathology and Laboratory Medicine, The University of Texas Medical School at Houston.)

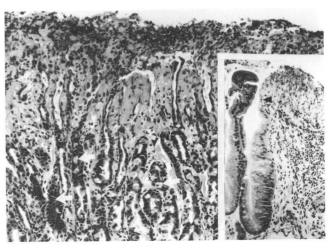

Fig 13–3.—Light micrograph of a gastric erosion. The most superficial portion of the mucosal surface is destroyed and replaced by a dense, mucopurulent material. Epithelium-lined glands still remain in the middle and lower regions of the mucosa *(arrows)*; ×100. *Inset:* Light micrograph showing destruction of the interfoveolar surface epithelium extending as deep as the level of the gastric glands. *Arrowheads* demarcate the zone where epithelial cells are replaced; ×100. (Courtesy of Karmen L. Schmidt, Department of Pathology and Laboratory Medicine, The University of Texas Medical School at Houston.)

mucosal lesion tends to develop during later convalescence as compared to the more typical stress erosions of the stomach that occur within three to five days following an acute major burn. Further, duodenal lesions are generally single and penetrate more deeply than the gastric lesions, which are multiple and shallower. Of interest, the ulcers first described in 1842 by Curling[9] in burn patients were duodenal in distribution.

Intracranial disease, trauma, or operations on the CNS are also associated with acute GI injury. Originally described by Harvey Cushing, and thus referred to as Cushing's ulcer, these lesions may be found in the esophagus, stomach, or duodenum. Morphologically, they differ from the stress ulcers associated with trauma, severe illness, or burns in that they tend to be deep and to extend well into the muscularis.[10] For this reason, they perforate more frequently than the true, more superficial, stress gastritis. Further, increased gastric acid and pepsin secretion is common in CNS-associated lesions, but is quite unusual in individuals with stress-induced acute mucosal injury.[11, 12] Such hypersecretion is particularly frequent in patients with CNS dysfunction, resulting in a decerebrate state.[13] Finally, in patients sustaining injuries to the CNS, serum gastrin levels are significantly elevated when compared with trauma patients without CNS injury.[10] In view of these distinctions, we feel that the Cushing ulcer is a separate entity that should be distinguished from classic stress erosive gastritis.

A variety of drugs may result in the development of acute gastric injury. Particularly noteworthy in this regard are alcohol and the nonsteroidal anti-inflammatory agents, such as acetylsalicylic acid and indomethacin. Endoscopic evidence of mucosal injury has also been observed in patients taking corticosteroids, but, compared with aspirin, the incidence of injury is considerably lower.[14] Furthermore, a dose of 10 mg of prednisone (or its equivalent) for periods in excess of six months appears to be necessary for damage to occur. Because drug-induced lesions are often indistinguishable from stress erosive gastritis in terms of morphological characteristics and anatomical distribution, these lesions have been grouped under the general heading of stress ulceration. While a common pathogenetic mechanism may ultimately be shown to be responsible for both drug- and stress-induced lesion formation, initial factors leading to damage appear to be different for the two kinds of gastric insults. Following ingestion of agents such as alcohol or salicylates, the permeability of the gastric epithelium to secreted acid is greatly increased, resulting in back diffusion of hydrogen ion and ultimate cellular death. A similar permeability disruption has been observed in stress ulcers induced experimentally. Stress erosive gastritis, however, appears to be related to a reduction in the ability of the gastric epithelium to withstand acid diffusing into the tissue (even that which occurs normally) rather than to an increase in the absolute amount of back-diffused hydrogen ion as seems to be necessary for drug-induced ulceration to occur. Further, massive bleeding from drug-induced lesions is rare, and the need for surgical intervention to control bleeding from these lesions is distinctly uncommon.

Finally, it must be emphasized that upper GI bleeding in critically ill patients may be caused by a preexisting chronic duodenal or gastric ulcer in contrast to stress erosive gastritis. Since about 10% of the population will develop a chronic gastric and/or duodenal ulcer,[15] it should not be surprising that activation of a chronic ulcer diathesis may be manifested during another acute illness. This has been noted especially in patients who have undergone a renal transplantation in which a previous history of peptic ulcer was obtained. When such a circumstance occurs, the reactivated ulcer is usually single in contrast to the multiple erosions observed in stress erosive gastritis. Although the factors that give rise to reactivation are not well understood, a distinction between this condition and acute erosive gastritis is necessary because the prognostic and therapeutic considerations are clearly different. For example, since vagotomy and pyloroplasty appears to be an effective procedure in controlling hemorrhage in patients with ulcer disease undergoing transplant operations,[16] it has been misconstrued by some surgeons that this is the operative procedure of choice in all clinical settings for the management of stress erosive gastritis. This assumption is not only unproved, it could be dangerous.

PATHOPHYSIOLOGY OF STRESS EROSIVE GASTRITIS

The precise mechanisms responsible for the development of stress erosive gastritis are unknown. Current knowledge would suggest that a number of etiologic factors may be contributory. The common thread underlying each of these factors is a resultant inability of the stomach to protect itself effectively against its own secreted acid. The more important contributing factors are discussed in some detail in the following section.

Gastric Acid

The presence of luminal acid appears to be necessary for the development of stress ulceration. This circumstance has not only been observed clinically but has also been noted in almost all experimental models of stress ulceration in which the conditions eliciting gastric damage resemble the clinical situation. In contrast to Cushing's ulcer, in which hypersecretion of acid is often observed,[10–13] there is no evidence that increased quantities of acid secretion are a prerequisite for stress ulcer formation. It would appear, therefore, that some critical concentration of luminal acid is necessary for ulceration to occur, which will vary depending upon the adequacy of gastric perfusion, the ability of the stomach to maintain acid-base balance, and the effectiveness of the stomach's own endogenous protective mechanisms.[4, 15, 17] Evidence supporting this contention has been demonstrated in a number of animal ulcer models including the stomachs of the rat, dog, and rabbit.[4, 15, 17] Thus, while the absolute concentration of acid eliciting gastric injury may vary, some luminal acid is required.[4, 15, 17]

Gastric Permeability Barrier

The luminal acid normally present in the stomach does not diffuse back into the gastric epithelium to any significant degree. This ability of the undamaged gastric mucosa to maintain a hydrogen ion gradient between lumen and tissue has been termed the gastric mucosal barrier.[18] If this barrier is disrupted, as may occur when certain liposoluble substances such as aspirin, alcohol, and bile salts are topically applied to the gastric epithelium, a change in gastric mucosal permeability results.[18, 19] Such disruption allows hydrogen ions to diffuse back into the mucosa with a concomitant outpouring of water, sodium, potassium, and protein into the gastric lumen. Paralleling these permeability changes is a reduction in the transmucosal electrical potential difference, suggesting that normal electrochemical gradients between mucosa and gastric lumen have been altered. The ultimate outcome of these events, if not reversed, is direct damage to the gastric mucosa with rupture of mucosal capillaries, interstitial hemorrhage, and the formation of frank mucosal lesions that may bleed into the gastric lumen. Because barrier disruption is often accompanied by both gross and microscopic evidence of mucosal damage, this gastric barrier has been thought to be an important self-defense mechanism against autodigestion by luminal acid.[18, 19]

Although abundant experimental evidence is available suggesting that drug-induced ulceration is a consequence of barrier disruption,[15, 17–19] the role that the gastric mucosal barrier plays in stress-induced gastric injury is uncertain. It would appear from available information that disruption of this mucosal permeability barrier is not essential for the development of stress ulceration. Experimentally induced stress ulcers in both dogs and subhuman primates in response to shock caused by hemorrhage, vasopressin infusion, or *E. coli* endotoxin are not associated with the disruption of the mucosal barrier despite the development of acute gastric erosions.[15, 17] In contrast to these findings, studies in rabbits have demonstrated that some back-diffusion of hydrogen ion, albeit small, is essential for the development of ulceration in the shock-like state.[20]

Although overt barrier disruption may not be a direct cause of stress erosive gastritis, it may be an associated factor through bile reflux into the stomach from the duodenum. Several clinical reports suggest that bile reflux is more common in critically ill patients, probably due to the adynamic ileus, than in normal control patients.[17] Various experimental studies in animals have also emphasized the role that duodenal reflux of bile may play in the development of gastric injury. In both rats and dogs, acute ulceration of the stomach in response to sustained hypovolemic shock could be reversed with pylorus ligation.[17] In studies using the dog stomach, it was noted that ischemia and bile in the presence of acid by themselves were not ulcerogenic, but in combination produced severe mucosal lesions.[21] Since bile salts are known to disrupt the mucosal barrier and increase mucosal permeability,[18, 19, 21] the increased loss of luminal hydrogen ion induced by this damaging agent may be an important contributing factor in the development of stress ulceration in the critically ill patient. Another mechanism by which bile may mediate its damaging effects is through inhibition of active transport mechanisms within the gastric epithelium. This could severely hamper the ability of the mucosa to tolerate the back-diffusion of luminal hydrogen ion.[22, 23]

Of equal interest is the observation that stress ulceration often occurs in the severely ill patient with multisystem organ dysfunction including renal failure. Like bile, urea is also injurious to the gastric barrier.[24] The elevated urea levels in uremic patients gain access to the stomach as a consequence of diffusion from the blood.[15] Although it is not proved, disruption of the barrier by urea may be a contributing factor in the development of stress ulcer formation in the critically ill patient with renal failure.

Mucosal Ischemia

There is general agreement among clinicians and investigators that a common ingredient necessary for stress ulceration to occur is mucosal ischemia.[15, 17] Clinically, virtually all patients who develop stress ulcers have experienced some period of shock (hemorrhagic, cardiogenic, or septic in origin), even if only transient. Gastric damage produced in animal models simulating the stress gastritis seen clinically requires some form of experimental manipulation to decrease gastric mucosal blood flow. In rats, the severity of mucosal ischemia has been shown to correlate directly with the magnitude of gastric injury.[25] Similarly, an increase in mucosal perfusion by intra-arterial infusion of an agent such as isoproterenol can prevent hemorrhagic shock-induced ulcerations in dogs.[26] On the basis of these observations, there seems to be little question that mucosal ischemia is a prerequisite for the development of stress ulceration. How ischemia alters events at the cellular level to initiate ulceration remains to be defined.

One explanation offered by Menguy[27] is that ischemia may cause ulceration through an energy deficit in the gastric epithelium. Using a hemorrhagic shock model, his investigations have demonstrated a profound reduction in gastric mucosal adenosine triphosphate levels in the rat following hemorrhage that coincided with the development of mucosal ulcerations. This energy deficit was much greater in the gastric fundic mu-

cosa than in the antrum, liver, or muscle. Feeding animals prior to hemorrhage significantly lessened the magnitude of gastric injury when compared with fasting, presumably because of the greater availability of energy sources. It was also observed that such energy deficits occur whether or not luminal acid is present.[15] These findings were interpreted as indicating that cellular necrosis results from a deficit in mucosal energy metabolism secondary to the hemorrhagic shock and that the integrity of the gastric epithelium requires a constant and consistent supply of glucose and oxygen to prevent an anaerobic state.[27] The differential energy deficit which was observed between fundus and antrum provides a possible explanation for the susceptibility of the human fundus to develop stress ulceration more commonly than the antrum. Although a correlation between the status of mucosal energy metabolism and the presence or absence of ulceration is convincingly demonstrated in these studies, they do not explain other clinical and experimental findings where mucosal ulceration can be largely prevented by luminal neutralization of acid despite the metabolic status of the gastric epithelium.[15, 17]

Another explanation whereby ischemia may cause ulceration is through a disruption in the normal mechanisms by which the stomach maintains an acid-base balance.[15, 17] Normally, the gastric epithelium possesses a pH of 7.1 to 7.4 that is dependent upon the rate of mucosal blood flow as well as the pH of arterial blood perfusing the stomach. Since ischemia secondary to shock or sepsis is commonly associated with disturbances in the acid-base balance, it is not surprising that the pH of the gastric mucosa may be altered and thereby diminish the ability of the gastric lining to protect itself against luminal acid. As early as 1948, the importance of acid-base balance in the stomach was emphasized by Cummins and associates.[28] These investigators observed that the production of gastric and duodenal ulcers by systemic acidosis was induced by constant intragastric infusion of acid. Yet, these experimental lesions could be prevented by IV administration of sodium bicarbonate. The importance of acid-base balance in frog gastric mucosa was reported by Davies and Longmuir in the same year.[29] More recently, Cheung and associates,[30, 31] using the canine stomach, have shown that acidification of arterial blood significantly enhanced gastric mucosal injury induced by topical bile salts and that the injury induced by hemorrhagic shock and topical bile salts could be prevented by IV infusion of sodium bicarbonate. In a hemorrhagic shock model, Kivilaakso and associates,[20] using a microelectrode technique, noted that the pH of the lamina propria of both the rabbit and dog fundic mucosa bathed with acid solution dropped quickly during shock. In the rabbit gastric mucosa, which is a relatively permeable epithelium, this pH drop coincided with the development of severe lesion formation. Although the intramural pH decreased more slowly in the canine fundic mucosa, which has a more impermeable epithelium than that of the rabbit, disruption of the mucosal barrier by 5 mM of taurocholate resulted in a rapid and profound decrease in intramural pH, with concomitant development of extensive mucosal lesion formation. It was concluded from this study that a critical determinant of whether gastric ulceration will occur relates to the capacity of the mucosa to remove or buffer the influx of hydrogen ion, which is adversely affected in the ischemic state. It was also emphasized in this study that the absolute luminal loss of hydrogen ion in the ischemic stomach may be no greater than in the well-perfused organ, but that in the presence of ischemia, decreases in intramural pH and the extent of ulceration are far more profound. Further studies in this laboratory using isolated amphibian gastric mucosa have shown that a reduction in nutrient bicarbonate severely impairs the protective mechanisms of the stomach against ulceration.[32]

The role that acid-base balance may play in influencing mucosal protection has also been emphasized in studies of gastric epithelium during active secretion of acid. Hersey[33] was the first to observe that intracellular pH approached 8.0 in actively secreting gastric mucosa as compared with a pH of 7.1 to 7.4 in the resting or inhibited state. Further observations by Silen and associates[34, 35] have shown that the actively secreting histamine-stimulated stomach is much more resistant to injury than the metiamide-inhibited or resting stomach. Since the amount of bicarbonate given off within the tissue corresponds exactly to the amount of acid secretion into the gastric lumen, these investigators proposed that the alkaline tide released within the epithelium during active acid secretion is of importance in protecting the mucosa against ulceration. Similar observations have been made by Cheung and Sonnenschein[36] in the dog stomach, where the significant increase in intramural pH induced by histamine infusion could be prevented by the secretory inhibitor cimetidine. Taken together, these experimental findings emphasize the importance of intramural pH in mediating the protective mechanisms whereby the stomach prevents ulceration, and the necessity of establishing acid-base balance and an adequate circulating blood volume in the patient with shock or sepsis.

Alterations in Endogenous Defense Mechanisms

THE ROLE OF MUCUS.—The gastric epithelium is normally covered by a thin layer of mucous gel that is closely adherent to its entire surface. Recent evidence suggests that it may play a role in mucosal protection.[19, 37] The properties of this mucus have been extensively studied. It has been observed to consist of a matrix of glycoprotein molecules which form a gel that is joined together by physical noncovalent interactions, making it particularly suitable to support hydrogen and bicarbonate ion gradients. Recent *in vitro* studies indicate that the diffusion of hydrogen ion across this mucous gel is markedly slowed.[19] Further, this mucous gel is also capable of maintaining a pH gradient in several experimental animals, as well as the human stomach, so that the pH of the cell membrane is slightly alkaline (approximately 7.3) on the epithelial side of the mucous layer and acidic (approximately 2.3) on the luminal side.[19, 37] Since the gastric epithelium normally secretes a small amount of bicarbonate, the pH gradient induced by mucus could play an important role in enhancing the efficiency of acid neutralization at the cell membrane by the secreted bicarbonate. This factor may help maintain a neutral pH at the luminal cell membrane, even though the pH of the luminal bulk solution may be less than 2.0.[19, 37]

What role alterations in this mucus-bicarbonate barrier may play in stress erosive gastritis is unknown. Since the hexosamine content (a major component of gastric mucus) of gastric juice and gastric mucosa is lower in fasted animals developing experimental ulcers and appears to precede the formation of such ulcers,[38] the fasted state of most critically ill or traumatized patients may influence the composition and content of gastric mucus and thereby play a contributory role in stress ulcer formation. Further, bile salts have been shown to reduce the pH gradient across gastric mucus, probably by inhibiting bicarbonate secretion, although a direct effect on mucus production itself has not been excluded.[19, 37] Corticosteroids have also been shown to decrease the concentration of hexosamines in the gastric mucosa prior to the development of experimental animal ulcers.[38] Since circulating levels of steroids may be greatly increased in patients subjected to physical stress,[39] human gastric mucus may likewise be altered in such a clinical situation.

EPITHELIAL RENEWAL.—Studies also suggest that the rate of epithelial renewal may affect mucosal resistance. In several experimental animal models, the gastric mucosa has been shown during stress to have a decreased rate of cellular proliferation and DNA synthesis and an overall loss of RNA.[40] These findings have suggested that inhibition of DNA and RNA synthesis and mitosis, with the resultant inability of the epithelium to replace extruded cells, may contribute to the development of stress erosions. In support of this hypothesis is the further observation that agents such as pentagastrin, growth hormone, and epidermal growth factor, which stimulate protein and DNA synthesis as well as cell division, can prevent formation of restraint (stress) ulcers.[38, 40] To what extent these animal studies can be extrapolated to the human situation remains uncertain. Fasting is known to decrease DNA, RNA, and protein synthesis in gastric epithelium.[40] Thus, it is conceivable that in the critically ill or injured state in which patients generally have an adynamic ileus and are fed primarily intravenously, the decreased synthesis of macromolecules such as DNA may affect the ability of the gastric epithelium to withstand injury. This circumstance, coupled with poor perfusion, acid-base imbalance, and a deficit in energy metabolism may, either alone or in concert, make the gastric epithelium more susceptible to injury.

ENDOGENOUS PROSTAGLANDINS.—An abundant literature has demonstrated that prostaglandins are capable of preventing gastric mucosal injury induced by a variety of experimental ulcer preparations independent of their known ability to inhibit gastric acid secretion.[19] This protective phenomenon has been called "cytoprotection." Since prostaglandins are present in relatively large quantities in the gastric epithelium of man and animals, it has been proposed that they may play a role in maintaining gastric mucosal integrity.[19] In support of this hypothesis is the observation that aspirin-like drugs, which block the biosynthesis of prostaglandins in tissue, elicit gastric mucosal injury. How this occurs is not entirely known, but a deficiency of endogenous prostaglandins may result in a decreased mucosal resistance to contents within the gastric lumen, including acid, pepsin, and various barrier-breaking agents, such as refluxed bile from the duodenum. Whether endogenous prostaglandins play any significant role in the pathogenesis of stress ulceration is unknown and must await further study. Interestingly, stress ulcers induced in animals by pylorus ligation, restraint, glucocorticoid administration, hypothermia, and water immersion stress can all be prevented by exogenous prostaglandin administration.[19] It is tempting to speculate that each of these circumstances may somehow deplete endogenous prostaglandin levels (which is reversed by exogenous prostaglandins) and thereby decrease gastric mucosal resistance to injury.

HYPOTHESIS TO EXPLAIN THE ETIOLOGY OF STRESS EROSIVE GASTRITIS

It seems clear from the foregoing discussion that much needs to be learned about the underlying events that are responsible for the development of stress erosive gastritis. Nonetheless, several factors are sufficiently common in patients who suffer from this disease, which have been shown experimentally to induce stress ulcer formation, that a scenario on how stress gastritis might develop clinically can be formulated. Moody and Larsen[4] have summarized this quite well in the following way:

Consider a potential victim driving home on the freeway after an evening of alcohol and eating. He or she encounters an immovable object that contributes to severe blunt trauma. Visualize then at that point in time the stomach is secreting acid from the stimulus of food. The barrier to hydrogen ions, mildly disturbed by alcohol, may be further disrupted by duodenogastric reflux of bile salts. Gastric mucosal blood flow is decreased by the adrenergic response of impact, or the shock of blood loss from external or internal injury. The ratio of back-diffusion of hydrogen ions to mucosal blood flow increases, acidifying the epithelium, and setting into motion a sequence of deleterious effects that lead to cell destruction. The rapid extrusion of the mucus from the apex of surface epithelial cells, and the secretion and filtration of buffers and water are attempts to neutralize hydrogen ions and wash deleterious substances from the lumenal surface of the epithelium. These events may attenuate the process of injury or contribute further to it if excessive.

Taking into consideration the multiple factors that may play a role in the etiology of stress erosive gastritis, a schematic representation of these various components is summarized in Figure 13–4.

PROPHYLAXIS OF STRESS GASTRITIS

Based on the various derangements identified experimentally as responsible for the pathogenesis of stress gastritis, a variety of prophylactic measures can be instituted in patients at risk for this disease to lessen the likelihood of its development. Since mucosal ischemia may alter a number of mechanisms by which the stomach normally protects itself from injury, vigorous efforts should be made to correct any shock-like state resulting from blood loss and/or sepsis (see discussion under Medical Treatment). Of equal importance is adequate neutralization of intraluminal acidity. The efficacy of this maneuver has been supported by several recent controlled studies in which instillation of topical antacids has been shown to be highly effective in preventing stress gastritis.

In a prospective, randomized, controlled trial of 100 critically ill patients, Hastings and associates[41] assessed the role of topical antacids in patients who were at risk for the development of stress bleeding. In 51 patients, 30 ml of topical antacid (Mylanta II) was administered initially and 30 ml at hourly intervals if the pH of the gastric luminal contents was greater than 3.5. In patients in whom the pH was lower than 3.5, 60 ml was given. During the hour interval between antacid administrations, the nasogastric tube was clamped. In the 49 other patients in this study, no antacid therapy was rendered and the nasogastric tube was connected continuously to intermittent suction. Of the 51 patients receiving antacid therapy, only two (4%) bled. In contrast, 12 of the 49 patients (25%) bled who did not receive antacid therapy. When both groups were matched for such risk factors as sepsis, respiratory failure, jaundice, peritonitis, renal failure, and hypotension, a positive correlation was found between the number of risk factors and the incidence of GI bleeding.

Another study[42] assessed the role of topical antacids in the prevention of gastric bleeding in patients sustaining burns to more than 35% of the total body surface area. Twenty-four patients were randomly selected to receive antacid therapy which was administered in 60 ml aliquots to keep the gastric pH at 7 or above. Twenty-four other patients received no antacid therapy. Six of the 24 patients not receiving antacid therapy developed stress bleeding, and one other suffered a gastric perforation, for a 29% incidence of complications. Only one of the 24 patients (4%) receiving antacid treatment developed GI hemorrhage.

Histamine H_2-receptor antagonists (i.e., cimetidine) have also been purported to be useful in the prophylaxis of stress ulceration. In a study[43] involving 75 patients with fulminant hepatic failure, cimetidine was compared with topical antacids on the basis of ability to prevent upper GI bleeding; cimetidine was found to be more effective. Unfortunately, in the group of patients receiving topical antacids, the antacid dose schedule was administered at four-hour intervals rather than hourly, which may provide insufficient protection against bleeding and make comparison of the two regimens inappropriate. In another study involving renal transplant patients,[44] the effectiveness of cimetidine as a prophylaxis against GI bleeding was assessed. In the 35 patients treated with cimetidine, no episodes of upper GI hemorrhage occurred as compared with six of 33 patients (18%) developing hemorrhage who did not receive this drug. In contrast to these findings, Teres and associates[45] conducted a double-blind control trial in patients bleeding from acute mucosal lesions. They observed no difference between the effectiveness with which hemorrhage was controlled in patients receiving cimetidine in conjunction with topical antacid therapy and those treated with antacids alone. However, when the effect of preventing further hemorrhage after its initial cessation was compared, no bleeding was observed in 18 patients receiving cimetidine and topical antacid in combination, while six of 20 patients who received antacid alone experienced further hemorrhage during the subsequent two weeks. In yet another study, Priebe and colleagues[46] reported that cimetidine did not adequately protect seriously ill patients from acute upper GI bleeding and that topical antacid therapy was more effective in this regard. Similar findings were reported by Weigelt and associates[47] and Zinner and colleagues.[48] Taken together, these studies suggest that cimetidine may play a role as adjunctive therapy in the management of stress ulcer bleeding when administered in combination with topical antacid therapy, but when given alone, it does not appear to provide the

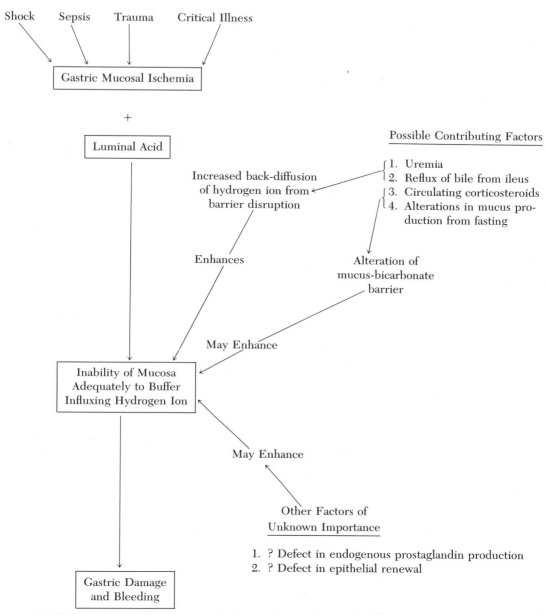

Fig 13–4.—Schema of the various factors in the pathogenesis of stress erosive gastritis.

same degree of protection against mucosal injury as topical antacids.

Intragastric prostaglandin treatment as a prophylaxis for patients at risk for stress ulceration has also been evaluated. The preventive effect on GI bleeding of 15(R)-15-methyl prostaglandin E_2 (100 μg) was studied in 46 patients admitted to a respiratory-surgical intensive care unit.[49] This substance was instilled every four hours by nasogastric tube and compared with hourly titration of the gastric juice to a pH greater than 3.5 using a standard antacid (usually Mylanta II). In contrast to only three of 22 patients in the antacid group who bled, 12 of 24 patients in the prostaglandin group bled (a highly significant difference). The major problem in interpreting these results is that the prostaglandin used in this study must be epimerized in acid medium (below pH 3) to 15(S)-15-methyl

prostaglandin E_2 to elicit any appreciable antisecretory (and presumably antiulcer) effects.[50] It is entirely possible that such epimerization did not consistently occur in the stomach which accounts for its relative ineffectiveness in preventing stress bleeding when compared with topical antacids. Thus, no firm conclusions can be reached at this time regarding the role of prostaglandins in prophylaxis against stress bleeding. Further studies are clearly needed to define this role, using prostaglandins that do not depend upon the pH of the stomach to influence their activity.

Based on the findings enumerated in the preceding discussion, we feel that a strong argument can be made for early and aggressive neutralization of intragastric acidity in patients at risk for the development of bleeding from stress gastritis. Since available studies suggest that H_2 blockers are not as effective as antacids in this regard, our initial approach is topical antacid administration at a sufficient rate to keep the intragastric pH above 5.0. At this pH, 99.9% of gastric acid is buffered and the activity of the proteolytic enzyme, pepsin, is virtually abolished.[51] If not previously placed, a nasogastric tube is inserted into the stomach of the patient at risk, and the pH of the recovered aspirate checked at periodic intervals with pH-sensitive paper. Initially, we lavage the stomach with 30 ml of antacid to adequately coat the epithelial surface. Several minutes later, this volume is evacuated, 30 ml of fresh antacid is instilled into the stomach, and the nasogastric tube is clamped for 30 minutes. The tube is then unclamped, the gastric contents aspirated, and a sample of aspirate checked for acidity. If the pH is above 5.0, the pH is then checked 30 minutes later; and if it remains above 5.0, 30 ml of antacid is instilled into the stomach, and the same process repeated at hourly intervals. If the pH is below 5.0, 60 ml of antacid is instilled and the process repeated. If sufficient neutrality can be maintained with this additional volume of antacid, 60-ml aliquots of antacid are then administered on an hourly schedule. If the pH is still below 5.0 with this additional volume of antacid, we add cimetidine in standard IV doses (300 mg every six hours). Although we usually use Mylanta II as our antacid of choice, aluminum hydroxide is substituted in the rare patient whose renal failure results in the develop ment of hypermagnesemia. The prophylactic treatment just described is continued until the patient sufficiently recovers from illness to commence oral alimentation. A schema for prophylactic management is presented in Figure 13–5.

CLINICAL PRESENTATION AND DIAGNOSIS OF STRESS GASTRITIS

The prophylactic measures outlined above will prevent the development of bleeding from stress ulceration in the large majority of patients at risk. In the rare individual who fails to respond to such preventive measures or in whom prophylaxis was not instituted, the only consistent clinical sign suggesting the presence of stress erosive gastritis is painless GI bleeding. Although the initial bleeding may be rapid, resulting in a bloody vomitus or the passage of gross blood per rectum, characteristically the hemorrhage from the superficial lesions of stress gastritis is slow. Often the first indication that stress ulceration is present is the appearance of flecks of blood within the nasogastric aspirate or an unexplained guaiac-

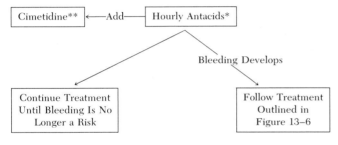

*Keep pH above 5.0; **If antacids alone cannot keep pH above 5.0.

Fig 13–5.—Schema of the prophylactic management of stress erosive gastritis.

positive stool. On occasion, an unexplained fall in the hematocrit may be the presenting sign. Because the loss of blood is frequently so subtle, vital signs may be relatively stable; at worst, a slight tachycardia may be present. When hemorrhage is more rapid and massive, the clinical presentation becomes more dramatic, with obvious tachycardia, restlessness, systemic arterial hypotension, and a pale, cool, moist skin. Patients who are at risk for erosive gastritis are those who have sustained trauma, burns, sepsis, shock, or some form of organ failure. Therefore, any evidence of GI bleeding or unexplained blood loss in such clinical settings should be considered as arising from stress gastritis until proved otherwise.

Although erosion formation can often be demonstrated by gastroscopy within 24 hours after severe trauma, actual evidence of clinical bleeding usually does not occur until three to seven days after the initial insult.[1-3, 7] Massive hemorrhage may be delayed even longer. In any patient suspected of having stress gastritis, endoscopic visualization of the GI tract is the mainstay in diagnosis. If bleeding has been massive prior to undertaking this diagnostic maneuver, it is important first to evacuate blood from the stomach. This can be accomplished with a large-bore tube, preferably an Ewald tube. A thorough endoscopic examination should include visualization of the esophagus, stomach, and duodenum, since the bleeding may be the result of esophageal varices, a Mallory-Weiss tear, or a chronic gastric or duodenal ulcer rather than stress gastritis. If stress gastritis is present, usually numerous, small, well-delineated punctate lesions can be identified along the crests of the rugae within the acid-secreting portion of the stomach. The size of these erosions will vary greatly, but usually they are only several millimeters in length.

If the diagnosis is in doubt after endoscopic visualization, selective visceral angiography is the next procedure to perform. This is particularly important if bleeding continues. Through percutaneous insertion of a catheter into the left or right femoral artery, cannulation of the left gastric artery can easily be accomplished under fluoroscopic control. Contrast material is then introduced into the left gastric arterial system. A blush or seepage of contrast material into the gastric lumen indicates the site of the bleeding erosion.

Barium contrast examination of the stomach and duodenum is usually of little value in the diagnosis of stress erosive gastritis, since the lesions are so superficial with no significant penetration into the gastric wall. Thus, unless other diagnostic modalities have failed to reveal the source of bleeding, we virtually never resort to this type of examination. Gastric analysis is also of no help in the diagnosis of stress erosions because of the large variation in hydrochloric acid output. Although hypersecretion of acid can be demonstrated in patients sustaining head trauma, the hydrogen ion concentration may be high, low, or normal in other clinical settings.

NONOPERATIVE TREATMENT

Medical Treatment

In the treatment of patients with stress erosive gastritis, the importance of prompt and adequate supportive care for shock and sepsis cannot be overemphasized (Fig 13–6). Hypovolemic shock should be adequately corrected to restore intravascular blood volume using whole blood replacement. If the

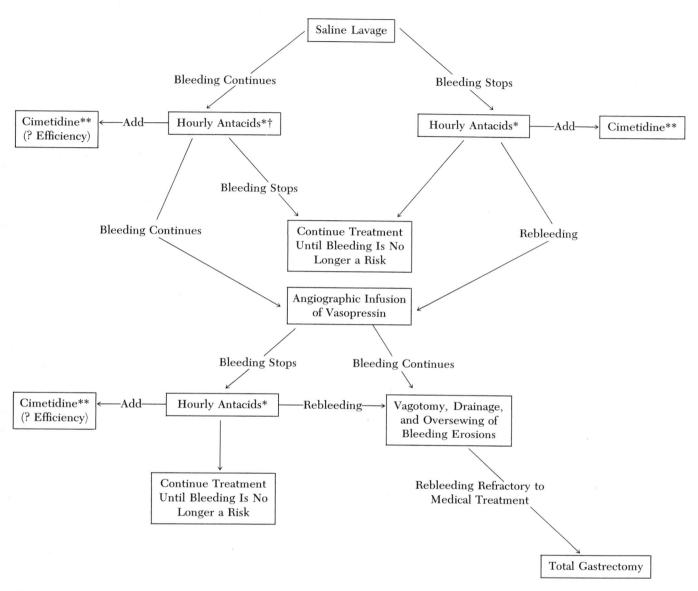

*Keep pH above 5.0; **If antacids alone cannot keep pH above 5.0; †Usually increased dosages needed.

Fig 13–6.—Schema of therapeutic management of stress erosive gastritis.

magnitude of bleeding necessitates multiple blood transfusions, fresh whole blood should be given with every fourth or fifth unit of banked blood. Any coagulopathy should be identified early and corrected. This may necessitate the use of fresh frozen plasma and platelet packs. In those patients in whom sepsis appears to be a contributing factor in the development of stress ulceration, vigorous efforts should be undertaken to identify the source of infection. Appropriate antibiotic therapy should be instituted in this circumstance and surgical drainage of the infected focus performed when it can be identified.

To gain information about the rate of bleeding and to provide a means by which blood and/or clots can be evacuated from the stomach, a large-bore nasogastric tube should be inserted that is at least a size 30 French or greater. The Ewald

tube best accomplishes this purpose. Lavage of the stomach is then carried out with solutions of either water or saline. Although no controlled trials are available using room-temperature solutions for comparison, it is the empirical impression of most clinicians that iced solutions of saline or water are best suited to bring about cessation of bleeding. Generally, we lavage the stomach with 60-ml aliquots of saline solution at a time. This approach provides for adequate fragmentation of clots and aids in the evacuation of any blood remaining in the stomach to reduce fibrinolysis at bleeding sites. In addition, by totally clearing the stomach, gastric distention is prevented, thereby eliminating the stimulus to secrete acid via gastrin release. Using this approach, greater than 80% of patients will stop bleeding. Although other agents administered through nasogastric tubes, such as topical thrombin and intragastric norepinephrine, have been advocated for the control of stress bleeding, published reports using these therapeutic approaches have involved only small series of patients without adequate controls.[4, 38] As we have not enjoyed success with either of these agents, we do not recommend their routine use in the control of stress bleeding. Similarly, the use of anticholinergics in the treatment of bleeding stress erosions appears to be of little, if any, value.

If bleeding has ceased with saline lavage, management should next be aimed at providing adequate intragastric neutralization of acid. This is accomplished by administering sufficient quantities of antacids to keep the intragastric pH above 5.0. Clinical support for this recommendation has been obtained in patients with stress-induced acute gastric ulceration, where it was shown that instillations of antacid therapy were effective in controlling the incidence of rebleeding once initial hemorrhage had ceased.[52, 53] This therapeutic approach is further supported by a number of recent controlled studies[41, 42, 45–48] detailing the efficacy of topical antacids in the prevention of stress ulcer bleeding as reviewed in an earlier section of this chapter. The volume and frequency of antacid administration is identical to that previously outlined in the section on prophylaxis.

If bleeding does not cease after saline lavage, instillation of antacids through the nasogastric tube may still be helpful in the attempt to arrest hemorrhage. In one study, successful control of acute bleeding with antacid therapy in stress gastritis was obtained in 89% of patients.[53] Generally, when treating stress bleeding with antacids, the volumes required are much larger and may be twice those normally employed for prophylaxis.[4] If hemorrhage continues despite vigorous antacid therapy, we proceed to angiography (see following discussion) as a possible therapeutic measure. Although cimetidine treatment has been tried in this clinical setting, we are unaware of any controlled studies demonstrating its efficacy in arresting established bleeding. Only one controlled study is available[54] evaluating prostaglandins in arresting established bleeding from stress ulcers. When administered intragastrically, 15(R)-15-dimethyl PGE_2 (50 µg every six hours) was found to be no more effective than placebo. Since the prostaglandin used in this study was the same as the one used in the Skillman study,[49] similar criticisms (as discussed under Prophylaxis) with regard to its findings and interpretation apply.

Endoscopic Therapy

The cauterization of bleeding erosions through the endoscope has emerged as a potentially effective way to control hemorrhage from the gastric mucosa. Techniques for the treatment of stress gastritis via endoscopy include either electrocoagulation or laser photocoagulation. Experience with each of these techniques experimentally has been reported, using various animal ulcer models.[4, 38, 55] Such studies have demonstrated the efficacy of these two methods in controlling hemorrhage and their safety in terms of depth of tissue injury when employed. Initial clinical experience with electrocoagulation suggests a hemostatic efficacy approaching 95%.[4, 38, 55] However, its ultimate role in the management of hemorrhage from stress ulceration in the human stomach awaits further evaluation. If endoscopic electrocoagulation

turns out to be useful in the management of stress bleeding, it will find its greatest application in areas of hemorrhage confined to small punctate lesions. Larger areas of bleeding mucosa will be difficult to control with electrocoagulation because of the small size of the current source that can be generated with this form of therapy and the obfuscating nature of a more diffuse hemorrhagic area. In this clinical setting, laser photocoagulation has a much higher probability of controlling bleeding. This relates to the unique aspects of laser energy. It can be "sprayed" onto a large surface area without the necessity of physical contact as is needed with electrocoagulation, and the carbon dioxide gas which jets forth from the laser itself displaces blood from the target area as the laser light is applied.[4, 55] Further, the ability to control the intensity and duration of the light energy from the laser enables the depth of coagulation to also be controlled, a circumstance which cannot be duplicated with routine electrocoagulation. Studies in various animal models have shown that laser photocoagulation has a success rate in controlling bleeding from experimental ulcers approaching 100%.[4, 38, 55] Whether similar success rates can be achieved in the human stomach remains to be determined. In the few preliminary studies available, laser photocoagulation has been reported to be 90%–96% effective in controlling GI bleeding in humans, with a 1%–2% incidence of perforation.[4, 38, 55]

Angiographic Therapy

The ability to selectively catheterize various branches of the splanchnic arterial circulation using angiographic methods represents an additional therapeutic modality which can be considered for the control of bleeding when more conventional forms of treatment have failed. Rosch and colleagues[56] were the first to show that gastric bleeding can be successfully controlled by selective infusion of vasopressor agents into the splanchnic circulation. A subsequent study by Nusbaum and associates[57] clearly established that vasopressin infusion into the left gastric artery could control hemorrhage from erosive gastritis. In yet another study, Athanasoulis and associates[58] noted that selective infusion of vasopressin into the left gastric artery permanently controlled bleeding from acute gastric mucosal lesions in 31 of 37 patients (84%). The success of this therapy appeared to be related to the successful catheterization of the left gastric artery and infusion of vasopressin for a prolonged period well beyond the point when the bleeding actually ceased. Since this original study was not randomized, one might argue that a number of patients would stop bleeding spontaneously without vasopressin therapy. Thus, to evaluate that consideration, a follow-up study[59] was conducted in a randomized fashion and demonstrated that initial control of bleeding still occurred in 80% of patients, but permanent control could only be achieved in 67%. In another randomized study by Conn and associates,[60] vasopressin was found to reduce massive upper GI hemorrhage, but no improvement in patient survival rate could be demonstrated.

It would appear from these observations that vasopressin therapy is a useful adjunct in the control of bleeding from stress erosive gastritis if more conventional therapy proves unsuccessful. If angiographic facilities and trained personnel are available, this approach to therapy should be tried prior to subjecting a patient to operative intervention. In patients found suitable for this therapy, vasopressin is administered as a continuous infusion at a rate of 0.2–0.4 units per minute following intra-arterial celiac or left gastric artery catheterization.[59] This treatment is generally continued for a period of 48–72 hours with tapering of the dose before its discontinuation. If this form of therapy is successful, it is usually associated with a prompt reduction in blood loss. Although a variety of side effects has been reported with the use of vasopressin therapy, they generally are infrequent, since this drug is metabolized by the liver.[59] Caution, however, should be exercised in using this treatment modality in patients suffering from ischemic heart disease.

An alternative angiographic technique for the control of bleeding in stress gastritis is occlusion of the bleeding artery by transcatheter embolization. The embolus used may be autologous blood clot, Gelfoam, or metal coils. In a patient with persistent bleeding from a gastric erosion, contrast medium is injected into the left gastric artery, where it puddles in the gastric lumen at the bleeding site. It is postulated that the pressure in this arterial branch is lower than that in other branches, and therefore that thrombin clots or other emboli injected into the system will be attracted to this site of bleeding.[4, 38, 59] The optimal situation in which this approach to hemorrhage would prove successful is in the circumstance where one major artery is responsible for the bleeding. In the stomach, however, this situation is distinctly unusual. The rich, anastomosing network of submucosal arterial vessels is so extensive that no gastric artery is an end vessel. In addition, since ischemia appears to be an etiologic factor in the pathogenesis of stress erosive gastritis, embolization of a bleeding vessel could further compromise nutrient blood flow and result in ischemic necrosis of the gastric wall. Although transarterial embolization has been reported to be a useful adjunct for the control of upper GI bleeding, no controlled studies have been conducted, and the number of cases which have been studied employing this tecnique are too few to permit adequate evaluation of its therapeutic usefulness at this time.

OPERATIVE TREATMENT

Although the large majority of patients who hemorrhage from stress erosive gastritis will respond to nonoperative therapy, approximately 10%–20% of them will continue to bleed despite aggressive medical management and require some type of operative intervention (see Fig 13–6). This therapeutic approach becomes necessary in one of two clinical situations. The first is the patient who presents with an unusually aggressive hemorrhage from the outset and in whom the persistent hypotension becomes a serious management problem. The second involves the patient who bleeds more slowly, and may even stop for a period, but in whom continued bleeding occurs necessitating in excess of 5 units of blood over 24–48 hours (or longer if bleeding has stopped for several days) to maintain an adequate circulating blood volume. It is often a tendency to prolong attempted medical management in patients with stress erosive gastritis with the hope of preventing surgical intervention. However, clinical experience with this entity suggests that the earlier operation is performed in the clinical settings enumerated above, the more favorable will be the outcome.

Because the incidence of stress erosive gastritis has markedly decreased over the past decade and no single surgeon has a sufficiently large experience with this entity, a multiplicity of operations has been proposed for its management, resulting in considerable controversy as to the best procedure to use to control hemorrhage[61–63] (Table 13–1). Although the goal of operation is quite clear—namely, to arrest hemorrhage with the lowest possible mortality—no single operation has emerged as the procedure of choice, and proponents of a wide variety of operative approaches can be found on review of the literature. Menguy and associates[64] have proposed the use of total gastrectomy in the surgical management of stress erosive gastritis because of the high rebleeding rate associated with lesser procedures. In their series of 12 patients, ten survived the operation (for a mortality of 17%) with no rebleeding. Although these results are as good as any published for this disease, others have had much less success with total or near-total (95%) gastrectomy and have encountered mortality as high as 100%.[62, 63] It is for this reason that most surgeons advocate the use of vagotomy in conjunction with gastric drainage, usually pyloroplasty, or hemigastrectomy as the procedure of choice in these critically ill patients. The collected experience with each of these procedures is virtually the same in terms of mortality and rebleeding rate (see Table 13–1). An alternative approach, advocated by Richardson and Aust,[65] is that of gastric devascularization in which both the right and left gastric arteries and the right and left gastroepiploic arteries are ligated near their respective origins, leaving the entire blood supply to the stomach dependent upon the short gastric vessels via the splenic artery. Although their experience with this procedure resulted in excellent control of recurrent hemorrhage (9%), the mortality still approached 40%, similar to that of other procedures.[61–63] Finally, even suture ligation alone of bleeding erosions without vagotomy and pyloroplasty has been employed by some surgeons, with varying degrees of success in terms of rebleeding and mortality.[61, 63]

Accepting the fact that there are no prospective, randomized, clinical trials to substantiate the superiority of one form of surgical therapy over another, and that the results with most operations are comparable, we believe that the treatment of choice in most instances should be vagotomy and pyloroplasty in combination with oversewing the bleeding erosions. The operative procedure we use is carried out through a midline abdominal incision. Once the abdomen has been entered, a generous longitudinal gastrotomy in the anterior wall of the stomach is performed. Any blood and/or clots are evacuated to provide better visualization of the mucosal surface. Any bleeding erosions are then secured with deep suture ligatures in a figure-of-8 fashion using fine, nonabsorbable material such as silk. The operation is then completed by a truncal vagotomy and pyloroplasty following closure of the gastrotomy incision. If the bleeding mucosal surface is found to have more diffuse, rather than discrete, identifiable bleeding points, a partial gastric resection (usually 40%–60%) and truncal vagotomy is performed, utilizing a Billroth I gastroduodenal reconstruction.

Because infection commonly occurs following these procedures, we generally begin broad-spectrum antibiotic coverage preoperatively, which is continued for 24–48 hours following operation. In addition, vigorous antacid therapy plus cimeti-

TABLE 13–1.—RESULTS OF VARIOUS OPERATIVE APPROACHES TO THE CONTROL OF BLEEDING FROM STRESS EROSIVE GASTRITIS

OPERATIVE PROCEDURE	NO. OF PATIENTS	REBLEEDING (%)	DEATHS (%)	REFERENCE NO.
Total or near-total (95%)	12	0	17	62 (Literature review, 1949–71)
gastrectomy (n = 18)	1	0	100	63 (Personal series, 1977)
	5	0 (Av. 0%)	100 (Av. 44%)	64 (Personal series, 1980)
Subtotal gastrectomy	95	51	38	62 (Literature review, 1949–71)
(n = 121)	10	40	60	62 (Personal series, 1973)
	7	57	43	63 (Personal series, 1977)
	9	33 (Av. 49%)	44 (Av. 40%)	64 (Personal series, 1980)
Vagotomy and partial	54	17	24	62 (Literature review, 1949–71)
gastrectomy (n = 71)	1	100	100	62 (Personal series, 1973)
	7	28	57	63 (Personal series, 1977)
	9	44 (Av. 23%)	33 (Av. 30%)	64 (Personal series, 1980)
Vagotomy and drainage (suture	177	29	23%	62 (Literature review, 1949–71)
ligation of bleeding erosions	19	47	32%	62 (Personal series, 1973)
either not done or not	16	25	38	63 (Personal series, 1977)
mentioned) (n = 214)	2	50 (Av. 30%)	50 (Av. 31%)	64 (Personal series, 1980)
Vagotomy and drainage (with	21	9.5	24	62 (Personal series, 1973)
suture ligation of bleeding	21	43 (Av. 26%)	62 (Av. 43%)	64 (Personal series, 1980)
erosions) (n = 42)				
Gastric devascularization	21	9	38	65 (Personal series, 1977)

dine is administered during the postoperative period to insure that the intragastric pH is maintained above 5.0. If recurrent bleeding from stress ulcers occurs postoperatively, vigorous medical management should again be employed using iced saline lavage. In addition, angiographic placement of a catheter in the left gastric artery should be undertaken for vasopressin infusion. If these measures fail to control bleeding, the patient is returned to the operating room, and a total gastrectomy is performed.

SUMMARY

Although bleeding from stress erosive gastritis continues to be seen in critically ill and injured patients, its incidence has decreased dramatically over the last decade. The explanation for this is not entirely certain, but probably relates to our increased knowledge of its pathophysiology. This new understanding has resulted in the nearly routine use of prophylactic antacid therapy to buffer adequately intragastric acidity (luminal acid being a prerequisite for stress ulceration to occur), coupled with improved techniques for the treatment of shock and the accompanying gastric mucosal hypoperfusion (another prerequisite for the formation of stress ulcers). If bleeding occurs despite these prophylactic measures, vigorous medical management with saline lavage and hourly antacid therapy to keep the intragastric pH above 5.0 will stop the hemorrhage in over 80% of patients. In the few patients requiring surgery to control bleeding, no operation has emerged as the recognized procedure of choice. For that reason, we believe that a conservative approach is indicated and recommend vagotomy and pyloroplasty with oversewing of the bleeding erosions as appropriate therapy for most patients requiring operation.

REFERENCES

1. Lucas C.E., Sugawa C., Riddle J., et al.: Natural history and surgical dilemma of "stress" gastric bleeding. *Arch. Surg.* 102:266, 1971.
2. Lucas C.E.: Stress ulceration: The clinical problem. *World J. Surg.* 5:139, 1981.
3. Czaja A.J., McAlhany J.C., Pruitt B.A. Jr.: Acute gastroduodenal disease after thermal injury: An endoscopic evaluation of incidence and natural history. *N. Engl. J. Med.* 291:925, 1974.
4. Moody F.G., Larsen K.R.: Acute erosions and stress ulcer, in *Bockus' Gastroenterology*, 4th ed. Philadelphia, W.B. Saunders Co. In press.
5. Priebe H.J., Skillman J.J.: Methods of prophylaxis in stress ulcer disease. *World J. Surg.* 5:223, 1981.
6. Skillman J.J., Bushnell L.S., Goldman H., et al.: Respiratory failure, hypotension, sepsis and jaundice: A clinical syndrome associated with lethal hemorrhage from acute stress ulceration of the stomach. *Am. J. Surg.* 117:523, 1969.
7. Stremple J.F., Mori H., Lev R., et al.: The stress ulcer syndrome. *Curr. Probl. Surg.* 20:1–64, 1973.
8. Greenburg A.G.: Invited commentary on stress ulceration. *World J. Surg.* 5:148, 1981.
9. Curling T.B.: On acute ulceration of the duodenum, in cases of burn. *Medico-Chir. Trans.* (London) 25:260, 1842.
10. Bowen J.C., Fleming W.H., Thompson J.C.: Increased gastrin release following penetrating central nervous system injury. *Surgery* 75:720, 1974.
11. Gordon M.J., Skillman J.J., Zervas N.T., et al.: Divergent nature of gastric mucosal permeability and gastric acid secretion in sick patients with general surgical and neurosurgical disease. *Ann. Surg.* 178:285, 1973.
12. Norton L., Greer J., Eiseman B.: Gastric secretory response to head injury. *Arch. Surg.* 101:200, 1970.
13. Watts C., Clark K.: Gastric acidity in the comatose patient. *J. Neurosurg.* 30:107, 1969.
14. Caruso I., Porro G.B.: Gastroscopic evaluation of anti-inflammatory agents. *Br. Med. J.* 1:75, 1980.
15. Silen W., Merhav A., Simson J.N.: The pathophysiology of stress ulcer disease. *World J. Surg.* 5:165, 1981.
16. Kyriakides G.S., Najarian J.S.: Operation for the prophylaxis of stress ulceration in transplant patients, in Najarian J.S., Delaney J.P. (eds.): *Gastrointestinal Surgery.* Chicago, Year Book Medical Publishers, 1979, pp. 291–301.
17. Cheung L.Y.: Pathophysiology of stress-induced gastric mucosal erosions: An update. *Surg. Gastroenterol.* 1:235, 1982.
18. Davenport H.W.: Back diffusion of acid through the gastric mucosa and its physiological consequences, in Glass G.B.J. (ed.): *Progress in Gastroenterology.* New York, Grune & Stratton, 1970, vol. II, pp. 42–56.
19. Miller T.A.: Protective effects of prostaglandins against gastric mucosal damage: Current knowledge and proposed mechanisms. *Am. J. Physiol.* 245:G601, 1983.
20. Kivilaakso E., Fromm D., Silen W.: Relationship between ulcer-

ation and intramural pH of gastric mucosa during hemorrhagic shock. *Surgery* 84:70, 1978.

21. Ritchie W.P. Jr.: Role of bile acid reflux in acute hemorrhagic gastritis. *World J. Surg.* 5:189, 1981.
22. Silen W., Forte J.G.: Effects of bile salts on amphibian gastric mucosa. *Am. J. Physiol.* 228:637, 1975.
23. Kuo Y.-J., Shanbour L.L.: Inhibition of ion transport by bile salts in canine gastric mucosa. *Am. J. Physiol.* 231:1433, 1976.
24. Davenport H.W.: Destruction of the gastric mucosal barrier by detergents and urea. *Gastroenterology* 54:175, 1968.
25. Mersereau, W.M., Hinchey, E.J.: Effect of gastric acidity on gastric ulceration induced by hemorrhage in the rat utilizing a gastric chamber technique. *Gastroenterology* 64:1130, 1973.
26. Ritchie W.P. Jr., Shearburn E.W. III.: Influence of isoproterenol and cholestyramine on acute gastric mucosal ulcerogenesis. *Gastroenterology* 73:62, 1977.
27. Menguy R.: Role of gastric mucosal energy metabolism in the etiology of stress ulceration. *World J. Surg.* 5:175, 1981.
28. Cummins G.M., Grossman M.I., Ivy A.C.: An experimental study of the acid factor in ulceration of the gastrointestinal tract in dogs. *Gastroenterology* 10:714, 1948.
29. Davies R.E., Longmuir N.M.: Production of ulcers in isolated frog gastric mucosa. *Biochem. J.* 42:621, 1948.
30. Cheung L.Y., Toenjes A.A., Sonnenschein L.A.: Acidification of arterial blood enhances gastric mucosal injury induced by bile salts in dogs. *Am. J. Surg.* 143:74, 1982.
31. Cheung L.Y., Porterfield G.: Protection of gastric mucosa against acute ulceration by intravenous infusion of sodium bicarbonate. *Am. J. Surg.* 137:106, 1979.
32. Schiessel R., Merhav A., Matthews J.B., et al.: Role of nutrient HCO_3^- in the protection of amphibian gastric mucosa. *Am. J. Physiol.* 239:G536, 1980.
33. Hersey S.J.: Intracellular pH measurements in gastric mucosa. *Am. J. Physiol.* 237:E82, 1979.
34. Kivilaakso E., Fromm D., Silen W.: Effect of the acid secretory state on intramural pH of rabbit gastric mucosa. *Gastroenterology* 75:641, 1978.
35. Smith P., O'Brien P., Fromm D., et al.: Secretory state of gastric mucosa and resistance to injury by exogenous acid. *Am. J. Surg.* 133:81, 1977.
36. Cheung L.Y., Sonnenschein L.A.: Effect of cimetidine on canine gastric mucosal pH and blood flow. *Am. J. Surg.* 145:24, 1983.
37. Allen A., Garner A.: Mucus and bicarbonate secretion in the stomach and their possible role in mucosal protection. *Gut* 21:249, 1980.
38. Robert A., Kauffman G.L. Jr.: Stress ulcers, in Sleisenger M.H., Fordtran J.S. (eds.): *Gastrointestinal Disease*, ed. 3. Philadelphia, W.B. Saunders Co., 1984, pp. 612–625.
39. Moore F.D.: Homeostasis: Bodily changes in trauma and surgery, in Sabiston D.C. Jr. (ed.): *Davis-Christopher Textbook of Surgery*, ed. 12. Philadelphia, W.B. Saunders Co., 1981, p. 41.
40. Takeuchi K., Johnson L.R.: Pentagastrin protects against stress ulceration in rats. *Gastroenterology* 76:327, 1979.
41. Hastings P.R., Skillman J.J., Bushnell L.S., et al.: Antacid titration in the prevention of acute gastrointestinal bleeding: A controlled randomized trial in 100 critically ill patients. *N. Engl. J. Med.* 298:1041, 1978.
42. McAlhany J.C., Czaja A.J., Pruitt B.A.: Antacid control of complications from acute gastroduodenal disease after burns. *J. Trauma* 16:645, 1976.
43. McDougall B.R.D., Bailey R.J., Williams R.: H$_2$-receptor antagonists and antacids in the prevention of acute gastrointestinal hemorrhage in fulminant hepatic failure. *Lancet* 1:617, 1977.
44. Jones R.H., Rudge C.J., Bewick M., et al.: Cimetidine: Prophylaxis against upper gastrointestinal haemorrhage after renal transplantation. *Br. Med. J.* 1:398, 1978.
45. Teres J., Bordas J.M., Rimola A., et al.: Cimetidine in acute gastric mucosal bleeding: Results of a double-blind randomized trial. *Dig. Dis. Sci.* 25:92, 1980.
46. Priebe H.J., Skillman J.J., Bushnell L.S., et al.: Antacid versus cimetidine in preventing acute gastrointestinal bleeding: A randomized trial in 75 critically ill patients. *N. Engl. J. Med.* 302:426, 1980.
47. Weigelt J.A., Aurbakken C.M., Gewertz B.L., et al.: Cimetidine versus antacid in prophylaxis for stress ulceration. *Arch. Surg.* 116:597, 1981.
48. Zinner M.J., Zuidema G.S., Smith P.L., et al.: The prevention of upper gastrointestinal tract bleeding in patients in an intensive care unit. *Surg. Gynecol. Obstet.* 153:214, 1981.
49. Skillman J.J., Lisbon A., Long P.C., et al.: 15(R)-15-methyl prostaglandin E$_2$ does not prevent gastrointestinal bleeding in seriously ill patients. *Am. J. Surg.* 147:451, 1984.
50. Robert A., Yankee E.W.: Gastric antisecretory effect of 15(R)-15-methyl PGE$_2$, methyl ester and of 15(S)-15-methyl PGE$_2$, methyl ester (38707). *Proc. Soc. Exp. Biol. Med.* 148:1155, 1975.
51. Morrissey J.F., Barreras R.F.: Drug therapy: Antacid therapy. *N. Engl. J. Med.* 290:550, 1974.
52. Curtis L.E., Simonian S., Buerk C.A., et al.: Evaluation of the effectiveness of controlled pH in management of massive upper gastrointestinal bleeding. *Am. J. Surg.* 125:474, 1973.
53. Simonian S.J., Curtis L.E.: Treatment of hemorrhagic gastritis by antacid. *Ann. Surg.* 184:429, 1976.
54. Levine B.A., Sirinek K.R., Gaskill H.V.: A prospective, randomized, double-blind study of topical prostaglandin E$_2$ in the treatment of acute upper gastrointestinal hemorrhage. *Arch. Surg.* In press.
55. Silverstein F.E., Gilbert D.A., Auth D.C.: Endoscopic hemostasis using laser photocoagulation and electrocoagulation. *Dig. Dis. Sci.* 26:31S, 1981.
56. Rosch J., Gray R.K., Grollman J.H. Jr., et al.: Selective arterial drug infusions in the treatment of acute gastrointestinal bleeding: A preliminary report. *Gastroenterology* 59:341, 1970.
57. Nusbaum M., Baum S., Blakemore W.S., et al.: Clinical experience with selective intra-arterial infusion of vasopressin in the control of gastrointestinal bleeding from arterial sources. *Am. J. Surg.* 123:165, 1972.
58. Athanasoulis C.A., Baum S., Waltman A.C., et al.: Control of acute gastric mucosal hemorrhage: Intra-arterial infusion of posterior pituitary extract. *N. Engl. J. Med.* 290:597, 1974.
59. Athanasoulis C.A.: Medical progress: Therapeutic application of angiography. *N. Engl. J. Med.* 302:1117, 1980.
60. Conn H.O., Ramsby G.R., Storer E.H., et al.: Intra-arterial vasopressin in the treatment of upper gastrointestinal hemorrhage: A prospective controlled clinical trial. *Gastroenterology* 68:211, 1975.
61. Wilson W.S., Gadacz T., Olcott C. III., et al.: Superficial gastric erosions: Response to surgical treatment. *Am. J. Surg.* 126:133, 1973.
62. Cody H.S., Wichern W.A.: Choice of operation for acute gastric mucosal hemorrhage: Report of 36 cases and review of literature. *Am. J. Surg.* 134:322, 1977.
63. Hubert J.P. Jr., Kiernan P.D., Welch J.S., et al.: The surgical management of bleeding stress ulcers. *Ann. Surg.* 191:672, 1980.
64. Menguy R., Gadacz T., Zajtchuk R.: The surgical management of acute gastric mucosal bleeding: Stress ulcer, acute erosive gastritis, and acute hemorrhagic gastritis. *Arch. Surg.* 99:198, 1969.
65. Richardson J.D., Aust J.B.: Gastric devascularization: A useful salvage procedure for massive hemorrhagic gastritis. *Ann. Surg.* 185:649, 1977.

14

Duodenal Ulcer

DAVID FROMM, M.D.

HISTORICAL ASPECTS

Gastric surgery apparently had its origins in Prague, when a knife was removed from the stomach of a professional knife thrower in 1612. However, it was not until the late 1800s that major advances were made. The standard operative procedures used today for duodenal ulcer involve a combination of separate procedures for the most part used initially for other diseases.

Gastrojejunostomy was first performed for obstructing carcinoma by Wölfler in 1881 and three years later by Rydygier for gastric outlet obstruction as a result of duodenal ulcer disease. The success of gastrojejunostomy for peptic ulcer disease, as well as its relative simplicity and safety, led to its widespread adoption. However, it was not until the 1920s that the high incidence (in excess of 30%) of recurrent ulcer was realized. As a result, gastric resection slowly became more popular, eventually becoming the standard procedure.

Partial gastrectomy, initially little more than a pylorectomy, was first used for the treatment of gastric carcinoma. The first survivor of pylorectomy with anastomosis of the stomach to the duodenum was reported by Billroth in 1881. Four years later, he performed a partial gastrectomy with anastomosis of the gastric stump to the jejunum.

The early years of gastrojejunostomy and gastrectomy were associated with a great many reports, as almost every conceivable modification was tried in order to minimize a number of complications. Laboratory studies were used to perfect the multitude of techniques rather than to try to understand the physiologic consequences of the operations.

Vagotomy was performed in the early 1900s and was based on Pavlov's studies showing a cephalic phase of gastric secretion. Concerns were expressed over delays in gastric emptying, and in 1922 Latarget suggested that gastrojejunostomy accompany vagotomy. However, vagotomy only started to be accepted as a standard procedure in 1943, when Dragstedt and Owen reported two cases of duodenal ulcer treated by transthoracic vagotomy without drainage. Gastrojejunostomy was subsequently added, and the combination became popular because of what appeared to be a reasonable alternative to subtotal gastrectomy that was associated with an apparent lower morbidity and mortality. Vagotomy with drainage became even more popular in the early 1960s, when Weinberg reported the use of the Heineke-Mikulicz pyloroplasty as the drainage procedure. Pyloroplasty was performed by Heineke in 1886 and by Mikulicz in 1888 for congenital hypertrophic pyloric stenosis but was unpopular at the time because of the high operative mortality. Three years after the clinical introduction of vagotomy, Smithwick and associates began to perform vagotomy with hemigastrectomy, a combined procedure that had great appeal in terms of classic gastric physiology.

Although a constellation of symptoms had been recognized in a small percentage of patients who had excision or bypass of the pylorus, the dumping syndrome did not receive appropriate emphasis until 1920 when Andrews, Andrews, and Mix published their paper describing the syndrome. As technical details and acid secretory consequences of the various operative procedures became better understood, greater emphasis was placed on determining the incidence of dumping and other long-term sequelae of peptic ulcer surgery. The frequency of various syndromes occurring after gastrectomy and/ or vagotomy ranged from practically none to virtually always. These figures were used to support use of one operation over others, but agreement was far from uniform. However, it remained for the Leeds/York prospective study, published in 1968, to put the problem in perspective.[1] As the incidence of sequelae related to removal or destruction or bypass of the pylorus and vagotomy became better appreciated, interest in the 1970s gravitated toward an acid-reducing operation which could safely permit leaving the pylorus intact, proximal gastric (or highly selective) vagotomy. This partial vagotomy was applied clinically in the 1960s by Holle and Hart, who also did a concomitant pyloroplasty. However, Johnston reported in 1969 that an accompanying drainage procedure was not necessary, thereby realizing the full potential of Griffith and Harkins' experimental work reported in 1957.

Just as enthusiasm for proximal gastric vagotomy was increasing in the United States, cimetidine became clinically available in 1977. Although the incidence of peptic ulcer surgery had been progressively declining since 1973, this decrease became more noticeable the year after the introduction of a practical H_2-receptor antagonist.[2] The decline continued its previous straight-line course thereafter (Fig 14–1). Reasons for the continuing decline in peptic ulcer disease requiring operation are speculative, although obviously are related to the decreasing incidence of ulcer. The incidence of peptic ulcer disease as a whole has decreased from 1968 to 1975 in the United States. Along with this trend, there has been a decline

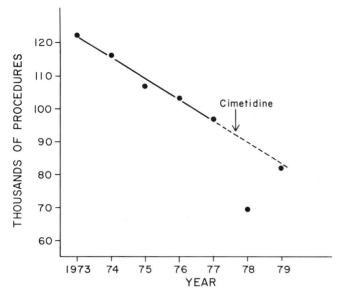

Fig 14–1.—Yearly incidence of vagotomy and partial gastrectomy in the United States. Cimetidine was approved by the Food and Drug Administration in August 1977. (Modified from Fineberg and Pearlman.[2])

in hospitalization rates for uncomplicated peptic ulcer disease. This is at least in part due to changes in criteria for admission, coding practices, and diagnostic procedures. Yet, there has been little or no change in hospitalization rates for perforated duodenal ulcer and only a slight decrease in admissions for hemorrhage. Deaths from peptic ulcer, both as an underlying and contributing cause, also have been declining since 1962.

In addition to the H_2-receptor antagonists, newer classes of medications for the treatment of peptic ulcer disease have been introduced recently. Current non-antacid medications taken for relatively short periods can be very effective, but there is concern about their as yet unknown long-term side effects. Even if it can be shown that these medications are safe when taken for the prolonged periods necessitated by the natural history of peptic ulcer disease, it appears unlikely that they will have a significant long-term impact on the indications for operation. The same may be true for the ever-increasing variety of invasive but nonoperative methods for the treatment of complications of peptic ulcer. These methods still have not been convincingly shown to be definitive or even effective therapeutic modalities.

INDICATIONS FOR OPERATION

The indications for operation are intractability, hemorrhage, obstruction, and perforation. The latter three conditions present less of a problem than intractability in making a decision about the timing of operation.

Intractability

Peptic ulcer disease seems to be a lifelong phenomenon, marked by periodic healing and recurrence. The majority of recurrences respond to repeated courses of nonoperative treatment. Prolonged antacid use is impractical for many pa-

tients, and the long-term effects of H_2-receptor antagonists and other more easily taken medications are unclear. Nevertheless, an important benefit of effective medications taken more readily than frequent antacids is that they notably decrease failure of compliance as an indication for operation.

Frequently it is helpful to make a distinction between asymptomatic and symptomatic recurrence, since symptomatic patients are more likely to opt for operation, especially when symptoms interfere with their daily activities. However, asymptomatic ulcers also present a threat, as illustrated by the patient whose first manifestation of the disease is perforation or bleeding. While many such patients, on careful history, have premonitory symptoms, they are often mild enough that patient and physician pay little attention.

Certain types of ulcers are notorious for failure to heal or tendency to recur. Examples include giant duodenal, pyloric channel, and postbulbar ulcers. Whereas in the past, patients with these types of ulcers were advised to undergo early operation, the situation is less clear today, because such ulcers can heal with cimetidine treatment. Although conclusive data are not currently available, one of the advantages of a well-accepted medication such as an H_2-receptor antagonist may be that it selects those patients who are prone to frequent, threatening recurrences despite adequate nonoperative treatment.

Obstruction

A distinction should be made between chronic and acute obstruction. Little is gained by postponing operation in the patient with chronic symptomatic obstruction, since the scarring causing the obstruction will not be relieved by medication. Particular attention should be paid to patients with gastric outlet obstruction during the induction of anesthesia to avoid aspiration.

In the case of acute obstruction, a limited trial of nonoperative treatment is begun. If the patient is unable to take a liquid diet at the end of 72 hours of nasogastric suction, operation is performed; longer periods of treatment are seldom beneficial. When a longer period is necessary to control other problems preoperatively, parenteral nutrition can be given. However, the patient becomes exhausted both emotionally and physically during the prolonged nonoperative treatment associated with unrelenting obstruction. Parenteral nutrition in this circumstance is reserved for the preoperative course, not used as a convenient vehicle to prolong nonoperative treatment, except in unusual circumstances. Parenteral nutrition should be tapered prior to operation, since maintenance of a high glucose load intraoperatively and in the immediate postoperative period can lead to significant CO_2 retention. The patient may be unable to blow off the increased CO_2 load that results from the oxidation of glucose.

Perforation

Although there are advocates of nonoperative treatment for perforated ulcer, it is generally accepted that immediate operation is preferable for acute perforation. Nonoperative treatment can be used in selected circumstances, provided radiographs using water-soluble contrast material show that the perforation has sealed, the abdominal findings improve within 3–5 hours, and there is no increasing pneumoperitoneum, severe aerophagia, or deterioration after a period of improvement.[3] This approach may play a role in those cases with underlying medical problems that make the risk of operation prohibitive. However, the nonoperative approach to perforation requires careful surveillance, since the fibrin seal of the perforation can subsequently break down.

Bleeding

While about 70% of patients with upper GI hemorrhage spontaneously stop bleeding, and while it is safer to operate on a patient who is not bleeding, certain circumstances require an early, aggressive operative approach because of a low chance of spontaneous cessation of hemorrhage. Many surgeons recommend operative therapy for the patient who bleeds into shock while under observation. The nonoperative mortality is greater in these patients as well as those with continuous bleeding. There is a relationship between the magnitude of the hemorrhage and mortality, which is lower if the patient has lost 6 or fewer units of blood.[4]

Age also is an important factor relating to mortality. The mortality for bleeding from either a duodenal or gastric ulcer more than doubles after age 60. Some continue to take a different approach to bleeding duodenal and gastric ulcers, being less aggressive about advising early operation for the former. This is based on the erroneous belief that the mortality in patients with bleeding gastric ulcer is twice that for bleeding duodenal ulcer. However, this does not appear to be the case when age and other factors are matched.

There are at least three other groups of patients who are presumably at greater risk with continuation of nonoperative treatment. One includes those being intensively treated for ulcer disease in the hospital who during the course of such treatment develop hemorrhage requiring transfusion. Another group consists of those who initially respond to nonoperative treatment and, after a period of apparent cessation of bleeding, have recurrence. The third group involves those patients with a remote history of hemorrhage requiring transfusion who rebleed. The incidence of rebleeding ranges from about 30% to 50%, but the long-term risk of this event's occurring for any given patient is difficult to predict. On one hand, there are data indicating that the incidence of rebleeding is relatively constant after a first, second, or third episode. Other data suggest that the chance of bleeding a third time is more than twice that of bleeding a second time.

Many surgeons feel that early endoscopy is an important procedure in the patient with upper GI hemorrhage, despite several prospective studies indicating that early endoscopy with definition of the bleeding site has little or no influence on mortality. Criteria for management and/or timing of operation were not firmly established in these studies. The major issue, however, is related to what one does with the endoscopic information. For example, the presence of a visible vessel in the ulcer bed should lead to urgent operation, because more than half (56%) of these patients will rebleed in contrast to 8% of those with other stigmas of recent hemorrhage.[5]

Another reason for early endoscopy is that the results of the procedure may help to plan the operative approach. Knowledge of the absence of certain lesions or normal areas of mucosa can lead to a more expeditious exploration and earlier control of the bleeding site. For example, a high gastrotomy can be avoided if it is known that the patient is not bleeding from a Mallory-Weiss tear or the proximal stomach. On the other hand, one should not be misled by erroneous endoscopic information if a more distal lesion is not found.

There are no universally accepted criteria relating to the timing of operation for the acutely bleeding patient. There is, however, near-consensus that an aggressive approach should be taken. Many of the criteria proposed by various groups incorporate an aggressive scheme, thus agreeing in principle but differing in details. My preference is for the approach proposed by Enquist and associates.[6] If the blood volume is not initially restored with 3 units of whole blood or its equivalent, or if the patient's requirement is greater than 500 ml of whole blood or its equivalent in any subsequent eight-hour period, the patient undergoes immediate operation. The advantage of this approach is that it limits the number of transfusions before there is dilution of clotting factors. Implicit in the success of this scheme, however, is that the patient is taken immediately to the operating room once the criteria have been met. The same is true for the previously mentioned high-risk patients; we have yet to regret the aggressive approach of immediate operation. However, there is little question that elective operation is associated with a lower mortality than emergent operation in the presence of active bleeding; this line of reasoning should not be used to cause unnecessary delay when indications for emergent operation are evident.

There remain in some circles beliefs that elderly patients should be given the benefit of the doubt and receive more transfusions and that younger patients can tolerate hypovolemic insults much better. An aggressive approach to patients over age 60 is supported by a recent prospective study in which the criteria for early operation included 4 units of blood or plasma expander within 24 hours, or one rebleed, or endoscopic evidence of recent bleeding, or a previous episode of bleeding and two-year history of dyspepsia.[7] Using this scheme, the mortality was 2% compared with less stringent criteria that were followed by a 13% mortality. It is the elderly patient with significant, other diseases that is least likely to withstand an episode of hypovolemic shock. While there is little doubt that younger patients do better in this situation, one should not underestimate the morbidity of this event in such patients.

A trap to avoid in dealing with upper GI hemorrhage is the patient who has been taking aspirin or other drug(s) that interfere with platelet function. This can be readily diagnosed by obtaining a bleeding time, which, if significantly prolonged, should be treated with platelet transfusions. This approach has been followed, either by association or fortuitously, by prompt cessation of hemorrhage in four of our patients with bleeding duodenal ulcer.

Particular attention to preoperative respiratory care should be given to patients with upper GI hemorrhage. The incidence of pulmonary aspiration is higher than generally appreciated—as a result of manipulation of an endoscope or a nasogastric tube; or during induction of anesthesia; or even hospital personnel's not helping the patient to turn on his side during emesis.

PREOPERATIVE CONSIDERATIONS

It is helpful to have certain information about the serum gastrin, location of the ulcer, and perhaps the level of gastric secretion. Considering the use of antibiotic(s) prior to operation also contributes to proper preoperative planning, thus minimizing morbidity.

Serum Gastrin

With the widespread availability of immunoassay of serum gastrin, there is little reason why this measurement should not be done preoperatively. While it may be argued that the incidence of gastrinoma or antral G-cell hyperfunction (a term preferable to antral G-cell hyperplasia because not all agree that there are an increased number of G cells) is rare relative to ordinary peptic ulcer disease, significant morbidity can occur as a result of incorrect operative treatment. An operation with less than complete removal of the antral mucosa (anatomical antrectomy) is insufficient for the treatment of antral G-cell hyperfunction, and not knowing that the patient has a gastrinoma usually leads to inaccurate exploration and operation, even though the approach to such patients is controversial. The majority of patients with gastrinoma seen today have ulcer disease that is difficult to distinguish, on the basis of history or location, from "garden variety" disease.

Serum gastrin measurements are frequently neglected in patients who present with an acute complication of peptic ulcer disease such as obstruction, bleeding, or perforation. While awaiting the result of this measurement will unnecessarily delay an urgent or emergent operation, full treatment with an H_2-receptor antagonist can be continued postoperatively until the gastrin value is known. An abnormal serum gastrin measurement demands further study using the secretin, and perhaps calcium, as well as protein stimulation tests. Gastric analysis is not a substitute for serum gastrin measurement, as the analysis often is inaccurate, and overlap of secretory values is not unusual.

Location of the Ulcer

It is generally accepted that different operative concepts apply to ordinary gastric as opposed to duodenal ulcer. Yet, controversy continues about the correct approach to the treatment of ulcers in certain specific locations.

A prepyloric ulcer, while in the stomach, is believed to be more akin to a duodenal ulcer than ordinary gastric ulcer. Data regarding this point are unclear primarily because of the overlap of acid secretory values between gastric and duodenal ulcers, the location of the prepyloric ulcer with respect to the antral and parietal bearing cell mucosa,[4] and the variable definition of "prepyloric." The last has ranged from those presenting to the right of the gastric angulus to within 2–3 cm of the pylorus.[4] Accepted operative treatment is to deal with a prepyloric ulcer like a duodenal ulcer, even though the adequacy of proximal gastric vagotomy for such an ulcer has been questioned by at least one report.[8] However, the lack of precise definition, acceptable control patients, and adequate prospective study compounds the issues involved.

Those with ulcer of both the stomach and duodenum are believed generally to belong to a hypersecretory group that acts primarily like duodenal ulcer patients. The majority of such patients are believed to have an element of pyloric stenosis and large, deep gastric ulcers. Epidemiologic data, however, indirectly suggest that the gastric ulcer precedes duodenal ulcer more frequently than the reverse.[9]

Until data further clarify whether or not prepyloric ulcers behave like gastric or duodenal ulcers, it is best to continue to treat them as if they were duodenal. In the case of combined ulcers, elements of treatment of both (antrectomy for the gastric ulcer and vagotomy for the duodenal ulcer) should be incorporated into the operative procedure.

Gastric Analysis

It is tempting to think that an operative procedure for duodenal ulcer can be tailored to the individual patient based on preoperative acid secretory studies. The premise of selective surgery is that an operation associated with a greater, or perhaps more lasting, reduction in acid secretion (for example, vagotomy with antrectomy) is necessary for those with high acid secretory rates, whereas a less radical procedure (for example, vagotomy without resection) will suffice for those with normal or low acid secretory rates. While there are data to support such an approach, the bulk of clinical experience does not. The concept of selective surgery implies that there is an acid secretory threshold necessary for ulceration, but this threshold must vary to accommodate a large amount of data. Furthermore, the selective operative approach based on acid secretory levels does not encompass certain features about the pathophysiology of ulcers such as the extent of mucosal permeability to acid, the degree of bicarbonate and mucous secretion, and the ability of the mucosa to buffer diffusing acid. Presumably, these and perhaps other factors may explain why some patients with acid hypersecretion do not ulcerate and others with normal secretory rates do ulcerate.

Antibiotic Treatment

There is nothing particularly specific about the immediate preoperative preparation of a patient other than a consideration of antibiotic treatment to minimize the incidence of wound infection. Prior to the availability of an H_2-receptor antagonist, it was unnecessary to give antibiotics to patients undergoing gastric surgery because of the presence of acid in the gastric lumen. Today, however, many patients are given an H_2-receptor antagonist up to the time of operation. As the luminal pH increases from about 3 to 7, the chances of harboring a significant colony count also progressively increases. Thus, in this situation, antibiotics directed at the oral flora are administered. Antibiotic coverage should also be considered for those with upper GI hemorrhage, as the incidence of wound infection is much greater in such patients after the lumen has been exposed.

CHOICE OF OPERATION

Before undertaking operation, it is helpful to know the advantages and disadvantages of the currently accepted operative approaches.

Truncal vagotomy with drainage, truncal vagotomy with antrectomy, and subtotal gastrectomy are the three generally accepted operative procedures for peptic ulcer disease of the duodenum. For the purposes of the discussion that follows, it makes no difference whether the drainage is a pyloroplasty or gastrojejunostomy, or whether the reconstruction after resection involves a gastroduodenostomy (Billroth I) or gastrojejunostomy (Billroth II). Unless stated otherwise, antrectomy as used here (in contrast to anatomical antrectomy) refers to what some consider a hemigastrectomy, but reference to antrectomy is frequently made in the literature. This loose definition does not imply that all of the antral mucosa is removed (Fig 14–2). Subtotal gastrectomy refers to excision of 70%–75% of the distal stomach.

Prospective studies indicate that there are no significant differences in operative mortality among the three operative procedures,[1, 10–12] which is in contrast to suggested differences reported by retrospective studies. Two studies, in fact, reported no mortality.[1, 10] The reason is that the prospective studies not only were performed under elective circumstances, but the protocols also contained an escape clause that permitted rejection of a specific operative procedure if it was not technically safe to perform. This feature is of prime importance in minimizing operative mortality and morbidity. In one prospective study, the operative complications related to the specific procedure were not significantly different,[10] but in another, the incidence of complications was significantly lower following vagotomy with drainage.[11]

Prospective studies comparing the three standard operative procedures indicate that while the majority of patients are pleased with the results of their operations, new symptoms can occur as a consequence of the operation (Table 14–1). Such symptoms include epigastric fullness, heartburn, abdominal pain, nausea, regurgitation, bile vomiting, food vomiting, dumping syndrome, flatulence, diarrhea, and hypoglycemia (sometimes referred to as late dumping). The incidence

	%	%	%
TABLE 14–1.—COMBINED RESULTS OF THREE PROSPECTIVE TRIALS OF STANDARD ULCER OPERATIONS[1, 10–12]			
RESULT	V AND D*	V AND A*	STG*
Fullness	14–40	29–36	16–37
Heartburn	20	16	8
Abdominal pain	19–30	20–29	19–24
Nausea	13–20	17–24	23–31
Reflux	4	7	4
Regurgitation	3	12	4
Bile emesis	15	14	13
Food emesis	4	10	6
Dumping	9–27	9–33	22–42
Flatulence	18	23	20
Diarrhea	14–26	21–23	7–17
Hypoglycemia	6–12	4–16	1–12
Operative death	0–2	0–3	0–2
Operative complications	6	6–12	8–9
Recurrence	6–10	1–4	2–5
Overall result			
Excellent-good	70–83	78–91	77–90
Fair	12–19	7–14	7–17
Poor	5–11	2–8	3–6

*V and D = vagotomy with drainage; V and A = vagotomy with antrectomy; STG = subtotal gastrectomy.

of these side effects of operation varies from series to series, in part owing to definition. A number of claims have been made suggesting that the incidence of certain symptoms are greater or lower after one of three standard operative procedures, but by and large this is not substantiated by prospective studies.

The most common long-term symptom is the sensation of epigastric fullness. This is not usually incapacitating, and its etiology is speculative. It is probably related to the loss of receptive relaxation of the fundus following vagotomy, and in the case of subtotal gastrectomy without vagotomy, to the reduced size of the gastric pouch. The incidence of fullness is not significantly different among the three standard operative procedures.[1]

The most frequent troublesome sequela is the dumping syndrome, the incidence of which is confusing because of its variability. For example, the incidence of dumping was significantly lower after vagotomy with drainage in the Minnesota study,[10] whereas there was a significant increase in severity of dumping as the amount of stomach excised increased in the VA study.[11, 12] In contrast, the incidence of dumping was significantly lower after vagotomy with antrectomy in the Leeds/York study during the 5–8-year follow-up,[1] but this difference was no longer significant with further follow-up, 10–16 years postoperatively.[13]

A major difficulty in determining the true incidence of dumping is that the diagnosis usually is based on history rather than on the oral administration of a standard osmotic load, and other postgastrectomy disorders are erroneously labeled as part of the dumping syndrome. A hypertonic glucose load given orally provokes dumping symptoms in 20% of duodenal ulcer patients prior to operation, in 73% of patients with truncal vagotomy with pyloroplasty, in 80% of patients with selective vagotomy with pyloroplasty, and in 47% of pa-

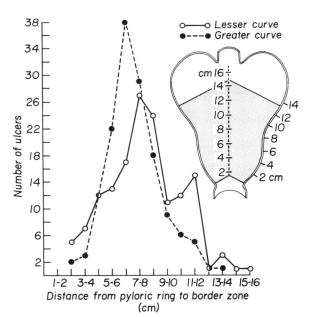

Fig 14–2.—Variable distance between the pylorus and 2-cm border zone between antral and parietal cell bearing mucosa. (The Y-axis indicates the number of gastric ulcers found in the border zone at various distances from the pyloric ring.) (From Fromm D.[4] and modified from Oi et al.[19] Used by permission.)

tients with proximal gastric vagotomy.[14] Since these figures are higher than those generally encountered clinically, it is likely that patients do not ordinarily ingest a similar hypertonic load and that in time they consciously or unconsciously adjust their diets.

Many still believe that diarrhea is not a significant problem following operation. The Minnesota and VA data suggest that the occurrence of postvagotomy diarrhea has been overemphasized, because the incidence following vagotomy was not significantly different from that occurring after subtotal gastrectomy.[10, 11] Others argue that little attention usually is paid to preservation of the vagal divisions during subtotal gastrectomy.[17] The incidence of diarrhea was significantly lower after subtotal gastrectomy in only one study.[1] However, prospective data for selective vagotomy leave little doubt that there is an increased incidence of diarrhea after truncal vagotomy (Fig 14–3).[15, 16] For reasons that are unclear, the differing incidence of diarrhea following gastric resection without vagotomy and vagotomy without resection in the Leeds/York study disappeared with longer follow-up.[13]

The etiology of postvagotomy diarrhea is poorly understood. However, it appears that the incidence is much greater in patients who have undergone or who will undergo cholecystectomy, and it has been suggested that preservation of the hepatic division of the left anterior vagus nerve minimizes the incidence of diarrhea.[17] Diarrhea tends to be ignored postoperatively because it is usually not a severe problem in the majority of patients. However, as many as 5%–10% find it troublesome, but in less than 1% the diarrhea is disabling.

Prospective studies indicate that the major difference between vagotomy with drainage, vagotomy with antrectomy, and subtotal gastrectomy relates to the incidence of recurrent ulceration. The incidence of recurrent ulcer ranged from 7%

to 10% after vagotomy with drainage in four prospective studies.[4] This is in contrast to a 1%–4% incidence after vagotomy with antrectomy and a 2%–5% incidence after subtotal gastrectomy.[4] Although some data suggest otherwise,[13] it is generally accepted that the incidence of recurrent ulcer is least after vagotomy with antrectomy. This is most likely due to the dual protective nature of the operation: antrectomy compensates for an incomplete vagotomy, and vagotomy compensates for an incomplete antrectomy.[18] While it is clear that residual antral mucosa in the duodenal stump of a Billroth II reconstruction places the patient at great risk for a recurrent ulcer, the role of residual antrum in the gastric stump is not clear. It cannot be assumed that the operation of hemigastrectomy always removes the antrum, since the proximal extent of the antrum varies from patient to patient on both the greater and lesser curve aspects of the stomach (see Fig 14–3).[19] Conceptually, it appears that if gastric resection is done, an anatomical antrectomy (which removes all of the antral mucosa) should be done (Fig 14–4).[4] That this is accomplished can be verified by histologic examination of both greater and lesser curves of the proximal aspect as well as the most distal aspect of the specimen.

The most important observation emerging from the prospective studies of the three standard operations for duodenal ulcer is that there is no significant difference in terms of long-term sequelae. However, the incidence of recurrent ulcer is least with vagotomy and antrectomy but still within an acceptable range following vagotomy with drainage. Furthermore, given appropriate anatomical circumstances, any one of the three standard operations can be done with minimal immediate postoperative morbidity and mortality. Thus, if one plans a vagotomy with antrectomy preoperatively and the duodenum is found to be markedly scarred or edematous, one need not undertake a potentially hazardous resection. Furthermore, there are no substantive data indicating any long-term differences between the various types of drainage procedures accompanying vagotomy. Thus, if the duodenum is

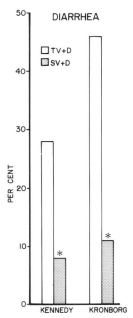

Fig 14–3.—Incidence of diarrhea following truncal vagotomy with drainage (TV+D) and selective vagotomy with drainage (SV+D). (Data are from the prospective studies of Kennedy et al.[15] and Kronborg et al.[16])

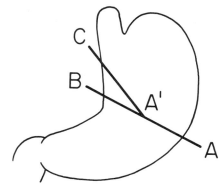

Fig 14–4.—Because of the variable extent of the antral mucosa (see Fig 14–2) and because it may extend to near the esophagogastric junction on the lesser curvature side, transection of the stomach perpendicular to greater and lesser curves (line AB) may leave antral mucosa on the lesser curve side of the gastric pouch. Retention of antral mucosa on the lesser curve side is less likely if a Schoemaker resection is done: the stomach is divided first along line AA' and then resected in a more proximal plane along line A'C.

scarred or edematous, a gastroenterostomy as a drainage procedure can be done without hesitation.

My preference is generally to avoid subtotal gastrectomy because of my impression that while the incidence of associated symptoms is not greater than that of the other standard procedures, the severity is. Subtotal gastrectomy, however, can be a useful procedure in the presence of severe portal hypertension, a situation in which one may want to avoid dissection around the esophagus. Some continue to do truncal vagotomy along with subtotal gastrectomy, but this combination usually is unnecessary and may increase the risk of diarrhea.

Selective Vagotomy With Drainage

The incidence of diarrhea can be minimized by doing a selective vagotomy. The only major difference between truncal and selective vagotomy in two prospective studies was a significantly lower incidence of diarrhea with the selective technique (see Fig 14–3).[15, 16] Selective vagotomy has not caught on as a standard operative procedure for duodenal ulcer disease, because the overall results of the technically more difficult selective and less difficult truncal techniques combined with drainage are not different. Yet, there is a role for selective vagotomy in those patients who are prone to diarrhea. For example, those with a prior cholecystectomy, or who require gastroenterostomy as a result of Crohn's disease or chronic pancreatitis and are prone to diarrhea from differing etiologies, may benefit from selective as opposed to truncal vagotomy.

DRAINAGE PROCEDURE.—Truncal vagotomy classically involves division of the vagal trunks proximal to the celiac and hepatic divisions and thus also interrupts vagal flow to the nerves of Latarget innervating the parietal cell bearing and antral mucosa (Fig 14–5,A and B). Selective vagotomy, on the other hand, involves division of the nerves of Latarget at their origins, thereby preserving the hepatic and celiac divisions (Fig 14–5,C). Since both types of vagotomy interrupt the parasympathetic flow to the antrum, there is impairment of emptying of solids from the stomach. However, it appears that only about 20% of patients will have clinically significant impaired gastric emptying if truncal or selective vagotomy is done without an accompanying drainage procedure. While this figure invites the tempting possibility of doing a truncal vagotomy without an accompanying drainage procedure, insufficient information is available for the group of patients absolutely requiring drainage. It is doubtful that scarring from the ulcer alone is the sole determinant of the necessity for drainage, because at least 20% of patients following esophagoproximal gastrectomy without a drainage procedure have impaired gastric emptying. The drainage procedure is in itself a cause of morbidity, especially dumping, hypoglycemia, and bilious vomiting. The majority of patients either do not have the symptoms to a significant degree or are able to cope with them. Nevertheless, there remains a group of patients that is difficult to treat, which has led to enthusiasm for proximal gastric vagotomy.

Proximal Gastric Vagotomy Without Drainage

Proximal gastric vagotomy differs from the other types of vagotomy in that the nerves of Latarget innervating the an-

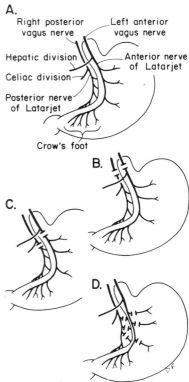

Fig 14–5.—Schematic representation of the different types of vagotomy. *A,* vagal anatomy (note, in contrast to Figure 14–6, that the hepatic division of the left vagus is represented as a single branch; the number of hepatic division branches is variable). *B,* truncal vagotomy. *C,* selective vagotomy. *D,* proximal gastric vagotomy.

trum remain intact, whereas the branches of these nerves innervating the parietal cell mass are severed. Thus, the celiac and hepatic divisions also remain intact (Fig 14–5,D). Because the antral mill is preserved, it is unnecessary to do a drainage procedure with proximal gastric vagotomy. It is generally agreed that all symptoms, with the exception of epigastric fullness, are decreased in incidence following proximal gastric vagotomy. However, prospective studies indicate that the major difference between proximal gastric vagotomy and selective vagotomy relates to the dumping syndrome,[20–24] the incidence of which is lower after proximal gastric vagotomy, both by history and after a standard osmotic load given orally. The incidence of dumping reported by prospective studies comparing selective to proximal gastric vagotomy ranges from 28% to 59% for the former and 4% to 17% for the latter. Even though the pylorus is intact with this procedure, dumping may occur because of the faster emptying of liquids as a result of the loss of receptive relaxation in the fundus.

The operative mortality of proximal gastric vagotomy is not significantly different from that of other procedures. On a retrospective basis, however, proximal gastric vagotomy is associated with a lower operative mortality, 0.3% in over 5,500 operations.[25] This figure for mortality is less than that reported by other retrospective series involving gastric resection or vagotomy with drainage.

The major question concerning proximal gastric vagotomy is its durability in terms of recurrent ulceration. In the relatively short follow-up available from most prospective studies, the incidence of recurrence is not significantly different from that following other forms of vagotomy. However, it is clear that lack of attention to technical details of the procedure will result in an unacceptably high recurrence rate.[4] Now that greater emphasis has been placed on the periesophageal dissection of the vagal branches, the incidence of postoperative dysphagia appears to have increased, but this is usually mild and rarely permanent.

Proximal gastric vagotomy usually is begun 7 cm proximal to the pylorus. This landmark generally corresponds to being just proximal to the so-called crow's feet of the nerves of Latarget (see Fig 5,A). The results using the 7-cm landmark do not differ from the antral mapping technique, which is perhaps a more physiologic approach. However, a potential problem with proximal gastric vagotomy is that the extent of antral mucosa may differ from the external landmark(s) of the antrum. It has been suggested that as many as 20% of patients may not have complete denervation of the distal fundic mucosa.[26] This consideration has not yet been shown to be clinically significant, but it may account for some of the recurrences after a technically well-performed operation. Many surgeons believe that the incidence of incomplete truncal vagotomy also is about 20%.

In the absence of outlet obstruction, I prefer to do proximal gastric vagotomy for duodenal ulcer because the incidence of side effects is lower than that associated with other procedures, but realize that the incidence of recurrent ulcer is the same as for other forms of vagotomy unaccompanied by resection.

OPERATION FOR SPECIFIC COMPLICATIONS OF PEPTIC ULCER
Gastric Outlet Obstruction

Many continue to believe that vagotomy with drainage (gastrojejunostomy) or vagotomy with resection is not a good procedure for the relief of gastric outlet obstruction, mainly because of postoperative difficulties with gastric emptying. This problem has been ascribed to gastric atony (a situation also used to explain clinically significant impaired emptying following truncal vagotomy in the absence of obstruction). Careful analysis of such patients, however, suggests that in the majority of instances, the so-called postoperative gastric atony is related to inadequate preoperative decompression and/or, more likely, a technical problem associated with the drainage procedure. Many cases of "atony" that I have seen following operations for a variety of different indications are in fact related to mechanical problems observed either endoscopically or radiographically. Even an atonic or denervated stomach should empty by gravity, provided there is no mechanical problem at the outlet. These views probably oversimplify a complex situation, the physiology of immediate postoperative gastric emptying being poorly understood. Edema at the anastomotic site is a continuing problem, and even though temporary, it may last four weeks or longer.

Those who subscribe to the premise that vagotomy contributes to greater emptying problems after operation on a patient with obstruction prefer to do a subtotal gastrectomy without vagotomy. However, this approach is not essential, as

antrectomy with vagotomy works well, just as does vagotomy with gastrojejunostomy.

There are advocates of proximal gastric vagotomy in the presence of gastric outlet obstruction. The pylorus in this instance is mechanically dilated at operation, but perforation can result. It is possible that many of the favorable results are a consequence of doing an operative procedure primarily in the presence of edema as the cause of obstruction, whereas the unfavorable results may be due to primarily dealing with scar tissue. My experience with proximal gastric vagotomy and dilatation in six patients has been unfavorable in two. While both patients are improved compared to their preoperative conditions, one has clinically apparent impairment of gastric emptying and the other has recurring gastric ulcers that are most likely a result of persisting, mildly symptomatic obstruction, whereas preoperatively he had duodenal ulcer.

My choice of operative procedure depends on anatomical circumstances and overall condition of the patient, but I give preference to vagotomy with antrectomy, since it is followed by the lowest incidence of recurrent ulcer. However, vagotomy with drainage (usually gastroenterostomy in this circumstance) is a very good alternative.

Perforation

While the primary goal of operation is the control of the perforation, there is controversy about definitive treatment. Although figures vary somewhat from series to series, 70%–75% of patients remain asymptomatic after closure of the perforation provided they have an acute history (shorter than three months) of ulcer symptoms. In contrast, only 25%–30% of patients remain asymptomatic after closure if they have a chronic history (longer than three months) of symptoms prior to perforation. Thus, there are advocates of definitive operation in addition to closure of the perforation in patients with a chronic history. However, the arbitrary division of ulcer symptoms into acute and chronic has been questioned. Consequently, others conclude that there are no good guidelines for selecting patients for definitive operation at the time of closure of the perforation. Those who favor simple closure only point out that the majority of patients who have recurrent ulcer symptoms postoperatively do so within one year and can be considered for definitive operation at that time. A factor that has not been studied in detail is whether the patient has been receiving adequate treatment for the ulcer up to the time of perforation. Such patients are presumably at greater risk for recurrent perforation.

A rigid policy toward perforation is not supported by factual data, but where the situation is appropriate, there need be no fear for definitive surgery. However, an operative procedure done to control the ulcer disease, in contrast to closure of the perforation, is not done as an immediate lifesaving procedure but to avoid future complications.

Those undergoing definitive operation at the time of closure of the perforation are a select group, only 30% of the patients in most series. This may be a reflection of the degree of peritoneal contamination. The concept of a "golden period" relative to the time of perforation and operation has been nearly replaced by the importance of the extent of contamination. However, the degree of spillage is difficult to predict prior to operation and shows little correlation with positive cultures, even though a higher incidence of postoperative complications occurs in those with marked as opposed to moderate or slight contamination. In patients considered to be good candidates for definitive surgery, contamination is associated with a mortality of less than 3%, which compares favorably with figures for simple closure only.

My approach depends on the history and stability of the patient and the degree of contamination. If a patient has been treated for peptic ulcer disease prior to perforation, I do not hesitate to perform proximal gastric vagotomy in addition to simple closure, provided the patient is reasonably healthy, stable, free of obstruction, and has minimal contamination. Proximal gastric vagotomy has the advantage that there are no suture lines. Although there has been fear of causing mediastinitis as a result of the dissection around the esophagus, this complication has not been reported in a large series. In other circumstances, I prefer simple closure only, since nonoperative treatment with an H_2-receptor antagonist thereafter is fairly effective long enough to determine whether there is an unusual etiology of the ulcer, while the patient recovers from the consequences of perforation and operation per se.

Care must be taken to insure, insofar as possible, that the closure does not result in obstruction, a situation that is more likely with perforated pyloric channel ulcers. Gastrojejunostomy with vagotomy may be necessary.

A small percentage of patients present with perforation and bleeding, the latter being due to a synchronous posterior ulcer. The only reliable sign of the second ulcer is the presence of preoperative hemorrhage. Although this may be due to perforation itself, a synchronous posterior ulcer must be diagnosed at the time of operation. If inspection or palpation do not reveal another ulcer in the bleeding patient with perforation, the perforated area should be opened to inspect directly and to palpate the posterior duodenal wall. An additional ulcer should be treated as if it were the site of a significant hemorrhage.

Hemorrhage

The site of a bleeding duodenal ulcer frequently is indicated by the external appearance of the duodenum. If the surgeon is accustomed to performing proximal gastric vagotomy, a transverse duodenotomy can be made. A longitudinal duodenotomy, however, is used when the precise location of the ulcer is uncertain. This need not be converted into a pyloroplasty, since precise closure of the longitudinal duodenotomy can be accomplished without causing obstruction, provided there is not significant scarring. In either case, since most patients present acutely, without benefit of studies to determine outlet obstruction, at the time of operation a judgment must be made by luminal palpation to determine the potential presence of obstruction within the duodenum as the result of dense scarring.

Most cases of massive hemorrhage involve penetration of the gastroduodenal arterial complex which requires complete control and may involve several sutures.[4] I believe that a three-point ligation that encompasses the gastroduodenal artery proximal and distal to the penetration as well as the transverse pancreatic artery originating from the gastroduodenal is essential for preventing rebleeding in the immediate postoperative period.[27]

The method of closure of the duodenum will depend on the type of vagotomy and gastrectomy to be performed. If a vagotomy with Heineke-Mikulicz pyloroplasty is preferred, closure of the duodenum may be less than perfect, especially when a duodenotomy longer than 2 cm beyond the pylorus is made.[4] In this instance and in cases where there is distortion of the duodenum as a result of scarring, it is far better to close the duodenum in the safest manner, not worry about obstruction, and perform a gastrojejunostomy. If a drainage procedure has been performed, truncal vagotomy is done. Vagotomy with antrectomy is another option depending on the circumstances. Proximal gastric vagotomy is acceptable if the pylorus can be preserved and the duodenum can be closed without causing obstruction.

In the elderly unstable patient, one must make a value judgment after controlling the hemorrhage as to the merits of continuing the operative procedure and doing something definitive for the ulcer disease. The majority of patients will stabilize once control of hemorrhage is obtained. The judgment to continue in the relatively unstable patient must be weighed against the concept that these are precisely the patients who cannot tolerate a postoperative hemorrhage. This is not always prevented by intensive treatment with medication(s).

Some reports emphasize that there is a high incidence of recurrent bleeding within five years of definitive treatment for bleeding peptic ulcer disease, this figure approaches 20% or greater in at least one series.[4] Such figures should be cautiously interpreted, since authors have not always distinguished between the causes. Part of the problem with recurrence may be a reflection of a hastily done, and thus likely inadequate, operation. For example, if truncal vagotomy is done, only transecting the vagal trunks might be an inadequate procedure, because there may remain branches originating proximal to the point of transection and innervating the fundus (Fig 14–6).

RECURRENT ULCER

It is essential that the etiology of recurrent ulcer be determined so that appropriate treatment is given. Factors that must be excluded include antral stasis, drainage procedure without vagotomy, inadequate gastric resection, retained excluded distal antrum, hypergastrinemia of antral origin, gastrinoma, hyperparathyroidism, suture erosion, and drug-induced ulcer. Some believe that the incidence of recurrent ulcer is greater after a Billroth I than after a Billroth II reconstruction, but this is not substantiated by available data.

Acid secretory studies reportedly directed at testing the integrity of the vagi are plagued by so much overlap that interpretation is impractical for individual patients. A serum gastrin measurement is essential, and all other causes of an elevated gastrin level must be excluded before it is concluded that an abnormal value is the result of vagotomy. Retained excluded antrum, a cause of hypergastrinemia, can be easily diagnosed by reviewing the original pathologic slides, provided adequate sections were made. Sometimes it is not appreciated that the antrum may extend 0.5 cm beyond the pylorus. A technetium scan often is helpful in diagnosing the presence of antral mucosa in the duodenal stump of a Billroth II anastomosis.

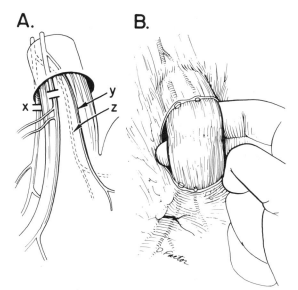

Fig 14–6.—*A*, if the vagal trunks are divided only at point *X*, branches originating more proximally *(Y and Z)* and innervating a portion of the parietal cell mass will remain intact. *B*, a complete vagotomy necessitates stripping the esophagus of areolar tissue lying over its longitudinal muscle for 5–7 cm. (The latter should also be done for selective and proximal gastric vagotomy.)

The mortality for nonoperative treatment of recurrent ulcer was 11% and the relapse rate was 42% before the era of H_2-receptor antagonists. These figures are in contrast to an operative mortality of 4% and a postoperative relapse rate of 14%.[28] This relapse rate is high, because it includes inadequate operative procedures as judged by current standards.

The role and efficacy of H_2-receptor antagonists in the treatment of recurrent ulcer is still unclear. Patients appear to require more prolonged treatment than if they had not had prior operation and require more than the usual maintenance dose once healing has occurred. A 71% recurrence rate has been reported after cessation of maintenance treatment for one year.[29] Certainly, failure to heal and recurrence during maintenance medication or after cessation of maintenance treatment are indications for operation. That a marginal ulcer is still present but not symptomatic during or following treatment should not dissuade one from recommending operation, since silent ulcers belie their potential danger. Repeated endoscopy may be necessary to make the sometimes difficult distinction between a recurrent ulcer and an erosion associated with postoperative gastritis.

In the absence of a specific cause other than a prior inadequate operation, the principal in treatment usually involves the next greater magnitude of operation to reduce acid secretion (Fig 14–7). Thus, most instances of recurrence require resection or re-resection with vagotomy or revagotomy. Recurrence following vagotomy with drainage or following gastroenterostomy or partial gastrectomy either with or without vagotomy is treated by (re-) vagotomy and anatomical antrectomy. Recurrence following proximal gastric vagotomy should be treated by at least anatomical antrectomy, which in itself suffices for the short term. Some would also do truncal vagot-

omy in this circumstance. If a patient with a prior proximal gastric vagotomy needs to undergo partial gastrectomy because of recurrent ulcer, the original operative report should be carefully studied to insure that the left gastroepiploic vessels are intact. These may have been unknowingly sacrificed during an unplanned splenectomy; an arteriogram may resolve the question. Since proximal gastric vagotomy by necessity involves sacrifice of the left gastric artery and vein, the left gastroepiploic vessels are the major remaining vascular supply to the gastric pouch after distal resection.

Those who have had prior antrectomy or hemigastrectomy with vagotomy should undergo subtotal gastrectomy. If the patient has had an adequate prior subtotal gastrectomy without vagotomy, vagotomy is done through an abdominal or thoracic approach. The latter frequently is easier because one is dealing with a virgin operative field. If revagotomy is done transabdominally, redivision of only the vagal trunks is insufficient, since the problem may be due to intact vagal branches originating proximal to the trunks and innervating a portion of the parietal cell mass (see Fig 14–6). About 90% of patients will be cured of their recurrent ulcer. The 10% failure rate is unexplained. These cases have not been completely analyzed as to the adequacy of reoperation or etiology of recurrence.

TECHNICAL COMPLICATIONS

The most common problems occurring in the postoperative period are suture line or anastomotic leakage, bleeding, and obstruction. The incidence of leakage varies considerably and is based on technical error(s). Disruption of the duodenal stump in a Billroth II anastomosis may occur for reasons that any anastomosis leaks. It also may be the result of trying to

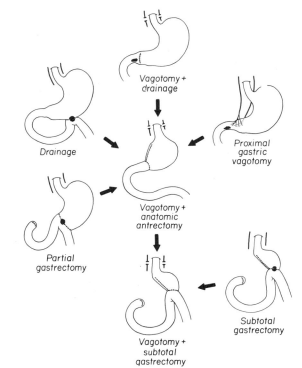

Fig 14–7.—Treatment of recurrent ulcer. (From Fromm D.[4] Used by permission.)

close a scarred, edematous duodenal stump or occur as a result of obstruction of the afferent limb, particularly at the gastrojejunal anastomosis from angulation or twisting. The lack of normal duodenum or the presence of tension can lead to disruption of a Billroth I reconstruction. Such complications usually become manifested within the first seven days of operation. The principles of treatment are those involved in management of any intestinal fistula: control of the fistula, then control of sepsis, and provision of nutrition.

Bleeding can occur from the anastomotic site acutely or a week later, the latter being frightening but usually less serious than the former. Anastomotic bleeding in the immediate postoperative period generally does not require reoperation but may necessitate transfusion of 2 or 3 units of blood. In contrast, anastomotic bleeding one week postoperatively usually requires no treatment but reassurance. Caution should be used in ascribing postoperative bleeding to the suture line when the indication for original operation was a bleeding duodenal ulcer. Either endoscopy or angiography can be useful in the distinction. Should reoperation for bleeding be necessary, it is helpful to know the site beforehand, because reoperation can be extraordinarily difficult if there are thick, inflamed adhesions, especially when a gastrectomy has been performed.

Anastomotic obstruction continues to be a source of major morbidity. Although the figure for such obstruction is usually stated to be 5%, it is greater. Many cases that have been ascribed to postvagotomy atony are more than likely due to obstruction as a result of anastomotic edema. This is probably a universal phenomenon in GI anastomoses, and while poorly understood, it probably is not clinically evident in intestine-to-intestine anastomoses because of the presence of proximal peristalsis. The majority of obstructions following gastroduodenal or gastrojejunal anastomosis will resolve but can take as long as four to six weeks. Another cause of obstruction is adherence of the anastomosis to the anterior abdominal wall, which causes the anastomotic lumen to be eccentrically placed and distorted. Evidence for this is more readily obtained by endoscopy than radiography using contrast material. Most cases of anastomotic obstruction, or "dysfunction," are deceptive in their initial presentation. The typical patient has resolution of the ileus as expected; nasogastric losses (if a tube is used) are minimal and contain bile; heartburn begins on about the fifth postoperative day; and vomiting occurs about two days later. Upper GI radiographs may demonstrate reasonable gastric emptying on the fifth day only to show worse emptying a few days later.

There is a unique complication that is rare after proximal gastric vagotomy. Necrosis of the lesser curve has been reported to occur in 0.15% of an international collection of patients.[25] This complication becomes clinically manifested by the fourth or fifth postoperative day. Some of the reported cases involved a focal area of necrosis and conceivably were due to the manner of securing lesser curve vessels if a portion of gastric wall was included in the ligature.[4] Other cases, however, involved an extensive area of necrosis. This might be the combined result of sacrifice of the left gastric arterial arcade, leaving an avascular corridor[30] and a temporary decrease in mucosal blood flow as a consequence of the vagotomy per se.

Some rare but nonetheless important anatomical complications can present in the acute or remote postoperative period. They can be avoided by attention to details during the operation. A long afferent limb is predisposed to volvulus, torsion, or kinking. Failure to suture the transverse mesocolon to the gastric pouch in a retrocolic anastomosis can result in external compression of the jejunum by scarring of the mesocolic opening. Retroanastomotic hernia can occur following a gastrojejunal anastomosis if the space behind the anastomosis is not closed with suture (Fig 14–8). Jejunogastric intussusception can occur acutely or chronically and be avoided only by doing a Billroth I reconstruction. These complications present as obstruction acutely, chronically, or even intermittently. The chronic forms can present as a malabsorption syndrome caused by bacterial overgrowth. The acute forms which cause a closed-loop obstruction of the afferent limb can be deceptive because such an obstruction mimics acute pancreatitis.

Too narrow an anastomosis between the stomach and small intestine will result in enhancement of symptoms of early satiety as well as outlet obstruction. A good rule of thumb is that the width of the anastomosis should be equal to the transverse diameter of the intestine. A larger anastomosis will not provide better emptying since the transverse intestinal diameter governs the rate of emptying. The misadventure of gastroileostomy can present acutely with symptoms of malabsorption or be more elusive, being relatively asymptomatic for

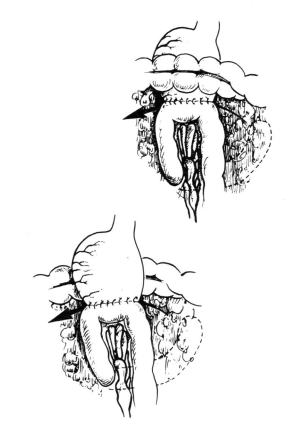

Fig 14–8.—A space for potential herniation of the small bowel exists behind the gastrojejunal anastomosis of a Billroth II reconstruction, be it retrocolic or antecolic. (From Fromm D.[17] Used by permission.)

some time after operation. This complication is easily avoided by being certain that the ligament of Treitz is identified at operation.

REFERENCES

1. Goligher J.C., Pulvertaft C.N., de Dombal F.T., et al.: Five-to eight-year results of Leeds/York controlled trial of elective surgery for duodenal ulcer. *Br. Med. J.* 2:781, 1968.
2. Fineberg H.V., Pearlman L.A.: Surgical treatment of peptic ulcer in the United States. *Lancet* 1:1305, 1981.
3. Berne C.J., Rosoff L. Sr.: Acute perforation of peptic ulcer, in Nyhus L.M., Wastell C. (eds.): *Surgery of the Stomach and Duodenum.* Boston, Little, Brown & Co., 1977, p. 449.
4. Fromm D.: Peptic ulcer, in Fromm D. (ed.): *Gastrointestinal Surgery.* New York, Churchill-Livingstone, 1984, pp. 233–323.
5. Storey D.W., Bown S.G., Swain C.P., et al.: Endoscopic prediction of recurrent bleeding in peptic ulcers. *N. Engl. J. Med.* 305:915, 181.
6. Enquist I.F., Karlson K.E., Dennis C., et al.: Statistically valid ten-year comparative evaluation of three methods of management of massive gastroduodenal hemorrhage. *Ann. Surg.* 162:550, 1965.
7. Morris D.L., Hawker P.C., Brearley S., et al.: Optimal timing of operation for bleeding peptic ulcer: Prospective randomized study. *Br. Med. J.* 288:1277, 1984.
8. Andersen D., Amdrup E., Hostrup H., et al.: The Aarhus County vagotomy trial. *World J. Surg.* 6:86, 1982.
9. Bonnevie O.: Gastric and duodenal ulcers in the same patient. *Scand. J. Gastroenterol.* 10:657, 1975.
10. Howard R.J., Murphy W.R., Humphrey E.W.: A prospective randomized study of the elective surgical treatment for duodenal ulcer: Two- to ten-year followup study. *Surgery* 73:256, 1973.
11. Postlethwait R.W.: Five year follow-up results of operations for duodenal ulcer. *Surg. Gynecol. Obstet.* 137:387, 1973.
12. Price W.E., Grizzle J.E., Postlethwait R.W., et al.: Results of operation for duodenal ulcer. *Surg. Gynecol. Obstet.* 131:233, 1970.
13. Goligher J.C., Feather D.B., Hall R., et al.: Several standard elective operations for duodenal ulcer: Ten to 16 year clinical results. *Ann. Surg.* 189:18, 1979.
14. Humphrey C.S., Johnston D., Walker B.E., et al.: Incidence of dumping after truncal and selective vagotomy with pyloroplasty and highly selective vagotomy with drainage procedure. *Br. Med. J.* 3:785, 1972.
15. Kennedy T., Connell A.M., Love A.H.G., et al.: Selective or truncal vagotomy? Five-year results of a double-blind randomized, controlled trial. *Br. J. Surg.* 60:944, 1973.
16. Kronborg O., Malmstrom J., Christiansen P.M.: A comparison between the results of truncal and selective vagotomy in patients with duodenal ulcer. *Scand. J. Gastroenterol.* 5:519, 1970.
17. Fromm D.: *Complications of Gastric Surgery.* New York, John Wiley & Sons, 1977.
18. Stempien S.J., Lee E.R., Dagradi A.E.: The role of distal gastrectomy, with and without vagotomy, in the control of cephalic secretion and peptic ulcer disease. *Surgery* 71:110, 1972.
19. Oi M., Oshida K., Sugimura S.: The location of gastric ulcer. *Gastroenterology* 36:45, 1959.
20. Amdrup E., Andersen D., Hostrup H.: The Aarhus County vagotomy trial: I. An interim report on primary results and incidence of sequelae following parietal cell vagotomy and selective gastric vagotomy in 748 patients. *World J. Surg.* 2:85, 1978.
21. Andersen D., Hostrup H., Amdrup E.: The Aarhus County vagotomy trial: II. An interim report on reduction in acid secretion and ulcer recurrence rate following parietal cell vagotomy and selective gastric vagotomy. *World J. Surg.* 2:91, 1978.
22. Faxen A., Kewenter J., Stockbrugger R.: Clinical results of parietal cell vagotomy and selective vagotomy with pyloroplasty in the treatment of duodenal ulcer. *Scand. J. Gastroenterol.* 13:741, 1978.
23. Jordan P.H. Jr.: A prospective study of parietal cell vagotomy-antrectomy for treatment of duodenal ulcer. *Ann. Surg.* 183:619, 1976.
24. Kennedy T., Johnston G.W., Macrae K.D., et al.: Proximal gastric vagotomy: Interim results of a randomized controlled trial. *Br. Med. J.* 2:301, 1975.
25. Johnston D.: Operative mortality and postoperative morbidity of highly selective vagotomy. *Br. Med. J.* 4:545, 1975.
26. Nielsen H.O., Monoz J.D., Kronborg O., et al.: The antrum in duodenal ulcer patients. *Scand. J. Gastroenterol.* 16:491, 1981.
27. Berne C.J., Rosoff L.: Peptic ulcer perforation of the gastroduodenal artery complex. *Ann. Surg.* 169:141, 1969.
28. Stabile B.E., Passaro E. Jr.: Recurrent peptic ulcer. *Gastroenterology* 70:124, 1976.
29. Koo J., Lam S.K., Ong G.B.: Cimetidine versus surgery for recurrent ulcer after gastric surgery. *Ann. Surg.* 195:406, 1982.
30. Thomas D.M., Langford R.M., Russel R.C.G., et al.: The anatomical basis for gastric mobilization in total oesophagectomy. *Br. J. Surg.* 66:230, 1979.

15

Gastric Ulcer

CHARLES M. SHEAFF, PH.D., M.D.
LLOYD M. NYHUS, M.D.

GASTRIC ULCERS are a unique subset of peptic ulcers. In fact, the term "peptic ulcers" should probably be used as little as possible because gastric ulcers and duodenal ulcers differ so much in their etiology and mode of treatment. Their natural histories follow different courses and their malignant potential is markedly different. There should probably even be a third subset of this disease for prepyloric ulcer based on difficulty of treatment. Gastric ulcers occur in the general population with a frequency of 0.4%,[1] and although not nearly as frequent as duodenal ulcers, nevertheless represent a major source of economic loss in the United States today. In the United States in 1967, including loss of personal income, loss of expected aggregate income owing to premature death, and cost of medical care for the totally disabled, such loss was $1 billion.[2] Noting that there has been no change in the incidence of gastric ulcer, unlike duodenal ulcer, which has decreased considerably in frequency over the past decade,[3] extrapolation can be made from old figures that the economic loss each year now is approximately $3 billion.

COMPARISON OF GASTRIC AND DUODENAL ULCER

There have been a number of empirical observations on the differences between gastric ulcers and duodenal ulcers. First, patients with gastric ulcers tend to have much lower acid secretory rates than patients with duodenal ulcers. The overnight collection of acid in a gastric ulcer patient will average 1.2 mEq/hour vs. 4.0 mEq/hour in a duodenal ulcer patient.[4] What is fascinating is that the epidemiology of duodenal ulcers has changed in the past 10–15 years, there being a higher incidence of duodenal ulcers 15 years ago than there is now. Also, the male-female ratio has changed, from men being four times more likely to have duodenal ulcers to a nearly equal incidence in men and women.[3] In gastric ulcers, the male-female ratio has not changed in the past 15 years.

One interesting and inexplicable observation is the difference in blood types in the two different diseases. Patients with blood in group O have a 30% higher risk of having a duodenal ulcer. Patients whose reaction to Lewis factor "a" is positive do not secrete blood group antigens in their gastric juice; they are also at increased risk for duodenal ulcer. A combination of these two genes increases the risk of duodenal ulcer threefold.[5] Such observations do not hold true for gastric ulcers.

There is some difference in the age distribution of duodenal ulcer and gastric ulcer, the latter occurring in an older population.[6] The peak occurrence of gastric ulcers is between the ages of 55 and 65 years. Gastric ulcers are generally considered unusual in the pediatric population. Nord and associates[7] found, however, that gastric ulcers occurred more frequently than duodenal ulcers in children. The ratio of duodenal to gastric ulcers was 11:17 in a group of 32 children with ulcer disease. Twelve percent of the children with gastric ulcers had relapses, whereas 45% of the children with duodenal ulcers had recurrences.

CLINICAL PRESENTATION

Most of the patients who present with simple, uncomplicated gastric ulcers complain of a characteristic pain pattern. The pain is dull, poorly localized, and centers around the midline. It is relieved by meals and recurs one to three hours after eating. It is common for the person with a gastric ulcer to be awakened at night by epigastric pain. A small number of patients have no relief of the pain by food ingestion or have actual exacerbation of the pain by food. An even smaller number will not have any pain and have their ulcer discovered when they have an acute hemorrhage or perforation. Generally, once treatment is started, the pain resolves quickly, long before the ulcer has healed.

A pain pattern that is constant, sharply localized, or acute usually indicates parietal pain caused by a complicated gastric ulcer. The classic pattern of food-induced relief is not invariable. One study found no relief with food in more than half the patients and exacerbation of pain in 25%.[8] Nocturnal pain occurs in 30% of patients. Weight loss is common, but nausea and vomiting are not.

The natural history of gastric ulcers has been documented by several studies comparing placebo and medical managements. Pain disappears in two weeks in 30%–40% of placebo-treated patients and in six weeks in 60%.[9] Ulcers treated with placebo heal in 12 weeks in 68% of patients.

The risk of malignant tumors is high in gastric ulcers. Kukral[10] reviewed 21 series and found an average incidence of malignant tumors of 10.02% in medically and surgically treated ulcers. The total number of patients in this combined review was 9,710, and the range of reported rates varied from 1.6% to 18.0%. This finding emphasizes the importance of adequate diagnostic studies, including biopsies, before therapy is initiated.

Unfortunately, the recurrence rate for gastric ulcers is extremely high. Once administration of histamine antagonists has been stopped, the ulcer disease is likely to recur. The recurrence rate is approximately 30% at one year and 50%–75% within two years.

Barr and associates[11] studied the effect of long-term maintenance cimetidine therapy and found no statistically significant reduction in the recurrence rate at two years, although there was a significant reduction at one year. Marks and co-workers[12] followed up 112 patients with duodenal and gastric ulcers treated with sucralfate or cimetidine. They found a 70% relapse rate at one year regardless of therapy. Richardson[13] noted that it is unusual to see patients with more than two or three recurrences of gastric ulcers. He suggested that this was because of either ultimate surgical referral or a propensity of gastric ulcers to "burn out," or behave as a self-limited disease. There are no experimental data to support this view, nor are there any clinical studies whose results support this hypothesis. Experimental data suggest that the damaged stomach will form a hyalinized substratum that is prone to future ulcers, and results of all clinical studies have shown high rates of recurrence.

Although the incidence and prevalence of gastric ulcer have not changed in the United States in the past few decades, the prevailing methods of treatment have changed substantially in the past decade with the advent of endoscopy and the histamine antagonists. Two decades ago, the approach to gastric ulcer therapy commonly resulted in an operation. Because of the risk of malignant disease and the lack of good peroral endoscopy, gastric ulcers were operated on if they were not 50% healed after three weeks of medical management or completely healed by eight weeks as judged by a barium study. The first recurrence of a gastric ulcer was always an indication for operation, and in many medical centers still is. The past decade, however, has shown a trend from aggressive surgical management toward long-term medical management. That long-term medical management does not prevent recurrence has been shown,[11] and perhaps there will be a swing back to early surgical therapy to prevent complications.

ETIOLOGY

Exogenous Factors

Multiple factors, including numerous ulcerogenic drugs and smoking, can contribute to a propensity for ulceration. Alcohol use and stress have been thought to be factors, but this has not been documented. Smoking has been demonstrated to prolong the time required to achieve healing and to reduce the ultimate healing rate from 80% to 50% for a six-week course of cimetidine.[14] Ulcer rates are higher in smokers than in nonsmokers. Piper and associates[15] found that smoking increased by 3.3 times the chances of a gastric ulcer's developing. In a case-controlled study of the association of smoking, alcohol, and heavy analgesic ingestion with the development

of gastric ulcer, Piper and co-workers found heavy analgesic use to increase the risk of ulcers by 5.3-fold. Smoking plus heavy alcohol use and heavy analgesic use led to an increased risk of 7.5-fold. Alcohol use alone was not a risk factor. Results of other studies have also shown no increased risk with the use of alcohol.[16, 17] When analgesics were analyzed separately, increased risk was found with acetaminophen-containing drugs as well as with aspirin and dextropropoxyphene.

The effect of various exogenous influences on the location and size of gastric ulcers was studied by Thomas and associates.[18] They found little effect of exogenous influences on ulcer size or location, except smoking, which favored location in the lower third of the stomach.

Few studies have addressed stress. Thomas and co-workers[19] looked at stress in patients with gastric ulcers during the two years before their diagnosis and the two years after their diagnosis and compared them to community controls. There were no differences in temporal stress patterns and no differences with respect to controls.

The effect of personality was investigated by Berndt,[20] who found a slight increase in neuroticism and introversion in patients with duodenal ulcers compared to controls. Gastric ulcer patients and gastric cancer patients, on the other hand, had highly stable personalities.

Endogenous Factors

The classic theory of Dragstedt states that gastric ulcers form in response to antral stasis—secondary either to previous duodenal ulcer disease or to vagomotor dysfunction. There is little doubt that in fact different pathogenetic mechanisms are at work at different sites, and different mechanisms may pertain in different individuals.

DRAGSTEDT.—Dragstedt and associates[21] proposed that gastric ulcers are usually caused by hypersecretion of gastric juice of humoral or hormonal origin. Duodenal ulcers, on the other hand, are caused by hypersecretion of acid of nervous origin. Hence, the explanation for higher *fasting* acid production in duodenal ulcer patients. Gastric ulcer patients produce the high quantities of acid necessary for ulcer production in response to food stimuli. The reason for both the higher acid production and the location of the ulcer is gastric stasis. The stasis can be secondary to either pyloric scarring from previous duodenal ulcer disease or to vagal hypofunction.

The Dragstedt theory is supported empirically by the excellent results of antrectomy alone for gastric ulcer.[22] In Dragstedt's words:

The concept that gastric ulcers are due to a hypersecretion of gastric juice of hormonal origin dependent upon prolonged or excessive liberation of the gastric secretory hormone, gastrin, is supported by the following evidence. A hypersecretion of gastric juice due to excessive or prolonged liberation of gastrin can be induced in dogs by the transplantation of the antrum of the stomach into the colon as a diverticulum. This hypersecretion is sufficient in degree to produce typical ulcers in previously normal mucosa. Stasis of food in the stomach, either as a result of pyloric stenosis or gastric atony, can cause a hypersecretion of gastric juice of humoral origin sufficient in degree to produce gastric ulcers in experimental animals and in man. The response of gastric and duodenal ulcers to gastric surgery supports these concepts of their origin. Thus, complete gastric vagotomy has been found effective in the treatment of duodenal ulcers, but not in gastric ulcers. Antrum resection which abolishes the humoral phase of gastric secretion is followed by a high incidence of marginal ulceration when done for patients with duodenal ulcer but is rarely followed by this complication when done for patients with gastric ulcer. Gastroenterostomy which relieves the stasis of food in the stomach is seldom followed by marginal ulceration when done for gastric ulcer but is frequently followed by marginal ulceration when done for the treatment of duodenal ulcer.

Documentation of gastric stasis has been difficult in patients with gastric ulcer and has been disputed. Mangold,[23] using roentgenography, noted delayed emptying in only 19% of gastric ulcer patients. Miller and associates[24] found that gastric emptying is delayed in most gastric ulcer patients. As noted earlier, there are probably several subsets of gastric ulcers based on varying etiologies. The mechanism proposed by Dragstedt is probably quite accurate for one of these subsets of patients.

MUCOUS BARRIER DEFICIENCY.—Controversies exist in where to draw the line among ulcers of different etiologies. It is generally agreed that ulcers that occur near the pylorus have the same pathophysiologic basis as ulcers that occur in the duodenum. What does not fit perfectly with this theory, however, is the large amount of data that show that pyloric channel and prepyloric ulcers are much more refractory to therapy than purely duodenal ulcers. It may be simply added mechanical factors related to emptying that increase intractability when the pylorus is involved with the ulcerative process, but the fact remains that responses to therapy and recurrence rates differ in that region, suggesting a need for modification of therapy and close follow-up study. Johnson[25] has nicely divided gastric ulcers into three categories: (1) prepyloric gastric ulcer—essentially the same disease as duodenal ulcer; (2) gastric ulcer associated with pyloric stenosis of duodenal ulcer origin; and (3) gastric ulcer associated with deficiency in mucous secretion. Johnson suggests no operation that is specific for control of either hypersecretion or hyposecretion should be adopted as a routine procedure for all gastric ulcers on an anatomical basis alone, without regard to ulcer type.

That Johnson's third category exists has been supported by analysis by Younan et al.[26] of mucus from gastric ulcer patients. Compared to normal persons, gastric ulcer patients have mucus with lower molecular weight glycoproteins. Whether this indicates an inferior or weaker mucus is not known but is presumed.

The role of gastric mucus is believed to be severalfold. It acts as a lubricant for the gastric mucosal cells, preventing abrasion and mechanical trauma. It also acts as a buffer zone between the acidic luminal environment and the mucosal cells. The quality of this barrier helps to maintain a hydrogen ion gradient that prevents or slows back-diffusion. The mucus is helped in this regard by the secretion of nonparietal bicarbonate-rich fluid into the mucous gel.[27] Factors that contribute to the production of weak or defective mucus, or factors that damage the existing mucus, are thought to include analgesic abuse, gastric mucosal ischemia (as in stress syndromes), and bile reflux.

PREPYLORIC GASTRIC ULCERATION.—Johnson was probably wrong in classifying prepyloric ulcers together with duodenal ulcers. Prepyloric ulcers are much more difficult to treat and have a higher recurrence rate regardless of surgical therapy. Especially high recurrence rates have been noted when parietal cell vagotomy has been used to treat prepyloric ulcers.[28] Lawson[29] studied the microscopic anatomical detail of 15 prepyloric ulcers and found prepyloric chronic gastritis in all patients. He proposed that prepyloric ulcers are a particularly intractable disease in which chronic mucosal damage and acid hypersecretion are important. For surgical management to be effective, both components should be treated, i.e., both a gastric resection and a vagotomy should be performed.

DIAGNOSTIC APPROACH

The diagnosis of gastric ulcer should be suspected from the history. The first test to be done when one suspects a gastric ulcer is endoscopy rather than a barium study. The reason for this is simply cost-benefit ratio. If one does an upper GI roentgenographic study and finds a gastric ulcer, endoscopy is warranted to obtain a biopsy specimen. On the other hand, if one does the roentgenographic study and it is normal, but the patient has symptoms suggestive of a gastric ulcer, endoscopy is also warranted because roentgenographic studies are only 75%–80% accurate. For gastric ulcers the accuracy of endoscopy approaches 100%. For duodenal ulcers, it is about 95%, which is still much better than roentgenography.

This recommendation can be thought through a little more carefully. If there is 80% confidence that a patient has a gastric ulcer, and one uses a barium swallow as the first step in the diagnostic study, then a gastric ulcer will be found 80% of 80% of the time, or 64% of the time. In that group, gastroscopy is done immediately for the purpose of a biopsy. The remaining 36% of the time, other tests will probably be done to find the cause of the epigastric pain. A few patients will have their diagnoses established by such a test, and the rest will ultimately need endoscopy. Endoscopy will confirm the 16% of gastric ulcers missed on barium meal examination. Following this algorithm, roughly 90% of patients will come to endoscopy, 100% will have a barium study, and 36% will have additional testing.

Following an algorithm of using endoscopy first when a gastric ulcer is suspected, 100% of patients would undergo endoscopy—which would identify the 80% of patients with gastric ulcers and would establish another diagnosis in half of the others—10% would have a barium meal, and probably 5% would receive additional tests. Even without including the substantial savings in hospitalization from making the diagnosis earlier, there is a substantial savings from performing fewer tests.

The same conclusion was reached by Kiil and Andersen,[30] who stated: "When both costs and diagnostic yield are considered, endoscopy seems to be the examination of choice, with x-ray examination reserved for exceptional cases when endoscopy for one reason or another cannot be carried out."

Roentgenography

Arguments have been made that roentgenographic examination need be the only diagnostic test used, especially if double contrast examinations are used. Thompson and associates[31] reviewed 7,600 double contrast barium meals and reported that 221 gastric ulcers were reported as benign by roentgenographic criteria. Follow-up data were available on 199 and all proved to be benign. The authors concluded that, when roentgenography shows a gastric ulcer as clearly benign on double contrast examination, there is no need for endoscopic confirmation of the diagnosis. Montesi and co-workers[32] examined 4,538 double contrast studies and found eight early gastric cancers. An additional four instances of early gastric cancer were found by endoscopy or at operation among the ulcers reported as benign. The authors concluded that, although double contrast examinations are helpful in identifying early gastric cancer, integration of radiologic, endoscopic, and cytologic data with accurate histopathologic study of the surgical specimen is necessary. Gelfand and Ott[33] challenged the usefulness of double contrast barium meals. In reviewing the statistics in Western publications with regard to sensitivities of simple and double contrast examinations, they found an advantage only in the detection of colonic polyps. There was no advantage to a double contrast technique for detection of gastric cancer, gastric ulcer, or duodenal ulcer. Clearly, the issue of sensitivity of roentgenographic examinations is not resolved, and endoscopic examinations of roentgenographically diagnosed gastric ulcers will remain the gold standard for some time to come.

Endoscopy

Before the routine use of endoscopy with biopsy, most gastric ulcers were operated on to rule out malignant tumors. The number of operations for suspicion of malignant disease has decreased with refinement in diagnostic methods. In a three-year study of endoscopy in gastric ulcer patients, Malmaeus and Nilsson[34] noted this decrease and also found 4 of 120 ulcer patients who had a cancer diagnosed on a routine follow-up endoscopy. In all instances, the endoscopist was suspicious of the ulcer at the initial endoscopy, but biopsy results were normal. This finding emphasized the importance of appropriately taken biopsy specimens and the macroscopic appearance of the ulcer. Clemencon[35] reiterated the importance of follow-up endoscopy not only because of the risk of malignancy, but also because one third of ulcer recurrences are asymptomatic. The application of endoscopy in gastric ulcer disease should clearly follow a popular perception of the Chicago voting rule: It should be done early and often.

Serum Tests

Gastrin levels are usually mildly elevated in gastric ulcer patients, but this is hardly a diagnostic test for the condition. In a few patients, markedly elevated gastrin levels may be found—notably in patients with Zollinger-Ellison syndrome or achlorhydria. Achlorhydria was considered a hallmark of malignant tumors of the stomach, but many patients with achlorhydria have benign gastric ulcers. Serum gastrin measurements are therefore not valuable unless the patient has symptoms or a history suggestive of a gastrinoma.

Serum pepsinogen I level is increased in the sera of duodenal ulcer patients but not in that of gastric ulcer patients,[36] if prepyloric ulcers are excluded. Serum pepsinogen I levels are low in patients with atrophic gastritis and therefore may be useful in screening for patients at risk for cancer. Serum levels of pepsinogen I are directly related to peak pepsin output and peak acid output. Serum levels are therefore thought to reflect chief cell mass.[37]

Serum oncofetal antigen is found in 8.8% of the normal population, 20% of duodenal ulcer patients, 54% of gastric ulcer patients, and 91% of patients with gastric cancers.[38] As yet it has no clinical relevance.

MEDICAL THERAPY

The mainstay of medical therapy has always been combating the effects of acid. Although there have been reports of benign gastric ulcers in the presence of achlorhydria, these are rare, and the classic teaching of "no acid, no ulcer" holds true more than 99% of the time. Dietary restrictions in an attempt to avoid secretagogues alone will cause ulcers to heal. Healing can be enhanced, however, by pharmacologic manipulations, including not only antacids, but many new drugs that work in a variety of ways against the ulcer diathesis.

Antacids

Antacids alone are generally as effective as the H_2-receptor antagonists in curing both gastric and duodenal ulcers. The therapy must be intensive, requiring 30 ml of antacid one and three hours after meals as well as at bedtime. The calculated cost of such a regimen is generally equal to or greater than that of most of the newer medicines and certainly requires a higher degree of compliance; hence, the shift by most practitioners to other regimens.

Cimetidine

Cimetidine was the first of a new class of drugs, the H_2-receptor blockers, to be released for public use. It competitively inhibits the action of histamine H_2 receptors of the parietal cell and thereby blocks basal and stimulated acid secretion. A single, 300-mg dose will block basal acid secretion for $2\frac{1}{2}$–4 hours in a normal individual. Higher or more frequent doses may be required in patients with gastrinomas. It is currently approved for use in the treatment of acute gastric ulcers, but not for long-term prophylaxis against recurrent gastric ulcer.

Several studies have been done to determine the usefulness of cimetidine for prophylaxis against recurrent gastric ulcer. In 25 patients who had healed gastric ulcers, cimetidine was significantly more effective than placebo in preventing recurrence of the gastric ulcer. Recurrence rates in 11 months were 86% in a placebo group and 19% in a group receiving cimetidine (1 gm/day).[39] It should be noted that this is nevertheless a rather high recurrence rate on a high dose of cimetidine for continuous prophylaxis. A similar long-term trial in Austria examining healed gastric ulcers revealed that 86% of the ulcers showed continued remission with 400 mg of cimetidine per night compared with 45% in the placebo group.[40] A two-year study from Australia examined the same question, but used 400 mg twice a day of cimetidine, and showed significant differences at one year but insignificant differences at two years. Cumulative two-year recurrence rates were 52% in the placebo group and 33% in the cimetidine-treated group.[41]

Concerns that must be remembered in the long-term treatment of patients taking cimetidine include side effects and potential side effects. Some investigators have voiced a concern that long-term use of cimetidine may place patients at increased risk for gastric cancer by increasing gastric bacteria, nitrates, and nitrosamines. It is known that these compounds are increased in the stomachs of patients with atrophic gastritis and pernicious anemia and that these patients are at high risk of gastric cancer. It is also known that cimetidine therapy raises the concentration of these compounds in the stomach. Whether or not this is of any long-term clinical significance remains to be seen.[42, 43] Other side effects of cimetidine use include CNS disturbances, gynecomastia, hepatotoxicity, interstitial nephritis, bradycardia, hypotension, and thrombocytopenia. Cardiac arrest has been reported with rapid bolus injection. All of these side effects have been reported with low frequency.[44]

Ranitidine

Ranitidine is an H_2-receptor blocker. Like cimetidine, ranitidine causes an increase in intragastric nitrate-reducing organisms. It appears to have some advantages over cimetidine in that it has a longer half-life and fewer side effects. In all studies that have compared ranitidine to placebo for the treatment of acute gastric ulcer, there has been a statistically significant improvement in healing rates.[45–49] When ranitidine was compared to cimetidine, healing rates were equal[50–52] whether patients received 1.2 gm of cimetidine per day or 150 mg of ranitidine twice daily. Based on one study, ranitidine seems to be particularly effective at reducing the recurrence of gastric ulcer when taken continuously in a maintenance dose of 150 mg per night. Only one of 15 gastric ulcer patients had a relapse on this regimen in a trial of one year. This compared to a placebo group relapse rate of 15 of 17.[53]

Sucralfate

Sucralfate is basic aluminum sucrose sulfate and seems to work in the healing of gastric ulcers, as well as duodenal ulcers, by a cytoprotective mechanism. When exposed to acid, sucralfate hydrolyzes, releasing aluminum ions and generating sucrose octasulfate. This will bind to the positively charged proteins found in the ulcer base. This makes an insoluble, viscous coating that protects the tissue against diffusion of acid and bile acids. The response rates to sucralfate therapy (1 gm, four times per day) are equal to those to cimetidine therapy at 12 weeks.[54, 55] Although some studies have suggested that the recurrence rate after sucralfate therapy is less than with cimetidine therapy, these studies were done on both duodenal and gastric ulcers analyzed together. Further, this effect seems to disappear after more than a year of follow-up study. Recurrence rates of about 70% are seen by two years after discontinuation of therapy with either regimen.[56–58] One study that examined relapse rates for patients treated with sucralfate compared to placebo found no differences.[59] In summary, sucralfate appears to be as effective as cimetidine in healing gastric ulcers acutely, and may be safer, but there is no selective advantage in terms of recurrence rates.

Pirenzepine

Pirenzepine is a new antimuscarinic agent that has been shown to be effective in healing both gastric and duodenal ulcers when used in a dose of 150 mg/day. The achieved short term success rate with gastric ulcers was 72%.[60] Pirenzepine acts apparently more selectively on the stomach than on other organ systems, although at dosages above 100 mg per day, parasympatholytic effects are reported in an incidence of 13%–18%. These effects include a dry mouth and visual disturbances. Cardioacceleration is not produced.[61]

Bismuth

Tripotassium dicitrato-bismuthate is not a new drug. It has been used for many years in Europe and works well in healing peptic ulcers. It works by chelating with proteins at acidic pH levels, thereby providing a cytoprotective barrier against acid. It is not absorbed systemically, and its only adverse effects seem to be its odor and a darkening of the stools. In one study comparing the effectiveness of bismuth to placebo for treatment of gastric ulcer, 72% of the ulcers in the bismuth group healed compared with 36% in the placebo group. The patients in the bismuth group experienced significantly less pain. The relapse rate was 27% at three months and 41% at two years.[62] This rate compares favorably with that for other therapies.

Carbenoxolone

Carbenoxolone seems to work by a mechanism separate from that of all the other agents. It stimulates mucous secretion from the stomach and decreases hydrogen ion back-diffusion. It is not available in the United States and probably will not be for some time because of side effects resembling hyperaldosteronemia. Patients have experienced hypertension, hypokalemia, and sodium retention. These effects can be blocked by giving spironolactone, but this also blocks the effect of ulcer healing.

Carbenoxolone has been used successfully in conjunction with cimetidine to enhance healing rates, and it has been reported anecdotally to be effective for a gastric ulcer that was refractory to cimetidine.[63, 64] Ganguli and Mohamed[65] used a course of carbenoxolone tapered over six months on 140 gastric ulcer patients and found a greatly reduced three-year recurrence rate of 26.7%. They gave 300 mg/day for one week, 150 mg/day for 5 weeks, 100 mg/day for 6 weeks, and 50 mg/day for the last three months. All side effects were successfully treated with diuretics and potassium supplements.

Prostaglandins

Another approach to cytoprotection involves the use of new prostaglandin derivatives, most notably 15, 15-dimethyl-PGE_2. This drug was shown in rats to protect the stomach against mucosal erosions when acid was infused into the stomach exogenously. Under these conditions, cimetidine would not protect the stomach. This drug is thought to work by stimulating the secretion of gastric bicarbonate as well as generating enhanced mucous production.[66] It has been found to be effective clinically when used to treat intractable gastric ulcers. A dosage of 3.0 mg/day caused healing in 65% of patients within 4–14 weeks.[67]

INDICATIONS FOR SURGICAL THERAPY

Hemorrhage

Approximately 12% of gastric ulcer patients will present with hemorrhage, and of that group, 30% will rebleed in the future. It is interesting that it is not possible to predict the risk of rebleeding from age, type of ulcer, or amount of bleeding. In general, most patients with hemorrhage can be managed by medical therapy consisting of gastric lavage, IV cimetidine, and blood replacement. The decision of when to go to the operating room should be made when it is apparent that the bleeding is not going to stop. That decision should be tempered by several factors, including the age of the patient, prior history of chronic ulcer trouble, and endoscopic examination. The rule followed in most medical centers mandates operative intervention if the patient is still bleeding after 5 units of blood have been transfused. For the average 70-kg man, this represents 40% of the circulating blood volume. If the person is much larger than 70 kg, or young and vigorously healthy, waiting out a 6–8-unit bleed may be acceptable without increasing the surgical risk. However, if the person is small or elderly, compensation should be made the other way. For example, an 80-year-old person should probably be operated on when 30% of the circulating volume has been transfused. This would translate to 1,080 ml.

Another factor modulating the timing of surgical intervention is endoscopic diagnosis. All patients with upper GI bleeding should undergo endoscopy within 24 hours of admission to the hospital to establish a diagnosis. Considering all patients, 50% will be found to be bleeding from ulcer disease; 15%–20% will be bleeding from gastric ulcers; and 3%–9% will be bleeding from gastric cancer.[68-70] The subsequent therapy and timing of surgical treatment will depend on the diagnosis. If endoscopy reveals a bleeding ulcer, the usual medical management should be tried first, unless the ulcer has a visible vessel in its base. In that case, early operative intervention should be pursued, because there is a high probability of failure of conservative therapy.

It should be mentioned that this doctrine has been challenged by Peterson and associates.[71] They randomized 206 patients to either routine early endoscopy or endoscopy alone if bleeding recurred during hospitalization or if roentgenograms disclosed gastric ulcer or suggested neoplasia. All patients were empirically treated with antacids. In comparing the two groups, there were no significant differences in deaths, recurrent bleeding, units of blood transfused, or length of hospital stay. The authors concluded that endoscopy should not be a routine procedure in patients with upper GI tract bleeding that ceases during treatment.

From a surgical standpoint, preoperative endoscopy, preferably viewed or performed by the operating surgeon, is mandatory. The intraoperative approach and the ultimate surgical therapy are expedited by knowing the diagnosis ahead of time, as is the decision of when to operate. From a medical standpoint, it may be difficult to show advantages in therapy or outcome, but a procedure that establishes the diagnosis early will certainly make therapeutic decision making more comfortable for the physician. This difference alone, in the absence of any other marked measurable benefit, supports early endoscopy.

Perforation

Perforation of a gastric ulcer is, like uncontrollable bleeding, an indication for emergency operation. Mortalities from perforated gastric ulcers are about 20%. The diagnosis can usually be suspected from the history, sudden onset of pain being a prominent feature. The pain is usually constant, severe, boring, and unrelenting. Confirmation of the diagnosis depends on roentgenographic studies. When the diagnosis is suspected, it is sometimes helpful to instill 200–300 ml of air into the stomach through a nasogastric tube before obtaining upright or decubitus positioned roentgenograms. Optimal therapy includes resection of the ulcer and resection of the distal stomach. When the condition of the patient mandates closure of the ulcer only, it is important to obtain a biopsy of the ulcer with at least a full-thickness wedge.

Large Gastric Ulcer

The larger the gastric ulcer, the more prone that ulcer is to malignancy, and the less likely it is to heal. The malignant potential of the ulcer can be investigated by endoscopy with biopsies, and the expected rate will exceed 10% in ulcers over 2.0 cm in diameter. The VA study showed that the recurrence rate is higher in these large ulcers and the healing time is much longer. In most patients of good surgical risk, an operation should be the first choice of therapy for large gastric ulcers. In poor-risk patients, medical therapy could be pursued only if an adequate initial study indicated the ulcer to be benign. It could be expected that only 70% of ulcers larger than over 2.0 cm would be healed by 24 weeks.

Recurrent Ulcer

As indicated in the introduction, the recurrence of a gastric ulcer is no longer uniformly considered to be an indication for surgical intervention. The argument has been advanced that most index ulcers are in themselves recurrent ulcers and are usually easy to heal with medical therapy. When an ulcer recurs, it is usually smaller than the index ulcer, and is therefore easier to heal. The reason for the smaller size is the greater awareness of the problem and closer monitoring. Some studies have appeared advocating chronic maintenance histamine antagonists to prevent recurrence.[72]

Others have noted no effect on recurrence rates of as much as 800 mg/day of cimetidine for two years.[73] Perhaps the pendulum will start to swing back to a more surgically oriented approach as more studies examine the therapeutic efficacy of the histamine antagonists for long-term maintenance therapy. Also worth mentioning again is the concern of some investigators over the increase in nitrate-reducing gastric flora provoked by the histamine antagonists. This is thought to increase the potential for the development of gastric cancer. Whether this will evolve into a legitimate clinical concern awaits several more years of long-term maintenance use.

Malignant Tumors

It is almost a moot point to advocate surgical intervention when biopsies have proved malignancy. Unfortunately, 10%–15% of all malignant tumors are not diagnosed at the first biopsy. When there is a suspicion of malignancy, the diagnosis must be vigorously pursued. The incidence of gastric cancer in gastric ulcers is commonly cited to be 5%, but is probably double that. Kukral[10] reviewed 21 studies from 1941 to 1967 and found a mean incidence of gastric cancer of 10.02% among 9,710 gastric ulcer patients. Mountford and associates[74] examined all instances of gastric ulcer diagnosed between 1974 and 1976 at Bristol and found 14% (37 of 265) to be malignant. A group from the Soviet Union[75] examined 1,237 patients at high risk for stomach cancer and found a 32.7% incidence of cancer. Among their high-risk groups were included 669 patients with chronic gastric ulcer, 78 with polyps, 382 with chronic gastritis, and 108 who had undergone gastric resection more than ten years before. Patients with chronic ulcers had a 17% incidence of malignant tumors.

Gastrocolic Fistula

A rare complication of benign gastric ulcer disease is the development of a gastrocolic fistula. This is more usually a complication of surgical therapy with marginal ulceration occurring in Billroth II anastomoses eroding into the colon. It is uncommon in that setting, but it is rare in the patient who has not undergone an operation. It presents with the same triad of symptoms—diarrhea, weight loss, and fecal breath or vomiting. The diarrhea is severe and debilitating. Originally the diarrhea was considered a result of dumping gastric contents into the colon. Pfeiffer and Kent[76] were the first to postulate that the diarrhea was caused by the presence of feces in the upper GI tract. This concept was proved correct by the remarkable improvement in these patients after proximal colostomy or ileosigmoidostomy, and it has been substantiated experimentally.[77]

Karakousis and Greenberg[78] reported on three patients with gastrocolic fistula as a complication of benign gastric ulcer. They confirmed the experience in gastrocolic fistulas of other etiologies that barium meal examination disclosed only 70% of the fistulas, while barium enema revealed all of them. They recommended a one-stage resection with appropriate reconstruction of GI continuity when possible. That same recommendation was also made by Lundell and Svartholm[79] and Simpson and White.[80] Ekbom and Lieberg[81] reported on the successful treatment of two patients with cimetidine. It must be emphasized that before either medical or surgical therapy is undertaken, the presence of malignant tumors must be carefully ruled out.

SURGICAL THERAPY

The decision about which operation to choose for therapy for gastric ulcer disease must be predicated on an understanding of the etiology of gastric ulcer disease, as well as on technical factors faced at the time of the operation. The operation of choice will depend on the location of the ulcer, not only because this implies much about the underlying pathophysiology, but also because it dictates the technical considerations.

Lesser Curve Ulcers

Since the single most important component in the etiology of lesser curve ulcers is a mucosal defect, the surgical therapy is directed at removal of the diseased stomach. A partial gastrectomy (antrectomy) that removes the diseased mucosa with the ulcer is sufficient to prevent recurrence in 98% of all instances without the addition of a vagotomy. The type of gastrectomy depends on the preference of the surgeon, but physiologic and functional results should be carefully weighed against technical considerations.

BILLROTH I PARTIAL GASTRECTOMY.—This is the classic operation for uncomplicated chronic benign gastric ulcer. The best results obtained with any operation have been reported with this procedure. Tanner[82] reported a recurrence rate of 0.2% in a series of 1,000 patients.

Departure from this procedure has been stimulated by long-term follow-up studies of functional results. Several studies have been done with five- to ten-year follow-up periods on patients after Billroth I gastrectomy. Duthie and Branson[83] reported that only 75% of these patients had good to excellent functional results. Side effects that are frequent include diarrhea, dumping, early satiety, and vomiting. On the other hand, Rehnberg[84] reported only a 3% Visick grade 3 or 4 rate with antrectomy, and Thomas and associates[85] reported 84% good to excellent results on clinical Visick grading. Comparative studies with other operative procedures have not yet shown any clear advantage in the use of any other procedure.[86]

BILLROTH II PARTIAL GASTRECTOMY.—Billroth II partial gastrectomy is the procedure of choice if a Billroth I anastomosis cannot be done. A Billroth I procedure disturbs the physiology and anatomy less than a Billroth II; a gastrojejunostomy, however, may be preferable in certain patients from a technical standpoint. When the duodenum cannot be mobilized enough, or the gastric stump will not reach the duodenum without undue tension, a gastrojejunostomy is preferable. Attempting a tenuous gastroduodenal anastomosis will surely lead to an anastomotic leak, probably at the infamous Jammerecke or "corner of misery."

A good summary of the indications for the Billroth II operation was put forth by Maingot:[87]

The Billroth I operation is indicated in cases of chronic gastric ulcer *where the duodenum is normal.* When a duodenal ulcer is present in addition to a gastric ulcer (i.e. combined ulcers) the Schoemaker-Billroth II procedure is to be preferred; it is also preferred in those cases in which the first and second parts of the duodenum appear to be unduly shortened and narrowed or show evidence of fibrotic distortion from past or present ulceration.

PARIETAL CELL VAGOTOMY WITH ULCER RESECTION.—This is a procedure that has been used by Johnston since 1969 with good results.[88] He has reported on the treatment of 100 patients with gastric ulcer with 2% operative mortality, 4% recurrent ulceration, and a considerable decrease in the incidence of side effects, such as dumping, compared with the incidence that is recorded after partial gastrectomy. Another similar study was reported by Jordan,[89] who followed up 22 patients for two to five years. Results were excellent to good in 87% and fair in 5%. Nine percent of the procedures were failures. The trials, however, were not prospective and randomized. Three such trials have now been reported, and the results are not quite as encouraging. In all three trials, the randomization was Billroth I vs. parietal cell vagotomy with ulcer excision. None of them demonstrated a significant difference between ulcer recurrence rates. The study by Reid and colleagues[90] showed some symptomatic advantage to the parietal cell vagotomy, but also had high recurrence rates for the partial gastrectomy group (16%). Taking all three studies together, the recurrence rate for parietal cell vagotomy with excision is 17.8% (11 of 62) and for partial gastrectomy it is 9.4% (6 of 64, five of the recurrences being from the Reid et al. series).[90-92] It appears that partial gastrectomy may suffer some disadvantage with respect to the production of dumping and diarrhea, but is still a superior operation from the respect of ulcer recurrence.

VAGOTOMY AND PYLOROPLASTY WITH ULCER EXCISION.—This has been proposed not only as a less morbid approach to acutely bleeding gastric ulcers,[93] but also as an elective procedure. Cade and Allen[94] reported their experience with 90 patients operated on between 1963 and 1975. The mean follow-up time was 7.5 years. Only two patients had recurrent ulcers. These figures are at variance with the experience reported by others, who generally found 10% recurrence rates after this operation.[95]

Prepyloric Ulcers

A study by Andersen and associates[96] has highlighted the prepyloric ulcer as a particularly difficult entity to treat, having a high recurrence rate. Rehnberg[84] also noted an 18% recurrence rate when pyloric or prepyloric ulcers were treated by antrectomy alone. Andersen's study noted a high recurrence rate for this class of ulcer when treated by highly selective vagotomy. Studies by Lawson[29] showed that the histopathology of juxtapyloric ulcers includes features of both duodenal and gastric ulcers. The therapy therefore should include antral resection as well as vagotomy. The improvement in results over either antrectomy or vagotomy alone was shown by Rehnberg, who found only a 2% recurrence rate with the combined approach.

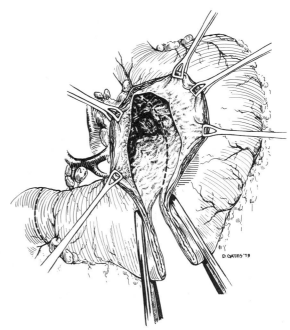

Fig 15–2.—Pauchet gastrectomy. The distal stomach is divided, and the proximal stomach opened for freehand division around the exposed ulcer.

High Lesser Curve Ulcer

Several approaches have been recommended for high-lying gastric ulcers. Leaving the ulcer in place and performing a distal gastric resection with or without vagotomy (Kelling-Madlener procedure) has been advocated by some. Unfortunately, this operation does not allow exclusion of the diagnosis of malignant disease. A four-quadrant biopsy of the ulcer may decrease the chances of a later malignant tumor, but the operation still suffers from a high persistence of gastric ulceration. We believe that the Kelling-Madlener operation should be abandoned in favor of the Pauchet procedure, which combines distal resection of the stomach in continuity with a

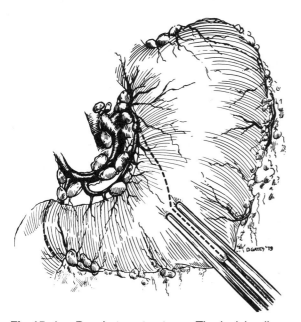

Fig 15–1.—Pauchet gastrectomy. The incision line.

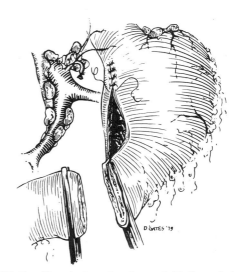

Fig 15–3.—Pauchet gastrectomy. Initiation of closure.

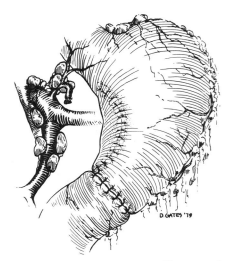

Fig 15–4.—Pauchet gastrectomy. The completed anastomosis. (From Donahue P.E., Nyhus L.M.: Surgical excision of gastric ulcers near the gastroesophageal junction. *Surg. Gynecol. Obstet.* 155:85, 1982. By permission of *Surgery, Gynecology & Obstetrics*.)

tongue of tissue along the lesser curvature.[97] The design of this tongue is such that the ulcer is near its tip, usually with equal amounts of the anterior and posterior walls of the lesser gastric curvature. Because the operation removes the ulcer, there is no role for vagotomy in this procedure. The technical aspects are outlined in Figures 15–1 to 15–4.

REFERENCES

1. Rudick J.: Gastric ulcer, in Nyhus L.M., Wastell C. (eds.): *Surgery of the Stomach & Duodenum*. Boston, Little, Brown & Co., 1977.
2. Blumenthal I.S.: *Social Cost of Peptic Ulcer*. Santa Monica, Calif., Rand Corporation, 1967.
3. Elashoff J.D., Grossman M.I.: Trends in hospital admissions and death rates for peptic ulcer in the United States from 1970 to 1978. *Gastroenterology* 78:280, 1980.
4. Dragstedt L.R., Oberhelman H.A. Jr., Evans S.O., et al.: Antrum hyperfunction and gastric ulcer. *Ann. Surg.* 140:396, 1954.
5. Menguy B.: Genetics and secretion of Lewis factor, in Schwartz S.E. (ed.): *Principles of Surgery*. New York, McGraw-Hill Book Co., 1979.
6. Nyhus L.M.: Gastric ulcer. *Scand. J. Gastroenterol.* [*Suppl.*] 6:123, 1970.
7. Nord K.S., Rossi T.M., Lebenthal E.: Peptic ulcer in children: The predominance of gastric ulcers. *Am. J. Gastroenterol.* 75:153, 1981.
8. Edwards F.C., Coghill N.F.: Clinical manifestations in patients with chronic atrophic gastritis, gastric ulcer, and duodenal ulcer. *Q. J. Med.* 37:337, 1968.
9. Freston J.W.: Cimetidine in the treatment of gastric ulcer. *Gastroenterology* 74:426, 1978.
10. Kukral J.C.: Gastric ulcer: An appraisal. *Surgery* 63:1024, 1968.
11. Barr G.D., Kang J.V. Canalese J., et al.: A two-year prospective controlled study of maintenance cimetidine and gastric ulcer. *Gastroenterology* 85:100, 1983.
12. Marks I.N., Lucke W., Wright J.P., et al.: Ulcer healing and relapse rates after initial treatment with cimetidine or sucralfate. *J. Clin. Gastroenterol.* 3(suppl. 2):163, 1981.
13. Richardson C.T.: Gastric ulcer, in Sleisenger M.H., Fordtran J.S. (eds.): *Gastrointestinal Disease*. Philadelphia, W.B. Saunders Co., 1983.
14. Da Silva E.P., Zaterka S.: Long-term treatment of gastric ulcer with cimetidine. *Clin. Ther.* 4:24, 1981.
15. Piper D.W., McIntosh J.H., Greg M., et al.: Environmental factors and chronic gastric ulcer. *Scand. J. Gastroenterol.* 17:721, 1982.
16. Friedman G.D., Siegelaub A.B., Seltzer C.C.: Cigarettes, alcohol, coffee, and peptic ulcer. *N. Engl. J. Med.* 290:469, 1974.
17. Paffenbarger R.S., Wing A.L., Hyde R.T.: Chronic disease in former college students XIII. Early precursors of peptic ulcer. *Am. J. Epidemiol.* 100:307, 1974.
18. Thomas J., Greig M., McIntosh J., et al.: The location of chronic gastric ulcer: A study of the relevance of ulcer size, age, sex, alcohol, analgesic intake and smoking. *Digestion* 20:79, 1980.
19. Thomas J., Greig M., Piper D.W.: Chronic gastric ulcer and life events. *Gastroenterology* 78:905, 1980.
20. Berndt H.: Untersuchungen zur Personlichkeitsstructur nach Eysenck an Magenkranken. *Dtsch. Z. Verdau Stoffwechselkr.* 40:7, 1980.
21. Dragstedt L.R., Oberhelman H.A. Jr., Smith C.A.: Experimental hyperfunction of the gastric antrum with ulcer formation. *Ann. Surg.* 134:332, 1951.
22. Dragstedt, L.R.: A concept of the etiology of gastric and duodenal ulcers. *Gastroenterology* 30:208, 1956.
23. Mangold R.: Combined gastric and duodenal ulceration: Survey of 157 cases. *Br. Med. J.* 2:1193, 1958.
24. Miller L.J., Malagelada J.R., Longstreth G.F.: Dysfunctions of the stomach with gastric ulceration. *Dig. Dis. Sci.* 25:857, 1980.
25. Johnson H.D.: Etiology and classification of gastric ulcers. *Gastroenterology* 33:121, 1957.
26. Younan F., Pearson J., Allen A., et al.: Charges in the structure of the mucous gel on the mucosal surface of the stomach in association with peptic ulcer disease. *Gastroenterology* 82:827, 1982.
27. Flemstrom G.: Gastric secretion of bicarbonate, in Johnson L.R., (ed.): *Physiology of the Gastrointestinal Tract*. New York, Raven Press, 1981, pp. 603–616.
28. Anderson D., Hostrup H., Amdrup E.: Aarhus County Vagotomy Trial II. *World J. Surg.* 2:91, 1978.
29. Lawson H.H.: Prepyloric gastric ulceration. *Surg. Annu.* 16:229, 1984.
30. Kiil J., Andersen D.: X-ray examination and/or endoscopy in the diagnosis of gastroduodenal ulcer and cancer. *Scand. J. Gastroenterol.* 15:39, 1980.
31. Thompson G., Somers S., Stevenson G.W.: Benign gastric ulcer: A reliable radiologic diagnosis? *A.J.R.* 141:331, 1983.
32. Montesi A., Graziani L., Pesaresi A., et al.: Radiologic diagnosis of early gastric cancer by routine double-contrast examination. *Gastrointest. Radiol.* 7:205, 1982.
33. Gelfand D.W., Ott D.J.: Single- vs. double-contrast gastrointestinal studies: Critical analysis of reported statistics. *A.J.R.* 137:523, 1981.
34. Malmaeus J., Nilsson F.: Endoscopy in the management of gastric ulcer disease. *Acta Chir. Scand.* 147:551, 1981.
35. Clemencon G.H.: Die konservative Therapie des peptischen Ulkus. *Schweiz. Med. Wochenschr.* 110:1474, 1980.
36. Peyre S., Di Napoli A., Pelissero A., et al.: Diagnostic usefulness of serum group I pepsinogen determination. *Gastroenterol. Clin. Biol.* 7:793, 1983.
37. Nakanome C., Akai H., Goto Y., et al.: Serum group I pepsinogen levels in patients with peptic ulcer and normal subjects. *J. Exp. Med.* 139:151, 1983.
38. Hakkinen I.P., Heinonen R., Inberg M.V., et al.: The use of oncofetal antigen FSA in discrimination between benign and malignant gastric ulceration. *Acta Chir. Scand.* 146:507, 1980.
39. Machell R.J., Ciclitira P.J., Farthing M.J., et al.: Cimetidine in the prevention of gastric ulcer relapse. *Postgrad. Med. J.* 55:393, 1979.
40. Hentschel E., Schutze K., Weiss W., et al.: Effect of cimetidine treatment in the prevention of gastric ulcer relapse: A one year double blind multicentre study. *Gut* 24:853, 1983.
41. Barr G.D., Kang J.Y., Canalese J., et al.: A two-year prospective controlled study of maintenance cimetidine and gastric ulcer. *Gastroenterology* 85:100, 1983.

42. Stockbrugger R.W., Cotton P.B., Eugenides N., et al.: Intragastric nitrites, nitrosamines, and bacterial overgrowth during cimetidine treatment. *Gut* 23:1048, 1982.

43. Bartholomew B.A., Hill M.J., Hudson M.J., et al.: Gastric bacteria, nitrate, nitrite and nitrosamines in patients with pernicious anaemia and in patients treated with cimetidine. *IARC Sci. Publ.* 31:595, 1980.

44. Freston J.W.: Cimetidine: II. Adverse reactions and patterns of use. *Ann. Intern. Med.* 97:728, 1982.

45. Gibinski K., Nowak A., Gabryelewicz A., et al.: The treatment of duodenal and gastric ulcer with ranitidine: A controlled multicentre clinical trial. *Dtsch. Z. Verdau Stoffwechselkr.* 42:64, 1982.

46. Ashton M.G., Holdsworth C.D., Ryan F.P., et al.: Healing of gastric ulcers after one, two, and three months of ranitidine. *Br. Med. J.* 284:467, 1982.

47. Forssell H., Koch G.: Effects of H2-receptor blockade by ranitidine on ulcer healing and gastric acid secretion in patients with gastric and duodenal ulcers. *Eur. J. Clin. Pharmacol.* 25:195, 1983.

48. Leroux P., Farley A., Archambault A., et al.: Effect of ranitidine on healing of peptic ulcer: A 2-month study. *Am. J. Gastroenterol.* 78:227, 1983.

49. Takemoto T., Okazaki Y., Okita K., et al.: Ranitidine: A pilot study in Japan. *Scand. J. Gastroenterol. [Suppl.]* 69:125, 1981.

50. Barbara L., Corinaldesi R., Dobrilla G., et al.: Ranitidine vs cimetidine: Short-term treatment of gastric ulcer. *Hepatogastroenterology* 30:151, 1983.

51. Kellow J.E., Barr G.D., Cowen A.W., et al.: Comparison of ranitidine and cimetidine in the treatment of chronic gastric ulcer: A double-blind trial. *Digestion* 27:105, 1983.

52. Wright J.P., Marks I.N., Mee A.S., et al.: Ranitidine in the treatment of gastric ulceration. *S. Afr. Med. J.* 61:155, 1982.

53. Alsted E.M., Ryan F.P., Holdsworth C.D., et al.: Ranitidine in the prevention of gastric and duodenal ulcer relapse. *Gut* 24:418, 1983.

54. Lahtinen J., Aukee S., Miettinen P., et al.: Sucralfate and cimetidine for gastric ulcer. *Scand. J. Gastroenterol. [Suppl.]* 83:49, 1983.

55. Martin F., Farley A., Gagnon M., et al.: Short-term treatment with sucralfate or cimetidine in gastric ulcer: Preliminary results of a controlled randomized trial. *Scand. J. Gastroenterol. [Suppl.]* 83:37, 1983.

56. Marks I.N., Wright J.P., Lucke W., et al.: Relapse rates following initial ulcer healing with sucralfate and cimetidine. *Scand. J. Gastroenterol. [Suppl.]* 83:53, 1983.

57. Marks I.N., Lucke W., Wright J.P., and Girdwood A.H.: Ulcer healing and relapse rates after initial treatment with cimetidine or sucralfate. *J. Clin. Gastroenterol.* 3(suppl. 2):163, 1981.

58. Miyake T., Ariyoshi J., Suzaki T., et al.: Endoscopic evaluation of the effect of sucralfate therapy and other clinical parameters on the recurrence rate of gastric ulcers. *Dig. Dis. Sci.* 25:1, 1980.

59. Classen M., Bethge H., Brunner G., et al.: Effect of sucralfate on peptic ulcer recurrence: A controlled double-blind multicenter study. *Scand. J. Gastroenterol. [Suppl.]* 83:61, 1983.

60. Bianchi Porro G., Petrillo M.: Pirenzepine in the treatment of peptic ulcer disease: Review and commentary. *Scand. J. Gastroenterol.* 72(suppl. 17):229, 1982.

61. Texter, E.C. Jr., Reilly, P.A.: The efficacy and selectivity of pirenzepine: Review and commentary. *Scand. J. Gastroenterol.* 72(suppl. 17):237 1982.

62. Sutton D.R.: Gastric ulcer healing with tripotassium dicitrato bismuthate and subsequent relapse. *Gut* 23:621, 1982.

63. Lewis J.R.: Carbenoxolone sodium in the treatment of peptic ulcer. *J.A.M.A.* 229:460, 1974.

64. Simon B., Kather H., Kommerella B.: Treatment of cimetidine-resistant gastric ulcer with carbenoxolone-sodium. *Med. Klin.* 74:1250, 1979.

65. Ganguli P.C., Mohamed S.D.: Long-term therapy with carbenoxolone in the prevention of recurrence of gastric ulcer: Natural history and evolution of important side-effects and measures to avoid them. *Scand. J. Gastroenterol.* 15(suppl. 65):63, 1980.

66. Marti-Bonmati E., Alino S.F., Lloris J.M., et al.: Effects of cimetidine, atropine and prostaglandin E2 on rat mucosal erosions produced by intragastric distention. *Eur. J. Pharmacol.* 68:49, 1980.

67. Kobayashi K., Arakawa T., Nakamura H., et al.: Role of prostaglandin E2 on human gastric ulcers. *Gastroenterol. Jpn.* 17:21, 1982.

68. Correia J.P., Cruz A.G., Batista M.R., et al.: Endoscopy in the upper G.I. bleedings. *Arq. Gastroenterol.* 16:119, 1979.

69. Baccaro J.C., Gonzalez B.A., Cupula C.A.: Value of endoscopy in the diagnosis of upper digestive tract hemorrhage. *Acta Gastroenterol. Latinoam.* 9:209, 1979.

70. Khachiev L.G., Kalish Iu.I., Malikov Iu.R., et al.: Bleeding gastric ulcer. *Vestn. Khir.* 124:44, 1980.

71. Peterson W.L., Barnett C.C., Smith H.J., et al.: Routine early endoscopy in upper-gastrointestinal-tract bleeding: A randomized, controlled trial. *N. Engl. J. Med.* 304:925, 1981.

72. Hentschel E., Schutze K., Weiss W., et al.: Ulcer relapse: A one year double blind multicentre study. *Gut* 24:853, 1983.

73. Barr G.D., Kang J.Y., Canalese J., et al.: A two-year prospective controlled study of maintenance cimetidine and gastric ulcer. *Gastroenterology* 85:100, 1983.

74. Mountford R.A., Brown P., Salmon P.R., et al.: Gastric cancer detection in gastric ulcer disease. *Gut* 21:9, 1980.

75. Khonelidze G.B., Iakovleva I.A., Koshchug G.D., et al.: Groups at high risk for stomach cancer morbidity and the effectiveness of dispensary care. *Vopr. Onkol.* 28:62, 1982.

76. Pfeiffer D.B., Kent E.M.: The value of preliminary colostomy in the correction of gastrojejunocolic fistula. *Am. Surg.* 110:659, 1939.

77. Jew P.W. Jr., Lavowitz B.S., Fisher B.: Alteration of the effects of jejunocolic fistula: An experimental study. *Am. Surg.* 155:175, 1962.

78. Karakousis C.P., Greenberg P.H.: Gastrocolic fistula as a complication of benign gastric ulcer. *Arch. Surg.* 114:1426, 1979.

79. Lundell L., Svartholm E.: Gastrocolic fistula: A rare complication of benign gastric ulcer. *Acta Chir. Scand.* 146:213, 1980.

80. Simpson E.T., White J.A.: Gastrocolic fistula complicating benign gastric ulcer: A case report and review of the literature. *S. Afr. Med. J.* 61:717, 1982.

81. Ekbom A., Lieberg G.: Gastrocolic fistula: Report on two cases healed by medical treatment. *Acta Chir. Scand.* 148:551, 1982.

82. Tanner N.C.: Surgical aspects of gastric and duodenal ulceration (excluding complications). *Postgrad. Med. J.* 30:124, 1954.

83. Duthie H.L., Branson C.J.: Highly selective vagotomy with excision of the ulcer compared with gastrectomy for gastric ulcer in a randomized trial. *Br. J. Surg.* 66:43, 1979.

84. Rehnberg O.: Antrectomy and gastroduodenostomy with or without vagotomy in peptic ulcer disease: A prospective study with a 5-year follow-up. *Acta Chir. Scand. [Suppl.]* 515:1, 1983.

85. Thomas W.E., Thompson M.H., Williamson R.C.: The long-term outcome of Billroth I partial gastrectomy for benign gastric ulcer. *Ann. Surg.* 195:189, 1982.

86. Tanner N.C.: Billroth II gastrectomy, in Nyhus L.M., Wastell C.W. (eds.): *Surgery of the Stomach and Duodenum.* Boston, Little, Brown & Co., 1977, pp. 355–385.

87. Maingot R.: The Billroth I operation, in Maingot R. (ed.): *Abdominal Operations.* New York, Appleton-Century-Crofts, 1980.

88. Johnston D.: Chronic gastric and duodenal ulcer, in Maingot R. (ed.): *Abdominal Operations.* New York, Appleton-Century-Crofts, 1980, pp. 211–254.

89. Jordan P.H. Jr.: Treatment of gastric ulcer by parietal cell vagotomy and excision of the ulcer: Rationale and early results. *Arch. Surg.* 116:1320, 1982.

90. Reid D.A., Duthie H.L., Bransom C.J., et al.: Late follow-up of highly selective vagotomy with excision of the ulcer compared with Billroth I gastrectomy for treatment of benign gastric ulcer. *Br. J. Surg.* 69:605, 1982.

91. Emas S., Hammarberg C.: Prospective randomized trial of selective proximal vagotomy with ulcer excision and partial gastrectomy with gastroduodenostomy in the treatment of corporeal gastric ulcer. *Am. J. Surg.* 146:631, 1983.

92. Becker H.D., Lehmann L., Lohlein D., et al.: Selective proximal vagotomy with ulcer excision or Billroth I resection in

chronic stomach ulcer: A prospective randomized multicenter study. *Chirurgie* 53:773, 1982.

93. Gayral F., Ghouti A., Salmon R., et al.: Gastric ulcer: Conservative surgical treatment in 100 patients. *Nouv. Presse Med.,* 8:3131, 1979.

94. Cade D., Allen D.: Long-term follow-up of patients with gastric ulcers treated by vagotomy, pyloroplasty and ulcerectomy. *Br. J. Surg.* 66:46, 1979.

95. Madsen P., Schousen P.: Long-term results of truncal vagotomy and pyloroplasty for gastric ulcer. *Br. J. Surg.* 69:651, 1982.

96. Andersen D., Amdrup E., Hostrup H., et al.: The Aarhus County vagotomy trial: Trends in the problem of recurrent ulcer after parietal cell vagotomy and selective gastric vagotomy with drainage. *World J. Surg.* 6:86, 1982.

97. Donahue P.E., Nyhus L.M.: Surgical excision of gastric ulcers near the gastroesophageal junction. *Surg. Gynecol. Obstet.* 155:85, 1982.

16

Gastric Cancer

Daniel G. Coit, M.D.
Murray F. Brennan, M.D., F.A.C.S.

PREVALENCE AND INCIDENCE

In 1985 there will be 25,000 new cases of gastric cancer in the United States, 15,000 male and 10,000 female. There will be 14,300 deaths from gastric cancer in 1985.*

There has been a progressive decline in the incidence of gastric cancer for both males and females. For females, in 1930 it was 30/100,000 of population and in 1980, it was 5/100,000 of population. For males, the same figures were 38/100,000 in 1930 and 10/100,000 in 1980.

A recent analysis has questioned whether this decline is due to changes in diagnosis or classification.[1] From 1935 to 1979, a statistically significant decline was noted, regardless of whether diagnosis was limited to clinical diagnosis, confirmed by tissue biopsy, or both. This decline in mortality due to gastric cancer is seen in most countries of the world except Japan, where only minimal change has been seen in recent years.

Other analyses have suggested a change in the type and presentation of gastric cancer. Proximal (cardia) lesions are now more common than they were 40 years ago, and there is both an increase of mean age of diagnosis (from 58 to 68 years) and an increase in the prevalence of predominantly signet ring cell histopathology.[2]

This increase in signet ring cell neoplasms was particularly noted in the distal gastric lesions and in younger women. The increase in cardia lesions has occurred mainly in men, and the lesions show a paucity of signet ring cells.[3]

CLASSIFICATION AND STAGING

There have been multiple classifications of gastric cancer, based on gross appearance and macroscopic features, in an effort to define prognosis at various stages and to help define optimal treatment regimens.

In 1926, Borrmann[4] devised a gross classification with four types: I—polypoid, II—ulcerated, III—ulcerated and infiltrating, and IV—infiltrating. McNeer and Pack,[5] in their review, found determinant five-year survivals of 45%, 45%, 20%, and 6% for types I–IV, respectively.

In 1954, Hoerr[6] described a system which incorporated

both depth of tumor penetration and the presence or absence of metastases (Table 16–1).[5] Hoerr used these two prognostic indicators to select that group of patients who could be potentially cured by operation. In 1970, following a multicenter field trial involving over 1,200 patients, Kennedy[7] published a staging system which incorporated depth of primary invasion, presence and extent of nodal metastases, and presence or absence of distant metastases, as determined by clinical and pathologic criteria with the TNM system. This classification was adopted by the American Joint Committee on Cancer (AJC) Staging and End Results in 1972. The system correlated well with prognosis, as shown in Figure 16–1. Within stage I, the depth of the primary lesion was also identified as a significant and independent determinant of survival. Diffusely infiltrating tumors and nodal metastases further compromise prognosis, and survival beyond two years in patients with distant metastases was rare.

This original AJC classification has since been modified to describe stage I and stage II patients as earlier disease without nodal metastases. The current stage I embraces only T_1N_0 lesions, whereas previously it included $T_{1-3}N_0$ lesions. Stage II now includes $T_{2-3}N_0$ lesions, while originally it was described as T_4N_0 or $T_{1-3}N_1$. The most recent staging system is shown in Table 16–2. It is important, when comparing results of various series, to review the TNM status that each stage describes, as some of the more recent papers still employ the older TNM staging system.

Japanese investigators report most of their results using the Union Internationale Contre le Cancer (UICC) TNM staging system. There is a primary difference between this and the AJC system. In describing the tumor, an initial separation between mucosal and submucosal lesions (T_1), and lesions with deep infiltration is further subdivided into those lesions occupying less than one half of a region (cardia, upper third, middle third, lower third, and pylorus) (T_2), more than one half but not more than one region (T_3), and more than one region or extending to neighboring structures (T_4). This system emphasizes size of the primary lesion as a prognostic variable as well as depth. Nodal classification is largely the same. A staging system is not described by the UICC, which rather relies on the TNM description of individual lesions.

Efforts have been made to devise a histologic grading system. Broders[8] graded progressively anaplastic cytologic

---

*Data from *A Cancer Journal for Clinicians*. 35(1):26–27, 1985.

239

TABLE 16–1.—GASTRIC CANCER: CLASSIFICATION
OF HOERR*

A—No metastases	I—Inner gastric layers
B—Regional metastases	II—All gastric layers
C—Distant metastases	III—Extension to contiguous structures
	NX—Not explored

*Modified from reference 5.

changes I through IV. McNeer and Pack[5] found a correlation between five-year determinant survival and Broder's histologic grade, with 66%, 39%, 30%, and 11%, respectively, for classes I through IV.

In 1965, Lauren[9] described a division of gastric carcinoma into intestinal and diffuse types. This division has not only prognostic significance, with improved survival in patients with the intestinal type[10]; there is considerable epidemiologic appeal to this division, as intestinal metaplasia is frequently associated with the intestinal type of cancer, especially in high risk populations, with the degree of metaplasia often paralleling the incidence of clinical carcinoma.[11] Most investigators feel that there are common exogenous antecedents to both conditions with metaplasia as a direct premalignant precursor of intestinal-type cancer. The diffuse type of cancer carries a poorer prognosis, does not seem to be especially prominent in high-risk populations, and may well be related to more endogenous factors.[3] Ming[12] proposed a similar histologic division into expanding and infiltrating growth patterns, that closely parallels Lauren's system. Both systems emphasize that epidemiologically, histologically, and biologically, gastric cancer is not a single, uniform entity, with prognosis determined solely on the basis of depth of primary and extent of nodal and visceral metastases. There are at least two distinct types of tumor, each with its own set of behavioral patterns. While this histologic classification is less important for therapeutic decisions, it is central to understanding etiology.

PREMALIGNANT CONDITIONS

A variety of abnormalities of the gastric mucosa occur in association with gastric cancer. Atrophic gastritis, intestinal metaplasia, gastric polyps, the postgastrectomy gastric rem-

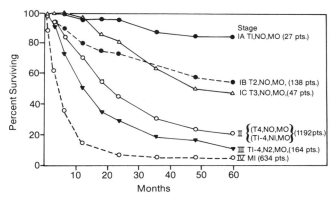

Fig 16–1.—Survivorship of 1,241 patients with stomach cancer according to this TNM classification, excluding operative mortality. (Reproduced with permission from *Cancer* 26:971–983, 1979.)

TABLE 16–2.—STAGE
GROUPING OF CARCINOMA
OF THE STOMACH*

Stage 0	Tis, N_0, M_0
Stage I	T_1, N_0, M_0
Stage II	T_2, T_3; N_0, M_0
Stage III	T_1–T_3; N_1, N_2; M_0
	T_{4a}, N_0–N_2; M_0
Stage IV	T_1–T_3; N_3, M_0
	T_{4b}, any N, M_0
	Any T, and N, M_1

*From American Joint Committee on Cancer: *Manual for Staging Cancer*, 1983, p. 69.

nant, pernicious anemia, and gastric ulcer have all been implicated as possible premalignant lesions. All have been extensively studied, but proof that any is a predictable precursor of gastric carcinoma is lacking.

Atrophic Gastritis

The incidence and prevalence of chronic atrophic gastritis and gastric carcinoma both increase with age. Despite their frequent coexistence, a causal relationship has yet to be established. Efforts to look at the etiologies of chronic gastritis and to correlate the subsequent incidence of cancer have resulted in its classification into three major subtypes: autoimmune, hypersecretory, and environmental.[13] Autoimmune chronic gastritis (type A), the model of which is pernicious anemia, tends to occur in the proximal stomach as a result of antibodies against intrinsic factor and parietal cells. Hypersecretory chronic gastritis is common, usually antral in distribution, associated with peptic ulcer disease, rarely associated with atrophy or intestinal metaplasia and is not felt to be a cancer precursor. Environmental chronic gastritis (type B) is most prevalent in those populations at high risk for gastric cancer; distribution in the stomach is more random and multifocal, with intestinal metaplasia and dysplasia frequent cofeatures.

Despite epidemiologic data to suggest a relationship, it was not until recently that an increased risk for carcinoma was demonstrated in patients with chronic gastritis.[14] Comparing a population of patients with carcinoma to an age- and sex-matched set of noncancer controls, Sipponen et al. demonstrated a similar prevalence of chronic gastritis in patients with and without malignancy when tumor histology and location were ignored. However, they found the progression of gastritis to be more severe in the cancer-afflicted areas than in noncancer afflicted areas. There was a clear correlation between the intestinal type of gastric cancer and areas of high prevalence and progression of chronic gastritis. This correlation was less distinct with the diffuse type of gastric cancer. While not conclusive, the association of degree of chronic gastritis with location and histology of gastric cancer supports the common pathway theory of gastric cancer development.

Intestinal Metaplasia

Sipponen and associates[14] further elaborated on this common pathway by demonstrating a positive correlation between the extent and distribution of intestinal metaplasia and intestinal gastric carcinoma. These anatomical data support epidemiologic data on populations in Colombia and Japan at high risk for gastric cancer in whom there is a marked increase in the prevalence of intestinal metaplasia.

Histochemical analysis defines categories of complete and incomplete intestinal metaplasia.[15] The former type reveals disappearance of the antral glands and replacement of gastric epithelium with orderly and mature absorptive and goblet cells. Incomplete metaplasia is characterized by fewer goblet cells and less well-developed columnar cells with incomplete biochemical profiles. Iida and Kusama[15] were able to demonstrate a close relationship between incomplete intestinal metaplasia and small, well-differentiated carcinomas. Relationships between larger or poorly differentiated carcinomas were not apparent, probably due to neoplastic overgrowth of the transition zones.

Correa[16] has proposed a sequence of events that would unite much of what is known about epidemiologic associations and experimental exogenous precursors. He postulates an initial nonspecific injury to normal gastric mucosa (age, bile, chronic aspirin, alcohol, sodium chloride, autoimmune factors), possibly compounded by inadequate repair secondary to nutritional deficiencies. This could lead to a progressive, superficial to chronic atrophic gastritis of the several subtypes mentioned, with intestinal metaplasia ensuing as a normal adaptive and reparative mechanism. This would lead to an increase in the gastric microenvironmental pH with bacterial overgrowth. The ensuing production by these bacteria of nitrate reductases would catalyze conversion of dietary nitrates to nitrites. These nitrites are known to react with a large number of compounds (bile acid, fish, fava beans, and multiple drugs) to form nitroso compounds, which are known mutagens in animal models. This would promote incomplete intestinal metaplasia, progressive dysplasia, and finally carcinoma. While appealing from many standpoints, proof of this pathway is lacking, as the sequence of metaplasia to dysplasia to carcinoma in situ to frankly invasive carcinoma has yet to be convincingly demonstrated.

Gastric Polyps

The risk of gastric cancer in the presence of gastric polyps has varied from 0% to 50%. The retrospective observation by Tomasulo,[17] that 35% of stomachs removed for carcinoma have polyps vs. 5% of stomachs removed for benign conditions having polyps, suggests that this is more than idle association. Efforts to define the risk of cancer in gastric polyps have looked at polyp histology, size, shape, and number. Longitudinal studies have tried to estimate the risk of carcinoma developing in polyps over time. Variations in the ratio of these factors are responsible for the broad range of risk as initially cited.

Epithelial polyps can be divided into two categories: hyperplastic and adenomatous. The former are more numerous in all series and have a much lower risk of cancer occurring within them or in association with them (Table 16–3). Adenomatous polyps, on the other hand, while less numerous, have a distinctly higher risk of carcinoma, both within the polyp or elsewhere within the stomach. Laxen et al.[20] demonstrated carcinoma in situ in five of 23 adenomas and adenomatous polyps at the margin of 34 invasive carcinomas.

Size is a reliable predictor of the malignant potential of a polyp (Table 16–4). The fact that hyperplastic polyps are rarely greater than 2 cm in diameter, while adenomatous polyps frequently are larger than 2 cm, obscures size as an independent predictor of malignancy. The Japanese have found that type 2 and type 3 polyps, sessile lesions greater than 2 cm in diameter, have a 70% and 94% chance of harboring carcinoma, respectively.[23]

Yamagata and Hisamichi[23] found that less than 1% of over 1,600 patients with gastric polyps of all types followed over time subsequently developed carcinoma. However, adenomatous polyps followed over time have a higher malignant potential, 11%–18%, often preceded by dysplasia and carcinoma in situ.[24] Laxen et al.[20] found, in following 357 patients for six to 18 months, an 18% incidence of intestinal type carcinoma developing outside of the polyp elsewhere in the stomach.

Multiplicity of polyps may increase the risk of cancer, depending on size and histology. Hamartomatous polyps as seen in the Peutz-Jeghers syndrome are thought to have a very low malignant potential, as are multiple hyperplastic polyps. Multiple adenomas such as with familial polyposis may pose a risk high enough to justify prophylactic total gastrectomy.

It seems clear that the malignant potential of gastric polyps is confined primarily to the adenomas which should be vigorously pursued with serial endoscopic biopsies. Any lesion greater than 2 cm in diameter should be removed entirely. Continued surveillance of these patients is mandatory.

Gastric Remnant Cancer

The first case of adenocarcinoma occurring in the gastric remnant following resection for benign peptic ulcer disease was reported by Balfour in 1922.[25] By 1980 an excess of 2,000 cases had been reported, and the association of prior gastric resection with subsequent malignancy had assumed the status of a clinical entity. A great deal of interest has been devoted to trying to establish a relationship between the two, with efforts directed at trying to define a relative risk and interval for the development of gastric cancer following gastric resection.

Initial efforts were retrospective, looking at the relative prevalence of prior gastric surgery in large groups of patients with an established diagnosis of gastric cancer (Table 16–5). These retrospective studies give no indication of the expected

TABLE 16–3.—MALIGNANT POTENTIAL OF GASTRIC POLYPS—HISTOLOGY

AUTHOR	YEAR	N	% HYPERPLASTIC	% ADENOMA	% CA IN ADENOMA	% CA WITH ADENOMA	% CA WITH HYPERPLASTIC
Ming and Goldman[18]	1965	49	79	21	40	30	8
Tomasulo[17]	1971	97	76	24	22	49	28
Remine et al.[19]	1981	43	58	24	17		
Laxen et al.[20]	1982	357				38	5

TABLE 16–4.—MALIGNANT POTENTIAL OF GASTRIC POLYPS—
SIZE

AUTHOR	YEAR	N	% MALIGNANT >2 CM	% MALIGNANT <2 CM
Hay[21]	1956	96	55	1.2
Eklof[22]	1962	221	33	5
Tomasulo[17]	1971	97	24	4
Ming and Goldman[18]	1965	49	27	0

prevalence of gastric cancer in the population, but do emphasize that it composes a small subset of patients with gastric
cancer.

Prospective studies have examined populations of patients
undergoing gastric surgery who subsequently developed gastric cancer. These studies require a defined population to be
followed up over a long period; the majority of such studies
are hampered by incomplete follow-up. Recently, however,
three studies have provided meaningful data. Welvart and
Warnsinck[39] found a 1.9% cumulative incidence (5 of 257 patients, 97% follow-up, minimum of 26 years), and Fisher et
al.[40] found a 1.3% cumulative incidence (13 of 1,000 patients,
95% follow-up, 22- to 30-year interval) of gastric cancer following gastric resection in Holland and Denmark, respectively. Comparing these figures to a regional cumulative incidence of 3% of patients aged 0 to 74 years developing
gastric cancer, they concluded that there was no increased
risk of gastric cancer in patients treated surgically for peptic
ulcer disease. A comparable study in the United States was
reported by Schafer et al. in 1983,[41] with an observed-to-ex-
pected ratio of 2.0–2.6 patients developing gastric cancer out
of a cohort of 338 patients, 17 to 19 years after gastric resection with 100% follow-up.

Thus, although attractive etiologic hypotheses can be devised to explain an increased susceptibility of the gastric remnant mucosa to undergo malignant transformation, critical statistical assessment would suggest that there is no significant
increased risk of gastric cancer subsequent to gastric resection. In practical terms, this implies that routine endoscopic

screening programs for patients with a history of prior gastric
resection are unwarranted. However, it also suggests that,
following resection of one half to two thirds of the stomach
most prone to develop cancer, the subsequent risk of gastric
malignancy is no lower. We may yet be able to define a population of gastric remnant patients at risk, based on more critical evaluation of the postgastrectomy mucosa (degree of intestinal metaplasia and dysplasia as defined by histochemical
profile, for example), who might benefit from closer surveillance.

Pernicious Anemia

The relative risk of gastric carcinoma in patients with pernicious anemia has been established to be three to 21 times
that of the normal population. Gregor[42] reported a 50% incidence of gastric cancer in patients with pernicious anemia followed up 15 years or longer. It seems that patients with pernicious anemia, composing 3% of people over 60 years of age,
would then represent a high risk group who might benefit
from screening programs. Eriksson et al.[43] in a large Swedish
autopsy series, however, found that only 19 of 917 patients
(2%) who died with gastric cancer had antecedent pernicious
anemia, a prevalence in pernicious anemia not statistically different from a control population dying of other causes. The
incidence of gastric cancer was only statistically increased, to
about twofold over control patients, when the pernicious anemia had been present for five to 15 years. It would seem prudent to investigate aggressively any symptoms in patients
with longstanding pernicious anemia; routine endoscopic
screening based on a two- to three-fold risk cannot be advocated at this time.

Gastric Ulcer

The issue of carcinoma arising at the site of benign gastric
ulcer has been long debated. Studies reporting a 2%–30%
incidence of gastric cancer in series of patients operated on
for benign disease reflect selection bias and problems with
defining "ulcer cancer."[23, 44] Morson et al.[45] would require

TABLE 16–5.—PREVALENCE OF GASTRIC REMNANT CANCER

AUTHOR	YEAR	PTS WITH CA	REMNANT CA	INCIDENCE (%)	INTERVAL (YR)
Helsingen and Hillenstrad[26]	1956	229	11	4.8	20
Krause[27]	1958	361	28	7.8	24
Saegesser and James[28]	1972	653	18	2.7	19
Domellof and Janunger[29]	1977	676	14	2.0	12+
Peitsch and Becker[30]	1979	302	27	8.9	12-GU 27-DU
Nichols[31]	1979	1,473	36	2.4	11.3
Karfeld and Resnick[32]	1979	100	7	7.0	21.6
Papachristou et al.[33]	1980	1,496	30	2.0	9.0-GU 24.5-DU 15-PG 28-V/GJ
Lygidakis[34]	1981	2,473	32	1.3	12
Orlando and Welch[35]	1981	678	17	2.5	18.7
Perez et al.[36]	1982	319	16	5.0	17.4
Dougherty et al.[37]	1982	1,079	21	1.9	24-PG
Totten et al.[38]	1983	1,092	40	3.8	8.5-V/GJ

DU = duodenal ulcer, GU = gastric ulcer, PG = partial gastrectomy, V/GJ = vagotomy and
gastrojejunostomy.

definitive evidence of a preexisting ulceration with complete destruction of the muscularis propria, the mucosa replaced by fibrous and granulation tissue with fusion of the muscularis propria and muscularis mucosa around the edge, with a surrounding zone of obliterative endarteritis as well as evidence of malignancy at the edge of the ulcer to define ulcer cancer. Based on these criteria, Morson and co-workers believe that the incidence of carcinoma developing in a previous peptic ulcer and of peptic ulceration at the edge of proved carcinoma are probably both less than 1%. The remainder of gastric ulcers associated with cancer are most likely malignant from the time of onset, their diagnosis confounded by their "malignant cycle" of regression and recurrence. Nonhealing gastric ulcers should always be viewed with suspicion and pursued aggressively with serial endoscopy, cytology, and multiple biopsies.

Summary

The attention focused on premalignant states is important as we try to define a population at risk for gastric cancer. Patients with active, incomplete intestinal metaplasia need closer surveillance than those with mild hypersecretory chronic gastritis. Patients with adenomatous polyps are at higher risk than those with hyperplastic polyps for carcinoma, both within the polyp and elsewhere in the stomach. The return on screening patients with pernicious anemia and postgastrectomy is less well defined, though any symptoms in those groups should be aggressively evaluated.

In evaluating the spectrum of mucosal abnormalities—from superficial gastritis to chronic atrophic gastritis, to intestinal metaplasia, to incomplete intestinal metaplasia, to dysplasia, to carcinoma in situ, to frankly invasive carcinoma—we have begun to understand potential mechanisms for the development of gastric cancer which, if confirmed, could result in prophylactic measures aimed at populations at risk.

DIAGNOSIS AND MANAGEMENT

Diagnosis and Screening

The importance of the evolution of techniques to diagnose gastric cancer is seen in the success of the mass screening programs of populations at risk. With increasing application and sophistication in diagnostics, the Japanese have significantly improved their overall five-year survival statistics in recent decades. They have proceeded from the investigation of advanced symptomatic patients to the detection of early and minute gastric cancers, usually asymptomatic, and not always clearly visible to the naked eye.

The standard barium upper GI series has been the mainstay of diagnosis in gastric cancer. With an overall accuracy of over 80% in gastric cancer, and a false negative rate of less than 20%,[46] it is an effective first step. However, it is less accurate in the diagnosis of early lesions. Air contrast hypotonic upper GI series with thin barium has increased the accuracy to over 90%.[47, 48]

Fiberoptic endoscopy has further increased the accuracy of diagnosis in gastric cancer. Endoscopy alone is accurate in 71%–98% in assessing the malignancy of a gastric lesion, depending on the skill and experience of the endoscopist. False negative impressions are recorded in 1.3%–28%, while false positive impressions appear in 2%–5% of cases. Endoscopic biopsy techniques reinforce the clinical appearance of malignant lesions with a similar accuracy of 75%–95%. Graham et al.[49] showed in a prospective fashion that accuracy was improved progressively from 70%–98% when the number of biopsies taken was increased from one to seven. False positive results are rare (0%–4%), while false negative results occur in 4%–21% of patients, depending on the biopsy techniques employed.

Direct brush cytology further increases the yield in diagnosis of gastric cancer with an accuracy of 75%–90%. False negative results are seen in 9%–17% of patients and false positive results are extremely rare, seen in 0%–8% of patients. Winawer et al.[50] have found that cytology is often not helpful in the recurrent infiltrating tumors and in the submucosal linitis plastica-type lesions.

The combination of endoscopic appearance, histology, and cytology have been found to be superior to any one method, with a diagnostic accuracy of 87%–100% of gastric cancer (Table 16–6).

Refinement in endoscopic techniques has been of particular value in early gastric cancer. Ikida et al.[57] described the enhancement of mucosal abnormalities with intraceliac Evans blue, with or without vasomotor drugs. Tatsuta et al.[58] described a less cumbersome method with improved delineation of both minute and early gastric cancer using an endoscopic combination of Congo red and methylene blue staining techniques, revealing the extent of lesions often beyond areas of unenhanced visual abnormality. Gilen and associates[59] demonstrated a similar technique using tolonium chloride to help distinguish between benign and malignant gastric ulcers.

Gastric juice analysis, first reported by Piper et al. in 1963,[60] has recently been reexamined. Mitti et al.[61] has found a higher gastric juice carcinoembryonic antigen (CEA) in patients with moderate to severe atrophic gastritis or gastric cancer than in those with minor mucosal abnormalities. Graffner and Hultberg[62] have reported gastric juice levels of CEA, β-hexosaminidase, and lysozyme levels to be significantly

TABLE 16–6.—DIAGNOSTIC ACCURACY IN GASTRIC CANCER
(% TRUE POSITIVES)

AUTHOR	YEAR	PTS WITH CA	ENDOSCOPY	BIOPSY	CYTOLOGY	ALL
Moshakis and Hooper[51]	1978	44	93	95	88	100
Puig-Lacalle et al.[52]	1980	93	71	85	90	—
Shanghai Study Group[53]	1982	155	—	74	77	88
Moreno-Ortero et al.[54]	1983	194	88	79	91	95
Gupta et al.[55, 56]	1983	60	—	75	85	93
Sekons et al.[46]	1984	165	99	96	—	99

higher in patients with gastric cancer than in a control group. Furthermore, while he found no difference in CEA and β-hexosaminidase levels between those patients with gastric cancer and those following resection for benign disease, lysozyme levels were significantly higher in the gastric cancer group. A role for use of these gastric juice markers is suggested as an alternative to endoscopic screening of early mucosal abnormalities.

While the diagnosis of advanced symptomatic gastric cancer rarely presents a problem to the astute clinician, efforts at identifying patients with early lesions continue. Current screening programs are cost-effective in populations at high risk but cannot be justified in a Western population. Until a method is found that is noninvasive, easily and widely applicable, sensitive, specific, and inexpensive, we will continue to be confronted by a spectrum of gastric cancer that is heavily weighed in favor of its systemic form.

Early Gastric Cancer

Early gastric cancer (EGC) is defined as a cancer confined to the gastric mucosa and/or submucosa, regardless of size or presence of lymph node metastases. In terms of the natural history of the disease, the term "early" may be a misnomer; the term does define a pathologic stage in the development of gastric cancer, a stage at which the vast majority of patients are surgically curable.

Incidence

The incidence of EGC is directly related to the diligence with which it is sought. In the pre-endoscopy era, EGC composed less than 5% of all gastric cancers. With increasing refinements in diagnostic techniques, including more frequent use of higher quality fiberoptic endoscopes, multiple biopsies, often directed by mucosal staining techniques and augmented by brush cytology, EGC now composes 15%–20% of gastric carcinoma in most Western series. Japanese investigators have increased the yield of EGC to 30%–40% of all gastric cancers through the use of mass screening programs in a population at high risk.

Pathology

The pathology of EGC has been extensively studied. It has a predilection for the distal half of the stomach and lesser curvature in all series. There are several schemas of macroscopic classification, the most common of which originated from the Japanese Gastroenterological Endoscopy Society as shown in Figure 16–2, dividing the lesion into type I (protruded), type II (superficial), and type III (excavated), with combinations of each possible. Kodama et al.[63] defined another system, based on growth patterns, and tried to correlate the types with prognoses. The superficial spreading type, a lesion of greater than 4 cm in diameter, had a favorable prognosis with low incidence of lymphatic or hematogenous metastases. The penetrating type B, a lesion of less than 4 cm in diameter infiltrating with fenestrations into the submucosa, had similar characteristics. However, they were able to identify a penetrating type A, a lesion of less than 4 cm with extensive infiltration and destruction of the submucosa, usually a well-differentiated lesion, with a high incidence of venous invasion and lymphatic metastases and a correspondingly poor

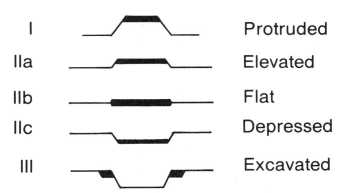

Fig 16–2.—The Japanese classification of early gastric cancer (*bold segments* indicate cancer).

prognosis. While over 90% of patients with the former two patterns survived five years in that study, only 65% of those with the penetrating type A pattern survived five years.

Despite its defined superficial nature, EGC has a small but finite incidence of lymph node metastases, 8%–15% in most series. This incidence correlates with the depth of penetration of the primary lesion, being two to five times more frequent with primary lesions extending into the submucosa as with those confined to the mucosa alone (Table 16–7). Bearzi and Rinaldi[68] confirmed this and also noted a higher incidence of lymph node metastases with the diffuse as opposed to intestinal type of primary lesion. Interestingly, Murakami[69] found that in contrast to advanced gastric cancer, the presence of N_1 disease alone was not a major determinant of five-year survival; it was only when N_2 and N_3 groups were involved that five-year survival declined.

EGC has been found to be multicentric in 9% to as many as 29% of cases.[68] This multicentricity does not seem to correlate with histologic type. It is thought to account in part for the local recurrence rate of 3% following seemingly adequate resection of the primary lesion. It would not seem high enough, however, to justify total gastrectomy in all instances of EGC.[70, 71]

Finally, patients with EGC have a marked tendency to develop a second malignancy. These malignancies are often those that determine the ultimate survival of these patients. The rate of second primary has been reported as high as 32% and mandates long-term close surveillance of these patients.[72]

Surgery

The surgical approach to EGC is derived from an understanding of the pathology. With a 15% incidence of lymph node metastases, a thorough lymph node dissection needs to be considered. The Japanese report up to 50% five-year survival with N_2 disease with complete lymphatic clearance to the level of N_3 in all patients. Fujita et al.,[64] however, found no difference in age-corrected, five-year survival rates among R_1, R_2, and R_3 resections for early gastric cancer despite a lymph node positivity of 1% for mucosal lesions and 19% for submucosal lesions. The issue of multicentricity and extent of surgical resection has not been directly addressed. A proximal or distal subtotal gastrectomy would be adequate in the absence of any mucosal abnormality in the gastric remnant. If

TABLE 16–7.—EARLY GASTRIC CANCER: INCIDENCE OF LYMPH NODE METASTASES (%)

| | | | LEVEL OF NODAL METASTASES | | | | | | | |
| | | | Mucosa | | | | Submucosa | | | |
AUTHOR	YEAR	N	N_1	N_2	N_3	All	N_1	N_2	N_3	All
Kodama et al.[63]	1981	109	6	0	2	8	10	3	2	15
Fujita et al.[64]	1983	184	1	0	0	1	16	3	0	19
Soga et al.[65]	1979	80	8.8	2.9	0	11.7	17.4	4.3	0	21.7
Gebhardt et al.[66]	1981	130	—	5.8	—	5.8	—	9.6	—	9.6
Miyake[67]	1979	126	—	3	—	3	—	16	—	16

multiple gastric cytologies are positive for carcinoma, but no specific lesion can be demonstrated on repeated endoscopic examination, a total gastrectomy is warranted in the good-risk patient. In the poor-risk patient, promising results with neodymium-yag laser ablation have been described.[73]

Prognosis

Enthusiasm for the prognosis of EGC should be tempered with an understanding of the natural history of the disease if left untreated. Tsukuma et al.[74] estimated a determinant five-year survival of 64.5% in patients with early gastric cancer in whom no therapeutic intervention was undertaken, with an estimated median survival of 77 months. He estimated a median time of progression of early gastric cancer to advanced gastric cancer of 37 months. Although there is bias in this retrospective review, which selected the slower-growing lesions, the indolent nature of the disease at this stage is in sharp contrast to the rapidly accelerating course of node-positive advanced gastric cancer.

Murakami,[69] in his review of 570 patients with EGC, found a 90%–100% determinant five-year survival excluding operative mortality in those patients with lesions confined to the mucosa only. With submucosal involvement, the five-year survival drops to 80%–85% (Table 16–8). These figures correlate well with those in the review by Gebhardt et al.[66] of 130 cases from northern Europe. The influence of lymph node involvement was examined by Murakami, noting an 86% five-year survival with N_1 and a 50% five-year survival with N_2. In lymph node-positive patients, there was no worsening of prognosis with submucosal lesions.

Kodama et al.[63] looked at morphological correlates of prognosis and found that patients with a "penetrating type A" had a high incidence of venous invasion and lymph node metas-

TABLE 16–8.—EARLY GASTRIC CANCER AND % FIVE-YEAR SURVIVAL

| | | | DEPTH OF PRIMARY | |
AUTHOR	YEAR	N	% Mucosa	% Submucosa
Gentsch et al.[76]	1981	113	96	79
Piper[77]	1978	2,751	93	85
Hirota and Sano[78]	1975	600	97	83
Soga et al.[65]	1979	80	91	91
Gebhardt et al.[66]	1981	130	96	85
Kishimoto[79]	1976	510	97	96
Iwanaga et al.[70]	1976	229	96	94
Kodama et al.[63]	1981	126	97	91
Fujita et al.[64]	1983	152	96	95

tases with a 65% five-year survival. He contrasted this to the prognosis of patients with small mucosal lesions, superficially spreading or penetrating type B where he found an excess of 95% ten-year survival (age-adjusted excluding operative mortality). In contrast to the advanced gastric lesions, penetrating type A lesions were usually well differentiated histologically, corresponding to Lauren's intestinal type.

Cause of Death in Early Gastric Cancer

The main sites of recurrence following adequate surgical intervention remain the gastric remnant and the liver. Kodama et al.[63] noted that gastric remnant recurrences tend to occur more often in the superficial spreading type, and often more than five years after the original surgical intervention. This biological fact would support the indolent and multifocal nature of the disease at this stage. Liver metastases tend to occur earlier, within three years in Kodama's series, and often in association with the penetrating type A primary. Finally, Green et al.,[72] in their series of 28 patients, noted only one death from recurrent gastric cancer. Five patients in the series, however, died within five years of metastases from a second, nongastric malignancy, underscoring the importance of this propensity for second nongastric neoplasms.

Summary

Early gastric cancer represents an invasive carcinoma of the stomach at a curable stage. The frequency with which it occurs depends directly on the diligence with which it is sought. In populations at risk high enough to justify mass screening, the yield of early gastric cancer has had significant impact on the overall prognosis of gastric cancer.[75] For the most part, it appears to be a biologically indolent stage, though up to 15% of patients have lymph node metastases at the time of operation. Furthermore, there does seem to be a subset of patients at higher risk for liver metastases. The presence of nodal metastases does not preclude reasonable survival and, accordingly, surgery should include wide resection of the primary lesion; the role of extensive regional lymph node dissection is less well defined. Long-term surveillance of these patients for both recurrent gastric carcinoma and second nongastric malignancies is mandatory, as, if discovered early enough, many will still be at a treatable stage.

Advanced Gastric Cancer

Surgery

The surgical objectives in advanced gastric cancer include maximizing the potential for cure in patients with localized lesions, while offering the most effective palliation to the remainder. As a local-regional measure, resection offers the only hope of cure in gastric cancer. The results in treating patients with early gastric cancer are excellent. The majority of unscreened patients, however, present at a late stage, as manifested by the consistently poor results reported in multiple large U.S. series, with generally fewer than 10% of all patients with gastric cancer surviving five years. Surgical objectives in symptomatic patients with advanced disease often equate with the most efficient palliation. Given the overall results and pessimistic outlook for the patient with gastric cancer, many questions arise with regard to surgical management. What should be the extent of surgery aimed at cure? What are the roles of extensive lymphadenectomy and splenectomy in curative procedures? Does adjacent organ involvement preclude curative surgery, or should aggressive wide en bloc resection be pursued? What constitutes an adequate proximal or distal margin, and what are the implications of histologically positive margins? If cure is not possible, what procedure or procedures afford optimal palliation with the least operative morbidity and mortality?

EXTENT OF OPERATION.—Theodor Billroth performed the first successful subtotal gastrectomy for cancer in 1881; his patient subsequently died of disseminated cancer 14 months later.[80] Since that time, with refinements in operative technique and perioperative care, efforts have been made to perform progressively larger resections in an attempt to circumscribe the limits of tumor and improve survival. Total gastrectomy was the operation of choice in the 1940s and '50s,[81] but could not withstand comparison with subtotal resection, as the increase in operative morbidity and mortality was not matched by improved survival.[82] Extended radical gastrectomy, to include en bloc removal of the spleen and body/tail of the pancreas, was proposed in an attempt at en bloc resection of the celiac and splenic hilar nodes.[5] Gilbertsen[83] found that these more extensive operations increased operative mortality, again, without improving survival.

From these and other series have evolved the generally accepted approach as espoused by Cady et al.,[84] Remine,[85] and Dupont et al.,[86] of radical distal subtotal gastrectomy to include 80%–85% of the stomach, for antral and small midstomach tumors, reserving total gastrectomy and esophagogastrectomy only for large midstomach or more proximal lesions. Most would advocate inclusion of the greater and lesser omenta as a routine, but extensive and systematic lymph node dissection is not thought necessary by most Western authors, given the increased morbidity and poor prognosis of lymph node-positive patients. Routine splenectomy has been a matter of debate, to be addressed below. This general approach would accede to the presence of nodal metastases as denoting incurable disease; in the absence of nodal metastases these operations are curative, and in their presence they are palliative.

In trying to determine the goals of a planned surgical approach to gastric cancer, Papachristou and Fortner[87] looked at the question of whether or not the tumor had already spread beyond the limits of curative resection at the time of operation. They reviewed autopsy data of 21 patients who died within two weeks of their "curative" surgery. They found that of eight patients with T_{1-4}, N_{0-1}, M_0 lesions, none had evi-

dence of systemic disease. Of interest, however, was the fact that ten of 13 patients with T_{1-4}, N_2, M_0 lesions; i.e., those patients with metastases to removed regional nodes or nodes on both gastric curvatures had evidence of residual nonresected disease, again, despite surgery of curative intent for apparently localized lesions ($P < .01$). These data help to explain the dismal results obtained with surgery alone for advanced disease. It provides some rationale for a more aggressive surgical approach in earlier-stage lesions and a more conservative approach to advanced disease.

Papachristou and Fortner[87–89] and Shiu et al.[90] expanded further on this point in their retrospective analyses of the results of various surgical procedures as applied to carcinoma of the gastric cardia, fundus, midbody, and antrum, analyzed by stage for operative mortality, local recurrence, and survival (Table 16–9). For lesions of all areas, patients with advanced disease (T_x, N_2, M_{0-1}) did poorly regardless of the extent of surgery. However, for early lesions (T_{1-4}, N_{0-1}, M_0) patients fared significantly better both in terms of local recurrence and survival at five years without increase in operative mortality when extended total gastrectomy was compared to proximal or distal subtotal resection. The explanation put forward was that the wider resections included submicroscopic spread that would have been left behind with lesser procedures. In these four studies from the same institution, there were too few total gastrectomies in early-stage lesions to allow comparison with lesser and greater procedures. Regardless of the small numbers, survival in early-stage tumors undergoing total gastrectomy was intermediate between a lesser and greater operation, except for body lesions where total gastrectomies were better, but, again, only small numbers of patients received total gastrectomy. The operative mortality was not statistically different among these procedures, calculated at overall 8.5% from 1970 to 1975.

In these retrospective studies, a group of patients with body lesions was identified who underwent deliberate or "elective" extended total gastrectomy (i.e., patients could have had a lesser operation, considered curative) that had a 93% five-year survival. This survival was higher despite poorer prognostic indicators in these patients than those receiving lesser operations. These data suggest that in early lesions, an extended operation in experienced hands may well influence survival.

LYMPHADENECTOMY.—The Japanese have made a most important contribution to the field of gastric cancer with re-

TABLE 16–9.—FIVE-YEAR SURVIVAL FOR STAGES I AND II*

	EXTENDED TOTAL GASTRECTOMY		SUBTOTAL GASTRECTOMY		
	N	%	N	%	P
Fundus	93	68	48	13	0.01
Cardia	7	83	17	PSG 16†	0.03
Midstomach	36	42	12	17	NS
Antrum	11	100	37	37‡	.02

*Adapted from Shiu M., Papachristou D., Kosloff C., et al.: Selection of operative procedure for adenocarcinoma of the midstomach. *Ann. Surg.* 192(6):730–737, 1980.[90]
†P 0.05.
‡ = Projected five-year survival (operative mortality excluded).

gard to extent of procedure in their painstakingly complete analysis of the extent of surgery and lymphadenectomy for various stage lesions. Their terminology has been summarized recently.[91] They divide the regional nodes into perigastric and extragastric groups, as described in Table 16–10. The extent of resection, termed R_0 (incomplete group 1), R_1 (complete group 1), R_2 (complete group 1 and group 2), and R_3 (complete groups 1, 2, and 3), is based on the location of these nodes relative to the location of the primary tumor, as shown in Table 16–11.

Mine et al.[92] examined the end results of 408 patients undergoing operation for gastric cancer; 277 patients underwent gastrectomy, of whom there were 63 five-year survivors, 23% of those resected and 15% of all patients studied. Operative mortality was 6% for R_1 and R_2 procedures, and 10.5% for R_3 procedures. As the majority of their R_1 resections were palliative, results between these and the more extensive procedures for cure could not be compared. They were unable to demonstrate a statistically significant survival advantage at five years between R_2 and R_3, stratified by stage, presence or absence of lymph nodes, and presence or absence of serosal invasion, though there seemed to be at least a trend in favor of the more aggressive R_3 procedures.

Kodama et al.[93] described 454 patients undergoing curative resection, including extensive lymph node dissection (R_2 and R_3) from 1964 to 1972, comparing end results to a historical control cohort of 254 patients undergoing curative, simple resection (R_{0-1}) from 1950 to 1957. Despite more extensive surgery, there was an improvement in operative mortality from 3.7% to 1.7% (Table 16–12). These deaths were excluded from further analysis. Somewhat contrary to the Memorial data, Kodama and associates found no difference in survival between the limited and aggressive lymph node dissections for those patients without lymph node metastases or in those patients with mucosal and submucosal or muscularis tumors, suggesting that R_1 resections are adequate for stage I and all early gastric cancers. (This occurred despite lymph node metastases in 8% of the mucosal lesions and 16% of submucosal

TABLE 16–10.—REGIONAL LYMPH NODES OF THE STOMACH*

PERIGASTRIC LYMPH NODES
1. Right pericardial
2. Left pericardial
3. Lesser curvature
4. Greater curvature
5. Suprapyloric
6. Infrapyloric
EXTRAPERIGASTRIC LYMPH NODES
7. Left gastric artery
8. Common hepatic artery
9. Celiac artery
10. Splenic hilus
11. Splenic artery
12. Hepatic pedicle
13. Retropancreatic
14. Mesenteric root
15. Middle colic artery
16. Periaortic

*Adapted from the Japanese Research Society for Gastric Cancer: The general rules for gastric cancer study in surgery and pathology. *Jpn. J. Surg.* 11:127–145, 1981.[91]

TABLE 16–11.—GROUPING OF REGIONAL LYMPH NODES IN RELATIONSHIP TO THE PRIMARY SITE OF CARCINOMA OF THE STOMACH*

PRIMARY SITE OF CARCINOMA	GROUP 1	GROUP 2†	GROUP 3†	GROUP 4
Lower third	3,4,5,6	1,7,8,9	11,12,13,14 (2) (10)	15,16
Middle third	1,3,4,5,6	7,8,9,11 (2) (10)	12,13,14	15,16
Upper third	1,2,3,4	7,8,9,10,11 (5) (6)	12,13,14	15,16
Whole stomach	1,2,3,4,5,6	7,8,9,10,11	12,13,14	15,16

*Adapted from Japanese Research Society for Gastric Cancer: The general rules for gastric cancer study in surgery and pathology. *Jpn. J. Surg.* 11:127–145, 1981.[91]
†Parentheses indicate nodes that need not necessarily be dissected.

lesions.) Furthermore, they found no difference in survival between limited and aggressive lymph node dissection in patients with total gastric involvement (linitis plastica) or adjacent organ invasion, or in patients with distant lymph nodes positive, with poor prognoses prevailing in all groups. However, in the patients with serosal invasion or with only regional lymph nodes positive (i.e., the majority of patients), there was a clear survival advantage when comparing extensive lymph node dissection vs. simple resection in this retrospective study. The improvement in survival was in the range of 20%–27% and could not be explained simply on the basis of improved perioperative care. The authors concluded that if extended lymphadenectomy could be performed in patients with tumors invading the serosa but not adjacent organs, with regional but not distant lymph nodes involved, with an operative mortality approaching 3% or less, significant survival advantages should accrue over those patients treated with simple resection alone. Prospective data to establish this point are lacking.

SPLENECTOMY.—The issue of elective splenectomy in patients undergoing total gastrectomy has recently been reexamined. Based on pathoanatomical data revealing a high incidence of clinically occult but histologically positive nodes along the splenic artery and in the splenic hilum, routine splenectomy, or pancreaticosplenectomy had been advised for lesions at risk.[94, 95] There is a significant body of information

TABLE 16–12.—FIVE-YEAR SURVIVAL PATIENTS SUBJECTED TO CURATIVE OPERATION*

DEPTH	(R_{0-1})† Simple Resection N	%	(R_{2-3}) EXTENSIVE REGIONAL Lymph node Dissection N	%
Mucosa	7	100	51	96
Submucosa	10	100	58	90
Muscularis	46	74	55	80
Serosa	179	18	251	45‡
Adjacent	12	8	39	18
Nodes				
Negative	73	73	209	81
Positive	181	18	245	39‡

*From Kodama Y., Sugimachi K., Soejima K., et al.: Evaluation of extensive lymph node dissection for carcinoma of the stomach. *World J. Surg.* 5:241–248, 1981.[93]
†Historical controls.
‡$P < 0.001$.

now accumulating that, despite the anatomical data, patients undergoing prophylactic splenectomy or pancreaticosplenectomy fare no better and possibly worse than similarly staged patients whose spleens are left intact.[96, 97] The splenic and splenic hilar nodes may be of prognostic rather than therapeutic importance. Prospective data are not available to answer this question.

ADJACENT ORGAN RESECTION.—In the assessment of gastric cancer, adjacent organ invasion is clearly a poor prognostic indicator. Surgery to attain clear margins is technically difficult and potentially morbid even if indicated, yet long-term survivors are reported. A report from our institution of 72 patients with en bloc multiple organ resection for carcinoma of the stomach found a 31% five-year survival in those patients with T_4 N_{0-1} lesions, not statistically different from a concurrent population of patients without organ invasion (T_{1-3} N_{0-1}), with an operative mortality of 25% vs. 17% for those lesions showing no local organ invasion. The patients with advanced stage disease did poorly, with a high operative mortality of 40% and no long-term survivors. The number and type of organ resections did not seem to affect the outcome in this series. For early-stage disease, adjacent organ resection should be performed when necessary to achieve adequate margins.[98]

MARGINS AND RECURRENCE.—Defining an adequate margin of normal tissue in gastric resection to decrease in the incidence of local recurrence and increase survival is difficult. Bizer[99] found that 14 of 15 patients with positive margins with stage I, II, and III disease died with early recurrence, with a mean survival of only nine months. Bozzetti et al.[100] looked at both proximal and distal margins; proximally, with gross margins of greater than or equal to 6 cm, no histologically positive margins were found. Distally, there were occasional positive histologic margins despite gross margins of 6–7 cm. Microscopically positive margins distant from gross margins correlated with the presence of serosal infiltration, prompting the suggestion that for early gastric cancer; i.e., without serosal invasion, a gross margin of 3 cm was adequate, while for advanced gastric cancer penetrating the serosa, 6-cm margins should be sought. Of note, however, Bozzetti et al. found the five-year survival of patients with histologically positive proximal margins to be 28% with a median of 12 months. Only 23% of his patients with positive margins subsequently died from local recurrence alone. Fortner and Papachristou[101, 102] have reported evidence to suggest that a macroscopic proximal margin of greater than 6 cm will reduce the incidence of subsequent esophageal anastomotic recurrence (Table 16–13). In this study of 351 patients, there was an overall operative mortality of 21%. However, it should be noted that histologically positive margins, again, were associated with only one third of all anastomotic recurrences. Clearly, there are other factors which influence the probability of local recurrence. The implications of these last two studies should be evident: escalating the magnitude of operative morbidity in an attempt to secure wide, histologically negative margins should be tempered by assessment of other possibly predominating prognostic variables such as serosal invasion, nodal metastases, and the overall general condition of the patient.

TABLE 16–13.—ANASTOMOTIC RECURRENCE OF GASTRIC CANCER*

SURGICAL MARGIN cm	ESOPHAGEAL RECURRENCE No.	(%)
All patients	35/278†	(13)
0	2/16	(12)
<2	10/61	(16)
2–4	18/134	(13)
4–6	5/50	(10)
≥6	0/17	(0)
Microscopic margin +	12/53	(23)
Microscopic margin −	23/225	(10)

*Adapted from Papachristou D., Agnanti N., D'Agostino H., et al.: Histologically positive esophageal margin in the surgical treatment of gastric cancer. *Am. J. Surg.* 139:711–713, 1980.[102]
†73 operative deaths not included.

PALLIATIVE RESECTION.—While the trend toward operability has been increasing in gastric cancer, the proportion of patients resected for cure remains in the 25%–50% range in most Western series, limited again by the predominance of advanced lesions. This leaves a large number of patients for whom less extensive procedures must be considered with the objective of patient comfort, optimal survival, minimal operative mortality and morbidity.

Results of bypassing distally obstructing lesions with gastrojejunostomy have been generally disappointing, with fair to good palliation of symptoms in approximately one third of patients; results in the remainder are limited by short mean survivals of two to six months.[86, 103] Prophylactic gastrojejunostomy seems to have no role, since no improvement in survival in 93 patients undergoing this procedure over a comparable group of patients without gastroenterostomy has been described.[104]

No prospective data prove that palliative resection improves survival. There is suggestive information based on retrospective reviews that, stage for stage, survival is improved with little or no increase in operative mortality when resection is compared to bypass of lesions that are technically removable. Lawrence and McNeer[105] found good symptomatic relief in over half of 57 patients undergoing palliative subtotal resection with a mean survival of 9.5 months vs. 4.5 months for those patients undergoing laparotomy alone. Stern et al.[106] found a significant increase in survival in stage III and stage IV patients resected vs. those who underwent laparotomy alone, and a marked improvement in survival following resection of patients with linitis plastica, although the number of such patients was not specified.

In patients undergoing gastric resection in the face of documented hepatic metastases, dividing patients into H_1 (single lobe metastasis), H_2 (bilobar metastases), H_3 (diffuse bilateral hepatic metastases) groups, Koga et al.[107] found a significant improvement in survival in H_1 and H_2 patients undergoing resection vs. laparotomy alone. No patient with peritoneal metastases of adjacent organ invasion survived more than one year. Unlike Kobayashi et al.,[108] Koga and associates were unable to demonstrate a survival advantage in resected patients with H_3 disease.

While the results of subtotal gastrectomy for palliation are encouraging in terms of possibly prolonging survival, there is considerably less enthusiasm for total gastrectomy or esophagogastrectomy. In most series, the operative mortality is sufficiently high (18%–20%), and the anticipated survival sufficiently short to contraindicate the procedure.[104, 109] Two recent series are more optimistic. Ellis et al.[110] has reported a personal series of 167 esophagogastrectomies performed between 1970 and 1983 for carcinoma of the gastric cardia and esophagus. They report a 1.3% operative mortality and 83% relief of dysphagia. Seventeen percent of the procedures were palliative, and half of the patients had lesions of the gastroesophageal junction, although morbidity figures are not broken down specifically to address these patients. At our institution, in a series of 147 patients undergoing esophagogastrectomy performed using the EEA stapler, there was only a 4% leak rate, with no deaths attributable to leak alone (M. Bains, personal communication, 1984). In carefully selected symptomatic patients with obstruction or bleeding, it may be that total gastrectomy and esophagogastrectomy have a place in safe palliation. In the absence of these firm indications, however, these procedures are to be avoided, as no improvement in survival has been demonstrated.

In poor-risk patients with obstructing lesions of the GE junction, good palliation with acceptable morbidity has been reported with silastic stents, placed either operatively or endoscopically. The Atkinson tube, placed endoscopically, with a distal "shoulder" to prevent its being dislodged, would seem to be the prosthesis of choice where clinically indicated and technically feasible.[111]

In general, unless outpatient nutritional support is required as part of a planned nonoperative approach that includes active treatment with chemotherapy or radiotherapy, feeding tube procedures such as gastrostomy or jejunostomy should be avoided.

In the preoperative setting of clinically widespread disease, as defined by palpable pelvic or rectal shelf disease, palpable hepatomegaly, supraclavicular or inguinal adenopathy, malignant ascites or bone metastases, Choi et al.[109] reported an operative mortality of 19% and a resectability of 26%, with median survival of 11 weeks following palliative resection. The survival was equal to that of patients unresected. Elective surgical intervention in this group of patients is inappropriate.

Summary

The surgical approach to the patient with gastric cancer should be a product of a thorough understanding of patterns of spread and potential for cure of the disease at various stages. While it seems clear that extensive radical lymphadenectomy is not necessary in early gastric cancer, and probably superfluous in far advanced disease, it may have a role in the intermediate stages. The advantages of including microscopic lymphatic disease with routine splenectomy may be counterbalanced by the immunologic deficit of routine prophylactic splenectomy. En bloc resection of adjacent organ invasion does have a place in otherwise localized disease. The issue of adequate surgical margins must be viewed in the context of the overall disease, as histologically positive margins are no guarantee of either local recurrence or death from local recurrence. Finally, the goals of palliative surgery must be well-defined preoperatively; while most would agree that subtotal gastric resection for distal lesions is indicated if technically feasible, total or proximal esophagogastrectomy should be reserved for those patients with specific complaints and performed with the minimal morbidity and mortality. Until significant numbers of patients are seen with earlier disease, however, surgery will only be part of the answer in the management of gastric cancer; effective adjuvant programs of chemotherapy and/or radiotherapy need to be developed to improve our results in advanced disease.

Patterns of Recurrence

Recurrent disease in gastric cancer following curative surgery is a major problem, the incidence of which varies inversely with the success of the original intervention. Thus, Iwanaga et al.[112] reported 230 of 924 patients, 25%, had recurring cancer after curative surgery following a minimum of five years. More pessimistic figures approaching 80% of patients autopsied following surgery for gastric cancer in the McNeer series,[113] and 60%–80% of patients subjected to second-look operations as reported by Gunderson and Sosin,[114] reflect, in part, the more advanced spectrum of disease seen in the Western world.

Eighty to ninety percent of recurrences occur within the first five years following surgery, and their distribution is somewhat different from those occurring after five years. Gunderson and Sosin[114] analyzed a series of 105 patients subjected to second-look operations and found a preponderance of local and regional as opposed to distant metastases, with an overall 80% (86/105) failure rate after curative operation. Local recurrence and regional lymph node metastases occurred as the only site of failure in 53.7% of the group. Kano et al.[115] also noted a preponderance of local and regional failure in the early recurrent group. Papachristou and Fortner[116] found 25% of patients from our institution with recurrence had a component of local disease.

Later recurrences, defined as those occurring five or more years following resection, were found by Koga et al.[117] to occur more often after resection of well-differentiated Borrmann type I and II lesions, not invading the serosa with a relative predominance of hematogenous or gastric stump recurrences. Iwanaga et al.[112] confirmed the emergence of stump recurrences over peritoneal metastases in patients with disease reappearing more than five years following original surgery. Kano et al.[115] found late recurrences to occur more often after stage I and II lesions, and more often to be resectable.

The incidence and pattern of recurrence is related to the stage of the original lesion. Matsusaka et al.[71] found recurrent cancer as a cause of death in only seven of 220 cases of early gastric cancer, occurring as hepatic or gastric remnant tumors in six of the seven cases. Gunderson and Sosin[114] found that ten of 12 patients whose lymph nodes were negative at the original surgery had no evidence of disease on reexploration, while 72 of 89 patients with lymph nodes involved at the original surgery had evidence of recurrent disease. There was a trend in his series for a lesion that extended through the wall to recur more frequently.

The histologic characteristics of the tumor are thought to influence the subsequent pattern of recurrence with poorly differentiated, infiltrated lesions recurring early and locally while well-differentiated and localized lesions tended to recur later, either as stump recurrences or liver metastases.[115, 117]

Management of local recurrence is discouraging, with only 18%–22% of local recurrences found to be resectable, usually those occurring within the gastric remnant, often after initial stage I and stage II well-diffentiated lesions. Following resection, Papachristou and Fortner[116] found a 62% long-term survival with a median survival of 18 months vs. less than two months for those patients whose lesions were unresectable. Kano et al.[115] confirmed this with a median survival of 21 months following resection. However, this represents a very small fraction of patients with recurrence; the remainder of the prognosis is poor.

Adjuvant Studies of Chemotherapy for Gastric Cancer

A number of prospective, randomized studies using chemotherapy as an adjuvant to resection for gastric cancer have been completed. Nonsignificant studies have examined the benefit of thiotepa, floxuridine (FUDR), mitomycin C, with a study approaching significance using fluorouracil (5-FU) and lomustine (methyl-CCNU) (Table 16–14). This latter study, involving several organizations, was well-controlled and was stratified for resection site, proximal or total versus distal, cardia versus all others, the extent of the neoplasm, confined to the gastric wall versus adjacent invasion, the presence or absence of positive lymph nodes, histopathology, and linitus plastica versus other. Recurrence rates favored the treatment group at the $P < 0.07$ level. Median survival in the treatment group was 48-plus months when compared to 33 months in the control group using all 71 patients in each arm. This is significant at the $P \leq 0.03$ level (Table 16–15). There was no survival difference in the first year, but there was a 20% improvement at four years. The operative mortality was significantly higher when total and proximal subtotal were compared to the distal subtotal procedure. In patients with positive lymph nodes, the operative mortality was greater ($P < 0.07$) than in those patients with negative lymph nodes.

These encouraging results are somewhat surprising since, in advanced disease, methyl-CCNU and 5-FU have activity in the 25% range. In a study using the identical chemotherapy, the Eastern Cancer Oncology Group (ECOG) has now reported, in abstract form, no impact on disease-free or total survival. Thus, there is no clear evidence that this type of therapy is of benefit.

In addition to the studies using methyl-CCNU and 5-FU, several adjuvant trials using the apparently more active 5-FV,

TABLE 16–15.—CONTROLLED TRIAL OF ADJUVANT CHEMOTHERAPY FOLLOWING CURATIVE RESECTION FOR GASTRIC CANCER*

RECURRENCE RATE		CONTROL	TREATMENT
Resection			
Distal—subtotal		18/47	14/41
Total—proximal subtotal		20/24	14/30
Lymph nodes			
Negative		6/27	5/27
Positive		32/44	23/44
Depth of invasion			
Submucosa, muscularis, serosa		24/52	18/51
Adjacent tissue		14/19	10/20
Sex			
Male		26/50	22/50
Female		12/21	6/21
Overall recurrence rate	$P = 0.07$		
Overall recurrence adjusted	$P = 0.01$		

*GITS = 1982.[121]

Adriamycin, cisplatinum (FAM) regimen are also under way. Only one of these has been reported, in abstract. The Southwestern Oncology Group (SWOG) notes no improvement in the treated arm, which received 12 months of FAM therapy, when compared to the control group.

Chemotherapy for Advanced Gastric Cancer

Several recent studies have been reported. In a series of 25 patients treated with FAM regimen, two patients had partial remission, and three minor remissions were seen. Median survival in the nonresponders was 2.5 months compared to 13 months in the responders.[122]

A randomized comparison of 5-FU vs. 5-FU plus doxorubicin (Adriamycin) vs. 5-FU plus Adriamycin and mitomycin C showed FAM to be the least favorable regimen with survival curves of all three treatment arms being identical.[123] Median survival was seven months in all groups.

Trials adding cisplatinum (DDP) to 5-FU and Adriamycin have been performed.[124] In 17 patients with gastric carcinoma, nine objective responses were seen, with three complete responses and a median survival for all treated patients of ten months. The addition of the newer agent, triazinate (TZT) has been examined by the GITS, where, in studies of advanced gastric cancer, a comparison of 5-FU, Adriamycin and TZT (FAT) to 5-FU, Adriamycin and DDP (FAD) was performed.[124] Ten patients were treated in either group with

TABLE 16–14.—GASTRIC CANCER: ADJUVANT TRIALS—CONTROLLED AND RANDOMIZED*

AUTHOR	YEAR	COUNTRY	CONTROL		TREATMENT		DRUG
			n	5-yr Surv	n	5-yr Surv	
Hattori et al.[118]	1976	Japan	278	50%	343	37%	Mitomycin C
Serlin et al.[119]	1977	U.S.	146	20%	130	22%	FUDR
Huguier et al.[120]	1980	France	26	15%	27	18%	5-FU
GITS[121]	1982	U.S.	71	MST = 33 mo	71	MST = 48 mo	5-FU + MeCCNU
VASOG	1971	U.S.	97	34%	97	26%	Thiotepa
VASOG	1969	U.S.	138	21%	138	24%	FUDR

*MST = Mean survival time; VASOG = Veterans Administration Surgical Oncology Group; GITSG = Gastrointestinal Tumor Study Group.

median survival of 15 months for the FAT regimen and 11 months for the FAD regimen. This was compared to a six-month median survival in previous GITSG studies with FAM.[125] A 22% response rate for a FAT regimen has been reported with the conclusion that the addition of the triazinate has not significantly increased the response rate from that previously reported for the FAM regimen.[127]

Radiation Therapy in the Treatment of Gastric Cancer

Technical advances in radiation therapy have led to an expansion of applications. Intraoperative radiation by external beam or interstitial temporary or permanent implants are being investigated. Carcinoma of the stomach provides some unique features that make radiation therapy difficult and less applicable than some other fixed solid tumors.

Historically, gastric adenocarcinoma is thought to be radioresistant. For the application of radiation therapy in unresectable gastric carcinoma, a single report has suggested that 7% of patients with gastric carcinoma who receive radiation to doses of 6,000 rad will survive for more than five years.[126]

Combination of radiation therapy and fluorouracil has been reported effective in many clinical trials. Two-year survival rates of 25% have been reported in a series of 32 cases treated with radiation therapy alone or the combination of radiation therapy and fluorouracil.[126] In a group of 23 patients with locally advanced unresectable carcinoma, doses of 3,500–4,000 rad over four weeks was compared to a historical control group of 43 patients to whom no treatment was given; no benefit from the radiation therapy could be shown.[128] In another study, a statistically significant survival advantage was seen for patients in the combination radiation and chemotherapy arm.[129]

A more recent study by the GITS group examined patients with unresectable and locally advanced gastric cancer who were randomized to receive fluorouracil and semustine or radiation therapy and fluorouracil followed by fluorouracil and semustine.[130] An initial therapeutic advantage for the chemotherapy alone was observed; but with longer-term follow-up, there was a statistically significant increase in survival in the patients receiving both chemotherapy and radiation therapy, with eight of 45 patients disease-free at two years. It would appear that lesser doses of radiation are ineffective, as 2,000 rad delivered over ten days was no different from a no-treatment arm in the treatment of both operable and inoperable gastric cancer.[131]

INTRAOPERATIVE RADIATION THERAPY.—Intraoperative radiation has received great emphasis. Theoretical advantages of delivering defined high-dose radiation to a particular area has been repetitively emphasized. There is little constructive critical information that would address its value in carcinoma in the stomach. The widest application of the technique has been in Japan, with more than 700 patients being treated with a variety of diseases.[132] Unfortunately, no comparative data exist from those studies to allow meaningful evaluation. An attempt by this group to examine the value of intraoperative radiation for carcinoma of the stomach treated by resection vs. intraoperative radiation therapy alone has demonstrated an increase in survival when compared with a historical group treated by operation alone. In the United States, several authors have examined the technique.[133] There are controlled prospective randomized studies currently ongoing, but it is too early to determine their value. In many institutions, there are great technical difficulties. The radiation therapy suite is remote from the operating room suite. The positioning of the patient, incision, and the presence of the rib cage all make accurate application of intraoperative radiation therapy limited. The majority of studies employed 1,000–3,000 rad in a single fraction with 2,000 rad being the most commonly employed fraction, delivered at approximately 250–300 rad/minute.[133]

Animal studies on toxicity have been performed in dogs.[134] These studies suggest that vascular structures can tolerate 5,000 rad without loss of structural integrity. The ureter develops stenosis at approximately 3,000 rad, arterial anastomosis can heal after doses of 4,500 rad, but usually are associated with fibrosis. Intestinal suture lines will still heal after doses of 4,500 rad and bile duct stenosis develops at 2,000 rad or greater. Almost all biliary enteric anastomoses fail to heal at any dose of radiation therapy.

For the meantime, intraoperative radiation therapy needs to be limited to a few select centers who are developing prospective and evaluable trials of the modality. Uniform application as either adjuvant therapy following resection or as primary treatment for unresectable carcinoma of the stomach cannot be recommended.

OTHER GASTRIC NEOPLASMS

Gastric Lymphoma

Primary gastric lymphoma composes 1%–5% of all gastric neoplasms. The stomach is the most common site of extranodal lymphoma, accounting for over one half of all primary GI lymphomas. Extremely rare in childhood, this is a disease primarily of the sixth and seventh decades, with a slight male preponderance in most series. The clinical presentation is virtually indistinguishable from gastric adenocarcinoma with symptoms of weight loss, early satiety, dyspepsia, and epigastric pain predominating. Approximately two thirds of the patients present with anemia. Upper GI series has been found to be sensitive but not specific in diagnosis. Endoscopic biopsy has led to preoperative diagnosis in 33%–80% of cases.

Treatment

Though prospective data are lacking, a multimodality treatment philosophy has evolved in the management of this unusual disease, with conservative resection of gross local disease followed by local radiotherapy for regional control with ultimately improved survival rates. The role of primary chemotherapy as the primary approach has been tempered by concern about complications of uncontrolled GI bleeding or perforation of transmural disease at a time of nadir counts in patients experiencing good response. Fleming et al.[135] found four or five patients treated with cytoxin, Adriamycin, Oncovin, and Prednisone (CAOP) requiring emergency surgery for massive GI hemorrhage, but no perforation in 11 of 15 patients treated with chemotherapy for nonresected tumors. Similarly, Mittal et al.[136] found the rate of gastric perforation to be 4% in a collected series of 700 gastric lymphoma patients, occurring with equal frequency before any treatment or after radiotherapy as a planned multimodality approach. With the demonstration by Shimm et al.[137] that involvement of surgical margins did not affect prognosis in those patients receiving postoperative radiotherapy, there would seem to be little rationale for extended radical resections with their attendant higher morbidity and mortality.

Following surgical resection, most authors have found in retrospective analyses significant improvement in local and regional control and in five-year survival with postoperative radiotherapy (Table 16–16). Shiu et al.[141] advocates a minimum of 2,000 rad over two and one half to three weeks to the gastric bed with periportal, splenic, and celiac extensions to achieve an 85% local control rate. Shimm et al.[137] found local failures only in patients receiving less than or equal to 4,000 rad following resection, though the benefits accrued by this increase in radiation dosage need to be balanced against the potential additive GI complications in the postgastrectomized patient.

The role of adjuvant radiotherapy in favorable lesions, less than 7 cm in greatest dimension with only serosal involvement and negative nodes, is unclear; in the Shimm series,[137] there were six patients with negative margins, negative nodes, and serosal disease only. All patients were disease-free at five years, three following adjuvant radiotherapy and three without adjuvant radiotherapy.

The role of adjuvant chemotherapy in unfavorable lesions—i.e., node-positive, transserosal, or greater than 7 cm in diameter—is unclear, though it would appear to be more rational. The predominance of distant failure, approaching 30% in some series, following adequate local surgery and radiotherapy and the attendant 60% mortality in stage II disease would both argue for aggressive adjuvant systemic therapy in advanced lesions.

Prognosis

The prognosis of gastric lymphoma is significantly better than that of adenocarcinoma, with overall five-year survival in excess of 50%. The primary prognostic variable is the stage of disease at presentation, with many series reporting in excess of 80% five-year survival for stage I disease and approximately half that for stage II disease. Nodal involvement, increasing depth of penetration, size of primary, and adjacent organ invasion all carry poorer prognoses. There is a trend toward poorer prognosis with diffuse vs. nodular histology. Although the consensus is not uniform, most series have found that patients with histiocytic lymphoma fare worse than those with lymphocytic lymphoma.[142, 143]

Summary

Gastric lymphoma is an unusual, though not rare, condition that lends itself ideally to a planned multimodality approach. This should include conservative surgical resection, with its limited morbidity and mortality, more important than the need for negative surgical margins. Retrospective data would suggest that planned postoperative radiotherapy improves local control and ultimate survival, though its role in the early favorable lesions is as yet unclear. In more advanced disease, the rationale exists for planned adjuvant systemic chemotherapy.

Gastric Pseudolymphoma

Gastric pseudolymphoma is thought to be a benign proliferation of lymphoid tissue that occurs in the stomach and resembles malignant lymphoma in both presentation and histopathology. The condition is uncommon and its natural history is largely unknown. The evidence for the lesion's being premalignant is questionable, although one of 11 patients in a recent report developed Hodgkin's disease 35 months after a subtotal gastrectomy for pseudolymphoma; another one of 11 developed recurrence in the proximal gastric stump.[144] Unfortunately, a diagnostic biopsy at the time of endoscopy is rarely obtained, as the gastroscopic appearance can range from superficial ulceration to large rugae or mass lesions thought to be ulcerated carcinomas. Because of the difficult histopathologic diagnosis, long-term follow-up is required to rule out conventional lymphoma. Surgical treatment is controversial. Usually the diagnosis is not made preoperatively, and the surgeon appears to be dealing with either benign gastric ulcer or a malignant lesion. Frozen-section diagnosis is difficult and is usually unrewarding. Gastric pseudolymphoma usually presents in the antrum and a distal subtotal gastrectomy usually suffices.[145, 146]

Gastric Sarcoma

Excluding lymphoma, sarcomas comprise 1%–3% of all gastric malignancies, of which the vast majority are leiomyosarcomas. Other types of gastric sarcomas include angiosarcoma, fibrosarcoma, and liposarcoma, of which only case reports can be found.

The relatively more frequent leiomyosarcomas usually present in the sixth or seventh decades of life, with equal-sex incidence. Their clinical presentation is nonspecific, with weight loss, epigastric fullness, and upper GI bleeding predominating; symptoms tend to be late in onset and correlate with the relative exogastric or endogastric component of the tumor. Specific diagnosis is rarely made preoperatively.[147]

Pathology

Grossly, these tumors are firm, smooth, yellow-white masses presenting intraluminally as ulcerated lesions or extraluminally as invasive or displacing tumors. They can be separated into a spectrum of low- to high-grade lesions, based on a number of histologic criteria.[148] Of these, mitotic rate is

TABLE 16–16.—GASTRIC LYMPHOMA FIVE-YEAR DISEASE-FREE SURVIVAL

AUTHOR	YEAR	SURGERY ALONE No.	(%)	SURGERY & RADIATION THERAPY No.	(%)
Burnett and Herbert[138]	1956	7	(43)	9	(62)
Connors and Wise[139]	1974	27	(37)	11	(45)
Hermann et al.[140]	1980	10	(50)	10	(90)
Shiu et al.[141]	1982	15	(33)	21	(67)
Shimm et al.[137]	1983	8	(25)	20	(60)
Mittal et al.[136]	1983	11	(45)	12	(75)
Mean			38		66

the most widely accepted and reproducible index, with tumors containing more than 5–10 mitoses/10 high-powered fields behaving in an aggressive fashion. Heterogeneity within a tumor must be compensated for by examination of multiple fields. Leiomyoblastoma is a morphological variant of leiomyosarcoma, which is thought by some to behave more aggressively, though this is not unanimous.

Progression of disease in patients with leiomyosarcoma is almost always intra-abdominal, with local recurrences and peritoneal sarcomatosis more frequent than hematogenous spread to the liver. Lung and distant metastases are uncommon. Lymphatic metastases are distinctly unusual, occurring in less than 10% of patients, either at presentation or late in the course of advanced disease.[149, 150]

Surgery

At presentation, approximately two thirds of leiomyosarcomas are resectable for cure, the remainder being limited by encasement of vital vascular structures, or peritoneal/systemic metastases. Surgical procedures advised range from simple wedge excisions of smaller lesions to wide en bloc resection of stomach with adjacent invaded organs for the more advanced lesions; the object remains to obtain histologically free margins. Lymph node dissection is not felt necessary, but omentectomy is advised, as several authors have documented omental metastases; the influence of omentectomy on survival is not clear.[147, 151]

Prognosis

Prognostic factors in gastric leiomyosarcoma include histologic grade, size of primary, and the depth of primary.[148, 152] Shiu et al. found an 81% five-year survival for low-grade lesions but only 32% five-year survival for high-grade tumors. Lindsay et al.[152] confirmed this with no difference among epithelioid, pleomorphic, or spindle cell-type tumors. Shiu et al.[148] found a 100% five-year survival with lesions less than or equal to 5 cm in diameter regardless of histologic grade, and a 57% five-year survival in patients with tumors over 5 cm in diameter. In the Lindsay series, transmural involvement was a poor prognostic indicator, with a median survival of 14 months, as opposed to 84 months when the tumor was confined to the stomach alone. Shiu et al. had no five-year survivors of six patients undergoing extensive en bloc resection for adjacent organ invasion.

Overall survival following resection should approach 50%, substantially better than that for gastric carcinoma. With none of the unfavorable prognostic indicators of high-grade, large tumor, or extragastric extension, Shiu et al.[148] found a five-year survival of 100%. With one factor present, this fell to 77%; with two factors present, only 19% of patients survived five years. Adjuvant radiotherapy or chemotherapy has not been shown to improve these figures.

Of uncertain biologic significance, there appears to be an unduly high incidence of associated neoplasms; as many as 27% of patients reported by Shiu et al.[148] were found to have second or even third synchronous or metachronous malignancies. As a further biologic curiosity, Carney[153] described a series of 24 patients, primarily young women, in whom multiple gastric epithelioid leiomyosarcomas occur as the most frequent manifestation of a triad that includes pulmonary chondromas and functioning extra-adrenal paraganglionomas. Genetic and immunologic studies of this syndrome have been inconclusive.

Squamous Carcinoma of the Stomach

Adenosquamous and squamous cell carcinoma of the stomach are both exceedingly rare. There are fewer than 100 cases reported in the English literature at present. It is difficult to evaluate the multiple case reports, but it would appear that the lesion most often develops as a polypoid lesion, localized, without metastases until late in the course. Theories as to the cell of origin are variable, most authors favoring the squamous metaplasia rather than the presence of congenital ectopic squamous cell rests. Meaningful survival data following surgical resection are not available.[154]

Gastric Carcinoids

Gastric carcinoids are uncommon, occurring in two of our recent 129 GI carcinoids seen over a ten-year period. This compares with ten of 155 seen in a previous report from this institution.[155] In a collective series, they make up 61 of 2,439[156] and 94 of 3,684[157] cases of GI carcinoid. This extraordinarily rare occurrence of gastric carcinoids makes any attempts at preoperative diagnosis difficult unless open endoscopic biopsy is confirmatory. The prognosis is associated with depth of penetration of the primary lesion and the presence of nodal and disseminated disease, as with other GI carcinoids.

Surgery remains the treatment of choice with radical removal of the primary lesion curative in those that have not extended outside the stomach wall. Because of the possibility of prolonged survival, aggressive surgery is indicated and should be considered in all cases.

CONCLUSIONS AND FUTURE CONSIDERATIONS

Only minimal progress has been made in the understanding and the treatment of gastric cancer in the past 25 years. We are still at a loss to be certain if, indeed, the true incidence is falling, or if we are seeing a redistribution in stage, presentation, and site of the lesions. No significant screening program has been implemented in the United States, and it seems unlikely in the near future, given the calculated cost and anticipated yield. Many of the suggested premalignant lesions, when examined critically, are found to have only minimal influence in the development of gastric cancer. The apparent major advances identified by the Japanese are difficult to interpret and hard to translate into the North American experience. The disparity between their results and ours seems to be based mainly on the fact that the Japanese authors report the number of resections rather than the number of presentations; the prevalence in their series of intestinal types, the greater preponderance of early gastric cancer, and, perhaps, the greater nodal dissection are all factors which, if translated to the North American experience, might result in similar end results.

Prospective studies are needed to identify a real benefit of more extensive surgical resection and should be vigorously encouraged. In the absence of more effective agents for the treatment of advanced disease, it is difficult to propose meaningful prospective adjuvant trials of modalities other than surgery. Every effort should be emphasized to embark on prospective, documented studies of the appropriateness, effectiveness, morbidity, and mortality of various surgical procedures. The development of such a data base would allow for meaningful examination of adjuvant therapies as more effective therapies are identified for advanced disease.

REFERENCES

1. Nobregra F.T., Sedlack J.O., Sedlack R.E., et al.: A decline in carcinoma of the stomach: A diagnostic artifact. *Mayo Clin. Proc.* 58:255–260, 1983.
2. Antonioli D.A., Goldman H.: Changes in the location and type of gastric adenocarcinoma. *Cancer* 50:775–781, 1982.
3. Cady B., Ramsden D.A., Stein D.O., et al.: Gastric cancer: Contemporary aspects. *Am. J. Surg.* 133:423–429, 1977.
4. Borrmann R.: In Handbuch der Speziellen Pathologischen. *Anat. Histol.* 4 (pt. 1):812, 1926.
5. McNeer G., Pack G.: *Neoplasms of the Stomach.* Philadelphia, J.B. Lippincott, 1967.
6. Hoerr S.: A surgeon's classification of carcinoma of the stomach. *Surg. Gynecol. Obstet.* 99:281, 1954.
7. Kennedy B.: TNM classification for stomach cancer. *Cancer* 26:971–983, 1970.
8. Broders A.C.: The microscopic grading of cancer. *Surg. Clin. North Am.* 21:947–983, 1941.
9. Lauren P.: The two histological main types of gastric carcinoma: Diffuse and so called intestinal type carcinoma. *Acta Pathol. Microbiol. Scand.* 64:31–49, 1965.
10. Stemmerman G., Brown C.: A survival study of intestinal and diffuse types of gastric carcinoma. *Cancer* 33:1190–1195, 1974.
11. Munoz N., Correa P., Cuello C., et al.: Histologic types of gastric carcinoma in high and low risk areas. *Int. J. Cancer* 3:809–818, 1968.
12. Ming S.: Gastric carcinoma—A pathobiological classification. *Cancer* 39:2475–2485, 1972.
13. Correa P.: Precursors of esophageal and gastric carcinoma. *Cancer* 50(suppl.):2560–2565, 1982.
14. Sipponen P., Kekki M., Sivrala M.: Atrophic chronic gastritis and intestinal metaplasia in gastric carcinoma. *Cancer* 52:1062–1068, 1983.
15. Iida F., Kusama J.: Gastric carcinoma and intestinal metaplasia. *Cancer* 50:2854–2858, 1982.
16. Correa P.: The gastric precancerous process. *Cancer Surveys.* 2(3):437–450, 1983.
17. Tomasulo J.: Gastric polyps; histologic types and their relationship to gastric carcinoma. *Cancer* 27:1346–1355, 1971.
18. Ming S.C., Goldman H.: Gastric polyps: A histogenetic classification and its relation to carcinoma. *Cancer* 18:721–726, 1965.
19. Remine S., Hughes R., Weiland L.: Endoscopic gastric polypectomies. *Mayo Clin. Proc.* 56:371–375, 1981.
20. Laxen F., Sipponen P., Ikamaki T., et al.: Gastric polyps; their morphologic and endoscopic characteristics and relation to gastric carcinoma. *Acta Pathol. Microbiol. Immunol. Scand.* 90(sect. A):221–228, 1982.
21. Hay L.J.: Surgical management of gastric polyps and adenomas. *Surgery* 39:114–119, 1956.
22. Eklof O.: Benign tumors of stomach and duodenum. *Acta Chir. Scand. Suppl.* 100:561, 1962.
23. Yamagata S., Hisamichi S.: Precancerous lesions of the stomach. *World J. Surg.* 3:671–673, 1979.
24. Kamiya T., Morishita T., Asakura H., et al.: Long term follow-up study on gastric adenoma and its relationship to gastric protruded carcinoma. *Cancer* 50:2496–2503, 1982.
25. Balfour D.C.: Factors influencing the life expectancy of patients operated on for gastric ulcer. *Ann. Surg.* 76:405–408, 1922.
26. Helsingen N., Hillenstrad L.: Cancer development in the gastric stump after gastrectomy for ulcer. *Ann. Surg.* 143:173–179, 1956.
27. Krause U.: Late prognosis after partial gastrectomy for ulcer. *Acta Chir. Scand.* 114:341–354, 1957.
28. Saegesser F., James D.: Cancer of the gastric stump after partial gastrectomy (Billroth II principle) for ulcer. *Cancer* 29:1150–1159, 1972.
29. Domellof L., Janunger K.: The risk for gastric carcinoma after partial gastrectomy. *Am. J. Surg.* 134:581–584, 1977.
30. Peitsch W., Becker M.D.: Frequency and prognosis of gastric stump cancer. *Front. Gastrointest. Res.* 5:170–177, 1979.
31. Nichols J.: Stump cancer following gastric surgery. *World J. Surg.* 3:731–736, 1979.
32. Karfeld J., Resnick G.: Gastric remnant carcinoma. *Cancer* 44:1129–1133, 1979.
33. Papachristou D., Agnati N., Fortner J.: Gastric carcinoma after treatment of ulcer. *Am. J. Surg.* 139:193–196, 1980.
34. Lygidakis N.: Gastric stump carcinoma after surgery for gastroduodenal ulcer. *Ann. R. Coll. Surg. Gynecol.* 63:203, 1981.
35. Orlando R., Welch J.: Carcinoma of the stomach after gastric operation. *Am. J. Surg.* 141:487–490, 1981.
36. Perez D., Narayasar C., Russell J., et al.: Gastric carcinoma after peptic ulcer surgery. *Curr. Surg.* 40:117–119, 1983.
37. Dougherty S., Foster C., Eisenberg M.: Stomach cancer following gastric surgery for benign disease. *Arch. Surg.* 117:294–297, 1982.
38. Totten J., Burns H., Kay A.: Time of onset of carcinoma of the stomach following surgical treatment of duodenal ulcer. *Surg. Gynecol. Obstet.* 157:431–433, 1983.
39. Welvart K., Warnsinck H.: The incidence of carcinoma of the gastric remnant. *J. Surg. Oncol.* 21(2):104–106, 1982.
40. Fisher A.S., Graham N., Jensen O.N.: Risk of gastric cancer after Billroth II resection for duodenal ulcer. *Br. J. Surg.* 70(9):552–554, 1983.
41. Schafer L., Larsen D., Melton J., et al.: The risk of gastric carcinoma after surgical treatment of benign ulcer disease. *N. Engl. J. Med.* 309:1210–1213, 1983.
42. Gregor O.: Gastric cancer detection among risk groups and their longitudinal follow-up (Abstract). *X Int. Cong. Gastroenterol. in Budapest.* 10:349, 1976.
43. Eriksson S., Clase L., Moquist-Olsson I.: Pernicious anemia as a risk factor in gastric cancer. *Acta Med. Scand.* 210:481–484, 1981.
44. Haukland H., Johnson J., Eide J.: Carcinoma diagnosed in excised gastric ulcers. *Acta Chir. Scand.* 147:439–443, 1981.
45. Morson B.C., Sobin L.M., Grundman E., et al.: Precancerous conditions and epithelial dysplasia in the stomach. *J. Clin. Pathol.* 33:711–721, 1980.
46. Sekons D., McSherry C., Calhoun W., et al.: Contribution of endoscopy to diagnosis and treatment of gastric cancer. *Am. J. Surg.* 147:662–665, 1984.
47. Keto P., Suoranta H., Ikamaki T., et al.: Double contrast examination of the stomach compared with endoscopy. *Acta Radiol. Diagn.* 20:762–768, 1979.
48. Laufer I., Mullens J., Hamilton J.: The diagnostic accuracy of barium studies of the stomach and duodenum—correlation with endoscopy. *Radiology* 115:569–573, 1975.
49. Graham D., Schwartz J., Cain G., et al.: Prospective evaluation of biopsy number in the diagnosis of esophageal and gastric carcinoma. *Gastroenterology* 82:228–231, 1982.
50. Winawer S., Posner G., Lightdale C., et al.: Endoscopic diagnosis of advanced gastric cancer: Factors influencing yield. *Gastroenterology* 69:1183–1187, 1975.
51. Moshakis V., Hooper A.: The accuracy of endoscopic diagnosis of gastric carcinoma and the conventional barium meal. *Clin. Oncol.* 4:359–368, 1978.
52. Puig-Lacalle J., Lluis F., Gastell E., et al.: Surgical treatment of gastric cancer—Evaluation of 596 cases. *International Congress Series No. 542: Diagnosis and Treatment of Upper Gastrointestinal Tumors.* 196–206, 1980.
53. Shanghai Gastrointestinal Endoscopy Cooperative Group, Peoples Republic of China: Value of Biopsy and Brush Cytology in the Diagnosis of Gastric Cancer. *Gut* 23:774–776, 1982.
54. Moreno-Ortero R., Martinez-Raposo A., Cantero J., et al.: Ex-

foliative cytodiagnosis of gastric adenocarcinoma—comparison with biopsy and endoscopy. *Acta Cytol.* 27(5):485–488, 1983.

55. Gupta J., Jain A., Agrawal B., et al.: Gastroscopic cytology and biopsies in diagnosis of gastric malignancies. *J. Surg. Oncol.* 22:62–64, 1983.

56. Gupta J., Rogers K.: Endoscopic cytology and biopsy in the diagnosis of gastroesophageal malignancy. *Acta Cytol.* 27:17–22, 1983.

57. Ikida K., Sannohe Y., Araki S., et al.: A new trial in endoscopic diagnosis for stomach cancer—Intraarterial dye method. *Gastrointest. Endosc.* 26(1):1–4, 1980.

58. Tatsuta M., Okuda S., Tamura M., et al.: Endoscopic diagnosis of early gastric cancer by the endoscopic congo red—methylene blue test. *Cancer* 50:2956–2060, 1982.

59. Gilen S., Kadish U., Urca I.: Use of tolonium chloride in the diagnosis of malignant gastric ulcer. *Arch. Surg.* 113:136–139, 1978.

60. Piper D.W., Macoun M.L., Broderick F.L., et al.: The diagnosis of gastric carcinoma by the estimation of enzyme activity in gastric juice. *Gastroenterology* 45:614–620, 1963.

61. Mitti D., Farini R., Grassi F., et al.: CEA in gastric juice collected during endoscopy. *Cancer* 52:2334–2337, 1983.

62. Graffner H., Hultberg B.: CEA and lysosomal enzymes in gastric juice as an aid in the diagnosis of gastric cancer. *J. Surg. Oncol.* 24:233–235, 1983.

63. Kodama Y., Inokuchi K., Soejima K., et al.: Growth patterns and prognosis in early gastric carcinoma. *Cancer* 51:320–326, 1983.

64. Fujita Y., Nishicka B., Sakita M., et al.: Conservative surgery for (sic) regional lymphadenectomy in the treatment of early gastric carcinoma. *Jpn. J. Surg.* 13(3):184–190, 1983.

65. Soga J., Kobayashi K., Saito J., et al.: The role of lymphadenectomy in curative surgery for gastric cancer. *World J. Surg.* 3:701–708, 1979.

66. Gebhardt C., Husemann B., Hermanek P., et al.: Clinical aspects and therapy of early gastric cancer. *World J. Surg.* 5:721–724, 1981.

67. Miyake M.: Occurrence of lymphogenic metastasis of gastric cancer with special reference to early carcinoma of the stomach. Juntendo University Medical Bulletin 1980.

68. Bearzi I., Rinaldi R.: Early gastric cancer: A morphologic study of 41 cases. *Tumori* 68:223–233, 1982.

69. Murakami T.: Early cancer of the stomach. *World J. Surg.* 3:685–692, 1979.

70. Iwanaga T., Furukawa M., Kosaki G.: Relapse of early gastric cancer and its prevention. *J. Clin. Surg. (Rinsho Geka)* 31:29, 1979.

71. Matsusaka T., Kodama Y., Soejima K., et al.: Recurrence in early gastric cancer—a pathological evaluation. *Cancer* 46:168–172, 1980.

72. Green P., O'Toole K., Weinberg L., et al.: Early gastric cancer. *Gastroenterology* 81:247–256, 1981.

73. Sakita T., et al.: Early cancer of the stomach treated successfully with an endoscopic neodymium-yag laser. *Am. J. Gastroenterol.* 76(5):441–445, 1981.

74. Tsukuma M., Mishima T., Oshima A.: Prospective study of "early" gastric cancer. *Int. J. Cancer.* 31:471–476, 1983.

75. Douglas M.O.: Potentially curable cancer of the stomach. *Cancer* 50:2582–2589, 1982.

76. Gentsch H.H., Groitl H., Gield J.: Results of surgical treatment of early gastric cancer in 113 patients. *World J. Surg.* 5(1):103, 1981.

77. Piper D.W. (ed): *Stomach Cancer U.I.C.C.* Technical Report Series, vol. 34, report no. 6. Geneva, U.I.C.C. 1978, pp. 35–40.

78. Hirota T., Sano R.: The pathology of early gastric cancer: Development and progress of early gastric cancer. Presented at the 14th Congress of Pan American Gastroenterology, Caracas, Venezuela, November 1975.

79. Kishimoto H., Fujii T., Adachi H., et al.: Resection line and long-term results in early cancer of the stomach. *J. Clin. Surg. (Rinsho Geka)* 31:45, 1976.

80. Dupont J., Cohn I.: Gastric carcinoma. *Curr. Probl. Cancer* 4:1–46, 1980.

81. Longmire W.: Total gastrectomy for carcinoma of the stomach. *Surg. Gynecol. Obstet.* 84:21, 1947.

82. Bush B., Brown M., Ravitch M.: Total gastrectomy: An evaluation of its use in the treatment of gastric cancer. *Cancer* 13:643, 1960.

83. Gilbertsen V.: Results of treatment of stomach cancer: An appraisal of efforts for more extensive surgery and a report of 1938 cases. *Cancer* 23:1305–1308, 1969.

84. Cady B., Ramsden D., Choe D.: Treatment of gastric cancer. *Surg. Clin. North. Am.* 56(3):599–605, 1976.

85. Remine W.: Indications and contraindications for surgery in gastric carcinoma. *World J. Surg.* 3:709–714, 1979.

86. Dupont J., Lee J., Burton G., et al.: Adenocarcinoma of the stomach: Review of 1,497 cases. *Cancer* 41:941–947, 1978.

87. Papachristou D., Fortner J.: Is gastric cancer generalized at the time of surgery? *J. Surg. Oncol.* 18:27–29, 1981.

88. Papachristou D., Fortner J.: Adenocarcinoma of the gastric cardia—choice of gastrectomy. *Ann. Surg.* 192(1):58–64, 1980.

89. Papachristou D., Fortner J.: Selection of gastrectomy for adenocarcinoma arising in the gastric fundus. *J. Surg. Oncol.* 21:165–169, 1982.

90. Shiu M., Papachristou D., Kosloff C., et al.: Selection of operative procedure for adenocarcinoma of the midstomach. *Ann. Surg.* 192(6):730–737, 1980.

91. Japanese Research Society for Gastric Cancer: The general rules for gastric cancer study in surgery and pathology. *Jpn. J. Surg.* 11:127–145, 1981.

92. Mine M., Majima S., Harada M., et al.: End results of gastrectomy for gastric cancer effect of extensive lymph node dissection. *Surgery* 68(5):753–758, 1970.

93. Kodama Y., Sugimachi K., Soejima K., et al.: Evaluation of extensive lymph node dissection for carcinoma of the stomach. *World J. Surg.* 5:241–248, 1981.

94. Fujimaki M., Soga J., Wada K., et al.: Total gastrectomy for gastric cancer. 30(3):660–664, 1972.

95. Sunderland D., McNeer G., et al.: The lymphatic spread of gastric cancer. *Cancer* 6:987–996, 1953.

96. Koga S., Kaibara N., Kimura O., et al.: Prognostic significance of combined splenectomy or pancreaticosplenectomy in total and proximal gastrectomy for gastric cancer. *Am. J. Surg.* 142:546–550, 1981.

97. Sugimachi K., Kodama Y., Kuimashiro R., et al.: Critical evaluation of prophylactic splenectomy in total gastrectomy for stomach cancer. *Gann* 71:704–709, 1980.

98. Papachristou D., Shiu M.: Management by en bloc multiple organ resection of carcinoma of the stomach invading adjacent organs. *Surg. Gynecol. Obstet.* 52:483–487, 1981.

99. Bizer L.: Adenocarcinoma of the stomach: Current results and treatment. *Cancer* 51:743–745, 1983.

100. Bozzetti F., Bonfanti G., Bufalino R., et al.: Adequacy of margins of resection in gastrectomy for cancer. *Ann. Surg.* 196(6):685–690, 1982.

101. Papachristou D., Karas M., Fortner J.: Anastomotic recurrence in the oesophagus complicating gastrectomy for adenocarcinoma of the stomach. *Br. J. Surg.* 66:609–612, 1979.

102. Papachristou D., Agnanti N., D'Agostino H., et al.: Histologically positive esophageal margin in the surgical treatment of gastric cancer. *Am. J. Surg.* 139:711–713, 1980.

103. Ekbom G., Gleysteen J.: Gastric malignancy: Resection for palliation. *Surgery* 88(4):476–481, 1980.

104. Remine W.: Palliative operations for incurable gastric cancer. *World J. Surg.* 3:721–729, 1979.

105. Lawrence W., McNeer G.: The effectiveness of surgery for palliation of incurable gastric cancer. *Cancer* 11:28–32, 1958.

106. Stern J., Denman S., Elias E., et al.: Evaluation of palliative resection in advanced carcinoma of the stomach. *Surgery* 77(2):291–298, 1975.

107. Koga S., Kawaguchi H., Kishimoto H., et al.: Therapeutic significance of noncurative gastrectomy for gastric cancer with liver metastases. *Am. J. Surg.* 140:356–359, 1980.

108. Kobayashi K., Hojo K., Miwa K., et al.: Operability of gastrointestinal cancer with hepatic metastases. *Surg. Ther.* 34:352, 1976 (in Japanese).

109. Choi T., Koo J., Wong J., et al.: Survival after surgery for advanced carcinoma of the stomach other than cardia. *Am. J. Surg.* 143:748–750, 1982.

110. Ellis F., Gibb P., Watkins E.: Esophagogastrectomy, a safe, widely applicable and expeditious form of palliation for patients with carcinoma of the esophagus and cardia. *Ann. Surg.* 4:531–540, 1983.

111. Atkinson M., Ferguson R., Ogilvie A.: Management of malignant dysphagia by intubation at endoscopy. *J. R. Soc. Med.* 72:894–897, 1979.

112. Iwanaga T., Koyama H., Furukawa H., et al.: Mechanisms of late recurrence after radical surgery for gastric carcinoma. *Am. J. Surg.* 135:637–640, 1978.

113. McNeer G., Vandenberg H., Donn F., et al.: A critical evaluation of subtotal gastrectomy for the cure of cancer of the stomach. *Ann. Surg.* 134:2–7, 1951.

114. Gunderson L., Sosin H.: Adenocarcinoma of the stomach; areas of failure in a reoperation series (second or symptomatic look); Clinicopathological correlations and implications for adjuvant therapy. *Int. J. Radiat. Oncol. Biol. Phys.* 8:1–11, 1982.

115. Kano T., Kusmashiro R., Masuda M., et al.: Recurrent gastric carcinoma—Analysis of 100 inpatients. *Jpn. J. Surg.* 13:106–111, 1983.

116. Papachristou D., Fortner J.: Local recurrence of gastric adenocarcinomas after gastrectomy. *J. Surg. Oncol.* 18:47–53, 1981.

117. Koga S., Kishimoto H., Tanaka K., et al.: Clinical and pathological evaluation of patients with recurrence of gastric cancer more than five years postoperatively. *Am. J. Surg.* 136:317–321, 1978.

118. Hattori T., Mari A., Hirata K., et al.: Five year survival rate of gastric cancer patients treated by gastrectomy, large dose of mitomycin C and or/allogeneic bone marrow transplantation. *Gann* 63:517–522, 1972.

119. Serlin O., Keehn R.J., Higgins G.A., et al.: Factors related to survival following resection for gastric carcinoma. *Cancer* 40:1318, 1977.

120. Huguier M., Destroyes J.P., Baschet C., et al.: Gastric carcinoma treated by chemotherapy after resection. A controlled study. *Am. J. Surg.* 139:197–199, 1980.

121. G.I.T.S. Gastrointestinal Tumor Study Group. Controlled trial of adjuvant chemotherapy following curative resection for gastric cancer. *Cancer* 49:116–122, 1982.

122. Biran H., Sikes: A possible dose response relationship in "FAM" chemotherapy for advanced gastric cancer. ASCO Abstract-C,515, 1984.

123. Cullinan S., Moertel C., Fleming T., et al.: A randomized comparison of 5-FU alone, 5-FU plus Adriamycin and 5-FU plus Adriamycin plus Mitomycin C in gastric and pancreatic cancer. ASCO Abstract-C,536, 1984.

124. Moertel C., Fleming T., O'Connel M., et al.: A phase II trial of combined intensive course of 5-FU Adriamycin and Cisplatinum in advanced gastric and pancreatic carcinoma. ASCO-Abstract-C,535, 1984.

125. Bruckner H.W., Stablein D.M.: Single arm trials of Triazinate, Cisplatinum, and Methotrexate combinations in advanced cancer. ASCO-Abstract C-562, 1984.

126. Ahlgren J.D., Smith F.P., Harvey J., et al.: A phase II study of FAM plus Triazinate for advanced measurable gastric carcinoma. ASCO Abstract-C,565, 1984.

127. Weissberg J.B.: The role of radiation therapy in gastrointestinal cancer. *Arch. Surg.* 118:96–104, 1983.

128. Child D.S., Moertel C.G., Holbrook M.A., et al.: Treatment of unresectable adenocarcinoma of the stomach with a combination of 5-Fluorouracil and radiation. *A.J.R.* 102:541–544, 1968.

129. Moertel C.G., Childs D.S., Reitemeir R.J., et al.: Combined 5-Fluorouracil and supervoltage radiation therapy of locally unresectable gastrointestinal cancer. *Lancet* 2:865–867, 1969.

130. Schein P.S., Stablein D.M., Novak J.W., et al.: A comparison of combination chemotherapy and combined modality therapy for locally advanced gastric carcinoma. *Cancer* 49:1771–1777, 1982.

131. Dent D.M., Werner I.D., Novis B., et al.: Prospective randomized trial of combined oncological therapy for gastric carcinoma. *Cancer* 44:385–391, 1979.

132. Abe M., Takahashi M.: Intraoperative radiotherapy: The Japanese experience. *Int. J. Radiat. Oncol. Biol. Phys.* 7:863–868, 1981.

133. Tepper J., Sindelar W.F.: Summary of the workshop on intraoperative radiation therapy. *Cancer Treat. Rep.* 65:911–918, 1981.

134. Sindelar W.F., Kinsella T., Tepper J., et al.: Experimental and clinical studies with intraoperative radiation therapy. *Surg. Gynecol. Obstet.* 157:205–219, 1983.

135. Fleming I., Stone M., Dilawari R.: The role of surgery in the management of gastric lymphoma. *Cancer* 49:1135–1141, 1982.

136. Mittal B., Wasserman T., Griffith R.: Non Hodgkins lymphoma of the stomach. *Am. J. Gastroenterol.* 78:780–787, 1983.

137. Shimm D.S., Dosoretz D., Anderson T., et al.: Primary gastric lymphoma—an analysis with emphasis on prognostic factors and radiation therapy. *Cancer* 52:2044–2048, 1983.

138. Burnett M., Herbert E.: The role of irradiation in the treatment of primary malignant lymphoma of the stomach. *Radiology* 67:723–728, 1956.

139. Connors J., Wise L.: Management of gastric lymphoma. *Am. J. Surg.* 127:102–108, 1974.

140. Hermann R., Panalion A., Barcos M., et al.: Gastrointestinal involvement in nonHodgkins lymphoma. *Cancer* 46:215–212, 1980.

141. Shiu M., Karas M., Nisce L., et al.: Management of primary gastric lymphoma. *Ann. Surg.* 195:196–202, 1982.

142. Sandler R.: Primary gastric lymphoma: A review. *Am. J. Gastroenterol.* 79:21–25, 1984.

143. Brooks J., Enterline H.: Primary gastric lymphoma: A clinicopathologic study of 58 cases with long term follow up and literature review. *Cancer* 51:701–711, 1983.

144. Orr R.K., Lininger J.R., Lawrence W.: Gastric pseudolymphoma: A challenging clinical problem. *Ann. Surg.* 200:185–194, 1984.

145. Smith J.L., Helwig E.B.: Malignant lymphoma of the stomach: Its diagnosis, distinction and biological behavior (abstract). *Am. J. Pathol.* 34:553, 1958.

146. Jacobs D.S.: Primary gastric malignant lymphoma and pseudolymphoma. *Am. J. Clin. Pathol.* 40:379–394, 1963.

147. Skandalakis J., Gray S., Sheperd D.: *Smooth Muscle Tumors of the Alimentary Tract.* Springfield, Ill., Charles C Thomas Publishers, 1962.

148. Shiu M., Farr G., Papachristou D.: Myosarcomas of the stomach; natural history, prognostic factors and management. *Cancer* 48(1):177–187, 1982.

149. Lee M.Y.T.: Leiomyosarcoma of the gastrointestinal tract: Should we consider metastases to regional lymph nodes? *J. Surg. Oncol.* 15:319–321, 1980.

150. Lee M.Y.T.: Leiomyosarcoma of the gastrointestinal tract: General pattern of metastases and recurrence. *Cancer Treat. Rep.* 10:91–101, 1983.

151. Stavorsky M., Morag B., Stavorsky H., et al.: Smooth muscle tumors of the alimentary tract. *J. Surg. Oncol.* 22:109–114, 1983.

152. Lindsay P., Ordonez N., Raaf J.: Gastric leiomyosarcoma: Clinical and pathological review of fifty patients. *J. Surg. Oncol.* 18:399–421, 1981.

153. Carney J.: The trial of gastric epithelioid leiomyosarcoma, pulmonary chondroma and functioning extra adrenal paraganglionoma: A five year review. *Medicine* 62(3):159–169, 1983.

154. Cox C.: Epidermoid carcinoma of the stomach. *J. Med. Assoc. State Ala.* 49(5):41–45, 1979.

155. Hajdu S.I., Winawer S.J., Myers W.P.L.: Carcinoid tumors: A study of 204 cases. *Am. J. Clin. Pathol.* 61:521–528, 1974.

156. Godwin J.D.: Carcinoid tumors: An analysis of 2837 cases. *Cancer* 26:560–569, 1975.

157. Wilson J.M., Melvin D.B., Gray G.F., et al.: Primary malignancies of the small bowel: A report of 96 cases and review of the literature. *Ann. Surg.* 180:175–179, 1974.

17

Surgical Management of Morbid Obesity

WARD O. GRIFFEN, JR., M.D., PH.D.

IT HAS BECOME increasingly evident that the following non-operative therapies for morbid obesity generally fail to produce permanent weight reduction: various diets; anorexic or hypermetabolic medication; psychotherapy in the form of rational behavior therapy, hypnotherapy, and long-term psychological counseling; acupuncture; and enforced fasting, usually involving something akin to incarceration. Therefore, surgical approaches to therapy for this disease have become popular. Morbid obesity is defined in a variety of ways, the most popular being 100 lb above the ideal body weight (IBW). Other definitions include double the IBW and more than 100% above the IBW.[1, 2] While there may be some debate as to whether morbid obesity represents a disease entity in itself, several studies on health and obesity clearly demonstrate that at weights 30% or greater above the IBW, life-threatening ailments occur.[3] These conditions include hypertension, diabetes mellitus, pulmonary insufficiency, arthritis, and cardiac disease.

The first surgical approaches to morbid obesity utilized methods of reducing absorption of calories. The jejunocolostomy was the first of such procedures, but early disastrous results led to quick abandonment of that operation. Jejunoileal bypass, either end-to-side (Fig 17–1, left), or end-to-end (Fig 17–1, right), then became extremely popular.[4] However, as patients undergoing this procedure were followed up over a long period, significant serious sequelae were noted. Although adequate weight reduction was achieved, the metabolic consequences were such that the operation has been abandoned by most bariatric surgeons.[5]

The other serious approach to achieving permanent weight reduction by surgical means is a reduction of caloric intake. Quite early in the development of procedures for reduction of intake, jaw wiring or dental occlusion was used as a relatively simple technique. Although many patients lost weight while their jaws were wired together, as soon as the wires were removed, they almost invariably became morbidly obese again.[6] Therefore, this approach is no better than the many nonoperative means of treating morbid obesity.

Gastric bypass was probably the first intake-reducing operation on the stomach designed to manage morbid obesity. It was described by Mason and Ito in 1969,[7] about the same time as the first reports on jejunoileal bypass were appearing. However, the seemingly enormous technical difficulties associated with any gastric procedure, as compared to the simpler

small-bowel operation, led to slow acceptance of gastric bypass. Over the years, there have been many modifications of the original technique, but the term "gastric bypass" is used to denote those procedures which separate the stomach into two portions, an upper pouch and a lower segment, the upper pouch being drained into the small bowel. Because of the physiologic alterations inherent in the gastric bypass, the concept of creating a partial division of the upper and lower stomach, so that food still traveled from stomach to duodenum to small bowel, became popular. These procedures, informally known as gastroplasty, at first were not as effective in producing permanent weight reduction. However, they have become popular as modifications have made the operation more successful in achieving permanent weight reduction.

More recently a procedure has been described which combines reduced intake with attenuated absorption to achieve permanent weight reduction. It was first described by Scopinaro et al. in 1979[8] and has been advocated in the United States by Holian and Clare.[9] The operation consists of a gastric resection and division of the small intestine at its midpoint, with anastomosis of the proximal end of the distal limb to the gastric remnant and the distal end of the proximal limb to the small intestine, 50 cm proximal to the ileocecal valve, in an end-to-side manner (Fig 17–2).

This chapter addresses the various approaches to the surgical management of morbid obesity, with emphasis on the gastric reduction procedures. Some of the procedures are mentioned only very briefly for obvious reasons. The results of other operations are summarized with some appropriate comments, and other approaches described in some detail, since they represent the current major surgical techniques used for the morbidly obese patient.

JEJUNOILEAL BYPASS

Payne and Dewind[10] described an end-to-side jejunoileal bypass in a series of morbidly obese patients with satisfactory results in terms of weight reduction. Some patients failed to lose weight, and because it was believed that this was due to reflux of nutrients, other surgeons described an end-to-end jejunoileal bypass, draining the bypassed small intestine into the cecum[4] or the sigmoid colon.[1] As long-term follow-up of these patients continued, a variety of untoward sequelae was

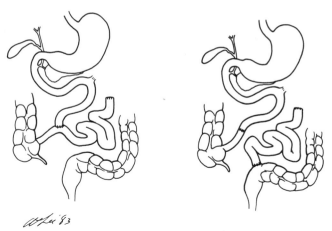

Fig 17–1.—Jejunoileal bypass. *Left,* end-to-side anastomosis; *right,* end-to-end anastomosis. (From Griffen W.O., Bell R.M.: Surgical approaches to morbid obesity. *Contemp. Surg.* 23:15, 1983. Used by permission.)

described.[11–14] The list grew longer, more varied, and of greater severity. The most serious problem was hepatic dysfunction to the extent of cirrhosis and even death.[12] Other problems included electrolyte imbalance, vitamin deficiencies, renal abnormalities, arthralgias, enteritis, and general lassitude. Despite an occasional encouraging report on the efficacy of the small-bowel bypass in the treatment of morbid obesity here and abroad,[15] most bariatric surgeons have abandoned the procedure as an acceptable method of management of morbid obesity.

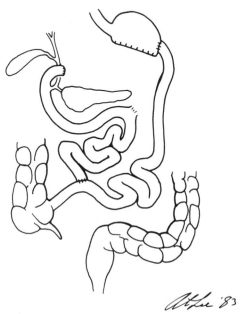

Fig 17–2.—Biliopancreatic bypass. Note three gastrointestinal pathways: (1) gastroileal, (2) biliopancreatic jejunal, and (3) combined (distal 500 cm). (From Griffen W.O., Bell R.M.: Surgical approaches to morbid obesity. *Contemp. Surg.* 23:15, 1983. Used by permission.)

BILIOPANCREATIC BYPASS

This procedure can be considered an attempt to capitalize on the best features of decreasing caloric intake and absorption while minimizing the negative features of the two approaches. The gastric reduction is not so severe as to greatly restrict intake, while the intestinal bypass is not so drastic as to produce the significant, serious postoperative derangements observed following jejunoileal bypass. The originator of the procedure, Scopinaro, and his associate Holian have reported on fewer than 400 patients. However, their results at two years indicate a maintained weight loss of 70% of excess weight and none of the serious adverse sequelae seen after small-bowel bypass.[16] Because of the Roux-en-Y reconstruction in the absence of a vagotomy, stomach ulceration has been observed, but apparently responds to nonoperative therapy in the majority of cases.

UNPROVED GASTRIC APPROACHES TO MORBID OBESITY

Three procedures fall into this category, two of which are mentioned only for completeness' sake, since the number of patients involved is small. One of the procedures, although described in at least 100 patients, has had little follow-up reporting, making the results both incomplete and difficult to interpret.

One gastric operation theoretically reduces food intake by increasing transit time. This procedure, described by Kral[17] in 1979, consisted of a bilateral truncal vagotomy without a drainage procedure. Thirteen morbidly obese patients were described, with a two-year follow-up. During that time, an average weight loss of 20–30 kg was described, but since the weight loss of each patient was not given, it is impossible to determine the percent of excess weight lost. Moreover, two of the 13 patients failed to lose any weight. These preliminary results, along with the fact that nothing has been reported since regarding the procedure, leads to the conclusion that it is probably not a reasonable approach to the problem. This approach has also been reported in children with the Prader-Willi syndrome and had the same inconclusive results.[18]

A similar fate has been reported with the placement of an intragastric prosthesis.[19, 20] While this is theoretically attractive for its simplicity and the possibility that it could be used intermittently, the small number of patients and experimental animals reported has been associated with both technical failure and lack of permanent weight loss. It has been abandoned as a recommended gastric procedure.

In 1981 Wilkinson and Peloso[21] described the operation of gastric wrapping (Fig 17–3). In this operation the lesser curve from the gastroesophageal junction to the incisura is inverted on itself. The distal esophagus and the entire stomach are then wrapped in a "coat" of polypropylene mesh in a way that prevents expansion of the stomach as a meal is consumed. Theoretically, this should reduce intake and permit satisfactory and permanent weight reduction. In the original report, 100 patients were described, and it was stated that only one patient had not lost weight satisfactorily. Essentially, however, the paper describes a technique only and does not give

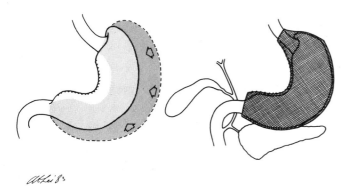

Fig 17–3.—Gastric wrapping procedure. (From Griffen W.O., Bell R.M.: Surgical approaches to morbid obesity. *Contemp. Surg.* 23:15, 1983. Used by permission.)

sufficient numerical data to make any sound conclusions regarding the operation. It is attractive, since it does not require opening of the bowel or stapling of the stomach. On the other hand, recognizing the eating habits of these patients and the fact that they cannot control their intake of calories, the procedure appears doomed to failure. Even in the preliminary paper, the authors admit that "patients can defeat the purpose of the operation by the almost continuous ingestion of high calorie liquids."

PROVED GASTRIC OPERATIONS FOR MORBID OBESITY

The two operations that have proved to be successful in achieving permanent weight reduction are known by the generic names of gastric bypass and gastroplasty. The concepts of the two operations are similar. The essence of success with either procedure is the development of a small upper pouch or reservoir into which food is delivered and the creation of an outlet or stoma that is maintained at a diameter small enough to delay emptying of the reservoir sufficiently to reduce caloric intake, but not so great as to produce outlet obstruction. For permanent weight reduction, most failures have been in the creation of too large a pouch, or, more often, either initial creation of too large a stoma or dilatation of the stoma over time.

Gastric Bypass

The first gastric bypass, described by Mason and Ito,[7] was one in which the stomach was transected to create an upper pouch capable of containing a volume of 50–60 ml. This pouch was drained into a loop of jejunum brought up in a retrocolic fashion, with a measured anastomosis of 1.2 cm. Variations on the theme have included an antecolic position for the loop of jejunum,[22] a Roux-en-Y configuration rather than a loop gastrojejunostomy,[23] a lesser curvature position for the gastrojejunostomy,[24] and abandonment of the transection of the stomach. Today, gastric bypass consists of the placement of a single or double complete line of staples to create a pouch with a volume of no greater than 50 ml. Some authors describe upper reservoirs of only a 30-ml volume. The pouch is then drained by means of a loop gastrojejunostomy, which can be placed on the greater curvature side or anteriorly, but with a measured stoma of no greater than 1.2

cm (Fig 17–4). The other configuration drains the upper pouch by means of a Roux-en-Y limb of jejunum, which can be placed either in the retrocolic or antecolic position (Fig 17–5).

Gastroplasty

Because of the recognized physiologic derangement produced by gastric bypass, the concept of gastroplasty was first described by Printen and Mason.[25] In the early operation, the stomach was only partially transected, leaving an opening on the greater curvature side. Unfortunately, the stoma enlarged in the majority of patients, and the procedure was abandoned as a failure. Pace et al.[26] in 1979 then described what appeared to be a very simple technique of removing several staples from the stapler and then applying a single or double partial staple line across the stomach in a horizontal fashion. The staples could be removed on the greater curvature side or in the middle of the staple equipment. Other variations were described by Gomez,[27] particularly when it was recognized that some form of restriction of the stoma was necessary to achieve permanent weight reduction. All of these procedures were accomplished by placing the staple line in a horizontal position with relation to the long axis of the stomach (Fig 17–6). These operations proved to be less satisfactory, predominantly because of enlargement of the stoma or breakdown of the staple line. Because it was thought that the incomplete staple line was the reason for failure, both Herbst and Jewell independently described the formation of a complete horizontal staple line or lines to separate the stomach into a small upper pouch and a larger lower segment, in combination with the creation of an anterior gastrogastrostomy of no greater than 1.2 cm in diameter as the outlet.[28, 29] The latter procedure has been much more satisfactory in terms of achievement of permanent weight reduction.

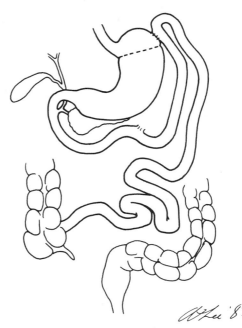

Fig 17–4.—Gastric bypass with loop gastrojejunostomy. (From Griffen W.O., Bell R.M.: Surgical approaches to morbid obesity. *Contemp. Surg.* 23:15, 1983. Used by permission.)

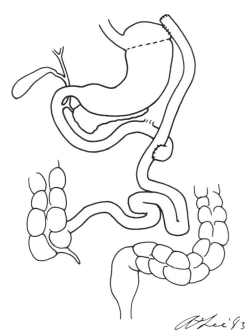

Fig 17–5.—Gastric bypass with Roux-en-Y gastrojejunostomy. (From Griffen W.O., Bell R.M.: Surgical approaches to morbid obesity. *Contemp. Surg.* 23:15, 1983. Used by permission.)

As dissatisfaction with the horizontal gastroplasty grew, other means of performing gastroplasty were sought. Eckhout and Prinzing[30] and Laws[31] in 1980–81 described the formation of a vertical staple line from the angle of His toward the lesser curvature. The stoma from upper pouch to distal stomach was then on the lesser curve side of the stomach, and in both instances was reinforced with some form of foreign body sutured into or through the stomach. In 1982 Mason described the vertical banded gastroplasty.[32] In this operation a complete through-and-through stapled opening is made on the

lesser curvature side of the stomach using an EEA stapler. A complete staple line is then created between this opening and the angle of His, creating an upper pouch of no greater than 50 ml volume. The resulting stoma between upper pouch and lower pouch on the lesser curvature is then reinforced with a collar of polypropylene mesh, which is not sutured to the stomach in any fashion (Fig 17–7). This operation is the culmination of the search for a satisfactory gastroplasty procedure. Two-year results are encouraging, and the final verdict awaits a longer follow-up period.

WEIGHT REDUCTION

Gastric Bypass

As indicated above, the standard gastric bypass procedure today does not involve transection of the stomach. For emptying of the upper pouch, there are several variations, but for purposes of analyzing the weight reduction results, all gastric bypasses—i.e., any procedure where a small upper pouch of stomach is drained into the small intestine—have been put together to show the potential for full weight reduction. Unfortunately, some of the studies cannot be used, because they reported the number of pounds or kilograms lost, rather than the percent of excess weight lost or the percent overweight of the patients after having had the gastric bypass. Obviously, a percentage evaluation is preferable in terms of reporting, because patients can be compared one to another. Moreover, an agreed upon definition of success following any operation for morbid obesity has never been established. Perhaps the best tabulation of success is that used by Linner,[33] who describes the following weight loss categories:

Excellent	0%–25% Overweight
Good	26%–50% Overweight
Fair	51%–75% Overweight
Poor	76%–100% Overweight
Failure	Over 100% Overweight

Using that scale, Linner's data, and our own, and having

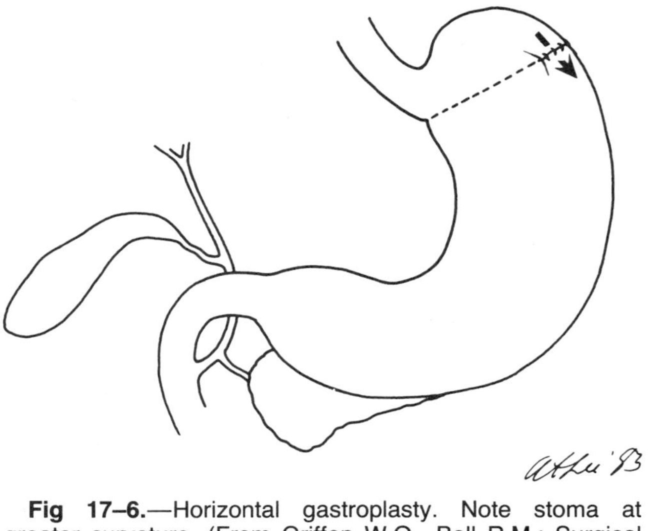

Fig 17–6.—Horizontal gastroplasty. Note stoma at greater curvature. (From Griffen W.O., Bell R.M.: Surgical approaches to morbid obesity. *Contemp. Surg.* 23:15, 1983. Used by permission.)

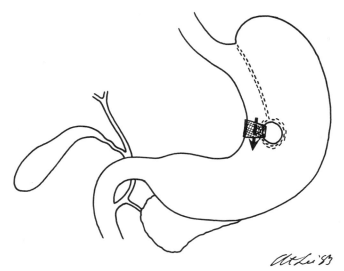

Fig 17–7.—Vertical banded gastroplasty. (From Griffen W.O., Bell R.M.: Surgical approaches to morbid obesity. *Contemp. Surg.* 23:15, 1983. Used by permission.)

contacted several surgeons known to be using gastric bypass almost exclusively,[34-36] the weight reduction appears to be excellent in about 60% of the patients and either good or excellent in 85%–90%. Basically, these results involve over 8,000 patients and were obtained at two years or longer. Since the "good group" represents patients who are between 26% and 50% overweight, this could mean that the majority of the patients in the "excellent" and "good" groups are within 30% of their IBW, or at the level where their risk for life-threatening diseases is small.

Gastroplasty

At present, two forms of gastroplasty are available. They are the horizontal gastroplasty (an incomplete staple line placed across the stomach in a horizontal fashion) or the complete staple line placed across the stomach, with a complementary anterior gastrogastrostomy for drainage. The former type of gastroplasty has not been successful in terms of weight reduction because of a high rate of staple line disruption. In several series comparing gastric bypass and gastroplasty, gastric bypass has been much better in terms of weight reduction.[37-40] Since the incomplete staple line may be the Achilles heel of that operation, the complete staple line with an anterior gastrogastrostomy may be a better procedure. Both Herbst and Jewell, reporting about 200 cases, have documented a success rate as defined above or about 80%.

A more recent form of gastroplasty has been termed the vertical or vertical-banded gastroplasty. This operation, in contrast to the horizontal gastroplasty, places the opening between the upper and lower stomach on the lesser curvature side, with the staple line from the angle of His toward the lesser curvature in a more or less vertical position. This operation, since it is a new procedure, has neither the numbers nor the years of follow-up of the gastric bypass operation. However, several bariatric surgeons have reported that at least at two years, the vertical types of gastroplasty appear to be as successful as gastric bypass in achieving permanent weight reduction.

COMPLICATIONS OF GASTRIC OPERATIONS FOR MORBID OBESITY

Early Complications

Postoperative mortality is at an acceptable level in the reported series, being less than 5% in all series and less than 2% in most.[41] Early complications following gastric operations for morbid obesity include all of the expected complications from any major surgical procedure. However, the incidence of wound infection, urinary tract infection, atelectasis and pneumonia, pulmonary embolism, and other complications is surprisingly low considering the seemingly high risk of many of these patients for receiving general anesthesia. For example, in several reported series, the incidence of wound infection is not above 4%.[41] Pulmonary embolism is likewise low whether the surgeons use minidose heparin or not. Specifically, the incidence of splenectomy has been relatively low and tends to decrease dramatically as the technique is learned. On the other hand, looking at all complications, at least one complication occurs in a high percentage (35%–40%) of patients.[41, 42]

One early complication after gastric bypass deserves special mention. Anastomotic leak has been reported in several series at a rate of approximately 2.5%.[41] The leak usually is detected between the second and fifth postoperative day. Tachycardia out of proportion to the temperature is the hallmark of making the diagnosis. Shoulder pain and fever are the next most common. The leak usually occurs at the anastomosis, but has been reported from both the upper and lower segments of the stomach. A leak following a loop gastrojejunostomy is usually more catastrophic than a leak following a Roux-en-Y procedure, because the leaking fluid is more likely to contain bile and pancreatic juice in the former. Usually a leak requires a second operation with appropriate drainage and establishment of a feeding mechanism distal to the leak.

Almost all of the patients undergoing gastric bypass or gastroplasty have some difficulty adjusting to the reduced reservoir capacity. Since they have been used to eating large meals and eating them quickly, the tendency is for the patient with a new gastric procedure in place to overeat, become uncomfortable, and to experience some dumping, especially with gastric bypass procedures. While not a true complication, because it is an expected side effect, a small number of patients have persistent vomiting, and some have required stoma revision to avoid the continuing difficulty of postprandial vomiting. If the patients are instructed preoperatively on the need to eat small meals, take small bites which are chewed thoroughly, and eat slowly, many of these difficulties can be lessened if not eliminated. There is no question that dumping is seen more frequently after gastric bypass than after gastroplasty. Some surgeons believe that it is the dumping syndrome that makes the gastric bypass a better weight reduction operation than the gastroplasty. Patients usually have dumping after eating highly concentrated foods, including ice cream, cookies and cakes, and other high-caloric nutrients.

Late Complications

A variety of late complications is now coming to the fore. Hair loss following gastric bypass and gastroplasty has been well recognized for some time. It is related to a specific protein lack and generally is self-limited, since that particular protein is reintroduced into the diet after the patient's original marked caloric deprivation in the early postoperative period. Sophisticated metabolic studies performed by McLean et al.[43] have clearly shown that there is loss of lean body mass and therefore protein deprivation in the early months following gastric exclusion. However, within six to nine months this protein lack has been corrected, and there are very few difficulties thereafter. Notably different from the jejunoileal bypass is the incidence of liver derangement following gastric bypass. Most studies indicate improvement of liver morphology after gastric bypass. However, recently, a case was reported of hepatic failure following a gastroplasty in which biopsy of the liver showed alcoholic injury.[44] Certainly, however, that is uncommon. Similarly, electrolyte abnormalities are also uncommon following gastric bypass, unlike the situation following the small-bowel bypass procedures.

Increasing but small numbers of patients have been described who have developed dizziness, motor weakness, gait problems, double vision, peripheral neuropathy, impaired position sense, and other evidence of polyneuropathy.[45]

While the exact cause of this is unknown, it is suspected to be vitamin B deficiency. Administration of vitamin B complexes, especially thiamine and niacin, will usually reverse the condition. These complications are almost always seen in patients who have greatly reduced postoperative intake either because of some stomach narrowing that produces excessive vomiting or because of voluntary intake restriction. In many ways the classic picture resembles that described many years ago in association with starvation.[46] The surgeons must be alert to this possibility and investigate the circumstances when the patient shows excessive or early weight loss (3 kg/month). Most bariatric surgeons do give their patients oral medication or preparations postoperatively as a prophylaxis.

A more challenging and perplexing problem is the development of deficiency anemia even in the absence of excessive weight loss. Iron deficiency and vitamin B_{12} deficiency anemias appear to be present in about 25% of the patients undergoing gastric bypass.[47] The mechanism of iron deficiency anemia in the gastric bypass operation seems fairly straightforward. Since the duodenum, where most iron is absorbed, is bypassed, absorption of iron will be deficient, and patients might be expected to develop iron deficiency anemia. Most of these anemias are readily treated by increasing the iron intake, although the amount of medication required may be two or three times that required by an individual with a normal GI tract.

The vitamin B_{12} deficiency represents a fascinating problem, not yet totally solved.[48] Vitamin B_{12} absorption requires an intrinsic factor, a glycoprotein elaborated by the parietal cells, and an intact ileum. Since vitamin B_{12} is plentiful in most foods and the ileum is intact in patients undergoing gastric bypass, the presumption must be that the intrinsic factor is lacking to account for postoperative vitamin B_{12} deficiency. Does that mean that the parietal cell mass in the bypassed stomach is decreased or even absent? This question has not been answered adequately until now. However, Flickinger et al.[49] examined the bypassed stomach through an endoscope and discovered intestinal metaplasia in a number of these individuals, which could account for a loss of parietal cell mass. At any rate, vitamin B_{12} deficiency, which occurs in about 5% of the patients, responds well to parenteral vitamin B_{12} given on a monthly basis.

Gastroplasty

The theoretical advantage of the gastroplasty procedures over gastric bypass is that the food stream is "normal." Therefore, in addition to being an easier procedure from a technical standpoint, in that the stomach does not have to be opened (unless one is doing a vertical banded gastroplasty), the postoperative metabolic consequences should be less evident. Although it is a little early to grant a clean bill of health to gastroplasty, it appears that the metabolic deficiencies associated with gastroplasty are not as significant as with gastric bypass, at least at two years.

Finally, a word must be said about a postoperative lack of weight loss or weight gain. Surgical mishaps account for early difficulty with weight reduction. Too large an original stoma or pouch or staple line disruption can result in inadequate weight loss or in fairly rapid weight gain after initial weight loss. In long-term follow-up, late weight gain almost invariably has been associated with some dilatation of the stoma. This permits either the jejunal limb or the distal stomach to act once again as a reservoir, allowing patients to ingest more calories than they consume on a daily basis. It is too early in the gastroplasty story to determine whether late weight gain will be a problem. Obviously, for the horizontal gastroplasties it was a problem early in the postoperative period, but was associated with technical difficulties. However, in the case of gastric bypass, it is now evident that late weight gain does occur in about 10% of the patients and may be significant enough to remove the patient from the "good" or "excellent" category to only a "fair" result at the end of five to ten years.[47]

BENEFITS OF GASTRIC EXCLUSION PROCEDURES

The benefits derived from undergoing these operations are easily recounted and are what have made the procedures so popular with surgeons and patients alike. When most patients first think about a major operation to achieve permanent weight reduction, they are concerned about the risks involved. However, by the time they have decided that an operation is the only way to achieve permanent weight reduction, the major motivating factor in their life has become weight reduction. For the majority of these patients weight reduction is a reality, and therefore the patients are willing to tolerate many difficulties to achieve that goal. Thus, some of the metabolic and other consequences of the gastric exclusion operations seem minor to the patient, even though they are of great concern to the surgeon. Parenthetically, it is the achievement of the relatively permanent weight reduction that also makes this group of patients a most grateful one.

In patients with established disease entities, such as hypertension, diabetes mellitus, arthritis, and hypertriglyceridemia, the benefits derived from weight reduction produced by gastric bypass have been dramatic. In one recent series, hypertension was eliminated in 96% of the patients, diabetes mellitus in 100%, gouty arthritis in a similar percentage, and hypertriglyceridemia in 92%.[42] Similar results have been reported by many bariatric surgeons. It is our own contention that if the hypertension has been present for less than five years, the likelihood is that the patient, after satisfactory weight reduction, will become normotensive without medication. If the hypertension has been present between five and 10 years, there is about a 50% chance of achieving the normotensive state. Even for those whose hypertension has been present for a decade or longer, the likelihood is that the hypertension will be controlled with much less medication. Diabetes has a similar pattern. If the diabetes has not been established for a long period, the likelihood is that the patient will once again achieve a normal blood glucose status. In general, most insulin-dependent diabetics will require less insulin for control once weight reduction has been achieved.

For the future, reporting of results should be made in terms of percentage of excess weight lost or percentage overweight, so that individuals and series can be compared to each other. In addition, patient follow-up must approach 100%. Series in which 10%–25% are "lost to follow-up" are scientifically worthless. Finally, long-term follow-up is essential, so that the final answers may be obtained regarding this approach to the morbidly obese patient.

CONCLUSION

It is apparent that nonoperative therapy for morbid obesity is ineffective, achieving permanent weight reduction in fewer than 5%. The gastric exclusionary procedures appear to achieve success in over 80% of the patients, with an acceptable mortality and morbidity both early and late in the postoperative period. While modifications continue to be made on the reported operations, the basic concept of any successful gastric procedure for morbid obesity is the creation of a very small reservoir, with a small outlet to encourage slow emptying of the reservoir. It is essential that complete and long-term reporting be done to ascertain the value of these procedures for this disease.

REFERENCES

1. Scott H.W. Jr., Law D.H. IV, Sandstead H.H., et al.: Jejunoileal shunt in surgical treatment of morbid obesity. *Ann. Surg.* 171:770, 1970.
2. Payne J.H., Dewind L.T., Schwab C.E., et al.: Surgical treatment of morbid obesity. *Arch Surg.* 106:432, 1973.
3. VanItallie T.B.: "Morbid" obesity: A hazardous disorder that resists conservative treatment. *Am. J. Clin. Nutr.* 33:358, 1980.
4. Buchwald H., Schwartz M.Z., Varco R.L.: Surgical treatment of obesity. *Adv. Surg.* 7:235, 1973.
5. Griffen W.O. Jr., Bivins B.A., Bell R.M.: The decline and fall of the jejunoileal bypass. *Surg. Gynecol. Obstet.* 157:301, 1983.
6. Kark A.E.: Jaw wiring. *Am. J. Clin. Nutr.* 33:420, 1980.
7. Mason E.E., Ito C.: Gastric bypass in obesity. *Ann. Surg.* 170:329, 1969.
8. Scopinaro N., Gianetta E., Civalleri D., et al.: Biliopancreatic bypass for obesity: II. Initial experience in man. *Brit. J. Surg.* 66:618, 1979.
9. Holian D.K., Clare M.W.: Biliopancreatic bypass for morbid obesity: Late results and complications. *Clin. Nutr.* In press.
10. Payne J.H., Dewind L.T.: Surgical treatment of obesity. *Am. J. Surg.* 118:141, 1969.
11. Jewell W.R., Hermreck A.S., Hardin C.A.: Complications of jejunoileal bypass for morbid obesity. *Arch. Surg.* 110:1039, 1975.
12. O'Leary J.P.: An appraisal of the status of small bowel bypass in the treatment of morbid obesity. *Clin. Endocrinol. Metab.* 5:481, 1976.
13. Halverson J.D., Schiff R.J., Gentry K., et al.: Jejunoileal bypass: Late metabolic sequelae and weight gain. *Am. J. Surg.* 140:347, 1980.
14. Hocking M.P., Duerson M.C., O'Leary J.P., et al.: Jejunoileal bypass for morbid obesity: Late follow-up in 100 cases. *N. Engl. J. Med.* 308:995, 1983.
15. Dewind L.T., Payne J.H.: Intestinal bypass surgery for morbid obesity: Long-term results. *J.A.M.A.* 236:2298, 1976.
16. Scopinaro N., Gianetta E., Civalleri D., et al.: Partial and total biliopancreatic bypass in the surgical treatment of obesity. *Int. J. Obesity* 5:421, 1981.
17. Kral J.G.: Vagotomy as a treatment for morbid obesity. *Surg. Clin. North Am.* 59:1131, 1979.
18. Fonkalsrud E.W., Bray G.: Vagotomy for treatment of obesity in childhood due to Prader-Willi syndrome. *J. Pediatr. Surg.* 16:888, 1981.
19. Miller J.D.: Intragastric prosthesis for management of obesity. *World J. Surg.* 6:492, 1982.
20. Nieben O.G., Harbor H.: Intragastric balloon as an artificial bezoar for treatment of obesity. *Lancet* 1:198, 1982.

21. Wilkinson L.H., Peloso O.A.: Gastric (reservoir) reduction for morbid obesity. *Arch. Surg.* 116:602, 1981.
22. Alden J.F.: Gastric and jejunoileal bypass. *Arch. Surg.* 112:799, 1977.
23. Griffen W.O. Jr., Young V.L., Stevenson C.C.: A prospective comparison of gastric and jejunoileal bypass for morbid obesity. *Ann. Surg.* 186:500, 1977.
24. Torres J.C., Oca C.F., Garrison R.N.: Gastric bypass Roux-en-Y gastrojejunostomy from the lesser curvature. *South. Med. J.* 76:1217, 1983.
25. Printen K.J., Mason E.E.: Gastric surgery for relief of morbid obesity. *Arch. Surg.* 106:428, 1973.
26. Pace W.G., Martin E.W. Jr., Tetrick C.E., et al.: Gastric partitioning for morbid obesity. *Ann. Surg.* 190:392, 1979.
27. Gomez C.A.: Gastroplasty in the surgical treatment of morbid obesity. *Ann. J. Clin. Nutr.* 33:405, 1980.
28. Herbst C.A., Buckwalter J.A.: Weight loss and complications after four gastric operations for morbid obesity. *South. Med. J.* 75:1324, 1982.
29. Peltier G., Hermreck A.S., Moffat R.E., et al.: Complications following gastric bypass procedures for morbid obesity. *Surgery* 86:648, 1979.
30. Eckhout G.V., Prinzing J.F.: Surgery for morbid obesity: Comparison of gastric bypass with vertically stapled gastroplasty. *Colo. Med.* 78:117, 1981.
31. Laws H.L.: Standardized gastroplasty orifice. *Am. J. Surg.* 141:393, 1981.
32. Mason E.E.: Vertical banded gastroplasty for obesity. *Arch. Surg.* 117:701, 1982.
33. Linner J.H.: *Surgery for Morbid Obesity.* New York, Heidelberg, Berlin, Springer-Verlag, 1984.
34. Alden J.F.: Unpublished data, 1984.
35. Lechner G.W.: Unpublished data, 1984.
36. Vaughn R.H.: Unpublished data, 1984.
37. Freeman J.G., Burchett H.J.: A comparison of gastric bypass and gastroplasty for morbid obesity. *Surgery* 88:433, 1980.
38. Linner J.H.: Comparative effectiveness of gastric bypass and gastroplasty, a clinical study. *Arch. Surg.* 117:695, 1982.
39. Pories W.J., Flickinger E.G., Meelheim H.D., et al.: The effectiveness of gastric bypass over gastric partitioning in morbid obesity. *Ann. Surg.* 196:389, 1982.
40. Lechner G.W., Elliott D.W.: Comparison of weight loss after gastric exclusion and partitioning. *Arch. Surg.* 118:685, 1983.
41. Thompson W.R., Amaral J.F., Caldwell M.D., et al.: Complications and weight loss in 150 consecutive gastric exclusion patients. *Am. J. Surg.* 146:602, 1983.
42. Amaral J.F., Thompson W.R., Caldwell M.D., et al.: Prospective metabolic evaluation of 150 consecutive patients who underwent gastric exclusion. *Am. J. Surg.* 147:468, 1984.
43. McLean L.F., Rhode B.M., Shizgal H.M.: Nutrition following gastric operations for morbid obesity. *Ann. Surg.* 198:347, 1983.
44. Hamilton D.L., Vest T.K., Brown B.S., et al.: Liver injury with alcoholiclike hyalin after gastroplasty for morbid obesity. *Gastroenterology* 85:722, 1983.
45. Carey L.C., Martin E.W. Jr., Mojziski C.: The surgical treatment of morbid obesity. *Curr. Probl. Surg.* 11:57, 1984.
46. Denny-Brown D.: Neurologic conditions resulting from prolonged and severe dietary restriction. *Medicine* 26:41, 1947.
47. Halverson J.L., Zuckerman G.R., Koehler R.E., et al.: Gastric bypass for morbid obesity: A medical surgical assessment. *Ann. Surg.* 194:152, 1981.
48. Crowley L.V., Olson R.W.: Megaloblastic anemia after gastric bypass for obesity. *Am. J. Gastroenterol.* 78:406, 1983.
49. Flickinger E.G., Pories W.J., Meelheim H.D., et al.: The Greenville gastric bypass: Progress report at three years. *Ann. Surg.* 199:555, 1984.

18

Postgastrectomy Syndromes

Wallace P. Ritchie, Jr., M.D., Ph.D.
Alice R. Perez, M.D.

INTRODUCTION

All operative procedures designed to ameliorate the peptic ulcer diathesis have a common and rational basis: reduction in the capacity of the stomach to secrete acid. This goal is accomplished by interrupting the celiac phase of secretion, by ablating the cephalic and gastric phases of secretion simultaneously, or by eliminating a significant portion of the parietal cell mass itself. Unfortunately, each of these approaches may be attended by untoward sequelae known collectively as the postgastrectomy syndromes: a group of conditions, each with unique pathophysiologic features and distinctive clinical signs and symptoms, which result from loss of gastric reservoir function, from bypass or ablation of the pylorus, or from parasympathetic denervation, either alone or in combination. The essence of the surgeon's dilemma is that those procedures with the highest potential for cure are also those most frequently associated with undesirable side effects. As is her wont, Mother Nature always exacts a price.

EARLY POSTPRANDIAL DUMPING SYNDROME

The existence of the early postprandial dumping syndrome was recognized as early as 1913; however, it was not until 1922 that it was given its colorful and appropriate appellation by Mix.[1] The syndrome consists of a constellation of GI and vasomotor signs and symptoms which occur early (within the first half hour) after ingestion of a meal, particularly when the meal is rich in carbohydrate. The GI components of the syndrome include a sensation of epigastric fullness, nausea, crampy abdominal pain, vomiting, and explosive diarrhea.[1] Vasomotor components of the syndrome include diaphoresis, weakness, dizziness, pallor followed by flushing, blurred vision, palpitations, and tachycardia.[1] In severe cases, weight loss may be considerable because of the fear of eating. The exact incidence of the syndrome is unknown but may occur in up to 50% of patients after partial gastrectomy, in 30% of patients after truncal vagotomy combined with a drainage procedure, and in 5% of patients following parietal cell vagotomy.[2] It should be emphasized that the complete expression of the syndrome is rarely present in any given patient and that its GI components are more common than its vasomotor ones.

Pathophysiology

Although the precise sequence of events responsible for the development of early postprandial dumping is incompletely defined, general agreement exists that the sine qua non of the syndrome is rapid emptying of hyperosmotic chyme from the residual stomach into the small intestine. Rapid gastric emptying, in turn, is the consequence of division of the pylorus or of resection or bypass of the distal stomach with loss of the capacity to triturate (mix and grind) ingesta and to deliver it to the small intestine in the form of small particles in isoosmotic solution. Vagotomy may aggravate the situation by impairing receptive relaxation of the proximal stomach, resulting in rapid emptying of liquids. Gravity also contributes to rapid gastric emptying following gastrectomy or pyloroplasty.

Once in the small intestine, hyperosmotic chyme induces a shift of extracellular fluid into the intestinal lumen in an attempt to achieve isotonicity. The resultant decrease in circulating plasma volume has been postulated to be responsible for the vasomotor components of the syndrome. Evidence to this effect includes the facts that oral hypertonic solutions produce a fall in plasma volume that is greater in patients with symptoms than in normal individuals and that the assumption of a supine position not only relieves symptoms but also prevents decreases in plasma volume.[3] On the other hand, the change in plasma volume observed in severe dumpers is frequently small, the correlation between the magnitude of altered plasma volume and the severity of symptoms is poor, and the onset of symptoms often precedes the change in plasma volume.[4]

It is paradoxical that, despite contracted blood volume, many patients with classic dumping demonstrate increased blood flow to the extremities. This circumstance suggests that additional factors may be involved in the development of the symptom complex—most probably humoral substances released in response to intestinal distention. This hypothesis is reinforced by the demonstration that a syndrome resembling dumping can be produced in normal dogs after transfusion with portal venous blood from dogs subjected to a dumping stimulus.[5] A variety of amines has been implicated, including serotonin, bradykinin, and enteroglucagon. Of these, serotonin has been studied most extensively; however, its exact role in the production of symptoms remains unclear. Serotonin is released in response to intestinal distention, elevated levels are found in the portal venous blood of postgastrectomy patients following a glucose challenge, and some patients benefit from the use of serotonin antagonists.[6] Hyperserotonanemia is not invariably present during attacks of dumping; even when present, elevated plasma serotonin levels do not always coincide with the onset of symptoms, and exogenous administration of serotonin does not reproduce all of the elements of the syndrome. On the other hand, it seems likely that a bradykinin-like peptide is at least partially responsible for the vasomotor components of dumping, as such a kinin is released during attacks (circulating kinin precursors fall at the same time),[7] and, when given exogenously, bradykinin does reproduce the vasomotor components of the syndrome. Enteroglucagon may also be involved in some of the symptomatology. Compared with preoperative levels or to nondumping controls, symptomatic postgastrectomy patients demonstrated significantly greater plasma enteroglucagon concentrations following a glucose challenge.[8] It has been suggested that excessive enteroglucagon release may be responsible for the diarrhea of early dumping because of its capacity to inhibit the absorption of sodium and water from the small intestine. The role of enteroglucagon in late postprandial dumping is discussed below.

Diagnostic Tests

The diagnosis of early dumping is usually made on clinical grounds alone: characteristic postprandial symptoms relieved by assuming a supine position. In most instances, sophisticated diagnostic evaluation is unnecessary—a fortunate circumstance, since no sensitive or specific test is currently available. However, in patients so incapacitated by dumping that an aggressive operative approach is contemplated, prudence dictates that some attempt be made to substantiate the diagnosis.

Routine upper GI series will delineate the appropriate anatomy and may demonstrate the presence of rapid gastric emptying of liquids. More important, the rate of gastric emptying of solids can be assessed using currently available radionuclide techniques. Obviously, the diagnosis is untenable if either rate is normal. The use of venous occlusion plethysmography and mercury strain gauge manometry, both of which detect changes in peripheral blood flow, may also be helpful,[9] particularly in patients who demonstrate the vasomotor components of the syndrome. Increases in either of these parameters above 200% of baseline are said to separate clearly classic dumpers from normal controls and from patients with other postgastrectomy syndromes. Provocative testing can also be undertaken. Hypertonic glucose solution is instilled directly into the residual stomach. The test should be controlled with isotonic saline lavage, and both observer and patient should be "blinded" as to the nature of the solution being used. Reproduction of symptoms with glucose but not with saline constitutes a positive response, said to occur more frequently in dumpers than in nondumpers. Although this type of testing is popular, it is not entirely specific, since several investigators have shown that many normal (i.e., nonoperated) individuals may exhibit typical symptoms when challenged in this manner.

Nonoperative Therapy

When questioned carefully in the early postoperative period, most patients will complain of some symptoms compatible with early dumping. However, over the course of several months, more than 80% will experience spontaneous relief.[1] Of the remainder, the vast majority can be adequately managed with dietary measures alone. These include frequent feeding of small meals, rich in protein and fat and low in carbohydrate, and the avoidance of liquids with meals (solutes require solvents). In some patients, the ingestion with the meal of the gel-forming carbohydrate pectin is of added benefit.[10] Posture may also be incorporated into the regimen, since the assumption of the recumbent position slows gastric emptying, minimizes plasma volume changes, and alleviates several of the symptoms of the syndrome.[11]

In intractable cases, a variety of drug treatments have been advocated, including the use of antihistaminics, ganglionic blockers, sedatives, parasympathomimetics, and anticholinergics. None has achieved striking success. Possible exceptions are the serotonin antagonists, which may offer temporary relief on occasion. Unfortunately, the large doses required frequently produce disagreeable side effects and, in any case, often fail to achieve permanent improvement. In such patients (approximately 1% of all those undergoing gastric surgery), an operative approach should be contemplated.

Operative Therapy

If the dumping syndrome is a consequence of loss of gastric reservoir function associated with rapid gastric emptying, logical operative approaches to the problem should aim at correcting one or both of these abnormalities. Conversely, operations which accomplish neither are doomed to failure. Conversions of Billroth II gastrojejunostomies to Billroth I gastroduodenostomies and narrowing revisions of the anastomotic stoma are examples of the latter category.[12, 13] On the other hand, expanding the gastric reservoir using plicated interposed pouches has inherent attraction.[14] Unfortunately, while pouches of this type appear to give good initial results, they dilate and elongate with time and create a new problem, gastric outlet obstruction. An alternative approach is to interpose a 10–20-cm isoperistaltic loop of jejunum between stomach and small intestine.[15] The loop promotes reservoir function, as it also dilates with time. In addition, even though it is isoperistaltic, it does delay gastric emptying, at least of liquids. Unfortunately, most long-term results have proved disappointing.

In contrast, the interposition of an antiperistaltic jejunal segment has been attended by considerable success. In theory at least, the antiperistaltic nature of the segment permits it to act as a substitute pylorus, slowing the rate of gastric emptying, refluxing chyme cephalad, and allowing more time for trituration and controlled delivery of that chyme to the small intestine.[16] It should be emphasized that the optimal length of the jejunal segment is 10 cm. Shorter segments are ineffective, while longer segments produce gastric outlet obstruction. In addition, to avoid marginal ulceration, vagotomy should be performed, if not previously performed, or completed if previously performed and found to be incomplete. Long-term follow-up studies have demonstrated that such segments are functional for up to ten years postoperatively and are associated with partial or complete remission of symptoms in more than 90% of patients.[16]

Recently, interest has been rekindled in the efficacy of a long-limbed Roux-en-Y anastomosis as therapy for dumping. The rationale for this approach is that, in the presence of truncal vagotomy, creation of a Roux limb significantly delays gastric emptying. Early results in a small group of patients have been encouraging.[17] It should be noted, however, that this procedure may not provide a satisfactory long-term solution: preliminary studies indicate that gastric emptying returns to normal (i.e., pre-Roux values) within 36 months after construction of the limb. An intriguing experimental variation on this theme has recently been reported. In dogs with vagotomy and distal gastrectomy reconstructed as a Roux gastrojejunostomy, retrograde electrical pacing of the loop not only slowed gastric emptying but also diminished postcibal hemoconcentration and hyperglycemia following a glucose challenge.[18] It is possible that Roux gastrojejunostomy and retrograde pacing with implantable units may play a role in the treatment of this vexing clinical problem in the future.

LATE POSTPRANDIAL DUMPING SYNDROME

The late postprandial dumping syndrome is less common than its early counterpart, affecting fewer than 2% of postgastrectomy patients. Those who have undergone extensive resection seem to be at greatest risk. As the name implies, symptoms occur much later than those of early dumping, usually one and one-half to three hours following the ingestion of a carbohydrate-rich meal. The syndrome may occur in association with early dumping or as in an isolated entity. Typically, patients complain of diaphoresis, tremulousness, tachycardia, and light-headedness.[12] In severe cases, they may experience difficulty in thinking, confusion, and even bizarre behavior. These symptoms are characteristically ameliorated by the ingestion of carbohydrates.

Pathophysiology

The basic defect responsible for late postprandial dumping is the same as that for early dumping: rapid gastric emptying. In this instance, however, a specific foodstuff, carbohydrate, is clearly incriminated. When sugars are delivered to the small intestine as a bolus, they are rapidly absorbed, resulting in a marked increase in blood glucose. Hyperglycemia triggers the release of large amounts of insulin, which, over the course of the next one to two hours, not only normalize blood sugar, but also in symptomatic patients "overshoot" the end point so that a profound hypoglycemia develops.[12] This circumstance, in turn, activates adrenal catecholamine secretion, with the end result that symptoms indistinguishable from insulin shock are produced. Postgastrectomy patients with hypoglycemia of this magnitude demonstrate higher peak glucose and insulin levels in response to a glucose challenge than do asymptomatic controls.[10] However, increased insulin sensitivity has not been demonstrated. Rather, enteroglucagon, liberated in response to intestinal distention, may be the real culprit, because it may promote excessive insulin secretion.[19]

Treatment

The aim of therapy in patients with late dumping is to normalize the glucose tolerance curve. It has been shown in postgastrectomy subjects that the addition of 10–15 gm of pectin to a glucose challenge prevents the occurrence of hypoglycemic symptoms and maintains blood sugar levels well above those observed in the same patients subjected to the same challenge without pectin.[10] Coincidentally, breath H_2 production, an index of bacterial fermentation of glucose, is markedly reduced.[10] Although the precise mechanism of action of pectin in this regard is unclear, it is likely that its gelling properties prolong the absorption of carbohydrate by increasing the viscosity of intraluminal content.[10] Unfortunately, this dose of pectin is usually intolerable on a long-term basis. An alternative and effective approach is to ingest, with meals, 5 gm of pectin in combination with 50 mg of acarbose, an α-glucoside hydrolase inhibitor.[20] This compound impairs intraluminal digestion of starch and sucrose and therefore delays carbohydrate absorption.[20] Additional nonoperative measures of value include the use of frequent, small feedings of carbohydrate-poor meals and the ingestion of carbohydrate when symptoms begin. Should these approaches fail, the interposition of a 10-cm antiperistaltic loop between residual gastric pouch and intestine has been shown to delay gastric emptying, to flatten the glucose tolerance curve, and to alleviate symptoms in the majority of patients in whom it has been employed.[21] Reversed segments placed distal to the ligament of Treitz seem less efficacious in this regard.[21]

THE AFFERENT LOOP SYNDROME; EFFERENT LOOP OBSTRUCTION

The afferent loop syndrome, first described by Wells and Welborne in 1951,[22] is the consequence of obstruction of an afferent limb; therefore, it can only occur following gastrectomy with reconstruction as a Billroth II gastrojejunostomy. Two forms are distinguished: chronic and acute, the chronic form being more common. The reported incidence of the syndrome varies from less than 1% to almost 20%.[23] The lower figure is probably more accurate.

The basic defect in the *chronic afferent loop syndrome* is intermittent obstruction of the limb after eating. Although the causes of obstruction may be diverse (retroanastomotic hernia, anastomotic kinking, adhesions, stomal obstruction, and volvulus of the afferent limb), the syndrome is almost always associated with the presence of a long (greater than 30–40 cm) afferent loop which has been anastomosed to the residual gastric pouch in an antecolic, antiperistaltic, manner using a Hofmeister valve.[24] Typically, patients complain of epigastric fullness and crampy abdominal pain shortly after the ingestion of a meal. The symptoms are readily relieved by vomiting. The vomitus is usually projectile and almost invariably contains bile but no food.

The pathogenesis of the chronic form of the syndrome correlates closely with the clinical picture. After eating, stimulation of hepatobiliary and pancreatic secretion results in the delivery of large volumes of bile and pancreatic juice to the duodenum. In the presence of partial or complete obstruction of the afferent loop, regardless of etiology, the limb rapidly distends, resulting in epigastric discomfort and cramping. Once the pressure in the loop is great enough to overcome the obstruction, it decompresses into the stomach, resulting in projectile vomiting and the immediate relief of symptoms. The vomitus lacks food because the ingested meal has already passed into the efferent limb.

Chronic afferent loop obstruction may be aggravated by the development of the blind loop syndrome. In this condition, bacteria characteristic of colonic flora proliferate in the static afferent limb with a variety of untoward results: bacteria compete for and bind vitamin B_{12}, resulting in systemic deficiency and megaloblastic anemia; they also deconjugate bile acids, resulting in inefficient micellization of fat which, in turn, produces steatorrhea; finally, deconjugated bile acids can cause diarrhea because of their capacity to inhibit water absorption in the colon. Thus, in severe cases, malnutrition, volume deficits, and anemia may be encountered.

The *acute form of afferent loop obstruction* occurs early (one to two days) after operation and is far less common than the chronic form, a fortunate circumstance because it is also far more lethal. This is so because the acute form is the consequence of complete blockage of the afferent limb, resulting in a closed-loop type of obstruction. Initially, the patient's complaints are nondescript, consisting of constant abdominal pain, most severe in the epigastric region and occasionally radiating to the back. Vomiting is common, but the volume of vomitus is usually small and it may not contain bile. The only specific physical finding is a palpable abdominal mass, which is found in fewer than one third of cases.[24] Delay in diagnosis is common. Not only is the physical examination of the postoperative patient difficult to interpret, but the condition is also often misdiagnosed as postoperative pancreatitis. Indeed, pancreatic inflammation and hyperamylasemia are commonly seen, because the increased hydrostatic pressure in the obstructed loop may cause reflux of duodenal content into the pancreatic duct and may drive intraluminal amylase into the systemic circulation. As the obstruction persists, the afferent loop may strangulate with catastrophic results.

Diagnosis

Although the diagnosis of the chronic afferent loop syndrome can be strongly suspected on clinical grounds alone, documentation of the abnormality is often difficult. A dilated afferent limb is seen on plain films of the abdomen in only 25% of instances.[24] Similarly, routine contrast studies are nonspecific, since the afferent loop frequently fails to fill with barium in asymptomatic postgastrectomy patients. Upper endoscopy may be helpful in suggesting the diagnosis if the endoscopist has difficulty visualizing the afferent limb.

A variety of more specific diagnostic maneuvers has been devised. One such test estimates the amount of bile found in the efferent loop. After passing a nasogastric tube into the limb, the patient is given a liquid fatty meal.[25] Limb content is then intermittently aspirated. In normal individuals, bile should always be found in the aspirate. In the presence of afferent loop obstruction, however, the aspirate consists of fatty meal only, until decompression through vomiting occurs, at which time bile reappears in the efferent limb.[25] It has

been suggested recently that hepatocystic radionuclide imaging techniques may be helpful. Following administration of the nuclide and satisfactory visualization of the hepatobiliary tree, the patient is given either a fatty meal or cholecystokinin. The radionuclide is then rapidly excreted into the afferent limb, where in the presence of obstruction it fails to pass either into the stomach or into the distal bowel until the obstruction is relieved. Although promising, only limited experience as yet has been gained with this methodology. A provocative test using exogenous secretin and cholecystokinin to reproduce symptoms has also been described, but its specificity and sensitivity are unknown.[26] In contrast, the concomitant presence of a blind loop syndrome can be confirmed readily using standard laboratory techniques. A Schilling test is first performed, assessing urinary excretion of radiolabeled vitamin B_{12}. The addition of intrinsic factor will not normalize the Schilling test under these circumstances; however, a brief (three- to six-day) course of a broad-spectrum antibiotic, usually tetracycline, will decrease intestinal flora sufficiently so that absorption of B_{12} returns toward normal.

Treatment

The presence of both the acute and chronic form of the afferent loop syndrome is an indication for operation. In most instances, an excessively long afferent limb is the root cause of the obstruction. The most expeditious and successful method of correcting this problem is to eliminate the loop. A variety of procedures have been devised to accomplish this, including conversion of the gastrojejunostomy to a gastroduodenostomy and the creation of a distal Braun enteroenterostomy.[24] In the experience of the authors, the creation of a long limb Roux loop with implantation of the afferent limb 45 cm distal to the gastroenteric anastomosis has been associated with an excellent outcome and is currently our procedure of choice. The existence of the acute afferent loop syndrome may present special problems because, if the loop is gangrenous, a pancreaticoduodenectomy is required. Fortunately, this situation is rarely encountered.

EFFERENT LOOP OBSTRUCTION

The efferent limb of a gastrojejunostomy may also obstruct. As with the acute form of afferent loop obstruction, efferent limb obstruction usually occurs in the immediate postoperative period. In contrast to the acute form, however, the pain associated with efferent loop obstruction is less well localized, is colicky, and is associated with copious, bilious vomiting. In addition, the abdomen is usually distended, and a mass is rarely felt. The most common cause of efferent loop obstruction is herniation of the limb behind the anastomosis in a right-to-left direction.[24] On occasion, the hernia may obstruct the afferent limb as well, in which instance bilious vomiting will be absent. The herniated segment of bowel is usually jejunum; however, more distal bowel may also act as the lead point.

Diagnosis of efferent loop obstruction may be difficult. Abdominal x-rays are often normal, particularly if the obstruction is at the level of the jejunum. Contrast studies may be helpful if barium fails to fill the efferent limb. Upper endoscopy appears to be of little value. Operative therapy is almost always indicated. If, as is usually the case, a retroanastomotic hernia is found, this must be reduced by pushing the bowel back through the neck of the hernia. It is then essential that the retroanastomotic space is securely closed. With such an approach, recurrence of this rare condition is distinctly unusual.

ALKALINE REFLUX GASTRITIS

Epigastric pain associated with bilious vomiting as a sequel of gastric surgery is a clinical problem as old as the discipline itself: Billroth reported a case in 1885.[27] Seventy years later, the pathophysiology of chronic intermittent obstruction of the afferent limb was delineated. Thereafter, the afferent loop syndrome was usually deemed responsible for these symptoms. In 1965, however, Toye and Williams[28] challenged this concept. They demonstrated that when the duodenal content from a patient who had suffered from bilious vomiting and epigastric pain for years following gastrectomy with Billroth II reconstruction was instilled into the residual stomach, the patient's symptoms were regularly and predictably reproduced. To shunt content away from the pouch, an isoperistaltic loop was interposed between stomach and duodenum, and the patient was "delighted with the result."

Subsequently, numerous series have appeared in the surgical literature suggesting that excessive reflux of upper intestinal content into the residual gastric pouch after gastrectomy or pyloroplasty is responsible for a specific complex, now commonly referred to as alkaline reflux gastritis. A recent review of more than 300 patients described in the largest and/or best studied of these series indicates that two most common presenting complaints were abdominal pain (89%) and vomiting (94%).[29-38] The vomitus was described as bilious in 62% of instances.[39] Signs said to be specific included a decreased capacity of the residual stomach to secrete HCl (*alkaline* gastric content), endoscopic gastritis associated with bile *reflux*, histologic *gastritis*, weight loss, and anemia. Most important, none of the patients to whom the diagnosis was assigned had evidence of recurrent ulcer, afferent or efferent loop obstruction, or cholelithiasis, findings which emphasize the exclusionary nature of the diagnosis.

In the majority of patients, the index procedure consisted of gastric resection with restoration of GI continuity as a Billroth II gastrojejunostomy. The syndrome was encountered less frequently in patients reconstructed as a Billroth I gastroduodenostomy and in patients undergoing truncal vagotomy with drainage. The addition of vagotomy to resection appeared to be of little consequence, since equivalent numbers of resected patients developed the syndrome without concomitant vagal interruption. The exact incidence of the syndrome is unknown, but is probably fewer than 3% of all patients undergoing gastric surgery. Parenthetically, it is for this reason that primary reconstruction via a Roux-en-Y limb following gastrectomy is not usually advised; the risk of marginal ulceration likely outweighs any anticipated benefit. In the series reviewed, a wide variety of operative procedures was employed to shunt upper intestinal content away from the residual gastric pouch.[29-38] Of these, creation of a Roux-en-Y limb ranging from 10 to 80 cm was the most popular. Although the results reported may represent the expectation of the surgeon

as much as the experience of the patient, they were quite salutary: satisfactory to excellent in more than 80% of instances.

Unfortunately, more recent and more carefully analyzed reports have failed to substantiate these results. In one study, only two thirds of patients subjected to remedial operation had complete or even partial relief of symptoms.[30] Furthermore, when symptomatic, endoscopic, or histologic predictors of success or failure were sought, few could be reliably identified on a statistical basis. In fact, outcome seemed almost random in this regard. In a second study, even worse outcomes were reported; only 47% of patients achieved a satisfactory result from diversion.[33] Those with impaired gastric emptying preoperatively fared especially poorly, undoubtedly because, as previously indicated, a Roux limb can itself cause marked and troublesome delays in gastric emptying.[17] This is particularly true if concomitant vagus section is performed. It is also increasingly apparent that the objective indices that many accept as being specific for the syndrome may not be as specific as previously claimed. The typical endoscopic findings of mucosal edema and erythema almost invariably disappear following diversion, but, as noted, patients do not invariably improve. In those who do, the histologic features of the residual gastric pouch have been reported to revert toward normal, to remain the same, or to worsen, depending upon the histologic criteria used. The capacity of the residual gastric pouch to secrete HCl, bile staining of the mucosa, even the demonstration of enterogastric reflux during endoscopy are equally inaccurate predictors of outcome. Given these ambiguities and discrepancies, it is not surprising that many have questioned the postulated pathophysiology of the syndrome, and some doubt its very existence.

At the heart of the controversy lie two basic questions. The first is: Does exposure of gastric mucosa to upper intestinal content on a chronic basis result in the development of gastritis? Experimental and clinical evidence exists to suggest that the answer to the question is almost certainly "yes." When acid peptic secreting mucosa is interposed into the proximal jejunum in the form of a pouch, it rapidly and predictably develops an active atrophic gastritis.[40] In contrast, pouch mucosa exposed to its own endogenous secretions remains histologically normal.[40] It is noteworthy that these experimental alterations are worsened in the absence of the antrum and its trophic hormone, gastrin.[41] Furthermore, a recent clinical study of postgastrectomy patients demonstrated that a strong correlation exists between intragastric bile-acid concentration and the severity of histologic gastritis in biopsies obtained from a constant location away from the region of the gastroenteric anastomosis.[42] Following conversion to a Roux, all patients demonstrated a significant improvement in the appearance of the gastric mucosa. The factors in upper intestinal content responsible for these alterations have not been completely identified, although the bile acids and lysolecithin are reasonable candidates.[43-46] Whether or not gastritis, per se, is in any way responsible for the typical symptoms of the syndrome is unknown.

The second and more important question is this: Does a relationship exist between excessive enterogastric reflux and symptoms? It is important to recognize that mild, burning epigastric pain and bilious vomiting are the only symptoms regularly induced when endogenous upper intestinal content from typically symptomatic patients is instilled into their residual stomach or are predictably relieved when reflux has been quantitatively eliminated by operation. Using these symptoms as an end point, several studies do, in fact, indicate that a rough correlation exists between their presence and greater than normal enterogastric reflux.[42, 47–49] For example, in one study, the finding of a net bile acid reflux of greater than 120 μM per hour was said to be 100% sensitive and specific for patients with epigastric pain coupled with "bile regurgitation."[49] Similarly, in the second study, all patients with the principal complaints of epigastric pain and bilious vomiting demonstrated significantly elevated intragastric bile acid concentration both in recumbency and postprandially.[42] In seven of nine additional patients whose pain was unassociated with bile vomiting, however, the magnitude of enterogastric reflux was not significantly different from that observed in asymptomatic postgastrectomy subjects.[47, 48]

An alternative approach to the question under consideration is to determine the effect of quantitative elimination of reflux on symptoms. Three studies have adopted this approach.[42, 50, 51] In one, a five- to thirteen-fold decrease in intragastric bile acid concentration resulted in partial symptomatic improvement in 12 of 13 patients.[51] A second study clearly demonstrated that a 45-cm Roux limb completely eliminated reflux of bile acids and that, concomitantly, epigastric pain and bilious vomiting were abolished.[42] In a third study, a Roux limb of similar length reduced net bile acid reflux to less than 120 μM per hour in 16 subjects.[50] Of the eleven who had demonstrated a net reflux per hour greater than that amount preoperatively, ten experienced marked symptomatic improvement compared to only one patient of the five with a preoperative value less than that amount. It requires reemphasis that the only symptoms regularly affected were those of mild continuous epigastric pain, bile regurgitation, and bilious vomiting. Finally, it has been demonstrated that instillation of autologous upper intestinal content from typically symptomatic patients is capable of reproducing symptoms in most, whereas instillation of normal saline usually elicits no response.[52] Taken together, these data are sufficiently compelling to suggest that the existence of the syndrome, as well as its postulated relationship to reflux, should not be dismissed out of hand. Without doubt, the syndrome has been overdiagnosed, symptoms ascribed to reflux have been uncritically defined, and objective indices of reflux have been sought too infrequently. Nevertheless, it is difficult to ignore the objective information available or to discount completely the widespread clinical impression that a substantial number of patients have improved with remedial operation.

Diagnosis

For the reasons indicated above, only those individuals complaining of mild, continuous, burning epigastric pain associated with nausea and bilious vomiting should be considered as potential candidates for remedial operation. An assiduous search for other causes of epigastric pain and vomiting must be undertaken, including scintigraphic assessment of the rate of gastric emptying of solid food. This is of critical importance, because a poor result is virtually guaranteed when a patient with delayed gastric emptying is converted to a Roux.

Endoscopy is often helpful in evaluating the presumed effects of reflux: mucosal erythema involving more than the peristomal region (i.e., most, if not all, of the surface area of the residual gastric pouch) coupled with mucosal biopsies of the mid-portion of the pouch to assess histology. Mucosal bile staining and endoscopically observed enterogastric reflux should be ignored, as they probably represent artifacts of endoscopy. Most important, direct assessment of reflux should be sought by determining intragastric bile acid concentration and content on at least two occasions, and by developing an enterogastric reflux index using technetium Tc 99m sulfur colloid.[42, 53] The methods for accomplishing both are well described. Normal values for asymptomatic postgastrectomy patients have also been published.[42]

Treatment

In patients deemed to have "excessive" reflux, a several-month trial of nonoperative therapy should be undertaken if not previously attempted. The regimen should include cimetidine, aluminum-containing antacids (they absorb bile salts), and, in patients who can tolerate the drug, metoclopromide, which is designed to enhance gastric clearance of refluxate.[39] The use of cholestyramine to bind bile acids should be discouraged, as it is demonstrably impotent. An occasional patient may respond to the regimen outlined, but its efficacy has not been overly impressive.[39] When operative therapy is required, the preferred approach is to create a 45-cm Roux limb.[39] If previous vagus section has been undertaken and is shown to be complete, the stoma is left undisturbed, if it is patent.[39] If vagus section is required, however, considerable delay in gastric emptying can be anticipated postoperatively.[39] Therefore, if stoma diameter is less than 3–4 cm at the time of operation, it may be advisable to revise the anastomosis to a Pólya gastrojejunostomy coincident with fashioning the Roux.[39] In view of the substantial vagaries that surround this supposed disease entity, such a rigorous approach to diagnosis and management seems most appropriate and, in our hands, has brought salutary results: improvement in histologic gastritis, recovery of the capacity to secrete HCl, and permanent elimination of reflux. Complications have been few (marginal ulceration, significant delays in gastric emptying), bilious vomiting has been completely eliminated, and two thirds of patients remain free of epigastric pain at least three years postoperatively.[39]

EARLY SATIETY

Early satiety, also known as the small-stomach syndrome, is the consequence of excessive loss of gastric reservoir function. The greater the magnitude of resection, the greater the likelihood the syndrome will develop. Characteristically, patients complain of an extremely unpleasant sensation of fullness after ingesting only small amounts of food. Vomiting usually ensues if the patient attempts to increase oral intake. In severe cases, only small liquid meals are tolerable. Anemia and malnutrition frequently develop in such instances.

Pathophysiology

Both the proximal and distal portions of the stomach play an important role in initiating digestion. Following ingestion of a bolus of food, the proximal stomach dilates to receive it, a vagally mediated process known as receptive relaxation. Distention is accomplished without increasing intragastric pressure, a property of the proximal stomach known as accommodation in which the vagus also plays a part. The distal stomach serves to mix and grind solid food, ultimately delivering ingesta to the duodenum as small particles in isotonic solution. This process is controlled by a proximal pacemaker and by the vagus nerves. Following extensive resection, particularly if combined with vagotomy, all of these properties are lost, with the end result that even small amounts of solid food greatly increase intragastric pressure, which, in turn, produces the sensation of epigastric fullness.

Treatment

The principal difficulty experienced by patients with early satiety is maintenance of adequate nutrition. A variety of nonoperative measures has been advocated, including the use of frequent small feedings, largely liquid diets, and even parenteral or enteral nutrition. None has achieved conspicuous success or patient acceptance. In fact, it has been estimated that early satiety is the postgastrectomy syndrome most refractory to nonoperative therapy. When operation is undertaken, the aim of the procedure should be to create an adequate substitute gastric reservoir. Both doubly plicated and triply plicated pouches, interposed between stomach and intestine, are available for this purpose and have proved reasonably satisfactory in the long term if the initial resection was extensive.[54] An alternative is to use a reservoir jejunal interposition with an isoperistaltic conduit, as described by Cuschieri.[55] On median follow-up of more than four years, improvement in hemoglobin and serum albumin levels was noted in all patients. However, only one third were capable of achieving ideal body weight, and no patient was rendered symptom free. The most common residual symptoms were heartburn and postprandial epigastric fullness (the symptoms for which the procedure was undertaken in the first place). Fortunately, these appeared to improve somewhat with metaclopramide therapy.

It is apparent that no surgical procedure can completely ameliorate the symptoms of early satiety. The best treatment of the syndrome is to avoid it in the first place.

POSTVAGOTOMY DIARRHEA

Increase in stool frequency may be experienced by as many as 30% of patients following transection of the vagus nerves.[2] Fortunately, the condition is either self-limiting or easily managed nonoperatively in the majority of instances. Four main varieties have been distinguished.[56] The first and most common occurs in the immediate postoperative period. Patients experience urgency followed by loose watery motions two to eight times per day. This form of diarrhea usually subsides spontaneously within a few months of operation. The second form is similar to the first except that resolution of the problem does not occur. This constant form of diarrhea can be incapacitating and is difficult to treat. A third variety takes the form of episodic attacks occurring at one- to three-month intervals and lasting a few days only. Between attacks, bowel movements are normal. It is not uncommon for patients with this variant of diarrhea to experience a prodromal syndrome

which is clinically similar to a mild virus infection. The fourth form of postvagotomy diarrhea is also intermittent but, in contrast to the third, it occurs without warning. The patient experiences sudden urgency, explosive incontinence, and soiling. Again, bowel movements are normal between attacks.

Pathophysiology

Although disabling diarrhea is relatively uncommon after vagotomy, its pathogenesis has elicited considerable interest. It seems reasonably clear that interruption of cholinergic innervation to some or all of the GI tract is, in some way, responsible for a type of diarrhea which is distinct from that associated with dumping. For example, in the Leeds/York Trial, 7% of patients developed diarrhea following subtotal gastrectomy compared to 23% who underwent resection of the same magnitude but in whom a truncal vagotomy was added.[57-59] It is also clear that afflicted patients are not psychiatrically disabled, do not have sprue, and are not lactase deficient.[60, 61] Beyond these observations, however, little agreement exists as to the pathophysiology of the syndrome.

Overgrowth of bacteria in the upper GI tract has frequently been proposed as one cause of postvagotomy diarrhea. Indeed, several studies indicate that colonization of the jejunum with aerobic and anaerobic bacteria is common following vagotomy; unfortunately, no differences in this regard have been observed between vagotomized patients with diarrhea and those who are symptom free.[62] A reduction in epithelial enzyme content in the small bowel and a decrease in mesenteric blood flow have also been proposed as mechanisms but are unlikely to be involved, since alterations in these parameters are transient and disappear within several months of vagus section.[63]

The possibility that denervation of the extrahepatic biliary tree or of the intestine might be responsible has received much attention. It has been shown in dogs, for example, that the "damming" effect of the ileocecal valve is lost following truncal vagotomy, permitting small intestinal content to move rapidly into the colon.[64] Whether this is of any consequence and, if so, whether a similar circumstance occurs in man is unknown. It has also been suggested that the denervated gallbladder, which is atonic and discoordinate, may play a role by delivering large quantities of bile salts into the small intestine at a time when maximal admixture between chyme and bile cannot be achieved. Unabsorbed bile salts enter the colon, where they are deconjugated and dehydroxylated, resulting in inhibition of water absorption. Under these conditions, cholecystectomy should ameliorate postvagotomy diarrhea.[65] It does not: removal of the gallbladder usually aggravates the problem.[63]

If, in fact, extragastric visceral denervation is responsible for postvagotomy diarrhea, preservation of cholinergic innervation to these organs should reduce or eliminate the complaint. Early clinical reports suggested that this was the case. Selective vagotomy, in which only the stomach is denervated, appeared to provide significantly greater protection against severe diarrhea than did truncal vagotomy. However, subsequent trials involving larger numbers of patients indicated a similar incidence of diarrhea following both types of vagus section.[56] Of parenthetical interest is the assertion by Burge and co-workers[66] that diarrhea can be eliminated by performing a total vagotomy of the right (celiac) vagus and a selective vagotomy of the left (hepatic) vagus (a claim that has never been independently corroborated).

Nevertheless, owing to the therapeutic efficacy of the cholestyramine in postvagotomy diarrhea, it is certain that the bile acids are somehow involved in the pathogenesis of the problem, most probably by virtue of their capacity to inhibit colonic water absorption. A variety of postvagotomy alterations in bile acid metabolism has been identified: the total body pool of taurocholate is reduced, while the fractional deconjugation and dehydroxylation rates of the bile acid are increased; total bile salt excretion in the feces of vagotomized patients is significantly greater than in normal individuals (although no differences have been found between those with and those without diarrhea); when individual bile acids are measured, a highly significant increase in the excretion of deconjugated chenodeoxycholic acid, a secondary (dehydroxylated) bile acid, is noted in afflicted patients; significantly, the effect of deconjugated secondary bile acids on colon function is far more profound than that of their conjugated primary counterparts.[64] All of these findings are compatible with excessive bacterial overgrowth in a relatively static denervated small intestine. As noted previously, however, the single study addressing this problem found no differences between patients with and without diarrhea.[62] In our opinion, these studies require repetition using modern bacteriologic techniques and H_2 breath analysis.

Treatment

In only 5%–10% of cases of postvagotomy diarrhea will symptoms be severe enough to require active intervention. The mainstay of nonoperative therapy is the bile salt binding agent cholestyramine. Cholestyramine is an anionic exchange resin which adsorbs bile salts, rendering them unabsorbable and inactive. Compared to placebo, the active drug significantly decreases urgency, frequency, and severity of diarrhea in vagotomized subjects.[67] Initially, the patient is given 4 gm with each meal. As early withdrawal is almost invariably followed by recurrence, and a prolonged course at these dosages (at least 12 weeks) is required, after which reduction can be attempted until an appropriate maintenance dose is found. Long-term cholestyramine therapy is not without hazard. Prothrombin times may be elevated, megaloblastic anemia due to folate deficiency may develop, and constipation is common.[61]

Remedial surgery is reserved for that small group of patients (approximately 1% of all those undergoing vagotomy) who, despite cholestyramine therapy, continue to suffer from incapacitating diarrhea for at least one year following the initial operation. Although an occasional good result has been reported following pyloric reconstruction, the procedure of choice is to interpose a 10-cm reversed jejunal segment 70 to 90 cm from the ligament of Treitz.[68] When segments of this length are used, most patients experience immediate and sustained relief from diarrhea without evidence of intestinal obstruction. The efficacy of this approach may be related to the fact that the reversed segment decreases the intestinal transit time, allowing for better admixture between chyme and pancreaticobiliary secretions, which, in turn, reduces the amount of bile salt delivered to the colon.

MISCELLANEOUS CONDITIONS
Metabolic Abnormalities

The excretion of greater than normal amounts of fat in the stool is relatively common following all types of operative procedures designed to attack the peptic ulcer diathesis. In most instances, the absolute magnitude of fecal fat loss is small and of no clinical consequence. In a few cases, however, fat malabsorption may lead to a fatty acid-induced diarrhea and to significant deficiencies in fat-soluble vitamin uptake. Steatorrhea may be the consequence either of inadequate micellization of ingested fat or to the development of the blind loop syndrome. When the latter is suspected, it must be treated as outlined above. Otherwise, therapy consists of feeding median-chain triglycerides, which do not require emulsification and micellization for absorption.

Resective procedures of the stomach in particular may be associated with the development of osteomalacia. Clinically, afflicted patients exhibited a negative calcium balance, increases in serum ATPase and hypophosphatemia. Steatorrhea is an important predisposing condition because free fatty acids bind calcium, rendering it unabsorbable, and because fat malabsorption results in hypovitaminosis D. In severe cases, spontaneous fractures may develop. Most patients can be adequately treated by increasing vitamin D intake.

If searched for carefully, a microcytic hypochromic anemia can be uncovered in more than 50% of patients following gastrectomy. The cause is unclear but may relate to impaired iron absorption or to subliminal blood loss from the perianastomotic region. On rare occasions, a megaloblastic anemia may develop. Maturation of red cells in marrow requires both vitamin B_{12} and folate, as these elements are essential for nucleic acid synthesis. Available intrinsic factor may be diminished, particularly in patients who have undergone a high subtotal gastrectomy, resulting in B_{12} malabsorption. Folate deficiency, which is usually a consequence of inadequate oral intake, may also contribute. Treatment consists of providing B_{12} and folate parenterally.

A few patients will develop lactose intolerance following gastrectomy. It is thought that these individuals have an intrinsic but unrecognized lactase deficiency which, for reasons that are unclear, becomes manifest only in the postoperative period. Treatment consists of avoiding lactose-containing foodstuffs.

Gastric Stump Carcinoma

It is now well established that, although infrequent, carcinoma of the gastric stump occurs in approximately 3% of patients undergoing gastrectomy. This represents a far greater incidence than that observed in age- and sex-matched patients not undergoing operation. Some series suggest that those patients whose index disease was gastric rather than duodenal ulcer are at greatest risk.[69] Males are more commonly afflicted than females, reflecting the fact that males are more commonly operated on for peptic ulcer.[69] A latent period of seven to 20 years is common. Patients usually present with symptoms indistinguishable from those of recurrent ulcer. Diagnosis is best established by endoscopy, since evaluation of the anastomosis by routine upper GI contrast studies is difficult.

In animals, the incidence of experimentally induced carcinoma is greatest following gastroenterostomy alone, less common following resection with Billroth II gastrojejunostomy, and least common following resection with Billroth I gastroduodenostomy.[69–72]

Although the pathogenesis of stump cancer remains obscure, reflux of bile acids, induction of hypochlorhydria, and ingestion of nitrates may all play a role. As noted previously, reflux of upper intestinal content into the residual gastric pouch can promote the development of an atrophic gastritis, a potentially premalignant lesion. In the face of hypochlorhydria or achlorhydria, the normally sterile upper GI tract is colonized with bacteria, particularly anaerobes, which have the capacity to convert ingested nitrates to nitrites, which, in turn, can combine with ingested protein to form potent carcinogens, the nitrosamines.[69, 70] The concomitant presence of a susceptible membrane and a potent carcinogen may be the sine qua non for the induction of malignancy. Operative therapy is mandatory; unfortunately, survival is poor, almost without exception. It is for this reason that many recommend lifelong follow-up for resected patients in an effort to detect malignancy early.

Jejunogastric Intussusception

Intussusception of the afferent or efferent limb into the residual gastric pouch is a rare (fewer than 200 cases reported) postgastrectomy condition which can occur after gastrojejunostomy, resection with Billroth II reconstruction, or creation of a Roux-en-Y limb. Two clinical variants are recognized: acute and chronic.[73] In the acute variety, the patient experiences severe, colicky, epigastric pain associated with vomiting, hematemesis, and a palpable abdominal mass. The intussusception almost invariably involves the efferent limb, and operation is mandatory to prevent its strangulation. In the chronic form, the patient experiences recurrent episodes of vague, upper abdominal discomfort which are exacerbated by meals. Generally, the pain subsides shortly after eating, coincident with reduction of the intussuscepted limb. The efferent limb is the most common intussuscipiens (80%), followed by both efferent and afferent limbs (10%) and by the afferent limb alone (10%).[73] Diagnosis is usually established by upper GI contrast studies which demonstrate an ovoid mass within the gastric lumen. In general, no effective medical treatment exists for this unusual condition.[73] Surgical options include reduction, resection, revision of the anastomosis, and takedown of the anastomosis. Fixation of the jejunum to adjacent tissue, mesocolon, colon, or stomach may be added. Under any circumstance, recurrence is rare.

Postvagotomy Dysphagia

Dysphagia is an unusual, yet well-recognized complication of bilateral vagotomy. It is more common after the transthoracic than the transabdominal approach, a consequence perhaps of denervation of the lower esophageal sphincter. Two forms are distinguished.[74] In the painless variety, the sphincter fails to relax with deglutition. The second form, dysphagia combined with odynophagia, is usually associated with normal sphincter manometry and is probably a consequence of periesophageal edema or fibrosis. Symptoms usually begin within two to six weeks of vagotomy and almost always subside spontaneously.[74] In a few instances, one or two esophageal dilations may be required before complete relief is achieved.

REFERENCES

1. Silver D., McGregor F.H. Jr., Porter J.M., et al.: The mechanism of the dumping syndrome. Surg. Clin. North Am. 46:425–439, 1966.
2. Becker J.M.: Complications of gastric surgery. Prac. Gastro. 8(S4):17, 1984.
3. Roberts K.E., Randall H.T., Farr H.W., et al.: Cardiovascular and blood volume alterations resulting from intrajejunal administration of hypertonic solutions to gastrectomized patients: The relationship of these changes to the dumping syndrome. Ann. Surg. 140:631–640, 1954.
4. Betz R.: Dumping syndrome studied during maintenance of blood volume. Ann. Surg. 154:225–234, 1961.
5. Johnson L.P., Sloop R.D., Jessep J.E., et al.: Serotonin antagonists in experimental and clinical "dumping." Ann. Surg. 172:585–594, 1970.
6. Reichle F.A., Brigham M.P., Reichle R.M., et al.: The effect of gastrectomy on serotonin metabolism in the human portal vein. Ann. Surg. 172:585–594, 1970.
7. Wang P.Y., Talamo R.C., Babiori B.M., et al.: Kalli krein-kinin system in postgastrectomy dumping syndrome. Ann. Intern. Med. 80:577–581, 1974.
8. Bloom S.R., Rorpton C.M.S., Thomson J.P.S.: Enteroglucagon release in the dumping syndrome. Lancet 2:789–791, 1972.
9. Creaghe S.B., Saik R.P., Pearl J., et al.: Noninvasive vascular assessment of dumping syndrome. J. Surg. Res. 22:328–332, 1977.
10. Jenkins D.J.A., Gassull M.A., Leeds A.R., et al.: Effect of dietary fiber on complications of gastric surgery: Prevention of postprandial hypoglycemia by pectin. Gastroenterology 72:215–217, 1977.
11. Amdrup E., Jorgensen J.B.: The influence of posture on the "dumping" syndrome. Acta Chir. Scand. 112:307–312, 1956.
12. Fromm D. (ed.): Complications of Gastric Surgery. New York, John Wiley & Sons, 1977, pp. 7–34.
13. Borg I., Borgströn S.G., Haeger K.: The value of the Billroth II-Billroth I conversion operation in the treatment of the postgastrectomy syndrome. Acta Chir. Scand. 134:655–659, 1968.
14. Kennedy C.S., Reynolds R.P., Cantor M.D.: A study of the gastric stoma after partial gastrectomy. Surgery 22:41–47, 1947.
15. Henley F.A.: Gastrectomy with replacement. Br. J. Surg. 40:118, 1952.
16. Sawyers J.L., Herrington J.L. Jr.: Superiority of antiperistaltic jejunal segments in management of severe dumping syndrome. Ann. Surg. 178:311–321, 1973.
17. Hocking M.P., Vogel S.B., Falasca C.A., et al.: Delayed gastric emptying of liquids and solids following Roux-en-Y biliary diversion. Ann. Surg. 194:494–501, 1981.
18. Cranley B., Kelly K.A., Go V.L.W., et al.: Enhancing the antidumping effect of Roux gastrojejunostomy with intestinal pacing. Ann. Surg. 198:516–524, 1983.
19. T.R. Harrison (ed.): Principles of Internal Medicine. New York, McGraw-Hill Book Co., 1983.
20. Speth P.A.J., Jansen J.B.M.J., Lammers C.B.H.W.: Effect of acarbose, pectin, a combination of acarbose with pectin, and placebo on postprandial reactive hypoglycemia after gastric surgery. Gut 24:798–802, 1983.
21. Fink W.J., Heicke S.T., Gray T.W., et al.: Treatment of postoperative reactive hypoglycemia by a reversed intestinal segment. Am. J. Surg. 131:19–22, 1976.
22. Buskin F.L., Woodward E.R.: Postgastrectomy Syndromes. Philadelphia, W.B. Saunders Co., 1976, pp. 34–48.
23. Mitty W.E. Jr., Grossi C., Nealon T.F. Jr.: Chronic afferent loop syndrome. Ann. Surg. 172:996–1001, 1970.
24. Fromm D. (ed.): Complications of Gastric Surgery. New York, John Wiley & Sons, 1977, pp. 35–49.
25. Jordon G.L. Jr.: The afferent loop syndrome. Surgery 38:1027–1035, 1955.
26. Dahlgren S.: The afferent loop syndrome. Acta Chir. Scand. [Suppl.] 327:1, 1964.

27. Billroth T.: *Clinical Surgery* (translated by Dent C.T.). London, New Sydenham Society, 1885.
28. Toye D.K.M., Williams J.A.: Postgastrectomy bile vomiting. *Lancet* 1:524–526, 1965.
29. Berardi R.S., Siroospour D.L., Ruiz R., et al.: Alkaline reflux gastritis: A study in forty postoperative duodenal ulcer patients. *Am. J. Surg.* 132:552–557, 1976.
30. Boren C.H., Way L.H.: Alkaline reflux gastritis: A re-evaluation. *Am. J. Surg.* 140:40–46, 1980.
31. Buskin F.L., DeFord J.W., Wickbom G., et al.: A clinical evaluation of postoperative alkaline reflux gastritis. *Am. Surg.* 41:88–93, 1975.
32. Coppinger W.R., Job H., Delauro J.E., et al.: Surgical treatment of reflux gastritis and esophagitis. *Arch. Surg.* 106:463–468, 1973.
33. Davidson E.D., Hersh T.: The surgical treatment of bile reflux gastritis: A study of 59 patients. *Ann. Surg.* 192:175–178, 1980.
34. Drapanas T., Bethea M.: Reflux gastritis following gastric surgery. *Ann. Surg.* 179:618–627, 1974.
35. Joseph W.L., Rivers R.A., O'Kieffe D.A., et al.: Management of postoperative alkaline reflux gastritis. *Ann. Surg.* 177:655–659, 1973.
36. Sawyers J.L., Herrington J.L., Buckspan D.S.: Remedial operation for alkaline reflux gastritis and associated postgastrectomy syndromes. *Arch. Surg.* 115:519–524, 1980.
37. VanHeerden J.A., Phillips S.F., Adson M.A., et al.: Postoperative reflux gastritis. *Am. J. Surg.* 129:82–88, 1975.
38. Zimmerman G.J., Westbrook K.C., Thompson D.W.: The surgical management of reflux gastritis. *Am. J. Surg.* 132:787–789, 1976.
39. Ritchie W.P. Jr.: Alkaline reflux gastritis: A diagnosis in search of a disease. *J. Clin. Surg.* 1:414–424, 1982.
40. Cheng J., Ritchie W.P. Jr., Delaney J.P.: Atrophic gastritis: An experimental model. *Fed. Proc.* 28:513, 1969.
41. Witt T.R., Roseman D.L., Banner B.F.: The role of the gastric antrum in the pathogenesis of reflux gastritis. *J. Surg. Res.* 26:220–232, 1979.
42. Ritchie W.P. Jr.: Alkaline reflux gastritis: An objective assessment of its diagnosis and treatment. *Ann. Surg.* 192:288–298, 1980.
43. Ritchie W.P. Jr.: Role of bile acid reflux in acute hemorrhagic gastritis. *World J. Surg.* 5:189–198, 1981.
44. Delaney J.P., Cheng J.W.B., Butler B.A., et al.: Gastric ulcer and regurgitation gastritis. *Gut* 11:715–719, 1970.
45. Orehard J.P., Reynolds K., Fox B., et al.: Effect of lysolecithin on gastric mucosal structure potential difference. *Gut* 18:457–464, 1977.
46. Kivilaasko E., Ehnholm C., Kalima T.V., et al.: Duodenogastric reflux of lysolecithin in the pathogenesis of experimental porcine stress ulceration. *Surgery* 76:65–69, 1976.
47. Ludwig S., Ippoliti A.: Objective evaluation of symptomatic bile reflux after antrectomy (abstract). *Gastroenterology* 76:1187, 1979.
48. Gadacz T.R., Zuidema G.D.: Bile acid composition in patients with and without symptoms of postoperative reflux gastritis. *Am. J. Surg.* 135:48–52, 1978.
49. Hoare A.M., Keighley M.R.B., Starkey B., et al.: Measurement of bile acids in fasting gastric aspirates: An objective test for bile reflux after gastric surgery. *Gut* 19:166–169, 1978.
50. Hoare A.M., McLeish A., Thompson H., et al.: Selection of patients for bile diversion surgery: Use of bile acid measurement in fasting gastric aspirates. *Gut* 19:163–165, 1978.
51. Malagelada J.R., Phillips S.F., Higgins J.A., et al.: A prospective evaluation of alkaline reflux gastritis: Bile acid binding agents and Roux-Y diversion (abstract). *Gastroenterology* 76:1192, 1979.
52. Meskinpour H., Marks J.W., Schoenfield L.J., et al.: Reflux gastritis syndrome: Mechanism of symptoms. *Gastroenterology* 79:1283–1287, 1980.
53. Tolin R.D., Malmud L.S., Stelzer F., et al.: Enterogastric reflux in normal subjects and patients with Billroth II gastroenterostomy. *Gastroenterology* 77:1027–1033, 1979.
54. Sawyers J.L.: Surgical management of postgastrectomy syndrome. *J. Miss. State Assoc.* 14:281–284, 1974.
55. Cuschieri A.: Long term evaluation of a reservoir jejunal interposition with an isoperistaltic conduit in the management of patients with small stomach syndrome. *Br. J. Surg.* 69:386–388, 1982.
56. Fromm D. (ed.): *Complications of Gastric Surgery.* New York, John Wiley & Sons, 1977, pp. 67–75.
57. Goligher J.C., Pulvertaft C.N., Irwin T.T., et al.: Five to eight years results of truncal vagotomy and pyloroplasty for duodenal ulcer. *Br. Med. J.* 1:7, 1972.
58. Goligher J.C., Pulvertaft C.N., DeDombal F.T., et al.: Five to eight years results of Leeds/York controlled trial of elective surgery for duodenal ulcer. *Br. Med. J.* 2:781, 1968.
59. Goligher J.C., Pulvertaft C.N., DeDombal F.T., et al.: Clinical comparison of vagotomy and pyloroplasty with other forms of elective surgery for duodenal ulcer. *Br. Med. J.* 2:787, 1968.
60. Johnstone E.C., Allan J.C., Geraghty B.P., et al.: Psychiatric disturbance and postvagotomy diarrhea. *J. Psychosom. Res.* 18:205–208, 1974.
61. Duncombe V.M., Bolin T.D., Davis A.E.: Double-blind trial of cholestyramine in postvagotomy diarrhea. *Gut* 18:531–535, 1977.
62. Browning G.G., Buchan K.A., Mackay C.: Clinical and laboratory study of postvagotomy diarrhea. *Gut* 15:644–653, 1974.
63. Ballinger W.F. II: Postvagotomy changes in the small intestine. *Am. J. Surg.* 114:382–387, 1967.
64. Allan J.C., Gerskovitch V.P., Russell R.I.: The role of bile acids in the pathogenesis of postvagotomy diarrhea. *Br. J. Surg.* 61:516–518, 1974.
65. Condon J.R., Robinson V., Suleman A.L.I., et al.: The cause and treatment of postvagotomy diarrhea. *Br. J. Surg.* 62:309–312, 1975.
66. Burge H., Lond M.B., Hutchinson J.S.F.: Selective nerve section in the prevention of postvagotomy diarrhea. *Lancet* 1:577–579, 1964.
67. Ayulo J.A.: Cholestyramine in postvagotomy syndrome. *Am. J. Gastroenterol.* 57:207–225, 1972.
68. Herrington J.L., Edwards W.H., Carter J.H., et al.: Treatment of severe postgastrectomy diarrhea by reversed jejunal segment. *Ann. Surg.* 168:522–541, 1968.
69. Orlando R. III, Welsh J.R.: Carcinoma of the stomach after gastric operation. *Am. J. Surg.* 114:487–491, 1981.
70. Eherlein T.J., Lorenzo F.V., Webster M.V.: Gastric carcinoma following operation for peptic ulcer disease. *Ann. Surg.* 187:251–256, 1978.
71. Domellof L., Jananger K.G.: The risk for gastric carcinoma after partial gastrectomy. *Am. J. Surg.* 134:581, 1977.
72. Papachristou D.N., Agnanti N., Fortner J.G.: Gastric carcinoma after treatment of ulcer. *Am. J. Surg.* 139:193–196, 1980.
73. Wait J.O., Beart R.W., Jr., Charboneau W.: Jejunogastric intussusception. *Arch. Surg.* 115:1449–1452, 1980.
74. Anderson H.A., Schlegel J.F., Olsen A.M.: Postgastrectomy dysphagia. Reprinted from *Gastrointest. Endosc.* May 1966.

PART IV

Gallbladder-Biliary Tract Disease

19

Gallstones and Cholecystitis

LAWRENCE DENBESTEN, M.D.
JOEL J. ROSLYN, M.D.

INTRODUCTION
Background

Overview

The management of human gallstone disease had its humble beginning over 1,500 years ago, when a Greek physician, Alexander Trallianus, first noted calculi within the hepatic radicals of a human liver.[1] Since that time, the many treatment recommendations for this most common of intra-abdominal disorders have paralleled our evolving understanding of the pathogenesis of cholelithiasis. The student of history may note that the cycle of management for gallstone disease has completed a full circle. The earliest attempts at therapy for gallstone disease were medical and included the prevention of bile stasis within the gallbladder by drinking spa waters that were rich in magnesium sulfate.[1] During that period, surgical intervention for gallstone disease was rarely considered. The only operative procedure available was cholecystolithotomy, and even this was not attempted unless there was definite evidence of adherence between the gallbladder and abdominal wall.

Successful elective cholecystostomy was first performed by an Indiana surgeon, John S. Bobbs, in 1867.[2] The modern era of biliary surgery was ushered in by a German surgeon, Carl Langenbuch, who in 1882 performed the first successful cholecystectomy.[3] During the past 100 years, cholecystectomy has remained the "gold standard" for the management of gallstone disease.

Recently, considerable time and effort have been expended in the evaluation of new ways to dissolve or to prevent gallstones. Most of these efforts have been aimed at cholesterol gallstones, which are the most prevalent type in the United States. The numerous agents tested for the dissolution of gallstones have had varying degrees of success. Interest in gallbladder stasis as an etiologic factor in the pathogenesis of cholesterol gallstones has been renewed and has prompted studies to evaluate the role of periodic gallbladder emptying as a means of reducing the incidence of gallstone formation. This concept has been verified in experimental models[4, 5] and awaits confirmation in humans at high risk for the formation of stones.

The history of gallstone disease and the evolution of its management illustrate the principle that improved patient care can be achieved through a better appreciation of the pathophysiology of disease processes. With our current understanding of the important roles of altered hepatic bile composition and gallbladder motility in the pathogenesis of gallstone disease, new therapeutic options for the management of this common disease will almost certainly be forthcoming.

Incidence

Gallstone disease is an international health problem of varying proportions throughout the world. The incidence of cholelithiasis in the United States is reported to be 10%. In addition to these 20 million people, another 800,000 new cases are discovered annually. The higher incidence of gallstone disease in women persists until the seventh or eighth decade of life, when it approaches 20% in both sexes. The myth that most patients with gallstone disease are "female, fat, forty, and fertile" is an oversimplification. Cholesterol and noncholesterol stones occur in both children and adults and in a variety of clinical settings. The incidence of cholelithiasis is particularly high in Indians of the Southwestern United States. A recent study revealed a 73% incidence of gallstones in Pima Indian females between the ages of 25 and 34 years.[6] For reasons that are still not clear, the incidence of cholelithiasis also varies greatly among countries. In certain African countries, for example, the incidence of gallstones is lower than 5%.[7] In contrast, the incidence and variety of gallstone disease constitutes a problem of considerable magnitude throughout the Far East. Traditionally, calcium bilirubinate stones were considered to be the predominant type of stone found in this region. In recent years, the incidence of pigment stones has steadily decreased, while that of cholesterol stones has increased.

An unfortunate byproduct of our advancing medical technology has been an increased incidence of both calculous and acalculous gallbladder disease in certain clinical settings. With our improved ability to care for the critically ill patient has come an increased incidence of acalculous cholecystitis, as well as a new clinical entity, total parenteral nutrition (TPN)-induced gallbladder disease.

Gallstone Classification

Although the color, size, shape, and configuration of gallstones are myriad, there are essentially three basic types: (1)

cholesterol; (2) pigment; and (3) mixed cholesterol and pigment stones. Using this simple classification, approximately 10% of all stones are pure cholesterol stones, 15% are pigment stones, and the remaining 75% are mixed. The unique composition of gallstones from an individual patient is a manifestation of the varying etiologies. The number, size, and shape of gallstones vary from patient to patient and are determined by factors that have not yet been elucidated. Irregularly shaped or faceted stones usually are seen with multiple stones as a result of contact between individual stones.

Biliary Physiology

Composition of Normal Bile

Normal bile is a complex solution which is isotonic with plasma and is composed primarily of water, electrolytes, and organic solutes. The three main solutes accounting for 80% of the dry weight of bile are bile salts, cholesterol, and phospholipids. Normally these substances are fully solubilized in bile. The primary bile acids, chenodeoxycholic acid and cholic acid, are synthesized from cholesterol and then conjugated with taurine or glycine in the liver. Most of the cholesterol found in bile is synthesized de novo in the liver, and dietary cholesterol contributes an insignificant amount to this pool. More than 90% of the phospholipid content found in human bile is lecithin.[8] The hepatic synthesis and the biliary secretion of lecithin is coupled with the hepatic secretion and enterohepatic circulation of bile acids.

A critical factor in the normal physiology, as well as in cholesterol gallstone formation, is the solubilization of cholesterol in bile. Cholesterol is virtually insoluble in a water medium and is therefore dependent on some other mechanism for its solubilization. The key to maintaining cholesterol in solution is the formation of mixed bile acid-lecithin-cholesterol micelles. Bile acids are amphipathic compounds containing both hydrophilic polar groups and hydrophobic nonpolar portions. In very dilute solution, bile acids exist as individual ionized molecules. However, when the bile acid concentration is above a certain level, the critical micellar concentration, the molecules tend to aggregate in small clusters, with the more polar hydrophilic group oriented outward and the hydrophobic group inward. The ability of a pure bile acid micelle to solubilize cholesterol is greatly enhanced by the incorporation of lecithin into the micellar structure. Water penetrates the crystalline structure of lecithin, causing swelling of the micelle. This mixed micelle is now capable of transporting cholesterol within the hydrophobic center and facilitates cholesterol solubilization (Fig 19–1).

Cholesterol solubility in bile is dependent on the relative concentration of cholesterol, bile acids, and lecithin. In a series of clinical and in vitro studies, Admirand and Small[9] first described the relationship between these three biliary lipids in health and during cholesterol gallstone formation. Their data on the cholesterol solubility limits in ideal solutions and in humans with and without gallstones has been displayed using triangular coordinates and is an expression of the degree of cholesterol saturation (Fig 19–2). More recently, Carey and co-workers[10] developed a mathematical model to express the limits of cholesterol solubility as influenced both by the relative concentrations of the lipid components and the total lipid

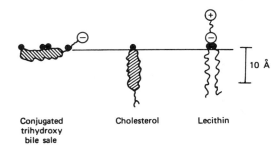

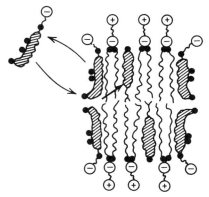

Fig 19–1.—Mixed bile acid-lecithin micelle. In the upper part of the diagram, the three lipid molecules are oriented such that their hydrophilic segments are above the line and their hydrophobic segments are below the line. Bile acids are amphiphaths and in aqueous solution form cylindrical aggregates (seen in cross section in the lower part of the diagram) wherein the hydrophilic groups point outward and the hydrophobic portion is oriented inward. Lecithin is penetrated by water and causes swelling of the micelle. Thus, cholesterol (arrow), which is virtually insoluble in water, is transported within the hydrophobic center of the mixed micelle in bile, an aqueous solution. (Courtesy of Dr. Donald Small.)

composition. A numerical value can therefore be derived for each solution to express the relative degree of cholesterol saturation or lithogenicity. This number, or lithogenic index, when greater than one, denotes a bile solution which is saturated with cholesterol. Alterations in the capacity of the mixed micelles to solubilize cholesterol occur when the relative concentration of bile acids, cholesterol, or phospholipids increases or decreases, resulting in a change in the lithogenic index of the solution.

Enterohepatic Circulation of Bile Acids

The two primary bile acids, cholic and chenodeoxycholic acid, are synthesized from cholesterol in the liver. Following conjugation with either taurine or glycine, these conjugated bile acids are then secreted by the liver into the extrahepatic biliary tract. As the result of a very efficient enterohepatic circulation, the bile acid pool is relatively stable, and in normal man, 95% of the bile acids are reabsorbed in the intestine and available for recirculation. During the interdigestive period, bile salts and other solutes are sequestered and concen-

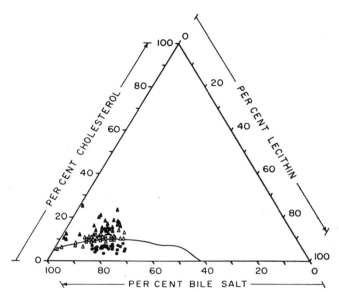

Fig 19–2.—The composition of gallbladder bile from normal subjects and patients with gallstones compared with the limits of cholesterol solubility as determined from a model system. The composition of bile from normal subjects *(closed circles)* is such that all circles fall within the micellar zone. The bile samples from patients with cholesterol or mixed gallstones in which no microcrystals were present *(open triangles)* fall on or very near the line, indicating maximum cholesterol solubilization. The biles from gallstone patients, which contain microcrystals of cholesterol *(closed triangles)*, fall well above the line of maximum saturation.

trated 20- to 30-fold in the gallbladder. During meals, cholecystokinin is released from the proximal small bowel and, in a manner not yet entirely clear, stimulates gallbladder contraction with release of bile into the small intestine. While there is some passive absorption of conjugated bile acids along the whole length of the small intestine, over 80% of these bile acids are absorbed in the terminal ileum. The remainder of the circulating bile salt pool is subject to enzymatic deconjugation by bacteria in the terminal ileum and colon. A portion of these unconjugated bile acids is also absorbed in the distal small bowel colon. Bacteria in the colon enzymatically dehydroxylate the unconjugated cholic and chenodeoxycholic acids that were not absorbed more proximally, resulting in the formation of the secondary bile acids, deoxycholic and lithocholic acids. These secondary bile acids are again partially absorbed in the colon by passive diffusion. This recycling system allows a small pool of bile salts to recirculate six to 15 times a day, with a loss of only 3%–5% of bile salts during each recirculation. There is a negative feedback system between the recirculation of bile acids and the regulation of hepatic synthesis of bile acids. In addition, bile acids are the most important regulators of hepatic synthesis and biliary secretion of lecithin.

Pathogenesis of Cholesterol Gallstones

Perspective

In recent years the focus of research on the pathogenesis of cholesterol cholelithiasis has completed a full circle,[11] one be-

gun more than 120 years ago. Early investigators implicated stasis of bile in the gallbladder as the primary etiologic factor in cholesterol gallstone formation. The description in 1968, by Admirand and Small,[9] of the physicochemical basis of cholesterol gallstone formation initiated a long series of clinical and laboratory investigations testing the hypothesis that altered hepatic secretion of biliary lipids is the primary cause of cholesterol cholelithiasis. The additional observation that humans with established cholesterol gallstones have a decreased bile salt pool size[12] suggested that alterations in the hepatic secretion of cholesterol saturated bile was a prerequisite for cholesterol gallstone formation. More recently, alterations in gallbladder motility have again become the focal point of clinical and experimental investigations. Compelling data have emerged which suggest that neither the liver nor the gallbladder alone has an exclusive etiologic role in the formation of cholesterol gallstones. Cholesterol gallstones are almost certainly the end product of a series of dynamic interactions between the liver and the extrahepatic biliary system, wherein increased biliary cholesterol alters gallbladder motility and altered motility in turn increases cholesterol concentration in hepatic bile. In addition, the experimental observations that there is altered mucus production and gallbladder absorption during early gallstone formation further suggest that the pathogenesis of this disease is multifactoral.

Cholesterol Saturation

The hepatic secretion of cholesterol supersaturated bile is a prerequisite for cholesterol gallstone formation. As stated earlier, the mathematical expressions of cholesterol saturation are based on percent molar concentrations of lecithin, cholesterol, and bile acids. A lithogenic index of 1 or greater suggests that the cholesterol content of the bile is in excess of its solubilizing capacity. Theoretically, altered secretion of any of the three biliary lipids might account for the increase in cholesterol concentration relative to bile acids and lecithin observed in subjects with cholesterol gallstones.

Current studies suggest two common causes for the secretion of cholesterol supersaturated bile: increased hepatic secretion of cholesterol and decreased secretion of bile acids. Excess hepatic cholesterol secretion has been clearly established as the cause of lithogenic bile in the increased incidence of cholesterol gallstones in obese humans.[13] In these patients bile acid secretion is also increased, but fails to keep pace with the increase in cholesterol secretion. Normal humans with established cholesterol gallstones have a decreased bile salt pool size. Early investigators suggested that this observed decrease in bile salt pool size was a cause of gallstone formation rather than an effect.[12] More recent studies in the prairie dog gallstone model demonstrate that the bile salt pool size is normal during early cholesterol gallstone formation and decreases only after the chronic presence of stones has induced physiologic, anatomical, and microscopic changes typical of chronic cholecystitis.[14] These findings suggest that the decreased bile salt pool size associated with chronic cholelithiasis is a result rather than a cause of gallstones.

Normal humans, without gallstones, secrete lithogenic bile during periods of fasting.[15] This observation suggests that factors other than saturation of bile are important in the formation of cholesterol crystals and gallstones. Recent studies have demonstrated an increased nucleation time in gallbladder bile from gallstone patients compared with nongallstone patients, despite similar lithogenic indices.[16] It would appear that there is a potent nucleating factor released by the gallbladder which induces this rapid nucleation.[17] Further studies are clearly needed to define the factors leading to cholesterol crystallization.

Gallbladder Stasis

The importance of gallbladder stasis as an etiologic factor in the pathogenesis of cholesterol gallstones was first suggested by Meckel von Helmsbach in 1856.[18] Despite the fact that gallstones form predominantly in the gallbladder, these early theories were ignored until recent times. Numerous current clinical and experimental studies have demonstrated stasis of bile within the gallbladder during gallstone formation and have suggested that stasis is the critical link between the hepatic secretion of cholesterol saturated bile and gallstone formation.

The demonstration of the significance of gallbladder stasis as an etiologic factor in the pathogenesis of gallstones has been facilitated by the development of an animal gallstone model. The prairie dog has biliary lipid composition and extrahepatic biliary physiology similar to those of humans and has been verified as a suitable model for cholesterol gallstone disease in numerous investigations.[19–21] In this model, stasis of bile in the gallbladder is present as soon as bile becomes saturated with cholesterol, antedating the presence of stones, and actually increases as stones become more well established.[22] Specific alterations in gallbladder motor function develop concurrently with biliary cholesterol crystallization but before gallstone formation. These include increased resistance to outflow through the cystic duct[23] and decreased gallbladder emptying.[24] Defects in gallbladder contractility have also been observed in other animal models during cholesterol gallstone formation.[25] Further evidence for the significance of gallbladder stasis as an etiologic factor in the pathogenesis of cholesterol gallstones comes from animal studies in which the incidence of cholelithiasis has been significantly reduced by the prevention of stasis by daily gallbladder stimulation.[4, 5]

Biliary scintigraphic studies in humans have demonstrated altered gallbladder response to cholecystokinin in gallstone patients.[26] In addition, patients with cholesterol crystals in their bile, but without gallstones, have impaired gallbladder emptying.[27] The mechanism by which gallbladder stasis promotes cholesterol gallstone formation is still the subject of continuing research. Presumably, stasis of bile within the gallbladder results in sequestration of bile acids and a reduction in the circulating bile salt pool available for cholesterol solubilization. In addition, the resultant gallbladder stasis provides an ideal milieu for the precipitation and agglomeration of cholesterol crystals and gallstone formation. Increased exposure time of the gallbladder mucosa to cholesterol-saturated bile may affect gallbladder absorptive and secretory function.

Altered Gallbladder Secretion

There is now ample evidence to suggest that there is increased gallbladder mucus secretion during experimental gallstone formation. Recent studies by Lee and co-workers[28] in-

dicate that cholesterol saturation of bile stimulates gallbladder mucus secretion and that gallbladder mucus gel is a nucleating agent for gallstone formation. Using the prairie dog gallstone model, Doty et al.[29] demonstrated that gallbladder bile mucus concentration is elevated prior to cholesterol precipitation and increases progressively with the formation of cholesterol crystals. Furthermore, these agglomerations of crystals increase cystic duct resistance resulting in gallbladder stasis. A self-perpetuating cycle of mucus hypersecretion, cholesterol crystallization and agglomeration, and gallbladder stasis ensues, culminating in the formation of gallstones. More recent studies have demonstrated that human gallbladder mucin enhances the in vitro nucleation of cholesterol crystals.[30] Pharmacologic doses of aspirin significantly reduce the incidence of gallstone formation by inhibiting mucus secretion without altering the degree of cholesterol saturation of bile.[31, 32] On the basis of these studies, it has been suggested that increased gallbladder mucus secretion may be an important etiologic factor in the pathogenesis of cholesterol gallstones.

A Unified Hypothesis for the Pathogenesis of Cholesterol Gallstones

It is now clear that the pathogenesis of cholesterol gallstones is multifactoral. Depending on the clinical situation, numerous etiologic factors are present in varying degrees and act in concert to promote the hepatic secretion of cholesterol saturated bile, gallbladder stasis, and altered gallbladder secretory function. Cholesterol supersaturated bile is a prerequisite of cholesterol gallstone formation, and supersaturation in hepatic bile may result from metabolic or genetic alterations acting directly on the hepatocyte, the enterohepatic circulation, or both. In addition, stasis of bile within the gallbladder leads to sequestration of bile acids with a resultant increase in the relative secretion of cholesterol and ultimately supersaturated bile. The presence of supersaturated bile in the gallbladder promotes stasis by mechanisms which remain unclear. Presumably there are factors present in the bile which induce gallbladder stasis as manifested by: (1) altered response to cholecystokinin, (2) increased cystic duct resistance, and (3) decreased gallbladder emptying. It also seems that factors present in cholesterol saturated bile induce gallbladder mucus hypersecretion. The combination of cholesterol supersaturated bile and the presence of increased amounts of mucus in a poorly emptying gallbladder provides an excellent milieu for nucleation and stone formation.

Pigment Gallstones

Perspective

The predominance of cholesterol gallstones in this country has traditionally relegated pigment gallstones to a second-class status. However, the recent observations that pigment gallstones form in a variety of clinical settings, heretofore unsuspected, has led to a resurgence of interest. Although early studies suggested that pigment stones accounted for only 10% of all gallstones,[33] more recent investigations suggest that this figure is closer to 30%.[34] Of interest is the shifting pattern in the Orient during the past 30 years, with a decline in the incidence of pigment vs. cholesterol stones. The realization that calcium bilirubinate stones form in patients with TPN-induced gallbladder disease[35] and in experimental animals following ileal resection[36] has led to a reevaluation of the pathogenesis of calcium bilirubinate stone formation.

Characterization of Pigment Stones

Pigment stones are not nearly as well defined as cholesterol gallstones. The broad term "pigment gallstones" encompasses a heterogeneous group with varying etiologies. In general, pigment stones are characterized by their relatively high concentration of bilirubin (usually in excess of 40%) and their low cholesterol content. While some of these stones may be composed purely of pigment, the vast majority are mixed and contain calcium bilirubinate. The typical calcium bilirubinate stones are small, multiple, dark reddish or brown, and are usually fragile. Although these stones form most commonly in the gallbladder, in the Far East intrahepatic cholelithiasis is a common problem.

Pathogenesis of Pigment Stones

The classic theory for the pathogenesis of calcium bilirubinate gallstone disease, expressed by Maki,[37] emphasizes the role of infection of bile with stagnation and the enzymatic hydrolysis of bilirubin glucuronide into free bilirubin and glucuronic acid. It has been suggested that this free unconjugated bilirubin, which is insoluble in water, then combines with calcium in the bile to produce a calcium bilirubinate matrix which is a component of most pigment stones. This single theory, however, would not explain the higher incidence of pigment stones which has been observed in cirrhotics,[38] in patients receiving long-term TPN,[35] following ileal resection[36] or hemolytic disorders,[39, 40] and in the general population.[34] It has recently been suggested that unconjugated bilirubin may be secreted directly into hepatic bile where, in the presence of increased amounts of cholesterol or calcium, it may be driven out of the micelle and be available for precipitation with calcium.[41] The role of calcium binding and ionized calcium as a nucleating agent has been the subject of recent investigations.[42, 43] Calcium binding in bile appears to be dependent on the presence of bile salt and the mixed micelles. Alterations in this homeostasis can result in calcium precipitation and may be an important nucleating factor in the pathogenesis of pigment gallstones.

Early studies suggested that increased absorption of water by the gallbladder wall occurred in certain noncholesterol gallstone animal models.[44] This has recently been verified in an ileal resection animal model which forms calcium bilirubinate stones.[45] The mechanism by which this altered absorption occurs and its impact on calcium bilirubinate stone formation is the subject of current investigation. Stasis of bile within the gallbladder has been shown to be a critical factor in the pathogenesis of experimentally induced cholesterol gallstones[22] and is considered to be an important etiologic factor in the pathogenesis of gallstones as observed during pregnancy,[46] following truncal vagotomy,[47] and most recently during long-term administration of TPN.[48] The finding that this last group of patients forms predominantly calcium bilirubinate stones suggests that stasis of bile within the gallbladder may be an important etiologic factor in the pathogenesis of both cholesterol and pigment gallstone disease. The ultra-

sonographic finding of gallbladder sludge has been assumed to be the result of stasis of bile in the gallbladder. Allen and his group[49] have verified this hypothesis and have demonstrated that sludge is composed of calcium bilirubinate crystals. Further refinement of a recently established animal model for pigment stones[50] should help to elucidate the mechanism by which these stones form.

FACTORS PREDISPOSING TO GALLSTONE FORMATION

Age

Epidemiologic studies have shown a linear relationship between increasing age and the incidence of gallstones.[51] Gallstones occurring in children and adolescents are distinctly uncommon and are usually associated with either congenital anomalies or hemolytic disorders.[52] Recent studies, however, have shown that the incidence of gallbladder disease in children maintained on TPN is 43%.[53] In healthy children and in those with ileal disorders, the degree of cholesterol saturation of bile is significantly lower than in their adult counterparts.[54] This finding may explain in part the reduced incidence of cholesterol gallstone disease seen in the young population and the fact that children with TPN-induced gallbladder disease develop calcium bilirubinate and not cholesterol stones.

Heredity and Ethnic Factors

Heredity has long been considered an important etiologic factor in the pathogenesis of gallstones, despite the fact that convincing evidence is at best circumstantial. Although there do appear to be some familial tendencies for cholesterol gallstone formation, such findings are not supported by studies of identical twins. Certain population groups with an inordinately high incidence of cholesterol gallstones have been identified; whether this is due completely to hereditary, genetic, environmental, or dietary factors is not clear. One of the most well-studied groups is the Pima Indians of the Southwest United States. These individuals tend to have extremely high lithogenic indices, even in the absence of gallstones. The specific defects responsible for these observations include an increase in hepatic biliary cholesterol secretion as well as a decrease in bile acid secretion.[55] The incidence of gallstones in Pima women between the ages of 25 and 34 years is over 70%.[6] In contrast, a group of Masai in East Africa has been characterized as having a high biliary ratio of phospholipid to bile acid to cholesterol; and, as one might expect, their incidence of gallstone disease is extremely low.[7]

Sex and Hormones

The adage that many patients with gallstones will be "female, fat, fertile, and fortyish" is still a reasonable generalization. The higher incidence of cholesterol gallstones among women compared to men has been well known for many years. Emerging data suggest that this increased incidence of stones is due to both alterations in hepatic biliary metabolism and gallbladder motility. The administration of exogenous estrogens to pre- and post-menopausal women,[56, 57] as well as to men,[58] significantly increases the incidence of cholesterol gallstone formation. Nearly 100 years ago, Heinrich Schroeder[58] observed that 90% of the women who had gallstones in an autopsy study had been pregnant. Studies suggest that estrogen administration leads to a decrease in bile acid synthesis and secretion and a secondary reduction in lecithin secretion.[60] The net effect is a relative increase in cholesterol secretion. The administration of estrogen to animals decreases the activity of the enzyme which regulates the conversion of cholesterol to bile acids and leads to cholesterol-saturated bile.[61] Braverman and co-workers[46] have used real-time ultrasonography to evaluate gallbladder kinetics in pregnant and nonpregnant women. The results of their studies demonstrate that pregnancy is associated with an increase in absolute and residual gallbladder volume after contraction. In addition, the rate of emptying and the percentage of the initial volume emptied are also diminished. The net effect of these alterations is incomplete gallbladder emptying and stasis of bile.

Obesity

Clinical studies suggest that there is an increased incidence of cholesterol gallstone disease among obese patients. Analysis of biliary lipid composition from obese and nonobese patients has demonstrated an increase in absolute and relative hepatic secretion of cholesterol as compared to bile acid and lecithin secretion.[62, 63] Until recently, jejunoileal bypass surgery was used to deal with morbid obesity. It is now well known, however, that in addition to myriad metabolic derangements, this operation also results in alterations in the enterohepatic circulation, a reduction in bile acid pool size, and a markedly increased incidence of cholesterol gallstone disease in an already high-risk population. Further studies are needed to evaluate the effects of the more recently used gastric reduction procedures for treatment of morbid obesity on the incidence of gallstone disease.

Post-truncal Vagotomy

Early clinical studies suggested that truncal vagotomy led to an increased incidence of gallstone disease. Clave and Gaspar[64] reported a 23% incidence of gallstone disease developing in 116 patients who had undergone vagotomy and pyloroplasty for peptic ulcer disease. The significance of vagotomy as a factor in stone formation has been further defined by the recent study in which 21% of patients undergoing gastric resection and vagotomy developed gallstone disease, as compared to only 6% in whom only resection without vagotomy was performed.[65] Altered gallbladder motor activity has been implicated in the pathogenesis of gallstones after vagotomy.[66] Experimental studies have suggested that stones forming after vagotomy may be noncholesterol.[67]

Long-term Administration of Total Parenteral Nutrition

Total parenteral nutrition is being used with increasing frequency throughout the country for an expanding number of indications. Recent studies have demonstrated that these patients are at increased risk for developing gallbladder disease.[53, 68, 69] The incidence of this complication is especially significant in those patients who are already at risk for gallstone formation on the basis of an ileal disorder. Calcium bilirubinate stones have been found in 11 of 12 (90%) patients in whom gallstone analysis has been performed.[35] Although the pathogenesis of gallstone formation in this setting has not

been defined, stasis of bile as a result of decreased gallbladder emptying appears to be a critical factor.[48]

MEDICAL TREATMENT OF GALLSTONES

Gallstone Dissolution

The medical dissolution and prevention of gallstones has been a goal of clinicians dating to ancient times. Throughout the years, numerous agents have been employed in the attempt to dissolve cholesterol gallstones. The present era of gallstone dissolution was initiated in the early 1970s by Thistle and Schoenfield[70] and Danzinger and colleagues,[71] who suggested that the administration of a primary bile acid, chenodeoxycholic acid (CDCA), was effective in dissolving cholesterol gallstones. Numerous studies have examined the efficacy and safety of this substance as an agent for dissolution. The most complete study was a multicenter trial sponsored by the National Cooperative Gallstone Study Group.[72] In this randomized, prospective, double-masked study of over 900 patients, varying doses of CDCA and placebo were evaluated. There was complete gallstone dissolution in only 14% of patients receiving the high-dose CDCA and partial dissolution in 41% of patients. In addition to this disappointingly low success rate, other problems with the use of CDCA include: (1) the need for lifelong therapy to prevent the recurrence of stones (50% of patients), (2) the need to limit dietary cholesterol, especially in obese patients, and (3) the potential toxicity and side effects. More recently, ursodeoxycholic acid (UDCA), a close analogue of CDCA, has been the focus of extensive investigation as an agent for dissolution. This substance is reported to have increased efficacy and reduced toxicity compared to CDCA.[73] Although these preliminary results are encouraging, prospective studies are lacking, and at present this drug remains primarily investigational.

Chenodeoxycholic acid reduces bile lithogenicity by selectively decreasing the rate-limiting enzyme for cholesterol synthesis, HMGCoA reductase.[74] The expansion of the bile salt pool size associated with CDCA therapy is not a factor in its ability to alter bile lithogenicity. The administration of UDCA also causes a fall in the cholesterol saturation of bile by a mechanism other than a simple expansion of the total bile acid pool. Presumably UDCA suppresses hepatic cholesterol synthesis in a manner comparable to that of CDCA.[75]

The efficacy of both agents is dependent on careful patient selection. The ideal patient is thin and has a functioning gallbladder on oral cholecystography, which contains multiple, small, floating, radiolucent, noncalcified gallstones. Even in these carefully selected patients, the efficacy of either agent is 40%–50%. Our interpretation of the available data is that there are limited indications for the use of dissolution agents in the management of patients with cholelithiasis. The long-term therapy required and the high recurrence rate when therapy is discontinued make this therapeutic modality undesirable in most instances. At least for the time being, cholecystectomy remains the gold standard to which all other treatment modalities should be compared.

Gallstone Prevention

With our evolving understanding of the pathogenesis of gallstone disease has come renewed attempts at gallstone prevention. The prevention of gallstone disease by the reduction of gallbladder stasis was first proposed during the Middle Ages.[2] More recently, daily stimulated gallbladder emptying, either by a lipid protein gavage[4] or exogenously administered cholecystokinin,[5] has been shown to prevent gallbladder stasis and significantly to reduce the incidence of gallstone disease in an animal model. In addition, Lee et al.[32] and others[31] have shown that the administration of aspirin-like compounds reduces the mucus hypersecretion which has been observed during formation of gallstones and thereby significantly reduces the incidence of stone formation. The ultimate value of these modalities in the prevention of gallstones in certain high-risk groups of patients awaits the completion of further studies.

GALLSTONE DISEASE AND CHOLECYSTITIS

A Problem in Perspective

Despite intense efforts to establish medical regimens for the prevention and dissolution of gallstones, cholecystectomy remains the cornerstone of treatment for patients with cholelithiasis. Although the morbidity and mortality after cholecystectomy are minimal, both internists and surgeons recognize several unresolved issues regarding this operation, including the natural history of gallstone disease, the pathogenesis of cholecystitis, and indications for elective and urgent cholecystectomy, to name a few.

Silent Gallstones: Fact or Fiction?

Recommendations for the management of patients with silent or asymptomatic gallstones continue to be debated. Should cholecystectomy be performed or should a period of watchful waiting be instituted? Reliable, definitive data to answer this question are not currently available. Those who recommend watchful waiting point to the frequency with which gallstones are found at autopsy, suggesting that many patients live with silent gallstones. However, such studies are of little benefit in establishing the natural history of patients with silent stones who continue living. The definition of asymptomatic or silent stones is difficult. When one hears that gallstones were picked up accidentally in a patient who is asymptomatic, one must consider why that study was being done and whether that patient was truly asymptomatic. Classically we think of biliary colic as being the only manifestation of gallstone disease. It is clear that a significant number of patients do not have postprandial pain, but instead have dyspepsia, vague epigastric discomfort, and perhaps even mild, increased flatulence as the primary manifestation of biliary lithiasis.

An issue of equal importance to that of the natural course of asymptomatic gallstone disease is the increased risk of eventual operation if essential on an elderly patient or on an emergency basis. Wenckert and Robertson[76] reported a series of 781 patients from Sweden with documented gallstones who were followed up for at least one year without cholecystectomy. During the follow-up period of 11 years, 35% of these patients developed complications including severe cholecystitis, jaundice, cholangitis, or such severe pain that elective cholecystectomy was performed. Similarly, in a series of 150 patients with known gallbladder disease but who refused cho-

lecystectomy, the incidence of patients requiring urgent operation for serious complications of biliary tract disease within two years was 27%.[77] Advocates of cholecystectomy, even for so-called silent gallstones, point out that the operative mortality for elective cholecystectomy in patients under 50 years old is 0.3%.[78] In sharp contrast is the 5% mortality reported in over 25,000 patients 65 years or older undergoing elective cholecystectomy.[78] Based on these data, it seems that elective cholecystectomy is safe and desirable in younger patients. However, if the patient with asymptomatic gallstones is observed until complications develop, mortality from operation increases tenfold. Such complications develop in 35%–50% of patients. Recent data have been reported from a linear study of a medical school faculty who were examined for cholelithiasis as part of a comprehensive medical evaluation program.[79] Oral cholecystography showed one hundred twenty-five patients to have silent gallstones. Thirty-five underwent prophylactic cholecystectomy, presumably for asymptomatic stones. Of the remaining 80, 16 developed symptoms of biliary colic or one of the many complications of gallstone disease, including pancreatitis and cholecystitis, with a mortality and morbidity equal to that of elective cholecystectomy. These authors concluded that routine prophylactic cholecystectomy for asymptomatic gallstone disease is unnecessary. Clearly, further such studies are needed to determine with a reasonable degree of certainty the natural history of asymptomatic gallstone disease. In the interim, we believe that the decision to perform a cholecystectomy in a patient with gallstone disease must be individualized. Clearly, the mortality and morbidity for cholecystectomy is significantly increased in those patients who have an emergency operation, an operation for one of the complications associated with calculous gallbladder disease, and those who are older than 65 years of age. Our current algorithm for "asymptomatic stones" is to recommend elective cholecystectomy for: (1) healthy patients less than 65 years old; (2) higher-risk or elderly patients undergoing laparotomy for other reasons; (3) patients who are candidates for renal or heart transplant; and (4) patients who will be receiving TPN indefinitely. Patients over 65 years old with asymptomatic stones are considered to be as much at risk from cholecystectomy as they are from watchful waiting, and operation is not routinely recommended.

Symptomatic Gallstones

The spectrum of clinical syndromes associated with gallstone disease is as varied in its manifestations as in its potential for morbidity and mortality. Many patients will have recurring bouts of biliary colic, often triggered by the ingestion of a large meal. These episodes of discomfort, lasting 30 minutes to a few hours, may be painful and disabling and perhaps result in loss of time from employment, but are not associated with a significant morbidity. Other than biliary colic, acute cholecystitis is the most common complication associated with gallstone disease, occurring in approximately 50% of patients with symptomatic gallstone disease. Without warning, a significant number of patients may develop gallstone pancreatitis, cholecystoenteric fistulas, empyema of the gallbladder, or choledocholithiasis with cholangitis. These complications can be devastating and life-threatening and frequently require urgent operation.

Pathogenesis of Cholecystitis

Classically, acute cholecystitis is associated with cystic duct obstruction. Cholecystitis is self-limiting and resolves in three to four days in over 75% of patients, suggesting that this obstruction is reversible. Cystic duct occlusion may result from impaction of a stone or sludge in the duct or in Hartmann's pouch, or from obstruction secondary to edema, fibrosis, or the congenital presence of a long, tortuous cystic duct of small diameter. The clinical observation that chronic cystic duct obstruction often leads to hydrops of the gallbladder rather than acute cholecystitis[80] suggests that factors other than obstruction are critical in the pathogenesis of calculous cholecystitis. Although numerous theories have been proposed and countless experiments performed, the mechanism by which cholecystitis develops in patients with gallstones remains unclear. The first successful induction of experimental cholecystitis was produced in an animal model by Mann in 1921, after the IV injection of Dakin's solution.[81] A series of classic studies by Womack and Bricker in 1942[82] demonstrated that complete obstruction of the cystic duct in a dog resulted in cholecystitis when the gallbladder was filled with native bile, but not when the gallbladder was filled with saline. These and other, later studies suggested that the course of events in the pathogenesis of acute cholecystitis could be summarized as follows[83]: "Obstruction of the cystic duct is followed by a destructive action of bile on the gallbladder wall, the severity and speed of this reaction probably being influenced by the concentration of the bile and state of the gallbladder circulation." In 1923 William Boyd[84] stated, "Too much stress has been laid upon the presence of calculi. Calculi are incidental, not essential, to gallbladder disease." These early perspectives—that the role of gallstones in the pathogenesis of cholecystitis was to obstruct the cystic duct and that the rest of the process had to do with bile within the gallbladder—have stood the test of time and careful scrutiny. Numerous substances in bile have been proposed as potential etiologic factors in the pathogenesis of cholecystitis, including pancreatic enzymes, lysolecithin, leukocytic proteases, and prostaglandins. While the role of bacteria as a primary etiologic factor in the pathogenesis of cholecystitis is attractive, there are, nonetheless, little data to support this concept.

In 1931 Wolfer[85] first proposed that the regurgitation of pancreatic enzymes into the biliary tree via a common channel might predispose to biliary inflammation. More recent studies have demonstrated elevated bile amylase and lipase levels in patients with cholecystitis, suggesting reflux of pancreatic enzymes.[86] Whether or not this truly represents reflux of pancreatic enzymes and of what etiologic significance this might be in initiating inflammatory changes in the gallbladder are still the subject of much debate. Phospholipase A, an acid hydrolase, is present within the human gallbladder epithelium.[87] It has been proposed that this enzyme may play an important etiologic role in the pathogenesis of cholecystitis by impairing the structural integrity and function of membranes in the gallbladder epithelium,[88, 89] as well as by catalyzing the formation of lysolecithin from bile lecithin. Support for this theory also comes from a series of experiments which have demonstrated both an increase in the ratio of lysolecithin to

lecithin in gallbladder bile of patients with aseptic cholecystitis,[88] as well as the ability of lysolecithin to induce an inflammatory reaction in rabbit gallbladders[90] which is identical to that observed in patients with cholecystitis. Based on these findings, the following cascade of events has been suggested by Sjodahl and co-workers to explain the pathogenesis of cholecystitis: Impaction of a stone in the cystic duct causes damage to the epithelium with the result that lysosomal enzymes are released from the epithelium and enter the gallbladder lumen. Phospholipase A is released and converts lecithin to lysolecithin. This substance causes further injury to the integrity of the epithelial membrane of the gallbladder with a further increase in permeability and further release of lysosomal enzymes occurring. This theory implies that cholecystitis is a localized inflammatory process mediated by local factors. The role of leukocytic proteases[91] and prostaglandins as mediators of this process remains speculative.

Fifty years ago, Andrews[92] found that the degree of gallbladder inflammation correlated closely with the absence of cystic duct patency rather than with the presence or absence of gallstones. All experimental models of acute cholecystitis have required an insult to the gallbladder in addition to cystic duct occlusion. Recent studies in the prairie dog gallstone model suggest that the two elements essential for the induction of acute cholecystitis are the chronic presence of cholesterol saturated bile and impaired gallbladder emptying.[93] The observations that stasis of bile in the gallbladder is critical in the pathogenesis of both calculous and acalculous cholecystitis and that the latter is histologically indistinguishable from calculous disease[94] suggest that the pathogenesis of these two disease entities may be related. Altered gallbladder motor activity has been demonstrated in patients with acalculous cholecystitis using biliary scintigraphy.[95] Increased absorption of water by the gallbladder epithelium during prolonged periods of stasis may predispose to alterations in gallbladder bile composition, which could initiate a cascade of events described previously, resulting in acalculous cholecystitis.

Although the pathogenesis of calculous and acalculous cholecystitis is still not clear, it seems that the disease entities are related and that their etiologies are multifactoral. Cystic duct occlusion, either mechanical or functional, in combination with alterations in gallbladder biliary lipid composition, seem to initiate a series of events that culminates in the local release of inflammatory agents resulting in acute cholecystitis.

Clinical Manifestations of Gallstone Disease

Biliary Colic

Biliary colic is the most important and most widely known symptom of cholelithiasis. Unfortunately the term "biliary colic" is misleading. Unlike other types of colicky pain, which are usually spasmodic and intermittent, biliary pain is generally characterized by a rapid increase in intensity, with a plateau of discomfort lasting for several hours, followed by a gradual decrease in intensity. The onset of pain is usually associated with impaction of a stone in the cystic duct or passage of a stone through this same structure. Classically, the pain is in the right upper quadrant or midepigastrium and may radiate into the back, usually in the inferior medial aspect of the scapula. If the pain lasts more than eight hours, one should consider an alternative diagnosis such as cholecystitis, pancreatitis, or other abdominal disorders. These episodes of pain may be postprandial and are often associated with nausea; however, the traditional notion that these attacks are precipitated by a fatty meal is probably more fiction than fact.

Nonspecific Symptoms

Although biliary colic is the classic symptom associated with cholelithiasis, many patients will have a chronic history of vague abdominal discomfort or dyspepsia without pain. Often these patients will complain of vague, poorly localized abdominal discomfort that occurs at some indeterminate time after a meal. They may complain of increased flatulence, eructations, or perhaps even heartburn. In this group of patients, the role of gallstones in producing the perceived symptoms is difficult to establish, and cholecystectomy may have an uncertain effect.[96]

Acute Cholecystitis

The clinical and pathologic entity of acute cholecystitis is generally initiated by a stone becoming impacted in the cystic duct or in Hartmann's pouch, causing cystic duct occlusion. The onset and character of the pain associated with cholecystitis is similar to that initially observed in individuals with biliary colic. However, the pain of acute cholecystitis persists and is generally unremitting for several days. With time and progression of the inflammatory process, the gallbladder becomes more distended, inflammation develops in the contiguous parietal peritoneum, and the patient complains of more localized right upper quadrant pain. This sometimes subtle change in pain patterns reflects the shift from visceral to parietal pain. Most often these patients will have anorexia, nausea, and vomiting, associated with a low-grade temperature. During physical examination, the patient is reluctant to move, reflecting the peritoneal component to his discomfort. Palpation will elicit localized tenderness in the right upper quadrant associated with guarding and rebound. The classic physical finding of acute cholecystitis is a Murphy's sign. This refers to inspiratory arrest during deep palpation in the right upper quadrant. It is important to note, however, that the patient's complaints and physical findings vary considerably, and often it is only the persistence of right upper quadrant discomfort that suggests the diagnosis of cholecystitis.

Most patients with uncomplicated acute cholecystitis have a mild leukocytosis, in the range of 12,000–15,000/cm mm. Mild jaundice may be present in up to 20% of patients and is usually due to contiguous inflammation, not common bile duct obstruction. Elevated alkaline phosphatase and transaminase levels may also be found.

Cholecystitis results from the action of inflammatory agents on the lining of an obstructed gallbladder. Bacterial infection probably plays a minor role in the early pathogenesis of this disease. For these reasons, the process is generally self-limited, if conservative management is instituted. Most patients will have significant diminution of their symptoms within three to four days and complete resolution of the inflammatory process within a week. Between 5% and 10% of patients will go on to develop one of the numerous complications of cholecystitis, including gangrene, empyema, perforation, and cholangitis.

Diagnosis of Gallstones and Cholecystitis

Until recent times, oral cholecystography has been the primary means for diagnosing cholelithiasis. During the past 15 years, new diagnostic modalities have been introduced which have revolutionized the approach to the patient with suspected gallstones or inflammatory disease of the gallbladder. The value of and indications for the use of these new modalities are still evolving as our experience with each of them increases.

Abdominal Radiography

Supine and upright radiograms of the abdomen may be useful in the overall evaluation of patients with abdominal pain, but are rarely diagnostic in patients with either cholelithiasis or cholecystitis. Visualization of gallstones or a plain abdominal radiogram is possible in the 20% of patients whose stones are partially calcified. Occasionally, gas may be trapped in the center of a cholesterol gallstone during formation, the resulting appearance on x-ray mimicking a Mercedes Benz sign.[97] In addition, plain radiograms of the abdomen may demonstrate air in the wall and lumen of the gallbladder as seen in emphysematous cholecystitis, or air in the biliary tree as a result of a cholecystoenteric fistula. Calcium in the gallbladder wall or its lumen is referred to as a porcelain gallbladder and milk of calcium bile, respectively, and may be observed on an abdominal radiogram. In general, plain abdominal radiograms continue to be ordered routinely, but are of limited value in the diagnosis and management of patients with cholecystitis.

Oral Cholecystography

Since its introduction by Graham and Cole[98] over 50 years ago, the oral cholecystogram has been the gold standard for the diagnostic evaluation of patients with cholelithiasis. The success of this test is dependent on excretion of hallogenated dyes by the liver into the bile and on the concentrating ability of the gallbladder. When used in appropriate clinical situations, the reported accuracy for oral cholecystography is 95%–99%.[99] However, several specific limitations apply to this test: (1) Generally it is not appropriate in the acutely ill patient; (2) Recent studies have documented a significant false negative rate that was previously not appreciated; (3) Patients who are noncompliant or who have emesis, malabsorption, diarrhea, jaundice, or any significant hepatic dysfunction will have a significant chance of a false negative study. Because of these limitations and the advances in ultrasonography and cholescintigraphy, the oral cholecystogram is being used with decreasing frequency.

Intravenous Cholangiography

With the advent of ultrasonography and biliary scintigraphy, IV cholangiography has become a test whose time has passed. The accuracy, sensitivity, and specificity of this examination are all suspect. Currently there is little indication for its use, and it is mentioned only to emphasize the superiority of the other diagnostic modalities.

Abdominal Ultrasonography

During the past several years abdominal ultrasonography has become a mainstay in the evaluation of suspected cholelithiasis or cholecystitis. This tool has significant advantages over oral cholecystography. There is no radiation to the patient; it is not dependent on patient compliance; and intestinal absorption, hepatic secretion, and gallbladder concentration of a dye are not required. An additional advantage is the information provided regarding the anatomy of the bile ducts and pancreas.

Cholecystosonography is most accurate in diagnosing cholelithiasis. Chronic and acute cholecystitis and choledocholithiasis may be diagnosed as well, but with less accuracy. The diagnostic potential of ultrasonography has been significantly enhanced by the use of real-time sonography. In a series of over 300 patients, the diagnostic accuracy for cholelithiasis exceeded 96%, and sensitivity and specificity were greater than 95%.[100] There are now many reports of calculi demonstrated on abdominal ultrasound and at laparotomy in patients who had a normal oral cholecystogram.[101] The information available from ultrasonography has now been expanded to include the size and shape of the gallbladder, gallbladder wall thickness, and the presence of pericholecystic fluid collections. Recent studies have also emphasized the benefit of the ultrasonographer attempting to elicit the point of maximal tenderness and to correlate this with the location of the gallbladder. This sonographic Murphy's sign is reported to have an 85% accuracy rate in patients with acute cholecystitis.[102]

Abdominal ultrasonography has also been of great benefit in those patients with acalculous cholecystitis. Gallbladder wall thickening can be accurately determined. Although it is neither sensitive nor specific for cholecystitis, nonetheless it may be a helpful diagnostic marker in the appropriate clinical setting. Thickening of the gallbladder wall may be seen in a variety of conditions including congestive heart failure, hepatitis, hepatic parenchymal disease, hypoalbuminemia, and ascites. The finding must, therefore, be correlated with the clinical history, physical exam, and laboratory data. The presence of pericholecystic fluid collections is highly suggestive of severe cholecystitis with or without perforation.

Hepatobiliary Scintigraphy

Until 1975, cholescintigraphy had a rather limited role in the evaluation of patients with acute cholecystitis. At that time, Harvey et al.[103] introduced the technetium 99m Tc-labeled N-substituted iminodiacetic acid (HIDA) derivatives as new, improved agents to facilitate hepatobiliary scanning. Currently, a group of related analogues of technetium 99m Tc HIDA are being used. These radionuclide substances are administered IV, taken up by the liver, and then excreted unconjugated (and unchanged) by the hepatocytes into the biliary ductular system. This concept is similar to the previously used rose bengal scan, which employed radioactive-labeled iodine. The newer technetium scans have significant advantages over the rose bengal scan and provide much better imaging potential. One of the primary advantages of technetium

scan is its ability to demonstrate cystic duct obstruction despite serum bilirubin levels in excess of 15 mg/dl. Significant information regarding focal hepatic masses, parenchymal function, and gallbladder motor activity can be obtained using imaging techniques. In most patients with biliary disease, the intrahepatic bile ducts, gallbladder, common bile ducts, and duodenum can all be visualized within 15–30 minutes.

It should be emphasized that radionuclide imaging is not a suitable diagnostic test for cholelithiasis. However, it is a very accurate means of diagnosing cystic duct obstruction, which is a sine qua non of acute cholecystitis. Under these circumstances, one would see normal imaging of the liver and common bile duct with prompt visualization of the duodenum but no visualization of the cystic duct or gallbladder. Failure to opacify the gallbladder after 60 minutes is diagnostic of cystic duct obstruction and highly suggestive of cholecystitis. Delayed visualization of the cystic duct and gallbladder after four hours, even in patients with altered hepatic cellular function, is diagnostic of cholecystitis except in the few patients receiving TPN or who are on a prolonged fast.[104] Extreme caution must be exercised in the interpretation of a scan in which imaging of the liver is obtained with no evidence of radionuclide in any portion of the extrahepatic biliary system. While this occasionally may be due to complete extrahepatic obstruction, more frequently it indicates diffuse parenchymal disease.

Numerous studies have looked at the accuracy, sensitivity, and specificity of radionuclide imaging as compared to ultrasonography and more traditional means of diagnosing biliary tract disease. In 1980 Suarez and co-workers[105] reported a prospective evaluation of hepatobiliary scanning in conjunction with ultrasonography in patients presumed to have acute cholecystitis. In this series, HIDA scanning had a diagnostic accuracy for acute cholecystitis of 98% and a comparable sensitivity. Considerable experience has now been obtained with this diagnostic modality, and the early experience has been confirmed. The specificity of this examination (false positive rate) is dependent on the clinical situation in which this test is used. Recent studies have demonstrated a significant false positive rate in patients receiving TPN or who are fasting[104] as well as in alcoholics.[106]

The choice of whether to obtain an abdominal ultrasound or a hepatobiliary scan in a patient with right upper quadrant symptoms continues to be debated. It is important to reemphasize the fact that abdominal ultrasonography is an accurate tool for diagnosing cholelithiasis but is limited in its ability to diagnose acute cholecystitis. In contrast, radionuclide imaging as currently employed is a very accurate test for acute cholecystitis but does not detect gallstones. In many clinical situations, however, knowledge of the presence of gallstones is all that is needed. The presence of gallstones in a patient who has right upper quadrant tenderness, mild leukocytosis, and fever is sufficient to make the diagnosis of cholecystitis without the necessity for confirmation with a hepatobiliary scan. However, there are instances where gallstones are absent, or so small that they go undetected on ultrasound, and definitive diagnosis by radionuclide scan is essential. In addition, abdominal ultrasonography is less expensive, takes less time to perform, and can be used to examine other intra-abdominal organs as well. Other problems, such as hepatic abscesses, may be responsible for right upper quadrant symptoms even in a patient with gallstones. For these reasons whether to obtain an abdominal ultrasound or a HIDA scan should not be an "either/or" situation. There are specific indications for the use of each test, and the choice of which one to perform should be based on the individual clinical situation.

Combined Biliary Drainage and Cholecystokinin Cholecystography

One of the more challenging problems that clinicians face is the patient with classic symptoms of biliary tract disease who has a normal oral cholecystogram and abdominal ultrasonogram. Clearly, not all of these patients have biliary tract disease, and cholecystectomy, even for classic symptoms, is beneficial in fewer than one third of these patients. Duodenal drainage with examination of bile for cholesterol crystals was introduced[90] long before the introduction of oral cholecystography by Graham and Cole in 1924.[98] More recently, this study, in conjunction with cholecystokinin cholecystography, has been suggested as a suitable means for detecting which patients with symptoms of biliary tract disease and a negative oral cholecystogram who do in fact have small stones, cholesterolosis, or biliary dyskinesia.[107] Patients selected for this examination receive iapanoic acid (Telepaque) tablets the evening before the examination. After confirmation of gallbladder visualization by abdominal radiography the next day, a duodenal tube is inserted and, using fluoroscopic control, is placed in the second portion of the duodenum. Intravenous cholecystokinin is then administered, and bile is collected from the duodenum in conjunction with gallbladder radiograms performed at five-minute intervals. Specific criteria for a positive study include reproduction of pain, absence of visible gallbladder contractions, and abnormal bile containing cholesterol or calcium bilirubinate crystals. Over 80% of those patients with abnormal test results will have significant improvement of their symptoms following cholecystectomy.[107] The study is relatively simple to perform and provides a basis for identifying those patients with negative biliary studies who might benefit from cholecystectomy.

Delayed vs. Early Cholecystectomy

The optimal timing for cholecystectomy in patients with acute cholecystitis has long been an area of controversy. For many years, the standard of practice was to admit patients with acute cholecystitis to the hospital for a period of intense medical management. These patients would be allowed to "cool down" while in the hospital and then would be discharged home. They would return in approximately six to ten weeks for an elective cholecystectomy. The rationale for this mode of therapy was to allow resolution of the acute inflammatory process and to facilitate the operative procedure.

This approach was challenged by the findings of a controlled, prospective, randomized clinical study of 140 patients with acute cholecystitis.[108] In this study, half of the patients were randomly selected to undergo either early cholecystectomy (fewer than four days after the onset of symptoms) or an initial trial of medical management followed by elective cholecystectomy eight to ten weeks later. The significant findings were that the morbidity and mortality rates were similar for both groups of patients, and therefore early cholecystectomy

was recommended for the management of acute cholecystitis to reduce hospitalization time and expense as well as the potential for recurrent cholecystitis. Subsequent studies have confirmed these early observations and have identified a recurrence rate of 24% for patients undergoing delayed cholecystectomy.[109] In addition, it has been the impression of those authors and our own experience that, when performed early in the course of the clinical disease, the operation is in fact technically easier than when performed electively six to ten weeks later. Further support for early cholecystectomy for patients with acute cholecystitis is provided by the finding of significantly increased morbidity and mortality for those patients who fail a trial of conservative medical management and require emergency cholecystectomy five to ten days following the onset of their symptoms.[110] More recent prospective controlled clinical trials have established the safety and value for early cholecystectomy in patients with acute cholecystitis. One hundred sixty-five patients were randomly selected for either early or delayed cholecystectomy. In this series of patients the operative morbidity and mortality rates were comparable. However, a total of 28% of the patients who had been selected for delayed operations had recurrent symptoms during the period of "watchful waiting," 13% of whom required emergency cholecystectomy.[111] In addition, those who had early cholecystectomy had a significantly reduced hospitalization stay and were able to return to employment two weeks before those undergoing delayed operation.

Currently, it is our practice to perform urgent cholecystectomy on most patients with acute cholecystitis within three to four days after the onset of their symptoms. Following the diagnosis of acute cholecystitis, these patients are managed with IV hydration, nasogastric decompression, and broad-spectrum antibiotics. If they demonstrate signs of clinical improvement, we continue the period of observation and perform an urgent cholecystectomy within three to four days. However, if there is no evidence of improvement after 24 hours of medical management, or if there are signs of clinical deterioration, we will proceed with cholecystectomy. Occasionally, cholecystectomy may be ill-advised in extremely high-risk patients. In this clinical setting, we will not hesitate to perform a cholecystectomy using local anesthesia if necessary. The experience of Morrow and co-workers[112] that acute cholecystitis is rarely responsive to conservative measures in elderly patients has led us to extend our aggressive approach to patients with acute cholecystitis to this high-risk group of patients as well.

Intraoperative Cholangiography

The issue of routine intraoperative cholangiography is currently as controversial as is the timing of cholecystectomy. Numerous authors have suggested that operative cholangiography is mandatory, stating: "the indication for operative cholangiography is cholecystectomy."[113] The rationale for its use during cholecystectomy is to identify patients with common duct stones who would require choledochotomy and to avoid unnecessary common duct exploration. There are advocates for both routine and selective cholangiography. The latter group states that routine intraoperative x-rays result in unnecessary common duct explorations, as well as added expense.[114] They also point to the fact that unsuspected common duct stones found by cholangiography are frequently asymptomatic and rarely require removal. These authors claim that the incidence of clinically significant retained stones following cholecystectomy in which cholangiography was not performed is less than 0.5% and that unnecessary common bile duct exploration can be avoided in 5%–10% of patients who have false positive cholangiograms.[115] Efforts at cost benefit analysis have not produced convincing data. Recently a group from Manchester, England, using computer analysis, attempted to develop a statistical model to predict the presence of common bile duct stones without the use of cholangiography.[116] Their data suggest that a dilated common bile duct was the most significant indicator of the presence of stones. It should be noted, however, that this same group recommends routine operative cholangiography whenever possible. A retrospective review of 4,000 patients undergoing cholecystectomy over a 25-year period suggests that the decrease in unnecessary duct exploration resulting from routine intraoperative cholangiography is the single most important factor in reducing the overall mortality associated with cholecystectomy. Compared to a 13-year period during which cholangiography was not used in 1,000 patients, with a mortality of 3.6%, the mortality in a similar number of patients having routine intraoperative cholangiography was reduced to 1.5%.[117] During these same intervals, the stone recovery rate from common duct exploration has increased from 34% to 71%.[117] Although this study can be criticized because it is a retrospective analysis and compares the surgical management of patients over periods during which preoperative evaluation, antibiotic therapy, and perisurgical care have improved, it nonetheless demonstrates the significant benefits of intraoperative cholangiography.

Many of the arguments against the routine use of cholangiography have to do with the technical aspects of the procedure. The pitfalls in diagnosis and wasted time associated with conventional operative cholangiography can be prevented with the use of a movable C-arm and fluoroscopic cholangiography. This technique is now used routinely in many institutions, permitting definitive identification and evaluation of the biliary ductal system in a matter of minutes. If there are any suspicious areas, more contrast can be injected and the area carefully examined without waiting for films to be taken, processed, and then returned to the operating room for the surgeon's review. In our experience this new, advanced technology has clearly facilitated intraoperative cholangiography and made it more accurate. We therefore continue to recommend that all patients undergoing either emergency or elective cholecystectomy have intraoperative cholangiography performed. Our preference is to place a cholangiocatheter down the cystic duct and obtain a film in this manner, although we will not hesitate to perform a needle cholangiogram through the common bile duct if this is the only route available.

Intraoperative manometry has been suggested as an adjunct to cholangiography in attempts to further refine the need for common bile duct exploration.[118] Generally, common bile duct pressures greater than 16 cm of saline are abnormal and suggestive of distal common duct stones. We have not found this additional procedure to be of significant benefit and continue to rely on the cholangiographic findings.

Bacteriology of Cholecystitis

Septic complications continue to be a source of significant morbidity following cholecystectomy. In most cases the organisms leading to wound infection are similar to those found in the patient's bile.

In normal, healthy subjects without gallstones, the incidence of positive bile cultures is essentially zero.[119] In contrast, the incidence of positive bile cultures for patients with acute cholecystitis ranges between 30% and 70%.[120, 121] That these numbers are not higher provides further evidence that acute cholecystitis is primarily a chemically induced inflammatory process with bacteria playing a secondary role. The presence of bacteria in bile of patients with acute cholecystitis is a source of significant morbidity and mortality. Prospective studies have demonstrated that the incidence of positive bile cultures increases significantly with age. While the incidence of positive bile cultures in patients undergoing cholecystectomy is somewhere between 20% and 30% in patients under 50 years of age, it increases to over 50% in patients who are 70 years or older.[122] The most common organism cultured from gallbladder bile is *E. coli*. Other bacteria found are of enteric origin, such as *Enterobacter*, *Klebsiella*, and *Enterococcus*. As one would expect, the rate of positive bile cultures is higher in patients with acute cholecystitis (60%–70%) than it is in patients with chronic cholecystitis (20%–40%).[120, 122]

Antimicrobial Therapy

Septic complications associated with cholecystectomy can best be prevented by the judicious use of appropriate antimicrobial agents. Selection of patients undergoing cholecystectomy who require antibiotic coverage has been the subject of numerous investigations. Based on a retrospective evaluation of over 1,400 patients, Chetlin and Elliott[120] identified high-risk factors for the development of septic complications following cholecystectomy. These include: (1) patients over 70 years of age; (2) patients with acute cholecystitis; (3) history of obstructive jaundice; and, (4) the presence of common duct stones with or without jaundice. In a subsequent prospective study, patients falling into these high-risk groups received prophylactic antibiotic therapy. Despite the fact that the incidence of positive bile cultures remained high, the rate of septic postoperative complications was significantly reduced from 27% to 4%.[123] This observation has since been confirmed by others.[124] Furthermore, a randomized, controlled trial has demonstrated that adequate serum and tissue levels of an effective antibiotic are more important to the reduction of the incidence of septic complications following cholecystectomy than is the selection of an antibiotic which is excreted almost entirely into the bile.[125] The use of intraoperative Gram staining in selected patients requiring antibiotic therapy has been the subject of several studies. In a prospective study of 200 patients who received either selected antibiotics based on intraoperative Gram staining or no antibiotics at all, the incidence of wound sepsis was 7% in the antibiotic group and 22% in the control group.[126] These data demonstrate the efficacy of this type of program and lend credence to the concept that antibiotic coverage can be efficacious when administered shortly after the period of contamination. Intraoperative Gram staining of bile is particularly helpful in identifying the occasional patient who has *Clostridium perfringens*.[128]

Antibiotic prophylaxis is now an accepted aspect of biliary surgery. Not all patients require antibiotics for elective cholecystectomy, and we continue to adhere to the criteria previously established by Chetlin and Elliott.[123] We prefer to administer a broad-spectrum antibiotic (a second-generation cephalosporin) one hour preoperatively to all patients meeting the criteria previously established. An intraoperative Gram stain is generally performed only to identify those patients who may have a clostridial infection. It has been already demonstrated by Stone and co-workers[128] that there is no benefit to continuing prophylaxis beyond the day of operation. We generally give one or two doses of antibiotics postoperatively unless there are extenuating circumstances. Should there be a septic complication postoperatively, our choice of antibiotics would be based on operative cultures as well as cultures from the wound or intra-abdominal collection.

Intraperitoneal Drains Following Cholecystectomy

Few areas in biliary tract surgery have received as much attention in the literature as the rationale and types of drains used following cholecystectomy. The advocates of routine drainage cite the necessity to prevent accumulation of bile or blood after cholecystectomy. This position is stated most forcefully by Deaver[129]: "The cemetaries are filled with patients whose gallbladders were removed without drainage." More recent studies suggest that there are specific indications for intraperitoneal drains, but that their use has been vastly overemphasized. The proponents recommending selective drainage point to the numerous problems associated with the use of intraperitoneal drains. These include: (1) the migration of exogenous bacterial organisms into the abdominal cavity via drains; (2) the failure of drains to achieve their purpose; and, (3) the potential for a hernia at the drain site. Many of these concerns are more theoretical than practical. A prospective study of 100 patients undergoing routine drainage following cholecystectomy demonstrated that the wound infection rate was 31% in those patients who had positive bile cultures, but only 5.7% in patients from whom only exogenous organisms were cultured from the drains.[130] These data suggest that the primary cause of postoperative wound infections in patients with intraperitoneal drains is related to the positive bile culture and not to the drain itself. The concern over migration of bacteria can further be reduced, as can the incidence of hernias in drain sites, by the use of small sump tubes rather than the larger, traditional Penrose drains. Polk[131] in 1973 reported his experience over a seven-year period with the use of Penrose drains compared to sump tubes. This study, although nonrandomized, clearly demonstrated superior benefits from sump suction drainage of the subhepatic space when compared to the more traditional type of Penrose drainage. Furthermore, sump drains may be removed after 24–36 hours, thus decreasing hospital stay, compared to the traditional management of patients with Penrose drains in whom the drain is twisted on the second postoperative day and then slowly advanced out over the next several days. While there are numerous anecdotal and retrospective reports evaluating

cholecystectomy with or without drainage, there are a limited number of prospective, randomized studies examining this issue. Budd and co-workers[132] reported a series of 300 patients who were randomized into either no drain, Penrose drain, or sump drainage. Although there was a significantly higher incidence of postoperative fevers in the drainage group, there was no significant difference in morbidity, mortality, or length of hospital stay among the three groups. This study and others have failed to identify any significant benefit from intraperitoneal drainage in patients undergoing elective, uncomplicated cholecystectomy. If a surgeon does choose to place an intraperitoneal drain, it is crucial that this drain not be placed through the abdominal incision. The incidence of wound infection has been reported to be four times greater in those patients in whom drains were placed via the operative incision as compared to a group where the drain was placed by a separate stab incision.[133]

The decision about whether to place an intraperitoneal drain following an uncomplicated cholecystectomy is influenced by the individual surgeon's experience as well as the considerable folklore which has surrounded this issue for some years. It is our impression that the data available clearly suggest that the routine use of intraperitoneal drains following uncomplicated cholecystectomy with or without intraoperative cholangiography is not essential. However, whether or not there is any genuine clinical morbidity from the use of drains has not been resolved. We continue to use small sump drains in selected cases and have abandoned the use of Penrose drains. If there is no evidence of significant intra-abdominal fluid collections or bilious output through the drain after 36 hours, we will then completely remove the tube.

Cholecystectomy, Gallstones, and Colon Carcinoma

Recent preliminary clinical studies have suggested increased risk of colorectal cancer following cholecystectomy. The theoretical basis for this proposal is the alteration in the relative concentrations of primary and secondary bile acids which occur following cholecystectomy and the observation that the quantity of secondary bile acids (deoxycholic and lithocholic acids) seems to be increased among patients with colorectal cancer.[134] In a retrospective autopsy series 15% of 304 patients with colorectal cancer had undergone a previous cholecystectomy.[135] In a control group, age- and sex-matched, but without colorectal cancer, the incidence of previous cholecystectomy was 10.5%. Although these data were statistically significant suggesting an increased risk of cancer following cholecystectomy, one must wonder about the clinical and biologic significance of these numbers. Similar differences were observed in a retrospective clinical study of 305 patients with a diagnosis of colorectal cancer.[136] In this latter study a relationship between colorectal cancer and cholecystectomy was observed only in women and not in men. In contrast, a recent epidemiologic study of women with colorectal cancer failed to establish any significant relationship between the carcinoma and cholecystectomy.[137] The most convincing data to dispute the etiologic association between cholecystectomy and subsequent colorectal cancer comes from a prospective study of over 16,000 patients undergoing cholecystectomy in

Sweden.[138] In this large group of patients, the incidence of colorectal cancer was no greater after cholecystectomy when compared to the general population. Data currently available suggest that the decision for or against cholecystectomy in a patient with symptomatic biliary tract disease should not be influenced by this theoretical consideration.

Cholecystitis, Specific Clinical Settings

Acalculous Cholecystitis

Since the initial clinical report by Duncan in 1844[139] of perforated acalculous cholecystitis, there has been an increasing number of reports concerning this unusual but potentially catastrophic disorder. The pathogenesis of acalculous cholecystitis is unknown. Recent clinical and experimental studies, however, suggest a multifactoral etiology, with different factors playing greater or lesser roles depending on the clinical situation. Stasis of bile in the gallbladder secondary to ampullary spasm caused by narcotics, decreased gallbladder emptying due to fasting, or cystic duct occlusion secondary to edema, are potential etiologic factors in the pathogenesis of acalculous disease. Stasis of bile, dehydration, and perhaps multiple transfusions with an increased pigment load may predispose to increased gallbladder absorption of water and altered viscosity of the bile. This increased viscosity may lead to functional occlusion of the cystic duct and may also lead to irritation and inflammation of the gallbladder mucosa by the altered concentration of biliary lipid and pigment components. A cascade of events may then be initiated similar to that which has been proposed for acute calculous cholecystitis, with the final result being similar.

Diagnosis of acalculous cholecystitis poses a considerable challenge to the clinician. The problem often occurs in a clinical setting where the patient has multiple other medical and/or surgical problems. The key to an early diagnosis of acalculous cholecystitis, especially in the critically ill patient, is a high index of suspicion. Although these patients will often have signs and symptoms suggestive of gallstone disease, occasionally, the only manifestation may be that of generalized sepsis. Despite earlier reports to the contrary, oral cholecystography probably has no role in the diagnosis of acalculous disease. While cholecystokinin cholecystography is useful in the diagnosis of acalculous disease in the nonacutely ill patient,[140] it has no role in the evaluation of a patient who is acutely ill. As reported earlier, hepatobiliary scintigraphy may not be reliable in the evaluation of the patient with suspected acute acalculous cholecystitis. Currently, we recommend abdominal ultrasonography or CT scanning for the early diagnosis of acalculous cholecystitis.

The overall incidence of acalculous cholecystitis is between 5% and 7%. Acalculous cholecystitis has been reported as a complication following surgery,[141] trauma,[142, 143] burns,[144] collagen vascular disorders,[145] and, most commonly, in critically ill patients in intensive care units.[146] It is in this latter group of patients that the associated morbidity and mortality are so high. In a recent series of nine critically ill patients developing acute acalculous cholecystitis, the mortality was 67%.[146] As many of these patients already have single or multiple organ failure, early and expeditious treatment is essential for a successful outcome. Surgical management is warranted in all patients with acute acalculous cholecystitis. Cholecystectomy may be contraindicated because of the patient's unstable overall condition. Under these circumstances, a cholecystostomy, perhaps even performed using local anesthesia, may be the procedure of choice.

Total Parenteral Nutrition-induced Gallbladder Disease

Recent studies have demonstrated an increased risk of cholelithiasis and cholecystitis in patients being maintained on long-term TPN. The pathogenesis of gallbladder disease in this group of patients has yet to be elucidated, although stasis of bile within the gallbladder appears to be critical.[48] Prospective studies suggest that the incidence of asymptomatic and symptomatic gallstone disease in long-term TPN patients (both children and adults) is 40%–45%.[53, 68] Most of these patients will be quite symptomatic, although the diagnosis may not be readily apparent because of the complex underlying GI disorder often present. In a recent report, 40% of these patients required emergency cholecystectomy, and severe, acute cholecystitis was present in over half of them.[147] Performing cholecystectomy in this group of patients is a formidable task, associated with significant morbidity and mortality. Factors contributing to the reported morbidity of 54% and mortality of 11% include the sequelae of TPN-induced liver disease.[147] In this high-risk group of patients, early cholecystectomy is indicated when stones first appear and should be considered in those patients without stones who are committed to a long-term course of TPN or who are undergoing laparotomy for other reasons.

Diabetes and Gallstone Disease

It has long been suggested that diabetics have an increased incidence of cholesterol gallstone disease.[148] This conclusion has been based largely on autopsy data. Other authors, however, have been unable to confirm the alleged increased incidence of gallstones among diabetics.[149] Recently Bennion and Grundy[150] demonstrated that in a group of high-risk patients with diabetes, biliary lipid composition was altered during insulin treatment so as to predispose the patient to cholesterol precipitation and gallstone formation. Furthermore, studies have suggested that diabetics with gallstones are more likely to develop acute cholecystitis, with a greater associated incidence of complications.[151] However, in a recent prospective review of 175 diabetic and nondiabetic patients undergoing cholecystectomy, the incidence of gallbladder perforation, wound infection, and overall morbidity and mortality were not significantly different between the two groups.[152] The conclusion that diabetes itself is not a significant risk factor for severe biliary tract disease should be tempered, since the study cited was not controlled for timing of operation. It may well be that because of concern about the diabetes in patients with biliary tract disease, these patients underwent earlier cholecystectomy perhaps with different antibiotic coverage. Despite these recent findings, however, we continue to recommend that elective cholecystectomy be strongly considered in diabetics with cholelithiasis, whether or not they are symptomatic. In addition, our management of a diabetic with presumed acute cholecystitis is aggressive in terms of antibiotic coverage and early operation.

Cirrhosis and Gallbladder Disease

Autopsy studies have suggested that the incidence of cholelithiasis is significantly increased in patients with Laënnec's alcoholic cirrhosis.[153] Biliary lipid secretion studies have demonstrated that cirrhotic patients have bile with a greater cholesterol-holding capacity than bile from controls, and therefore they would not be expected to have a high prevalence of cholesterol gallstones. The implication is that there would be an increased incidence of pigment stones among alcoholic patients, and this has in fact been observed by numerous authors.[153] Recent studies have clearly demonstrated that cholecystectomy when performed in a cirrhotic patient is associated with significant morbidity and mortality. Schwartz[154] reported a 57% complication rate due primarily to excessive intraoperative bleeding in a group of 21 cirrhotic patients undergoing cholecystectomy for cholecystitis and cholelithiasis. The mortality rate in this group of patients was 10%, which is approximately 20 times that reported for noncirrhotic patients by McSherry and Glenn.[155] In a subsequent study, Aranha and co-workers[156] reviewed records from 55 cirrhotic patients undergoing cholecystectomy. They further divided these patients into three groups depending on their prothrombin time. There was a direct correlation between the degree of prolongation of prothrombin time and mortality. In those patients who had a slightly prolonged prothrombin time, the mortality was 26%, while in the group whose prothrombin time was prolonged more than 2½ seconds the mortality was 100%. Our experience with this group of patients has been equally dissatisfying. The difficulties encountered in these patients are due in large part to the associated portal hypertension, thrombocytopenia secondary to hypersplenism, and prolongation of the activated partial thromboplastin time and prothrombin time. The indications for cholecystectomy in a cirrhotic patient should be more rigid than in the noncirrhotic patient. Operation should only be undertaken in those individuals who are extremely symptomatic or who have developed one of the complications of gallstone disease including cholecystitis, perforation, fistula formation, or empyema of the gallbladder. Administration of IV pitressin perioperatively has been proposed as a mechanism to reduce intraoperative blood loss and to facilitate operation. In addition, if there is a significant intrahepatic portion to the gallbladder, it is not essential that the entire structure be removed. Much of the bleeding encountered during cholecystectomy in the cirrhotic patient is a result of trying to shell the gallbladder out of its hepatic bed. We feel it is quite acceptable to leave the posterior wall of the gallbladder in situ under these circumstances and to cauterize the mucosa.

Cholecystitis in the Elderly

With the increasing longevity of our population, the incidence of cholecystitis among the elderly has become an increasingly frequent problem. The natural history of gallstone disease in this group of patients is more virulent than seen in younger individuals and warrants a different management protocol. Morrow and associates[112] recently reported their experience with 88 patients older than 60 years of age who underwent cholecystectomy. In this group of patients the overall mortality was 70%. Medical therapy was attempted in 44%;

however, emergency cholecystectomy was necessary because of failure to respond to conservative supportive treatment in 97%. In those undergoing emergency cholecystectomy, the morbidity and mortality were 44% and 10%, respectively. In contrast, the morbidity and mortality in 49 patients undergoing elective cholecystectomy for chronic cholelithiasis was only 22% and 2%, respectively. Similarly, Glenn[157] has reported that elderly patients, 65 years of age and older, accounted for 70% of all the deaths at the New York Hospital resulting from acute cholecystitis. In his study, the two most common causes of death were sepsis and cardiovascular disease. Furthermore, recent studies have suggested that the incidence of complications from cholecystitis, gallbladder perforation and empyema, may be greater in the elderly patients.[158] The significant morbidity and mortality associated with cholecystectomy in the elderly, as well as the advanced nature of the disease that most of these patients have, mandates an aggressive but rational approach to the elderly patient with biliary tract disease. Conservative, supportive management in the elderly patient with acute cholecystitis should not be a consideration. These patients must have an early diagnosis, aggressive management to optimize their medical condition, and an early and uncomplicated surgical procedure.

Complications of Cholecystitis

Gallbladder Perforation

In 1934 Niemeier[159] presented his classic description of acute perforation of the gallbladder and reviewed his experience with this complication of acute cholecystitis. He concluded that although a relatively rare condition, "it demands eternal vigilance in the delayed treatment of acute cholecystitis. The mortality is extremely high . . . and it would appear from our series that proper recognition and treatment might lower this considerably." Despite this recommendation, gallbladder perforation continues to be a dilemma in early diagnosis and is associated with significant morbidity and mortality. The incidence of gallbladder perforation is between 3% and 10% of all patients with acute cholecystitis. Gallbladder perforation can be classified into three types: type 1, acute free perforation with bile-stained peritoneal fluid; type 2, a subacute perforation with pericholecystic or right upper quadrant abscess; and type 3, chronic perforation with formation of either cholecystoenteric or cholecystocutaneous fistula. The exact pathogenesis of gallbladder perforation remains to be elucidated. However, it would seem, as Glenn and Moore[160] wrote in 1942: "This process is closely associated with circulatory changes and infection." A review of the literature suggests that gallbladder perforation tends to occur in patients who are elderly and who have either diabetes or evidence of systemic vascular disease, or who are immunosuppressed due to immunosuppressive therapy or malignancy. Fortunately, free perforation of the gallbladder is less commonly seen than the other two types, for it is associated with significant morbidity and mortality. Diagnosis of gallbladder perforation may be difficult to make in that the symptoms are frequently comparable to those of patients with uncomplicated cholecystitis. The successful management of gallbladder perforation is based on early recognition. The clinical suspicion should prompt early evaluation with abdominal ultrasonography or cholescintigraphy. Aggressive treatment with fluid resuscitation, nasogastric decompression, and IV, broad-spectrum antibiotic therapy should be instituted and followed by an expeditious laparotomy.

Cholecystoenteric fistulas are a well-recognized complication of cholecystitis. They account for 30%–40% of all patients with gallbladder perforation. Depending on the size of the fistulous communication, a gallstone may pass through this tract. In most cases the stones will simply pass through the intestinal tract without any difficulties. However, if a stone is large (greater than 2 cm in diameter), it may become lodged in a portion of the GI tract and cause bowel obstruction. When this occurs it is referred to as "gallstone ileus." This condition is relatively rare and accounts for fewer than 5% of all causes of intestinal obstruction. However, in the elderly population, gallstone ileus accounts for 20%–25% of all cases of small-bowel obstruction. While the diagnosis of a mechanical small-bowel obstruction is generally easy, it is often not appreciated preoperatively that the cause is a gallstone impacted in the small bowel. One should be suspicious of this possibility when small-bowel obstruction occurs in a patient who has not undergone previous surgery, who has documented cholelithiasis, or in whom intrahepatic biliary air is noted on abdominal radiography.[161] These patients are best managed as if they had mechanical small bowel due to any cause, with aggressive fluid resuscitation, broad-spectrum antibiotics, and expeditious laparotomy. In most cases the diagnosis is made at the time of laparotomy when a gallstone is palpated at the site of the obstruction. The primary therapeutic goal at laparotomy in a patient with gallstone ileus is correction of the obstruction and removal of the offending stone. Frequently, the stone will be impacted in the terminal ileum and is best managed by milking of the stone proximally into the dilated small bowel. After occlusion of the bowel proximally and distally to prevent gross contamination, a small enterotomy can be made and the stone easily removed. Occasionally the stones will be found in the colon, and similar maneuvers can be employed. Depending on the clinical situation, removal of the stone in correction of the bowel obstruction may be all that is necessary. Since most of these patients are elderly and quite ill, cholecystectomy and takedown of the biliary enteric fistula probably should not be performed at this time. However, if all is well and the patient's general condition is satisfactory, then one might consider dealing with the underlying biliary tract disease at the same operation. Most series have reported that the associated mortality from surgery from gallstone ileus is between 13% and 15%.[162] A group from Sweden[163] recently reported that a series of 20 patients with gallstone ileus who were managed by an enterolithotomy alone without cholecystectomy had a mortality of 5%. In this select group no patient required elective cholecystectomy for recurrent symptoms. Our current practice is to deal with the bowel obstruction and the offending gallstone without attempts at cholecystectomy unless there is evidence of acute biliary tract disease or it appears to be technically quite easy.

Emphysematous Cholecystitis

Acute emphysematous cholecystitis was initially reported by Hegner in 1931.[164] This entity, defined by the radiographic demonstration of gas either within the gallbladder lumen or wall, is associated with significant morbidity and mortality.[165] Emphysematous cholecystitis is more common in elderly men and is associated with gangrene (74%) and perforation of the gallbladder (21%).[165] Clostridial organisms are present in almost 50% of these patients and account for the remarkable radiographic features of this disorder. Despite the severity of this problem and the magnitude of the associated complications, 30 patients with emphysematous cholecystitis do not appear overtly septic. In any event, the potential for serious morbidity and mortality is so great that prompt cholecystectomy is indicated.

Choledocholithiasis and Gallstone Pancreatitis

The reported incidence of common bile duct stones in patients with gallstones whether or not they have cholecystitis is 15%. Stones floating or impacted in the common bile duct can lead to jaundice, cholangitis, or occasionally pancreatitis. The presence of either of these three complications of gallstone disease will significantly alter the pre- and intraoperative management of patients. These subjects will be fully discussed in a subsequent chapter.

REFERENCES

1. Glenn F., Grafe W.R. Jr.: Historical events in biliary tract surgery. *Arch. Surg.* 93:848, 1966.
2. Thorbjarnarson B.: History of biliary tract surgery, in Thorbjarnarson B. (ed.): *Surgery of the Biliary Tract.* Philadelphia, W.B. Saunders Co. 1982, pp. 1–2.
3. Langenbuch C.: Ein Fall von Exstirpation der Gallenblase wegen chronisher cholelithiasis. *Berl. Clin. Wochenschr.* 19:725, 1882.
4. Roslyn J., DenBesten L., Thompson J.E. Jr.: The effect of periodic gallbladder emptying on gallbladder function and cholesterol gallstone formation. *Surg. Forum* 30:403, 1979.
5. Roslyn J., DenBesten L., Pitt H.A., et al.: Effects of cholecystokinin on gallbladder stasis and cholesterol gallstone formation. *J. Surg. Res.* 30:200, 1981.
6. Sampliner R.E., Bennett P.H., Comess L.J., et al.: Gallbladder disease in Pima Indians: Demonstration of high prevalence and early onset by cholecystography. *N. Engl. J. Med.* 283:1358, 1970.
7. Biss K., Ho K.J., Mikkelson B., et al.: Some unique biologic characteristics of the Masai of East Africa. *N. Engl. J. Med.* 284:694, 1971.
8. Nilsson S.: Synthesis and secretion of biliary phospholipids in man: An experimental study with special reference to the relevance for gallstone formation. *Acta Chir. Scand. [Suppl.]* 405:1, 1970.
9. Admirand W.H., Small D.M.: The physicochemical basis of cholesterol gallstone formation in man. *J. Clin. Invest.* 47:1043, 1968.
10. Carey M.D.: Critical tables for calculating the cholesterol saturation of native bile. *J. Lipid Res.* 19:945, 1978.
11. La Morte W.W., Schoetz D.J. Jr., Birkett D.H., et al.: The role of the gallbladder in the pathogenesis of cholesterol gallstones. *Gastroenterology* 77:580, 1979.
12. Vlahcevic Z.R., Bell C.C. Jr., Buhac I., et al.: Diminished bile acid pool size in patients with gallstones. *Gastroenterology* 59:165, 1970.
13. Bennion L.J., Grundy S.M.: Effects of obesity and caloric intake on biliary lipid metabolism in man. *J. Clin. Invest.* 56:996, 1975.
14. Roslyn J.J., DenBesten L., Thompson J.E. Jr., et al.: Chronic cholelithiasis and decreased bile salt pool size—cause or effect? *Am. J. Surg.* 139:119, 1980.
15. Northfield T.C., Hofmann A.F.: Biliary lipid output during

three meals and an overnight fast: I. Relationship to bile acid pool size and cholesterol saturation of bile in gallstone and control subjects. *Gut* 16:1. 1975.

16. Holan K.R., Holzbach T., Hermann R.E., et al.: Nucleation time: A key factor in the pathogenesis of cholesterol gallstone disease. *Gastroenterology* 77:611, 1979.

17. Burnstein M.J., Ilson R.G., Petrunka C.N., et al.: Evidence for a potent nucleating factor in the gallbladder bile of patients with cholesterol gallstones. *Gastroenterology* 85:801, 1983.

18. von Helmsbach M.: *Mikrogeologic.* Berlin, Reimer, 1956.

19. Brenneman D.E., Connor W.E., Forker E.L., et al.: The formation of abnormal bile and cholesterol gallstones from dietary cholesterol in the prairie dog. *J. Clin. Invest.* 51:1495, 1972.

20. DenBesten L., Safaie-Shirazi S., Connor W.E., et al.: Early changes in bile composition and gallstone formation induced by a high cholesterol diet in prairie dogs. *Gastroenterology* 66:1036, 1974.

21. Holzbach R.T., Corbusier C., Marsh M., et al.: The process of cholesterol cholelithiasis induced by diet in the prairie dog: A physicochemical characterization. *J. Lab. Clin. Med.* 87:987, 1976.

22. Meyer P.D., DenBesten L., Gurll N.J.: Effects of cholesterol gallstone induction on gallbladder function and bile salt pool size in the prairie dog model. *Surgery* 83:599, 1978.

23. Pitt H.A., Roslyn J.J., Kuchenbecker S.L., et al.: The role of cystic duct resistance in the pathogenesis of cholesterol gallstones. *J. Surg. Res.* 30:508, 1981.

24. Doty J.E., Pitt H.A., Kuchenbecker S.L., et al.: Impaired gallbladder emptying before gallstone formation in the prairie dog. *Gastroenterology* 85:168, 1983.

25. Fridhandler T.M., Davison J.S., Shaffer E.A.: Defective gallbladder contractility in the ground squirrel and prairie dog during the early stages of cholesterol gallstone formation. *Gastroenterology* 85:830, 1983.

26. Shaffer E.A., McOrmond P., Duggan H.: Assessment of gallbladder filling and emptying and duodeno gastric reflux. *Gastroenterology* 79:899, 1980.

27. Brugge W.R.: Detection of gallbladder dyskinesia in patients with biliary cholesterol crystals (abstract). *Clin. Res.* 30:686, 1982.

28. Lee S.P., LaMont J.T., Carey M.C.: Role of gallbladder mucus hypersecretion in the evolution of cholesterol gallstones. *J. Clin. Invest.* 67:1712, 1981.

29. Doty J.E., Pitt H.A., Kuchenbecker S.L., et al.: The role of gallbladder mucus in the pathogenesis of cholesterol gallstones. *Am. J. Surg.* 145:54, 1983.

30. Levy P., Smith B.F., Atkinson D., et al.: Human gallbladder mucin enhances *in vitro* nucleation of cholesterol monohydrate crystals (abstract). *Gastroenterology* 84:1382, 1983.

31. Kuchenbecker S.L., Doty J.E., Pitt H.A., et al.: Salicylate prevents gallbladder stasis and cholesterol gallstones in the prairie dog. *Surg. Forum* 32:154, 1981.

32. Lee S.P., Carey M.C., LaMont J.T.: Aspirin prevention of cholesterol gallstone formation in prairie dogs. *Science* 211:1429, 1981.

33. Van der Linden W., Nakayama F.: Gallstone disease in Sweden versus Japan: Clinical and etiological aspects. *Am. J. Surg.* 125:267, 1973.

34. Trotman B.W., Soloway R.D.: Pigment vs. cholesterol cholelithiasis: Clinical and epidemiological aspects. *Am. J. Dig. Dis.* 20:735, 1975.

35. Pitt H.A., Berquist W.E., Mann L.L., et al.: Parenteral nutrition induces calcium bilirubinate gallstones (abstract). *Gastroenterology* 84:1274, 1983.

36. Coyle J.J., Hoyt D.B., Sedaghat A.: Relationship of intestinal bypass operations and cholelithiasis. *Surg. Forum* 31:139, 1980.

37. Maki T.: Pathogenesis of calcium bilirubinate gallstone: Role of E. Coli, β-glucuronidase and coagulation by inorganic ions, polyelectrolytes and agitation. *Ann. Surg.* 164:90, 1966.

38. Davidson J.F.: Alcohol and cholelithiasis: A necropsy survey of cirrhosis. *Am. J. Med. Sci.* 244:730, 1962.

39. Bates G.L., Brown C.H.: Incidence of gallbladder disease in chronic hemolytic anemia (spherocytosis). *Gastroenterology* 21:104, 1952.

40. Jordan R.A.: Cholelithiasis in sickle cell disease. *Gastroenterology* 33:952, 1957.

41. Dutt M.K., Murray B., Thompson R.P.: Bilirubin solubilization by mixed micelles and interaction with cholesterol and calcium. *Gut* 21:A919, 1980.

42. Williamson B.W.A., Percy-Robb I.W.: Contribution of biliary lipids to calcium binding in bile. *Gastroenterology* 78:696, 1980.

43. Moore E.W., Celic L., Ostrow J.D.: Interactions between ionized calcium and sodium taurocholate: Bile salts are important buffers for prevention of calcium-containing gallstones. *Gastroenterology* 83:1079, 1982.

44. Lee S.P.: Enhanced fluid transport across gallbladder mucosa in experimental cholelithiasis. *Am. J. Physiol.* 234:E575, 1978.

45. Pitt H.A.: Unpublished data, 1984.

46. Braverman D.Z., Johnson M.L., Kern F. Jr.: Effects of pregnancy and contraceptive steroids on gallbladder function. *N. Engl. J. Med.* 302:362, 1980.

47. Ihasz M., Griffith C.A.: Gallstones after vagotomy. *Am. J. Surg.* 141:48, 1981.

48. Messing B., Bories C., Kunstlinger F., et al.: Does total parenteral nutrition induce gallbladder sludge formation and lithiasis? *Gastroenterology* 84:1012, 1983.

49. Allen B., Bernhoft R., Blanckaert N., et al.: Sludge is calcium bilirubinate associated with bile stasis. *Am. J. Surg.* 141:51, 1981.

50. LaMont J.T., Turner B.S., Bernstein S.E., et al.: Gallbladder glycoprotein secretion in mice with hemolytic anemia and pigment gallstones. *Hepatology* 3:198, 1983.

51. Friedman G.D., Kannel W.B., Dawber T.R.: The epidemiology of gallbladder disease: Observations in the Framingham study. *J. Chronic Dis.* 19:273, 1966.

52. Andrassy R.J., Treadwell T.A., Ratner I.A., et al.: Gallbladder disease in children and adolescents. *Am. J. Surg.* 132:19, 1976.

53. Roslyn J.J., Berquist W.E., Pitt H.A., et al.: Increased risk of gallstones in children receiving total parenteral nutrition. *Pediatrics* 71:784, 1983.

54. Heubi J.E., Soloway R.D., Balistreri W.F.: Biliary lipid composition in healthy and diseased infants, children, and young adults. *Gastroenterology* 82:1295, 1982.

55. Bell C.C. Jr., McCormick W.C. III, Gregory D.H., et al.: Relationship of bile acid pool size to the formation of lithogenous bile in male Indians of the southwest. *Surg. Gynecol. Obstet.* 134:473, 1972.

56. Boston Collaborative Drug Surveillance Program: Oral contraceptives and venous thromboembolic disease, surgically confirmed gallbladder disease and breast tumors. *Lancet* 1:1399, 1973.

57. Boston Collaborative Drug Surveillance Program: Surgically confirmed gallbladder disease, venous thromboembolisms and breast tumors in relation to postmenopausal estrogen therapy. *N. Engl. J. Med.* 190:15, 1974.

58. The Coronary Drug Project Research Group: Gallbladder disease as a side effect of drugs influencing lipid metabolism: Experience in the coronary drug project. *N. Engl. J. Med.* 296:1185, 1977.

59. Glenn F., McSherry C.K.: Pregnancy, cholesterol metabolism, and gallstones. *Ann. Surg.* 169:712, 1969.

60. Nilsson S., Schersten T.: Importance of bile acids for phospholipid secretion into human hepatic bile. *Gastroenterology* 57:525, 1969.

61. Bonorris G.G., Coyne M.J., Chung A., et al.: Mechanism of estrogen-induced saturated bile in the hamster. *J. Lab. Clin. Med.* 90:963, 1977.

62. Freeman J.B., Meyer P.D., Printen K.J., et al.: Analysis of gallbladder bile in morbid obesity. *Am. J. Surg.* 129:163, 1975.

63. Mabee T.M., Meyer P., DenBesten L., et al.: The mechanism of increased gallstone formation in obese human subjects. *Surgery* 79:460, 1976.

64. Clave R.A., Gaspar M.R.: Incidence of gallbladder disease after vagotomy. *Am. J. Surg.* 118:169, 1969.

65. Sapala M.A., Sapala J.A., Resto Soto A.D., et al.: Cholelithiasis following subtotal gastric resection with truncal vagotomy. *Surg. Gynecol. Obstet.* 148:36, 1979.

66. Pitt H.A., Doty J.E., DenBesten L.: Increased intragallbladder

pressure response to cholecystokinin-octapeptide following vagotomy and pyloroplasty. *J. Surg. Res.* 35:325, 1983.

67. Wilbur B.H., Gomez F.C., Tompkins R.K.: Canine gallbladder bile: Effects of proximal gastric vagotomy, truncal vagotomy, and truncal vagotomy with pyloroplasty on volume and concentration. *Arch. Surg.* 110:792, 1975.

68. Roslyn J.J., Pitt H.A., Mann L.L., et al.: Gallbladder disease in patients on long-term parenteral nutrition. *Gastroenterology* 84:148, 1983.

69. Pitt H.A., King W. III, Mann L.L., et al.: Increased risk of cholelithiasis with prolonged total parenteral nutrition. *Am. J. Surg.* 145:106, 1983.

70. Thistle J.L., Schoenfield L.J.: Induced alterations in composition of bile of persons having cholelithiasis. *Gastroenterology* 61:488, 1971.

71. Danzinger R.G., Hofmann A.E., Schoenfield L.J., et al.: Dissolution of cholesterol gallstones by chenodeoxycholic acid. *N. Engl. J. Med.* 286:1, 1972.

72. Schoenfield L.J., Lachin J.M., Baum R.A., et al.: Chenodiol (chenodeoxycholic acid) for dissolution of gallstones: The National Cooperative Gallstone Study. A controlled trial of efficacy and safety. *Ann. Intern. Med.* 95:257, 1981.

73. Nakayama F.: Oral cholelitholysis—cheno versus urso: Japanese experience. *Dig. Dis. Sci.* 25:129, 1980.

74. Coyne M.J., Bonorris G.G., Goldstein L.I., et al.: Effect of chenodeoxycholic acid and phenobarbitol on the rate-limiting enzymes of hepatic cholesterol and bile acid synthesis in patients with gallstones. *J. Lab. Clin. Med.* 87:281, 1976.

75. Salen G., Colalillo A., Verga D., et al.: Effect of high and low doses of ursodeoxycholic acid on gallstone dissolution in humans. *Gastroenterology* 78:1412, 1980.

76. Wenckert A., Robertson B.: The natural course of gallstone disease: Eleven-year review of 781 nonoperated cases. *Gastroenterology* 50:376, 1966.

77. Clagett O.T.: Diseases of the gallbladder: Diagnosis and management. *Surg. Clin. North Am.* 25:929, 1945.

78. Glenn F.: Silent gallstones. *Ann. Surg.* 193:251, 1981.

79. Gracie W.A., Ransohoff D.F.: The natural history of silent gallstones. The innocent gallstone is not a myth. *N. Engl. J. Med.* 307:798, 1982.

80. Gambill E.E., Hodgson J.R., Priestley J.T.: Painless obstructive cholecystopathy. *Arch. Intern. Med.* 110:442, 1962.

81. Mann F.C.: The production by chemical means of a specific cholecystitis. *Ann. Surg.* 73:54, 1921.

82. Womack N.A., Bricker E.M.: Pathogenesis of cholecystitis. *Arch. Surg.* 44:658, 1942.

83. Thomas C.G. Jr., Womack N.A.: Acute cholecystitis, its pathogenesis and repair. *Arch. Surg.* 64:590, 1952.

84. Boyd W.: Cholesterolosis of the gallbladder. *Br. J. Surg.* 10:337, 1923.

85. Wolfer J.S.: The role of pancreatic juice in the production of gallbladder disease. *Surg. Gynecol. Obstet.* 53:433, 1931.

86. Anderson M.C., Hauman R.L., Suriyapa C., et al.: Pancreatic enzyme levels in bile of patients with extrahepatic biliary tract disease. *Am. J. Surg.* 137:301, 1979.

87. Sjodahl R., Tagesson C.: On the mediation of inflammatory reaction in the human gallbladder epithelium. *Scand. J. Gastroenterol.* 11:321, 1976.

88. Sjodahl R., Wetterfors J.: Lysolecithin and lecithin in the gallbladder wall and bile; their possible roles in the pathogenesis of acute cholecystitis. *Scand. J. Gastroenterol.* 9:519, 1974.

89. Sjodahl R., Tagesson C.: The biochemical prerequisites for preventing pathogenic lysolecithin activity in the human gallbladder. *Scand. J. Gastroenterol.* 11:661, 1967.

90. Sjodahl R., Tagesson C., Wetterfors J.: Lysolecithin-mediated inflammatory reaction in rabbit gallbladder. *Acta. Chir. Scand.* 141:403, 1975.

91. Gonciarz Z., Trusz-Gluza M., Kusmieriski S., et al.: Leukocytic proteases in gallbladder pathology, experimental acute cholecystitis in dogs. *Digestion* 10:65, 1974.

92. Andrews E.: Pathologic changes of diseased gallbladders. A new classification. *Arch. Surg.* 31:767, 1985.

93. Roslyn J.J., DenBesten L., Thompson J.E. Jr., et al.: Roles of lithogenic bile and cystic duct occlusion in the pathogenesis of

acute cholecystitis. *Am. J. Surg.* 140:126, 1980.

94. Glenn F., Thorbjarnarson B.: The surgical treatment of acute cholecystitis. *Surg. Gynecol. Obstet.* 116:61, 1963.

95. Brugge W.B., Atkins H., Abel W.: Biliary dyskinesia in acalculous chronic cholecystitis (ACC) (abstract). *Gastroenterology* 84:1115, 1983.

96. Goldsmith J.J.: The results of cholecystectomy. *Guy's Hosp. Rep.* 106:80, 1957.

97. Hay H.R.C.: Gas in gallstones. A rare radiological sign in the acute abdomen. *Gut* 7:387, 1966.

98. Graham E.A., Cole W.H.: Roentgenologic examination of the gallbladder, preliminary report of a new method utilizing the intravenous injection of tetrabromophenolphthalein. *J.A.M.A.* 82:613, 1924.

99. Baker H.L., Hodgson J.R.: Further studies on the accuracy of oral cholecystography. *Radiology* 74:239, 1960.

100. Cooperberg P.L., Burhenne H.J.: Real-time ultrasonography. Diagnostic technique of choice in calculous gallbladder disease. *N. Engl. J. Med.* 302:1277, 1980.

101. deGraaff D.S., Dembner A.G., Taylor K.J.W.: Ultrasound and false normal oral cholecystogram. *Arch. Surg.* 113:877, 1978.

102. Ralls P.W., Halls J., Lapin S.A., et al.: Prospective evaluation of the sonographic Murphy sign in suspected acute cholecystitis. *J.C.U.* 10:113, 1982.

103. Harvey E., Loberg M., Cooper M.: 99Tc-HIDA, a new radio pharmaceutical for hepatobiliary imaging (abstract). *J. Nucl. Med.* 16:533, 1975.

104. Potter T., McClain C.J., Shafer R.B.: Effect of fasting and parenteral alimentation on PIPIDA scintigraphy. *Dig. Dis. Sci.* 28:687, 1983.

105. Suarez C.A., Block F., Bernstein D., et al.: The role of HIDA/PIPIDA scanning in diagnosing cystic duct obstruction. *Ann. Surg.* 191:391, 1980.

106. Shuman W.P., Gibbs P., Rudd T.G., et al.: PIPIDA scintigraphy for cholecystitis: False positives in alcoholism and total parenteral nutrition. *A.J.R.* 138:1, 1982.

107. Burnstein M.J., Vassal K.P., Strasberg S.M.: Results of combined biliary drainage and cholecystokinin cholecystography in 81 patients with normal oral cholecystograms. *Ann. Surg.* 196:627, 1982.

108. van der Linden W., Sunzel H.: Early versus delayed operation for acute cholecystitis. A controlled clinical trial. *Am. J. Surg.* 120:7, 1970.

109. Lahtinen J., Alhava E.M., Aukee S.: Acute cholecystitis treated by early and delayed surgery. A controlled clinical trial. *Scand. J. Gastroenterol.* 13:673, 1978.

110. Wright H.K., Holden W.D.: The risks of emergency surgery for acute cholecystitis. *Arch. Surg.* 81:341, 1960.

111. Jarvinen H.J., Hastabacka J.: Early cholecystectomy for acute cholecystitis, a prospective randomized study. *Ann. Surg.* 191:501, 1980.

112. Morrow D.J., Thompson J., Wilson S.E.: Acute cholecystitis in the elderly: A surgical emergency. *Arch. Surg.* 113:1149, 1978.

113. Saltzstein E.C., Evani S.V., Mann R.W.: Routine cholangiography. *Arch. Surg.* 107:289, 1973.

114. Skillings J.C., William J.S., Hinshaw J.R.: Cost effectiveness of operative cholangiography. *Am. J. Surg.* 137:26, 1979.

115. Gerber A., Apt M.K.: The case against routine operative cholangiography. *Am. J. Surg.* 143:734, 1982.

116. Taylor T.V., Torrance B., Rimmer S., et al.: Operative cholangiography: Is there a statistical alternative? *Am. J. Surg.* 145:640, 1983.

117. Doyle P.J., Ward-McQuaid J.N., McEven Smith A.: The value of routine preoperative cholangiography—a report of 4000 cholecystectomies. *Br. J. Surg.* 69:617, 1982.

118. White T.T., Waisman H., Hopton D., et al.: Radiomanometry, flow rates, and cholangiography in the evaluation of common bile duct disease: A study of 220 cases. *Am. J. Surg.* 123:73, 1972.

119. Csendes A., Fernandez M., Uribe P.: Bacteriology of the gallbladder and bile in normal subjects. *Am. J. Surg.* 129:629, 1975.

120. Chetlin S.H., Elliott D.W.: Biliary bacteremia. *Arch. Surg.* 102:303, 1971.

121. Fukunaga F.H.: Gallbladder bacteriology, histology and gall-

stones: Study of unselected cholecystectomy specimens in Honolulu. *Arch. Surg.* 106:169, 1973.

122. Reiss R., Eliashiv A., Deutsch A.A.: Septic complications and bile cultures in 800 consecutive cholecystectomies. *World J. Surg.* 6:195, 1982.
123. Chetlin S.H., Elliott D.W.: Preoperative antibiotics in biliary surgery. *Arch. Surg.* 107:319, 1973.
124. Keighley M.R.B., Baddeley R.M., Burdon D.W., et al.: A controlled trial of parenteral prophylactic gentamicin therapy in biliary surgery. *Br. J. Surg.* 62:275, 1975.
125. Keighley M.R.B., Drysdale R.B., Quoraishi A.H., et al.: Antibiotics in biliary disease: The relative importance of antibiotic concentrations in the bile and serum. *Gut* 17:495, 1976.
126. McLeish A.R., Keighley M.R.B., Bishop H.M., et al.: Selecting patients requiring antibiotics in biliary surgery by immediate gram stains of bile at operation. *Surgery* 81:473, 1977.
127. Beinfield M.S., Hayes R.L.: Use of intraoperative gram stain during cholecystectomy. *Am. J. Surg.* 137:773, 1979.
128. Stone H.H., Hooper C.A., Kolb L.D., et al.: Antibiotic prophylaxis in gastric, biliary and colonic surgery. *Ann. Surg.* 184:443, 1976.
129. Deaver J.B.: Quoted by Madding G.F.: *Trauma to the Liver.* Philadelphia, W.B. Saunders Co., 1964, p. 69.
130. Feigenberg Z., Wolloch Y., Sokolousky R., et al.: Routine drainage in cholecystectomy: A bacteriologic and clinical assessment. *Am. J. Surg.* 136:314, 1978.
131. Polk H.C. Jr.: Sump-suction drainage of the subhepatic space after cholecystectomy. *Surgery* 74:462, 1973.
132. Budd D.C., Cochran R.C., Fouty W.J. Jr.: Cholecystectomy with and without drainage: A randomized, prospective study of 300 patients. *Am. J. Surg.* 143:307, 1982.
133. Todd G.J., Reemtsma K.: Cholecystectomy with drainage: Factors influencing wound infection in 1000 elective cases. *Am. J. Surg.* 135:622, 1978.
134. Hill M.J., Drasar B.S., Williams R.E.O., et al.: Faecal bile acids and clostridia in patients with cancer of the large bowel. *Lancet* 1:535, 1978.
135. Turunen M.J., Kivilaakso E.O.: Increased risk of colorectal cancer after cholecystectomy. *Ann. Surg.* 194:639, 1981.
136. Turnbull P.R.G., Smith A.H., Isbister W.H.: Cholecystectomy and cancer of the large bowel. *Br. J. Surg.* 68:551, 1981.
137. Weiss N.S., Daling J.R., Chow W.H.: Cholecystectomy and the incidence of cancer of the large bowel. *Cancer* 49:1713, 1982.
138. Lowenfels A.B., Domellof L., Lindstrom C.G., et al.: Cholelithiasis, cholecystectomy, and cancer: A case-control study in Sweden. *Gastroenterology* 83:672, 1982.
139. Duncan J.: Femoral hernia: Gangrene of the gallbladder, extravasation of bile; peritonitis, death. *North J. Med.* 2:151, 1844.
140. Neschis M., King M.C., Murphy R.A.: Cholecystokinin cholecystography in the diagnosis of acalculous extrahepatic biliary tract disorders. *Am. J. Gastroenterol.* 70:593, 1978.
141. Ottinger L.W.: Acute cholecystitis as a postoperative complication. *Ann. Surg.* 184:162, 1976.
142. Lindberg E.F., Grinnan G.L.B., Smith L.: Acalculous cholecystitis in Viet Nam casualities. *Ann. Surg.* 171:152, 1670.
143. DuPriest R.W. Jr., Khaneja S.C., Cowley R.A.: Acute cholecystitis complicating trauma. *Ann. Surg.* 189:1, 1979.
144. Munster A.M., Goodwin M.N., Pruitt B.A. Jr.: Acalculous cholecystitis in burned patients. *Am. J. Surg.* 122:591, 1971.
145. Swanepoel C.R., Floyd A., Allison H., et al.: Acute acalculous cholecystitis complicating systemic lupus erythematosus: Case report and review. *Br. Med. J.* 286:251, 1983.
146. Orlando R. III., Gleason E., Drezner A.D.: Acute acalculous cholecystitis in the critically ill patient. *Am. J. Surg.* 145:472, 1983.
147. Roslyn J.J., Pitt H.A., Mann L.L., et al.: Parenteral nutrition induced gallbladder disease—A reason for early cholecystectomy. *Am. J. Surg.* 148:58, 1984.
148. Lieber M.M.: The incidence of gallstones and their correlation with other diseases. *Ann. Surg.* 135:394, 1952.
149. Feldman M., Feldman M. Jr.: The incidence of cholelithiasis, cholesterosis and liver disease in diabetes mellitus: An autopsy study. *Diabetes* 3:305, 1954.
150. Bennion L.J., Grundy S.M.: Effects of diabetes mellitus on cholesterol metabolism in man. *N. Engl. J. Med.* 296:1365, 1977.
151. Turrill F.L., McCarron N.M., Mikkelsen W.P.: Gallstones and diabetics: An ominous association. *Am. J. Surg.* 102:184, 1961.
152. Walsh D.B., Eckhauser F.E., Ramsburgh S.R., et al.: Risk associated with diabetes mellitus in patients undergoing gallbladder surgery. *Surgery* 91:254, 1982.
153. Nicholas P., Rinaudo P.A., Conn H.O.: Increased incidence of cholelithiasis in Laennec's cirrhosis. A postmorten evaluation of pathogenesis. *Gastroenterology* 63:112, 1972.
154. Schwartz S.J.: Biliary tract surgery and cirrhosis: A critical combination. *Surgery* 90:577, 1981.
155. McSherry C.K., Glenn F.: The incidence and causes of death following surgery for nonmalignant biliary tract disease. *Ann. Surg.* 191:271, 1980.
156. Aranha G.V., Sontag S.J., Greenlee H.B.: Cholecystectomy in cirrhotic patients: A formidable operation. *Am. J. Surg.* 163:55, 1982.
157. Glenn F.: Surgical management of acute cholecystitis in patients 65 years of age and older. *Ann. Surg.* 193:56, 1981.
158. Roslyn J., Busuttil R.W.: Perforation of the gallbladder: A frequently mismanaged condition. *Am. J. Surg.* 137:307, 1979.
159. Niemeier O.W.: Acute free perforation of the gallbladder. *Ann. Surg.* 99:922, 1934.
160. Glenn F., Moore S.W.: Gangrene and perforation of the wall of the gallbladder: A sequela of acute cholecystitis. *Arch. Surg.* 44:677, 1942.
161. Rigler L.G., Borman C.M., Noble J.F.: Gallstone obstruction: Pathogenesis and roentgen manifestation. *J.A.M.A.* 117:1753, 1941.
162. Kurtz R.J., Hermann T.M., Kurtz A.B.: Gallstone ileus: A diagnostic problem. *Am. J. Surg.* 146:314, 1983.
163. Heuman R., Sjodahl R., Wetterfors J.: Gallstone ileus: An analysis of 20 patients. *World J. Surg.* 4:595, 1980.
164. Hegner C.G.: Gaseous pericholecystitis with cholecystitis and cholelithiasis. *Arch. Surg.* 22:993, 1931.
165. Mentzer R.M., Golden C.T., Chandler J.G., et al.: A comparative appraisal of emphysematous cholecystitis. *Am. J. Surg.* 129:10, 1975.

20

The Postcholecystectomy Syndrome

FRANK G. MOODY, M.D.

CHOLECYSTECTOMY has been the treatment of choice by surgeons for the symptoms and complications of gallstones since its introduction by Langenbuch[1] more than 100 years ago. The early development of what is now accepted as safe and effective therapy was not without controversy and diverse opinion.[2] Surprisingly, surgical removal of the gallbladder is associated with few serious, late sequelae. Even the operative morbidity has been reduced to a fraction of a percent when performed in otherwise healthy individuals under the age of 60.[3] One in five patients, however, develops new GI complaints or has a recurrence of the symptoms for which cholecystectomy was recommended.[4] This unfortunate outcome has been referred to as the "postcholecystectomy syndrome."

It is my intent to provide a framework for understanding and effectively treating this ill-defined entity. Clearly, abdominal pain after cholecystectomy, the unique symptom of this syndrome, may be a manifestation of a misdiagnosis. Associated GI problems that may be the source of the patient's symptoms should be identified and treated prior to cholecystectomy thereby avoiding an unnecessary operation in some, and simplifying the identification of postcholecystectomy symptoms in others. The importance of precise identification of the source of a patient's complaints prior to cholecystectomy cannot be overemphasized.

PREVALENCE OF POSTCHOLECYSTECTOMY COMPLAINTS

The incidence of GI symptoms after cholecystectomy has been reported to be between 10% and 50%.[5-7] Fortunately, these complaints are usually mild and nonspecific and consist mainly of transient nausea, indigestion, belching, bloating, and flatulence. However, about 5% of patients after cholecystectomy experience severe episodes of upper abdominal pain similar to those that they had prior to cholecystectomy.[8] Womack and Crider[9] reported in 1947 their experience with six patients who after cholecystectomy complained of recurrent attacks of severe upper abdominal pain with no apparent cause. They were the first to mention "the so-called postcholecystectomy syndrome," which they believed was secondary to biliary dyskinesia or an abnormality of the periductal autonomic neural net. Pribram[10] in 1950 reported that 20% of the 1,370 patients on whom he had performed a cholecystectomy experienced attacks of biliary colic. He entitled his discussion

"Postcholecystectomy Syndromes." The frequency of the problem in his experience stimulated an extensive study of biliary manometry and of sphincter of Oddi function and the development of a cholecystocholedochal shunt in an attempt to avoid the postcholecystectomy pain by leaving the gallbladder in place. Bodvall,[5] however, was the first systematically to study the diverse etiologies of the postcholecystectomy syndrome. He and his colleagues evaluated 1,930 patients after cholecystectomy and observed that nearly 40% had symptoms after operation. The relative frequency of complaints is shown in Table 20–1. Complaints were twice as frequent in women as in men and more common in the younger age groups. Only 2.4% of patients had persistent episodes of pain that could not be explained on the basis of the presence or passage of stones.

Glenn and McSherry[11] approached the question of postcholecystectomy problems by analyzing the reasons for reoperation on 253 of 5,859 patients who had previously undergone a cholecystectomy (4.5%). The majority (65.6%) of these patients was found to have diseases of the bile ducts, liver, or pancreas. Stefanini and de Bardinis[12] found a similar incidence of poor results (4%), while nearly a third (217) of 800 patients had postcholecystectomy symptoms. They observed, as had others, that advanced and neglected gallbladder disease is most likely to be associated with problems in the late postoperative period. The ability to detect gallstones by oral cholecystogram and ultrasound in symptomatic patients and earlier removal of the gallbladder in this situation by well-trained surgeons may explain what appears to be a decreasing prevalence of postcholecystectomy problems. The current incidence of GI symptoms after cholecystectomy for stones is in the range of 10%; fewer than 1% of patients have severe, disabling symptoms.

PATHOGENESIS OF POSTCHOLECYSTECTOMY SYNDROMES

Conditions that might mimic the symptoms of biliary tract disease either prior to or following cholecystectomy are listed in Table 20–2. The irritable bowel syndrome is a commonly associated GI disturbance that may be accompanied by symptoms identical to those experienced with the passage of a gallstone. Pancreatitis, peptic ulcer, reflux esophagitis, and right-sided colonic diverticulosis are only a few of many GI diseases

TABLE 20–1.—Frequency of
Symptoms After Cholecystectomy, %
(n = 1,930)

Asymptomatic	60.4
Dyspepsia	10.7
Mild pain	23.5
Occasional severe pain	3.0
Severe with cholangitis	2.4

Adapted from Bodvall B.: The postcholecystectomy syndromes. *Clin. Gastroenterol.*
2(1):103–125, 1973.[5]

that are associated with dyspepsia and the nonspecific symptoms of belching, bloating, and flatulence.

Tondelli et al.[13] emphasized the importance of considering
all symptoms after cholecystectomy as being related to the
operation or the pancreaticobiliary tree until proved otherwise. In their view, the true cause of symptoms will escape
detection unless all possibilities are considered.

The major biliary-related causes for postcholecystectomy
problems are listed in Table 20–3. It is easy to understand
why a retained common duct stone, incomplete cholecystectomy, or a benign stricture with or without stones might be
associated with symptoms of abdominal pain and jaundice. It
is not clear how a cystic duct remnant might provoke episodes
of biliary colic except when a stone is impacted within its lumen. Numerous authors since the earlier work of Womack
and Crider[9] have attempted to implicate the cystic duct itself
in the episodic attacks of severe abdominal pain. Bodvall and
Overgaard[14] observed a 22% incidence of stones within a retained cystic duct or gallbladder remnant in 452 reported
cases. They established a strong correlation between the
length of the cystic duct stump and severity of GI symptoms
in their study of 500 patients after cholecystectomy by IV cholangiography. This led to the speculation that the retained
stump may be the source of recurrent stone formation, a sup-
position that would account for the high incidence (34%) of
common duct stones in 68 cases with recurrent episodes of
cholangitis. A high incidence of cystic duct remnant was also
found in asymptomatic and mildly symptomatic patients,
leading to the conclusion that a cystic duct remnant per se
does not necessarily lead to severe symptoms. Glenn and
Whitsell[15] reported a comparable experience in which 25 of
95 patients had stones with a cystic duct remnant; 19 patients
were found to have stones within the common duct.
Millbourn[16] reported on a pain-free one- to seven-year follow-
up interval on seven patients who had stones removed from

TABLE 20–2.—Nonbiliary Sources
of Gastrointestinal Symptoms
After Cholecystectomy

Irritable bowel syndrome
Peptic ulcer
Reflux esophagitis
Pancreatitis (nonbiliary)
Liver disease
Coronary artery disease
Intra-abdominal adhesions
Intercostal neuritis
Wound neuroma

TABLE 20–3.—Biliary Sources
of the Postcholecystectomy Syndromes

Common duct stone
Retained gallbladder
Traumatic stricture
Cystic duct remnant
Stenosing papillitis
Biliary dyskinesia

long cystic duct remnants, but the remnants were left in
place. It therefore appears that many patients with long cystic
duct remnants have stones, and that it is the stones that cause
symptoms, not the remnants.

Chronic inflammation, fibrosis, and neuroma formation are
also common pathologic findings on histologic examination of
excised remnants. The role of these findings in the clinical
syndrome is as yet undefined.

STENOSING PAPILLITIS

Fibrosis and inflammation of the papilla of Vater have been
commented on extensively by biliary surgeons since the time
of the first series of cholecystectomies by Langenbuch.
Flörcken[17] is credited with the first systematic description of
papillary fibrosis. Acosta and colleagues,[18] in their in-depth
study of the histologic changes associated with this entity,
pointed out the difficulties of histologic diagnosis in view of
the extensive amount of collagen that normally resides within
the papilla. In their study of 38 surgical biopsies of the papilla
of patients with symptoms of recurrent episodes of pancreatitis, they found fibrosis in ten and chronic inflammation in
nine. It is of interest that all eight biopsies from patients with
biliary tract disease had histologic abnormalities.

Hess[19] also observed a high incidence of stenosing papillitis
in patients with biliary tract disease (29.4%) in the relative
frequency (Table 20–4). Grage and colleagues[20] (1960) in an
earlier histologic study of 50 transduodenal biopsies of the papilla of Vater found abnormalities in 32. There was no correlation between the clinical symptoms of the biliary tract disease and the severity of histologic changes. Numerous
surgeons before and since have observed fibrotic changes
within the papilla of Vater at the time of transduodenal
sphincterotomy thereby lending credence to the existence of
stenosing papillitis. Skepticism persists, however, as to the
clinical importance and frequency of the lesion, and is enhanced by a general lack of understanding of the pathogenesis
of the disease process within the papilla of Vater.

TABLE 20–4.—Incidence of Stenosing
Papillitis in Biliary Lithiasis

	TOTAL CASES	STENOSING PAPILLITIS	%
Chronic acalculous cholecystitis	90	12	13
Cholelithiasis	819	186	23
Choledocholithiasis	311	161	52

Adapted from Hess W.: Stenosing papillitis, in
Hess W. (ed.): *Surgery of the Biliary Passages and
the Pancreas.* Princeton, D. Van Nostrand Co.,
1965.[19]

My colleagues and I in Salt Lake City embarked on a systematic prospective study of human papillary disease by performing a transduodenal exploration of the papilla of Vater in patients with presumed papillary disease.[21] We hypothesized that the study group had severe recurrent episodes of chronic abdominal pain on the basis of papillary stenosis. Furthermore, we considered that the pain was likely pancreatic in origin due to outflow obstruction of the duct of Wirsung from thickening and fibrosis of the transampullary septum within the papilla of Vater. The operation performed included a long anterior sphincteroplasty if not previously done and a transampullary septectomy. The pathologic findings from the first 28 patients operated on are shown in Table 20–5. A larger study involving 92 patients revealed two general categories of inflammatory disease, one that included the entire papilla and one that primarily involved the transampullary septum. The results as shown in Table 20–6 of the initial 28 postcholecystectomy patients at five to ten years revealed that the procedure could provide long-term pain relief in over half of the patients. The results were substantiated in the larger series, with the interesting finding that patients with prior adequate sphincteroplasty obtained the highest level of pain relief.[22] This observation provided strong support for the idea that the diseased septum and pancreatic outflow obstruction might have played a role in the pain experienced by these patients.

Our attention to the opening of the duct of Wirsung was not novel. Cole and Grove[23] had described in 1952 a case where the opening of the bile duct entered the pancreatic duct within the papilla. They devised a procedure where following anterior sphincteroplasty they "cut the bridge between the pancreatic and common bile duct." Bartlett and Nardi[24] and Warren and colleagues[25] have also described removal of the transampullary septum in selected cases where the opening of the duct of Wirsung was compromised by fibrosis.

These studies suggest that stenosing papillitis is primarily the consequence of the chronic passage of gallstones. Whether the inflammatory response can occur in the absence of an associated pancreatitis is unclear. The majority of the postcholecystectomy patients on whom I operated, however, had a normal-appearing pancreas at the time of exploration. On the other hand, Acosta and Ledesma[26] have clearly established the high incidence of stone passage in biliary pancreatitis (95%). The passage of stones into the gut was also significant in patients with gallstones but without pancreatitis who were used as controls in their study.

Some potential etiologic factors in stenosing papillitis are listed in Table 20–7. Cholesterolosis of the papilla of Vater was diagnosed on the basis of histologic evidence of acute in-

TABLE 20–6.—OPERATIVE FINDINGS: FIVE- TO TEN-YEAR FOLLOW-UP ON 28 POSTCHOLECYSTECTOMY PATIENTS

RESULT	PRIOR REPORT	PRESENT STUDY
Good	16	13
Fair	5	11
Poor	7	4

From Moody F.G., Becker J.M., Potts J.R.: Transduodenal sphincteroplasty and transampullary septectomy for postcholecystectomy pain. *Ann. Surg.* 197:627–636, 1983. With permission from *Annals of Surgery.*

flammation or the gross presence of yellow submucosal deposits within the papilla, giving a "strawberry" appearance similar to that seen in cholesterolosis of the gallbladder. Possibly stenosing papillitis on the basis of cholesterolosis is a primary lesion in the biliary tract disease of this subset of patients.

Only two patients were known to have had previous forceful dilatation of their papilla. It has been recognized since the early work of Branch and co-workers[27] that injury from overstretching the papilla will lead to inflammation and fibrosis. The placement of a long limb of rubber tube will also lead to papillary fibrosis. It will be of interest to learn whether the current practice of long-term intubation of the papilla by the transhepatic or transendoscopic route will provoke inflammation and fibrosis.

BILIARY DYSKINESIA

The sphincter of Oddi of man has long been suspect of being the source of abdominal pain after cholecystectomy. It has been known since the time of Gage[28] (1879) and Oddi[29] (1887) that the papilla of Vater contains a highly specialized mound of smooth muscle that is distinct from the muscular layers of the duodenal wall. This muscle serves to direct and meter the flow of bile from the liver and pancreatic juice from the pancreas. The anatomy of the muscle fibers, and their relationship to the bile and pancreatic ducts in man have been extensively studied by Boyden.[30] His concept of the sphincter of Oddi is revealed in elegant detail in Figure 20–1. Parvel[31] in France (1932) and Schmeiden and Niessen[32] in Germany described their experience with patients presumed to have spasm of the sphincter of Oddi. Schmieden and Niessen and shortly thereafter Ivy and Sandbloom[33] (1934) called the syndrome biliary dyskinesia. McGowan et al.[34] in 1936 reported on their radiographic and manometric studies of the biliary tree of eight patients who had T tubes placed at the time of

TABLE 20–5.—FINDINGS AT EXPLORATION IN 28 PATIENTS WITH POSTCHOLECYSTECTOMY PAIN

	PANCREAS	PAPILLA	SEPTUM
Normal	20	5	16
Abnormal	8	23	12

From Moody F.G., Berenson M.M., McCloskey D.: Transampullary septectomy for postcholecystectomy pain. *Ann. Surg.* 186:415–423, 1977. Used by permission.

TABLE 20–7.—SOME ETIOLOGIC FACTORS IN STENOSING PAPILLITIS

Choledocholithiasis
Instrumentation
Intubation
Cholesterolosis
Peptic ulcer
Pancreatitis
Ascariasis
Sclerosing cholangitis

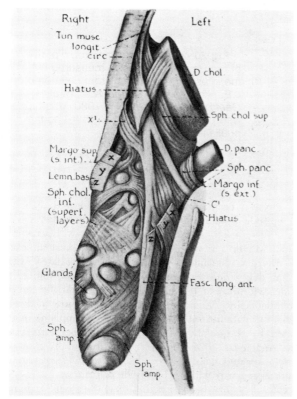

Fig 20–1.—Schematic of human papilla of Vater and its sphincter of Oddi represented in exquisite detail. Note that smooth muscle fibers envelop both the bile and pancreatic ducts. (Used with permission of *Surgery, Gynecology and Obstetrics.*[4])

cholecystectomy. They observed that morphine would provoke a rapid rise in intrabiliary pressure. In one patient, the rise in pressure was associated with severe epigastric pain similar to that experienced prior to cholecystectomy. Furthermore, recurrent episodes of pain without provocation were associated with a marked rise in intrabiliary pressure. A "few whiffs" of amyl nitrite completely relieved the pain produced by morphine and returned the elevated intrabiliary pressure to normal levels. These observations provide strong evidence for a relationship between increased biliary pressure and pain and suggest that the sphincter of Oddi may play a central role in the process.

Subsequently, Bachrach and colleagues[35] made the chance observation of a marked rise in intraductal pressure in a postcholecystectomy patient during a stressful episode, thereby suggesting that the autonomic nervous system may play a role in sphincter hypercontraction. The concept of biliary dyskinesia as a consequence of spasm of the sphincter of Oddi was reinforced by the results of Colp,[36] who in 1946 reported relief of biliary-type pain in six of eight postcholecystectomy patients by endocholedochal sphincterotomy. These earlier studies, however, did not distinguish whether the pain was from a spastic sphincter of Oddi or from the high pressures within the biliary tree. Dahl-Iversen et al.[37] concluded that the sphincter was the likely source of painful stimuli from their observation that patients would experience

episodic pain with presumed biliary dyskinesia even when a T tube within the common duct was left to dependent drainage. They further showed that static and perfusion pressures within the bile duct were no different from normal in patients with gallstones or postcholecystectomy biliary dyskinesia.

The failure of sphincterotomy to provide long-term relief of pain in postcholecystectomy patients raised serious doubts in the ensuing two decades as to whether biliary dyskinesia was a legitimate pathologic entity. The work of Steinberg et al.[38] added a further challenge to the concept of sphincter spasm as a clinical entity. They observed that 60% of healthy control subjects and patients with an irritable bowel syndrome would experience abdominal pain and an elevation of amylase and lipase on provocation with morphine and prostigmine, the so-called Nardi test.[39] Gregg and colleagues,[40] on the other hand, observed that 16 of 23 patients with abdominal pain and a positive Nardi test had moderate to marked signs of papillary stenosis by endoscopic evaluation. LoGuidice and colleagues[41] found results to the contrary. They could document no correlation between the extent of papillary stenosis at the time of operation and the results of the morphine-prostigmine test. There was a good correlation, however, between the pressure measurements of transpapillary manometry and the presence of papillary stenosis.

The development of transendoscopic papillary manometry has contributed a potential way to identify anatomical or functional defects of this area. The normal manometric profile of the transpapillary area as measured by the infusion technique of Geenen[42] is shown in Figure 20–2. The cyclical pressure waves observed in this short segment of the papilla (4 mm) represent contractions of the sphincter of Oddi. The manometric appearance of spasm of the sphincter of Oddi segment is shown in Figure 20–3. In this tracing, there is an elevation of the baseline pressure, and frequent, uncoordinated contractions. Csendes and colleagues[43] also observed higher peak Oddi pressures in patients after cholecystectomy compared to controls. In addition, they found no correlation between peak Oddi pressures and common bile duct pressures, further confirming the experience of others that the latter measurement is of little value in detecting papillary disease. On the contrary, transendoscopic, transpapillary manometry offers an opportunity to identify high pressures within the area of the sphincter of Oddi. It should be emphasized, however, that the perfusion technique cannot distinguish whether the channel within the papilla is narrowed from stenosis or from contraction of the sphincter of Oddi. Possibly this distinction is not important, since Bar-Meir and associates[44] observed that 10 of 14 patients with elevated basal pressures reported improvement in symptoms after transendoscopic sphincterotomy. Transpapillary manometry has emerged as a popular technique for evaluating postcholecystectomy pain. Unfortunately, uncertainty persists as to how to evaluate the results in a given patient, even though the group of patients with pain after cholecystectomy has higher pressures than control subjects. While the technique can be employed by cannulation of the common duct either directly or through the cystic duct, the operative state (anesthetic and dissection) makes interpretation difficult. Perfusion manometric studies are subject to the same reservations.

While the issue of biliary dyskinesia remains unresolved in

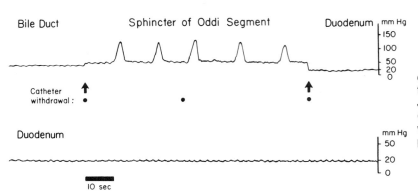

Fig 20–2.—Normal manotropic profile of the transpillary area is measured by the infusion technique. (From Geenen J.E., Hogan W.J., Dodds W.J., et al.: *Gastroenterology* 78:317, 1980. Used with permission from the author and the publisher.)

the human, there is one experimental circumstance where it can be produced without equivocation. The opossum, a third-order mammal, has a biliary sphincter that allows the easy insertion of extracellular electrodes. Becker and colleagues,[45] utilizing this model, demonstrated that in contradistinction to man, cholecystokinin is an agonist to the biliary sphincter of the opossum. Tooulli and associates[46] provided evidence that the opossum may lack a neural pathway to the papilla that is present in man. It is therefore possible that there are some individuals who lack this neural suppressive pathway and therefore may have a biliary sphincter that contracts, rather than relaxes, in response to cholecystokinin, thereby representing true biliary dyskinesia. Ono[47] has reported papillary myoelectric recordings in a patient in which there was an increase in burst spike potentials in response to exogenous cholecystokinin. Geenen and his colleagues[48] observed an increase in the frequency and amplitude of transpapillary pressures in a minority of patients studied by transendoscopic manometry. The majority have a complete cessation of contractions in response to cholecystokinin. The issue of the role of the sphincter of Oddi in the postcholecystectomy syndrome is therefore far from resolved.

CLINICAL MANIFESTATIONS

The abdominal pain of the postcholecystectomy syndrome is usually severe, episodic, and localized to the middle or right epigastrium. Eating may provoke the onset of pain in about 50% of patients. The variability in time of onset and the frequency of attacks makes diagnosis a difficult process. Often, the pain has subsided and physical and laboratory examinations are normal when the patient seeks medical atten-

tion. Physical examination, however, performed during an acute episode of pain will usually reveal upper abdominal tenderness. Nausea and occasionally vomiting will accompany the pain. Liver and pancreatic enzymes are normal, except when there is cholangitis or pancreatitis associated with a common duct stone. Fortunately, the pain is self-limited and subsides within 24 to 48 hours. Often, relief initially can only be obtained by the administration of narcotic analgesics. Work-up of patients with such nonspecific complaints is confounded by the relatively normal initial laboratory assessment. An elevation of the serum bilirubin or liver or pancreatic-associated enzymes occurs in about 20% of patients, but not necessarily with each episode of pain.

A careful history is an essential diagnostic tool. It is most important to ascertain the characteristics of the pain. Is it similar to that experienced prior to cholecystectomy? What are the circumstances of its onset and progression? What makes it worse or better? These are only a few of the questions that might provide useful clues to the underlying disease process.

It must be emphasized that there always is a reason for abdominal pain. The human mind is incapable of creating pain. Rather, the brain prefers to attenuate painful stimuli that are brought to it by peripheral receptors. Unfortunately, patients with chronic pain that remains undiagnosed become medical outcasts, estranged from society and eventually shunned by their physicians. Fortunately, the plight of the patient with chronic abdominal pain has attracted the interest of an increasing number of medical professionals. Chronic pain clinics that these specialists conduct are commonplace. Furthermore, remarkable developments in biliary and pancreatic imaging have offered precise tools for identifying anatomical defects in these organs. The application of ultrasonog-

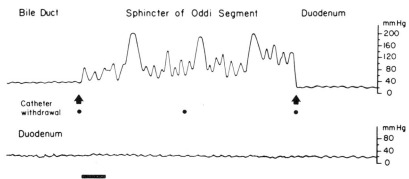

Fig 20–3.—Manometric appearance of spasm of the sphincter of Oddi segment. (From Geenen J.E., Hogan W.J., Dodds W.J., et al.: *Gastroenterology* 78:317, 1980. Used with permission from the author and the publisher.)

raphy, radionuclide scans, PTC, ERCP, CT, angiography, and transpapillary manometry should contribute to a better understanding of this elusive entity in the future.

ENTERTAINING THE DIAGNOSIS

Defining the cause of chronic postcholecystectomy abdominal pain is usually a difficult exercise in differential diagnosis. Having in mind a list of potential etiologic entities as shown in Table 20–3 can be most helpful as a starting point. For example, a history of the sudden onset of upper abdominal pain, accompanied by chills, fever, and jaundice, suggests the presence of a common duct stone. On the other hand, a long-standing history of recurrent episodes of moderately severe upper abdominal pain without associated symptoms or signs of hepatobiliary or pancreatic disease is more consistent with stenosing papillitis.

The presenting complaint and associated history and physical findings will therefore provide a working diagnosis. The value of a careful history cannot be overemphasized. Furthermore, it is of utmost importance to elicit details of the symptoms for which cholecystectomy was performed, and the extent to which the presence of gallstones or gallbladder disease was documented by preoperative studies, and morphological examination of the removed gallbladder. Hospital records including the operative note, pathology report, and discharge summary should be obtained from the patient's surgeon. A careful review should also be made of cholangiographic or other biliary imaging studies if available. While this advice appears self-evident, it is often omitted in the early phase of the assessment of postcholecystectomy pain.

DIAGNOSTIC SEQUENCE

The laboratory work-up should be based on the presumed diagnosis and the information gleaned from the hospital record, and the interval evaluation since cholecystectomy. As a general rule, I prefer to initiate a completely new diagnostic work-up with a few simple laboratory tests such as a urinalysis, stool guaiac, hemoglobin, WBC count, and serum analysis for bilirubin, albumin, alkaline phosphatase, and SGOT. In the usual case of chronic postcholecystectomy pain without associated signs, these tests are normal.

It is helpful to have the patient keep a pain diary in which the time, circumstances, severity, and duration of pain are carefully recorded. A parallel record is kept of what medications were used to gain relief. No effort should be made at this time to alter the patient's medications or diet unless narcotic analgesics are used on a constant basis. This situation requires a more urgent approach to diagnosis within a hospital setting. Most patients, however, seek parenteral narcotic analgesics only for severe attacks, and rely on oral analgesics such as acetaminophen (Tylenol) with codeine for daily or weekly pain control. In this situation, patients can be evaluated on an ambulatory basis until the pattern of their pain syndrome has been established.

The next step is predicated on the established or presumed diagnosis. Irritable bowel syndrome symptoms, for example, might be controlled by a mild sedative and the addition of bulk to the diet. An ultrasound study of the upper abdomen is often the best starting point for a more definitive diagnosis

of biliary tract or pancreatic disease. A barium roentgenogram of the upper GI tract should be obtained to rule out the presence of esophagogastric reflux or chronic duodenal ulcer. Persistent symptoms will require an upper GI endoscopy and ERCP. Transpapillary manometry is currently being refined and assessed as to its value in the detection of motor disturbances of the papilla of Vater, as discussed above.[42] I believe that this technique will emerge as the single best definitive way to diagnose benign disease of the papilla.

The results of attempts to identify vaterian disease by pharmacologic provocation of pain or pancreatic enzyme changes have been varied. The Nardi test, in which the papilla is stimulated to contract by morphine while the pancreas is induced to secrete by physostigmine, has predicted long-term pain relief in the hands of Nardi and Acosta.[39] Steinberg et al.[38] in a randomized control trial, however, were not able to distinguish patients with organic hepatobiliary or pancreatic disease from normal controls. Apparently, the combination of morphine and physostigmine can elicit intense spasm and pain from a viscera other than the papilla in patients without GI disease. The secretin-provocative test, in which the pancreas is stimulated to secrete at a maximal rate, is also of little discriminative value. One would expect that pain would be produced in patients in whom there was obstruction to the outflow of pancreatic juice in response to secretin stimulation, but the results are inconsistent. Patients have been identified in whom increments in pressure within the bile duct will induce severe upper abdominal pain. Possibly a choleretic provocative test should be developed in combination with biliary imaging by radionuclide scanning. While biliary imaging by radionuclide scan has been employed for a variety of diseases of the biliary tract, its use for this purpose has not been reported.

There appears to be little use for PTC, CT scanning, or angiography in the assessment of the postcholecystectomy patient if endoscopic retrograde biliary imaging is available. In the absence of ERCP, the demonstration of dilated ducts by ultrasound should be followed by radiographic imaging of the biliary tree by percutaneous thin-needle cholangiography. The characteristic radiographic findings of stenosing papillitis are shown in Figure 20–4.

CHARACTERISTICS AND TREATMENT OF SPECIFIC LESIONS
Biliary Tract Stones

The recognition of specific postcholecystectomy problems depends heavily on biliary imaging. Common duct lithiasis, the most common cause of postcholecystectomy pain in the early postoperative period, usually is suspected by the history of chills, fever, jaundice, and elevation of serum liver chemistries. Ultrasound will usually reveal dilation of the extrahepatic bile ducts. Endoscopic retrograde cholangiography is helpful in identifying the number and location of stones and provides a safe and convenient vehicle for their removal following endoscopic sphincterotomy.[44] In the absence of this technology, it is acceptable to move directly to a transabdominal operative approach. This is desirable in cases where there is distal stricture of the bile duct or stenosis of the papilla of Vater. If there is uncertainty as to diagnosis, a thin-needle

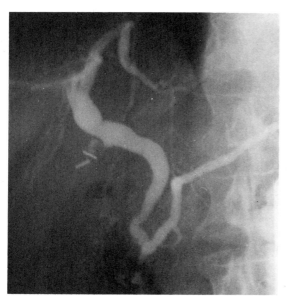

Fig 20–4.—Typical radiographic findings in stenosing papillitis. (With permission from Year Book Medical Publishers. Najarian J., Delaney J. (eds.): *Advances in Hepatic, Biliary, and Pancreatic Surgery.* In press.)

PTC is an appropriate diagnostic intervention. Radionuclide biliary scanning may also reveal useful information.

Bile duct strictures with or without proximal stones are associated with ultrasonic evidence of dilatation of the intrahepatic biliary tree. A PTC is required to identify the anatomy of the stricture and its relationship to the bifurcation of the primary biliary radicles. An endoscopic retrograde study is often of little value in this situation. Repair by a Roux-en-Y limb cholangiojejunostomy can be undertaken without further study.

The principles of surgical repair of benign strictures have been recently clearly elucidated by Warren et al.,[49] Bismuth,[50] and Moody.[51] In my experience, a successful repair requires a life-long follow-up, since stones may re-form within a proximal biliary tree that has been subjected to chronic obstruction and infection.

Retained Gallbladder—Cystic Duct Remnant

The ultrasonic or roentgenographic demonstration of a retained gallbladder in a patient with biliary colic provides a secure diagnosis. Excision of the gallbladder remnant will most surely lead to pain relief. Identification of a cystic duct remnant on contrast evaluation of the biliary tree is quite another matter. There is serious question as to whether even a long cystic duct remnant can contribute to biliary-associated pain.

In rare cases, a small stone that was undetected at the time of cholecystectomy will be retained within a cystic duct remnant of even a normal length (3–5 mm). This condition is difficult to recognize, since ultrasound and contrast imaging cannot demonstrate a stone in this position. It can only be found by mobilization of the cystic duct and careful palpation of its contents at the time of exploratory surgery. Often, the end of the cystic duct is fibrotic and is the site of accumulation of

fibrous and neural tissue. This entity, called a cystic duct neuroma, may suggest that a stone is present when in fact the lumen of the cystic duct is empty. The treatment of both entities is the same: excision of the cystic duct remnant, operative cholangiogram, and consideration of exploration of the bile duct if it is dilated. I usually perform the last to assess the caliber of the papilla of Vater and to search for stones within the bile duct. The inability to easily pass a 3-mm probe or catheter into the duodenum suggests the presence of stenosing papillitis. Hopton and White[52] found intraoperative manometry to be useful in detecting the presence of stones within the biliary tree. Manometric techniques have been employed extensively in Europe for many years to identify diseases of the papilla of Vater. I use a simple gravity flow technique described elsewhere, but do not depend on the results for making a decision about whether to explore the papilla. A transduodenal sphincteroplasty or choledochoduodenostomy should be performed as described below when the bile duct is dilated and thick-walled or when there is a long transmural component of the cystic duct that is not available for excision. The rationale relates to the possibility that small stones are being formed in the cystic duct remnant within the wall of the bile duct and that the passage of stones through the papilla of Vater is the source of the patient's pain.

Stenosing Papillitis

It should not be surprising that the papilla of Vater may contribute to biliary tract symptoms after cholecystectomy in view of its critical location at the confluence of the bile and the major pancreatic ducts within the duodenum.

The diagnosis, however, of benign diseases of the papilla remains difficult, even with the availability of sophisticated hepatobiliary-imaging technology. This diagnostic dilemma relates in part to an inability to precisely define papillary function and anatomy.[50] Even transpapillary manometry, when successful, provides ambiguous results that correlate poorly with the presence of overt disease and with clinical outcome. Furthermore, the papilla of Vater appears normal through the endoscope, even when its lumen is markedly deformed by scar tissue. Recent studies by us demonstrated that the major defect in 83 postcholecystectomy patients was confined to the transampullary septum at the opening of the duct of Wirsung at an anatomical point 1 mm or more within the channel of the papilla.[22] It is unfortunate that only 20% of patients with stenosing papillitis secondary to gallstone disease have liver or pancreatic enzyme elevations or dilatation of the bile or pancreatic ducts, since such changes would provide objective evidence of ductal obstruction and lead to earlier definitive therapy.

The diagnosis of stenosing papillitis in most patients is based on the clinical history and the failure to identify a reason for a patient's pain after cholecystectomy. The character of the pain is important. Chronic, severe, episodic pain in the middle or right upper abdomen in the absence of other demonstrable GI disease is most likely due to stenosing papillitis in a postcholecystectomy patient. Also, patients with occult biliary tract disease, i.e., cholesterolosis or multiple small stones, are more likely to develop the lesion, possibly because such patients are more prone to pass calcareous debris from their gallbladder into the bile duct.

The decision to pursue an operative approach is always difficult when objective evidence of a lesion is absent. These patients should be thoroughly assessed and followed up for a period by a gastroenterologist prior to surgical intervention. I prefer to educate thoroughly such patients as to the presumed nature of their illness, once referred to me. The discussion includes my uncertainty as to whether sphincteroplasty and septectomy will help relieve their pain. It is essential to gain their commitment to an in-hospital course of narcotic detoxification if they are medically addicted.

The details of the operative procedure have been described elsewhere.[21] They are of sufficient importance to the success of the procedure to repeat here. Preoperative antibiotics (second-generation cephalosporins) are employed for wound prophylaxis. I prefer to enter the abdomen through the incision used for cholecystectomy, if appropriately positioned. After careful exploration of the abdominal cavity without finding a cause for the patient's pain, the bile duct and stump of the cystic duct are exposed and the duodenum and the head of the pancreas mobilized by the Kocher maneuver. A small, anterior, longitudinal choledochotomy is performed in the lower bile duct, and exploration is performed with a biliary scoop. The passage of a 5 F catheter through the papilla helps to identify its precise location within the vertical limb of the duodenum.

The duodenum is entered through an anterior longitudinal duodenotomy that should be no more than 2 cm in length. The insertion of small loop retractors provides easy access to the papilla. Withdrawing and placing tension on the transpapillary catheter elevates the papilla so that traction sutures of 5–0 silk can be placed on either side of its opening. Progressive incisions at 3-mm intervals are made along its anterior border with iris scissors, and the bile duct mucosa is successively approximated to the duodenal mucosa with 5–0 polyglycolic acid sutures. The sphincteroplasty should be 1.5–2.0 cm long. A headlight and 2.0 magnification optics enhance the precision of the procedure. Clamps should not be placed on the papilla, and electrocauterization should be used sparingly.

The opening of the duct of Wirsung should be identified early in the procedure. An intraoperative pancreatogram is obtained if endoscopic retrograde study was unsuccessful. Stenosing wirsungitis from transampullary septitis presents a challenge, since in many cases the opening of the duct of Wirsung is obscured by scar tissue. The optical loops, a fine lacrimal probe, and patience will always yield a pinpoint opening that will enlarge with progressive dilatations. The septum is then incised for 1 cm and a small piece removed for histologic examination. The mucosa of the duct of Wirsung is approximated to the mucosa of the bile duct with polyglycolic acid sutures of 7–0 gauge. The appearance of the reconstructed papilla is shown schematically in Figure 20–5.

The duodenotomy is closed with a running 4–0 polyglycolic acid suture, and an outer row of 4–0 silk placed in interrupted fashion. A tag of omentum is placed over the closure. I have not had a duodenal dehiscence in 103 such closures. A small (10 or 12 F) T tube is secured in the bile duct, and Penrose drains are placed into the subhepatic space through a separate incision.

There have been no deaths, but a few serious complica-

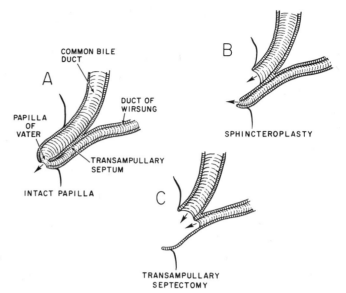

Fig 20–5.—Schematic of anatomic relationships within the papilla of Vater. Note the position of the ampullary septum forming the posterior wall of the bile duct and the anterior wall of the duct of Wirsung. (From Moody F.G., et al.[21] Used with permission of author and publisher.)

tions, as shown in Table 20–8. Only two of the eight patients with signs of acute pancreatitis (ileus, hyperamylasemia) had prolonged hospital courses, of three and four months, respectively. The late results for the initial postcholecystectomy patients operated on five to ten years ago are shown in Table 20–6. The outcome of a larger group of patients with a variety of benign lesions is shown in Table 20–9. Of interest is that patients with prior sphincteroplasty who only required septectomy appeared to have the best results. This suggests that either the septum or the pancreatic ductal system was the source of pain in those who gained relief from the procedure.

The ductal anomalies in this series were too few to be evaluated. The most frequent anomaly, pancreatic divisum, was treated by septectomy with dilatation of the duct of Wirsung and an accompanying Santoriniplasty in three patients.

The opening of the duct of Wirsung was below the papilla in two instances and on its anterior lip in one. Obviously,

TABLE 20–8.—MORBIDITY
IN 103 PATIENTS
FOLLOWING TRANSAMPULLARY
SEPTECTOMY*

Pancreatitis	8
Atelectasis	6
Cholangitis	4
Ileus	3
T-tube dysfunction	3
Bile drainage	3
Pneumonia	2
Skin rash	2
Wound infection	2
Pulmonary embolus	1
Upper GI bleed	1

*No mortality.

TABLE 20–9.—RESULTS FROM 83 PATIENTS
FOLLOWED UP FOR 1–10 YEARS

	RESULTS		
FINDINGS	Good	Fair	Poor
Papillitis	15	16	9
Septitis	17	10	9
Dysfunction	4	1	2
Overall (%)	36(43)	27(33)	20(24)
Prior sphincteroplasty	9	3	3
Papillary cholesterolosis	3	5	2
Anomaly	2	1	2
Concomitant cholecystectomy	2	5	6

Moody F.G., Becker J.M., Potts J.R.: Transduodenal sphincteroplasty and transampullary septectomy for postcholecystectomy pain. *Ann. Surg.* 197(5):627, 1983.[22] Used with permission of authors and publisher.

these are important aberrations to identify. Whether these anomalies or pancreatic divisum itself can produce the postcholecystectomy pain syndrome remains unproved. I remain skeptical as to their role in pancreatic disease.

Biliary Dyskinesia

It is appropriate to conclude a discussion of the postcholecystectomy syndrome with its most poorly understood potential cause—biliary dyskinesia. Is it possible that the giants of yesteryear were indeed correct in ascribing postcholecystectomy pain to an inappropriate response of the sphincter of Oddi to a neural or humoral stimuli?[9, 10] Unfortunately, the technology by which to study these questions in humans is still in an early stage of its development. Indiscriminate ablation of the papilla may lead to severe morbidity either at the time of the procedure or at a later date. There is a need for controlled trials of new therapies, which, with careful long-term follow-up, should help to resolve the occasionally severe and often mystifying symptoms that follow cholecystectomy.

Geenen et al.[48] at the University of Wisconsin in Milwaukee have made important contributions to our ability to identify sphincter of Oddi dysfunction by transendoscopic transpapillary manometry. This technology involves the retrograde passage of a 1.7-mm catheter with three side holes at 2-mm intervals. The catheter is perfused with degassed water at 0.5 ml/min by a low-compliance pneumatic pump (Andorfer Medical).[53] Meshkinpour and colleagues,[53] utilizing this technique, observed that patients with presumed biliary dyskinesia have elevated transpapillary pressures with a higher precentage of retrograde contractions than controls. The frequency and amplitude of contractions, however, were similar between patients and subjects. Hogan and colleagues identified a similar group of patients with persistent pain after cholecystectomy.[48] Forty-five patients were randomly assigned to endoscopic sphincterotomy or no sphincterotomy after ERCP. All patients demonstrated either elevation of liver function studies or delayed emptying of contrast from their bile ducts. Fifteen of 22 patients who underwent sphincterotomy (68%) were improved, while only seven of 23 (30%) of the controls had relief of their pain. The follow-up period was short, and the results thus far have been expressed only in abstract format. Transpapillary manometry nonetheless offers the possibility of identifying by an objective means those patients with motor abnormalities of the sphincter of Oddi or anatomical deformity of the papilla of Vater. Geenen and associates, using the technology that they developed, have clearly shown that endoscopic papillotomy reduces the pressure gradient across the papilla of Vater from duodenum to bile duct for up to two years of follow-up. They also observed that the size of the opening of the transsected papilla decreased from 11.0 ± 1.5 mm to 6.5 ± 0.7 mm in eight patients. There was no significant decrease in size from one to two years. A 6-mm opening should be more than adequate in the majority of patients who require free flow of bile from their biliary tree.

It now remains to improve our understanding of papillary function. The humoral and neural influences on sphincter function and the relationships between anatomical defects, congenital or acquired, and sphincter function need further study in humans and in the laboratory. Only in this way will our understanding of postcholecystectomy pain be enhanced to a point of more effective therapy and prevention.

REFERENCES

1. Langenbuch C.: Ein fall von exstirpation der gallenblase wegen chronischer cholelithiasis. Heilung. *Berl. Klin. Wochenschr.* 19:725–727, 1882.
2. Ammon H.V., Hofmann A.F.: The Langenbuch paper: I. An historical perspective and comments of the translators. *Gastroenterology* 85:1426–1433, 1983.
3. McSherry C.K., Glenn F.: The incidence and causes of death following surgery for nonmalignant biliary tract disease. *Ann. Surg.* 191:271–275, 1980.
4. Bodvall B., Overgaard B.: Computer analysis of postcholecystectomy biliary tract symptoms. *Surg. Gynecol. Obstet.* 124(4):723–732, 1967.
5. Bodvall B.: The postcholecystectomy syndromes. *Clin. Gastroenterol.* 2(1):103–125, 1973.
6. Christiansen J., Schmidt A.: The postcholecystectomy syndrome. *Acta Chir. Scand.* 137:789–793, 1971.
7. Ekdahl P.H.: On late distress following biliary tract operations. *Acta Chir. Scand.* 106:339, 1953.
8. Bar-Meir S., Halpern Z., Bardan E., et al.: Frequency of papillary dysfunction among cholecystomized patients. *Hepatology* 4(2):328–330, 1984.
9. Womack N.A., Crider R.L.: The persistence of symptoms following cholecystectomy. *Ann. Surg.* 126(1):31–55, 1947.
10. Pribram R.O.C.: Postcholecystectomy syndromes. *J.A.M.A.* 142:1262, 1950.
11. Glenn F., McSherry C.K.: Secondary abdominal operations for symptoms following biliary tract surgery. *Surg. Gynecol. Obstet.* 121:979–988, 1965.
12. Stefanini P., De Bernardinis G.: Factors influencing the long term results of cholecystectomy. *Surg. Gynecol. Obstet.* 139:735–738, 1974.
13. Tondelli P., Gyr K., Stalder G.A., et al.: The biliary tract. *Clin. Gastroenterol.* 8(2):487–505, 1979.
14. Bodvall B., Overgaard B.: Cystic duct remnant after cholecystectomy: Incidence studied by cholegraphy in 500 cases, and significance in 103 reoperations. *Ann. Surg.* 163:382–390, 1966.
15. Glenn F., Whitsell J.C.: The surgical treatment of cystic duct remnants. *Surg. Gynecol. Obstet.* 113:711–719, 1961.
16. Millbourn E.: On the importance of the remnant cystic duct in the development of post-operative biliary distress following cholecystectomy: A study partly based on a cholangiography series. *Acta Chir. Scand.* 100:448–465, 1950.
17. Flörcken H.: Gallenblasenregeneration mit steinrecidiv nach cholecystectomie. *Dtsch. Z. Chir.* 113:604, 1967.
18. Acosta J.M., Civantos F., Nardi G.L., et al.: Fibrosis of the papilla of Vater. *Surg. Gynecol. Obstet.* April 124:787–794, 1967.
19. Hess W.: Stenosing papillitis, in Hess W. (ed.): *Surgery of the*

Biliary Passages and the Pancreas. Princeton, N.J., D. van Nostrand Co., 1965, pp. 71–76.

20. Grage T.B., Lober P.H., Imamoglu K., et al.: Stenosis of the sphincter of Oddi: A review of 50 cases. *Surgery* 48(2):304–317, 1960.
21. Moody F.G., Berenson M.M., McCloskey D.: Transampullary septectomy for post-cholecystectomy pain. *Ann. Surg.* 186(4):415–423, 1977.
22. Moody F.G., Becker J.M., Potts J.R.: Transduodenal sphincteroplasty and transampullary septectomy for postcholecystectomy pain. *Ann. Surg.* 197(5):627–636, 1983.
23. Cole W.H., Grove W.J.: Persistence of symptoms following cholecystectomy with special reference to anomalies of the ampulla of vater. *Ann. Surg.* 136:73–82, 1952.
24. Bartlett M.K., Nardi G.L.: Treatment of recurrent pancreatitis by transduodenal sphincterotomy and exploration of the pancreatic duct. *N. Engl. J. Med.* 262(13):643–648, 1960.
25. Warren K.W., Veidenheimer M.: Pathological considerations in the choice of operation for chronic relapsing pancreatitis. *N. Engl. J. Med.* 266:323, 1962.
26. Acosta J.M., Ledesma C.L.: Gallstone migration as a cause of acute pancreatitis. *N. Engl. J. Med.* 290(9):484–487, 1974.
27. Branch C.D., Bailey O.T., Zollinger R.: Consequences of instrumental dilation of the papilla of Vater. *Arch. Surg.* 28:358, 1939.
28. Gage S.H.: The ampulla of Vater and the pancreatic ducts in the domestic cat. *Am. Q. Micro J.* 1:128–169, 1879.
29. Oddi R.: D'une disposition a sphincter speciale de l'ovverture du canal choledogue. *Arch. Ital. Biol.* 8:317–322, 1887.
30. Boyden E.A.: The anatomy of the choledochoduodenal junction in man. *Surg. Gynecol. Obstet.* 104(6):641–652, 1957.
31. Parvel I.: Ictete par obstacle functionnel du au spasme da sphincter d'Oddi avec examen anatomique. *Presse Med.* 2:1948–1950, 1932.
32. Schmieden V., Miessen H.: Dyskinesie der gallenwege (cholepathia spastica) and chirurgie. *M.M.W.* 80:247–250, 1933.
33. Ivy A.C., Sandbloom P.: Biliary dyskinesia. *Ann. Intern. Med.* 8(2):115, 1934.
34. McGowan J.M., Butsch W.I., Walters W.: Pressure in the common bile duct of man. *J.A.M.A.* 106(26):2227–2230, 1936.
35. Bachrach W.H., Smith J.L., Halsted J.A.: Spasm of the choledochal sphincter accompanying sudden stress. *Gastroenterology* 22:604–606, 1952.
36. Colp R.: The treatment of postoperative biliary dyskinesia. *Gastroenterology* 7:414–429, 1946.
37. Dahl-Iverson E., Sorensen A.H., Westengaard E.: Pressure measurement in the biliary tract in patients after cholecystolithotomy and in patients with dyskinesia. *Acta Chir. Scand.* 114:181–190, 1958.
38. Steinberg W.M., Salvato R.F., Toskes P.P.: The morphine-prostigmin test—is it useful for making clinical decisions? *Gastroenterology* 78:728–731, 1980.
39. Nardi G.L., Acosta J.M.: Papillitis as a cause of pancreatitis and abdominal pain: Role of evocative test, operative pancreatography and histologic evaluation. *Ann. Surg.* 164(4):611, 1966.
40. Gregg J.A., Taddeo A.E., Milano A.F., et al.: Duodenoscopy and endoscopic pancreatography in patients with positive morphine prostigmine tests. *Am. J. Surg.* 134:318–321, 1977.
41. LoGuidice J.A., Geenen J.E., Hogan W.J., et al.: Efficacy of the morphine-prostigmin test for evaluating patients with suspected papillary stenosis. *Dig. Dis. Sci.* 24(6):455, 1979.
42. Geenen J.E., Hogan W.J., Dodds W.J., et al.: Intraluminal pressure recording from the human sphincter of Oddi. *Gastroenterology* 78:317–324, 1980.
43. Csendes A., Kruse A., Funch-Jensen P., et al.: Pressure measurements in the biliary and pancreatic duct systems in controls and in patients with gallstones, previous cholecystectomy, or common bile duct stones. *Gastroenterology* 77:1203–1210, 1979.
44. Bar-Meir S., Geenen J.E., Hogan W.J., et al.: Biliary and pancreatic duct pressures measured by ERCP manometry in patients with suspected papillary stenosis. *Dig. Dis. Sci.* 24(3):209–213, 1979.
45. Becker J.M., Moody F.G., Zinsmeister A.R.: Effect of gastrointestinal hormones on the biliary sphincter of the opossum. *Gastroenterology* 1300, 1982.
46. Toulli J., Geenen J.E., Hogan W.J., et al.: Sphincter of Oddi motor activity: A comparison between patients with common bile duct stones and controls. *Gastroenterology* 82:111, 1982.
47. Ono K.: The discharge of bile into the duodenum and electrical activities of the muscle of Oddi and duodenum. *Nippon Heikatsukin Gakkai Zasshi* 6:123, 1970.
48. Geenen J.E., Toulli J., Hogan W.J., et al.: Endoscopic sphincterotomy: Follow-up evaluation of effects on the sphincter of Oddi. *Gastroenterology* 87:754, 1984.
49. Warren K.W., Christophi C., Armendariz R.: The evolution and current perspectives of the treatment of benign bile duct strictures: A review. *Surg. Gastroenterol.* 1:141, 1982.
50. Bismuth H.: Postoperative stricture of the bile duct, in Blumgart L.H. (ed.): *The Biliary Tract.* Edinburgh, Churchill Livingstone, 1982, vol. 5, p. 209.
51. Moody F.G.: Biliary pancreas and papilla of Vater interrelationships, in Blumgart L.H. (ed.): *The Biliary Tract.* New York, Churchill Livingstone, 1982, pp. 197–208.
52. Hopton D., White T.T.: An evaluation of manometric operative cholangiography in 100 patients with biliary disease. *Surg. Gynecol. Obstet.* 133:949–954, 1971.
53. Meshkinpour H., Mollot M., Eckerling G.B., et al.: Bile duct dyskinesia. *Gastroenterology* 87:795, 1984.

21

Common Duct Stones

ROSS E. J. STIMPSON, M.D.
LAWRENCE W. WAY, M.D.

CLINICAL AND MORPHOLOGICAL FEATURES OF DUCTAL STONES

Like gallbladder stones, common duct stones may be classified as cholesterol or pigment stones, depending on the amount of cholesterol they contain.[1] The few remaining stones are composed of inorganic calcium salts.[2] Though definitions vary, stones with more than 50% cholesterol are considered to be cholesterol stones and those with less are pigment stones. Pigment stones also contain varying amounts of soluble bilirubin (calcium bilirubinate), insoluble pigment (bilirubin polymers), and an unmeasured material.

The type of stone can be identified by its physical characteristics alone in most cases.[1] Cholesterol stones are usually light-colored (brown, tan, or yellow) and often display a radial crystalline structure internally. Pigment stones are dark brown, black, or earthy (claylike), and have a dull, laminated appearance. Pigment stones can be visually divided into tarry or earthy stones. Tarry stones are black, shiny, and amorphous, while earthy stones are clay-colored to dark chocolate brown, easily crushable, and lack a crystalline interior.

Pigment stones can be further subdivided chemically into stones with a predominance of soluble bilirubin (bilirubin stones) and those with a predominance of insoluble pigment residue (residue stones). Earthy stones tend to contain more cholesterol and less residue than do tarry stones. Pigment stones in the gallbladder generally contain more insoluble pigment residue and less soluble bilirubin than associated common duct stones. Cholesterol stones in the duct are chemically similar to their gallbladder counterparts.

PATHOGENESIS

Common duct stones may be classified as primary or secondary, depending on the site of origin. Primary stones are formed in the common duct, while secondary stones form in the gallbladder and pass to the common duct via the cystic duct. Although there is considerable debate on this subject, most authors believe the majority of common duct stones are of gallbladder origin.[1, 3–5] Epidemiologic evidence supporting this is as follows. Ninety-five percent of patients with common duct stones have gallbladder stones, while only 15% of patients with gallbladder stones have common duct stones.[5] In

patients with gallbladder stones, common duct stones are more common in the presence of small stones in the gallbladder,[6] a large cystic duct, long-standing disease, and old age.[3, 5, 7] These factors either facilitate stone passage from the gallbladder or allow more time for it to occur. The fact that cholecystectomy plus choledocholithotomy cures most patients with choledocholithiasis[8] (including those who are said by some criteria to have primary stones)[4, 9] suggests that the gallbladder is the source of the disease in most cases.

Stones may form primarily in the ducts as shown by their occurrence in 30% of cases of congenital absence of the gallbladder.[10, 11] Stasis of any cause predisposes to stone formation, and ductal stones may be found in association with biliary stricture,[1] congenital cystic dilatation of the intrahepatic ducts (Caroli's disease),[12] massive duct dilatation,[13] and experimentally induced partial obstruction of the bile duct in animals.[14] In these and other pathologic situations, the stones that form are invariably of the pigment variety.

The presence of bacteria may also play an etiologic role in primary choledocholithiasis. Bactobilia is common in patients believed to have primary stones,[13] and is invariably present in patients with recurrent pyogenic cholangitis (Oriental cholangiohepatitis).[15–17] In fact, bacterial invasion of the duct is thought to be the prime etiologic factor for stone formation in the latter disease. The mechanism is thought to involve deconjugation of bilirubin by β-glucuronidase secreted by bacteria.[18] The insoluble bilirubin then precipitates to form pigment stones. This disease is discussed further under the heading "Intrahepatic Stones."

The older Aschoff classification,[19] which relies on morphological criteria, has been used to identify primary stones on the basis of morphological criteria alone.[13, 20] Primary stones are described as being soft, brown, and easily crushable—in other words, earthy stones. Using these criteria, as many as 60% of patients with choledocholithiasis could be said to have primary stones.[9, 20] Clinical experience indicates, however, that this is far too high an incidence of primary stones,[4] which calls into question the validity of the Aschoff system for identification.

One study addressed this question in detail by comparing the physical characteristics and chemical composition of gallbladder and common duct stones from the same patient.[1] Cholesterol common duct stones were found to be virtually indistinguishable morphologically from their gallbladder counterparts, while substantial differences were noted between pigment gallbladder and common duct stones. The chemical composition of cholesterol common duct stones was identical to their gallbladder counterparts, while pigment common duct stones had relatively more soluble bilirubin and less insoluble pigment residue than their gallbladder counterparts. In only one of 58 patients was a pigment duct stone found in a patient with a cholesterol gallbladder stone.

Earthy stones in the duct were associated with earthy stones in the gallbladder. Pigment stones were present in 43% of the entire group of patients with common duct stones and in 36% of the patients who also had gallbladder stones (gallbladder intact). The high incidence of pigment common duct stones suggests that patients with pigment gallbladder stones may be more prone to common duct stone formation than are patients with cholesterol gallbladder stones. Common duct stones that developed proximal to a stricture or in a markedly dilated duct were invariably pigment stones.

These findings support the following conclusions. Because cholesterol stones from the gallbladder and duct of the same patient are chemically and visually indistinguishable, and because common duct stones that are definitely of ductal origin are always composed of pigment, cholesterol common duct stones are always or almost always secondary, having been formed in the gallbladder. The greater variability in appearance and chemical composition between the pigment stones from the gallbladder and those from the duct suggests that pigment common duct stones can form in either location, but it appeared that most of them occurring in patients who had gallbladder stones were secondary stones. Whether secondary pigment stones always passed into the duct in their final form was questioned. It seemed likely that in some cases pigment debris passed from the gallbladder into the duct where the stone was then formed. In other cases, ductal solids appeared to have coated stones that had originally come from the gallbladder.

Motor abnormalities in patients with common duct stones may contribute to primary stone formation. Using manometry, Toouli et al.[21] observed more retrograde wave sequences in the choledochal sphincter in patients with ductal stones than in asymptomatic controls. Whether these abnormalities were primary or secondary to the presence of the stones is uncertain. The resulting ductal stasis would be expected to promote stone formation. Other investigators have found no differences in basal pressures or wave amplitudes in the choledochal sphincters of patients with and without gallstones.[22] Ductal stasis would be expected to promote stone formation.

Lotveit[23] has noted a high incidence of juxtavaterian duodenal diverticula among patients with choledocholithiasis. The common duct stones in these patients are invariably pigment stones and are associated with positive bile cultures. Lotveit postulates that the diverticulum may interfere with function in the sphincter of Oddi, thereby promoting retrograde bacterial contamination of the duct, which then leads to pigment stone formation. Stone formation has also been reported in association with incrustation of suture material left behind at previous surgery,[2, 24] and while this may be a common cause in some places,[2] it is rare in the United States.

INCIDENCE AND NATURAL HISTORY

Common duct stones are found in about 15% of patients undergoing cholecystectomy for gallbladder stones, but the reported incidence varies from 7% to 20%, reflecting differences in the efforts to find common duct stones and characteristics of the patient populations cared for at the reporting institution. The incidence increases with the age of the patient, the frequency of operative cholangiography during cholecystectomy, and whether the patient population typically seeks medical care early or late.[5]

Little has been written on the natural history of choledocholithiasis, probably because there are few data on the subject. Millbourn[25] described the outcome of expectant management in 38 patients followed up for 6 months to 13 years. Symptoms appeared in 21 (55%) patients, and 17 patients (45%) remained asymptomatic. In an autopsy study, Kozoll et al.[26] noted that only 50% of patients with common duct stones had clinical manifestations of biliary disease. The morbidity among patients diagnosed at autopsy was high, however.[26, 27] The reports on the natural history of gallstone disease by Lund,[28] Wenckert and Robertson,[29] and Comfort and associates[30] cited manifestations of common duct disease in only one-third of affected patients. Finally, in an analysis of 105 patients with choledocholithiasis, we detected symptoms in only 40%.[5] These figures suggest that choledocholithiasis, like cholecystolithiasis, is characterized in many patients by prolonged asymptomatic periods, and even though the clinical manifestations are sometimes devastating, this is uncommon in relation to the prevalence of the disease.

PATHOPHYSIOLOGY

The major consequence of common duct stones is ductal obstruction, which gives rise to pain, infection, and jaundice. The obstruction is usually incomplete and remitting, unlike that of malignant bile duct obstruction. Clinically this is reflected by fluctuating symptoms and jaundice. The serum bilirubin usually remains below 15 mg/dl (averaging about 4 mg/dl) in choledocholithiasis, in contrast to malignant obstruction in which values above 15 mg/dl are typical.[31]

In the absence of obstruction, common duct stones do not cause resting ductal pressure to rise.[22] When obstruction occurs, changes are produced throughout the biliary tree and the hepatic parenchyma.[32] Normal pressure in the system is 10–15 cm H_2O. If obstruction causes the pressure to approach the maximum secretory capacity of the liver (about 30 cm H_2O), bile secretion will stop. The proximal bile ducts may dilate if the obstruction is prolonged and relatively complete. The presence of cholangitis and hepatic cirrhosis interferes with dilatation. Experimentally, the severity of pathologic changes in the liver parenchyma depends on the degree, duration and site of obstruction, although clinical studies do not confirm this.[31] However, the functional recovery of the liver after relief of obstruction tends to be poorer in patients with bilirubin levels above 10 mg/dl and those in whom jaundice has been present for more than four weeks.[31] Eventually with prolonged obstruction, permanent damage to hepatic function may ensue accompanied by connective tissue proliferation.[32] The end stage of complete or recurrent obstruction, particularly when complicated by cholangitis, is biliary cirrhosis. This is uncommon in societies where early access to medical care is a feature. It is more common in such conditions as recurrent pyogenic cholangitis, in which infection complicates intrahepatic stones and strictures, which may be difficult or impossible to eradicate.[16] In one study biliary cirrhosis was found in 8% of patients with choledocholithiasis,[33] but the current figure would be 1% or less in the average hospital in North America.

Bile cultures are positive in up to 90% of patients with choledocholithiasis.[13, 34] *Escherichia coli, Klebsiella, Enterobacter,* and *Proteus* are the aerobic bacteria most commonly isolated. Twenty percent of patients harbor anaerobic bacteria, with clostridia or *Bacteroides* being the most common.[34] Anaerobes are more common in patients who have had previous biliary surgery, particularly when a bilioenteric anastomosis has been performed.[35]

The incidence of bactobilia increases with age, previous surgery, number of stones present, duration of the disease, and height of serum bilirubin levels.[34, 36] In most cases, bacteria probably gain access to the biliary tree by ascending from the duodenum through the papilla of Vater.[37] Perhaps this is facilitated by the motor disturbances of the ampullary sphincter that have been found in this disease.[21] Duodenocholedochal reflux has been documented in common duct stone disease.[38] Once present, the bacteria are protected from the host's immune defenses by the foreign body effect of the calculi. The almost universal bactobilia in common duct stone disease contrasts sharply with the situation in malignant obstruction, where the incidence of positive bile cultures is low (10%), unless bacteria are introduced by surgical or other instrumental intervention.

Bactobilia is of no danger to the patient unless obstruction supervenes or high pressures are imposed by diagnostic cholangiography. When obstruction occurs, pressures may rise rapidly to levels of 20–30 cm H_2O,[39] producing the manifestations of acute cholangitis. Common duct pressures above 20 and 25 cm H_2O are associated with cholangiolymphatic and cholangiovenous reflux, respectively,[40] which lead to systemic dissemination of bacteria and their toxins. Cholangitis can be likened to any infection in a closed space, where resolution is unlikely in the absence of drainage. Formation of fibrin webs in the common duct may complicate efforts to obtain adequate drainage.[41] Because obstruction due to stones is usually incomplete, cholangitis resolves on medical therapy alone in many cases.[42]

CLINICAL FINDINGS

Common duct stones may remain asymptomatic for long periods, but with the onset of symptoms, further problems can be anticipated. The manifestations are pain, jaundice, chills and fever, and pancreatitis,[1, 5, 42] and may occur in any combination. The first three characterize cholangitis and are referred to as Charcot's triad. The most common syndromes are intermittent cholangitis, intermittent jaundice and pain, and acute pancreatitis. Nevertheless, an occasional patient presents with painless, feverless jaundice, or biliary colic without jaundice or fever. The pain is similar to that caused by gallbladder stones from which it cannot be differentiated. It is a deep-seated visceral pain with minor fluctuations in

intensity, usually felt in the midepigastrium or right upper quadrant with radiation to the back. The pain may be girdle-like, particularly if the stone is impacted in the ampulla of Vater.

The jaundice of calculous obstruction is characteristically mild and remitting.[31] The fever is usually intermittent, reflecting the intermittency of obstruction. More than 90% of patients with Charcot's triad have common duct stones, although only 25% of patients with choledocholithiasis present in this manner.[43] In patients with gallstone pancreatitis, the pain may be more typical of pancreatitis, being located in the epigastrium, back, left shoulder, and left upper quadrant.

In the absence of complications, physical examination of a patient with common duct stones is unlikely to reveal any abnormalities. In severe toxic cholangitis, however, the patient may be febrile, icteric, and in extremis. A distended, nontender, palpable gallbladder in a jaundiced patient suggests obstruction distal to the cystic duct, more likely secondary to a neoplasm rather than stones (Courvoisier's Law). The reason why Courvoisier's Law holds true is that patients with gallstone obstruction usually have a partial low-grade block,[44] and their gallbladders are more apt to be fibrotic and less distensible.[32]

LABORATORY INVESTIGATIONS

In the absence of clinical findings, laboratory values are usually normal. When obstruction occurs, serum levels of liver enzymes such as alkaline phosphatase, 5'-nucleotidase, and leucine aminopeptidase increase.[32, 45] SGOT and SGPT may also rise transiently with obstruction, but they are not specific,[32, 33] and if their elevation is prolonged, it usually reflects parenchymal liver disease. The level of alkaline phosphatase is the most sensitive index of ductal obstruction, as it rises early and rapidly, even in the absence of jaundice.[14, 31] Unlike the bilirubin level, it may increase in response to segmental obstruction in the liver.[32] Elevated intraductal pressure proximal to the obstruction stimulates increased hepatocyte synthesis of alkaline phosphatase with regurgitation into the hepatic sinusoids.[46] Bilirubin, on the other hand, increases as a result of blocked excretion, and in the absence of parenchymal disease, serum levels usually remain normal with obstruction of less than half of the biliary tree.[32]

The absolute level of alkaline phosphatase is of little value in predicting the cause or magnitude of obstruction. However, values greater than five times normal are more typical of malignant or benign stricture than of choledocholithiasis.[31] The absolute value of bilirubin is of diagnostic significance. Values above 15 mg/dl are rarely caused by common duct stones; the mean value in patients with jaundice caused by stones being 5.5 mg/dl.[31, 47]

In cholangitis, the WBC count is often elevated, but it does not correlate closely with the severity of the condition, and may be depressed in the most severe cases. Blood cultures are positive in most patients with cholangitis.[42]

SPECIALIZED DIAGNOSTIC PROCEDURES
Ultrasound

Ultrasound is useful as a screening test for obstructive jaundice if it demonstrates ductal dilatation. However, dilatation is absent in 35% of jaundiced patients with choledocholithiasis[48–50] due to the incomplete and fluctuating nature of the obstruction. Therefore, absence of dilatation does not rule out obstruction, especially obstruction due to common duct stones.

Ultrasound is about 90% accurate in diagnosing gallbladder stones.[47] If found, they are highly likely to be the cause of jaundice. The sensitivity of ultrasound in diagnosing common duct stones is reported to be about 25%,[47, 48, 51–53] with an overall accuracy (excluding false positives and false negatives) of about 20%.

For best results, high resolution, real-time scanners should be used. Gallbladder stones as small as 3 mm have been detected, as well as stones in a nondilated duct, although this is unpredictable.[54] Despite the enthusiasm of some ultrasonographers, we believe that ultrasound is not a clinically important test for common duct stones, because its reliability is too low.

Computerized Tomography

Reported results of CT scanning for detection of choledocholithiasis vary widely, but are better than those obtained using ultrasound. The sensitivity is about 50% and accuracy about 80%.[51, 55, 56] CT is less accurate in detecting gallbladder stones, the majority of which do not contain calcium. The accuracy of CT in detecting ductal dilatation exceeds 90%.[31]

CT is better than ultrasound in finding common duct stones because of better success in delineating the anatomy and lack of interference by gas or obesity. In one review, 100% of pigment common duct stones (which contain calcium) and 80% of cholesterol common duct stones were demonstrated by CT.[56]

When stones are not seen, their presence may be inferred from a picture of distal duct obstruction in the absence of a ductal stricture or a mass in that area. Both CT and ultrasound are reasonably successful in making the diagnosis of intrahepatic bile duct stones, which are usually pigment stones with a high calcium content.[57] Therefore, CT scanning is more apt to be clinically useful in the diagnosis of choledocholithiasis, although it should not be considered an important test in the evaluation of most patients with this disease.

Endoscopic Retrograde Cholangiopancreatography (ERCP) and Transhepatic Cholangiography (THC)

ERCP and THC provide the most accurate information about the presence of common duct stones, although they are indicated in only a minority of cases. For example, a cholangiogram would not be necessary preoperatively for a patient with intermittent jaundice, bilirubin levels in the 2–4 mg/dl range, and fever, whose ultrasound or oral cholecystogram showed gallbladder stones. In this kind of patient, the need for laparotomy is apparent and the surgeon can readily assess the duct (by direct inspection and cholangiography) at the time of surgery. On the other hand, ERCP or THC is indicated for the following kinds of patients: (1) those with known gallbladder stones who have high (>10 mg/dl) bilirubin levels, because of the risk of a neoplasm[47]; (2) symptomatic patients with a previous cholecystectomy; and (3) patients with biliary symptoms and inconclusive evidence of gallstone disease.

If the patient has clotting abnormalities, sensitivity to IV

contrast mediums, or nondilated intrahepatic ducts, an ERCP should be performed instead of a THC.[58] ERCP is also preferable if pancreatic or periampullary disease is suspected or if a concomitant sphincterotomy is being considered. On the other hand, THC is better if a previous Billroth II gastrectomy has been performed or if injection of the pancreatic duct might be hazardous (e.g., in patients with recent acute pancreatitis). Because of the risk of precipitating acute cholangitis, prophylactic antibodies should be used routinely when performing either of these tests. The risk of sepsis is proportional to the severity of the most recent attack of cholangitis. The pressures used to inject the contrast agent should be limited,[59] and the duct should be allowed to decompress afterwards.

ERCP successfully opacifies the biliary tree in 80% of cases, irrespective of whether the duct is dilated,[58] and it demonstrates over 90% of common duct stones.[60] Complications occur in 2% of patients, pancreatitis and sepsis being the most common.[58] When the ducts are dilated, THC can identify the level of obstruction in 90% of cases[47, 61] and more accurately defines the cause of obstruction than does ERCP. Even when thin needles are used for THC, bile may leak from the liver in some cases and require surgery.[45]

Intravenous cholangiography is only able to opacify the ducts in patients whose serum bilirubin values are below 3 mg/dl. Even then, inadequate opacification is common. Furthermore, stones are not seen on the films in as many as 40% of patients with common duct stones.[5, 43] Like ultrasound, it may give accurate measurements of common duct size. Because of its weaknesses and the occasional allergic reaction to IV contrast mediums, IV cholangiography has largely been replaced by ERCP and THC.

TREATMENT

Medical

Oral administration of chenodeoxycholate and ursodeoxycholate has been used to dissolve common duct stones. Cholic acid and deoxycholate are ineffective. In theory, enriching the bile with bile salts should reduce the lithogenic index and promote dissolution of cholesterol stones. The results have not been encouraging,[62, 63] however, as would be expected by the high proportion of common duct stones that are composed of pigment. At present, there are no oral agents capable of dissolving pigment stones. Ursodeoxycholate has generally been preferred over chenodeoxycholate because it causes less diarrhea and is less likely to disturb liver function.[62] Owing to the low response rate, bile acid therapy should probably be reserved for patients with mild or no symptoms who are poor candidates for other kinds of treatment. There is currently little enthusiasm for dissolving common duct stones with oral agents.

Surgical

Most patients with common duct stones should have them removed surgically or by endoscopic sphincterotomy. The aims of therapy include: (1) removal of all stones from the common duct; (2) removal of the gallbladder, the source of the stones; and (3) prevention of recurrent disease. Surgery accomplishes these aims and is indicated in most patients who have a gallbladder. Endoscopic sphincterotomy, which is discussed later, is most often the treatment of choice in patients who have had a cholecystectomy in the past.

PREOPERATIVE PREPARATION

Because the incidence of medical disease and choledocholithiasis increase with age,[64, 65] many patients undergoing common duct exploration have underlying medical problems that require attention before surgery. In patients with benign disease, operative mortality increases with the depth of jaundice.[36] Although most patients with ductal stones are not profoundly icteric, functional liver impairment may be present in 35% of them.[33, 59]

The serum albumin concentration is depressed in over 20% of patients with jaundice secondary to choledocholithiasis,[33] possibly as a result of decreased protein intake or diminished albumin synthesis. However, anorexia and weight loss are generally uncommon in jaundiced patients with benign disease. If the patient is dehydrated due to recent vomiting, low serum albumin levels will contribute to a decreased circulating volume and therefore to a diminished capacity to tolerate blood loss. Adequate oral protein intake with supplemental IV nutritional therapy, if necessary, should be ensured preoperatively. The prothrombin time is abnormal in about 30% of patients with choledocholithiasis.[33] Unless hepatic parenchymal damage is present, parenteral vitamin K preparations will usually restore the clotting factors to normal. Occasionally fresh frozen plasma may be required.

The incidence of bactobilia is high in patients with common duct stones, and correlates with old age, increasing jaundice, increased numbers of stones, and previous instrumental manipulation of the biliary tree.[34, 36] Infectious complications (cholangitis, septicemia, subphrenic abscess, and wound infection) are eight times more common in patients with positive bile cultures.[36, 66, 67] The offending organisms are usually the same as those cultured from the bile.[36]

In general, antibiotics that achieve high serum concentrations are more effective than those excreted in the bile. Cephalosporins (cefazolin, cephalothin, and cefamandole) are probably the best choice for prophylaxis at present. To be effective, the antibiotic must be given preoperatively, and it can be discontinued after 2–3 postoperative doses. In fact, a single 2-gm dose of cefazolin given preoperatively was reported to decrease infective complications tenfold in high-risk patients.[66] Aminoglycoside antibiotics should generally be avoided for prophylaxis because of their potential for renal toxicity, particularly in older patients.[67]

The high morbidity of surgery in jaundiced patients stimulated interest in decompressing the bile duct by inserting percutaneous transhepatic catheters preoperatively, in an attempt to decrease complications. Because bilirubin levels rarely exceed 10 mg/dl in patients with choledocholithiasis, this concern is more germane to those with neoplastic obstruction. Nevertheless, enthusiasm for this idea has waned as experience demonstrated no improvement in the outcome after preoperative decompression.[36, 68] If this approach is to be used at all, it should probably be reserved for severely jaundiced (bilirubin level >20 mg/dl), elderly patients (age >60 years), especially those with existing renal dysfunction.

INDICATIONS FOR COMMON DUCT EXPLORATION

Choledochotomy and choledocholithotomy are most commonly performed at the time of cholecystectomy in a patient with previously undiagnosed common duct stones. Since only 10%–15% of patients undergoing cholecystectomy have coexisting stones in the duct, the surgeon must have a strategy for deciding which ducts to explore. Presumably, the goal would be to explore the duct in every patient with stones and avoid unnecessary explorations in those whose ducts are clear. Although perfection cannot be attained with present diagnostic techniques, an efficient approach can be devised.

The clinical findings in this disease can be divided into those associated with a high (>50%) or a low (<50%) chance of stones being present in the duct. Those in the former category include: (1) palpable stones in the duct; (2) high (>7 mg/dl) bilirubin levels; (3) demonstration of common duct stones on preoperative cholangiograms; and (4) recent cholangitis. Manifestations of possible common duct stones associated with a lower incidence of stones include: (1) mild jaundice; (2) a history of pancreatitis; (3) the presence of a dilated duct; and (4) the presence of small stones in the gallbladder. Obviously, the incidence is low with this second group only when none of the first set of criteria is present.

To use traditional surgical terminology, these criteria constitute the "absolute" and "relative" indications for common duct exploration. The usual approach is to explore the duct in every patient with an absolute indication and to use operative cholangiography to exclude ductal stones and avoid exploration in the 60%–70% of patients with only relative indications, whose ducts actually contain no stones.[5, 64, 69] If one were to explore the duct in every patient who has relative indications, almost two thirds of explorations would be unproductive (i.e., exploration, not cholangiography, would be used for diagnosing stones). Exploring only patients with absolute indications would miss about half of the patients with common duct stones.

Patients who have gallbladder stones and bilirubin levels greater than 3 mg/dl have about a 70% chance of having ductal calculi,[5, 64] and those with bilirubin levels greater than 7 mg/dl almost invariably have stones.[5] The chances of finding choledocholithiasis on exploration also increases with the size of the common duct.[64, 65] Ducts greater than 13 mm have nearly a 70% chance of having stones,[64] but most of these patients also have one or more absolute indications for exploration. In the absence of other indications, an enlarged duct is associated with only a 30% incidence of stones. Patients having nonfunctioning gallbladders and an age greater than 60 have a high incidence of choledocholithiasis,[64, 65] but only because they tend to have larger ducts.[64]

The poor correlation between a history of pancreatitis and ductal stones[5, 64, 65] is not surprising, because it has been shown that the acute attack is generally associated with passage of a stone. Exploration in the first 48 hours of acute gallstone pancreatitis will uncover a common duct stone in 70% of cases, but the incidence falls to about 30% within a couple of days.[70–72] If the surgeon thinks he can feel stones in the duct, he will be correct in over 90% of cases.[5, 73] Palpation is not, however, a reliable method for excluding stones.

Other factors, including the number of gallbladder stones, a history of jaundice in the past, and the size of the cystic duct, correlate with the presence of common duct stones,[65] but the yield is not high enough to warrant exploration without first confirming their presence by cholangiography.

About 15% of patients with acute cholecystitis have common duct stones.[74, 75] Cholangiography should be performed during cholecystectomy in patients with this disease and the duct should be explored if stones are seen. If the inflammatory changes are especially severe, and exploration of the duct appears to be unusually hazardous, it may be preferable in the absence of cholangitis to treat the stone postoperatively by endoscopic spincterotomy. The mortality and morbidity of common duct exploration in patients with acute cholecystitis is not much different than in patients who are undergoing elective cholecystectomy,[75] although septic complications may be more frequent. Bile duct injury is rare.

OPERATIVE CHOLANGIOGRAPHY

Operative cholangiography is the best method for deciding when to explore the duct in patients with relative indications. Its overall accuracy is greater than 98%.[76–78] The major value of preexploratory cholangiography is to decrease the incidence of negative common duct explorations when only relative indications are present.[5, 69, 76, 79] About 75% of common duct explorations which are based on preexploratory cholangiography are positive.[5, 69, 76–78, 80, 81] Avoiding unnecessary duct explorations decreases operative morbidity.[71]

Operative cholangiography can also demonstrate stones in about 5% of patients undergoing cholecystectomy who have no indications for common duct exploration.[76, 77, 79, 80] Negative cholangiograms are thought to be highly predictive in ruling out stones.[80, 81]

Some surgeons believe that finding unsuspected stones benefits so few patients that it should be avoided in the absence of indications for ductal exploration.[78–80] Others perform operative cholangiography routinely during cholecystectomy for the reasons cited.[5, 76] The argument has sometimes been misconstrued to mean that operative cholangiography is being recommended as a mandatory procedure for all patients. What it really intends to say, however, is that a 5% incidence of unsuspected common duct stones is considered in the average patient to be worth the time, cost, and morbidity of performing cholangiography to find them. If the patient is unstable, however, or if technical problems interfere with obtaining a good study promptly, the efforts of getting a cholangiogram may not be worth the yield. The main point is that the surgeon should know the probability that the study will reveal new important information. Other benefits of routine cholangiography include the rare discovery of other ductal lesions (e.g., biliary or periampullary tumors), demonstration of anatomical variations and the precise localization of stones in the duct.[77]

The cholangiograms must be of good quality. As many as 40% of operative cholangiograms are technically inadequate,[82] which is undoubtedly the explanation of the false positive results.[64, 82] The exposure must take into account the build of the patient and the presence of colonic gas or surgical instruments. Usually the standard 50% concentration of contrast medium is diluted by one or two equal volumes of saline. Experience has shown that it may have to be as dilute as a 15% concentration to demonstrate small calculi in large ducts.[82] Injecting the contrast medium under manometric control may decrease septic complications.[59]

Postexploratory T-tube cholangiography decreases the incidence of retained stones by 75%.[5] Introduction of air bubbles and sphincter spasm produced by the preceding exploration may make interpretation difficult.[83] The use of choledochoscopy does not eliminate the need for completion cholangiography, because the latter will still show some stones missed by the former.[84–86] These procedures should be considered as complementary.

TECHNIQUE OF OPERATIVE CHOLANGIOGRAPHY

Preexploratory cholangiography is generally performed by a catheter inserted into the cystic duct at the time of cholecystectomy. If this is not technically possible, or if cholecystectomy has been performed previously, the contrast medium can be injected through a fine needle inserted directly into the common bile duct at the proposed site of choledochotomy.

After the cystic duct is isolated, a ligature is placed around the base of the gallbladder to prevent stone migration. A small incision is made in the cystic duct to allow advancement of a pre-filled polyethylene catheter into the common bile duct. The catheter is then secured in place by a ligature. Two films are generally taken: one using 2–5 ml of contrast medium and the other using 10–15 ml. The smaller-volume injection prevents small stones from being obscured, while the second injection uses larger amounts of contrast medium to fill the entire ductal system and demonstrate emptying into the duodenum. The patient may be tilted, with his left side elevated 15° to rotate the spine away from the plane of the distal common duct.

The injection should be done slowly to minimize the possibility of causing bacteremia. A third film may be taken after withdrawing the contrast medium in an attempt to collapse the duct around any stones. The films should be interpreted by a radiologist as well as the surgeon. All ducts, including the intrahepatic ducts, should be filled, and contrast medium should be seen entering the duodenum.

T-tube cholangiography is performed at the completion of common duct exploration. Before taking the films, the duct is flushed with saline in an attempt to remove any air introduced during the exploration.

OPERATIVE ULTRASOUND

Intraoperative ultrasonography has been proposed as an adjunct to preexploratory operative cholangiography to screen for common duct calculi. With the use of high-resolution, real-time B-mode scanners, ultrasound is about as sensitive and specific as cholangiography.[87, 88] However, the frequency of false positives caused by air bubbles may be lower than the 20%–30% incidence associated with cholangiography.[87]

Other advantages include the absence of radiation exposure, decreased time required, and the avoidance of allergic reactions caused by contrast material. Operative ultrasonography will probably have other worthwhile applications in general surgery,[89] and it is only a matter of time before the equipment becomes generally available and there has been enough experience to say just how valuable it is in detecting gallstones.

CHOLEDOCHOSCOPY

Choledochoscopy is now an established adjunct to cholangiography in the search for common duct stones. Two kinds of choledochoscopes are currently in use. The rigid Storz scopes have a 4- or 6-cm horizontal viewing arm and a glass lens system. The flexible scopes rely on fiberoptics. Both are valuable. The rigid scopes have a somewhat better image and are adequate for most cases. The fiberoptic scopes also give an excellent view and have the advantage of being flexible. Both accommodate a large variety of accessory tools, including Dormia baskets, Fogarty catheters, and stone-grasping and biopsy forceps.

Choledochoscopy should be performed routinely during common duct exploration, a practice that appears to decrease the incidence of retained stones from about 5% to about 2%.[84, 90–92] After instrumental exploration of the duct, choledochoscopy has been noted to locate additional stones in about one quarter of cases.[85, 86, 90, 91, 93] Many of these stones would be detected on subsequent cholangiography, but it simplifies the operation if they are found before the T tube is inserted. In instances where contrast medium fails to enter the duodenum (as a result of sphincteric spasm or edema) on completed cholangiography, choledochoscopy can eliminate stones as the cause. The initial reservations about the value of choledochoscopy and concern that it may be cumbersome have disappeared with time. Because choledochoscopy has a limited ability to investigate the intrahepatic ducts, postexploratory T-tube cholangiography should not be omitted.[84–86]

For those who use choledochoscopy regularly, it no longer seems to be a separate examination, but only one of the various tools used in the exploration. The choledochoscope should be the last instrument used before inserting the T tube, but it may also be used early in the exploration if this seems to be desirable. Biopsy specimens may be obtained in addition to removing stones. In the presence of ductal dilatation, the operator may be able to explore as high as the tertiary hepatic ducts. In general, the morbidity is not increased appreciably by choledochoscopy.[85, 91] One report noted a few more infectious complications,[92] which could probably be avoided by better aseptic technique when handling the scope.

TECHNIQUE OF COMMON DUCT EXPLORATION

A Kocher maneuver is usually performed to mobilize the second and third portions of the duodenum. This facilitates palpation of the duct for stones and enables the operator to guide instruments accurately into the distal duct. Sometimes it is easier to handle the duct if the operator stands on the left side of the patient. The choledochotomy is usually 1.5–2.0 cm long, with its lowest point being about 1.0 cm from the duodenum. The incision is made closer to the duodenum

if a choledochoduodenostomy is anticipated. The peritoneum and loose areolar tissue over the common duct are cleared for a short distance over the proposed site of choledochotomy. If any doubt exists, the location of the common duct can be confirmed by fine-needle aspiration.

After placing fine silk stay sutures, the duct is opened longitudinally. In widely dilated ducts, the incision may be horizontal or diagonal to the long axis of the duct to facilitate a choledochoduodenal anastomosis if required. Upon opening the duct, gentle milking in the direction of the choledochotomy may extrude stones. A scoop is then used to extract stones by trapping them between the instrument and the duct wall. The duct is then flushed with saline instilled through a rubber catheter introduced proximally and distally. The catheter or a small (e.g., 3-mm) Bakes dilator may be gently passed into the duodenum to confirm distal duct patency, but the use of larger dilators should be avoided, because they may cause a fistula or pancreatitis. The older practice of "dilating" the sphincter is definitely contraindicated, for it carries a high risk of producing pancreatitis—a potentially fatal complication. Therefore, if the sphincter is judged to be stenotic, either a sphincteroplasty or choledochoduodenostomy is indicated. If stenosis is not present—if the 3-mm dilator passes smoothly—there is no need for additional manipulations of the sphincter.

The choledochoscope is then introduced into the duct. Continuous saline irrigation through the instrument distends the duct and improves visability. The operator generally stands on the left side of the patient and guides the scope with his left hand, while using the controls with his right. A systematic examination is performed upstream and downstream, and any stones encountered are removed by a Dormia basket or biliary Fogarty catheter introduced through the scope. Alternatively, the scope can be removed and the stones extracted using direct vision. Fogarty catheters should be used cautiously, because it is difficult to judge the amount of pressure they exert on the duct wall.

After ensuring that all calculi have been removed, a T tube is inserted and the choledochotomy is closed around it, using 3–0 or 4–0 polyglycolic acid (Dexon) sutures. One should use as large a T tube as comfortably fits inside the duct, usually size 12 F, 14 F, or 16 F. Because there is always a possibility that there will be a reason for instrumenting the duct postoperatively, a Whalen T tube is recommended for all common duct explorations performed for gallstone disease. The Whalen tubes have larger vertical stems than horizontal bars (the portion that goes into the duct). The tubes with 12 F, 14 F, and 16 F horizontal bars have 18 F stems; the tubes with 18 F and 20 F horizontal bars have 22 F stems. The larger stem presents no disadvantages, while it ensures that the T-tube track will be large enough if retained stones require passage of instruments into the duct at some later date.

It is important to leave some slack in the tube between the duct and the point of skin fixation at the abdominal wall exit site. Also, the exit site should not be placed far caudad but preferably within 5 to 10 cm of the costal margin. Otherwise, there is a risk that as the patient begins walking postoperatively, and the abdominal wall fat shifts downward, the T tube will be pulled out of the duct. Every so often one hears of a case where the T tube stopped draining within several days of surgery, and it was eventually found to be dislodged from the duct. The above mechanism is nearly always the explanation.

DRAINAGE PROCEDURES

After common duct exploration, stones may remain in the duct, or additional stone formation may be likely. The addition of a drainage procedure is indicated in such patients. The term "drainage procedure" in this context means any maneuver that allows bile to flow into the gut without having to pass through an opening as narrow as the normal sphincter. The most commonly used surgical drainage procedures are transduodenal sphincteroplasty, side-to-side choledochoduodenostomy, end-to-side choledochoduodenostomy, and choledochojejunostomy (Roux-en-Y).

Stones that are left behind in the duct after a previous biliary operation are referred to as residual stones. Residual stones discovered on T-tube cholangiograms in the first two weeks after surgery are referred to as retained stones. Stones that are believed to have formed in the duct after exploration are referred to as recurrent (primary) stones. By making its junction with the intestine as wide as the duct itself and by eliminating stasis in a large duct, a drainage procedure should allow residual stones to pass and prevent formation of recurrent stones.

A drainage procedure is appropriate in about 15% of common duct explorations. The indications are as follows: (1) history of a previous choledocholithotomy; (2) the presence of many (more than 5–10) stones in the duct; (3) marked ductal dilatation (> than 2 cm); (4) known or suspected stones remaining in the duct; (5) stenosis of the ampulla; (6) stricture of the lower end of the duct; or (7) intrahepatic gallstone formation.

A previous independent choledocholithotomy is an indication for a drainage procedure because if one is not done, about 25% of patients manifest recurrent disease at a later date.[94–96] If choledocholithotomy is performed without a drainage procedure for patients who have had a previous postcholecystectomy choledocholithotomy (i.e., if this is the third or more operation for stone disease), the chance of symptoms appearing later from additional common duct stones exceeds 80%.[94]

Choledocholithotomy alone is unsuccessful in 35% of patients with ducts greater than 2 cm in diameter.[94] Dilatation is a response to anything that increases the resistance to bile flow, such as ampullary stenosis or bile duct stricture. It may also be a primary disease or it may just be a response to having housed large numbers of stones for many years. The large duct allows bile flow to become stagnant and pigment solids to precipitate and form new gallstones. The process can be successfully interrupted by a drainage procedure.

Duct dilatation may also be present in the absence of distal obstruction, usually in elderly patients with long-standing disease.[13, 97] The duct may be massively dilated (greater than 3 cm), and in contrast to cases with mechanical obstruction, is thin-walled.[13, 98] Many of these patients exhibit primary stone formation due to stasis. Choledochoduodenostomy is required to drain these large ducts. Sphincteroplasty is inadequate, because the lower end of the duct inevitably narrows as it passes through the pancreas, and the discrepancy between the large supraduodenal segment and the intrapancreatic segment still allows for stasis. The presence of a relatively patulous sphincter in many of these patients is another clue that sphincteroplasty would be ineffective.

Patients with intrahepatic gallstone disease must have a drainage procedure as part of their surgical treatment. This does not apply to patients with a single stone that has floated up into the proximal ducts, but rather to those with multiple stones, which are often difficult to remove. This condition is occasionally seen in Western countries, but is common in recurrent pyogenic cholangitis (Oriental cholangiohepatitis), the peculiar primary ductal disease that is largely confined to lower socioeconomic populations in some parts of Asia. Residual stones and recurrent stones are both almost inevitable in these patients.[16] Early cases respond to sphincteroplasty, but if intrahepatic stricture formation occurs, more extensive operations may be necessary. Intrahepatic gallstone disease is discussed further later in this chapter.

The presence of multiple stones (e.g., >5–10 stones) in the duct increases the likelihood that at least one stone will evade detection during exploration and also suggests the possibility of primary stone formation. The other indications for a drainage procedure are self-evident.

A drainage procedure is obviously indicated for primary ductal stones. However, there is no pathognomonic way to diagnose primary stones. Using a variety of criteria, different authorities have estimated the frequency to range from 4% to 60% of patients with choledocholithiasis.[4, 9, 13] Soft, brown, easily crushable earthy stones have been thought by many surgeons to always reflect primary stone formation,[9, 13] but recent evidence suggests that many earthy stones are actually secondary, having first formed in the gallbladder.[1] Nonetheless, when earthy stones are found in the presence of stasis, duct dilatation, and infection, it is likely that they are truly primary.[13] When stone extraction and T-tube drainage alone are performed in patients diagnosed as having primary stones (by various criteria), the recurrence rate is approximately 25%.[4, 9]

CHOICE OF A DRAINAGE PROCEDURE

The decision to use a particular drainage procedure depends on the patient's anatomy and other details of the disease. Choledochoduodenostomy and sphincteroplasty are the procedures used most often. In some circumstances one procedure is definitely preferred, but in others either would suffice.

A sphincteroplasty is generally the preferred drainage procedure for[94, 99, 100]: (1) a stone impacted in the distal common bile duct; (2) stenosis of the ampulla; or (3) when the duct is narrow (less than 1.5 cm). It is relatively contraindicated in the presence of a periVaterian diverticulum[101] or a long stricture of the distal duct.[99, 102] Recent pancreatitis is a contraindication because of the presence of inflammation and the possibility of causing a flare-up.[101] Nevertheless, emergency sphincterotomy and stone extraction has been performed safely in some patients with acute gallstone pancreatitis.[70, 103, 104]

In performing a sphincteroplasty, the entire sphincter is divided. The incision should extend from the papillary orifice to the top of the funnel-shaped portion of the duct, where the duct diameter reaches a maximum. The resulting incision will vary from 1 to 3 cm. In the surgical literature, the term "sphincterotomy" has been restricted to an incision that divides just the distal 1.0 cm,[105] which would not abolish the entire sphincter mechanism in many patients. A sphincterotomy may be enough to allow removal of an impacted calculus in the ampulla, but it may not provide adequate drainage over a long period.

Choledochoduodenostomy is probably easier to perform and has slightly lower morbidity and mortality rates than sphincteroplasty, particularly in the elderly.[95, 106] However, choledochoduodenostomy requires a large duct (1.5 cm at least or larger).[95, 107] The anastomosis can be performed in a side-to-side or end-to-side fashion.

One minor drawback of the side-to-side technique is the potential for developing the sump syndrome postoperatively, which consists of pain, jaundice, and cholangitis.[95, 108–110] The sump syndrome results from food particles entering the bile duct and lodging in the lower end, the segment between the anastomosis and the papilla of Vater. This produces a low-grade cholangitis. Anastomotic obstruction is present in some but not all cases.[96, 101, 110] In those instances without a fixed anastomotic narrowing, the duct probably fails to drain adequately because of the anatomical relationships between the duct and the duodenum. Backwash of duodenal contents, in the absence of some stasis-producing mechanism, is not a tenable explanation for the cholangitis in these cases. On upper GI series, barium passes readily into the ducts through widely patent anastomoses, in patients who have no symptoms.

ERCP, barium upper GI series, and direct endoscopic inspection may be useful in defining an anastomotic stenosis or debris in the blind distal segment.[109, 111] The syndrome may be treated by sphincteroplasty or by conversion to a Roux-en-Y choledochojejunostomy, although endoscopic sphincterotomy is usually the easiest.[109]

We prefer the end-to-side technique of performing a choledochoduodenostomy. It avoids the problem of the sump syndrome, provides streamlined drainage, and prevents the anastomosis from being compromised as a result of the distorted relationship created by the duodenum hitching up onto the anterior aspect of the duct.[112]

The mortality rate of common duct exploration with choledochoduodenostomy averages about 2%.[106, 110, 113–115] The drainage procedure is well tolerated in the elderly and adds little risk to common duct exploration alone. The mortality of sphincteroplasty (4%) is slightly higher than that of choledochoduodenostomy,[102, 104, 106] and postoperative pancreatitis remains the most frequent cause of death. Other complications, such as duodenal leak or cholangitis are infrequent. The long-term results of both procedures are excellent and similar. Owing to its lower immediate morbidity, choledochoduodenostomy should probably be performed in situations where either procedure is feasible.

Roux-en-Y choledochojejunostomy diverts intestinal contents from the biliary tree, thereby minimizing bacterial contamination. The practical importance of this is questionable, however, since cholangitis is generally believed to require biliary obstruction. Nevertheless, it may be of some significance in patients with chronic stasis and bactobilia who are prone to recurrent sepsis and stone formation (e.g., Caroli's disease, Oriental cholangiohepatitis). The Roux limb should be at least 45 cm long to provide adequate diversion. In young patients and in those with benign disease, where prolonged survival is anticipated, construction of an end-to-side anastomosis seems preferable. Drainage would be dependent and a defunctionalized distal segment of duct would be avoided. Because the procedure diverts alkaline bile from the duodenum, it probably should be avoided in patients with peptic ulcer disease.

TECHNIQUE OF SPHINCTEROPLASTY

It is usually best to open the supraduodenal portion of the common duct first, which allows one to pass instruments and catheters through the papilla of Vater, thus enabling the operator to locate the papilla in relation to the duodenal wall. After the duodenum is fully mobilized, a small (i.e., 1 cm) incision is made in the lateral wall of the duodenum opposite the papilla. A heavy silk thread is used to drag a 12 F rubber catheter through the papilla, and with the catheter in place, an incision is made with the electrocautery along the summit of the ridge produced by the catheter. The initial incision should be about 1 cm long. The catheter can be temporarily withdrawn to inspect the papilla (checking for signs of a tumor), and the orifice of the pancreatic duct can be identified. Sutures of 4–0 polyglycolic acid are used to approximate the duodenal and common duct mucosa on each side of the incision. The incision is then extended further up the duct, dividing all the sphincter muscle until the maximum diameter of the duct is reached. Additional interrupted sutures are used to secure the cut edges where duct and duodenum meet. It is important to place a stitch at the apex of the incision, for this is the point where the duct and duodenum are most likely to have lost a common wall. The length of the incision, which is determined by the intramural length of the sphincter, averages 2–3 cm. The duodenum is closed in two layers, a T tube is placed in the choledochotomy, and sutures of 3–0 or 4–0 polyglycolic acid are used to close the duct around the T tube.

TECHNIQUE OF END-TO-SIDE CHOLEDOCHODUODENOSTOMY

After mobilizing the duodenum, the peritoneum over the common duct is divided. Using blunt dissection, the common duct is mobilized from the portal vein and encircled by a sling. With traction on the sling, the duct can be mobilized until it passes behind the duodenum. The duct is transected at this point. The distal end of the duct is closed with a running suture of 2–0 polyglycolic acid. A layer of 4–0 or 5–0 silk interrupted sutures is used to approximate the lateral duodenal wall to the posterior side of the duct. Then the duodenum is opened and a two-layer anastomosis is completed using running or interrupted 3–0 or 4–0 polyglycolic acid sutures for the inner layer. Usually no T tube or other kind of stent is used for these large ducts.

POSTOPERATIVE MANAGEMENT

Prophylactic antibiotics are continued for several doses postoperatively. If drains are used, they should be of the closed variety (e.g., Jackson-Pratt). They should be removed as soon as the output drops below about 15 ml/12 hours. The T tube is left to gravity drainage for seven days, and then a T-tube cholangiogram is performed. The entire biliary tree including the intrahepatic ducts must be opacified. After the cholangiogram, the T tube should be left to gravity drainage for 12 hours; then, if the patient has no fever and there is no obstruction to bile flow, the tube may be plugged.

In the absence of abnormalities on the cholangiogram, the T tube is left in place for three weeks from the time of operation and then is removed. Although it is usually safe to remove the tube as soon as ten days after surgery, a contained bile leak will occasionally occur on this schedule, and there are really no drawbacks to leaving the tube in longer. The patient may be discharged home with the tube in place to have it removed later in the office. If the cholangiogram is equivocal, or blood clots or air bubbles are thought to be responsible for the abnormalities on the x-rays, the test can be repeated in a few days. The patient need not be kept in the hospital any longer than dictated by his general condition (i.e., in most cases no more than 7–8 days). If more cholangiograms are indicated, they can be obtained on an outpatient basis.

Accidental dislodgment of the T tube from the duct is potentially serious. Most commonly the extrusion is partial, with just one limb of the tube lying outside the duct.[116] If drains are in place and signs of peritonitis are absent, the patient may be observed.[3] If the bile leak is not adequately drained, however, this can usually be accomplished with percutaneous catheters placed by an interventional radiologist. Otherwise, reoperation will be required to replace the T tube. As mentioned previously, accidental dislodgment of the T tube is a preventable complication, caused by leaving too little slack in the tube between the duct and the skin and bringing the tube through the abdominal wall too far from the costal margin.

After the T tube is withdrawn, bile usually drains for 3–12 hours. Persistent drainage for more than three days suggests that something is amiss (e.g., distal obstruction or subhepatic abscess), and a fistulagram should be performed. If no evidence of obstruction or bile collection is found, the fistula will probably close in another day or so.

MORBIDITY AND MORTALITY

The mortality of elective cholecystectomy alone is about 0.5%. It varies with the age of the patient, being 0.1% and 1.0% in patients less than or greater than 50 years of age, respectively.[117] When common duct exploration is performed in addition to cholecystectomy, the mortality is increased by a factor of 3 to 4[69]; although this is a reflection of the more serious illness in many of these patients, not the choledochotomy itself.

In patients undergoing biliary tract surgery, infection as well as cardiovascular and hepatobiliary problems are the most frequent complications resulting in death.[117] The presence of preoperative cirrhosis and the development of postoperative cholangitis account for a large percentage of deaths in these cases.[117] The development of renal failure or upper GI hemorrhage is also associated with a substantial increase in mortality.[118] Severely jaundiced patients tend to have a higher mortality.[119]

The commonest complications after common duct exploration are minor respiratory problems and wound infection. Postoperative pancreatitis has resulted from dilatation of the sphincter of Oddi,[120, 121] operative cholangiography,[122] the use of a long-arm (Cattel) type of T tube,[3] and the performance of sphincterotomy or sphincteroplasty.

Limited amounts of bile leakage from the drain are common after common duct exploration. It usually stops in 2–3 days and poses no threat as long as drainage is adequate.

RETAINED STONES

Stones discovered postoperatively on the T-tube cholangiogram are referred to as retained stones. Expert use of operative choledochoscopy and postexploratory T-tube cholangiography reduces the incidence of overlooked stones to about 2%.[5, 84, 90–92] Operative ultrasound is a sensitive method for detecting choledocholithiasis[87, 88]; however, its value in checking postexploratory clearance of the ducts has not yet been demonstrated. It is unlikely that the incidence of retained stones will ever be reduced to 0.

Retained stones nearly always follow an exploration that produces stones, not a negative exploration. The incidence of retained stones is roughly proportional to the number of stones found in the duct.[5, 123] There will always be an occasional stone that defies removal by any means. If an impacted stone is encountered at the lower end of the duct, every attempt should be made to remove it, including a transduodenal sphincteroplasty.[124] However, in the presence of marked inflammation of the distal duct (e.g., recent pancreatitis), an unstable or fragile patient, it may be advisable to defer operative removal in favor of postoperative extraction through the T-tube tract or endoscopic sphincterotomy.

When stones are discovered postoperatively on the T-tube cholangiogram, the simplest and safest approach is to extract them via the T-tube tract under radiologic guidance. The patient is discharged home for at least six weeks, during which time inflammation from the operation is allowed to settle and time is permitted for a firm, fibrous tract to form around the T tube. The tube may be left clamped if bile flow into the duodenum is unobstructed. If there is distal obstruction, or if symptoms develop with clamping, the T tube should be connected to a drainage bag. The biliary output should be measured, and the patient should be encouraged to match this output with adequate intake of fluids and electrolytes. Fat-soluble vitamin supplements (A, D, E, and K) should be given if drainage continues for more than one month.[125] Patients should never be given their bile to drink or have it instilled down a feeding tube.

From time to time, arguments in favor of primary closure of the common duct are presented in the literature.[126–128] A decreased incidence of postoperative septicemia and a reduced hospital stay are cited as advantages over conventional T-tube drainage.[127, 128] However, this practice denies postoperative access to the biliary tree to perform cholangiography or stone extraction. If it is to be used at all, it should be restricted to patients with negative duct explorations and normal ducts in whom the incidence of retained stones is likely to be minimal.

Stone removal via the T-tube tract can be performed under radiologic[129] or endoscopic guidance. For either of these methods, the T-tube tract must be 14 F or larger. General use of the Whalen T tubes described earlier will ensure that the tract is adequate in all cases. A narrow tract may be dilated to accommodate an instrument or to permit removing larger stones. A 14 F T-tube tract will generally accommodate a 6-mm stone; larger stones can be fragmented in the duct and removed piecemeal.[129] Smaller tracts may be enlarged by replacing the indwelling tube with successively larger rubber catheters.

Under fluoroscopic guidance, steerable catheters are passed into the duct and stones are removed or fragmented using a basket. The procedure is generally performed on an outpatient basis with oral antibiotics being given for several days. The success rate exceeds 85%, but depends considerably on the skill and experience of the radiologist.[129] Complications include fever, sinus tract perforation, bile collection, and pancreatitis.

Experience with choledochoscopic removal is more limited. Stones are removed under direct vision with baskets and forceps using fluoroscopic guidance if necessary.[130] Success rates of 92%–95% have been reported,[130–133] with complications similar to those encountered using radiologic guidance.

Retained stones can also be dissolved in some cases by infusing gallstone solvents in the duct. Because the technique is more time-consuming, requires the patient to be hospitalized, and is less predictable, extraction is usually preferable as a first approach.

Numerous agents capable of gallstone dissolution in vitro have been described, but only a handful are used clinically. Chloroform and ethyl ether were the first gallstone solvents tried, but they are no longer used. Ethyl ether vaporizes at body temperature and has only a transient effect. Chloroform instilled down the T tube has produced an anesthetic effect on some patients and centrilobular hepatic necroses on laboratory animals. Heparin was thought on theoretical grounds to help disperse gallstone fragments,[134] but direct observations have shown little genuine effect on gallstones. Heparin cannot really be considered a gallstone solvent. What clinical success has been achieved with this agent is most likely secondary to mechanical flushing.[135, 136]

Cholic acid[5, 135] and mono-octanoin[136–139] are the gallstone dissolving agents that have had the greatest recent use. They only dissolve cholesterol stones, however, not pigment stones. It is advisable, therefore, to test stones removed at surgery to determine whether they respond in vitro before embarking on a dissolution regimen. Cholic acid (220 mM), a normal bile salt, is effective in about two thirds of patients.[5] Ten to fourteen days of therapy are often required. The major side effect is diarrhea, which can be controlled by the oral administration of cholestyramine. Pain or fever during infusion reflect obstruction to flow and a risk of potentially severe cholangitis, and these symptoms should be treated by halting therapy and allowing the T tube to drain.

Mono-octanoin (glycerol-1-mono-octanoate), a medium-chain diglyceride, is somewhat more potent as a cholesterol solvent in vitro (it dissolves cholesterol stones 2.5 times as rapidly as cholate).[137] In vitro studies suggest that if the cholesterol content of the stones is greater than 40%, dissolution should occur in over 90% of cases.[138] Stones with a high cholesterol content generally dissolve faster. In clinical studies,

response rates average about 70%.[136, 139] It is often successful in seven days, although large stones or those with a low cholesterol content may require longer therapy. Hepatic function is not impaired,[136, 139] although severe cholangitis has been reported in one patient.[140] The major side effects include abdominal discomfort, diarrhea, and vomiting, which can usually be controlled by decreasing the rate of infusion.

Both cholate and mono-octanoin are given by continuous infusion through the T tube. A manometric overflow system should be used to prevent the infusion pressure from exceeding 30 cm of H_2O. Cholate (200 mM) is usually administered at 30 ml/hr and mono-octanoin at 3–10 ml/hr. The patient should be observed closely for signs of cholangitis, pancreatitis, or severe pain, which will necessitate interrupting the therapy.

Most treatment failures using these solvents are due to the presence of pigment stones. EDTA solutions have been used to dissolve pigment stones, but the safety of this method is questionable. Therefore, no dissolution regimen is currently available for this problem.

Patients in whom extraction or dissolution fail may be treated by endoscopic sphincterotomy. Failing this, reoperation is required, but this is rare. However, when nonoperative methods fail, some asymptomatic high-risk patients may be managed by expectant observation only. Oral dissolution therapy with UDCA and CDCA has been tried, but the response rate is very low.[62]

INTRAHEPATIC STONES

Intrahepatic stones are uncommon in North America, but are present in 30% of patients with choledocholithiasis in Asia.[16] In Western countries, intrahepatic stones are in some cases primary, but are most often a manifestation of advanced secondary choledocholithiasis with superimposed intrahepatic stone formation from bile stasis. Primary intrahepatic stones are also seen in Caroli's disease.[12, 141]

The disease in Asia is most often a manifestation of recurrent pyogenic cholangitis (Oriental cholangiohepatitis), which is characterized by recurrent primary stone formation in response to stasis and infection.[142, 143] These patients manifest recurrent cholangitis, right upper quadrant pain, and fever. Several factors are thought to be responsible. Bactobilia may result from superinfection by bacteria in patients who harbor parasites in the common duct,[144] usually *Opistorchis (Clonorchis) sinesis* or *Ascaris lumbricoides*. Portal bacteremia may also contribute to bile colonization. The typical low-protein, low-fat diet consumed in endemic areas may serve as a poor stimulus for cholecystokinin release with resulting gallbladder stasis.[145] The relative absence of dietary glucuronolactone (a β-glucuronidase inhibitor) in the presence of β-glucuronidase-producing bacteria may foster deconjugation and precipitation of bilirubin. The stones found in this disease are invariably composed of calcium bilirubinate, and the gallbladder is free of calculi in many cases.[142]

In the presence of bacteria, stones may produce obstruction with resulting inflammation and eventually stricture formation. This in turn may lead to further stasis, and eventually a cycle of stasis, infection, and stone formation ensues. Large, stone-containing, cavernous areas of duct destruction with distal stricturing may occur. Intrahepatic abscesses may form, and, after many attacks, portal fibrosis and biliary cirrhosis may result. Hepatic failure and portal hypertension with bleeding varices may complicate long-standing disease. The disease tends to have a predilection for the left lobe, possibly due to anatomical factors that impair drainage of that lobe.

Clinically, most patients present with recurring attacks of right upper quadrant or epigastric pain with fever, chills, and jaundice.[17] The patients tend to be young and of lower socioeconomic status. In other patients, fever and chills are less prominent. Attacks may recur three to four times a year, but the early stages may be mild.[17] Transhepatic cholangiography is often useful in determining the extent of intrahepatic disease. Obtaining adequate opacification by intraoperative cholangiography or ERCP is often difficult because of intrahepatic strictures that limit ductal filling with contrast mediums. Liver function tests often demonstrate elevated levels of bilirubin, alkaline phosphatase, SGOT, and SGPT. The extent of the liver function abnormality is related to the degree of hepatic fibrosis and to the continuing presence of intrahepatic stones and cholangitis.[16]

Treatment is primarily surgical. The aims of surgery include complete removal of all stones and the correction of stasis to prevent further infection and stone formation. In the presence of tight intrahepatic strictures, stone extraction and establishment of adequate drainage are more difficult. Sato et al.[16] divided patients into four types: Type I patients have no bile duct stenosis. Type II patients were further classified into three types depending on the site of duct stenosis as follows: (a) intrahepatic, (b) upper bile duct (above cystic duct junction) and (c) lower bile duct.

Type I patients should be managed by choledochotomy, thorough removal of stones, and sphincteroplasty or Roux-en-Y choledochojejunostomy. In the absence of stenosis, the results are good.[143] This procedure should also be adequate for most type IIc patients. Patients having severe disease with intrahepatic stenosis (type IIa) are best managed by hepatic resection if the disease is confined to one (usually the left) lobe.[141, 143] Patients with upper duct stenosis (type IIb) are best managed by upper duct reconstruction, if feasible, or hepatic resection.[16] In patients in whom the upper ducts are inaccessible by choledochotomy alone, cholangiolithotomy may be required to remove stones from large dilated proximal ducts.

The use of transhepatic intubation and irrigation is a poor alternative to stone removal, but may be necessary when many stones are present in the smaller hepatic branches of patients who are unsuitable for hepatic resection.[143] It is also of value in flushing out retained stones postoperatively.[16] Strictures may be dilated to gain access to stones, but restenosis is likely to occur.[143] Choledochoscopy is useful for stone removal at surgery, if the scope is not impeded by the presence of strictures.

In difficult patients with many recurrent or retained stones, another technique may be tried. In performing a Roux-en-Y choledochojejunostomy, the blind end of the Roux-en-Y loop is left long and is secured to the posterior rectus sheath and marked with metal clips.[15] This will permit stones to be removed by periodic percutaneous passage of catheters and baskets into the Roux-en-Y limb. A technique of percutaneous

transhepatic removal using the choledochoscope has been reported.[146] This procedure has been recommended for poor-risk patients who have had multiple previous procedures and in whom stones cannot be removed by the T-tube tract due to the presence of strictures. In this procedure, transhepatic drainage is performed under ultrasonic guidance, and the drainage tract is dilated over several weeks. Choledochoscopy can then be performed through the dilated tract. Successful transhepatic removal of stones using various instruments has also been reported.[147, 148]

Operative mortality, which averages 5%, is related to the extent of the ductal and hepatic parenchymal changes, and the number of previous procedures.[16, 17, 143] It tends to be higher after emergency operations,[143] in which stone extraction and T-tube insertion alone is commonly performed. Complications include cholangitis and septicemia, stress ulceration and bleeding, bleeding varices, and hepatic failure.

ENDOSCOPIC SPHINCTEROTOMY

Endoscopic sphincterotomy is an effective method for treating common duct stones. Using a side-viewing duodenoscope to cannulate the papilla of Vater, a diagnostic ERCP is performed to confirm the diagnosis and assess the feasibility of sphincterotomy. The sphincterotome is passed into the distal common duct, and its position is confirmed radiographically. Depending on the size of stone to be removed, a 1–2-cm incision is made in the choledochal sphincter at the 11 o'clock position by passing a blended diathermy current through the sphincterotome wire. Stones pass spontaneously or are extracted with balloon catheters and Dormia baskets. More than one attempt at extraction may be required. The technique successfully clears ductal stones in 85% of selected cases.[149–153]

Endoscopic sphincterotomy is contraindicated if the patient has a coagulation disorder or a long distal common duct stricture (endoscopic sphincterotomy cannot exceed 2 cm). Perivaterian diverticula and recent pancreatitis are relative contraindications. Anatomical factors must be considered when choosing patients for endoscopic sphincterotomy. The procedure is usually impossible in patients who have had Billroth II gastrectomy. Stones smaller than 1 cm can generally be removed, but those bigger than 2 cm may defy removal.[149]

The mortality of endoscopic sphincterotomy is about 1% and the morbidity about 8%.[150, 152–154] The major complications are pancreatitis, cholangitis, bleeding, and retroperitoneal duodenal perforation. Though hyperamylasemia occurs in about 8% of patients, clinical pancreatitis develops in 2% of patients[152] and is the commonest cause of death. Endoscopic sphincterotomy is no riskier in the aged or those who have had previous biliary tract surgery[151, 153, 154] or acute biliary tract disease (pancreatitis, cholangitis).[103, 104, 153]

Late results demonstrate that recurrent symptoms due to new stone formation or stenosis of the sphincterotomy occur in about 10% of patients.[154] Recurrent symptoms are often heralded by the onset of cholangitis. The enlarged opening created by sphincterotomy has been shown to remain open for at least two years with elimination of the common duct-to-duodenum pressure gradient.[155]

Assuming none of the contraindications are present, endoscopic sphincterotomy is clearly the treatment of choice for patients with choledocholithiasis who have had a previous cholecystectomy. The morbidity of the procedure is at least as good as that of surgery, and the cost is much less. The patient can return to work within a few days.

Stones occasionally recur in association with restenosis of the sphincterotomy, which can be treated by another sphincterotomy. One must be alert to ampullary neoplasm as the explanation, however, and an endoscopic biopsy should be obtained in all cases where a previous sphincterotomy narrows and symptoms recur.

Endoscopic sphincterotomy also has a place in treating selected patients with intact gallbladders. The procedure can often be performed in those whose general condition is poor (e.g., due to cardiac or pulmonary disease) or who have severe cholangitis, in which case it is a simple solution to the problems posed by the common duct stones.[153] Whether an interval cholecystectomy should be performed later, after the patient becomes a better surgical candidate, is a subject now being studied. The classic idea that the gallbladder would soon develop acute cholecystitis in the absence of sphincter function has had to be revised, as more patients in this situation have been followed up expectantly. The risk seems to be low (e.g., 10% in five years),[103, 150] and the disease is relatively mild when it does occur. Of course, expectant management would not be advisable for patients who already have chronic symptoms from the disease in the gallbladder.

Percutaneous extraction of biliary calculi using the transhepatic route has been described.[147, 148] Stones can be snared and then passed into the duodenum. At present, it is uncertain how much of a role this technique will play in the management of patients with calculous disease. It could conceivably be useful in the management of stones that lie proximal to ductal strictures.

ACUTE CHOLANGITIS

Choledocholithiasis is the most common cause of cholangitis, and may be the initial manifestation of the disease. The pathophysiology involves proliferation of bacteria in an obstructed (usually partially obstructed) bile duct. Common duct calculi are associated with positive bile cultures in over 90% of cases even in the absence of symptoms.[34] The calculi probably act like foreign bodies, protecting the bacteria from the host's immune defenses. Despite this contamination, cholangitis does not result unless obstruction supervenes. This allows the bacteria to proliferate, and pressures in the duct rise to levels as high as 30 cm H_2O.[39] Reflux of infected bile into lymphatics and hepatic sinusoids results in bacteremia.[40] In severe cases, the end result may be the development of multiple hepatic abscesses with fulminant sepsis, resulting in death. With recurrent attacks or ongoing sepsis, biliary cirrhosis may eventually develop, leading to hepatic failure and portal hypertension.[156]

Clinically, patients with cholangitis usually present with right upper quadrant pain, fever and chills, and jaundice.[42, 157, 158] The presence of all three symptoms (Charcot's triad) is found in only 70% of patients.[42, 157] These symptoms in addition to mental obtundation and hypotension constitute

Reynold's pentad.[159] Renal shutdown, thrombocytopenia, and hypoglycemia may complicate severe cases.[160] Associated laboratory abnormalities usually include leukocytosis and elevation of serum bilirubin levels, alkaline phosphatase, SGOT, and SGPT.[158] Cholangitis in the presence of normal liver function tests is unusual.[157] Blood cultures are positive in over 40% of cases.[42] The organisms cultured are the same as those which colonize the biliary tree, with *E. coli, Klebsiella, Pseudomonas,* enterococci, and *Proteus* being the commonest. Anaerobic species, mainly *Clostridium* and *Bacteroides,* are found in 25% of cases. Ultrasound scans may demonstrate gallstones.

The term "suppurative cholangitis" has been used to denote patients with the severest form of cholangitis. However, analysis of clinical and laboratory findings has not revealed any features that are consistently present in this condition other than septic cholangitis.[42, 157] For example, patients in extremis may have normal-appearing bile (not pus) in the duct, while patients with less severe symptoms may have bile that looks like frank pus. The mortality of septic cholangitis is high. Leukocytosis, elevated bilirubin and BUN levels, and decreased hemoglobin are associated with a high mortality.[161]

The clinical severity of an attack generally determines the urgency for surgery.[42] Because the obstruction in gallstone disease is usually incomplete,[42, 157] about 80% of patients respond to medical therapy consisting of antibiotics and supportive measures such as IV fluids. Antibiotics that achieve adequate tissue levels are preferred over drugs that are excreted in the bile. Cephalosporins, such as cefazolin or cefamandole, are effective in most cases. An aminoglycoside antibiotic should be added in severe cases. If concomitant anaerobic infection is suspected, cefoxitin or clindamycin should be given.

After the acute manifestations resolve, further diagnostic studies, such as ERCP or THC, may be indicated to confirm the diagnosis and aid in surgical planning. These tests are not required in every case, however, and they are always risky in a patient who has recently recovered from severe cholangitis.

Some patients will present in extremis with severe sepsis and hypotension. Other patients, having initially presented with mild disease, will deteriorate despite medical therapy. These patients require urgent decompression of their bile ducts after a brief period of resuscitation. If the diagnosis of gallstone disease is relatively certain, biliary decompression in these severe cases may be most easily accomplished by endoscopic sphincterotomy.[153] The patient usually recovers rapidly, and a definitive operation consisting of cholecystectomy and common duct exploration may be scheduled a few days later under much more favorable circumstances.

The timing of therapy is critical, however, in septic cholangitis. If endoscopic decompression cannot be achieved quickly, surgical decompression must be performed. In the most severely ill patients, it is preferable just to open the duct, empty the bile, and insert a T tube, postponing time-consuming efforts to remove common duct stones and the gallbladder until the patient has recovered. Cholecystostomy is too often inadequate for draining the duct to rely on this procedure as treatment for cholangitis.[162] Most patients are not this critically ill, however, and a definitive operation is often possible.

GALLSTONE PANCREATITIS

Gallstones are the cause of 50% of cases of acute pancreatitis. The incidence varies inversely with that of alcoholic pancreatitis. Unlike alcoholic pancreatitis, gallstone pancreatitis tends to occur more commonly in patients of higher socioeconomic status.

Passage of a stone through the ampulla of Vater with obstruction of the bile and pancreatic duct is thought to be the initiating event in gallstone pancreatitis.[70, 71, 163] The obstruction may result from stone impaction[70] or the severe inflammatory reaction that results from stone passage.[163] Patients with gallstone pancreatitis more often have many small gallbladder stones and a wide cystic duct, factors that facilitate stone passage into the common duct.[70, 72] In patients who undergo surgery less than 48 hours after symptoms begin, a stone will be found impacted in the ampulla in 70% of cases.[70, 71] Furthermore, stones can be recovered from the stools of over 80% of patients recovering from an acute attack.[71]

Other factors may contribute to the pathogenesis of the disease. Simultaneous stimulation of the pancreas in association with partial pancreatic duct obstruction produces pancreatitis in animal studies.[164] Similarly, many patients give a recent history of dietary excess,[70] and postprandial release of cholecystokinin and secretin may stimulate gallbladder contraction and pancreatic secretion. Reflux of infected bile from the common duct into the pancreatic duct may also play a role.[165] For this to occur, there must be "common channel" draining the bile and pancreatic ducts, an anatomical finding in about 80% of humans. Cholelithiasis must be suspected in every patient with acute pancreatitis and is present in all but a few who give no history of alcohol abuse. Patients who harbor gallstones can be spared further attacks by cholecystectomy.[166]

Serum amylase levels greater than 1,500 IU are much more likely to be associated with gallstone pancreatitis than with alcoholic pancreatitis. Similarly, bilirubin and alkaline phosphatase values are more likely to be elevated, but are of less value in differentiating between the two diseases.[163] Urine amylase excretion is often greater than 10,000 IU in 24 hours. Ultrasound detects gallstones in 80% of cases[72, 163] and may demonstrate pancreatic edema. This means, however, that ultrasound misses gallstones in 20% of patients who actually have gallstone pancreatitis. In the presence of gaseous distention due to ileus, CT scanning may be of benefit. THC and ERCP may demonstrate choledocholithiasis or stone impaction in the ampulla. ERCP is safe if measures are taken to avoid introducing contrast material into the pancreatic duct.[103] As in all cases of pancreatitis, other causes of hyperamylasemia must be considered in the differential diagnosis.

In the majority of patients, gallstone pancreatitis is an acute self-limited condition that responds to the usual medical measures. In about 20% of cases, however, it will progress to severe forms, raising the question of whether early intervention is appropriate. Acosta et al.[70] claimed that early operation to remove an impacted common duct stone obviated complications in enough patients to warrant this approach as standard therapy. In their experience, the mortality of gallstone pancreatitis was 2% in patients operated on early and 16% in those who were operated on late. In the United States, Stone et al.[163] found no difference in mortality between early surgery (less than 72 hours) or operation performed three months after the attack. In general, expectant management is thought to be the safest approach by most experts.

While early surgery is not enthusiastically embraced, the weight of opinion favors performing the cholecystectomy during the same hospitalization, but after the patient's pain has resolved, amylase levels have returned to normal, and eating has resumed.[71, 167–170] Early surgery may be indicated for a few patients in whom the diagnosis is in doubt or deterioration necessitates surgical intervention. If surgery is delayed for a month or two after the acute attack has resolved, 40% of patients will have a recurrent attack in the interval.[166, 170, 171]

REFERENCES

1. Bernhoft R.A., Pellegrini C.A., Motson R.W., et al.: Composition and morphological and clinical features of common duct stones. *Am. J. Surg.* 148:77, 1984.
2. Wosiewitz U., Schenk J., Sabinski F., et al.: Investigations on common duct stones. *Digestion* 26:43, 1983.
3. Jordon G.L. Jr.: Choledocholithiasis. *Curr. Probl. Surg.* 19:723, 1982.
4. Saharia P.C., Zuidemia G.D., Cameron J.L.: Primary common duct stones. *Ann. Surg.* 185:598, 1977.
5. Way L.W., Admirand W.H., Dunphy J.E.: Management of choledocholithiasis. *Ann. Surg.* 176:347, 1973.
6. Mullen J.L., Rosato E.F., Ipsen J., et al.: Gallstone characteristics in the diagnosis of choledocholithiasis. *Ann. Surg.* 176:718, 1972.
7. Taylor V.T., Torrance B., Rimmer S., et al.: Operative cholangiography: Is there a statistical alternative? *Am. J. Surg.* 145:640, 1983.
8. Yamamoto K., Tsuchiya R., Ito T., et al.: Reoperative surgery in cholelithiasis. *Jpn. J. Surg.* 12:6, 1982.
9. Madden J.L.: Primary common bile duct stones. *World J. Surg.* 2:465, 1978.
10. Wahlby L.: Aplasia of the gallbladder with common duct stones. *Acta Chir. Scand.* 143:241, 1977.
11. Rogers A.I., Crews R.D., Kalser M.H., et al.: Congenital absence of the gallbladder with choledolithiasis. *Gastroenterology* 48:524, 1965.
12. Pridgen J., Bradley J., McInnis D.: Primary intrahepatic gallstones. *Arch. Surg.* 112:1037, 1977.
13. Lygidakis N.J.: Incidence and significance of primary stones of the common bile duct in choledocholithiasis. *Surg. Gynecol. Obstet.* 157:434, 1983.
14. Pikula J.V., Dunphy J.E.: Some effects of stenosis of the terminal common bile duct on the biliary tract and liver. *N. Engl. J. Med.* 260:315, 1959.
15. Nagase M., Tanimara H., Takenaka M., et al.: Treatment of intrahepatic gallstones. *Nippon Geka Hokan* 47:467, 1978.
16. Sato T., Suzuki N., Takahashi W., et al.: Surgical management of intrahepatic gallstones. *Ann. Surg.* 192:28, 1980.
17. Chang T., Passaro E.: Intrahepatic stones: The Taiwan experience. *Am. J. Surg.* 146:241, 1983.
18. Tabata M., Nakayama F.: Bacteria and gallstones—etiological significance. *Dig. Dis. Sci.* 26:218, 1981.
19. Ashchoff L.: *Lectures in Pathology.* New York, Paul B. Hoeber, 1924.
20. Madden J.L., Vanderheyden L., Kandalaft S.: The nature and surgical significance of common duct stones. *Surg. Gynecol. Obstet.* 126:3, 1968.
21. Toouli J., Geenen E., Hogan W.J., et al.: Sphincter of Oddi motor activity: A comparison between patients with common bile duct stones and controls. *Gastroenterology* 82:111, 1982.
22. Guelrud M., Mendosa S., Vicent S., et al.: Pressures in the

sphincter of Oddi in patients with gallstones, common duct stones, and recurrent pancreatitis. *J. Clin. Gastroenterol.* 5:37, 1983.

23. Lotveit T.: The composition of biliary calculi in patients with juxtapapillary duodenal diverticula. *J. Gastroenterol.* 17:653, 1982.

24. Orr K.B.: Suture material as a nidus for formation of common bile duct stones. *Aust. N.Z. J. Surg.* 50:493, 1980.

25. Millbourn E.: On re-operation for choledocholithiasis. *Acta Chir. Scand.* 99:285, 1950.

26. Kozoll D.D., Dwyer G., Meyer K.A.: Pathological correlation of gallstones: A review of 1,874 autopsies of patients with gallstones. *Arch. Surg.* 79:514, 1959.

27. Bateson M.C., Bouchier I.A.D.: Prevalence of gallstones in Dundee: A necropsy study. *Br. Med. J.* 4:427, 1975.

28. Lund J.: Surgical indications in cholelithiasis: Prophylactic cholecystectomy elucidated on the basis of long-term followup on 526 non-operated cases. *Ann. Surg.* 151:153, 1960.

29. Wenckert A., Robertson B.: The natural course of gallstone disease. Eleven-year review of 781 non-operated cases. *Gastroenterology* 50:376, 1966.

30. Comfort M.W., Gray H.K., Wilson J.M.: The silent gallstone: A ten to twenty year follow-up study of 112 cases. *Ann. Surg.* 128:931, 1948.

31. Pellegrini C.A., Thomas M.J., Way L.W.: Bilirubin and alkaline phosphatase values before and after surgery for biliary obstruction *Am. J. Surg.* 143:67, 1982.

32. Pellegrini C.A., Way L.W.: Biliary tract mechanisms, in Frolich E.D. (ed.): *Pathophysiology: Altered Regulatory Mechanisms in Disease.* Philadelphia, J.B. Lippincott Co., 1984, p. 581.

33. Lindenauer S.M., Child C.G.: Disturbances of liver function in biliary tract disease. *Surg. Gynecol. Obstet.* 123:1205, 1966.

34. Lygidakis N.: Incidence of bile infection in patients with choledocholithiasis. *Am. J. Gastroenterol.* 77:12, 1982.

35. Keighley M.R.: Preventing infection in biliary surgery. *Infections in Surgery* 1:711, 1982.

36. Armstrong C.P., Dixon J.M., Taylor T.V., et al.: Surgical experience of deeply jaundiced patients with bile duct obstruction. *Br. J. Surg.* 71:234, 1984.

37. Cetta F.: The route of infection in patients with bactobilia. *World J. Surg.* 7:562, 1983.

38. Larry M., Meier D.E.: Sphincter incompetence caused by common duct stones. *Surgery* 98:538, 1983.

39. Csendes A., Debandi A., Miranda M., et al.: Common bile duct pressures in patients with common bile duct stones with or without acute suppurative cholangitis. *Surg. Gastroenterol.* 2:273, 1983.

40. Huang T., Bass J., Williams R., et al.: The significance of biliary pressure in cholangitis. *Arch. Surg.* 98:629, 1969.

41. Schein C.J.: The Web factor in cholangitis. *Am. J. Surg.* 135:624, 1978.

42. Boey J., Way L.W.: Acute cholangitis. *Ann. Surg.* 191:264, 1980.

43. Rubin J.R., Beal J.M.: Diagnosis of choledocholithiasis. *Surg. Gynecol. Obstet.* 156:16, 1983.

44. Chung R.S.: Pathogenesis of the Courvoisier gallbladder. *Dig. Dis. Sci.* 28:33, 1983.

45. White T.T.: Obstructive biliary tract disease. *West J. Med.* 136:484, 1982.

46. Kaplan M.N.: Alkaline phosphatase. *N. Engl. J. Med.* 286:200, 1972.

47. Thomas M.J., Pellegrini C.A., Way L.W.: Usefulness of diagnostic tests for biliary obstruction. *Am. J. Surg.* 144:102, 1982.

48. Cronan J.J., Mueller P.R., Simeone J.F., et al.: Prospective diagnosis of choledocholithiasis. *Radiology* 146:467, 1983.

49. Beinart C., Efremidis S., Cohen B., et al.: Obstruction without dilatation: Importance in evaluating jaundice. *J.A.M.A.* 245:353, 1981.

50. Haubeck A., Pederson J.H., Burcharth F., et al.: Dynamic sonography in the evaluation of jaundice. *A.J.R.* 136:1071, 1981.

51. Mitchell S.E., Clark R.A.: A comparison of computed tomography and sonography for the diagnosis of choledocholithiasis. *A.J.R.* 142:729, 1984.

52. Einstein D.M., Lapin S.A., Ralls P.W., et al.: The insensitivity of sonography in the detection of choledocholithiasis. *A.J.R.* 142:725, 1984.

53. Gross B.H., Harter L.P., Gore R.M., et al.: Ultrasonic evaluation of common bile duct stones: Prospective comparison with endoscopic retrograde cholangiopancreatography. *Radiology* 146:471, 1983.

54. Parulekar S.G., McNamara M.P.: Ultrasonography of cholelithiasis. *J. Ultrasound Med.* 2:395, 1983.

55. Suzuki M., Takashima T., Funak H., et al.: CT diagnosis of common bile duct stones. *Gastrointest. Radiol.* 8:327, 1983.

56. Jeffrey R.B., Federle M.P., Laing F.C., et al.: Computed tomography of choledocholithiasis. *A.J.R.* 140:1179, 1983.

57. Itai Y., Araki T., Furui S., et al.: Computed tomography and ultrasound in the diagnosis of intrahepatic calculi. *Radiology* 136:399, 1980.

58. Shapiro H.A.: Endoscopic diagnosis and treatment of biliary tract disease. *Surg. Clin. North Am.* 61:843, 1981.

59. Lygidakis N.J.: Potential hazards of intraoperative cholangiography in patients with infected bile. *Gut* 23:1015, 1982.

60. Frey C., Burbige E., Meinke W., et al.: Endoscopic retrograde cholangiopancreatography. *Am. J. Surg.* 144:109, 1982.

61. Wild S.R., Cruikshank J.G., Fraser G.M., et al.: Grey-scale ultrasonography and percutaneous transhepatic cholangiography in biliary tract disease. *Br. Med. J.* 281:1524, 1981.

62. Dowling R.H.: Management of stones in the biliary tree. *Gut* 24:599, 1983.

63. Salvioli G., Salati R., Lugli R., et al.: Medical treatment of biliary duct stones: Effect of ursodeoxycholic acid administration. *Gut* 24:609, 1983.

64. Reiss R., Deutsch A.A., Nadelman I., et al.: Statistical value of various clinical parameters in predicting the presence of choledochal stones. *Surg. Gynecol. Obstet.* 159:273, 1984.

65. Taylor T.V., Torrance B., Rimmer S., et al.: Operative cholangiography: Is there a statistical alternative? *Am. J. Surg.* 145:640, 1983.

66. Lewis R.T., Allan C.M., Goodall R.G., et al.: Single preoperative dose of cefazolin prevents postoperative sepsis in high-risk biliary surgery. *Can. J. Surg.* 27:44, 1984.

67. Pitt H.A., Postier R.G., Cameron J.L.: Biliary bacteria. *Arch. Surg.* 117:445, 1982.

68. Hatfield A.R.W., Terblanche J., Fataar S.: Preoperative external biliary drainage in obstructive jaundice. *Lancet* 2:896, 1982.

69. Doyle P.J., Ward-McQuaid J.N., McEwen-Smith A.: The value of routine preoperative cholangiography—a report of 4000 cholecystectomies. *Br. J. Surg.* 69:617, 1982.

70. Acosta J., Pellegrini C., Skinner D.: Etiology and pathogenesis of acute biliary pancreatitis. *Surgery* 88:118, 1980.

71. Kelly T.: Gallstone pancreatitis: The timing of surgery. *Surgery* 88:345, 1980.

72. McMahon M., Shefta J.: Physical characteristics of gallstones and the calibre of the cystic duct in patients with acute pancreatitis. *Br. J. Surg.* 67:6, 1980.

73. Cassie F.G., Kapadia C.R.: Operative cholangiography or extraductal palpation: An analysis of 418 cholecystectomies. *Br. J. Surg.* 68:516, 1981.

74. Stryker S.J., Beal J.M.: Acute cholecystitis and common duct calculi. *Arch. Surg.* 118:1063, 1983.

75. Coelho J.C., Buffara M., Pozzobon C.E., et al.: Incidence of common bile duct stones in patients with acute and chronic cholecystitis. *Surg. Gynecol. Obstet.* 158:76, 1984.

76. Cheng F.C.Y., Shum D.W.P., Shum J.W.P., et al.: Operative cholangiography: Evaluation of its use in 569 cholecystectomies. *Aust. N.Z. J. Surg.* 50:484, 1980.

77. Pagana T.J., Stahlgren L.H. et al.: Indications and accuracy of operative cholangiography. *Arch. Surg.* 115:1214, 1980.

78. Stark M.E., Loughry C.W.: Routine operative cholangiography with cholecystectomy. *Surg. Gynecol. Obstet.* 151:658, 1980.

79. Gerber A., Malcolm K.: The case against routine operative cholangiography. *Am. J. Surg.* 143:734, 1982.

80. Levine S.B., Lerner H.J., Leifer E.D., et al.: Intraoperative cholangiography: A review of indications and analysis of age-sex groups. *Ann. Surg.* 198:692, 1983.

81. Rolfsmeyer E.S., Bubrick M.P., Kollitz P.R., et al.: The value of operative cholangiography. *Surg. Gynecol. Obstet.* 154:369, 1982.

82. Machi J., Sigel B., Spigos D.G., et al.: Critical factors in image clarity of operative cholangiography. *J. Surg. Res.* 35:480, 1983.

83. Millward S.F.: Post-exploratory operative cholangiography: Is it a useful technique to check clearance of the common bile duct? *Clin. Radiol.* 33:535, 1982.

84. Yap P.C., Atacador M., Yap A.G., et al.: Choledochoscopy as a complementary procedure to operative cholangiography in biliary surgery. *Am. J. Surg.* 140:648, 1980.

85. Rattner D.W., Warshaw A.L.: Impact of choledochoscopy on the management of choledocholithiasis: Experience with 449 common duct explorations at the Massachusetts General Hospital. *Ann. Surg.* 194:76, 1981.

86. Kappas A., Alexander-Williams J., Keighley M.R., et al.: Operative choledochoscopy. *Br. J. Surg.* 66:177, 1979.

87. Sigel B., Machi J., Beitler J.C.: Comparative accuracy of operative ultrasonography and cholangiography in detecting common duct calculi. *Surgery* 94:715, 1983.

88. Siegel B., Coelho J.C.U., Nyhus L.M., et al.: Comparison of cholangiography and ultrasonography in the operative screening of the common bile duct. *World J. Surg.* 6:440, 1982.

89. Sigel B., Coelho J.C.U., Spigos D.G., et al.: Ultrasonic imaging during biliary and pancreatic surgery. *Am. J. Surg.* 141:84, 1981.

90. Escat J., Glucksman D.L., Maigne C., et al.: Choledochoscopy in surgery for choledocholithiasis: Six year experience in 380 consecutive patients. *Am. J. Surg.* 47:670, 1984.

91. Bauer J.J., Salky B.A., Gelernt I.M., et al.: Experience with the flexible fiberoptic choledochoscope. *Ann. Surg.* 194:161, 1981.

92. Kappes S.K., Adams M.B., Wilson S.D.: Intraoperative biliary endoscopy: Mandatory for all common duct operations? *Arch. Surg.* 117:603, 1982.

93. Feliciano D.V., Mattox K.L., Jordan G.L.: The value of choledochoscopy in exploration of the common bile duct. *Ann. Surg.* 191:649, 1980.

94. Allen B., Shapiro H., Way L.W.: Management of recurrent and residual common duct stones. *Am. J. Surg.* 142:41, 1981.

95. Anderberg B., Bolin S., Heuman R., et al.: Choledochoduodenostomy for choledocholithiasis—indications and functional results. *Acta Chir. Scand.* 150:75, 1984.

96. Lygidakis N.J.: A prospective randomized study of recurrent choledocholithiasis. *Surg. Gynecol. Obstet.* 155:679, 1982.

97. Way L.W., Morgenstern L., Cameron J.L., et al.: Duct stone disease. *Contemp. Surg.* 18:83, 1981.

98. Lygidakis N.J.: Surgical approaches to postcholecystectomy choledocholithiasis. *Arch. Surg.* 117:481, 1982.

99. Thomas C.G., Nicholson C.P., Owen J.: Effectiveness of choledochoduodenostomy and transduodenal sphincteroplasty in the treatment of benign obstruction of the common duct. *Ann. Surg.* 173:845, 1971.

100. Stuart M., Hoerr S.: Late results of side to side choledochoduodenostomy and of transduodenal sphincterotomy for benign disorders. *Am. J. Surg.* 123:67, 1972.

101. Rutledge R.H.: Sphincteroplasty and choledochoduodenostomy for benign biliary obstruction. *Ann. Surg.* 183:476, 1976.

102. Jones S.A., Smith L.L.: A reappraisal of sphincteroplasty (not sphincterotomy). *Surgery* 71:565, 1972.

103. Rosseland A., Solhaug J.: Early or delayed endoscopic papillotomy in gallstone pancreatitis. *Ann. Surg.* 199:165, 1983.

104. Safrany L., Cotton P.: A preliminary report: Urgent duodenoscopic sphincterotomy for acute gallstone pancreatitis. *Surgery* 84:424, 1981.

105. Partington P.F.: Twenty-three years of experience with sphincterotomy and sphincteroplasty for stenosis of the sphincter of Oddi. *Surg. Gynecol. Obstet.* 145:161, 1977.

106. Lygidakis N.J.: Choledochoduodenostomy in calculous biliary tract disease. *Br. J. Surg.* 68:762, 1981.

107. Kraus M.A., Wilson S.D.: Choledochoduodenostomy—importance of duct size and occurrence of cholangitis. *Arch. Surg.* 115:1212, 1980.

108. Barkin J.S., Silvis S., Greenwald R.: Endoscopic therapy of the "sump" syndrome. *Dig. Dis. Sci.* 25:597, 1980.

109. Siegel J.: Duodenoscopic sphincterotomy in the treatment of the "sump" syndrome. *Dig. Dis. Sci.* 26:922, 1981.

110. Madden J.L., Gruwez J.A., Tan P.Y.: Obstructive (surgical) jaundice: An analysis of 140 consecutive cases and a consideration of choledochoduodenostomy in its treatment. *Am. J. Surg.* 109:89, 1965.

111. Akiyama H., Ikezawa H., Kameya S., et al.: Unexpected problems of external choledochoduodenostomy-fiberscopic examination in 15 patients. *Am. J. Surg.* 140:680, 1980.

112. Cushieri A., Wood R.A.B., Metcalf J.M., et al.: Long-term experience with transection choledochoduodenostomy. *World J. Surg.* 7:502, 1983.

113. de Almeida A.M., Cruz A.G., Aldeia F.J.: Side-to-side choledochoduodenostomy in the management of cholelithiasis and associated disease: Facts and fiction. *Am. J. Surg.* 147:253, 1984.

114. Moesgaard F., Nielsen M.L., Pedersen T., et al.: Protective choledochoduodenostomy in multiple common duct stones in the aged. *Surg. Gynecol. Obstet.* 154:232, 1982.

115. Schein C.J., Shapiro N., Gliedman M.L.: Choledochoduodenostomy as an adjunct to choledocholithotomy. *Surg. Gynecol. Obstet.* 148:25, 1978.

116. Ger R., Duboys E., Addei K.A.: The mechanism of T-tube dislocation and its prevention. *Surgery* 91:531, 1982.

117. McSherry C.K., Glenn F.: The incidence and causes of death following surgery for non-malignant biliary tract disease. *Ann. Surg.* 191:271, 1980.

118. Pitt H.A., Cameron J.L., Postier R.G., et al.: Factors affecting mortality in biliary tract surgery. *Am. J. Surg.* 141:66, 1981.

119. Blamey S.L., Fearon K.C.H., Gilmore W.H., et al.: Prediction of risk in biliary surgery. *Br. J. Surg.* 70:535, 1983.

120. Thorbjarnarson B., Glenn F.: Complications of biliary tract surgery. *Surg. Clin. North Am.* 44:431, 1964.

121. Heimbach D.M., White T.T.: Immediate and long-term effects of instrumental dilatation of the sphincter of Oddi. *Surg. Gynecol. Obstet.* 148:79, 1979.

122. Holm J.C., Edmunds L.H., Baker J.W.: Life threatening complications after operations upon the biliary tract. *Surg. Gynecol. Obstet.* 127:241, 1968.

123. Heuman R., Smeds S., Hellgren E., et al.: Evaluation of factors affecting the incidence of retained calculi in the bile ducts. *Acta Chir. Scand.* 148:185, 1982.

124. Leckie P.A., Schmidt N., Taylor R.: Impacted common bile duct stones. *Am. J. Surg.* 143:540, 1982.

125. Way L.W.: Retained common duct stones. *Surg. Clin. North Am.* 53:1139, 1973.

126. Vassilakis J.S., Chattopadhyay D.K., Irvin T.T., et al.: Primary closure of the common bile duct after elective choledochotomy. *R. Coll. Surg. Edinb.* 24:156, 1979.

127. Lygidakis N.J.: Choledochotomy for biliary lithiasis: T-tube drainage or primary closure—effects on postoperative bacteremia and T-tube bile infection. *Am. J. Surg.* 146:254, 1983.

128. Chande S., Devitt J.E.: T-tubes, the surgical amulet after choledochotomy. *Surg. Gynecol. Obstet.* 136:100, 1973.

129. Burhenne H.J.: Percutaneous extraction of retained biliary tract stones: 661 patients. *A.J.R.* 134:889, 1980.

130. Berci G., Hamlin A., Grundfest W.S.: Combined fluoroendoscopic removal of retained biliary stones. *Arch. Surg.* 118:1395, 1983.

131. Jakimowicz J.J., Mak B., Carol E.J., et al.: Postoperative choledochoscopy—a five year experience. *Arch. Surg.* 118:810, 1983.

132. Yamakawa T., Komaki F., Shikata J.: Experience with routine postoperative choledochoscopy via the T-tube sinus tract. *World J. Surg.* 2:379, 1978.

133. Birkett D.H., Williams L.F.: Postoperative fiberoptic choledochoscopy: A useful surgical adjunct. *Ann. Surg.* 194:630, 1981.

134. Gardner B., Dennis C.R., Patti J.: Current status of heparin dissolution of gallstones. *Am. J. Surg.* 130:293, 1975.

135. Way L.W., Motson R.W.: Dissolution of retained common duct stones. *Adv. Surg.* 10:99, 1976.

136. Velasco N., Braghetto I., Csendes A.: Treatment of retained

common bile duct stones: A prospective controlled study comparing monooctanoin and heparin. *World J. Surg.* 7:266, 1982.

137. Thistle J.L., Carlson G.L., Hofmann A.F., et al.: Monooctanoin, a dissolution agent for retained cholesterol bile duct stones: Physical properties and clinical application. *Gastroenterology* 78:1016, 1980.
138. Sharp K.W., Gadacz T.R.: Selection of patients for dissolution of retained common duct stones with mono-octanoin. *Ann. Surg.* 196:137, 1982.
139. Gadacz T.R.: The effect of monooctanoin on retained stones. *Surgery* 89:527, 1981.
140. Crabtree T.S., Dykstra R., Kelly J., et al.: Necrotizing choledochomalacia after use of monooctanoin to dissolve bile duct stones. *Can. J. Surg.* 25:644, 1982.
141. Adson M., Nagorney D.: Hepatic resection for intrahepatic ductal stones. *Arch. Surg.* 117:611, 1982.
142. Nagase M., Hikasa Y., Soloway R., et al.: Gallstones in western Japan—factors affecting the prevalence of intrahepatic stones. *Gastroenterology* 78:684, 1980.
143. Choi T., Wong J., Ong G.: The surgical management of primary intrahepatic stones. *Br. J. Surg.* 69:86, 1982.
144. Lam S.K., Wong K.P., Chan P.K.W., et al.: Recurrent pyogenic cholangitis: A study by endoscopic retrograde cholangiography. *Gastroenterology* 74:1196, 1978.
145. Nagase M., Tanimura H., Motoichi S., et al.: Present features of gallstones in Japan: A collective review of 2,144 cases. *Am. J. Surg.* 135:788, 1978.
146. Murata N., Beppu T., Bandai Y., et al.: Treatment of intrahepatic lithiasis using the choledochofiberscope. *Endoscopy* 13:240, 1981.
147. Clouse M., Falchuk K.: Percutaneous transhepatic removal of common duct stones: Report of 10 cases. *Gastroenterology* 85:815, 1983.
148. Ellman B., Berman H.: Treatment of a common duct stone via transhepatic approach. *Gastrointest. Radiol.* 6:357, 1981.
149. Mazzeo R.J., Jordan F.T., Strazius S.R.: Endoscopic papillotomy for recurrent common bile duct stones and papillary stenosis: A community hospital experience. *Arch. Surg.* 118:693, 1983.
150. Escourrou J., Cordova J.A., Lazorthes F., et al.: Early and late complications after endoscopic sphincterotomy for biliary lithiasis with and without the gallbladder "in situ." *Gut* 25:598, 1984.
151. Mee A.S., Vallon A.G., Croker J.R., et al.: Non-operative removal of bile duct stones by duodenoscopic sphincterotomy in the elderly. *Br. Med. J.* 283:521, 1981.
152. Ghazi A., McSherry C.K.: Endoscopic retrograde cholangiopancreatography and sphincterotomy. *Ann. Surg.* 199:21, 1984.
153. Neoptolemos J.P., Carr-Locke D.L., Fraser I., et al.: The management of common bile duct calculi by endoscopic sphincterotomy in patients with gallbladders in situ. *Br. J. Surg.* 71:69, 1984.
154. Cotton P.B.: Endoscopic management of bile duct stones; (apples and oranges). *Gut* 25:587, 1984.
155. Geenen J.R., Toouli J., Hogan W.J., et al.: Endoscopic sphincterotomy: Follow-up evaluation of effects on the sphincter of Oddi. *Gastroenterology* 87:754, 1984.
156. Dow R., Lindenauer S.: Acute obstructive suppurative cholangitis. *Ann. Surg.* 169:272, 1969.
157. Saharia P., Cameron J.: Clinical management of acute cholangitis. *Surg. Gynecol. Obstet.* 142:369, 1976.
158. Saik R., Greenburg A., Farris J., et al.: Spectrum of cholangitis. *Am. J. Surg.* 130:143, 1975.
159. Reynolds B., Dargan E.: Acute obstructive cholangitis. *Ann. Surg.* 150:299, 1959.
160. Hinchey E., Couper C.: Acute obstructive suppurative cholangitis. *Am. J. Surg.* 117:62, 1969.
161. O'Connor M., Schwartz M., McQuarrie D., et al.: Acute bacterial cholangitis: An analysis of clinical manifestations. *Arch. Surg.* 117:437, 1982.
162. Saik R., Greenburg G., Peskin G., et al.: Cholecystostomy hazard in acute cholangitis. *J.A.M.A.* 235:2412, 1976.
163. Stone H.H., Fabian T.C., Dunlop W.E.: Gallstone pancreatitis: Biliary pathology in relation to time of operation. *Ann. Surg.* 194:305, 1981.
164. Broe P.J., Cameron J.L.: Experimental gallstone pancreatitis—pathogenesis and response to different treatment modalities. *Ann. Surg.* 195:566, 1982.
165. Kelly T.R.: Gallstone pancreatitis: Pathophysiology. *Surgery* 80:488, 1976.
166. Paloyan D., Simonowitz D., Skinner D.B.: The timing of biliary tract operations in patients with pancreatitis associated with gallstones. *Surg. Gynecol. Obstet.* 141:737, 1975.
167. Ranson J.: The timing of biliary surgery in acute pancreatitis. *Ann. Surg.* 189:654, 1979.
168. Semel L., Schrieber D., Fromm D.: Gallstone pancreatitis—support for a flexible approach. *Arch. Surg.* 118:901, 1983.
169. Kim U., Sheth M.: Optimal timing of surgical intervention in patients with acute pancreatitis associated with cholelithiasis. *Surg. Gynecol. Obstet.* 150:499, 1980.
170. Mayer A.D., McMahon M.J., Benson E., et al.: Operations upon the biliary tract in patients with acute pancreatitis: Aims, indications and timing. *Ann. R. Coll. Surg. Engl.* 66:179, 1984.
171. Osborne D.H., Imrie C.W., Carter D.C.: Biliary surgery in the same admission for gallstone-associated pancreatitis. *Br. J. Surg.* 68:758, 1981.

22

Benign Strictures of the Bile Ducts

DAVID L. NAHRWOLD, M.D.

BENIGN strictures of the bile ducts are important because when unrecognized or treated improperly, they lead to biliary cirrhosis, portal hypertension, and death. Over 90% of benign strictures of the bile ducts occur following primary operations on the gallbladder or biliary duct system or after reconstructive surgery on the ducts. The remainder are associated with surgery on the liver, portacaval shunting, gastrectomy, or pancreatic surgery.[1, 2]

Less common causes of bile duct strictures are abdominal trauma, inflammation and fibrosis from a calculus impacted within a duct, chronic pancreatitis, and stenosis of the sphincter of Oddi. Finally, sclerosing cholangitis, a poorly understood condition manifested by multiple strictures in the intrahepatic and extrahepatic ducts, is encountered rarely.

STRICTURES ASSOCIATED WITH BILE DUCT INJURY

The incidence of injury to the bile ducts in the United States is not known. Nearly all biliary reconstructive operations at major centers are performed on patients referred from other institutions, so the number of strictures seen at a given institution is not reflective of the incidence of bile duct injury at that institution. In Finland and Sweden, studies reported over 20 years ago suggested that a bile duct injury occurred in about one of every 500 cholecystectomies.[3, 4] The present incidence probably is lower, due to larger numbers of trained surgeons, more rigid requirements for the granting of surgical privileges by hospital medical staffs, and the dissemination of knowledge about the prevention and treatment of bile duct injuries.

More than 80% of injuries occur after cholecystectomy, many of which can be prevented.[1, 5] The more obvious general causes are inadequate exposure and lighting and failure to identify structures before clamping, ligating, or dividing them. Undue haste or complacency also contribute. Failure to recognize congenital anomalies of the bile ducts and anomalous anatomical relationships between the bile ducts and the hepatic artery and its branches sometimes leads to confusion and errors. In fact, many bile duct injuries are unrecognized at the time of operation.[2] Many occur during the so-called difficult cholecystectomy. Often, these are in cases of acute cholecystitis, where omentum is adherent to the gallbladder, the neck of the gallbladder is adherent to the hilus of the liver, and the gallbladder is distended and tense, making exposure difficult.

The right hepatic duct or the common duct can easily be injured when significant bleeding occurs during dissection of Calot's triangle, and a hemostat is placed blindly to control it. Patients who have an aberrant right hepatic artery or whose right hepatic artery loops to the right in Calot's triangle are prone to this injury.[6, 7] The clamp may damage the duct by crushing it, and the injury is compounded by ligating beneath the clamp. A similar injury occurs when the cystic duct is tented outward by excessive traction and a ligature is placed too proximal, so as to encompass a portion of the medial wall of the common bile duct. Simultaneous ligation of the 9 o'clock artery may contribute to the formation of a stricture. Ligation of a portion of the circumference of a bile duct or complete ligation of the duct usually results in a narrow stricture without much proximal or distal fibrosis, a favorable circumstance from the standpoint of reconstruction.

Serious injury to the common bile duct may result from zealous attempts to separate a long cystic duct from the common duct, to which it may be fused for a variable distance. When fused, the two ducts share a common wall and are separated only by mucosa, so that attempts to separate them leaves a defect, most often in the common duct. If the injury is recognized immediately, the duct can be reconstructed over a T tube, but when it is not, a bile leak and probable stricture will result. The cystic duct has an abnormal termination in the common bile duct in about one third of individuals. Although the two ducts are not always fused, an anomalous course and termination of the cystic duct increases the possibility of bile duct injury and stricture. This is especially true when the cystic duct courses behind the common duct to enter posteriorly or on the left side. Attempts to ligate the cystic duct flush with the common duct should be avoided in these circumstances.

The most common as well as the most devastating injuries are those in which portions of or the entire hepatic, common hepatic, or common bile ducts have been excised. These injuries almost always result from the mistaken identification of another duct for the cystic duct. Those most frequently thought to be the cystic duct are the right hepatic, the common hepatic, and the common bile ducts. The circumstance often is the patient with a small, contracted gallbladder which has a very short, dilated cystic duct. Traction on the gallbladder pulls the common duct to the right, and, if unrecognized, the duct may be excised. Confusion also may arise when the right hepatic duct is absent, and its two branches, the anterior and posterior segmental ducts, enter the common hepatic duct separately. This occurs in about 25% of individuals.[8] One or both of these segmental ducts from the right lobe of the liver are often referred to as "accessory ducts." In fact, there are no accessory ducts from the liver, and this term should not be used. Rarely, the right hepatic duct enters the cystic duct, a situation which may give rise to its transection or ligation.

The keys to avoidance of bile duct injury during cholecystectomy are the complete dissection and identification of the cystic duct, the common bile duct, and common hepatic duct 1 cm above and below the entrance of the cystic duct, the division of the branches of the cystic artery at their entrance into the gallbladder, and the performance of operative cholangiography prior to the division of any structure. The cholangiogram, done by placing a catheter in the proximal end of the presumed cystic duct, should outline the anatomy of the entire biliary tract. If it does not, an anomaly or mistaken identification of the cystic duct should be suspected, and no structure should be divided until the problem is resolved (Fig 22-1). This added benefit of the operative cholangiogram is often overlooked. In cases of acute cholecystitis the gallbladder should be decompressed with a trocar placed into the fundus, and the omentum and other surrounding structures must be carefully and completely dissected free from the gallbladder and the porta hepatis. Special care must be taken in dissecting the cystic duct and its junction with the common bile duct and the common hepatic duct because it tends to be very friable and easily torn. If the ducts are especially friable, an

operative cholangiogram could be hazardous and should not be done.

Strictures secondary to injuries of the distal common bile duct usually arise during the course of common duct exploration. Probes, dilators, and forceps, inserted through a choledochotomy, may perforate the distal common duct, especially in its intrapancreatic portion, and create tracts which end blindly or communicate with the duodenum. This is most likely to occur in attempts to extract a stone impacted in the distal duct, where surrounding inflammation has made the duct friable. Fibrosis, resulting in a stricture, may occur when perforation of the duct is followed by abscess, severe inflammation, or pancreatitis. Stricture of the distal duct occasionally occurs following sphincterotomy or sphincteroplasty. The mechanism is not known.

The proximity of the common bile duct to the first portion of the duodenum, and the inflammation and fibrosis associated with duodenal ulcer makes the common duct vulnerable to injury during antrectomy. The duct may be transected, clamped, ligated, or incorporated into the sutures taken to close the duodenal stump or to approximate the posterior walls of the duodenum and stomach during gastroduodenostomy.

Very rarely, the extrahepatic duct system may be injured during hepatic lobectomy or portacaval shunting procedures.

Mechanisms of Stricture Formation

While all healing takes place by deposition of collagen and formation of scar, injuries to bile ducts appear to be unusually prone to scarring, with resultant stricture formation. The precise mechanism for this is unknown, but several factors probably contribute. First, the blood supply to the extrahepatic ducts superior to the duodenum, the "supraduodenal bile duct," is axial in nature. That is, the small vessels that supply the duct have their origins from two vessels that course alongside the duct at the 3 o'clock and 9 o'clock positions, respectively (Fig 22-2). These vessels, approximately named the 3 o'clock artery and the 9 o'clock artery by Northover and Terblanche,[9] could easily be transected or damaged by clamps. In general, about 60% of the arterial supply to the supraduodenal bile duct comes from below, 38% from above and 2% directly from the common hepatic artery in a nonaxial fashion. Thus, that portion of the supraduodenal bile duct

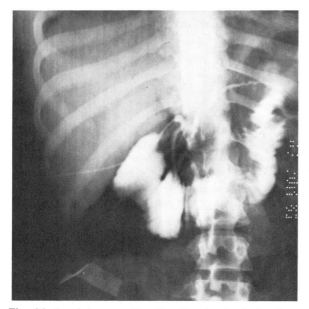

Fig 22-1.—Intraoperative "cystic duct" cholangiogram showing distal common bile duct, but nothing proximal to the entrance of the cystic duct. Common hepatic duct was mistaken for the cystic duct and cholangiogram prevented injury.

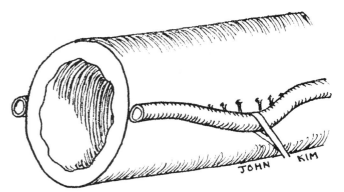

Fig 22-2.—Cross section of the common bile duct showing the 3 o'clock and 9 o'clock arteries.

proximal to the locus of transection or damage is vulnerable to ischemia, which may contribute to fibrosis and stricture formation during the healing.

Second, the presence of bile itself may predispose an injured duct to fibrosis because, in experimental bile duct anastomosis in the dog, fibrosis is minimized when bile is diverted proximally.[10] When bile has access to the collagen within the wall of the bile duct, rapid collagen turnover and fibrosis occurs.[11] Northover and Terblanche[9] have postulated that ischemia, caused by clamping of the duct or trauma to the blood supply of the duct, leads to mucosal damage, making it permeable to bile, which then induces inflammation and fibrosis within the wall of the bile duct. This theory could explain the fibrosis and virtual disappearance of a substantial segment of the supraduodenal bile duct following some injuries, and the occasional stricture of an end-to-end or end-to-side biliary-enteric anastomosis done at the distal portion of the common bile duct.[12] Theoretically, the propensity of the latter anastomosis to stricture would be increased if the proximal duct were skeletonized.

Finally, the nature of many duct injuries is such that leakage of bile occurs. Whether confined or removed by the presence of a drain, surrounding tissues become inflamed and subsequently fibrose, during the healing process. Bacteria are present in the bile in many patients who undergo biliary tract operations, so that leakage of bile is often associated with the development of a phlegmon or abscess, with scarring during the process of resolution or after drainage of pus. Thus, inflammation and fibrosis of tissues surrounding the ducts may be as important in the formation of strictures as the tissues of the ducts themselves.

Patterns of Location of Strictures

The location of strictures reflect their cause; most involve the common hepatic duct with or without involvement of the individual hepatic ducts. Table 22–1 shows the sites of strictures in 958 patients collected by Warren et al.[2] between 1940 and 1965. More than three-fourths of the strictures involved the hepatic ducts or the common hepatic duct. This is similar to the pattern observed by others.[13] Bismuth has classified strictures into five types according to the pattern of involvement, and the proximal level at which healthy mucosa may be found for an adequate reconstruction.[14] A modification of this classification is shown in Figure 22–3. This classification should prove to be very useful because the various op-

TABLE 22–1.—SITE OF STRICTURE
IN 958 PATIENTS

SITE	% OF PATIENTS
Right hepatic duct	2.8
Left hepatic duct	1.1
Bifurcation of hepatic ducts	6.2
Common hepatic duct	39.5
Common hepatic and common bile duct	27.7
Proximal common bile duct	21.2
Distal common bile duct	1.5

From Warren K.W., Mountain J.C., Midell A.I.: *Management of strictures of the biliary tract. Surg. Clin. North Am.* 51:711, 1971.

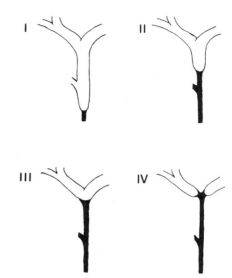

Fig 22–3.—Classification of strictures. (From Bismuth H.: Postoperative strictures of the bile duct, in Blumgart L.H. (ed.): *The Biliary Tract.* Edinburgh, Churchill Livingstone, 1982, pp. 209–218. Used by permission.)

erative procedures used can be applied to strictures which have been defined anatomically in a very specific manner. This will permit comparisons, which have not been possible to date, except in a very general manner.

Clinical Presentation

Strictures which result from bile duct injury present either during the immediate postoperative period or later, sometimes as long as 20 years after the operative procedure. The most common early postoperative sign is the development of jaundice, which usually is obvious by the second or third postoperative day. Failure of jaundice to resolve in the patient who was icteric preoperatively should arouse suspicion of a bile duct injury. In such cases, comparison of preoperative and postoperative bilirubin values may be necessary. Notation of the presence or absence of bile in the nasogastric aspirate, and the volume of bile from a T tube, if one is present, should be routine after biliary tract surgery. These observations are helpful in sorting out the various causes of postoperative jaundice, which include hemolysis from blood transfusions, sepsis, hepatic failure, and anesthetic agents, as well as bile duct injury.

Drainage of bile from the wound or through a drain is abnormal and may result from a bile duct injury. Occasionally, bile drainage occurs from the bed of the gallbladder, from a damaged subvesical duct,[15] the cystic duct stump, or from a minor leak in a choledochotomy suture line. Such drainage will almost always decrease and stop within a few days unless there is obstruction distal to the site of leakage. Continued drainage or leakage of bile from the wound beginning four to seven days after operation is an ominous sign, especially if the patient is jaundiced. Periodic opening and closing of the bile fistula with concomitant decrease and increase, respectively, in the degree of jaundice is also suggestive of major bile duct injury.

Patients who do not have a drain or in whom the drain has been removed may develop bile peritonitis or bilious ascites when a bile duct has been injured. The difference between the mere accumulation of bile as ascites and the development of peritonitis apparently is due to the presence of pathogenic bacteria in the bile in peritonitis. Jaundice accompanies both conditions owing to the absorption of bile pigments from the peritoneum. The onset of bilious ascites often is insidious, and gradual enlargement of the abdomen with mild jaundice may be the only signs.

Finally, postoperative sepsis may herald the presence of a bile duct injury. Fever, abdominal tenderness, paralytic ileus, and elevation of the WBC count or a shift to the left are findings that may be caused by a subhepatic or subphrenic collection of infected bile resulting from bile duct injury. The diagnosis may become obvious when the collection is drained and the egress of bile persists.

Recurring cholangitis is the most frequent finding in those patients whose stricture becomes evident months or years after operation. Only about 70% of patients have all the manifestations of cholangitis: chills and fever, abdominal pain, and jaundice (Charcot's triad).[16] Stricture is a rare cause of acute suppurative cholangitis, in which pus under pressure is present in the common bile duct. The development of jaundice without other symptoms or findings is a common mode of presentation. Formation of sludge or stones proximal to a stricture which had been adequately patent for many years may become manifest by jaundice, with or without the other symptoms of cholangitis. A few patients present with hepatosplenomegaly, ascites, and other signs of long-standing biliary cirrhosis. A history of prolonged drainage of bile or jaundice following a previous operation on the biliary tract is not unusual. Table 22–2 shows the frequency of the clinical findings in a large series of patients seen at the Lahey Clinic in Boston between 1940 and 1967.[2]

The interval between the surgical procedure and presentation of the patient with symptoms of stricture is shown for a large series of 104 patients at UCLA in Figure 22–4. The problem was suspected within one week of operation in 11 percent, and within 3 months in 60%. Symptoms did not develop for months or years in the remaining 40%.

During the early postoperative course after biliary tract surgery, the presence of jaundice, bile drainage through a

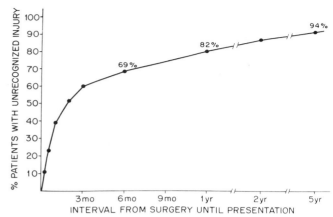

Fig 22–4.—Cumulative percentage of patients with bile duct stricture shown as a function of the interval between operation at which injury occurred and the development of symptoms. (From Pitt H.A., Miyamoto T., Parapatis S.K. et al.: Factors influencing outcome in patients with postoperative biliary strictures. *Am. J. Surg.* 144:14, 1982. Used by permission.)

drain or the wound, bile peritonitis, bilious ascites or sepsis, or combinations of these findings are not diagnostic of a bile duct injury; nor, when they result from an injury, do they always eventuate in a bile duct stricture. Similarly, the development of recurrent cholangitis, jaundice, or signs of biliary cirrhosis months or years after biliary tract surgery are not diagnostic of stricture. However, these symptoms or findings, whether they occur during the early postoperative period or years later, are indications for investigation, and traumatic injury and biliary stricture should be included in the differential diagnosis.

Diagnosis

The early development of jaundice or symptoms of cholangitis following biliary tract surgery is an indication for liver function tests, which, if a stricture is present, will show elevation of the serum bilirubin and the alkaline phosphatase. The development of ascites calls for paracentesis to confirm the presence or absence of bile. When there is uncertainty, the technetium 99m Tc IDA scan may show extravasation of radioactivity outside the biliary tract into the peritoneal cavity. A fistulagram should be done in patients who have bile drainage through a drainage tube or the wound. Injection of contrast material through the T tube may be helpful. The key to diagnosis of bile duct injury and stricture is a cholangiogram. The surgeon needs precise anatomical information to plan the repair, which can be provided only by cholangiography. Generally, percutaneous transhepatic cholangiography (PTC) is more valuable than endoscopic retrograde cholangiopancreatography (ERCP), because most duct injuries are in the proximal portion of the extrahepatic biliary tract, and it is the proximal extent of the stricture which determines the type of repair and, frequently, its degree of difficulty. Neither ultrasonography nor CT is useful in visualization of the stricture itself[18]; however, both are able to detect dilatation of bile ducts proximal to a stricture with a high degree of sensitivity.[19, 20] Ultrasonography usually is necessary prior to PTC to

TABLE 22–2.—CLINICAL FEATURES IN 987 PATIENTS WITH BILIARY STRICTURE (1940–67)

CLINICAL FEATURES	NO. OF PATIENTS	%
Chills and fever	632	64.0
Abdominal pain	482	48.8
Jaundice and pruritus	433	43.9
Hepatomegaly	369	37.4
External fistula	237	24.0
Portal hypertension	189	19.1
Hepatomegaly and splenomegaly	76	7.7
Splenomegaly	45	4.6
Ascites	24	2.4
None	9	0.9

From Warren K.W., Mountain J.C., Midell A.I.: Management of strictures of the biliary tract. *Surg. Clin. North Am.* 51:711, 1971.

determine whether the hepatic ducts are dilated, because PTC is not likely to be successful without ductal dilatation. In such cases, ERCP will be necessary. Dilatation of the intra-hepatic ducts may be absent during the early postoperative phase following a biliary tract injury, especially when a bile leak is present.

The differential diagnosis of obstructive jaundice or cholangitis which occurs months or years postoperatively includes stricture, stones, and malignant tumors of the bile ducts and pancreas. The choice of diagnostic procedures must be individualized according to the history, physical examination, and other circumstances surrounding each case. However, when stricture or stone is suspected, the most efficient diagnostic route is ultrasonography followed by PTC or ERCP, depending on the presence or absence of ductal dilatation, respectively. Patients who have had repeated episodes of cholangitis or those who have severe biliary cirrhosis may not have dilated ducts proximal to the stricture. PTC and ERCP should be used as complementary, rather than as competing, tests. When one fails to give a diagnosis and the other is used, the diagnostic accuracy approaches 100%.[21]

Preoperative Management

Patients who have strictures detected early in their post-operative course may be septic and have uncontrolled leakage of bile from the biliary tract. Sepsis must be controlled by percutaneous catheter drainage or operative drainage of abscesses, when appropriate, or in the absence of localization, by administration of antibiotics. Adequate drainage of bile leaks must be established. Once stabilization has occurred, the usual principles of preparation for a major surgical procedure apply, with attention to nutritional status, coagulation defects, anemia, and cardiopulmonary status.

Patients who present with strictures months or years after operation may need immediate percutaneous transhepatic drainage of the biliary tract if acute suppurative cholangitis is present. Nonsuppurative cholangitis can be managed with antibiotics effective against the flora of an infected biliary system. The presence of biliary cirrhosis with portal hypertension increases the mortality and morbidity of biliary tract surgery in general[22] and of bile duct reconstruction in particular.[23] Serious consideration should be given to preliminary portasystemic shunting in patients who require reconstruction. Preliminary splenorenal shunt has been advocated to avoid dissection in the hepatoduodenal ligament.[24, 25] This problem has received very little attention, and the possible application of the proximal splenorenal shunt of Warren in this situation has not been explored in depth.

The role of preoperative percutaneous transhepatic biliary catheter drainage in benign strictures of the biliary tract is not yet clear. Early reports suggested that the mortality of extra-hepatic bile duct obstruction was reduced by preoperative percutaneous drainage.[26, 27] Subsequent studies showed a reduction in morbidity but not mortality, and documented a significant mortality and morbidity from the procedure itself.[28, 29] At present, percutaneous drainage appears to be advantageous when the serum bilirubin is in excess of 25 or 30 mg/dl, when renal function is significantly compromised, in elderly patients, when sepsis or cholangitis are not controlled adequately, and when prolonged preoperative preparation is

necessary, such as for the administration of parenteral hyperalimentation to correct nutritional deficits. Future studies should define the specific indications and contraindications more clearly.

All patients with stricture should receive a course of antibiotic prophylaxis, which should begin preoperatively and continue for at least three days into the postoperative period. At this writing, a second-generation cephalosporin is adequate for this purpose.[30]

Surgical Therapy

The goals of treatment are to establish free drainage of bile into the GI tract in a manner that will prevent cholangitis, stone formation, restricture, and biliary cirrhosis. These goals are best met by the construction of a tension-free, mucosa-to-mucosa anastomosis between normal bile duct and intestine at least 18 in. from the flow of chyme.

While excision of the stricture and end-to-end anastomosis of the bile ducts is the most physiologic method of repair and was used extensively in early attempts to treat strictures,[31] complete excision of the stricture and an adequate anastomosis is almost never possible. The discrepancy in size between the two ends and the necessary tension on the anastomosis obviate its use for chronic strictures, and the long-term results now confirm the superiority of other procedures.[2] End-to-end anastomosis and plastic repairs of the bile ducts may be very useful in reconstruction at the time of the original injury. A thorough Kocher maneuver should be done to eliminate tension, and a large-bore T tube, inserted above or below the anastomosis or closure, should be used as a splint.

Anastomosis of the proximal bile duct to the superior aspect of the first portion of the duodenum is unwise for strictures which extend proximal to the retroduodenal portion of the common duct. For such lesions, the distance between the cut end of the duct and the duodenum is almost always too great for a tension-free anastomosis.

Bile duct strictures may be approached through an extended right subcostal or a long right paramedian incision. The choice will depend on the placement of previous incisions, the site of biliary fistulas or drainage tubes, and the body habitus of the patient. The hepatic flexure should be completely mobilized and all adhesions lysed. The duodenum should be completely mobilized by a Kocher maneuver, and both the stomach and duodenum separated from the inferior surface of the liver. Additional mobility can be gained by dividing adhesions of the liver to the anterior peritoneal surface, and the falciform ligament. Often, the best approach to the bile ducts is to follow the inferior border of the liver posteriorly to the hilum, where the confluence of the right and left hepatic ducts can be identified. In difficult cases, needle aspiration will confirm the location of bile ducts. Liberal use of operative cholangiography should be made to determine the precise location and especially the proximal extent of the stricture. However, the final level at which the duct is transected proximally must be based on visual inspection, with the principal concern that the duct be normal at the point of anastomosis. Compromise of this principle invites a high risk of recurrent stricture and an even more difficult and dangerous subsequent operation to correct it. When normal ductal tissue is found below the bifurcation of right and left hepatic ducts, a Roux-en-Y choledochojejunostomy or hepaticojejunostomy should be carried out. The end of the Roux limb should be closed and the anastomosis done 2 or 3 cm proximal to the closure, on the antimesenteric border. This permits the opening in the jejunum to be tailored to the size of the duct. The author prefers a two-layer anastomosis whenever possible, with an inner layer of 4–0 polyglycolic acid sutures to approximate mucosa to mucosa, and an outer layer of interrupted 4–0 silk sutures which do not penetrate the lumen. In some cases the caliber of the duct is too small for two layers, in which case a single layer of 4–0 polyglycolic acid sutures is used. Two layers are preferred because we feel it is important to prevent leaks at the suture line. While they usually close spontaneously after draining for a short time through the drain placed near the anastomosis, we believe that the healing of a leaking anastomosis probably contributes to reformation of a stricture. When the anastomosis is large, the duct tissue normal, and the apposition of mucosa to mucosa precise, a stent is not used. When the duct is small and a sufficient length of proximal duct is available, a T tube is inserted with the distal limb through the anastomosis. When the anastomosis is too high for this, a Silastic stent is placed through the anastomosis, through the right anterior segmental bile duct, the anterior surface of the liver, and the anterior abdominal wall. The other end of this transhepatic stent is brought through the Roux limb as a Witzel enterostomy and the abdominal wall. This U-tube stent is left in place for an arbitrary period of two or three months. It should be flushed with 20 ml of sterile normal saline daily to rid the system of debris.

Several options are available when the stricture involves the bifurcation and/or one or both hepatic ducts. In such cases the "hilar plate"—the thickening in Glisson's capsule which overlies the anterior aspect of the hilus of the liver and is confluent with the reflection of Glisson's capsule over the gallbladder on the right and the round ligament on the left—should be opened. This is done by incising Glisson's capsule at the posterior edge of the quadrate lobe, where the quadrate lobe is joined to the anterior aspect of the structures within the hilus of the liver. This incision then can be extended to the right immediately adjacent to the hepatic parenchyma, bringing the right and left hepatic ducts into view. This maneuver, described by Hepp and Couinaud[32] is essential for the proper surgical therapy of high strictures. When the bifurcation is involved to the extent that no communication exists between the right and left ducts, it may be possible to suture the left wall of the right duct to the right wall of the left duct, creating a new confluence, and then anastomosing this unit to the Roux limb. When this is not possible, two separate anastomoses must be done. In these cases, we prefer the use of two transhepatic U-tube stents, one through each major duct.[33]

An important alternative to end-to-side hepaticojejunostomy is a side-to-side anastomosis of the left hepatic duct to the Roux limb. In this technique, also described by Hepp and Couinaud,[32] a long opening (3–4 cm) along the anterior surface of the left hepatic duct is anastomosed to the side of the Roux limb 2 or 3 cm distal to its closed end. Because it is possible to dissect the anterior surface of the left hepatic duct high up into the hepatic parenchyma, this procedure permits an anastomosis to normal mucosa, even though there may be fibrosis and stricture at the bifurcation of the ducts and within the distal portions of each hepatic duct. Obviously, there must be some communication between right and left ducts for this procedure to drain the right lobe of the liver effectively.

Some have preferred to use a defunctionalized loop of jejunum, ranging from 15 to 50 cm long, between the proximal bile duct and the second part of the duodenum as originally described by Lopez.[34] Presumably, this method obviates some theoretical disadvantages of a Roux-en-Y reconstruction. Diversion of bile from the duodenum to the distal intestine increases gastric acid secretion in animals and causes peptic ulcers, and theoretically could contribute to malabsorption of fat. Pappalardo and associates[35] found that the jejunal segment had to be 50 cm long to obviate duodenal reflux to the hepaticojejunal anastomosis. They compared a group of patients with Roux-en-Y hepaticojejunostomy to a group with hepaticojejunoduodenostomy and found no difference in the restenosis rate, although follow-up was insufficiently long. Serum gastrin and basal acid secretion rates were the same in both groups, but the Roux-en-Y hepaticojejunostomy group had a significantly higher stimulated acid output. However, this does not prove that acid output in response to meals is higher after Roux-en-Y hepaticojejunostomy, or that these patients are predisposed to ulcer. In general, peptic ulcer after hepaticojejunostomy has not been a serious problem in most series unless patients with pancreatic disease have been included.[5, 36, 37] Thus, the logical notion that hepaticojejunoduodenostomy is the superior method of reconstruction remains unproved.

Smith and co-workers[38, 39] developed the technique of a jejunal "mucosal graft," in which a patch of the seromuscular wall of the Roux-en-Y jejunal limb is removed, and a percutaneous transhepatic catheter is placed into the jejunal limb through a small incision in the pouting jejunal mucosa. The mucosa is then anchored to the catheter and it, together with the tented mucosa, is pulled up into the lumen of the bile duct, where it apparently heals to the mucosa. The seromuscular surface of the jejunal limb is sutured to the scar about the duct and the hilus of the liver to reduce tension and hold the mucosal graft in position. Although the results reported by Smith[40] have been comparable to those using other techniques, this procedure is not based on the principle of a precise mucosa-to-mucosa apposition of normal duct tissue to jejunum and probably should be reserved for those cases in which it is truly impossible to get high enough in the hilum to find normal duct tissue.

The issue of when to place a stent in an anastomosis and how long to leave a stent in place is unresolved. As stated previously, we do not use stents for a large, secure anastomosis, but insert transhepatic U tubes whenever individual ducts are sutured to the jejunum, when the bile duct is small, or when a one-layer anastomosis is necessary. Stents are removed in two or three months, assuming a cholangiogram is normal. Many experts recommend that stents be left in place for at least six months, and some for a longer period,[2, 13, 41, 42] whereas others use no stent at all or leave them in place for only two or three months.[43, 44] The only solid data are from Pitt et al.,[17] who found significantly better results in patients whose stents were in place for more than one month compared with less than a month. The likelihood is that stenting will have no benefit when a large anastomosis that does not leak has been done to normal duct tissue, and primary healing takes place. On the other hand, there is no doubt that a stent will keep open a small anastomosis done to a scarred duct, which is likely to become more narrow as it heals.

Results and Complications

The operative mortality for groups of patients reported recently is under five percent.[13, 17, 35, 37, 41, 45] In general, both early and late deaths are related to hepatic failure, which results from preexisting biliary cirrhosis. This lends emphasis to the need for early repair of strictures, as well as the importance of not delaying reconstruction when a previous repair is not satisfactory.

Excellent results are obtained in 75%–90% of patients,[5, 13, 17, 37, 41, 46] meaning that strictures do not recur and that patients are asymptomatic. The percentage of good results appears to be related inversely to the number of previous repairs.[17] Length of follow-up is very important in analyzing the final results, because restenosis can occur up to 20 years after the original procedure.

Recurrent cholangitis is a frequent problem in those patients who do not have an excellent result. This may be caused by recurrent stricture, retained intrahepatic stones, or new stone formation. Our understanding of cholangitis and stone formation in patients who have had biliary tract reconstruction is incomplete. Clearly, the presence of a stricture predisposes to stone formation and cholangitis, but episodes of cholangitis and the formation of stones also occur in a small group of patients in whom no stasis or stricture is apparent.[37, 41, 47] Nevertheless, patients who have had reconstruction and who have chills, fever, abdominal pain, or jaundice should be investigated for the possibility of stones or restenosis, and operation should be done if either is present. To procrastinate invites additional liver damage and portal hypertension.

Serum bilirubin and alkaline phosphatase values have been used to monitor the relief of obstruction postoperatively. Serum bilirubin is useful when not increased from hepatic parenchymal disease, but the alkaline phosphatase is of questionable value.[48] The ^{99m}Tc IDA scan provides both anatomical and physiologic information and will probably prove to be the most valuable test in follow-up of reconstructions. The size of the anastomosis can be seen, and the rapidity with which the radioactivity enters the intestine also can be monitored. About two thirds of recurrent strictures will be evident within two years, and 90% within seven years.[49]

Alternatives to Surgical Therapy

Percutaneous transhepatic balloon dilatation of strictures has been used by some, as has the placement of indwelling stents.[50–52]

The preliminary experience with balloon dilatation of bile duct strictures has been made possible by the development of the side-viewing cannulating endoscope with a large biopsy channel. The balloon catheters are modified angioplasty catheters of the Gruntzig type. After a cannula has been placed in the bile duct, an ERCP is done to localize the stricture, and a guide wire is passed through the cannula, which is then removed. The balloon catheter is passed over the guide wire and the balloon is filled with contrast material to a predetermined pressure for several minutes. The dilatation is repeated twice at each endoscopy, and several sessions may be necessary. Geenen[53] summarized a worldwide experience in 1984. Fifteen of twenty attempts to dilate benign bile duct strictures were successful, and the complication rate was low. However, the follow-up period was very short; therefore, a valid assessment of this technique must await prospective studies with long-term follow-up.

Another new option is percutaneous placement of an endoprosthesis through the benign stricture, as has become popular for treatment of incurable malignant strictures. Indwelling stents become occluded periodically and are frequently complicated by recurrent episodes of cholangitis. Nevertheless, dilatation and stenting may prove to be useful in very old patients, and those in whom severe liver disease with portal hypertension or other concurrent disease obviates bile duct reconstruction.

STRICTURES ASSOCIATED WITH CALCULOUS DISEASE

Bile duct strictures may occur in association with impaction of a stone in the distal common duct or by erosion of a stone from the gallbladder into the common hepatic duct or the common bile duct.

Strictures due to stones impacted in the distal common bile duct are rare. Presumably, the mucosa of the distal duct is eroded, and the surrounding inflammation leads to fibrosis and stricture as it resolves. Because of the normal tapering of the distal portion of the common duct, nearly all impacted stones are found in the intrapancreatic portion of the duct. Localized pancreatitis may also contribute to the inflammation and subsequent fibrosis. The diagnosis of this stricture is always made after the stone has been removed. Extraction of an impacted stone often involves extensive manipulation with forceps, scoops, and catheters, which might easily traumatize the already friable distal duct. Furthermore, extraction of an impacted stone frequently necessitates duodenotomy and sphincterotomy. Thus, it is possible that the occasional stricture seen after disimpaction of a stone is as much the result of operative trauma or post-sphincterotomy stricture as the disease process itself.

Because these strictures become apparent after removal of the offending stone, the diagnosis often is made at postoperative T-tube cholangiography, done prior to planned removal of the tube. Late strictures become manifested by jaundice and cholangitis.

The treatment of distal duct strictures is a biliary enteric anastomosis, either Roux-en-Y choledochojejunostomy or choledochoduodenostomy (Fig 22–5). The theoretical disadvantage of the latter is the possibility of the "sump syndrome" in which food and debris fill the segment of the duct distal to the anastomosis and partially obstruct it, giving rise to cholangitis. This syndrome appears to be related to small anastomoses, so that a large choledochoduodenal anastomosis should be made. Unless this is not possible, we prefer the choledochoduodenostomy in patients with distal common duct strictures because it is simple and long-term results are excellent. Transduodenal sphincteroplasty is rarely successful, because

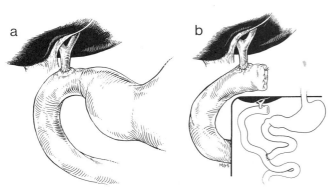

Fig 22–5.—Choledochoduodenostomy *(left)* and Roux-en-Y choledochojejunostomy.

distal strictures are too long to be opened adequately by this technique. Strictures in the distal duct associated with calculous disease should not be confused with ampullary stenosis, in which sphincteroplasty is the curative procedure.

A rare but vexing problem is stenosis of the common hepatic duct caused by a stone in the infundibulum of the gallbladder or the cystic duct. Several anatomical and pathophysiologic circumstances may produce this lesion. First, simple compression may occur when the infundibulum, containing a large stone, lies adjacent to the common hepatic duct, or when a stone is present in a long cystic duct which courses parallel to the common hepatic duct. Second, in either of these anatomical variants, inflammation of the gallbladder or of the cystic duct may produce contiguous inflammatory changes which involve the common hepatic duct and cause the lumen to be narrowed. In severe inflammation, the stone may erode through the infundibulum or the cystic duct into the common hepatic duct, causing obstruction and a fistula. Narrowing of the common hepatic duct associated with one of these circumstances has become known as the Mirizzi syndrome, even though Mirizzi described a narrowing of the common hepatic duct which he thought was a functional disorder of a sphincter-like mechanism.[54] He thought this disorder was brought on by the presence of an adjacent stone with or without contiguous inflammation. More recent investigations have demonstrated no evidence for a sphincter-like mechanism in the common hepatic duct, on either anatomical or physiologic grounds.[55] Thus, as the term is now used, the Mirizzi syndrome consists of a group of complications of cholelithiasis and cholecystitis.

The clinical manifestations are those of acute cholecystitis with jaundice or hyperbilirubinemia. The diagnosis is almost always made during cholecystectomy, either for acute cholecystitis or on an elective basis. When associated with acute inflammation, the size of the common hepatic duct almost always returns to normal after the offending stone has been removed by cholecystectomy and as the inflammatory process resolves. Sometimes a portion of the wall of the duct has been eroded by a stone, leaving a large defect in the duct at the time of cholecystectomy. This is best managed by placement of a T tube in the duct through the defect, and closure of the duct around the transcutaneous limb of the tube. This repair can be bolstered by omentum. The T tube should be left in place for about three months. Strictures which become man-

ifest months or years after the acute episode should be managed like those which occur after injuries to the bile ducts, usually with Roux-en-Y hepaticojejunostomy.

STRICTURES ASSOCIATED WITH CHRONIC PANCREATITIS

Chronic pancreatitis may result in a narrowing of the intrapancreatic portion of the common bile duct. The true incidence of stricture in chronic pancreatitis is not known, because not all patients have cholangiography; in one review some degree of bile duct obstruction was found in almost 30%.[56] The obstruction is usually caused by fibrosis from the pancreatitis, but occasionally results from compression by a pseudocyst located in the head of the pancreas.

The characteristic clinical finding is chronic upper abdominal pain that cannot be distinguished from that of chronic pancreatitis and may, in fact, be due to the pancreatitis. Jaundice may be present and is often intermittent. Frequently, the condition becomes manifest by the appearance of jaundice during an episode of pain in the patient with chronic pancreatitis, or by the development of cholangitis. The alkaline phosphatase is usually greatly elevated, but the bilirubin may be normal or only slightly elevated.

Cholangiography is the definitive test. ERCP is preferable if there is need for pancreatography to evaluate the pancreatic duct or the possibility of a pseudocyst. Otherwise, the percutaneous transhepatic route should be used. The cholangiogram reveals a long narrowing in the intrapancreatic portion of the duct that is almost never complete (Fig 22–6).

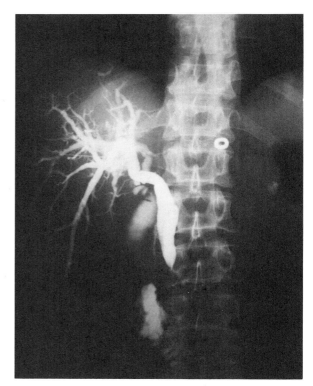

Fig 22–6.—Distal common duct stricture from chronic pancreatitis. Note calcium in the region of the tail of the pancreas.

The need for surgical therapy is obvious in patients who have recurrent attacks of cholangitis. In other patients, the goal of surgery is to prevent biliary cirrhosis and the development of portal hypertension and its complications. The persistently elevated alkaline phosphatase in the presence of a known stricture is an indication for operation. Edema within the head of the pancreas, caused by an exacerbation of the disease, may increase the alkaline phospatase temporarily, but this should not be taken as an indication for surgery. Obviously, patients who have evidence of bile duct obstruction or early cirrhosis on liver biopsy also are candidates for surgery.

The simplest and most effective procedure is choledochoduodenostomy, which may be carried out in conjunction with pancreaticojejunostomy, when the latter is indicated for treatment of chronic pancreatitis. The results are excellent. Sphincterotomy or sphincteroplasty should not be done, because the stricture extends too far proximally for these procedures to be effective.

SCLEROSING CHOLANGITIS

Sclerosing cholangitis, a rare condition, is a chronic inflammation of the bile ducts which leads to fibrosis, thickening, and strictures. The intrahepatic and extrahepatic ducts, as well as the gallbladder, may be involved, but occasionally only a single stricture may be present. As the disease progresses, obstruction of the bile ducts leads to cirrhosis, portal hypertension, and death. Many cases occur in association with other diseases and circumstances, so that efforts have been made to classify sclerosing cholangitis into primary and secondary types. In general, primary sclerosing cholangitis includes cases in which there is no associated condition, as well as those which occur in association with inflammatory bowel disease, including ulcerative colitis and Crohn's disease, retroperitoneal and mediastinal fibrosis, Riedel's thyroiditis, pancreatitis, pancreatic fibrosis, orbital pseudotumors, Peyronie's disease, and the familial immunodeficiency syndrome. The most frequent association, which accounts for about 70% of cases that have an association, is with inflammatory bowel disease. However, the incidence of sclerosing cholangitis in patients with inflammatory bowel disease is very low; fewer than 1% of patients with ulcerative colitis have sclerosing cholangitis.

Secondary sclerosing cholangitis is taken to include cases that occur in patients who have had previous biliary tract surgery or who have choledocholithiasis or cholangiocarcinoma. This classification is too rigid, but it arises from attempts to exclude from the diagnosis patients with sclerosing cholangitis who have bile duct strictures and chronic cholangitis with bile duct thickening and fibrosis from operative injuries, choledocholithiasis, and an inadequate biliary-enteric anastomosis. Clearly, primary sclerosing cholangitis can occur in an individual who previously underwent an unrelated and uncomplicated cholecystectomy for gallstones, and primary common duct stones may form proximal to strictures in a person who has sclerosing cholangitis. Cholangiocarcinoma may give a cholangiographic picture similar to that of sclerosing cholangitis, and when the carcinoma is well-developed, histological distinction between the two may be difficult. To further complicate matters, the two diseases may coexist, and sclerosing cholangitis may predispose patients to cholangiocarcinoma. Complete elucidation of the biliary tract problem in a given patient, including a search for associated diseases or conditions, is more useful than attempts to fit the patient into a classification system.

The etiology is unknown. Toxins, viruses, excess hepatic copper, altered immunity, and genetic factors have been implicated.[57]

Sclerosing cholangitis is more frequent in males (ratio 3:2) and usually becomes manifest before the age of 45. Fatigue, anorexia, nausea and vomiting, weight loss, and jaundice with pruritus are the usual symptoms. Although upper abdominal pain may be present, the other feature of cholangitis—chills and fever—usually is not. The diagnosis is established by cholangiography, which gives a characteristic pattern of short, anular strictures separated by ducts of normal or slightly enlarged caliber (Fig 22–7). Massive dilatation proximal to a strictured area is not characteristic. Occasionally, the extrahepatic duct system has a beaded appearance, with diverticular outpouchings. Liver biopsy is also helpful. The clinical course of the patient, cholangiography, and liver biopsy will establish the diagnosis in most patients.

Medical therapy has consisted of steroids, immunosuppressive agents, and penicillamine, but none has been proved to be efficacious. Cholestyramine is effective in relieving pruritus, and antibiotics are indicated during episodes of cholangitis, which are infrequent unless surgery has been done.

The role of surgery is not clear. A biliary-enteric anastomosis proximal to a stricture may provide palliation in the jaundiced patient. This is best done with the use of a Roux-en-Y anatomical arrangement, and often, the use of an intrahepatic U-tube stent is advisable.[58] Cameron and associates[59] believe that many patients have their most severe narrowing at or near the hepatic duct bifurcation, and they report good early results with excision of the bifurcation and the distal bile

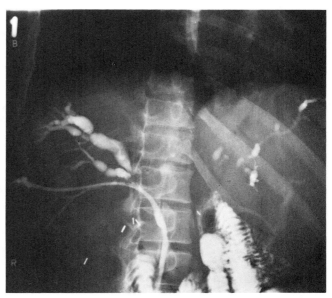

Fig 22–7.—Cholangiogram in a patient with sclerosing cholangitis.

ducts, dilatation of the intrahepatic ducts, and bilateral hepaticojejunostomies splinted by transhepatic U tubes.[59]

Our indications for surgery are quite specific. Laparotomy may be required if the diagnosis is uncertain; usually this is occasioned by concern over the possibility of cholangiocarcinoma. In established cases, operation is done when liver function tests, especially the alkaline phosphatase, are persistently elevated and cholangiography demonstrates that an anastomosis proximal to a stricture would provide better drainage. This includes patients with strictures in the area of the bifurcation of the hepatic ducts, in which case separate right and left Roux-en-Y hepaticojejunostomies, splinted by transhepatic U tubes, may be necessary. Insertion of a T tube in the common duct should not be done; instead, distal strictures should be bypassed by a biliary-enteric anastomosis. The presence of biliary cirrhosis and portal hypertension is a contraindication to operation because the course of the patient is not altered by a surgical procedure. Hepatic transplantation should be considered in such patients.

REFERENCES

1. Bismuth H., Lazorthes F.: *Les Traumatismes Operatories de la Voie Biliaire Principale*. Masson Ed., Paris, 1981, vol. 1.
2. Warren K.W., Mountain J.C., Midell A.I.: Management of strictures of the biliary tract. *Surg. Clin. North Am.* 51:711, 1971.
3. Viikari S.J.: Operative injuries to the bile ducts. *Acta Chir. Scand.* 119:83, 1960.
4. Rosenquist H., Myrin S.O.: Operative injury to the bile ducts. *Acta Chir. Scand.* 119:92, 1960.
5. Lindenauer S.M.: Surgical treatment of bile duct strictures. *Surgery* 73:875, 1973.
6. Benson E.A., Page R.E.: A practical reappraisal of the extrahepatic bile ducts. *Br. J. Surg.* 63:853, 1976.
7. Moosman D.A., Coller F.A.: Prevention of traumatic injury to the bile ducts. *Am. J. Surg.* 82:132, 1951.
8. Kune G.A.: The influence of structure and function in the surgery of the biliary tract. *Ann. R. Coll. Surg. Engl.* 47:78, 1970.
9. Northover J.M.A., Terblanche J.: A new look at the arterial supply of the bile duct in man and its surgical implications. *Br. J. Surg.* 66:379, 1979.
10. Douglas T.C., Lounsbury B.F., Cutter W.W., et al.: An experimental study of healing of the common bile duct. *Surg. Gynecol. Obstet.* 91:301, 1950.
11. Carlson E., Zukoski C.F., Campbell J., et al.: Morphological, biophysical and biochemical consequences of ligation of the common bile duct in the dog. *Am. J. Pathol.* 86:301, 1977.
12. Terblanche J., Allison H.F., Northover J.M.A.: An ischemic basis for biliary strictures. *Surgery* 94:52, 1983.
13. Kalman P.G., Taylor B.R., Langer B.: Iatrogenic bile-duct strictures. *Can. J. Surg.* 25:321, 1982.
14. Bismuth H.: Postoperative strictures of the bile duct, in Blumgart L.H. (ed.): *The Biliary Tract*. Edinburgh, Churchill Livingstone, 1982, pp. 209–218.
15. Healy J.E. Jr., Schroy P.C.: Anatomy of biliary ducts within the human liver: Analysis of prevailing pattern of branchings and major variations of biliary ducts. *Arch. Surg.* 66:599, 1953.
16. Boey J.H., Way L.W.: Acute cholangitis. *Ann. Surg.* 191:264, 1980.
17. Pitt H.A., Miyamoto T., Parapatis S.K., et al.: Factors influencing outcome in patients with postoperative biliary strictures. *Am. J. Surg.* 144:14, 1982.
18. Thomas M.J., Pelligrini C.A., Way L.W.: Usefulness of diagnostic tests for biliary obstruction. *Am. J. Surg.* 144:102, 1982.
19. Haubek A., Pedersen J.H., Burcharth F., et al.: Dynamic sonography in the evaluation of jaundice. *A.J.R.* 136:1071, 1981.
20. Goldberg H.I., Filly R.A., Korobkin M., et al.: Capability of CT body scanning and ultrasonography to demonstrate the status of

the biliary ductal system in patients with jaundice. *Radiology* 129:731, 1978.
21. Ginestal-Cruz A., Pinto-Correia J., Camilo E., et al.: Combined approach to the differential diagnosis of cholestatic jaundice with endoscopic retrograde cholangiopancreatography, percutaneous transhepatic cholangiography, ultrasonography and liver biopsy. *Gastrointest. Radiol.* 6:177, 1981.
22. Aranha G.V., Sontag S.J., Greenlee H.B.: Cholecystectomy in cirrhotic patients: A formidable operation. *Am. J. Surg.* 143:55, 1982.
23. Schwartz S.I.: Biliary tract surgery and cirrhosis: A critical combination. *Surgery* 90:577, 1981.
24. Sedgwick C.E., Hume A.: Management of bile duct structures with associated portal hypertension. *Surg. Gynecol. Obstet.* 108:627, 1959.
25. Sedgwick C.E., Poulantzas J.K., Kune G.A.: Management of portal hypertension secondary to bile duct strictures: Review of 18 cases with splenorenal shunt. *Ann. Surg.* 163:949, 1966.
26. Takada T., Hanuy F., Kobayshi S., et al.: Percutaneous transhepatic cholangial drainage: Direct approach under fluoroscopic control. *J. Surg. Oncol.* 8:83, 1976.
27. Nakayama T., Ikeda A., Okuda K.: Percutaneous transhepatic drainage of the biliary tract: Technique and results in 104 cases. *Gastroenterology* 74:554, 1978.
28. Denning D.A., Ellison E.C., Carey L.C.: Preoperative percutaneous transhepatic biliary decompression lowers operative morbidity in patients with obstructive jaundice. *Am. J. Surg.* 141:61, 1981.
29. Mueller P.R., van Sonnenberg E., Ferrucci J.T. Jr.: Percutaneous biliary drainage: Technical and catheter-related problems in 200 procedures. *A.J.R.* 138:17, 1982.
30. Keighley M.R.B: Infection and the biliary tree, in Blumgart L.H. (ed.): *The Biliary Tract*. Edinburgh, Churchill Livingstone, 1982, pp. 219–235.
31. Lahey F.H., Pyrtele L.J.: Experience with operative management of 280 strictures of the bile ducts with a description of a new method and a complete follow-up study of end results in 229 of the cases. *Surg. Gynecol. Obstet.* 91:25, 1950.
32. Hepp J., Couinaud C.: L'abord et l'utilisation du canal hepatique gauche dans les reparations de la voie biliare principale. *Presse Med.* 64:947, 1956.
33. Rossi R.L., Gordon M., Braasch J.W.: Intubation techniques in biliary tract surgery. *Surg. Clin. North Am.* 60:297, 1980.
34. Lopez G.J.: Interposicion de una ansa yeyunal excluida entro coledoco y duodeno para tratamiento de una estenosis biliar postgastrectomia. *Cir. Ginec. Urol.* 18:128, 1964.
35. Pappalardo G., Correnti S., Mobarhan S., et al.: Long-term results of Roux-en-Y hepaticojejunostomy and hepaticojejunoduodenostomy. *Ann. Surg.* 196:149, 1982.
36. McArthur M.S., Longmire W.P. Jr.: Peptic ulcer disease after choledochojejunostomy. *Am. J. Surg.* 122:155, 1971.
37. Bismuth H., Franco D., Corlette M.B., et al.: Long term results of Roux-en-Y hepaticojejunostomy. *Surg. Gynecol. Obstet.* 146:161, 1978.
38. Smith R.: Strictures of the bile ducts. *Proc. R. Soc. Med.* 62:131, 1969.
39. Wexler M.J., Smith R.: Jejunal mucosal graft. A sutureless technic for repair of high bile duct strictures. *Am. J. Surg.* 129:204, 1975.
40. Smith, Lord of Marlow: Obstructions of the bile duct. *Br. J. Surg.* 66:69–79, 1979.
41. Braasch J.W., Bolton J.S., Rossi R.L.: A technique of biliary tract reconstruction with complete follow-up in 44 consecutive cases. *Ann. Surg.* 194:635, 1981.
42. Cameron J.L., Skinner D.B., Zuidema G.D.: Long term transhepatic intubation for hilar hepatic duct strictures. *Ann. Surg.* 183:488, 1976.
43. Smith R.: Hepaticojejunostomy with transhepatic intubation. *Br. J. Surg.* 51:186, 1964.
44. Way L.W., Bernhoft R.A., Thomas M.J.: Biliary stricture. *Surg. Clin. North. Am.* 61:963, 1981.
45. Saber K., El-Manialawi M.: Repair of bile duct injuries. *World J. Surg.* 8:82, 1984.

46. Moreno-Gonzalez M., Sanmartin J.H., Azcoita M.M., et al.: Reconstruction of the biliary tract using biliary-duodenal interposition of a defunctionalized jejunal limb. *Surg. Gynecol. Obstet.* 150:678, 1980.

47. Goldman L.D., Steer M.L., Silen W.: Recurrent cholangitis after biliary surgery. *Am. J. Surg.* 145:450, 1983.

48. Pellegrini C.A., Thomas M.J., Way L.W.: Bilirubin and alkaline phosphatase values before and after surgery for biliary obstruction. *Am. J. Surg.* 143:67, 1982.

49. Pelligrini C.A., Thomas M.J., Way L.W.: Recurrent biliary stricture: Patterns of recurrence and outcome of surgical therapy. *Am. J. Surg.* 147:175, 1984.

50. Molnar W., Stockum A.E.: Transhepatic dilatation of choledochoenterostomy strictures. *Radiology* 129:59, 1978.

51. Pollock T.W., Ring E.R., Oleaga J.A., et al.: Percutaneous decompression of benign and malignant biliary obstruction. *Arch. Surg.* 114:148, 1979.

52. Teplick S.K., Goldstein R.C., Richardson P.A., et al.: Percutaneous transhepatic choledochoplasty and dilatation of choledochoenterostomy strictures. *J.A.M.A.* 244:1240, 1980.

53. Geenen J.E.: Balloon dilatation of bile duct strictures, in Classen M., Geenen J., Kawai K. (eds.): *Nonsurgical Biliary Drainage.* Berlin, Springer-Verlag, 1984, pp. 105–108.

54. Mirizzi P.L.: Sindrome del conducto hepatico. *J. Intern. Cir.* 88:737, 1948.

55. Didio L.J.A., Anderson M.C.: *The "Sphincters" of the Digestive System.* Baltimore, Williams & Wilkins Co., 1968, pp. 129–131.

56. Scott J., Summerfield J.A., Elis E., et al.: Chronic pancreatitis: A cause of cholestasis. *Gut* 18:196, 1977.

57. LaRusso N.E., Wiesner R.H., Ludwig J., et al.: Primary sclerosing cholangitis. *N. Engl. J. Med.* 310:899, 1984.

58. Pitt H.A., Thompson H., Tompkins R.K., et al.: Primary sclerosing cholangitis: Results of an aggressive surgical approach. *Ann. Surg.* 196:259, 1982.

59. Cameron J.L., Gayler B.W., Herlong H.F., et al.: Biliary reconstruction with Silastic transhepatic stents. *Surgery* 94:324, 1983.

23

Cystic Lesions of the Liver and Biliary Tree

Jeffrey E. Doty, M.D.
Henry A. Pitt, M.D.

Cysts of the liver and biliary tree are rare lesions that may appear in various forms and combinations. As a result, some confusion has occurred in their classification. In the liver they may be parenchymal, ductal, or combinations of both types. Liver cysts may also be congenital or acquired; solitary or multiple; traumatic or inflammatory; benign, premalignant, or malignant; and may or may not be associated with extrahepatic ductal cysts or cysts in other organs. To review these various lesions of the liver and bile ducts, the classification proposed in Table 23–1, which is based on whether the cysts are intrahepatic, extrahepatic, or combinations of both, will be followed.

CONGENITAL INTRAHEPATIC PARENCHYMAL CYSTS

Congenital intrahepatic cysts involving the liver parenchyma are benign and may be either solitary or multiple. These cysts are rare, having been reported to occur in 0.14%–0.30% of postmortem examinations.[1] In most series, solitary cysts are more common than polycystic disease. As the name implies, these cysts are thought to be congenital. Etiologic theories include: (1) defective development or faulty fusion of the intrahepatic bile ducts; (2) aberrant bile ducts that become stenosed as the result of inflammatory hyperplasia; or (3) congenital lymphatic obstruction. In most cases, cystic areas are associated with normal second-generation bile ducts elsewhere in the liver, and, therefore, biliary and hepatic function is usually normal.

Solitary Cysts

Congenital solitary cysts of the liver may present at any age but are most often observed in patients who are 40 or more years old. These cysts are seen three times more commonly in women than men. Solitary cysts usually occur in the right hepatic lobe but may arise from any area of the liver. Cysts vary considerably in size and may be wholly or partially intrahepatic or pedunculated. The largest solitary hepatic cyst described in the literature contained 17 L of fluid.

Solitary liver cysts grow very slowly and, therefore, usually do not cause symptoms until later in life. When symptoms do appear, the most common complaint is the presence of a painless, upper abdominal swelling. Alternatively, some of these lesions will be entirely asymptomatic or present only with fullness or heaviness in the upper abdomen. Other cysts are discovered on routine physical examination or because hepatomegaly is discovered on an abdominal roentgenogram performed for vague symptoms. Rarely, acute abdominal pain may be caused by hemorrhage into the cyst, secondary infection, or torsion of the pedicle of a pedunculated cyst. If a large, solitary cyst compresses the duodenum or stomach, nausea, vomiting, or early satiety may also be present. Jaundice is a presenting complaint in only a small percentage of patients.

As with all liver lesions, physical examination may reveal hepatomegaly or an upper abdominal mass. Liver function tests are usually normal in patients with solitary cysts. Barium studies of the upper or lower intestinal tract may be normal or may demonstrate extrinsic compression. Intravenous pylography (IVP) may be useful for differential diagnosis, especially in children, and may reveal caudad displacement of the right kidney by a large mass posteriorly in the right hepatic lobe. Liver scans may also detect cysts that are greater than 2.0 cm in diameter. However, with the advent of ultrasound and computerized tomography (CT), many of the previously mentioned tests have become unnecessary. Ultrasound and CT are now preferred because they are able to detect smaller defects and to differentiate cystic from solid lesions.

Cholangiography or cholecystography is usually not necessary but may be helpful in some cases of polycystic disease or to differentiate a solitary cyst from an intrahepatic gallbladder or a ductal cyst. Angiography will demonstrate the avascular nature of these lesions but should be reserved for cases where surgical excision is contemplated or diagnosis is still in question after ultrasound and CT. Laparoscopy is usually not required but can be diagnostic for cysts that are on the surface. If ultrasound demonstrates internal echoes, fine-needle aspiration with cytologic examination of fluid may be helpful in differentiating congenital from malignant cysts. Needle biopsy of the liver has proved to be safe in congenital cysts and will usually provide a portion of the cyst wall for histologic examination.

Complications of hepatic cystic disease, which include hemorrhage, rupture, torsion, erosion of adjacent organs, biliary obstruction, and, rarely, malignant degeneration, may require individual surgical intervention. However, since these

TABLE 23–1.—CLASSIFICATION OF CYSTIC LESIONS
OF THE LIVER AND BILIARY TREE

I. Intrahepatic cysts
   A. Parenchymal lesions
      1. Congenital intrahepatic parenchymal cysts
         a. Solitary cysts
         b. Polycystic disease
      2. Traumatic intrahepatic cysts
      3. Inflammatory intrahepatic cysts
         a. Echinococcal cysts
         b. Amebic abscesses
         c. Pyogenic abscesses
      4. Neoplastic intrahepatic cysts
         a. Malignant
         b. Benign
   B. Ductal lesions
      1. Congenital intrahepatic ductal cysts (Caroli's disease)
      2. Acquired intrahepatic ductal cysts
II. Extrahepatic cysts
   A. Cystic lesions of the gallbladder and cystic duct
   B. Congenital extrahepatic biliary cysts
      1. Choledochal cysts (Alonso-Lej type 1)
      2. Choledochal diverticulum (Alonso-Lej type 2)
      3. Choledochocele (Alonso-Lej type 3)
   C. Acquired extrahepatic biliary cysts
III. Combined intrahepatic and extrahepatic cysts
   A. Multiple saccular cysts
   B. Fusiform cysts

complications are unusual, an asymptomatic cyst that is found during an unrelated diagnostic evaluation should be observed by ultrasound for growth. If a cyst is found at laparotomy for another condition and is smaller than 10 cm, Hadad and associates[2] recommend aspirating the cyst dry, sending the fluid for culture and cytology, and leaving the cyst alone. The one exception to this rule would be the operative finding of a cyst on a pedicle, which could be excised with essentially no morbidity.

The operative approach to a large, symptomatic cyst of the liver may be through an extended right subcostal incision or an upper midline abdominal incision, depending on whether the cyst is in the right or left lobe, respectively. Rarely would it be necessary to enter the chest to manage a solitary cyst. At operation, the upper abdomen should be carefully walled off before aspiration to prevent problems if the lesion turns out to be an abscess or hydatid cyst. In excluding this and other possibilities, the character of the cyst's fluid is extremely important.

If the cyst's fluid is clear and Gram stain is negative, the cyst may be either totally or partially excised. This decision will be based on the degree of adhesion between the cyst wall and the adjacent liver parenchyma. If partial excision is contemplated, any papillary projections or irregularities of the cyst lining should be biopsied and sent for frozen section to be sure that the cyst is not neoplastic. Some authorities have recommended light cauterization of the retained cyst wall to diminish secretion. However, free drainage of this clear, uninfected fluid into the peritoneal cavity is generally of sufficiently low volume to be reabsorbed without causing any problems.

If the cyst contains cloudy fluid, pus, blood, or bile, neither total nor partial excision is indicated. If Gram stain of cloudy fluid gives any suspicion of infection, the cyst should be opened widely and either drained externally or marsupialized to the abdominal wall. Similarly, if the cyst contains pus or blood, external drainage is the preferred treatment. If bile is present within the cyst, operative cholangiography should be performed. If the biliary tree is normal except for communication with the cyst, internal drainage of the cyst to a Roux-en-Y limb of jejunum is the treatment of choice. In performing this procedure, only a small opening in the cyst wall is necessary.

Polycystic Disease

Polycystic liver disease, whether localized to one area or occurring throughout the liver, is always congenital. Depending on the extent of liver involvement, these lesions may present in childhood or adolescence but have a peak incidence in the third and fourth decades. Polycystic liver disease is associated with polycystic disease of the kidneys in approximately half of the patients; less commonly, it is also associated with congenital hepatic fibrosis. In a small percentage of cases, cysts may also be present in the pancreas, spleen, ovaries, or lung (Fig 23–1).

Depending on the number and size of cysts, the liver may be normal-sized or greatly enlarged. Cysts may vary in size from minute to quite large but rarely exceed 10 cm in diameter. Larger cysts are probably derived from degeneration of septa between adjacent cysts. As this process continues, a honeycomb pattern on cut section develops. These thin-walled cavities generally contain clear fluid and do not communicate with the biliary system.

In many patients without kidney involvement, asymptomatic cysts are discovered at laparotomy or autopsy. Others are found when ultrasound or CT scans are performed for unrelated abdominal complaints such as symptomatic gallstones. Still others are discovered incidentally after the patient has presented because of polycystic kidneys. Patients with symptoms and signs resulting directly from polycystic liver disease usually note a gradual swelling in the upper abdomen. Most of these patients have a feeling of heaviness or fullness in the epigastrium. As the disease progresses, the discomfort increases, the diaphragm becomes elevated, and some patients experience respiratory difficulties, nausea, and occasional vomiting. Rarely, loss of appetite, severe pain, and weight loss may occur.

On physical examination the liver may not be palpable or may be so large that it seems to fill the entire upper abdomen. The edge is usually firm, and nodules may be palpable. Associated polycystic kidneys may also be appreciated on physical examination. Liver function tests are usually normal, because hepatocytes and bile ducts are not involved. However, jaundice has been reported as a complication. Barium studies may show displacement resulting from hepatomegaly. Esophageal varices, however, are rare.

Ultrasound or CT scans should delineate the multiple liver cysts as well as associated cysts in the kidneys, pancreas, or spleen. Radionuclide scans will also demonstrate multiple filling defects. Needle biopsy has been proved to be safe but is usually not necessary when typical CT findings are present. If resection of a portion of the liver is contemplated, selective celiac and superior mesenteric angiography will define vas-

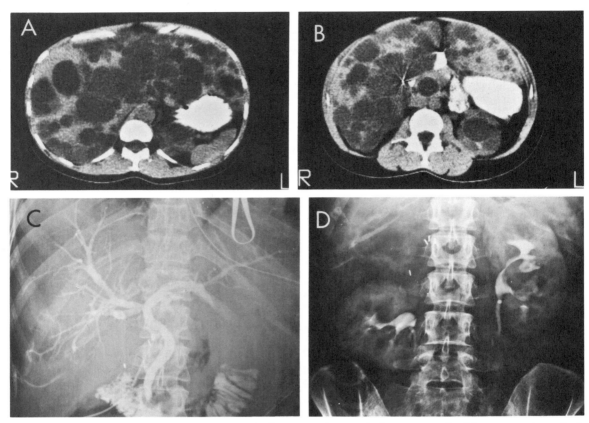

Fig 23–1.—A, CT scan of a patient with polycystic liver and kidney disease. Note the multiple hepatic cysts, left renal cysts, and compression of the stomach by the enlarged left hepatic lobe. **B,** CT scan of the same patient demonstrating a cyst in the pancreas *(center)* as well as multiple cysts in the liver and left kidney. **C,** operative chol-angiogram in the same patient from a previous cholecystectomy demonstrating normal biliary anatomy. Liver function tests were normal. **D,** intravenous pyelogram in the same patient demonstrating multiple kidney cysts and distortion of the right kidney by the enlarged liver.

cular anatomy and demonstrate branches of the hepatic artery stretched around avascular cysts.

Polycystic disease of the liver is compatible with long life. However, when associated with renal cysts, deterioration of renal function may alter the patient's prognosis. Operation for polycystic liver disease is indicated when extreme symptoms of abdominal fullness or pain or respiratory compromise are caused by massive hepatic enlargement. The choice of incisions, either a long, midline incision or bilateral subcostal incisions, is dictated by the patient's body habitus and the position of dominant cysts.

At operation as many of the cysts as possible should be unroofed or partially resected. If segments of the liver are extremely enlarged, these segments may be excised. Cysts that are deep within the liver may be aspirated to aid in decompression of the swollen liver. However, if aspiration reveals pus or old blood, external drainage is indicated. Complete hepatic lobectomy for relief of compressive symptoms is rarely necessary. Moreover, this procedure may be hazardous because normal anatomical landmarks are absent and because of concerns about hepatic reserve after resection. Following these guidelines, the risk of surgery in these patients should be low.

TRAUMATIC INTRAHEPATIC CYSTS

A traumatic intrahepatic cyst may occur after liver injury that has resulted in an intraparenchymal or subcapsular hematoma. As the hematoma resolves, fibrosis and cystic degeneration may result in a solitary cyst that is otherwise indistinguishable from a congenital, nonparasitic cyst. These patients with traumatic cysts, however, may remember an episode of relatively mild upper abdominal trauma in the distant past. As with congenital solitary cysts, traumatic cysts may be asymptomatic or present with fullness or heaviness in the upper abdomen. Other cysts will be discovered on routine physical examination or because ultrasound or CT is performed for vague upper abdominal symptoms.

Indications for operation are the same as those discussed above for solitary congenital cysts. At operation traumatic cysts may be differentiated by the fact that the cyst wall may be densely fibrosed and contain hemosiderin. Traumatic cysts are frequently found at the periphery of the liver, having resulted from a subcapsular hematoma. Cysts in this position can often be completely dissected away from the adjacent normal liver and totally excised. Complete excision is the operative treatment of choice. However, if dissection is difficult because of dense adhesion of the cyst to the adjacent liver, a portion of the cyst wall may be left behind. In this situation, however, frozen section should be performed to be sure that the cyst is not neoplastic.

INFLAMMATORY INTRAHEPATIC CYSTS

Inflammatory cysts of the liver fall into three categories, two of which are parasitic in origin and two of which are really liver abscesses. The two parasitic infestations that can cause cystic liver lesions are echinococcosis and amebiasis. Whereas echinococcal liver lesions are definite cysts, amebic liver infestations are generally called abscesses, partly because they have less well-defined walls and partly because they cause systemic manifestations that mimic a pyogenic infection. Although pyogenic liver abscesses are not true cysts, their clinical and roentgenographic presentation can closely mimic those of liver cysts, and therefore they will also be reviewed in this chapter.

Echinococcal Cysts

Echinococcal liver disease can be caused by either *Echinococcus granulosus* or *E. multilocularis*. *Echinococcus granulosus* is the most common form, giving rise to cysts primarily in the liver and lungs. *E. multilocularis* is much less common, which is fortunate because this species of cestode causes multilocular cysts that invade and replace liver tissue in a tumor-like fashion. As a result, complications and reoperations are much more frequent with cysts caused by *E. multilocularis*. However, because more than 95% of echinococcal cysts are caused by *E. granulosus*, the remainder of the discussion will focus on this more common variety.[3]

Hydatid disease of the liver occurs worldwide and is endemic in many areas where sheep are raised, such as Australia, New Zealand, South America, the Middle East, and those countries surrounding the Mediterranean and Baltic seas. Among these countries, Greece has perhaps the highest incidence, with approximately 500 patients operated on each year. In North America, the highest prevalence is in Alaska and in northwestern Canada. In the United States hydatid disease is rare except in immigrants who have harbored the parasite since childhood.

Echinococcus granulosus is a worm measuring 5–6 mm long whose life cycle depends on a definitive and an intermediate host. Adult worms usually inhabit the small intestines of dogs, foxes, wolves, and jackals. These definitive hosts pass *E. granulosus* eggs in their stool, which may then be ingested by sheep, cows, pigs, moose, caribou, and man (intermediate hosts). Fortunately, many swallowed ova do not hatch and are destroyed. However, alkaline digestive juices dissolve the rigid membrane of some ova, releasing the hexacanth embryo, so named because of the six spicules located on its head. This embryo bores through the mucosa of the upper intestine and enters the portal system.

As the liver is the first filter of parasitic embryos migrating from the intestine, this organ is the most frequent site of hydatid disease. Some embryos proceed to the lungs, where they are again trapped. As a result, relatively few embryos reach the general circulation. Approximately 65%–70% of echinococcal cysts are found in the liver, 20%–25% in the

lungs, and the remainder elsewhere in the body. Within the liver, 75%–80% of echinococcal cysts are found in the right lobe and 20%–25% in the left lobe. However, multiple cysts involving both lobes may occur in as many as 25%–30% of cases.

Within the liver many embryos are destroyed by the host's defense mechanisms. However, in three to four days, surviving embryos are transformed into tiny cysts, the acephalocyst. Growth of these cysts is very slow, taking 15 or more years to become large. As a cyst grows, it develops layers. The outer pericyst, or ectocyst, results from the host's foreign body response, which forms a protective layer around the cyst. On the inner surface of the pericyst is the endocyst, which is part of the parasite. Between these two layers is a potential space that permits their separation.

The inner layer of the endocyst has a granular surface which is the active, germinating part of the cyst. This surface produces crystal-clear, colorless, hydatid fluid as well as broad capsules, which are collections of scoleces. At this stage the cyst is no longer an acephalocyst, but is now a fertile cyst. The scolex is a miniature version of the adult worm's head, which is just visible to the naked eye. Collections of brood capsules and scoleces, which may layer within a fertile cyst, have been termed hydatid sand. As a cyst further matures, its germinal layer also produces daughter cysts that float within the mother cyst. Daughter cysts may also produce scoleces and even daughter cysts of their own. As a result, hydatid cysts may become large, containing liters of fluid and hundreds of daughter cysts.

Patients may be asymptomatic for years. When symptoms do develop, vague abdominal discomfort is the usual complaint. Fever, jaundice, productive cough, pruritus, urticaria, a rash, or anaphylactic shock occur in fewer than one quarter of patients and usually indicates secondary infection or rupture into the biliary tree, abdomen, or chest. On physical examination, hepatomegaly or a mass within the liver may be appreciated in as many as 50%–60% of cases. Abnormal liver function tests, including alkaline phosphatase, occur in only 20%–30% of patients. Eosinophilia of 5%–15% is present in approximately one third of the cases.

As hydatid disease progresses, an immune response develops that is dependent on parasitic antigens. This principle led to the development of the Casoni test, the injection of human or animal hydatid fluid into the dermis. The Casoni test, however, is no longer used because of nonspecificity, difficulty in obtaining satisfactory test fluid, and the development of more accurate serologic tests. The indirect hemagglutination (IHA) test has generally been found to be more sensitive and specific than the complement fixation test. Although the accuracy of the IHA test approaches 85%, recently developed immunoelectrophoretic tests may detect over 90% of proved cases.

Various imaging techniques have also been employed in the diagnosis of hydatid disease of the liver. Plain abdominal x-rays may demonstrate hepatomegaly, displaced viscera, or calcification of the cyst wall. This latter finding is present in 50%–60% of patients with echinococcal cysts of the liver. Scintillation scans of the liver may reveal a "cold" area due to decreased uptake of radionuclide. However, a positive scan cannot be distinguished from other cysts, tumors, or abscesses. Similarly, selective angiography will demonstrate an avascular, space-occupying mass that cannot be differentiated from other cysts or abscesses. Ultrasound and CT, on the other hand, are able to detect calcified walls and daughter cysts and therefore can establish a specific diagnosis. In cases of suspected rupture into the biliary tree, ERCP may also be diagnostic (Fig 23–2).

Control of human hydatid disease is really a public health problem. For example, reducing the number of stray dogs and strictly controlling the disposal of infected viscera from slaughtered animals would dramatically reduce the prevalence of this disease. Medical treatment of established echinococcal cysts through the use of antihelmintics remains disappointing. Mebendazole is one such medication that has been reported to be effective in small numbers of patients with relatively small, uncomplicated cysts. Albendazole is a similar agent recently reported by Saimot et al.[4] to be effective in 11 patients. Until further clinical trials are reported, however, these drugs should be reserved for patients who are at high risk during anesthesia.

Percutaneous aspiration or drainage of cysts in which echinococcosis is suspected should not be performed, because dissemination and anaphylaxis can occur. Thus, most workers in this field agree that the treatment of choice of hydatid cysts of the liver is surgical. The specific operation will depend on: (1) the size and anatomical location of the cyst, (2) whether the cyst is secondarily infected, and (3) whether the cyst has ruptured. Many operative procedures have been proposed for the management of echinococcal cysts. However, they all have the same objectives, which include (1) total removal of all parasitic elements, (2) avoidance of spillage of cyst contents, and (3) management of the residual pericystic cavity without development of secondary infection.

Hepatic lobectomy or partial hepatectomy may be indicated in selected cases; for example, isolated cysts in the lateral segment of the left lobe. In most cases, however, surgical treatment includes initial evacuation of the cyst followed by management of the pericyst cavity. In this approach, the upper abdomen is first walled off with large, moist packs to isolate the cyst from the peritoneal cavity. The cyst is then aspirated with a large-bore needle, connected to a three-way stopcock and syringe, and then instilled with a scolicidal agent. Aspiration should always precede instillation because intracyst pressures are usually quite high.

The ideal scolecidal agent should be able to kill scoleces with only a short period of contact and have minimal or no toxicity. Formalin was once the agent of choice. However, recent reports of biliary sclerosis and death following instillation contraindicate the use of formalin. Other agents include hypertonic saline (5%–20%), 90% ethyl alcohol, 0.5% silver nitrate, and cetrimide. Whichever agent is instilled should be left in place for approximately five minutes before being aspirated. Further evacuation may be done with a trochar connected to suction or by unroofing the cyst and directly suctioning residual daughter cysts.

In the process of evacuation of cyst contents, the endocystic lining should be removed. In performing this procedure, as much of the pericyst wall as possible should be removed, and the remainder cauterized. If no bile leak is present and the cyst is not secondarily infected, surgical options include closure of the cavity or packing with omentum. A recent report by Langer and co-workers[5] suggests that these options are preferable to external drainage or marsupialization.

If a bile leak is present, an attempt should be made to close it with absorbable sutures. In this situation cholangiography is also indicated to be sure that no element of biliary obstruction is present. Infected cysts, of course, should be drained externally. Cysts that have ruptured into the biliary tree may present with fever, jaundice, and pain, and, therefore, mimic acute cholangitis resulting from choledocholithiasis. Most of these patients will require surgery, cholecystectomy and common duct exploration being the usual treatment. Rupture into the abdomen or thorax are also indications for surgery, and medical therapy may also be necessary in these rare cases. In these situations mortality may be as high as 20%–30%, whereas mortality of only 2%–3% can be expected in uncomplicated cases.

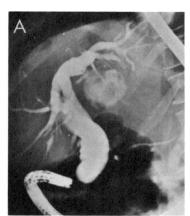
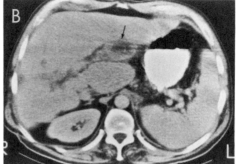
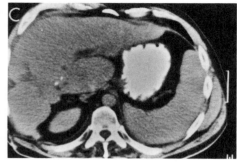

Fig 23–2.—A, ERCP demonstrating dilatation of the intrahepatic and extrahepatic biliary tree and an echinococcal cyst that had recently ruptured into the left biliary system causing "echinococcal cholangitis." **B,** CT scan in the same patient demonstrating the echinococcal cyst *(arrow)* in the left hepatic lobe. **C,** CT scan six months later in the same patient demonstrating resolution of the cyst after conservative therapy dictated by the patient's refusal to undergo surgery.

Amebic Abscess

Even before 1875, when Lösch discovered that *Entamoeba histolytica* was the causal agent of amebic dysentery, several European investigators had suggested a relationship between dysentery and liver abscess. In 1890, however, Sir William Osler first reported the presence of amebas in a liver abscess as well as in the stool of the same patient. In 1922, Sir Leonard Rogers documented that active amebas were rarely present in the "pus" of an amebic abscess but were present in the abscess wall.[6] By the 1930s Ochsner and co-workers[7] clearly demonstrated that mortality was greatly reduced when aspiration and emetine were used instead of surgical drainage. Since that time, several further advances in diagnostic techniques and the development of newer amebicidal drugs have led to earlier diagnosis and avoidance of aspiration in most cases.

Amebiasis has a worldwide distribution, the highest prevalence found in tropical and subtropical areas, where there is poor sanitation. The ease of world travel, recent immigration trends, and the U.S. military presence in tropical climates continue to contribute to a significant incidence of amebiasis in the United States. As a result, in southern states and in some northern U.S. cities the incidence of amebic abscesses is now similar to that of pyogenic abscesses.

In their cystic form, *Entamoeba histolytica* gain access to the body by oral ingestion, usually of contaminated water. In the small intestine, the cyst wall is digested by trypsin releasing four invasive trophozoites that live and multiply in the lumen of the colon, especially the cecum. Some trophozoites pass into the distal colon and change into cysts. These cysts, which are passed in the stool of human carriers, become the primary source of infection. Other amebic trophozoites may invade the cecal wall, enter the mesenteric venules and lymphatics, and are carried to the liver, lungs, and other organs.

When sufficient numbers of amebic trophozoites enter the liver and become lodged in smaller venules, thrombosis and infarction of small areas of hepatic parenchyma occur. An amebic abscess develops from coalition of several small areas of necrosis and amebic cytolytic destruction of hepatic tissue. An example of the ultrasonographic appearance of the progression from an early stage of infestation to abscess formation is presented in Figure 23–3.

The fluid contained within a mature amebic liver abscess is usually dark reddish brown and has been described as "anchovy paste" or sauce. Demonstration of amebic trophozoites within a liver abscess is more frequent during the early stages of development and less likely in an older abscess with a thick, fibrotic capsule. Abscess cavities can vary from 1 to 25 cm and, if untreated, can rupture into adjacent organs, the peritoneal or pleural cavities, the lung or pericardium.

Patients with an amebic liver abscess may present with either an acute inflammatory process or an indolent disease suggestive of a malignancy. The major complaint of patients with an amebic liver abscess is pain, usually localized to the right upper quadrant. In a collected series[6] of 954 recently published cases of amebic liver abscess, pain was the presenting symptom in 90% of patients. Almost three fourths of patients with an amebic hepatic abscess will have fever, and 20%–40% will also present with chills. Nausea, vomiting, anorexia, and weight loss are seen in 30%–40% of patients. Diarrhea will also be a symptom at the time of presentation in many patients and may help to differentiate on clinical grounds an amebic from a pyogenic abscess (Table 23–2).

On physical examination, upper abdominal tenderness and hepatomegaly are present in 75%–85% and 60%–80% of patients, respectively. These two findings are also seen more frequently in patients with amebic than in those with pyogenic liver abscesses (see Table 23–2). Jaundice, on the other hand, is present in only 5%–15% of patients with amebic abscesses compared to 30%–35% of patients with pyogenic abscesses. A palpable abdominal mass is an uncommon finding with either type of liver abscess but is seen more frequently with pyogenic abscesses.

The reported incidence of finding amebic cysts or trophozoites in the stool of patients with an amebic liver abscess varies considerably from 15%–55%. Since stool specimens are frequently not diagnostic, serologic tests are particularly useful in evaluating these patients. Numerous serologic tests for amebiasis have been developed. The IHA and gel diffusion precipitin (GDP) tests have been the most frequently employed. Several authors report the IHA test to be positive in

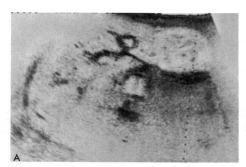
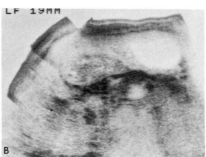
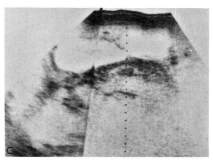

Fig 23–3.—A, transverse abdominal ultrasound demonstrating the early phase of an amebic abscess in the lateral segment of the left hepatic lobe. This segment is swollen, but no liquefaction is present. **B,** a repeat ultrasound of the same patient 13 days later reveals liquefaction and abscess formation of the lateral segment of the left lobe and the new appearance of a second area of early amebic involvement in the medial segment of the left lobe. **C,** a third ultrasound in the same patient after five days of metronidazole therapy shows slight diminution in the size of the lateral abscess and liquefaction of the medial abscess. (From Pitt[6] with permission of the author.)

TABLE 23–2.—DISTINGUISHING CLINICAL AND
LABORATORY CHARACTERISTICS OF HEPATIC ABSCESSES*

AMEBIC ABSCESS	PYOGENIC ABSCESS
Mexican ancestry	Age > 50 yr
Recent travel to or from an endemic area	Jaundice
	Pruritus
Abdominal pain	Sepsis/shock
Diarrhea	Palpable mass
Abdominal tenderness	↑ Bilirubin
Hepatomegaly	↑ Alkaline phosphatase
Positive serology	Abnormal abdominal x-ray

*Adapted from Conter et al.[8]

90%–95% of patients with an amebic liver abscess, whereas the GDP test is positive in 85%–90% of patients. One disadvantage of the IHA, however, is that it will frequently remain positive for many years after invasive amebiasis.

In a recent collected series of 592 cases of amebic liver abscess,[6] 71% of patients had a WBC count greater than 10,000/mm[3], and 49% were anemic. While 53% had an elevated alkaline phosphatase, only 34%–43% had elevations of serum transaminase levels, and 30% had a bilirubin greater than 2.0 mg/dl. Approximately two thirds of patients had abnormal chest x-rays. Several authors have reported that radionuclide scans of the liver identify amebic liver abscesses in 90%–95% of patients. Gallium scanning has also been reported to be able to differentiate amebic from pyogenic abscesses by demonstrating peripheral uptake around a central cold area of an amebic abscess.

In recent years, however, ultrasound has become the diagnostic method of choice for detecting amebic liver abscesses. Not only is ultrasound extremely accurate in detection, but in many cases this test can also differentiate amebic abscesses from other hepatic lesions. In addition to determining the number, size, and location of abscesses, ultrasound can be used to guide percutaneous aspiration and is a noninvasive, relatively inexpensive tool for follow-up. Although CT may be able to detect smaller lesions, most amebic abscesses are solitary and of sufficient size (> 2 cm) to be easily detected by ultrasound.

Even before the advent of ultrasound or CT-guided aspiration, most experts found diagnostic needle aspiration of amebic liver abscesses to be a safe procedure. The main reasons to aspirate amebic liver abscesses are (1) to establish a diagnosis and (2) to reduce the likelihood of rupture of a large abscess. The reported incidence of recovery of amebas from amebic abscess cavities varies tremendously, from 7% to 99%. Thus, failure to demonstrate amebic trophozoites does not rule out an amebic abscess. Moreover, the color of the fluid is not always the typical reddish brown; it may be white, yellow, or green. Absence of a foul odor and failure to demonstrate bacteria on Gram stain and culture are supportive evidence of amebic abscess.

The reported incidence of complications from an amebic hepatic abscess varies from 20% to 35%. The most common complications are those involving the pleura and lung, such as pleural effusion, empyema, perforated diaphragm, pneumonitis, and lung abscess. Rupture of an amebic abscess into the peritoneum has been reported to occur in as high as 20%–30% of patients. However, these series have generally been from areas of the world where medical aid is not readily available. In other series intraperitoneal rupture accounts for only 2%–3% of cases. In most reports, however, erosion of an amebic abscess into the intestinal tract or through the abdominal wall occurs in fewer than 1% of patients. Erosion, usually from the left lobe, into the pericardium is the most hazardous complication of an amebic hepatic abscess. Fortunately, this complication is rare, occurring in only 1%–2% of cases.

Treatment options in uncomplicated amebic liver abscess include amebicidal drugs, closed aspiration, percutaneous drainage, and surgical drainage. For many years, emetine was the only effective drug for the treatment of amebic hepatic abscesses. Chloroquine was the next amebicidal drug, which became available in 1948. While both of these agents have excellent initial response rates, the relapse rate of patients treated with chloroquine is significantly higher. Metronidazole was introduced in 1966 and has become the agent of choice because of a high probability of cure with a shorter course of treatment.

Considerable controversy exists regarding the role of closed needle aspiration in the management of patients with amebic hepatic abscesses. Some authors suggest that needle aspiration is rarely indicated. However, other authorities list several indications for aspiration, including: (1) persistence of symptoms despite appropriate drug therapy; (2) concern about rupture because of the size and/or location of the abscess; (3) suspicion that the abscess may be pyogenic or a secondarily infected amebic abscess; and (4) the presence of a large abscess in which a previous aspiration has yielded more than 250 ml.

While percutaneous catheter drainage of selected cases of pyogenic hepatic abscess is being reported with increasing frequency, this technique has not gained widespread popularity in the management of amebic liver abscesses. Similarly, since most patients with an amebic liver abscess respond to amebicidal drug therapy with or without closed needle aspiration, surgical drainage has generally been reserved for patients with complications. In patients with rupture into the peritoneal cavity, most authorities agree that surgical drainage is indicated. However, no clear consensus exists regarding the need for surgical drainage in patients whose abscess has ruptured into the pleura, lung, or pericardium.

Thus, considerable variation exists among reported series in the percentage of patients requiring surgical drainage. One of the largest surgical series was recently reported by Balasegaram[9] from Malaysia. He noted only six deaths among 269 surgically managed patients, a 2% mortality. On the other hand, numerous reports of large series of patients have been published in which nearly all patients were managed medically with similarly low mortality.

Pyogenic Abscess

Pyogenic hepatic abscesses have been the predominant form of liver abscess reported from medical centers in the more temperate climates found in the northern United States, England, and northern Europe. Hospital admission data suggest that the incidence of pyogenic hepatic abscess has changed very little over the past 80 years, varying from 0.013% to 0.035% of admissions. Both pyogenic and amebic liver abscesses are more common in men than in women. However, the mean age and percentage of patients older than 50 years is greater among patients with pyogenic abscesses (see Table 23–2).

The majority of pyogenic liver abscesses are caused by infections in the biliary tree or intestines. Several authors, therefore, have categorized pyogenic abscesses by the route of extension of infection. These etiologic categories include the following sources of infection: (1) biliary, from ascending cholangitis; (2) portal vein, as in pylephlebitis resulting from appendicitis; (3) hepatic artery, from septicemia; (4) direct extension, from a contiguous disease process; (5) traumatic, from blunt or penetrating injuries; and (6) cryptogenic, when no primary source of infection is found.

Prior to the introduction of antibiotics, pylephlebitis resulting from appendicitis was the leading cause of pyogenic liver abscesses. Moreover, this cause and other intra-abdominal infections resulting in pylephlebitis accounted for more than 40% of liver abscesses reported by Ochsner et al.[7] in the 1930s. In comparison, recent reports[6, 8] suggest that the biliary system is now the most common origin of pyogenic hepatic abscesses, accounting for approximately 35% of all cases. Moreover, further scrutiny of these reports suggests that approximately 40% of abscesses of biliary origin occur in patients with an underlying malignancy. The relative incidence of pyogenic abscesses resulting from systemic bacteremia, direct extension, trauma, and those in which no etiology could be determined has remained relatively constant.

The majority of both pyogenic and amebic liver abscesses are found in the right hepatic lobe. Only 10%–15% occur in the left lobe, whereas approximately 25% of pyogenic and 15% of amebic abscesses are bilateral. Approximately 45% of pyogenic abscesses are multiple, and mortality correlates closely with the number of abscesses (Fig 23–4). The multiplicity of abscesses also correlates with the origin, for example, 90% of abscesses of biliary origin are multiple. This association, therefore, helps to explain the continued high mortality of pyogenic abscesses.

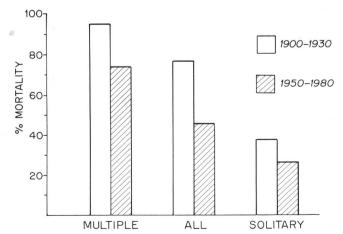

Fig 23–4.—Comparison of mortality from pyogenic hepatic abscesses among 479 cases collected by Ochsner et al.[7] from 1900 to 1930 and 598 collected cases treated between 1950 and 1980. (From Pitt[6] with permission of the author.)

In the preantibiotic era, gram-positive aerobes were the organisms most often isolated from pyogenic hepatic abscesses. In recent years, however, gram-negative aerobes have been isolated from 65%–70% of patients. Moreover, recent reports suggest that in 25%–30% of patients anaerobes are cultured. For many years *Escherichia coli* has been the organism most commonly isolated from hepatic abscesses. Various streptococcal species are the next most commonly cultured organisms, followed by *Klebsiella* and staphylococcal species. The most frequently isolated anaerobes are streptococcal and *Bacteroides* species.

The majority of patients with pyogenic hepatic abscesses will present with an acute illness of less than two weeks' duration. Occasionally, a patient will come to the hospital in septic shock, whereas, at the other end of the spectrum, approximately one third of patients will have had symptoms for a month or more. Fever and pain are the most common presenting symptoms, present in approximately 85% and 55% of patients, respectively. The most frequently physical finding in patients with pyogenic abscesses is an enlarged, tender liver, which is present in approximately 50% of patients. Jaundice is apparent on physical examination in approximately 30% of cases and may give a clue to the etiology.

The persistently high mortality of pyogenic hepatic abscesses attests to the difficulty in establishing the diagnosis on clinical grounds alone. Routine hematologic and liver function tests are abnormal in the majority of patients. Significant elevations of serum bilirubin and/or alkaline phosphatase may also help differentiate a pyogenic from an amebic liver abscess (see Table 23–2). Roentgenograms of the chest will be abnormal in slightly more than half of the patients. Abnormalities on plain abdominal x-rays, such as hepatomegaly or gas within the abscess, are seen less frequently. Preoperative and operative cholangiography have also become important aids in establishing the diagnosis in many cases where the underlying cause is biliary obstruction.

One of the important advances in improving mortality during the 1960s was the development of radionuclide hepatic scanning. Technetium sulfur colloid (^{99m}Tc), gallium citrate (^{67}Ga), and indium (^{111}In) WBC scans are currently being employed for detection of pyogenic liver abscesses. These scans can all provide useful information on the location, size, and number of abscesses as well as a mechanism for follow-up. Disadvantages of radionuclide scanning, however, are that lesions smaller than 2 cm cannot always be detected, and differentiation among abscesses, cysts, and tumors is not always possible.

Ultrasound is now able to delineate liver lesions as small as 2 cm and can usually differentiate cystic from solid masses. Another advantage of ultrasound is that it requires no ionizing radiation. Numerous reports have now documented that ultrasound is 80%–90% accurate in diagnosing liver abscesses. Ultrasound, however, may provide misleading information because of (1) difficulty visualizing lesions near the dome of the right lobe, (2) inability to detect multiple microscopic abscesses and those smaller than 2 cm, and (3) failure to visualize small abscesses when fatty infiltration is present.

Computerized tomography has the advantage over both radionuclide scanning and ultrasonography of being able to detect intrahepatic lesions as small as 0.5 cm (Fig 23–5). Moreover, the entire liver is visualized with CT, and fatty infiltration does not present a problem. Recent comparative studies suggest that CT may be the most accurate (90%–95%) diagnostic modality available for the detection of pyogenic hepatic abscesses. Nevertheless, CT also has occasional difficulty in differentiating abscesses from neoplasms or cysts.

Until recently, most authorities have not recommended diagnostic aspiration of pyogenic hepatic abscesses. However, with the advent of ultrasound and CT-guided aspiration, this diagnostic option has become safer and should be considered in selected cases where the usual diagnostic measures have failed. Percutaneous aspiration and catheter drainage may obviate operation, but this form of treatment is not applicable in many patients with pyogenic abscesses. To consider this option, the fluid collection should be unilocular and accessible by a safe approach. Moreover, in case of failure or complications, the patient should be prepared for surgery before aspiration, making surgical consultation mandatory in all cases.

Pyogenic hepatic abscess is almost uniformly fatal in patients in whom the disease is not diagnosed and appropriately treated. Obviously, early institution of antibiotic therapy is extremely important. Until specific bacteria have been isolated and sensitivities are known, broad antibacterial coverage is indicated. Various antibiotic options are now available, but whichever regimen is chosen should provide coverage for gram-negative aerobes, streptococci, and anaerobes. In choosing an agent for anaerobic coverage, metronidazole has the additional advantage of providing coverage for *Entamoeba histolytica* should there still be a suspicion that the lesion may be an amebic abscess.

Once sensitivities of the infecting organisms are known, appropriate adjustments should be made in the antibiotic regimen so that the least toxic agents are being employed. This principle is important because an extended period of antibiotic treatment is usually required to eradicate these infections. The exact length of antibiotic therapy should be individualized on the basis of the number of abscesses, the adequacy of drainage, the clinical response, and the toxicity of the required antibiotics.

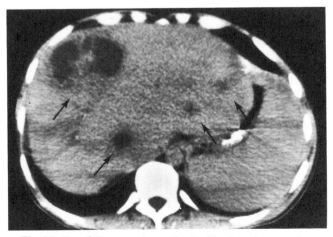

Fig 23–5.—CT scan of a patient with chronic granulomatous disease who had multiple recurrent pyogenic liver abscesses *(arrows)*. Note the thick wall of the abscesses on the *right.*

Several reports suggest that closed aspiration or percutaneous drainage and antibiotics can be successfully employed in selected cases; i.e., those who are relatively young, otherwise healthy, and have no other source of intra-abdominal infection. These are the very patients, however, who will tolerate a laparotomy without difficulty. Theoretically, open drainage in these patients should provide more adequate and dependent drainage with more rapid resolution of the abscess. Among the categories of patients in whom closed aspiration or percutaneous drainage should not be employed include those with: (1) multiple abscesses, (2) abscesses of biliary origin, and (3) abscesses with no known etiology. One or more of these categories, unfortunately, applies to most patients with pyogenic abscesses.

Prior to the introduction of antibiotics, the extraperitoneal approach to drainage of hepatic abscesses was recommended because of fear of contamination of the pleural or peritoneal cavities with the transthoracic or transperitoneal approaches. The obvious disadvantage of these techniques, however, is that they do not allow for adequate exploration of the entire liver or for recognition of an inadequately treated intra-abdominal source of infection. For these reasons, most authorities now advocate transperitoneal drainage. This approach has several advantages, including complete exposure of the liver so that the best drainage site can be determined, location of multiple abscesses, and exploration of the entire abdomen for an occult source.

In patients with a biliary source of infection, choledochotomy with insertion of a T tube is necessary to achieve adequate drainage. In this situation, extensive exploration of the duct, choledochoscopy, and completion cholangiography should be performed with caution and individualized on the basis of biliary pathology and the patient's stability. In other cases after needle aspiration to help localize the abscess, laparotomy pads are placed adjacent to the lesion. The surgeon then drains the abscess dependently by creating a tract through the liver. A biopsy should also be taken of the abscess wall to rule out an infected tumor and to search further for amebic trophozoites.

In patients with multiple microscopic abscesses no formal liver drainage is indicated, but a careful search for a biliary or intra-abdominal source should be undertaken. Infrequently, the only way to control multiple intrahepatic abscesses will be with a formal hepatic resection. This form of treatment is generally reserved for patients with long-standing biliary obstruction involving one hepatic lobe.

Mortality rates for patients with pyogenic hepatic abscess reported between 1950 and 1980 vary from as low as 24% to as high as 88%. The mortality rate for multiple hepatic abscesses has been and continues to be quite high (see Fig 23–5). Reasons for continued high mortality among these patients include: (1) failure to consider the diagnosis; (2) failure to detect small intra-hepatic abscesses; (3) ineffective surgical drainage; (4) failure to control the source of infection; and (5) an associated end-stage malignancy. Mortality is also affected by such factors as advanced age, the patient's immune status, and the presence of polymicrobial bacteremia. In comparison, the prognosis for a patient with a solitary abscess is quite good (see Fig 23–5). In these patients death generally occurs only when there is failure to establish a diagnosis and to achieve adequate drainage.

NEOPLASTIC INTRAHEPATIC CYSTS

In addition to congenital, traumatic, and inflammatory intrahepatic cysts, cystic lesions of the hepatic parenchyma may be neoplastic. Benign and malignant primary hepatic cystic tumors are termed cystadenomas and cystadenocarcinomas, respectively. Cystic liver metastases from cystadenocarcinoma or cystic neuroendocrine tumors of the pancreas have also been described (Fig 23–6). Perhaps more common than these rare lesions, however, are cystic degeneration and necrosis of primary liver tumors or of liver metastases from solid tumors originating in other organs. Tumor necrosis may also result in abscess formation, which may present as a cystic lesion.

Cystadenomas and cystadenocarcinomas of the liver are rare lesions, with only seven cases reported from the Cleveland and Mayo Clinics over a total of 60 years.[1] As with other cystic liver lesions, symptoms are usually vague and nonspecific. These lesions may be incidental findings during laparotomy for other diseases or may be detected by ultrasound or CT. If these studies suggest a cystic tumor, selective arteriography may help to confirm this impression and provide important anatomical information necessary for resection.

As with other cystic liver masses, operative approach will be dictated by the size and location of the lesion. At surgery the initial step should be to biopsy the cystic mass. If the diagnosis of cystadenoma or cystadenocarcinoma is confirmed, the lesion should be excised with a margin of adjacent normal liver. Depending on the size and location of the tumor, resection may require wedge resection, segmentectomy, or formal hepatic lobectomy. These cystic liver tumors have a relatively low-grade malignant potential and an excellent long-term prognosis when complete excision is performed.

INTRAHEPATIC DUCTAL CYSTS

Intrahepatic ductal cysts may be either congenital (Caroli's disease) or acquired and may or may not be associated with extrahepatic ductal dilatation. Congenital cystic malformations of the intrahepatic ducts were first described in 1906 by Vachel and Stevens but received little attention until the 1958 report by Caroli and colleagues.[10] Subsequent reports by Caroli and by others documented two types of congenital intrahepatic ductal dilatation, a "simple" type and a "periportal fibrosis" type.

The simple type is clinically significant because of recurrent cholangitis, liver abscess, pain, and fever but is not associated with hepatic fibrosis, cirrhosis, or portal hypertension. These latter manifestations of congenital hepatic fibrosis are present in the periportal fibrosis type. Unfortunately, more than half of the patients with Caroli's disease also have congenital hepatic fibrosis. In addition, approximately 20%–25% of patients with Caroli's disease will have extrahepatic cystic dilatation, and many patients will have both intrahepatic and extrahepatic ductal dilatation as well as hepatic fibrosis.

Caroli's disease has been reported in siblings but not in subsequent generations. Patients with congenital intrahepatic ductal cysts present most often with long histories of abdominal pain, fever, chills, and mild jaundice. These symptoms often begin in childhood, and the vast majority of patients become symptomatic before the age of 30. In those patients with congenital hepatic fibrosis, presenting symptoms may also include manifestations of portal hypertension such as variceal bleeding or hepatic encephalopathy.

Saccular dilatations of the intrahepatic ducts may also be acquired following prolonged, recurrent obstruction associated with biliary stasis and infection.[11] This situation may occur with a high stricture of the common hepatic duct resulting from either operative or blunt trauma. Another good example of acquired intrahepatic ductal dilatation are patients with recurrent pyogenic cholangitis or Oriental cholangiohepatitis. These patients can develop huge saccular and/or fusiform dilatations, usually of the left intrahepatic ducts. Patients with this disease also have multiple intrahepatic stones, and many, but not all, also harbor the parasites *Clonorchis sinensis* or *Ascaris lumbricoides*. In addition to a parasitic cause, some authorities have suggested that dietary insufficiencies may result in the multiple intrahepatic stones that develop in patients with recurrent pyogenic cholangitis.

Not long ago, the diagnosis of Caroli's disease and of recurrent pyogenic cholangitis was rarely made preoperatively. However, with the advent of ultrasound, CT, iminodiacetic acid scanning, thin-needle transhepatic cholangiography and ERCP, most cases are being diagnosed much earlier. After diagnosis and before surgery, ultrasound may be particularly useful for detection of intrahepatic stone formation. When surgery is contemplated, however, direct cholangiography, either by the transhepatic or retrograde route, is extremely important in planning the correct operative approach.

Patients with intrahepatic cystic dilation without evidence of obstruction, cholangitis, or intrahepatic stones should be

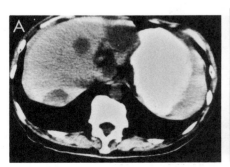
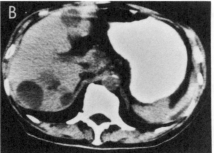
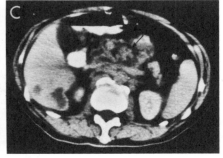

Fig 23–6.—A, a CT scan demonstrating multiple cystic metastases from a cystic pancreatic neoplasm. **B,** more caudad cut from the same CT demonstrating more cystic metastases in the same patient. **C,** more caudad cut from the same CT demonstrating both cystic hepatic metastasis and the primary pancreatic tumor *(arrow)*.

observed. However, when symptoms begin, treatment should be surgical, because several reports suggest that medical treatment results in a high mortality. The type of surgical procedure that will be necessary depends on the location and extent of disease. If the disease is confined to a local area peripherally, excision of the diseased area is the procedure of choice. Unfortunately, this configuration is not usually the case.

In patients with unilateral intrahepatic ductal dilatation, two treatment options are possible: (1) clean-out of all stones and debris, and (2) hepatic lobectomy. In patients with unilateral disease without severe congenital or secondary biliary cirrhosis, the authors usually recommend the former option. In general, our approach[13] has been to clean and drain by way of the common hepatic duct (Fig 23–7). The operative cholangioscope has proved to be extremely valuable in the operative clean-out process. However, even with this aid and an extensive operative effort, complete clean-out may not be possible.

Therefore, in these cases our policy has been to place a 16 or 20 F transhepatic Silastic stent through the dilated ductal system and into a Roux-en-Y limb of jejunum, which is sewn end-to-side to the common hepatic duct. This long-term indwelling tube is irrigated daily with sterile saline and changed every three months because of build-up of biliary sludge within the tube. At the time of tube change, the ductal system is reassessed for residual stones and debris which can be irrigated or manipulated into the Roux-en-Y limb of jejunum or extracted via the tube tract with the aid of a Dormier basket. Percutaneous cholangioscopy with the flexible cholangioscope can also be quite useful in retrieving retained intrahepatic stones.

Patients with unilateral Caroli's disease who continue to have cholangitis despite the above-described treatment should be considered for hepatic lobectomy. Moreover, in patients who present with severe, unilateral, lobar cirrhosis and atrophy, hepatic lobectomy may be appropriate as the initial surgical procedure. Most cases of congenital intrahepatic ductal dilatation, however, are bilateral. In these cases hepatic lobectomy is not an option; and therefore, bilateral clean-out with transhepatic stenting has been our usual initial treatment. If severe cirrhosis or unremitting cholangitis continues

to be a problem, hepatic transplantation must be considered.

In the past, long-term prognosis for patients with bilateral Caroli's disease has been poor. It is hoped that with the aggressive operative and postoperative approach described above as well as the option of transplantation, the outlook for these patients will be somewhat better. An additional problem that these patients face, however, is the potential development of cholangiocarcinoma. Dayton et al.[13] have recently described four cases of cholangiocarcinoma developing in patients with Caroli's disease. Six other cases complicated by bile duct tumors have been described. Thus, 10 of the 142 reported cases (7%) have developed cholangiocarcinoma, suggesting that Caroli's disease is a premalignant lesion. Whether biliary malignancies result from exposure to carcinogens present in bile, constant stone irritation, vitamin A deficiency, or a combination of these factors is unknown. However, if intrahepatic stones and stasis do play a role, treatment of these factors may also be important in preventing malignant deterioration.

CYSTIC LESIONS OF THE GALLBLADDER AND CYSTIC DUCT

Cystic anomalies of the gallbladder and cystic duct are rare. These lesions may be of little clinical significance except that they may result in altered gallbladder emptying and, therefore, predispose to gallstone formation. However, a number of developmental abnormalities of the gallbladder and/or cystic duct can occur. These anomalies include absence of the gallbladder, double gallbladder, bilobed gallbladder, left-sided gallbladder, accessory ducts to the gallbladder, hourglass gallbladder, intrahepatic gallbladder, Phrygian cap, and diverticulum of the gallbladder. This last anomaly may occur in the neck, body, or fundus of the gallbladder and might be considered a cystic lesion.

Similarly, many anomalies of the cystic duct have been described. These variations include entrance into the hepatic ducts, into the common duct in a spiral fashion or in a very low position, or directly into the duodenum at the ampulla. A congenital diverticulum or cystic dilatation of the cystic duct occurs much less frequently than the above-mentioned anom-

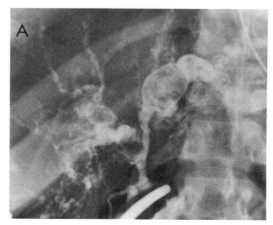
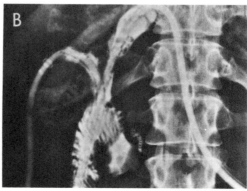

Fig 23–7.—A, intraoperative cholangiogram of a patient with bilateral Caroli's disease. Note the multiple intrahepatic stones. **B,** postoperative cholangiogram in the same patient after placement of bilateral Silastic transhepatic tubes. Note some reduction in the left intrahepatic dilatation.

alies. Acquired dilatation of the cystic duct secondary to impaction by a large stone may also occur. When this situation results in erosion of the stone into, or compression of, the common hepatic duct, this rare clinical entity is termed the Mirizzi syndrome. In general, when these various cystic anomalies of the gallbladder or cystic duct cause typical biliary symptoms or gallstones, they can easily be managed by cholecystectomy. The Mirizzi syndrome, on the other hand, frequently requires common duct exploration and careful reconstruction or biliary bypass.

CONGENITAL EXTRAHEPATIC BILIARY CYSTS

The first case of a choledochal cyst was described by Vates in 1723. Nearly 100 years later, Todd reported another case of "remarkable enlargement of the biliary duct." In 1852 Douglas was the first clinician clearly to document this entity in a 17-year-old girl. The first collected series of 28 cases was reported by Laverson in 1909. Since that time, the number of new cases has steadily grown. In 1959 Alonso-Lej[14] published a collected series of 393 cases and proposed a classification for choledochal cysts that is still used. In 1980 Yamaguchi[15] presented 1,433 collected cases, more than three quarters of which were Japanese. Over the past 25 years, significant advances have been made in the diagnosis and surgical management of choledochal cysts, new etiology theories have been proposed, and the premalignant potential of these lesions has been recognized.

Classification

A choledochal cyst is a localized dilatation of the bile duct and is not a true cyst per se. Most commonly, the dilatation is circumferential and in the supraduodenal common bile duct. The bile ducts above and below the cyst as well as the gallbladder are usually of normal caliber or slightly dilated proximally. This configuration distinguishes choledochal cysts from the diffuse dilatation of the biliary tree seen in biliary obstruction. However, choledochal cysts have been reported with diffuse fusiform dilation of both extrahepatic and intrahepatic ducts.

In 1959 Alonso-Lej proposed a classification of choledochal cysts, which included three types (Fig 23–8). Type I, cystic dilation of the common bile duct, is by far the most common. This dilation may be saccular (IA), localized (IB), or fusiform (IC), and may involve any or all of the common bile duct from the hepatic bifurcation to the duodenum. Most commonly, type I cysts are large and saccular, and type IA cysts involve most of the extrahepatic biliary system. Type I cysts can also be localized to a small segment of the duct as in the type IB cyst, or be quite diffuse with a fusiform configuration as in type IC. The common bile duct is usually narrowed distal to the cyst but on occasion may be of normal caliber. The remainder of the biliary tree is frequently normal in type I biliary cysts, but the intrahepatic bile ducts and biliary radicals may be dilated in as many as 20% of cases. The cystic duct may enter the cyst directly or enter a normal common bile duct uninvolved by the cyst. As described below, anomalies of the junction of the cyst or common bile duct with the pancreatic duct are frequent.

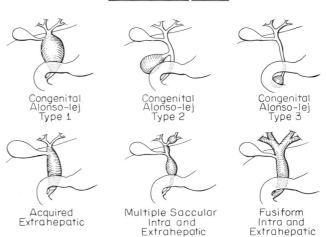

EXTRAHEPATIC CYSTS

Congenital Alonso-lej Type 1

Congenital Alonso-lej Type 2

Congenital Alonso-lej Type 3

Acquired Extrahepatic

Multiple Saccular Intra and Extrahepatic

Fusiform Intra and Extrahepatic

Fig 23–8.—Classification of extrahepatic *(top)* and combined intrahepatic and extrahepatic cysts *(bottom)*.

A type II choledochal cyst is essentially a congenital diverticulum which may arise from the common bile duct or the hepatic ducts (see Fig 23–8). Type III is a congenital choledochocele. The intraduodenal portion of the common bile duct is dilated, which may result in duodenal as well as biliary obstruction. These type III cysts are managed quite differently from type I or type II biliary cysts. In 1971, Longmire et al.[11] expanded on Alonso-Lej's original classification of biliary cysts and proposed two more groups. Longmire's type IV cyst has multiple intrahepatic and extrahepatic biliary dilations, and his type V cyst consists of fusiform intrahepatic and extrahepatic dilatation (see Fig 23–8).

The relative incidence of the different types of choledochal cysts depends on which classification is utilized. Yamaguchi[15] utilized Longmire's modification of Alonso-Lej's classification and reported that in 878 cases, 77.7% were type I; 2.0% were type II; 1.4% were type III; and 18.9% were type IV. Similarly, Flanagan[16] reported that 86.7% were type I; 3.1% were type II; 5.6% were type III; and 2.6% were type IV. Thus, most authors agree that approximately 80% of choledochal cysts are type I.

Histologically, biliary cysts consist of a 4–5-mm thick, fibrotic wall of dense collagenous connective tissue with occasional disrupted elastic fibers and smooth muscle. Frequently, a significant inflammatory reaction of either chronic or acute inflammatory cells is also present. The cysts are frequently denuded of any epithelial lining. The presence or absence of epithelial cells lining the cyst does not appear to correlate with a congenital or acquired etiology.[16] The size of a cyst may vary from quite small, measuring less than 1 cm to giant cysts that may contain up to 5,000 ml of fluid.

Most frequently, these cysts are sterile but may be superinfected by any variety of bacteria, most commonly gram-negative rods. Cysts that have been anastomosed to the biliary tract, however, are routinely infected with myriad organisms, including gram-negative rods, enterococci, staphylococci, and anaerobes. Congenital biliary cysts contain stones or concretions much less frequently than do acquired biliary dilatations proximal to iatrogenic biliary strictures.

Etiology

Numerous theories have been proposed to explain the pathogenesis of choledochal cysts. However, little experimental evidence has been published to support any of these theories. Most likely, the different forms of choledochal cysts are due to different pathogenic mechanisms. Type II cysts, which are a simple diverticulum of the common bile duct, are probably developmental anomalies similar to diverticula of the duodenum or small bowel. Type II choledochal cysts are not mucosal diverticula, as seen in colonic diverticulosis, which result from a degenerative aging process. Similarly, choledochoceles, type III choledochal cysts, are more similar to small-bowel diverticula in clinical presentation and histology than to choledochal cysts of the type I variety. Histologically, choledochoceles are lined by mucosa of the small intestine and lack the degenerative and inflammatory changes present in type I cysts. Type II and III cysts, therefore, appear to be secondary to an embryologic abnormality and not a developmental process. Very little is known regarding the etiology of type IV or V cysts. However, the presence of multiple saccular dilatations of the intrahepatic ductal system, with or without extrahepatic dilatation, in the absence of strictures or obstruction argues strongly for a congenital and not an acquired defect.

The greatest controversy surrounds the pathogenesis of type I cysts, perhaps because these cysts are considerably more common than the other types of choledochal cysts. The primary debate as to the pathogenesis of these lesions revolves around the question of whether they are congenital or acquired. Current theories include: (1) the possibility that there is an intrinsic abnormality in the wall of the extrahepatic bile ducts, (2) that they develop because of alterations in the arrangement of the choledochopancreatic duct junction, or (3) that these cysts result from distal obstruction. Numerous other theories have been proposed to explain the etiology of these cysts. Theories explaining the pathogenesis of choledochal cysts range from proposals that choledochal cysts are

analagous to achalasia of the sphincter of Oddi, resulting in a "megalocholedochus," to theories proposing that choledochal cysts are in fact accessory gallbladders.

Two quite different theories, however, are most popular. In 1936 Yotsuyanagi proposed that choledochal cysts resulted from an inequality of proliferation of the epithelial cells of the extrahepatic biliary ducts at the stage when the primitive choledochus is still a solid cord of cells. The extrahepatic common bile ducts form from a solid core of epithelial cells that first enter a proliferative stage and then develop a lumen. Yotsuyanagi proposed that patients with choledochal cysts had excessive localized proliferation with subsequent vacuolization, a weakness of the wall, and, as a result, cystic dilatation. Extensions of this theory have been suggested that propose that there may also be a distal obstructive element in addition to excessive localized proliferation.

A second, more current and quite popular theory to explain the pathogenesis of choledochal cysts was proposed initially by Babbitt in 1969.[17] On reviewing numerous cholangiograms of inpatients with choledochal cysts, Babbitt astutely observed that many—in fact, most—of these patients had an abnormal junction of the pancreatic and biliary ducts within the pancreas. Normally, the common bile duct joins the pancreatic duct within 5 mm, or at most 10 mm, of the duodenal lumen in adults and 4 mm in infants. Thus, in adults the common channel is normally shorter than 10 mm. The pancreatic and common bile duct, therefore, join within the muscular segment of the sphincter of Oddi, which prevents reflux of pancreatic juice into the common bile duct.

Babbitt and colleagues in subsequent publications and others[18, 19] have demonstrated that the common pancreatic-biliary channel is much longer (20–40 mm) in most patients with choledochal cysts (Fig 23–9). This congenitally high junction of the pancreatic duct and the bile duct causes a mixture of pancreatic juice and bile within the bile duct. This caustic mixture may destroy the epithelial lining and supportive structures of the bile duct resulting in cystic dilatation. This theory has been supported both by the observation that

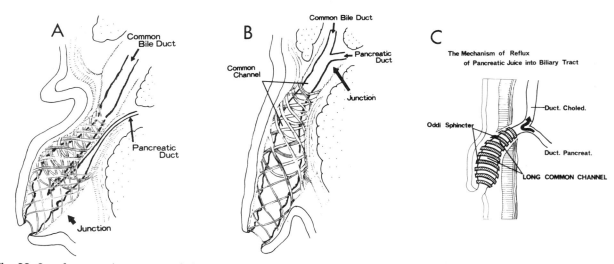

Fig 23–9.—A, normal anatomy of the pancreatic-biliary ductal junction. **B,** abnormal junction of the pancreatic-biliary ductal system. **C,** pancreatic juice regurgitates up the common bile duct extrasphincterically. (From Miyano et al.[19] with permission of the authors.)

an anomalous junction of the pancreatic and biliary ducts is frequently found in individuals with type I choledochal cysts[17-19] and also by the presence of high amylase levels in the cyst contents.[18, 19] However, experimental confirmation of this theory remains lacking, and it may be that these anomalies are simply associated developmental anomalies that are not pathologically related.

A third theoretical explanation for choledochal cysts argues that they occur proximal to an obstruction. Certainly, patients with distal biliary strictures or cancers of the bile duct and the pancreas and those with long-standing choledocholithiasis will develop progressive dilation of the extra- and intrahepatic biliary ducts. However, the dilatation under these circumstances involves the entire biliary ductal system in a fusiform fashion and is quite distinct from the usual choledochal cyst. Support for the obstructive theory, however, comes from the work of Caroli and Marculoides,[20] who demonstrated that there was increased outflow resistance from choledochal cysts into the distal bile duct.

Most likely, however, the outflow obstruction demonstrated in some patients with choledochal cysts is secondary to torsion and kinking at the junction of a large cyst and the distal duct. The observation that patients with jaundice generally have quite large cysts and, conversely, that patients with small cysts rarely present with jaundice supports the hypothesis that outflow obstruction is secondary to the mechanical effects of a large cyst, not a primary causative factor.

Clinical Presentation

Choledochal cysts may present clinically in several ways. Owing to earlier diagnosis with the aid of modern biliary imaging techniques, the classic presentation of right upper quadrant pain, jaundice, and a palpable abdominal mass inferior to the liver is now the exception rather than the rule. Recent studies[15, 16] suggest that this triad of symptoms may be present in 15%–40% of patients (Table 23–3). The earlier diagnosis of choledochal cysts has resulted in fewer patients presenting with complications, such as peritonitis secondary to spontaneous or traumatic rupture, liver failure due to secondary biliary cirrhosis, or sepsis resulting from cholangitis. In Yamaguchi's 1980 review,[15] abdominal pain was the most common presenting symptom (51%). Jaundice was observed in 45% of cases, and an abdominal mass was palpable in 37%. Fever, nausea, and vomiting have been observed in approximately 15% of cases. Less common presenting symptoms are alcoholic stools, anorexia, pruritus, and weight loss.

The pain from choledochal cysts is most frequently vague and dull, starting in the right upper quadrant and radiating to the epigastrium, right lower quadrant, or through to the back. The pain often mimics biliary colic or acute cholecystitis.

Jaundice may be intermittent or chronic and is commonly mild. A mass is of obvious diagnostic importance and is usually soft, mobile, and nontender, and may fluctuate in size between examinations. Vomiting may be due to compression of the duodenum by the cyst, infection, or rapid disgorgement of cyst contents into the duodenum. Symptoms tend to be more severe in children and infants. The clinical triad of pain, jaundice, and a mass is more common in children than adults. Children usually present with jaundice and a mass or the complete triad, whereas adults more commonly present with pain, an asymptomatic abdominal mass, or cholangitis. the duration of symptoms can range from several days to years (Table 23–4). Although generally much smaller than type I cysts, choledochoceles (type III cysts) often present with nausea, vomiting, and vague upper abdominal pain, and seldom with jaundice.

Diagnosis

Over the past 15 years, advances in imaging have provided the diagnostician with numerous, and frequently redundant, studies to confirm the diagnosis of choledochal cyst. Prior to the availability of these diagnostic modalities, the correct diagnosis of choledochal cysts was frequently not made preoperatively. Routine liver function tests do not distinguish choledochal cysts from other more common causes of biliary obstruction. In the past intravenous cholangiography, Rose bengal tests, and upper GI radiographs were seldom diagnostic of choledochal cysts. With the increased availability of ultrasonography, choledochal cysts can now be readily demonstrated in a painless, risk-free manner (Fig 23–10). In fact, ultrasonography has become a routine diagnostic test in evaluation of a patient with any one of the three classic signs for choledochal cysts—jaundice, pain, or right upper quadrant mass. Having demonstrated a thick-walled cyst in the right upper quadrant by ultrasound, its relationship to the biliary system can be investigated with more invasive studies. Computerized tomography provides essentially the same information as ultrasound but is generally more expensive and less readily available. While either study is generally sufficient to suggest the diagnosis, in combination they are redundant and not cost-effective.

Preoperative visualization of the biliary tract with either ERCP or percutaneous transhepatic cholangiography (PTC) is recommended (Fig 23–11): (1) to document a biliary origin of a right upper quadrant cystic mass, (2) to exclude other causes for a dilated common bile duct, such as a tumor or stricture

TABLE 23–3.—PRESENTING SYMPTOMS IN PATIENTS WITH CHOLEDOCHAL CYSTS

| AUTHOR | YEAR | % PATIENTS | | | % PATIENTS |
		Jaundice	Pain	Mass	The Triad
Alonso-Lej[14]	1959	73	65	60	21
Flanigan[16]	1975	64	55	58	38
Yamaguchi[15]	1980	45	51	37	13

TABLE 23–4.—DURATION OF SYMPTOMS BEFORE DIAGNOSIS IN PATIENTS WITH CHOLEDOCHAL CYSTS*

DURATION	% PATIENTS
< 1 wk	10
1–4 wk	9
1–5 mo.	33
½–4 yr	26
5–19 yr	18
> 20 yr	4

*Adapted from Flanigan.[16]

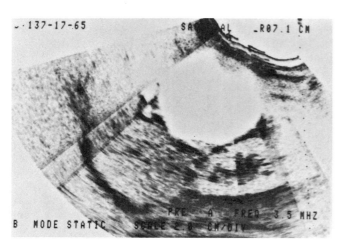

Fig 23–10.—Upper abdominal ultrasound of a large choledochal cyst. The liver is cephalad and posterior and the kidney is caudad and posterior to the cyst.

of the distal bile duct, and (3) to establish an operative plan. We generally prefer ERCP in patients in whom ultrasound suggests a choledochal cyst because: (1) cannulation rates are generally better than 90%; (2) the proximal biliary system is visualized in almost all patients, since there is seldom complete biliary obstruction; (3) the ampulla is visualized; and (4) the pancreatic-biliary junction is well demonstrated. Since stasis, superinfection, and partial biliary obstruction are common in choledochal cysts, antibiotics should be given immediately prior to ERCP. In the absence of jaundice and intrahepatic biliary ductal obstruction, PTC is successful in only 70% of cases and should be reserved for patients in whom ERCP has been unsuccessful or is unavailable. Percutaneous transhepatic cholangiography and ERCP are equally efficacious in jaundiced patients whose intrahepatic ducts are dilated on ultrasound or CT scan. Although successful ERCP in children as young as 18 months has been reported, the pres-

ence of an extrarenal cyst in the right upper quadrant on ultrasound or CT scan mandates surgical exploration even if cholangiography is unsuccessful. In these children, cholangiography can be performed intraoperatively.

Numerous other radiographic studies can suggest a choledochal cyst. On an upper GI roentgenographic study, the duodenum may be displaced inferiorly or to the left. On barium enema the hepatic flexure may be displaced inferiorly. The right kidney may also be displaced inferiorly on IVP, a study frequently obtained in children with an upper abdominal mass to exclude a nephroblastoma. Biliary scintigraphy with an iminodiacetic acid derivative will frequently demonstrate a dilated common bile duct, but does not provide any information in addition to an ERCP or PTC. Scintigraphy is most commonly obtained in a patient presenting with acute symptoms to exclude acute cholecystitis and will demonstrate filling of both the gallbladder and a large common bile duct, suggesting the diagnosis of a choledochal cyst. However, scintigraphy should be restricted to acutely ill patients and has little place in the evaluation of chronic complaints. Intravenous cholangiography and cholecystography are of no particular value in the evaluation of patients thought to have a choledochal cyst. Type III choledochal cysts, choledochoceles, are frequently not demonstrated by ultrasonography and appear as a polypoid mass near the ampulla of Vater on upper GI radiographic studies. The diagnosis is best confirmed by duodenoscopy.

Whether preoperative angiography is necessary in patients in whom resection of a choledochal cyst is contemplated is debatable. In adults, however, angiography may provide useful information regarding pericyst anatomy. Preoperative diagnosis of choledochal cysts has steadily increased over the past four decades. Prior to 1960, fewer than 40% of patients had the diagnosis of a choledochal cyst established preoperatively. Most recent publications, however, document a correct preoperative diagnosis in approximately 80% of cases. The value of correct preoperative diagnosis may influence surgical mortality.

Fig 23–11.—ERCP of the same patient shown in Figure 23–10. Note the large choledochal cyst, the long common channel, and the anomalous junction of the pancreatic and biliary ducts.

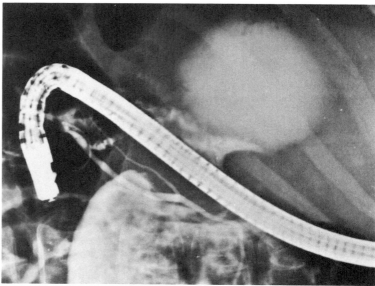

Surgical Management

Recent reviews primarily generated by the Japanese experience have clearly demonstrated that total excision of the choledochal cyst with reconstruction by a Roux-en-Y hepaticojejunostomy is the preferred surgical procedure for this entity. Previously this procedure was viewed with considerable reluctance, primarily by American surgeons, because of early reports of high mortality and morbidity associated with the excision of the cyst. Owing to local inflammation and involvement of associated portal structures, this procedure requires more technical expertise than simple bypass. However, with better understanding of the premalignant potential of these cysts and better preoperative demonstration of biliary and vascular anatomy, total excision has replaced simple drainage as the preferred method of surgical management.

Simple medical observation has been shown to be associated with almost universal mortality. In one series of 30 patients treated medically, 29 succumbed to their disease. External drainage is associated with almost equally dismal results. In one report external drainage resulted in an 83% mortality. In patients who are severely ill from sepsis and cannot tolerate a prolonged procedure, external drainage is a reasonable alternative but, understandably, is associated with up to a 30% mortality. In his classic review, Alonso-Lej[14] reported a 15%–40% mortality with excision of the cyst, which resulted in considerable reluctance on the part of American surgeons to attempt this procedure. As a result, for some time the greatest controversy was whether choledochal cysts should be drained into the duodenum or the jejunum. However, subsequent reports have shown that ascending cholangitis is not infrequent following either of these procedures. Sepsis may result from anastomotic stricture, stone formation, or after choledochocystduodenostomy with regurgitation of intestinal contents. The argument for choledochocystduodenostomy over Roux-en-Y diversion is that this latter procedure may be ulcerogenic. However, the incidence of morbidity after choledochocystduodenostomy has been reported to be as high as 55%.[16] Thus, when excision is not feasible for technical reasons, a Roux-en-Y choledochocystjejunostomy is preferable.

Despite early concerns with a high operative mortality from total excision of the choledochal cyst, recent reviews have clearly demonstrated that this procedure carries no greater operative mortality than simple drainage. Flanigan[16] reports a 7% mortality for excision compared to 17% for Roux-en-Y diversion and 5% for duodenal diversion. In another series by Klotz et al.,[21] postoperative mortality was 4%, 5%, and 2%, respectively, for these procedures. However, the incidence of stricture formation and cholangitis requiring reoperation is considerably lower for excision and hepaticojejunostomy than for choledochocystojejunostomy and choledochocystoduodenostomy. Similar figures have also been published by Flanigan.[16] One factor favoring excision of an extrahepatic biliary cyst is the presence of chronic inflammation, which may increase the incidence of stricture formation when the cyst itself is sutured to the jejunum or duodenum.

The critical aspect of excising a choledochal cyst is not to attempt to remove the entire cyst but to develop a plane between the lining of the cyst and its serosa which is often a relatively avascular plane.[22] Using this technique, injury to the portal vein and hepatic arteries, to which the cyst is often densely adherent on a serosal plane, can be avoided (Fig 23–12). The gallbladder should be removed in all operations, since it becomes physiologically defunctionalized by any of these procedures and hence has a high risk of developing acute cholecystitis postoperatively. Radiographic demonstration of the cyst's communications with the hepatic ducts and the pancreatic duct is critical and is preferably obtained preoperatively by ERCP. However, intraoperative cholangiography obtained by instilling contrast medium into the gallbladder or directly into the cyst with a small-caliber needle can frequently provide the surgeon with the prerequisite anatomical delineation to allow a safe procedure. Of critical importance is demonstration of the choledochopancreatic duct junction to avoid injury to this structure. To leave a small portion of the cyst distally is safer than attempting complete excision and causing injury to the pancreas or pancreatic duct.

The common hepatic duct is almost invariably dilated, although there may be a relative narrowing at the confluence of the right and left hepatic ducts. With careful dissection in the hilum of the liver, an adequate length of normal proximal common hepatic or hepatic duct can be isolated to allow direct anastomosis to a Roux-en-Y limb of jejunum. This anastomosis is usually stented with a Silastic tube, which is brought out either transhepatically or via the Roux-en-Y limb of jejunum. The route and length of time this stent remains

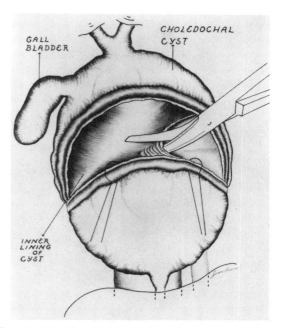

Fig 23–12.—Surgical technique for excision of choledochal cysts. The cyst has been opened by a transverse incision across the anterior, medial, and lateral walls. An arbitrary plane of dissection is selected in the back wall that separates it into two layers. After resection of the entire cyst anteriorly and the mucosal layer posteriorly, the outer wall remains adherent to the portal vein and hepatic artery. (From Lilly[21] with permission of the author.)

postoperatively is individualized on the basis of (1) the level and size of the anastomosis, (2) the degree of scarring, and (3) the early postoperative course. Although some experts would not stent these anastomoses, we recommend stenting to allow radiographical assessment of the anastomosis in the early postoperative period and to facilitate management if a bile leak or cholangitis occurs.

Management of the rare type II choledochal cysts is simple and entails ligation of the base of the stalk of the diverticulum and cholecystectomy. If the neck of the diverticulum is broad, however, care must be exercised in reconstructing the duct over a T tube that exits the duct via a separate choledochotomy. Choledochoceles are generally lined with duodenal mucosa and, as such, are not at risk for malignant degeneration as are the other types of choledochal cysts. Excision of the cyst is not mandated for this reason. Similarly, these cysts generally present as duodenal obstruction, and not biliary obstruction, and biliary diversion is seldom required. Simple drainage of the cyst by a long sphincteroplasty (internal marsupialization of the cyst), taking care to avoid the pancreatic duct, carries minimal risk and effectively prevents distention and compression of the duodenal lumen. If biliary obstruction is a problem and pancreatitis has occurred preoperatively, we recommend dividing the common duct above the cyst, oversewing the distal cut end and performing a Roux-en-Y choledochojejunostomy. This procedure is safer than total excision with reimplantation of the common and pancreatic ducts.

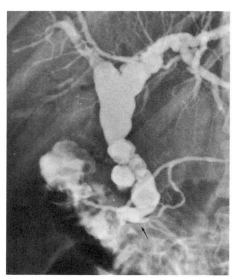

Fig 23–14.—Fusiform dilatation of the right, left, and common hepatic ducts. Note the multiple stones in the common bile duct and the anomalous junction of the biliary and pancreatic ducts *(arrow)*.

As with congenital intrahepatic ductal cysts, choledochal cysts are also premalignant lesions. Yamaguchi[15] noted 46 cases of biliary carcinomas among the 1,433 cases in his collected series, an incidence of 3.2%. Twelve of these cases (27%) were in men, and 33 were in women (73%). His data and other recent analyses suggest that the prevalence of malignant degeneration increases with age. This complication of choledochal cysts has been used as a strong argument for resection.

ACQUIRED AND COMBINED DUCTAL CYSTS

As mentioned above, extrahepatic cysts may also be acquired and may be found in combination with intrahepatic cysts (Longmire's types IV and V). Acquired extrahepatic cysts may be the result of distal obstructions from stones, tumors, chronic pancreatitis, or ampullary stenosis. The lack of intrahepatic ductal dilatation in some cases may be caused by secondary biliary cirrhosis. Presentation, diagnosis, and management of these lesions have been discussed in separate chapters.

Whether combined intrahepatic and extrahepatic cysts are a manifestation of Caroli's disease or of choledochal cysts is a matter of conjecture. The overlap in these two entities, of course, suggests that they may be related. As described by Longmire,[11] combined cysts may be saccular or fusiform (Figs 23–8, 23–13, and 23–14). Whether all of these lesions are congenital or some are acquired, however, is not known. In general, management of these combined lesions should follow the principles outlined above for treating intrahepatic ductal cysts and choledochal cysts. Extrahepatic cysts should be excised, and management of intrahepatic cysts will be dependent on whether they are bilateral and on the degree of cirrhosis.

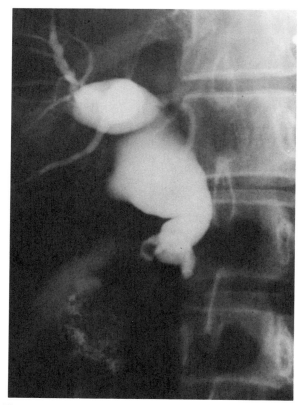

Fig 23–13.—Congenital saccular choledochal cyst with stones distally and an associated saccular dilatation of the right intrahepatic duct.

REFERENCES

1. Herman R.E.: Liver cysts, in Cameron J.L. (ed.): *Current Surgical Therapy*. Philadelphia, B.C. Decker, Inc., 1984, pp. 156–160.
2. Hadad A.R., Westbrook K.C., Graham G.G., et al.: Symptomatic nonparasitic liver cysts. *Am. J. Surg.* 134:739, 1977.
3. Dagher F.J.: Echinococcal liver disease, in Shackelford R.T., Zuidema G.D. (eds.): *Surgery of the Alimentary Tract*, ed. 2. Philadelphia, W.B. Saunders Co., 1983, pp. 498–512.
4. Saimot A.G., Meulemans A., Cremieux A.C., et al.: Albendazole as a potential treatment for human hydatidosis. *Lancet* 2:652, 1983.
5. Langer J.C., Rose D.B., Keystone, J.S., et al.: Diagnosis and management of hydatid disease of the liver. A 15-year North American experience. *Ann. Surg.* 199:412, 1984.
6. Pitt H.A.: Liver abscess, in Shackelford R.T., Zuidema G.D. (eds.): *Surgery of the Alimentary Tract*, ed. 2. Philadelphia, W.B., Saunders Co., 1983, pp. 465–497.
7. Ochsner A., DeBakey M., Murray S.: Pyogenic abscess of the liver. *Am. J. Surg.* 40:292, 1938.
8. Conter R.L., Pitt H.A., Tompkins R.K., Longmire W.P. Jr.: Differentiation of pyogenic from amebic liver abscesses. *Surg. Gynecol. Obstet.*, in press.
9. Balasegaram M.: Management of hepatic abscess. *Curr. Probl. Surg.* 18:282, 1981.
10. Caroli J., Soupalt R., Kossakowski J., Plocker L., et al.: La dilatation polycystique congenitale des voies biliaries intrahepatiques. Essai del classification. *Sem. Hop. Paris* 34:488, 1958.
11. Longmire W.P. Jr., Mandiola S.A., Gordon H.E.: Congenital cystic disease of the liver and biliary system. *Ann. Surg.* 174:711, 1971.
12. Tompkins R.K., Pitt H.A.: Surgical management of benign lesions of the bile ducts. *Curr. Probl. Surg.* 19:321, 1982.
13. Dayton M.T., Longmire W.P. Jr., Tompkins R.K.: Caroli's disease: A premalignant condition? *Am. J. Surg.* 145:41, 1983.
14. Alonso-Lej F., Rever W.B., Pessagno D.J.: Congenital choledochal cyst, with a report of 2, and an analysis of 94 cases. *Int. Abstr. Surg.* 108:1, 1959.
15. Yamaguchi M.: Congenital choledochal cyst: Analysis of 1,433 patients in the Japanese literature. *Am. J. Surg.* 140:653, 1980.
16. Flanigan D.P.: Biliary cysts. *Ann. Surg.* 182:635, 1975.
17. Babbitt D.P.: Congenital choledochal cysts. New etiological concept based on anomalous relationships of the common bile duct and pancreatic bulb. *Ann. Radiol.* 12:231, 1969.
18. Arima E., Hachinen A.: Congenital biliary tract dilatation and anomalous junction of the pancreatico-biliary ductal system. *J. Pediatr. Surg.* 14:9, 1979.
19. Miyano T., Suruga K., Suda K.: Abnormal choledocho-pancreatico ductal junction related to the etiology of infantile obstructive jaundice diseases. *J. Pediatr. Surg.* 14:16, 1979.
20. Caroli J., Marcoulides, G.: Study of the pathogenesis of congenital dilatation of the common bile duct. *Arch. Med.* 42:1045–1060, 1953.
21. Klotz D., Cohn B.D., Kottmeier P.K.: Choledochal cysts. Diagnostic and therapeutic problems. *J. Pediatr. Surg.* 8:271, 1973.
22. Lilly J.R.: The surgical treatment of choledochal cyst. *Surg. Gynecol. Obstet.* 149:36, 1979.

24

Cancer of the Gallbladder and Biliary Tree

RONALD K. TOMPKINS, M.D., M.SC., F.A.C.S.

GALLBLADDER

Malignant tumors of the gallbladder are notoriously poorly diagnosed and, when found, very often untreatable for cure. The very best results in these dismal tumors have been reported in those few patients in whom the cancer was an incidental finding by the pathologist after cholecystectomy for cholelithiasis.

Natural History

De Stoll[1] is reported to have made the first description of carcinoma of the gallbladder in 1777. The incidence of the disease has been reported to be 0.4% of all gallbladder operations done in Sweden.[2] If this figure were applied to the estimated 500,000 cholecystectomies done annually in the United States, about 2,000 cases of gallbladder cancer would be discovered each year.

Patients with gallbladder carcinoma are most likely to be in the seventh decade of life and are six times more likely to be female. Ninety-eight percent of these patients have associated gallstones.

Five-year survival rates are 3% or less.[3] The median survival in this series was 5.2 months. The stage of the disease has a definite influence on the postoperative survival rate (see Treatment) (Fig 24–1).

Gallbladder cancer spreads initially by direct extension into the liver rather than by hematogenous routes. Its early spread into regional lymphatics is along the cystic duct node to lower bile duct and superior and posterior pancreatoduodenal nodes. The hepatic artery nodes do not connect with gallbladder lymphatics and, like the celiac and superior mesenteric nodes, are involved only in the later states of the disease.[4]

Etiology

While the exact cause of gallbladder cancer is not known, there are several factors which have been implicated in the causation of the disease.

GALLSTONES.—It has been suggested that chronic irritation by gallstones predisposes to malignant degeneration of the gallbladder. Support for this theory comes from data collected by Diehl,[5] which has shown a decrease in the total deaths from gallbladder cancer since 1968 along with a decrease in crude mortality rates. This has been associated with a rise, during the same period, in the rate of cholecystectomies and suggests that the risk of dying of gallbladder cancer

may have been lowered by increasing the rate of removal of the gallbladder. This relationship has been most prominent in white females. There is no proof that these two observations are linked, however, and the association may be coincidental.

In a recent retrospective, case-control study, Diehl[6] found that the odds ratios (closely related to relative risk) for gallbladder cancer are directly related to size of gallstones. In patients with gallstones less than 1.0 cm, the odds ratio was 1.0. For gallstone size of 2.0–2.9 cm, the odds ratio was 2.4, and for stones greater than 3.0 cm, the odds ratio was 10.1. If this information is confirmed, it may provide another incentive for removing gallstones while they are still small.

RACIAL INFLUENCES.—Gallbladder cancer rates are lowest for American blacks. Whites in the United States have a 50% higher incidence of gallbladder cancer than blacks. The Southwestern American Indians have a rate of gallbladder cancer of 21.1/100,000/year—a rate twice that of Spanish Americans and 15 times that of Caucasians living in the same area.

CARCINOGENS.—As yet, no human carcinogens have been identified for the production of gallbladder cancer. Animal research has shown that dimethylnitrosamine given to hamsters with cholesterol pellets implanted in their gallbladders would result in cancer of the gallbladder. Chemical analogues of bile salts, α-toxin B_1, and other chemical agents have been shown to induce carcinoma in animal gallbladders. Speculation still exists on the roles of other factors such as bacteria, radiation, and industrial toxins.

Clinical Presentation and Evaluation

In the early stages, gallbladder cancer may cause no symptoms that are distinct from those associated with cholelithiasis. In the later stages, acute cholecystitis with or without jaundice is a common form of presentation. The very far advanced case may present with a palpable mass in the presence of pain and jaundice.

Preoperative evaluation by ultrasound may yield only gallstones in a thickened gallbladder. CT scans usually do not show a definite tumor pattern. Cholangiograms done percutaneously or endoscopically in the jaundiced patient will often show a lesion consistent with tumor obstruction or extrinsic pressure on the biliary ducts.

The definitive diagnosis is often made at operation and often has been unsuspected preoperatively.

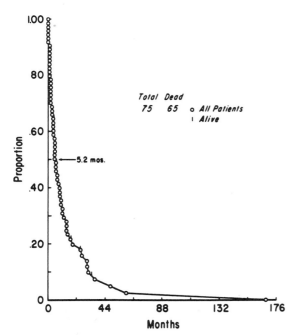

Fig 24–1.—Survival curve from diagnosis of gallbladder cancer—all patients. (From Perpetuo M.D., Valdivieso M., Heilbrun L.K., et al.: Natural history study of gallbladder cancer. *Cancer* 42:330, 1978. Used by permission.)

Treatment

In a review of the literature, Nevin and associates[7] found that two thirds of patients with gallbladder cancer had unresectable lesions at the time of operation. Nevin et al. retrospectively classified 399 patients with gallbladder cancers into five stages and analyzed their survival based on the stage (Fig 24–2). Stage I lesions were intramucosal only, and the five-year survival was 100% after cholecystectomy alone. Stage II lesions involved mucosa and muscularis, and the five-year survival rate was also 100% after cholecystectomy. Stage III lesions involved all three layers of the gallbladder, and survival rates following operation were 40.6% (1 year); 29.7% (2 years); 14.3% (3 years); 8.8% (4 years); and 6.6% (5 years). Stage IV tumors involved all layers of the gallbladder and the cystic lymph node, and three patients with this lesion all survived five years after operation. Stage V malignancies involved all areas of stage IV plus extension or metastasis to the liver or other organ. None of the 265 patients with this stage lesion survived to two years.

Bergdahl[8] divided 32 patients with microscopic gallbladder cancers found after cholecystectomy into two groups. Group A (11 patients) had lesions confined to mucosa and submucosa (Nevin's stage II). Group B (21 patients) had lesions involving the entire thickness of the gallbladder wall. Group B patients had an operative mortality of 14.3% including reoperations (one patient had a right hepatic lobectomy), and all were dead of carcinoma within two years and five months (Fig 24–3). Group A patients had a 63.6% five-year survival and a 45.5% ten-year survival. Thus, it is clear that if the lesion is able to be completely resected, the chance of survival is much improved. Palliative measures are technically difficult to perform in most advanced cases because of the bulk of the tumor and many of these patients are better managed by radiologic or endoscopic insertion of biliary stents for decompression.

This author's approach to the surgical management of gallbladder cancer is to begin by opening every gallbladder removed for stones and examining their linings in the operating room. A frozen section is requested on any suspicious-looking area. If an unsuspected carcinoma is found, a wide excision of gallbladder bed in the liver is done, along with a regional lymphadenectomy. If the lesion is so small as to be found only on microscopic examination some days after the operation, serious consideration must be given as to whether reoperation should be carried out. The data would suggest that for stage I and II lesions cholecystectomy alone is sufficient. For lesions beyond those stages, reoperation for wedge resection of the liver and lymphadenectomy should be urged.

Radical resections of the liver have not been shown to be beneficial over wedge resection of the gallbladder fossa and regional lymphadenectomy.[9] In more advanced lesions that cannot be resected, palliative decompressions are performed, either at operation or postoperatively, and the radiation and medical oncologists are consulted regarding further therapy.

Adjunctive Therapy

The most common type of gallbladder cancer is adenocarcinoma. Occasional cases of squamous cell carcinoma, either alone or combined with adenocarcinoma, have been found. There are reports of longer survival than nontreated patients

Stage	No. of patients	1	2	3	4	5
I	8					8
II	32					32
III	91	37	27	13	8	6
IV	3					3
V	265	265				

(header: Survival in years)

Fig 24–2.—Survival of gallbladder cancer patients by extent of lesion. (From Nevin J.E., Moran T.J., Kay S. et al.: Carcinoma of the gallbladder. *Cancer* 37:141, 1976. Used by permission.)

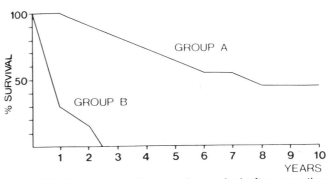

Fig 24–3.—Marked difference in survival after operation for gallbladder cancer is related to extension of lesion. (From Bergdahl L.: Gallbladder carcinoma first diagnosed at microscopic examination of gallbladder removed for presumed benign disease. *Ann. Surg.* 191:19, 1980. Used by permission.)

in those with advanced disease who receive chemotherapy, radiation therapy, or a combination. There are no good data to support adjunctive therapy in those patients whose tumors have been completely removed. Overall, there is no strong evidence that postoperative chemotherapy and/or radiation therapy have an effect on the prognosis of gallbladder cancer.

CARCINOMA OF THE CYSTIC DUCT

This rare lesion will doubtless be found at operation for an obstructed gallbladder or discovered incidentally in the cholecystectomy specimen. When advanced, it may not be discernible from carcinoma of the gallbladder or bile duct on a gross examination basis. The criteria for diagnosis of the lesion are (1) carcinomatous growth restricted to the cystic duct, and (2) absence of neoplasia in the gallbladder or hepatic or common ducts.

A review of 25 cases by Nishimura et al.[10] indicated that over half of the patients had undergone cholecystectomy and removal of the entire cystic duct. Additional resection of the common duct was done in 32% of the cases; 16% of the cases were diagnosed at autopsy. The lesions ranged from 0.4 cm to 3.2 cm, with an average of 1.3 cm.

The survival figures are not clearly delineated in the literature, but one third of the collected patients were alive 12 to 52 months postoperatively.

Gallstones were present in only 33% of the cases. Over 80% of the patients presented with right upper quadrant pain and 41% had a palpable mass.

The treatment of choice appears to be complete surgical removal of the gallbladder, cystic duct, and periductal lymphatics for the smaller localized lesions. If larger lesions involve the adjacent bile duct, radical resection of the duct and periductal tissue is included in the operative procedure. There are no data to support adjunctive therapy in these patients.

CANCER OF THE EXTRAHEPATIC BILE DUCTS

Introduction

Intrahepatic bile duct carcinoma, or cholangiocarcinoma, is beyond the realm of surgical management. The surgeon is called on most often to differentiate this lesion from extrahepatic bile duct cancer and, when the latter is confirmed, to decide on the best course of therapy. These often small lesions involve the adjacent major vascular structures early in their course and, hence, are often unresectable for cure. These lesions are being more frequently diagnosed and referred for treatment, probably due to better technology such as transhepatic cholangiography with the thin needle and the endoscopic retrograde cholangiogram (ERC). Some authorities have suspected that the incidence of the disease itself is on the rise.

Natural History

Clinically the extrahepatic bile duct cancers differ in several respects from gallbladder cancer. In the former, males are afflicted as often as females. Bile duct cancer is associated with gallstones in only 10%–30% of cases. The course of pa-

tients operated on for bile duct cancers is longer than that of patients with gallbladder cancer.

Etiology

While the exact cause of bile duct cancer is unknown, there are relationships between the disease and exposure to toxins and between associated diseases, such as ulcerative colitis and biliary tract malignancy. Aflatoxins have been shown to cause bile duct tumors in animals. Infestation with *Clonorchis sinensis* is found more frequently in Oriental patients with cholangiocarcinomas than in matched controls. Scattered reports of bile duct carcinomas in patients taking oral contraceptive steroids or anabolic steroids have stirred speculation on the role of these agents in development of bile duct cancers.

One of the strongest associations is that between ulcerative colitis and bile duct cancer. It has been shown that bile duct cancer occurs earlier in ulcerative colitis patients than in the normal population, and prior removal of the colon or successful medical management of the colitis does not prevent later occurrence of bile duct cancer. Finally, the tumors seem more aggressive when they arise in ulcerative colitis patients.

Chronic typhoid carriers died of hepatobiliary cancer six times more frequently than their matched controls in a retrospective study reported from New York.[11]

Cystic dilatation of the biliary tract has been found to be associated with development of bile duct cancer. Choledochal cyst has long been recognized to be a risk factor for carcinoma, while malignancy is rarely found in nonparasitic cysts of the liver or in polycystic liver disease. Bloustein[12] has analyzed these associations and found the risk of carcinoma to be 1% in congenital hepatic fibrosis, 4% in choledochal cysts, and 7% in congenital cystic dilatation of the intrahepatic ducts (Caroli's disease). Dayton and associates[13] reported four cases of carcinoma occurring in Caroli's disease and reviewed an additional 138 cases of Caroli's disease from the literature. The incidence of carcinoma was found to be 7% in that review also.

Anatomical Site

Longmire[14] has suggested the categorization of extrahepatic bile duct cancers into three anatomical regions. The upper third extends from the undersurface of the liver down to the junction of the cystic duct with the common hepatic duct, and this includes the bifurcation of the right and left hepatic ducts. The middle third is that portion of the bile duct which extends from the junction of the cystic and common hepatic duct down to the superior border of the pancreas. The lower third is the intrapancreatic portion of the bile duct. Ampullary tumors are not included as lower third bile duct lesions.

In our series of 96 patients at U.C.L.A.,[15] 49% of patients had upper third lesions, 25% had middle third lesions, and 19% of the lesions were in the lower third (Fig 24–4). Seven percent of the tumors were diffuse in the extrahepatic system, with multiple sites of tumor being identified. Operative cholangioscopy has been of great value in identifying these multicentric lesions.[16]

Clinical Presentation

Since pain is infrequently associated with bile duct cancer, most patients are seen first because of the onset of jaundice.

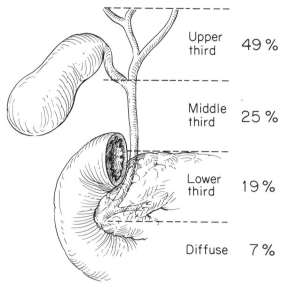

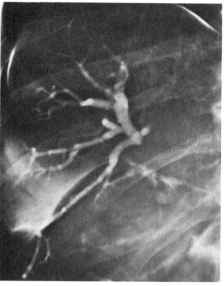

Fig 24–4.—Anatomical location of bile duct tumors in 96 patients treated at UCLA. (From Tompkins R.K., Thomas D., Wile A., et al.: Prognostic factors in bile duct carcinoma. *Ann. Surg.* 194:477, 1981. Used by permission.)

Fig 24–5.—Demonstration of proximal bile duct cancer by percutaneous "skinny" needle transhepatic cholangiography.

In our experience, 91% of patients have had serum bilirubin levels over 2.0 mg/dl, and 50% were greater than 13.0 mg/dl.[15] Alkaline phosphatase and transferase levels in the serum are uniformly elevated in these patients. Weight loss, pruritus, steatorrhea, and anemia are seen with varying frequency, and cholangitis is a distinct problem in some of these patients. The average age of the patient at presentation is 60 years.

Examination of the patient at presentation usually reveals, in addition to the icterus, the presence of an enlarged and occasionally mildly tender liver. Ascites is a grave sign, as is the presence of muscle wasting.

The patients with upper third lesions presented for definitive treatment on an average of 6.1 months after the onset of symptoms. This delay was almost twice that of the 3.2 months observed in patients with lower third bile duct lesions. Reasons for the delay in definitive management of the upper third lesion patients are not clear, but it is my opinion that many of these patients' tumors arise in the right or left hepatic duct initially and spread to the bifurcation area slowly, so that early symptoms are not associated with jaundice but may consist only of mild discomfort, itching, and be associated with only a mild elevation of the alkaline phosphatase.

Diagnostic Tests

In addition to the blood chemistry evaluation, definitive preoperative diagnosis can be made by radiologic means.

The most commonly utilized radiologic tests in evaluating the jaundiced patient are ultrasound, CT scanning, and cholangiography. The order of preference in my practice is to evaluate the liver, pancreas, and biliary system initially by ultrasound. If the biliary ducts are dilated in the intrahepatic portion, then a thin-needle transhepatic cholangiogram (THC) is performed (Fig 24–5). This is usually the test which definitely diagnoses the lesion. Occasionally, endoscopic retrograde cholangiopancreatography (ERCP) is utilized to visual-

ize the biliary system as well as to evaluate the ampullary region and the pancreatic duct (Fig 24–6).

The use of the CT scan is reserved for those cases in which the diagnosis is not clear by the above tests or in which additional evaluation of the pancreas or liver is needed. It is not routinely used in the work-up of these patients.

Preoperative attempts to establish a tissue diagnosis by means of fine-needle-guided percutaneous aspiration or by cytology on the bile obtained by percutaneous puncture or endoscopic cannulation of the bile duct have been reported. Success rates for these preoperative diagnostic efforts have been less than 50%.

Some authors have proposed an extensive preoperative work-up to assess resectability and thus exclude some patients from operation. Blumgart et al.[17] utilized percutaneous cholangiography to assess the extent of the biliary lesion and, if

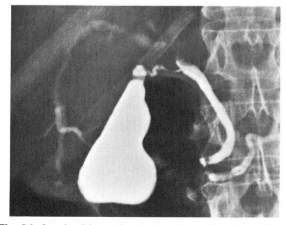

Fig 24–6.—In this patient a transhepatic cholangiogram had been unsuccessful and endoscopic retrograde cholangiogram has demonstrated the proximal bile duct lesion.

favorable, went on to study the patients with selective celiac and superior mesenteric arteriograms with indirect portography. In a series of 94 patients, angiography was done in 67. Forty-three of these (64%) were judged to have vessel involvement by tumor, most often the portal vein.

Operative Treatment

Because the practicing community surgeon sees so few of these patients in his career, the treatment has been confusing. Half of the patients in our series had had one or two previous operations before the definitive procedure was carried out at U.C.L.A. A total of 171 operations were done in 95 patients. Of the 95 definitive operations performed, 50 were for resection of the tumor and 45 for palliative purposes.

Upper third lesions were resected in 47% of cases with reconstruction by biliary-enteric anastomosis. Almost routinely, this anastomosis is a Roux-en-Y hepaticojejunostomy. The remaining 53% of patients received palliation by dilatation of the tumor and placement of indwelling tubes to maintain biliary patency. In the past eight to ten years these tubes have been of the transhepatic U or J type, which can be changed as necessary without need for anesthesia or reoperation. We recommend the use of a Roux-en-Y choledochojejunostomy for exiting the distal end of the U tube rather than simply bringing the tube out the side of the common duct to the skin. The latter procedure leads to a high rate of bile leak owing to the slow formation of fibrous tracts around silastic tubes and also to migration of the tube distally, allowing some holes to exit the duct.

Middle third lesions were resectable in 67% of the patients, with 10% undergoing Whipple procedures and the remainder having resection and biliary-enteric anastomosis; 33% of the patients had intubation for palliation.

Lower third lesions were resected in 71% of patients by Whipple procedure. The remaining 29% had palliative bypass with biliary-enteric anastomoses.

All patients with diffuse tumors had palliation by intubation.

Results of Operation

The overall 30-day postoperative mortality was 12%. The upper third lesion patients had the highest operative mortality: 23% for the resected patients and 16% for the palliative procedures.

There was no mortality in patients with middle third lesions. The operative mortality in the lower third lesion patients was 10% for the resections and zero for the palliative procedures.

Survival

The cumulative postoperative survival rate for the entire series of patients was 50% at nine months and 8% at five years (Fig 24–7).

The upper third lesion patients had the poorest survival of the three groups, with 50% dead at 8.9 months and all dead by 4.5 years. A few patients with resected upper third lesions lived a few months longer than those who had palliation but the difference was not significant.

Patients with middle third lesions had cumulative survival rates of 50% at 10.1 months and 12% at 5 years. Lower third

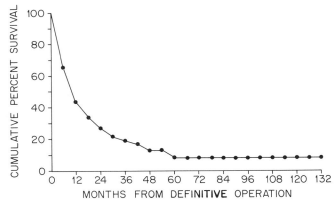

Fig 24–7.—Cumulative survival after operation in 96 patients treated at UCLA. (From Tompkins R.K., Thomas D., Wile A., et al.: Prognostic factors in bile duct carcinoma. *Ann. Surg.* 194:477, 1981. Used by permission.)

lesion patients had the best cumulative survival, with 50% still alive at 21.1 months and 28% surviving at five years (Fig 24–8).

The type of histology of the tumors also seemed to influence survival, with patients having papillary tumors having the best survival of the groups. The difference between the histologic groups was not significant, however (Figs 24–9,A and B, and Fig 24–10).

Postoperative Treatment

The role of adjunctive therapy in patients who have undergone resection of their tumors is not clear. Our tendency is not to treat patients with radiation therapy or chemotherapy after resection of their tumors.

It is more difficult to know the place of adjunctive radiation or chemotherapy in those patients whose tumors have been intubated or bypassed for palliation.

In the U.C.L.A. series of 96 patients, 68% of the patients received no postoperative adjunctive therapy; 19% received chemotherapy only; 8% received radiation therapy; and 5% received a combination of both. Thus, the numbers of pa-

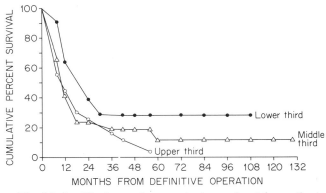

Fig 24–8.—Postoperative survival was best for patients with lower third of bile duct tumors and poorest for those with tumors in the proximal one-third. (From Tompkins R.K., Thomas D., Wile A., et al.: Prognostic factors in bile duct carcinoma. *Ann. Surg.* 194:477, 1981. Used by permission.)

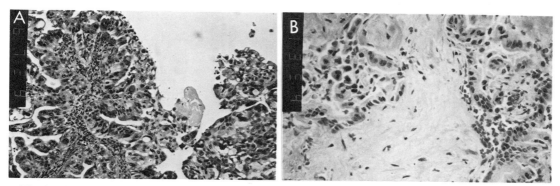

Fig 24–9.—**A,** histologic section of papillary type of bile duct tumor. **B,** histologic section of a sclerosing type of bile duct tumor.

tients receiving adjunctive therapy are not great enough to derive statistical information regarding the benefits or lack of benefits of treatment. Table 24–1 outlines the cases in which follow-up was available and compares their survival to patients not treated who had similar operations.

Other authors, notably Terblanche,[18] have recommended treating all proximal third cancers by U-tube intubation and radiotherapy. Others, such as Cameron and co-workers,[19] have utilized silastic stent tubes after resection as well as for palliation and followed up with either external radiation or a combination of external radiation with intraluminal radiation using iridium-192 seeds. Results in both of these series have been marked by occasional long-term survivals, but the overall figures are similar to those which we have reported.

A study carried out at the National Cancer Institute in dogs suggests that intraoperative radiation may not be well tolerated by the biliary tract.[20] Animals received laparotomy and dose levels of 2,000, 3,000, and 4,500 rad to a 5-cm-diameter circle, with the common duct as its center; 18-month follow-up was used. All animals surviving developed biliary cirrhosis. Ductal fibrosis, duodenal fibrosis, and biliary obstruction were seen in all animals. Consideration of radiation to the bile ducts during operation should be evaluated with these studies firmly in mind.

Recommendations for Treatment

Our approach to extrahepatic bile duct cancer is dependent on the anatomic region in which the tumor is found. In upper third lesions, unless the tumor is clearly localized and is resectable for cure, intubation with a transhepatic silastic tube is done. Usually a 12 F or 14 F tube is utilized. It is not necessary, and indeed may be undesirable, to attempt intubation of both right and left sides of the intrahepatic biliary system.[21] We have found that, most often, one or another main duct branch is virtually plugged (probably the side of origin of the tumor), and the other side is the only one which can be safely dilated. Enthusiastic dilation of these tumors may result in brisk bleeding due to injury of adjacent portal vein branches and hence should be avoided.

Recently, Blumgart et al.[17] reported on a large series of patients with proximal third tumors. From a group of 94 patients, 30 (32%) had preoperative tests suggesting resectability. At operation, only 18 of these patients (19% of total group) actually underwent a presumed curative resection. Six of these resections involved the bile ducts only, but the additional 12 required hepatic resections to clear the tumor. Nine of these were extended right hepatectomies, and three were left hepatectomies. Nine of the twelve resections required repair of the portal veins. The six patients who had

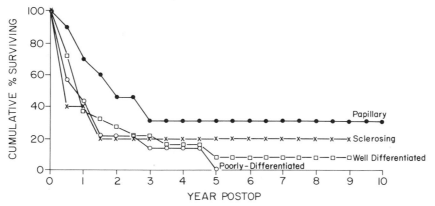

Fig 24–10.—Survival rates are best for patients who have the papillary (or exophytic) type of bile duct cancer. (From Tompkins R.K., Thomas D., Wile A., et al.: Prognostic factors in bile duct carcinoma. *Ann. Surg.* 194:477, 1981. Used by permission.)

TABLE 24–1.—SURVIVAL OF BILE DUCT CANCER PATIENTS RELATED
TO POSTOPERATIVE THERAPY

OPERATION	NO P.O. RX		CHEMOTHERAPY		RADIATION		COMBINATION	
	# Pts.	Mo.	# Pts.	Mo.	# Pts.	Mo.	# Pts.	Mo.
Intubation	22	9.8	6	18.6	2	24	—	—
Choledochojejunostomy	19	14.3	5	10.5	3	21	3	31.5
Cholangiojejunostomy	8	3.8	—	—	—	—	—	—
Whipple	7	21.0	2	18.0	1	42	1	9

local bile duct resections had no mortality, while two of the 12 hepatic resections died within 30 days (16.7%). One additional hepatic resection patient died after nine weeks of sepsis. The mean survival of all of the 15 surviving resected patients was 17 months, the longest survivor living 58 months.

The aggressive approach of Blumgart et al. to resection of these tumors will require longer follow-up to evaluate.

The U.C.L.A. approach to middle third and distal third cancers has been aggressive resection, unless they involve adjacent vascular structures. The Whipple procedure is most often necessary in the lower third lesions. In our hands this has been a low-risk procedure with no operative or postoperative mortality in the past ten years or so. There is no question that postoperative survival is greatest in those patients who have had their tumors resected (Fig 24–11). Surgical resection also offers the only chance for cure of these lesions.

Summary

Although extrahepatic bile duct cancer is infrequently seen by the average surgeon, there are increasing numbers of patients being diagnosed and referred for treatment to centers specializing in management of biliary tract lesions. Aggressive but thoughtful evaluation and operative therapy are indicated in these patients, especially those with lesions in the middle or lower third of the biliary tract.

Future advances in the management of these tumors will depend not only on earlier diagnosis by the rapidly improving technologies being utilized in liver and biliary tract diseases, but also on the more accurate preoperative and operative

staging of these lesions and the development of better non-surgical, adjuvant therapies for those patients whose lesions cannot be surgically removed.

REFERENCES

1. De Stoll M.: Rationis medendi in nosocomio practico vindobonensi. Quoted in Rolleston H.D., McNee J.S.: *Disease of the Liver, Gallbladder and Bile Ducts*, ed. 3. London, Macmillan, 1929, p. 691.
2. Wenckert A., Robertson B.: The natural course of gallbladder disease: Eleven year review of 781 non-operated cases. *Gastroenterology* 50:376, 1966.
3. Perpetuo M.D.C.M.O., Valdivieso M., Heilbrun L.K., et al.: Natural history study of gallbladder cancer. *Cancer* 42:330, 1978.
4. Fahim R.N., McDonald J.R., Richards J.C., et al.: Carcinoma of the gallbladder: A study of its modes of spread. *Ann. Surg.* 156:114, 1962.
5. Diehl A.K.: Epidemiology of gallbladder cancer: A synthesis of recent data. *J.N.C.I.* 65:1209, 1980.
6. Diehl A.K.: Gallstone size and the risk of gallbladder cancer. *J.A.M.A.* 250:2323–2326, 1983.
7. Nevin J.E., Moran T.J., Kay S., et al.: Carcinoma of the gallbladder. *Cancer* 37:141, 1976.
8. Bergdahl L.: Gallbladder carcinoma first diagnosed at microscopic examination of gallbladder removed for presumed benign disease. *Ann. Surg.* 191:19, 1980.
9. Adson M.A.: Carcinoma of the gallbladder, in Moody F.G. (ed.): *Advances in Diagnosis and Surgical Treatment of Biliary Tract Disease*. New York, Masson Publishing USA, 1983, pp. 93–101.
10. Nishimura A., Mayama S., Nakano K., et al.: Carcinoma of the cystic duct: Case report. *Jpn. J. Surg.* 5:109, 1975.
11. Welton J.C., Marr J.S., Friedman S.M.: Association between hepatobiliary cancer and typhoid carrier state. *Lancet* 1:791, 1979.
12. Bloustein P.A.: Association of carcinoma with congenital cystic conditions of the liver and bile ducts. *Am. J. Gastroenterol.* 67:40, 1977.
13. Dayton M., Longmire W.P. Jr., Tompkins R.K.: Is Caroli's disease a premalignant condition? *Am. J. Surg.* 145:41, 1983.
14. Longmire W.P. Jr.: Tumors of the extrahepatic biliary radicles, *Curr. Probl. Cancer* 1:1, 1976.
15. Tompkins R.K., Thomas D., Wile A., et al.: Prognostic factors in bile duct carcinoma. *Ann. Surg.* 194:477, 1981.
16. Tompkins R.K., Johnson J., Storm F.K., et al.: Operative endoscopy in the management of biliary tract neoplasms. *Am. J. Surg.* 132:174, 1976.
17. Blumgart L.H., Hadjis N.S., Benjamin I.S., et al.: Surgical approaches to cholangiocarcinoma at confluence of hepatic ducts, *Lancet* 1:66–70, 1984.
18. Terblanche J.: Carcinoma of the proximal extrahepatic biliary tree—definitive and palliative treatment. *Surg. Annu.* 11:249–265, 1979.
19. Cameron J.L., Broe P., Zuidema G.D.: Proximal bile duct tumors. *Ann. Surg.* 196:412–419, 1982.
20. Sindelar W.F., Tepper J., Travis E.L.: Tolerance of bile duct to intraoperative irradiation. *Surgery* 92:533–540, 1982.
21. Longmire W.P. Jr., Tompkins R.K.: Lesions of the segmental and lobar hepatic ducts. *Ann. Surg.* 182:478–495, 1975.

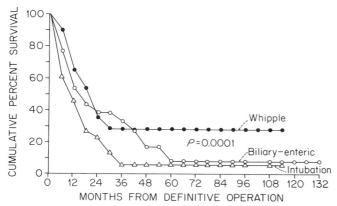

Fig 24–11.—The ability to resect bile duct cancers by Whipple's procedure significantly improved survival rates. (From Tompkins R.K., Thomas D., Wile A., et al.: Prognostic factors in bile duct carcinoma. *Ann. Surg.* 194:477, 1981. Used by permission.)

25

Biliary Sepsis and Suppurative Cholangitis

JOHN L. CAMERON, M.D.
HENRY A. PITT, M.D.

CHOLANGITIS is derived from the Greek words "chole," meaning bile, and "angeion," meaning vessel. Thus, the literal meaning of cholangitis is inflammation of a bile vesssel or bile duct. More accurately, however, cholangitis is an infection of the bile within the biliary ductal system.

The clinical entity of cholangitis has been recognized for just over 100 years. Charcot[1] in 1877 provided the first accurate and detailed description of cholangitis. He stated in his original paper that "intermittent hepatic fever" developed secondary to ". . . stagnant bile." Interestingly, he further remarked that stones, benign strictures, and malignancies were responsible for this clinical syndrome, a statement that has remained accurate to the present. Since Charcot's initial description, the triad of intermittent chills and fever, jaundice, and abdominal pain has become widely recognized as the hallmark of cholangitis. Cholangitis is a bacterial infection, in this country invariably associated with bile duct pathology producing some degree of biliary obstruction. Bacteria may be present in the biliary tree in large numbers in the absence of obstructive pathology. In this situation, however, the patient is asymptomatic and has no clinical signs of infection. Despite the time since the clinical entity of cholangitis was so accurately described by Charcot and the amount of clinical and experimental data accumulated, the source of the bacteria within the biliary tree is still unknown. Although the organisms are usually bowel organisms, the pathway by which they reach the biliary tree is still in question. There is clinical and experimental evidence to support the blood-borne, ascending biliary tree, and lymphatic pathways as the source of the biliary tree bacteria, but no conclusive evidence supports any of these possible routes.

What was probably the first attempt at surgical management of acute cholangitis was carried out by Rogers[2] in 1903. He reported removing stones from the common duct and draining the biliary tree with a glass tube in a patient who had cholangitis. The patient died, however, in the immediate postoperative period. The modern era of treatment of cholangitis began with the introduction of antibiotics. Although the management of cholangitis is still somewhat controversial, most physicians feel that the initial therapy should be with antibiotics. As with many disorders, there are all degrees of severity of bacterial cholangitis. In some instances the entity may be so mild and of such short duration that the episode resolves without the patient's seeking medical aid. At the opposite end of the spectrum is the patient who presents moribund, with a picture of septic shock and who, at the time of surgery or autopsy, is found to have gross pus under pressure in the bile ducts. These last patients have been categorized as having acute suppurative cholangitis. In all probability, however, this just represents one end of the particularly broad spectrum of pathology that cholangitis presents.

This chapter deals with the clinical presentation, diagnosis, and useful laboratory and radiographic tests for the work-up and initial management of patients with cholangitis. A discussion of the pathogenesis, treatment, and complications of cholangitis is also included, with a separate section on the most severe form of this bacterial disease, acute suppurative (or "toxic") cholangitis.

CLINICAL PRESENTATION

The clinical presentation of a patient with cholangitis can be quite variable. Not all patients with cholangitis present with the triad of fever and chills, jaundice, and abdominal pain, and not all patients with this triad have cholangitis. Pancreatitis, acute cholecystitis, pyelonephritis, or indeed sepsis from a variety of sources may at times present with fever and chills, jaundice, and some degree of abdominal pain. In addition, many patients with cholangitis present without one or more of the triad that is classically seen with cholangitis. Thus, as Rogers[2] pointed out in 1903, "This condition . . . is of considerable importance on account of the very great difficulty of diagnosis . . ." This difficulty in diagnosis is pointed out in a series of 180 hospitalized patients with the clinical diagnosis of cholangitis seen at The Johns Hopkins Hospital between 1952 and 1974.[3] On close inspection, only 78 of the 180 patients had enough clinical, laboratory, radiographic, operative, or postmortem data to support the diagnosis with any certainty. In other instances, the disease may also be under-diagnosed. In a series of 36 patients with cholangitis seen at the University of California at San Diego, the diagnosis was made prospectively in only 18 patients, the remaining being diagnosed at surgery or at autopsy.[4]

Very little has been written concerning the clinical presentation of cholangitis. In recent years authors have focused on the most severe form of cholangitis, acute suppurative cholangitis, and little attention has been paid to the less severe forms of the disease. The clinical spectrum of cholangitis varies widely. Just as the severity of other abdominal disorders such as pancreatitis can vary from mild, not requiring specific medical therapy, to a catastrophic episode, where the patient is dead within hours of admission, so may episodes of cholangitis vary. Often, in taking a history from a patient with gallstones, an episode of fever, chills, and jaundice is described. The patient may state that the episode lasted for 24 hours and abated without medical aid being sought. In addition, patients with benign strictures frequently will have recurrent episodes of cholangitis that are easily managed at home with oral antibiotics. Most patients with cholangitis, however, are ill enough to seek medical aid and are hospitalized. At the far end of the spectrum is the patient with "toxic" cholangitis who may be admitted in septic shock and die before surgery can be undertaken.

All patients who present with cholangitis have biliary tract pathology. In the Far East there is an entity variously called recurrent pyogenic cholangitis, Oriental cholangiohepatitis, or Hong Kong disease. In this disorder recurrent episodes of bacterial cholangitis can apparently occur in the absence, at least initially, of biliary tract pathology. However, in this country, biliary tract pathology with some degree of obstruction is always present. In a series of 78 patients presenting to The Johns Hopkins Hospital over a 22-year period with cholangitis, 48 (62%) had common duct stones[3] (Table 25–1). In 25 of the patients, no prior biliary tract surgery had been performed, and the stones were thought to be secondary common duct stones that had migrated from the gallbladder. However, in 23 of the patients with choledocholithiasis, prior biliary tract surgery had been carried out. Four of the 23 patients had undergone biliary tract surgery during the past year, and these patients probably had retained common duct stones. However, the remaining 19 patients had had their biliary tract surgery at least one year prior to presenting with acute cholangitis, and the average interval was nine years. Thus, this group of patients almost certainly had recurrent or primary common duct stones. These 19 patients represented almost one quarter of the entire series of patients presenting with acute cholangitis.

In a separate study of 30 patients seen at The Johns Hopkins Hospital, all of whom were thought to have primary recurrent common duct stones, 16 presented with acute cholangitis.[5] The soft brown primary or recurrent common duct stones that frequently present crumbled or as biliary mud must be conducive to episodes of cholangitis. Twelve of the

78 patients (15%) in the Hopkins series had total obstruction of the biliary tract secondary to a malignancy. Although cholangitis associated with complete obstruction from a malignancy is less common than partial obstruction secondary to calculous disease, it does occur. Nine patients had benign biliary tree strictures secondary to an operative injury, which is also a frequent setting for cholangitis. In the Hopkins series, patients were not included who developed cholangitis secondary to biliary tract manipulations. In recent years with the increased utilization of transhepatic, T tube, and ERCP as well as nonoperative biliary manipulations including percutaneous drainage and endoscopic sphincterotomy, cholangitis has been a fairly frequent complication. In a series of 100 consecutive T-tube cholangiograms performed at The Johns Hopkins Hospital, there were nine documented instances of bacteremia.[6] In a series of 75 patients undergoing transhepatic cholangiography presented by Flemma and colleagues,[7] five developed cholangitis. Cholangitis has also been reported following endoscopic retrograde cholangiography[8] and nonoperative extraction of biliary calculi through T-tube tracts.[9]

Patients who present with cholangitis tend to be in an older age group than is ordinarily seen with biliary tract disease. Average age of the 78 patients in the series from Hopkins was 61 years, with a range of 30 to 87 years.[3] In another series of 73 consecutive patients with choledocholithiasis seen at The Johns Hopkins Hospital, the mean age of the 33 patients presenting with cholangitis was 61 years.[10] In comparison, the mean age of the 40 patients with common duct stones and no preoperative cholangitis was only 48 years ($P < .001$). Among 36 patients with cholangitis reported from the University of California at San Diego (U.C.S.D.), 16 were older than 70 years of age and 11 were older than 80 years of age.[4] Despite the fact that biliary calculi occur more frequently in females than in males, the sex ratio of patients with cholangitis is approximately equal. Forty of the 78 patients in the series from Hopkins were males, and in the series from U.C.S.D., two thirds of the patients were males. The classic presentation of fever and chills, abdominal pain, and jaundice is by no means always present (Table 25–2). Although all of the 78 patients presenting to Hopkins had a history of recent fever, only 51 actually had a temperature of more than 100°F on admission. In 27 patients the admission temperature was between 97°F and 100°F, in 29 the temperature was greater than 102°, and

TABLE 25–1.—BILIARY TRACT PATHOLOGY IN 78 PATIENTS WITH ACUTE CHOLANGITIS—THE JOHNS HOPKINS HOSPITAL

BILIARY TRACT PATHOLOGY	NO. OF PATIENTS		%	
Common duct stones	48		62	
Secondary		25		32
Primary		19		25
Retained		4		5
Malignant stricture	12		15	
Benign stricture	9		11	
Biliary-enteric anastomosis	6		8	
Miscellaneous	3		4	

TABLE 25–2.—CLINICAL PRESENTATION OF 78 PATIENTS WITH ACUTE CHOLANGITIS—THE JOHNS HOPKINS HOSPITAL

SIGN	NO. OF PATIENTS	%
Fever	51	65*
Chills	58	74
Abdominal pain	62	79*
Nausea and vomiting	40	51
Jaundice	62	79*
Abdominal tenderness	63	81
Normal bowel sounds	76	97
Shock	4	5

*Charcot's triad present in fewer than 60% of patients with acute cholangitis.

in eight greater than 104°F. Chills were present by history in 58 (74%) of the patients. Spiking fevers were present in 94% and chills in 78% of the patients in the series from U.C.S.D. Abdominal pain was present in many of the patients in the Hopkins series (79%). However, in many instances the abdominal pain was mild, and in 16 patients there was no complaint of any abdominal discomfort. This is not unusual for cholangitis, and an initial complaint of severe abdominal pain should alert the clinician to consider other diagnoses in addition to cholangitis.

Nausea and vomiting were present in 40 of the 78 patients (51%). Sixty-two of the 78 patients (79%) presenting to Hopkins had clinical jaundice. Many authors have pointed out that this clinical sign of Charcot's triad is frequently absent and by no means rules out the possibility of bacterial cholangitis.

Physical examination of the abdomen can be quite variable. Sixty-three of the 78 patients in the Hopkins series had mild to moderate abdominal tenderness in the right upper quadrant.[3] However, 15 patients had no evidence of abdominal tenderness on exam. In addition, only 35 of the patients had evidence of peritoneal irritation. Nineteen patients had right upper quadrant guarding, and 16 patients had rebound tenderness in the right upper quadrant. In 76 of the 78 patients bowel sounds were recorded as normal. Thus, not only is severe abdominal pain unusual in cholangitis, but also marked generalized abdominal findings on physical examination are unusual. If generalized or severe abdominal findings are present, the physician should seriously consider other diagnoses in addition to acute cholangitis. Many of the errors in diagnosis of cholangitis hinge on the mistaken concept that patients invariably have severe abdominal pain and significant abdominal findings. In fact, the opposite is true. Four of the 78 patients (5%) in the Hopkins series were critically ill, in septic shock, with depressed mental function at the time of admission. These four patients were among the 11 patients (14%) in the series with the most severe form of cholangitis, acute "toxic" cholangitis.

In summary, the patient presenting with cholangitis will frequently be elderly, as often male as female, and be most likely to have a common duct stone. Fever will usually be present, mild abdominal pain is frequent, but abdominal tenderness is usually mild and may be absent. Many patients will have clinical evidence of jaundice, but this is by no means mandatory for diagnosis. An occasional patient may present in septic shock with CNS depression.

LABORATORY FINDINGS

As with most acute intra-abdominal disorders, the diagnosis of acute cholangitis cannot be made on the basis of laboratory findings. However, certain laboratory changes do occur and can add confirmatory evidence to support the clinical diagnosis (Table 25–3). Since cholangitis is an acute bacterial infection, leukocytosis is common. In a series of 78 patients presenting to The Johns Hopkins Hospital with acute cholangitis, 44 (57%) had leukocyte elevations greater than 10,000/cu mm.[3] Five of the patients (6%) had leukocyte counts greater than 20,000/cu mm. Twenty-seven of the patients had leukocyte counts in the normal range, between 5,000 and 10,000/cu mm. The remaining two patients (3%) came in markedly

TABLE 25–3.—LABORATORY FINDINGS IN ACUTE CHOLANGITIS—THE JOHNS HOPKINS HOSPITAL

STUDY	% RESULTS	% ABNORMAL
WBCs/mm^3		
< 5,000	3	
5–10,000	34	
10–20,000	57	
> 20,000	6	63
Bilirubin, mg/dl		
< 1	6	
1–2	13	
2–4	22	
> 4	59	94
SGOT, IU/L		
< 20	7	
20–100	64	
> 100	29	93
SGPT, IU/L		
< 20	3	
20–100	66	
> 100	31	97
Alkaline phosphatase		92
Amylase		35

leukopenic, with WBC counts below 5,000/cu mm. Therefore, the majority of patients in this series presented with either a leukocytosis, or a leukopenia suggesting sepsis. Those patients presenting with normal leukocyte counts in most instances had significant shifts to the left. This observation has also been made at the University of California at San Francisco by Boey and Way,[11] who noted that one quarter of their patients had a normal WBC count and a left shift. In a series of 36 patients presenting to the University of California at San Diego with acute cholangitis, 35 (97%) were found to have leukocyte counts in excess of 10,000/cu mm.

Even though most patients with acute cholangitis will have hyperbilirubinemia, the degree of bilirubin elevation is quite variable, and in some instances the serum bilirubin will be normal. Among the 78 patients presenting to Hopkins with acute cholangitis, five patients (6%) had normal serum bilirubin levels.[3] An additional 10 patients (13%) had minimal bilirubin elevations, between 1 and 2 mg/dl. Thus, almost 20% of the patients in this series had serum bilirubin levels of 2 mg/dl or less. In contrast, 46 of the patients (59%) had serum bilirubin levels greater than 4 mg/dl, and 12 of the 46 had bilirubin levels greater than 10 mg/dl. Most of the patients with markedly elevated serum bilirubin levels were among the patients with total biliary tract obstruction secondary to a malignancy. Longmire, in a series of 35 patients with acute nonsuppurative cholangitis seen at UCLA, stated that most patients had moderate elevations of the serum bilirubin, usually 5 mg/dl or below.[12] Boey and Way[11] reported that 16 of their 74 patients had a serum bilirubin of less than 2 mg/dl. Saik and colleagues[4] stated that three of 36 (8%) patients with acute cholangitis had normal serum bilirubins, whereas in the remaining 92% an elevated serum level was detected.

Alkaline phosphatase levels are usually elevated in patients with cholangitis. In the Hopkins series, 92% of patients with acute cholangitis had an elevated serum alkaline phosphatase level, and in the series from the U.C.S.D. recorded by Saik and colleagues,[4] 89% had alkaline phosphatase elevations.

The SGOT and SGPT levels are also elevated in the great majority of patients presenting with acute cholangitis. In the series of 78 patients at Hopkins, the SGOT levels were determined in 45 patients, and in only three (7%) were the serum levels normal. In 29 patients (64%) the serum transaminase was elevated between 20 and 100 units, and in 13 patients (29%) it was elevated greater than 100 units. The same held true for SGPT determinations. In the 35 patients from the Hopkins series in whom this determination was available, it was normal in only one (3%). In 23 patients the SGPT ranged between 20 and 100 units, and in 11 patients (31%) it was greater than 100 units. Thus, the trio of blood tests consisting of bilirubin, alkaline phosphatase, and transaminase levels may provide a degree of confirmatory evidence for the clinical diagnosis of acute cholangitis. As discussed subsequently in the section on pathogenesis, acute cholangitis in this country is invariably associated with some degree of partial obstruction of the biliary tract. Thus, elevations of these three serum tests would be expected. Among the 78 patients in the Hopkins series, 94% had bilirubin elevations, 92% had serum alkaline phosphatase elevations, 93% had SGOT elevations, and 97% had SGPT elevations. These tests in the clinical setting of acute cholangitis indicate biliary tract pathology. Although they by no means make the diagnosis of acute cholangitis, to see acute cholangitis in the absence of such serum abnormalities would be distinctly unusual. Serum amylase determinations were performed in 54 of the 78 patients in the Hopkins series. In 19 (35%), the serum levels were elevated, and in six (11%) the amylase was greater than 1,000 Caraway units/100 ml. Although not seen in many patients with acute cholangitis, a serum amylase elevation may provide clinical evidence of calculous disease in the common duct, and thus further support the clinical diagnosis of acute cholangitis.

The fever and chills associated with acute cholangitis in most instances signify a bacteremia. Many patients with cholelithiasis or with choledocholithiasis who are asymptomatic grow significant numbers of pathogenic bacteria when their common duct bile is cultured. Therefore, infected bile itself does not produce the picture of cholangitis. This will be discussed more thoroughly in the section on pathogenesis, but the clinical picture of acute cholangitis probably occurs when, in the face of some degree of biliary tract obstruction, the bile infection progresses resulting in a bacteremia. Blood cultures were obtained shortly following admission in 50 of the 78 patients presenting to Hopkins with acute cholangitis[3] (Table 25–4). In 20 patients (40%) the blood cultures were positive. In nine of the 20 patients (45%) *Escherichia coli* was the organism grown, and in eight patients (40%) *Klebsiella pneumoniae* was cultured. Thus, in 85% of the patients with positive blood cultures, the organisms were *E. coli* or *K. pneumoniae*. In one patient *Streptococcus faecalis* was cultured, in one a paracolon, and in one patient *Bacteroides fragilis* was cultured. Even though all of the patients in this series had a history of recent fever, only 65% were febrile at the time of admission. Furthermore, although 74% of the patients had a history of recent chills, in many instances the blood cultures were not drawn at the precise time of the chill. If one were to draw enough blood cultures and could time them appropriately, the incidence of a positive culture would probably approach 100% in acute cholangitis. Blood cultures

TABLE 25–4.—BACTERIOLOGY IN CHOLANGITIS—THE JOHNS HOPKINS HOSPITAL

	NO. POSITIVE	NO. OF PATIENTS	% POSITIVE
Blood cultures	20	50	40
Bile cultures	35	35	100
ORGANISMS	BLOOD (%)	BILE (%)	
Escherichia coli	45	74	
Klebsiella sp.	40	40	
Streptococcus faecalis	5	31	
Proteus sp.	–	14	
Pseudomonas sp.	–	11	
C. perfringins	–	11	
Paracolon sp.	5	6	
Bacteroides subtilis	–	3	
B. fragilis	5	–	

were positive in 36 of 84 patients (44%) reported from the University of California at San Francisco.[11] In the series of 36 patients with acute cholangitis from U.C.S.D., 17 (47%) had positive blood cultures.[4] In each of these three series, *E. coli* and *Klebsiella* sp. were the most frequent organisms obtained on blood culture.

At the time of surgery, bile cultures were obtained in 35 patients with acute cholangitis in the series of patients from Hopkins.[3] All cultures were positive. In 21 of the patients (60%), multiple organisms were found. However, as would be expected from the preoperative blood culture data, *E. coli* and *K. pneumoniae* were the most frequently cultured organisms. In 26 of the 35 patients (74%) *E. coli* was present in the infected bile, and in 14 (40%) *K. pneumoniae* was present. *Streptococcus faecalis* was cultured in the bile from 11 of the patients (31%). Bile cultures were positive in 79 of 86 patients (92%) studied by Boey and Way.[11] In 38 of their patients (48%) multiple organisms were isolated from the bile. In the series of 36 patients with cholangitis presented by Saik and associates,[4] 28 patients underwent surgery and had common duct cultures. In 26 patients (93%) the cultures were positive. In 16 of the 26 patients (61%) multiple organisms were grown. In 17 of the 26 positive cultures (65%) *E. coli* was grown. *Klebsiella pneumoniae* was present in 13 of the positive cultures (50%). *Streptococcus faecalis* was the next most commonly cultured organism, being found in seven bile samples (27%). Thus, the bile culture data from these three series are almost identical. In each of these series a large number of other organisms were infrequently cultured. However, *E. coli* and *K. pneumoniae* were the most common organisms found, with *Streptococcus faecalis* being cultured in a significant number. It is interesting that in each of these large series of patients with acute cholangitis, anaerobic organisms were only infrequently cultured in the blood or bile. One possible explanation is that anaerobic culturing techniques may not have been routinely employed during the period of these studies. In comparison, between 1976 and 1979, we isolated anaerobes from the bile of nine of 33 patients (27%) with choledocholithiasis and preoperative cholangitis.[10] During this same period, anaerobes were isolated from the bile of only two of 40 patients (5%) with common duct stones and no preoperative cholangitis ($P < .025$). The anaerobic organism most frequently recovered was *B. fragilis*.

RADIOGRAPHIC FINDINGS

Plain abdominal x-rays are generally not particularly helpful in evaluating acute cholangitis. In the series from The Johns Hopkins Hospital, 52 of the 78 patients had plain abdominal x-rays, and only eight abnormalities were seen.[3] In five of these eight patients the nonspecific finding of an ileus or a sentinel loop was present. In two patients radiopaque gallstones were seen, and in one patient air was noted in the biliary tree. In the remaining 44 patients the abdominal x-rays were normal or there were only nonspecific changes. This observation is further evidence of the minimal amount of peritoneal irritation that is present in many of these patients. Oral cholecystography is of no help in most patients with cholangitis because of hyperbilirubinemia at the time of presentation. Intravenous cholangiography may also not be possible for the same reason. In the Hopkins series 41 of the 78 patients had a bilirubin level greater than 5 mg/dl at the time of admission; as a result, only 38 patients underwent IV cholangiography. Of these 38 patients, 23 had nonvisualization of their bile duct; thus, the test was of no help. In 15 patients the biliary tree visualized and some abnormality was present. This was often only the presence of mild duct dilatation. In most instances adequate resolution to accurately define the biliary tract anatomy was not obtained. The use of ultrasound and CAT may be quite helpful in demonstrating the presence of stones or dilated bile ducts in those patients who present with a clinical picture of cholangitis. These techniques have the advantage of being noninvasive and may be quite helpful in confirming the diagnosis in an ill patient with a compatible clinical picture. Likewise, the use of radionuclide scanning of the biliary tree with ^{99m}Tc HIDA and other iminodiacetic acid derivatives has the advantage of being noninvasive. While these agents are quite useful in the diagnosis of acute cholecystitis, this technique lacks the resolution necessary to define biliary anatomy.[13]

As will be discussed later, most patients with acute cholangitis will eventually require surgery. Prior to surgery most patients will require cholangiography to adequately define the biliary tree anatomy. Intravenous cholangiography will usually not be adequate and a transhepatic (Fig 25–1) or endoscopic retrograde (Figs 25–2 and 25–3) cholangiogram will usually be necessary. While both of these techniques can very accurately define the biliary anatomy, they each are associated with a small incidence of complications. In performing either of these two procedures in a patient with a recent episode of cholangitis, the timing and antibiotic coverage are critical. Before a patient with a recent episode of cholangitis undergoes either of these procedures, he should have received an adequate course of systemic antibiotics and have been afebrile for at least several days. Transhepatic cholangiography is associated with approximately a 5% incidence of cholangitis and a 0.25% mortality. In a series of 75 patients undergoing transhepatic cholangiography with no antibiotic coverage, Flemma and colleagues reported a 7% incidence of cholangitis.[7] In a more recent series by Okuda and associates,[14] there was a 4% incidence of cholangitis among 315 patients undergoing transhepatic cholangiography with antibiotic coverage. The overall incidence of complications after ERC is approximately 3%, with a mortality of approximately

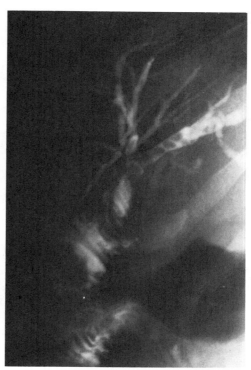

Fig 25–1.—Transhepatic cholangiogram (THC) of a 25-year-old male who presented with cholangitis seven years after a choledochojejunostomy performed for a benign stricture of the common bile duct. After responding to antibiotic therapy, the THC demonstrated not only an anastomotic stricture, but also multiple stones in the left hepatic duct.

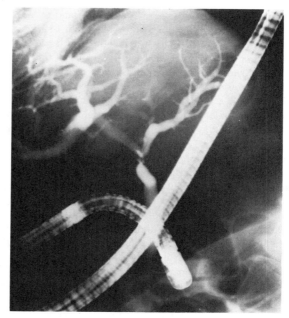

Fig 25–2.—Endoscopic retrograde cholangiogram (ERC) of a 55-year-old female who presented with fever and abdominal pain but no jaundice three months after cholecystectomy. The ERC demonstrated a stricture of the proximal common hepatic duct, presumably due to operative trauma.

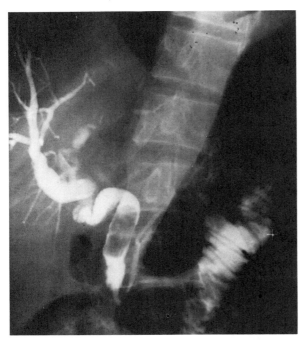

Fig 25–3.—Endoscopic retrograde cholangiogram (ERC) of a 60-year-old male who presented with cholangitis 15 years after a cholecystectomy. The ERC demonstrated partial common duct obstruction due to a large primary common duct stone.

0.2%. The incidence of cholangitis reported from The Johns Hopkins Hospital in 1975 following ERCP was 5% among 75 consecutive patients.[8] However, in a collected series of over 10,000 patients, Bilbao et al.[15] reported only 0.8% incidence of cholangitis. Other large series by Cotton[16] and by Zimmon et al.[17] confirm a 1% incidence of cholangitis. In the report by Zimmon et al.[17] cholangitis was not seen in those patients with a normal biliary tree, but occurred in 5% of the patients with an obstructed biliary tree. Kasagai and associates[18] performed ERC on 405 patients who were covered with systemic antibiotics with a 0.7% incidence of cholangitis. When they added thiamphenicol aminoacetate hydrochloride (Neomycin G) to the contrast medium, they experienced no cholangitis among 252 patients. These patients undergoing ERC were also covered with systemic antibiotics.

Therefore, either of these procedures can be performed reasonably safely in patients with a recent episode of cholangitis if adequate antibiotic therapy has been carried out prior to the performance of the cholangiogram, and if systemic antibiotic coverage is provided during the study. The addition of antibiotics to the contrast media in these high risk patients may also be indicated. Nakayama and colleagues[19] have recently reported 11 patients with acute obstructive suppurative cholangitis in whom percutaneous transhepatic drainage (PTD) was achieved. Two of these patients had multiple biliary liver abscesses. Only one of these 11 patients died. Percutaneous transhepatic drainage has been performed on 18 patients with biliary sepsis at The Johns Hopkins Hospital.[20] Fifteen of these patients had a favorable response; however, three elderly patients with carcinoma of the pancreas died.

At U.C.L.A., PTD has been performed in 24 patients with a temperature greater than 38°C, seven of whom had a bacteremia before the procedure. Complications following PTD were no higher when the 24 patients with pre-PTD fever were compared to 46 patients who were afebrile beforehand. However, complications were significantly higher in the patients with a documented bacteremia before PTD (unpublished data). Thus, this technique may prove to be quite useful in selected cases of acute cholangitis. In the absence of expert radiologists familiar with PTD, however, we recommend that surgery be scheduled shortly after either transhepatic or ERC in patients with a recent episode of cholangitis, because a second episode of cholangitis requiring surgical decompression may ensue despite apparently adequate antibiotic coverage.[8]

DIFFERENTIAL DIAGNOSIS

A variety of disorders in addition to acute cholangitis can present with fever and chills, abdominal pain, and jaundice (Table 25–5). The clinical entity that most frequently is confused with acute cholangitis is acute cholecystitis. As with cholangitis, patients who develop acute cholecystitis tend to be elderly, and both disorders are seen as frequently in men as in women.[21] While fever is seen in almost all patients with acute cholecystitis, chills are less common and more suggestive of cholangitis. Right upper quadrant pain and tenderness are present in almost all patients with acute cholecystitis but often are absent in cholangitis. Jaundice may be seen with both entities, but is more commonly seen with cholangitis. While hyperbilirubinemia may be present in as many as 20 to 25% of patients with acute cholecystitis, the level of bilirubin is usually less than 5 mg/dl.[21] In contrast, over 90% of patients who present with cholangitis have hyperbilirubinemia, and in 50% the bilirubin is greater than 5 mg/dl.[3] Nausea and vomiting may be seen with both illnesses and is not helpful in the differential diagnosis. Abdominal tenderness is present in the vast majority of patients with acute cholecystitis, and peritoneal signs are frequent. On occasion a palpable, tender

TABLE 25–5.—DIFFERENTIAL DIAGNOSIS OF CHOLANGITIS

Gallbladder
　Acute cholecystitis
　Empyema
Liver
　Hepatitis
　Pyogenic or amebic liver abscess
Pancreas
　Pancreatitis
　Pseudocyst
Stomach-duodenum
　Penetrating or perforated ulcer
Colon
　Right-sided diverticulitis
　Perforation
Appendix
　Appendicitis
Kidney
　Acute pyelonephritis
Lung
　Right lower lobe pneumonia
　Infarction
Heart
　Bacterial endocarditis

gallbladder or a positive Murphy's sign will also be present in acute cholecystitis. While the majority of patients with acute cholangitis have some abdominal tenderness, it is usually mild, and peritoneal signs are seen in less than half of the patients. The presence or absence of bowel sounds on physical examination does not differentiate between these two entities. The WBC count is frequently but not invariably elevated in both illnesses. A marked leukocytosis (> 20,000/cu mm) or a leukopenia suggests a septicemia and is most apt to be associated with acute cholangitis. The alkaline phosphatase is elevated in most patients with cholangitis, but as many as 40% of patients with acute cholecystitis will also have an elevated serum level.[21] Mild elevations in the SGOT or SGPT are seen in almost all patients with cholangitis; however, these enzymes are also elevated in approximately 50% of patients with acute cholecystitis.[21] The serum amylase may also be significantly elevated in both entities. Plain abdominal x-rays are normal in most patients with both acute cholangitis and acute cholecystitis, and the presence of gallstones on plain abdominal films does not differentiate between the two. The presence of air either within the biliary tree or within the gallbladder may be helpful, but these x-ray findings are rare. Intravenous cholangiography may differentiate the two illnesses if the common bile duct is visualized and appears normal without stones, and the gallbladder is not visualized. The differentiation between acute cholecystitis and cholangitis may be difficult and in some cases impossible. The two most important differentiating characteristics are the physical examination of the right upper quadrant and the level of bilirubin. The patient with true peritoneal signs in the right upper quadrant and a normal or only minimally elevated bilirubin is more likely to have acute cholecystitis. A patient presenting with less in the way of abdominal findings, but with a bilirubin of 5 mg/dl or greater, and with a septic picture, is most likely to have acute cholangitis.

Other diseases in and around the liver which might be confused with cholangitis are hepatitis, a liver abscess, and pancreatitis. Patients with viral or alcoholic hepatitis may present with fever, right upper quadrant abdominal pain, and jaundice. Differentiation between hepatitis and acute cholangitis can usually be made on the basis of a more chronic presentation, the absence of chills, and by the level of transaminase elevation. The presence of multiple microscopic liver abscesses may be an extension of acute suppurative cholangitis, discussed in the section on complications. However, liver abscesses of other than biliary tract origin may present in a fashion identical to cholangitis. The physical examination and laboratory findings may be very similar. These patients may be differentiated preoperatively with the use of ultrasound, radionuclide scanning, or computerized axial tomography. The clinical presentation of pancreatitis may also be very similar to that of acute cholangitis. Bilirubin elevations are common with both entities. Elevations in serum amylase are seen in most patients with pancreatitis, but also can be seen in as many as one third of patients presenting with acute cholangitis.[3] However, the abdominal findings in acute pancreatitis are almost always more severe than in acute cholangitis. Penetrating or perforated ulcers may also present with fever, right upper quadrant pain, hyperamylasemia, and a mild elevation in bilirubin secondary to sepsis.

Among other illnesses that might be confused with cholangitis are right-sided diverticulitis, appendicitis, right-sided pyelonephritis, a right lower lobe pneumonia, a pulmonary infarction, and bacterial endocarditis. While jaundice is generally not associated with diverticulitis or appendicitis, if sepsis occurs, mild bilirubin elevations can result. Also, rarely these diseases can result in pylephlebitis and multiple small liver abscesses. Patients with acute pyelonephritis or a right lower lobe pneumonia are also not generally jaundiced, but an elevated bilirubin may be seen secondary to hemolysis with severe sepsis. Patients with bacterial endocarditis can develop multiple abscesses in many organs, including the liver and spleen. Mild jaundice in these patients is common.

Usually, acute cholangitis can only be suspected at the time of presentation, and treatment will have to be initiated on the basis of this clinical suspicion. The clinical presentation and laboratory confirmation will usually be typical enough to make the diagnosis with a reasonable degree of confidence. The diagnosis can only be confirmed with certainty, however, when bile duct pathology is confirmed radiographically, at surgery, or at postmortem examination.

PATHOLOGY

Acute cholangitis implies bacterial infection within the bile ducts. In addition to the clinical criteria suggesting infection, bile duct pathology causing some degree of obstruction must be present to confirm the diagnosis of cholangitis. Stones within the biliary tree are the most common cause of cholangitis, accounting for 62% of the cases in the Hopkins series.[3] Malignant (15%) and benign (12%) extrahepatic strictures are present in most of the remaining patients, as Charcot pointed out in 1877.

The presence of an indwelling biliary tube is associated with positive bile cultures in over 90% of patients when the tube is in place for more than a week.[6] As a result, these patients are at a risk to develop cholangitis after cholangiography, particularly if the intraductal pressure is elevated during the examination. In the Orient the presence of the parasites *Clonorchis sinensis*, *Trichuris trichiura*, and *Ascaris lumbricoides* within the biliary tree is associated with cholangitis. These parasites cause obstruction of the intrahepatic duct system, and in association with secondary bacterial infection can cause repeated bouts of acute cholangitis. This may eventually lead to stenosis of the intrahepatic ducts.

Histologically, cholangitis is characterized by extrahepatic and intrahepatic bile ducts that contain numerous polymorphonuclear leukocytes and bacteria with inflammatory infiltrates in the surrounding portal triads. This process may extend to the surrounding liver parenchyma with formation of multiple liver abscesses, particularly in suppurative cholangitis. These may coalesce into one large abscess, but usually there are numerous small abscesses scattered throughout the liver near the termination of the bile canaliculi (Fig 25–4).

Suppurative cholangitis refers to gross purulence or pus in the bile ducts. This is often associated with complete biliary obstruction. Among 12 patients with acute suppurative cholangitis reported by Andrew and Johnson,[22] some degree of portal inflammatory changes were seen in 11 patients, and eight patients had a heavy portal infiltration with polymor-

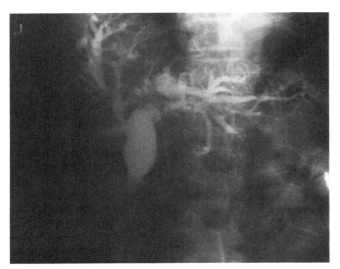

Fig 25–4.—Transhepatic cholangiogram (THC) of a 65-year-old female who presented with cholangitis one year following a choledochojejunostomy. The THC demonstrated multiple small sacculations of the biliary tree. The patient died of sepsis, and at postmortem the liver contained multiple microscopic and macroscopic abscesses thought to correspond to the sacculations.

phonuclear leukocytes. Six of the patients in this group also had portal fibrosis and proliferation of bile ducts, and five patients had microscopic liver abscesses. In a collected series of 86 patients with suppurative cholangitis from the literature, 69% developed liver abscesses.[22]

PATHOPHYSIOLOGY

The two factors that are necessary for the initiation of clinical cholangitis are the presence of significant numbers of bacteria within the biliary tree, and elevation of intraductal pressure sufficiently high to cause a reflux of bacteria into the bloodstream. Obstruction plays a key role in the pathogenesis of acute cholangitis because it has the dual effect of increasing the concentration of bacteria due to stasis, and of creating an increase in intraductal pressure. The presence of a foreign body such as a gallstone or parasite within the biliary tree is almost always associated with bacterial growth, can readily cause obstruction, and is responsible for most instances of cholangitis.

Cultures of normal gallbladder and common duct bile are almost always sterile. When gallbladder stones are present, however, gallbladder bile and gallbladder wall cultures are positive at least 50% of the time.[7, 23] In addition, when a stone is present in the common duct, cultures are positive in 75%–90% of patients, despite the fact that many of these patients may be asymptomatic.[10, 24–26] With partial common duct obstruction due to choledocholithiasis, benign biliary strictures, or a previous biliary-intestinal anastomosis, common duct bile cultures are also positive in 90%–100% of patients.[7, 24–26] However, with complete ductal obstruction, commonly seen with malignancy, only 25%–40% of bile cultures are positive.[26–28] Thus, infected bile appears to correlate with the presence of a foreign body (stones or parasites) and

partial obstruction. Complete obstruction in the absence of a foreign body (as with a malignant stricture) is less apt to be associated with infected bile or acute cholangitis. The incidence of positive bile cultures has also been shown to have a direct correlation with advancing age.[25, 26, 29, 30] The organisms most commonly cultured in the bile are *E. coli, K. pneumoniae,* and *Streptococcus faecalis.* These organisms are similar to those seen in the upper intestinal tract.[31] Prior to 1975 most published series described a striking absence of anaerobic bacteria cultured from the bile. This absence of anaerobes within the biliary tree may have been a reflection of (1) inhibition of their growth by bile salts[32, 33] or (2) inadequate culturing techniques. However, since 1975, numerous reports[6, 26, 34–38] have documented the presence of anaerobes, including *B. fragilis,* in bile from elderly patients with complex biliary problems, those most likely to develop cholangitis.

The pathway by which bacteria reach the biliary tree is still not entirely clear. Possibilities include: (1) the ascending route through the common duct from the duodenum; (2) through GI and biliary tract lymphatics; (3) via the hepatic artery; (4) via the portal vein; or (5) from a chronically infected gallbladder. The ascending route through the bile duct was proposed by Edlund et al.[24] in 1959 by a process of elimination, and because his work, that of Taylor,[39] and that of Orloff and associates[40] showed very little support for the portal vein bacteremia route. In addition, the fact that acute cholangitis is uncommon in the face of complete common duct obstruction is also supportive circumstantial evidence. Although the ascending route through the common bile duct from the duodenum at first seems quite logical, there is no experimental or clinical evidence to confirm reflux with a normal sphincter mechanism. Investigators have shown that Evans blue dye injected into the duodenum will extend along the common bile duct lymphatics to the gallbladder,[24] but there is no experimental evidence to suggest that bacteria can pass from ductal lymphatics back into bile. In addition, experimental work in guinea pigs by Dineen[41] demonstrated that the number of bacteria reaching the bile was insignificant if the bacteria were introduced via duodenal lymphatics. His studies showed that the flow of lymph around the common duct was away from the liver and toward periduodenal and celiac lymph nodes.

Multiple abscesses can develop within the liver in severe cases of sepsis, and presumably the bacteria reach the liver via the hepatic artery. However, there are no clinical or experimental data that suggest this route as a frequent source of biliary bacteria. Although Edlund and associates[24] initially thought that the portal vein was an unlikely source of bacteria in the bile, Dineen[41] showed that this pathway was by far the most significant and efficient mechanism for delivering bacteria to bile in his experimental model. Dineen's studies also showed that obstruction of bile flow increased the number of bacteria recovered from the bile after introduction of bacteria into the bloodstream via the portal route. Initial clinical studies showed a very low incidence of positive portal vein cultures in normal individuals. However, other studies have documented portal vein bacteremias in a variety of circumstances. Schatten and associates[42] in 1955 found a 32% incidence of positive portal vein cultures in patients undergoing upper abdominal operations. In 1958 Brooke and Slaney[43] showed a high incidence of portal vein bacteremia in patients with ulcerative colitis. In 1962 Ong[44] reported a 40% incidence of positive portal vein cultures from 33 patients with recurrent pyogenic cholangitis who were in an acute phase of the disease. Peripheral vein blood samples taken at the same time revealed only a 15% incidence of positive cultures. In contrast, portal vein cultures taken from patients operated on during a quiescent phase of recurrent pyogenic cholangitis were positive in only 6% of 64 patients.

The portal vein theory assumes that small numbers of enteric bacteria frequently enter the portal circulation. Some of these organisms are removed by the reticuloendothelial system within the liver, and some are excreted into the bile. With a normal biliary tree these organisms pass innocently back into the intestinal tract. However, in the presence of a foreign body such as a stone, and particularly with obstruction to the flow of bile, the bacteria that have survived this route will multiply. One objection to this theory is that the absence of anaerobes in biliary tract infections does not reflect the flora seen in the lower intestinal tract. However, the presence of bile salts which inhibit anaerobic growth seems to be a reasonable explanation. The other finding that is not entirely explained by the portal vein route is the low incidence of positive bile duct cultures in patients with complete obstruction secondary to a malignancy. Therefore, a foreign body, as well as obstruction is required to satisfactorily support this theory.

While most investigators feel that the portal vein is the most likely route of bacterial invasion of the biliary tree, Scott and Khan[45] in 1967 suggested that organisms in an infected common duct bile may be derived from a chronically infected gallbladder. They suggested that the gallbladder wall infection is initiated by the hematogenous route. Subsequently, others have suggested that these organisms reach the sluggish gallbladder bile and the gallbladder wall via the portal vein route. This combined theory is supported by the fact that the same organisms are invariably cultured from the gallbladder wall and the common duct bile in an individual patient. It also explains the low incidence of common bile duct infection seen with complete obstruction due to a tumor. The portal vein-infected gallbladder theory would be further supported if it could be shown that the 25%–40% of patients with complete obstruction due to a tumor who do have positive bile cultures also had gallstones or a chronically infected gallbladder.

Flemma and colleagues[7] demonstrated convincingly in 1967 that the presence of bacteria in the bile even in concentrations greater than 10^5/ml is not sufficient to produce cholangitis without concomitant obstruction. They demonstrated that cholangitis could be precipitated by cholangiography, and thought that the syndrome of clinical cholangitis with fever and chills was the result of disruption of the biliary tract mucosa with a direct entry of bacteria from the biliary system into the bloodstream, producing a septicemia. As early as 1947 Mixer and associates[46] demonstrated that particles the size of bacteria or viruses could be transferred to the bloodstream in association with cholangiography. They also observed that biliary pressures in the range of 20 cm of water were necessary to initiate reflux from the biliary system into the bloodstream. In 1953 Edlund and Hanzon[47] demonstrated

a direct communication between terminal bile duct canaliculi and liver sinusoids by fluorescent microscopic studies. The existence of this communication was also confirmed by electron microscopic studies done by Rouiller in 1956[48] and by Hampton in 1958.[49] Further support for the direct anatomical communication between biliary canaliculi and liver sinusoids came in 1962 when Hultborn and associates[50] demonstrated reflux of radioactive-labeled saline, dye, albumin, and gold when these substances were injected into an obstructed common bile duct. This reflux occurred so rapidly that these authors felt that the communication must have been a direct one with the venous system and not via the lymphatic system. The authors demonstrated that particles up to 200 or 300 Å, slightly larger than the size of a virus, could be regurgitated into the bloodstream at relatively low pressures. Further studies by Jacobsson et al.[51] in that same year demonstrated that radioactive-labeled bacteria refluxed into the bloodstream at pressures that were only slightly higher than the secretory pressure of the liver (15 cm of H_2O). In this experiment the majority of bacteria were filtered off in the liver, but approximately 10% of those injected entered the bloodstream. A further study in dogs by Huang et al.[52] in 1969 demonstrated that hepatic vein blood and thoracic duct lymph remained sterile if the pressure within an infected common bile duct remained less than 20 cm of H_2O. When pressures were raised above 25 cm of H_2O, organisms appeared rapidly in both the blood and lymph, and the concentrations of bacteria in both of these systems were directly proportional to the bile duct pressure. These authors stressed that increased biliary pressure associated with obstruction was the key factor in the pathogenesis of the bacteremia in cholangitis.

In 1952 Mallet-Guy[53] showed that normal biliary pressures ranged from 7 to 14 cm of H_2O. This finding was confirmed by Williams et al.[54] in 1967 in dogs. However, with partial common duct obstruction the average bile duct pressure increased to 18 cm of H_2O, and this pressure increased even further, to 29 cm of H_2O, with complete obstruction. Hopton and White[55] confirmed the presence of increased resting biliary tract pressures in patients with a diseased common bile duct. Although resting common bile duct pressures are higher with complete obstruction than with partial obstruction, cholangitis is more commonly associated with partial than with complete obstruction. This observation is explained by the fact that bile is infected more commonly in patients with partial obstruction, which is usually associated with calculi, than with total obstruction, which is often associated with tumor. In addition, acute cholangitis is more likely to occur when there is a sudden increase in intraductal pressure, as might occur more frequently with choledocholithiasis or during cholangiography, than with the gradual obstruction that accompanies a tumor.

Thus, the clinical symptoms of fever and chills associated with cholangitis are due to a systemic bacteremia caused by a cholangiovenous or a cholangiolymphatic reflux of organisms as a result of a rise in intrabiliary pressure. The presence of infected bile without obstruction or of obstruction without infection is not sufficient to produce clinical cholangitis. Both infection and obstruction are necessary, and the presence of a foreign body within the biliary tree enhances both of these factors.

TREATMENT

Once the clinical diagnosis of acute cholangitis is suspected, the initial treatment in most instances will be with antibiotics. Depending on the severity of the episode and the nature of the clinical presentation, other general supportive measures may be necessary. For the patient who presents with chills and a low-grade fever and no other systemic signs or symptoms, antibiotic therapy alone may be sufficient. For the patient who presents with fever and chills, vomiting, a tender abdomen, and absent bowel sounds, IV fluids and nasogastric decompression may be indicated as well as antibiotic therapy. For the infrequent patient who presents in septic shock, more intensive monitoring and therapy will be necessary. All such patients will require a central venous catheter, and some of them a Swan-Ganz catheter, to monitor the central venous and pulmonary wedge pressures. Volume therapy may be required to expand the patient's intravascular volume to compensate for peripheral vasodilatation. Steroid administration is advocated by many physicians for septic shock. Hypoglycemia is occasionally seen, and IV glucose should be administered, particularly if CNS depression is present. For the majority of patients presenting with acute cholangitis, however, antibiotic therapy will be the mainstay of treatment. There is no general agreement in the literature on the most appropriate antibiotic regimen in acute cholangitis. In recent years ampicillin has become a very popular drug for the treatment of biliary tract infections because it is secreted into the bile in fairly high concentrations. However, when one considers that the majority of patients with cholangitis will have *E. coli* or *K. pneumoniae* as the infecting organism, ampicillin is entirely inadequte. Approximately one half of the *E. coli* and most of the *Klebsiella* species seen in hospitals in this country are resistant to ampicillin. An aminoglycoside such as gentamicin, tobramycin, or amikacin provides excellent coverage for these two gram-negative aerobes.[6, 56–58] Approximately 30% of patients with cholangitis will also have *Streptococcus faecalis* (enterococcus) in their bile.[10] To cover this organism adequately a penicillin, which will be synergistic with an aminoglycoside in its effect against enterococcus, must be added. This combination will provide adequate antibacterial coverage for 85%–90% of patients with cholangitis.[6, 10] The addition of an antibiotic with coverage for *B. fragilis* will provide nearly complete antibacterial coverage for these patients (Table 25–6).

There has been a great deal written concerning the bile concentrations achieved with various antibiotics. Theoretically, the ideal biliary tract antibiotic would be one that not only covers the organisms found with biliary tract infections, but also one that is secreted in high concentration in the bile. Studies have identified that some of the newer penicillins and cephalosporins, the tetracyclines, the macrolides, and the rifamycins are secreted into bile in significant concentrations (Table 25–7). However, when choosing an antibiotic for the treatment of acute cholangitis, the most important factors are adequate coverage of the organisms and adequate serum or tissue levels. Concentration of an antibiotic in the bile is probably only of secondary importance. A controlled trial of parenteral prophylactic gentamicin therapy carried out by Keighley and associates[56] supports this concept. One hundred consecutive patients undergoing biliary tract surgery were randomly allocated to receive either gentamicin or no antibiotic. Among the patients receiving the antibiotic, twice the inhibitory concentration of gentamicin to biliary tract organisms was found to be present in the serum in 88%, but in the bile in only 18%. Despite this finding, gentamicin was effective in reducing wound sepsis from 21% to 6%, a reduction that was statistically significant. Furthermore, a bacteremia was demonstrated in only one patient receiving gentamicin, in contrast to five patients receiving no gentamicin. One patient in the control group died of sepsis. Finally, despite the fact that gentamicin was not secreted in the bile in significant concentrations in the majority of patients, the incidence of bacteria in the bile was only 25% as compared to 42% in the control group. This study suggests that the effectiveness of gentamicin in controlling and treating biliary tract infections is not dependent upon high concentrations in the bile.

A second study was performed by Keighley and associates[57] to further determine the relative importance of antibiotic concentrations in the bile and serum. A randomized prospective study was carried out in 150 patients undergoing biliary tract operations. Fifty patients received no antibiotic coverage, 50 patients received gentamicin, and 50 patients received rifamide, an antibiotic with good coverage of biliary tree organisms and one that is excreted almost entirely in bile. The study revealed that in the absence of biliary tree obstruction, rifamide achieved extremely high bile levels, but totally inadequate serum concentrations. However, in patients with biliary tract obstruction, not only serum levels, but also bile levels were totally inadequate. The study revealed that postoperative sepsis was not reduced by rifamide when compared to the controls. However, postoperative sepsis was significantly lowered in the patients receiving gentamicin. Adequate serum levels were achieved in 88% of the patients receiving gentamicin, but in most patients bile levels were low. Nevertheless, wound infection was decreased from 22% to 6%

TABLE 25–6.—SUSCEPTIBILITY OF VARIOUS BILIARY TRACT ORGANISMS TO COMMONLY USED ANTIBIOTICS, %*

ORGANISMS	GENTAMICIN	AMPICILLIN	CHLORAMPHENICOL	TETRACYCLINE
Escherichia coli	100	36	88	57
Klebsiella sp.	100	10	75	75
Streptococcus faecalis	56	93	93	58
Enterobacter sp.	100	10	93	86
Proteus sp.	100	100	100	11
Pseudomonas sp.	100	17	—	66

*Adapted from Keighley M.R.B., et al.[58]

TABLE 25–7.—BILIARY EXCRETION OF ANTIBIOTICS*

Amikacin	Amoxocillin	Ampicillin	Azlocillin
Bacitracin	Carbenicillin	Cefazolin	Cefamandole
Chloramphenicol	Cefonicid	Cefotaxime	Cefoperazone
Colistimethate	Methicillin	Cefoxitin	Mezlocillin
Gentamicin	Metronidazole	Cefuroxime	Nafcillin
Kanamycin	Oxacillin	Cephalothin	Piperacillin
Netilmycin	Penicillin	Cephradine	Rifamycins
Polymyxin	Sulfathiazole	Clindamycin	
Streptomycin	Sulfamethoxazole	Erythromycin	
Tobramycin	Ticarcillin	Moxalactam	
Vancomycin	Trimethoprim	Tetracyclines	

*Based on:

	LOW	MODERATE	HIGH	VERY HIGH
Peak bile/serum ratio:	< 1	1–2	2–20	> 20
Peak bile level (μg/ml):	< 5	5–20	20–100	> 100

and septicemia from 14% to 2% in the gentamicin group when compared to controls. Thus, these investigators have shown very nicely in two controlled prospective studies that it is far more important to have an antibiotic with good coverage and with adequate serum concentrations to prevent or treat bacteremias, than to have an antibiotic that is secreted in high concentrations into bile. This would be particularly true for patients with acute cholangitis since all of them have some degree of biliary tree obstruction which would likely inhibit secretion of any antibiotic into bile.

Therefore, when one is choosing an antibiotic to treat acute cholangitis, the antibiotic should be picked primarily for its ability to achieve adequate serum levels and to cover the organisms likely to be causing the infection. Most bacteriology studies, including those from The Johns Hopkins Hospital, the University of California, and the University of Birmingham in England, have shown that the three most common organisms cultured in biliary tract sepsis are *E. coli*, *K. pneumoniae*, and *Streptococcus faecalis*. In addition, recent studies[6, 26, 34–38] suggest that anaerobes including *B. fragilis* are frequently isolated from elderly patients with complex biliary problems, those most likely to present with cholangitis. Thus until very recently, "complete" antibacterial coverage for these patients will require the combination of an aminoglycoside, a penicillin, and an agent active against *B. fragilis*.

Until a few years ago, available antibiotic combinations that did not include an aminoglycoside provided antibacterial coverage for only 70%–75% of patients with cholangitis because of their failure to treat enterococcus. Neither chloramphenicol nor the second- or third-generation cephalosporins, with the possible exception of cefoperazone, provide protection from enterococcus. Some might argue that enterococcus is rarely isolated from the blood of these patients and, therefore, does not warrant specific coverage. However, now that newer antibiotics such as piperacillin, mezlocillin, and cefoperazone are available, this dilemma no longer exists. These agents provide antibacterial coverage for enterococcus as well as the gram-negative aerobes without the risk of nephrotoxicity associated with the aminoglycosides.

This risk may be particularly important in patients who present with cholangitis who, in addition to being septic, are frequently elderly, jaundiced, and have preexisting renal disease. In fact, in a recent analysis of 33 patients with cholangitis secondary to choledocholithiasis who were treated with

an aminoglycoside for a mean of 10 days, 11 (33%) developed a significant elevation of creatinine.[10] These renal problems, in turn, resulted in a significantly longer hospital stay for these patients.

Therefore, whenever any aminoglycoside is administered to a patient with cholangitis, very careful monitoring of serum antibiotic levels is mandatory. If blood or bile cultures indicate that less nephrotoxic agents will suffice, aminoglycoside therapy should be discontinued. In addition, prolonged postoperative administration of aminoglycosides to patients whose biliary obstruction has been alleviated and whose fever has abated is not warranted. Aminoglycosides should also be avoided in patients with cholangitis who present with only a transient fever and no other signs of sepsis. For these patients who are less severely ill, the newer antibiotics such as piperacillin, mezlocillin, or cefoperazone should provide adequate antibacterial coverage. Thus, we recommend that initial antibiotic therapy for patients with biliary sepsis should be individualized on the basis of the severity of the presenting symptoms.

The majority of patients presenting with acute cholangitis will respond to antibiotic therapy. Within 24–48 hours the fever will defervesce and liver function tests will return toward normal. For the infrequent patient who presents with acute suppurative cholangitis who does not respond to IV antibiotic therapy and general supportive methods, emergency decompression of the biliary tree needs to be performed. Generally, one should expect to see a response within 12–24 hours in a patient presenting with cholangitis. If a patient fails to show improvement, or shows signs of further deterioration, then emergency decompression should be carried out. In selected patients adequate decompression of these desperately ill patients can be obtained by the percutaneous transhepatic route. Whether endoscopic sphincterotomy is indicated in these patients has not yet been adequately answered. For the majority of patients, however, response to noninvasive therapy will be satisfactory. Since all patients will have some degree of obstruction secondary to biliary tract pathology, most patients will require workup of their biliary tract and subsequent surgery. For occasional patients, particularly those who have had multiple benign stricture repairs and in whom further biliary tract surgery would be risky and probably unsuccessful, one might choose to manage the patient nonoperatively, if the attacks of cholangitis are infrequent and mild. In such an instance, a choloretic agent to stimulate the flow of bile, along with the long-term administration of an antibiotic secreted in high concentration in bile, might be utilized. The combination of trimethoprim and sulfamethoxazole has been used in recent years because it is secreted in moderately high concentrations in the bile. Others have used ampicillin, tetracycline, or the cephalosporins with success despite their less than ideal coverage. When used as a chronic suppressant for biliary tract flora, an antibiotic secreted in high concentrations in bile has a theoretical advantage.

The majority of patients presenting with acute cholangitis, however, will have biliary tract pathology that requires surgical intervention. Once the patient has responded adequately to the initial antibiotic therapy, the biliary tract pathology should be accurately defined prior to carrying out biliary tract surgery. In recent years with the widespread availability of ERCP and transhepatic cholangiography, there is no longer any need to explore a patient following an episode of acute cholangitis without knowing the anatomical pathology with a great deal of accuracy. Intravenous cholangiography is rarely adequate in providing the type of resolution that one requires to define the biliary tract anatomy. The importance of accurately defining the obstructive pathology following an attack of acute cholangitis, but prior to operative intervention, was demonstrated in a series of 78 patients presenting with acute cholangitis to The Johns Hopkins Hospital.[3] There were 11 deaths in this series. Six of the 11 deaths were secondary to continuing or recurrent cholangitis and sepsis following surgery, often after an initial period of improvement. An autopsy was performed in each of the six patients, and in each patient retained stones or a persistent stricture inadequately stented was found. Thus, in this series of patients with acute cholangitis, the most frequent cause of death was recurrent sepsis following an unsuccessful operative procedure. In each instance the unsuccessful biliary tract procedure was secondary to incomplete information concerning the biliary tract pathology. If a patient with acute cholangitis does not respond rapidly to initial antibiotic therapy, then emergency surgical decompression of the biliary tree should be carried out. However, for the vast majority of patients who do respond, one has adequate time to subsequently define the patient's biliary tract pathology. Sixty-four of the 78 patients in the series from The Johns Hopkins Hospital underwent surgical intervention. In only 13 patients was the surgery carried out within the first 48 hours of admission. In 33 patients the surgery was carried out between two and ten days after admission, and in 18 patients a lapse of over ten days occurred before the corrective biliary tract surgery was carried out. In none of the patients in whom surgery was delayed for two or more days following admission to the hospital did a recurrent attack of cholangitis develop prior to surgery's being performed. Thus, one can proceed with the biliary tract workup without the threat of recurrent sepsis. This workup should proceed under the continuing coverage of antibiotics with a broad spectrum against the common biliary organisms. In addition, one has to be cautious that the biliary tree pressure is not elevated excessively during transhepatic or ERCP. If obstructive pathology is demonstrated and there is not adequate drainage of contrast medium from the biliary tree postcholangiography, surgery should be performed on an urgent basis to avoid sepsis.

Response to therapy for most patients with acute cholangitis is prompt and gratifying. The overall mortality in the group of patients from The Johns Hopkins Hospital was 14%.[3] Two of these 11 deaths were in patients who were admitted to the hospital in a state of severe septic shock and died within eight hours of admission without being stabilized to the point where an operation seemed reasonable. Six patients, previously mentioned, died of recurrent cholangitis following surgery because of inadequate surgical decompression. The development of an hepatic abscess, discussed later, considerably worsens the prognosis, and four of the 11 deaths in this series were in patients who developed this complication. The overall mortality in the group of 36 patients from the U.C.S.D. was 22%.[4] Sixteen of the 99 patients (16%) with

acute cholangitis reported by Boey and Way[11] died. If one extracts from these series, however, patients who present in septic shock with suppurative cholangitis, the mortality of acute cholangitis is much less.

Occasional patients presenting with acute cholangitis may in the future be managed routinely without the need for surgery. A significant number of patients presenting with acute cholangitis will have recurrent or primary common duct stones. Among the 78 patients in the series from The Johns Hopkins Hospital, 25% were thought to have recurrent or primary common duct stones.[3] These patients in most instances will already have undergone cholecystectomy and will present with a dilated common duct containing one or more primary common duct stones, or sludge.

Recently, some of these patients are being managed with endoscopic papillotomy and stone extraction, thereby avoiding the need for surgery. This approach may be appropriate for elderly patients with primary common duct stones presenting with acute cholangitis who may not tolerate a general anesthetic.

COMPLICATIONS

The two most common severe complications of cholangitis are acute renal failure and intrahepatic abscesses. Both of these complications contribute heavily to the mortality seen in acute cholangitis. Acute cholangitis implies a bacteremia of biliary tract origin. The bacteremia may be transient and of little systemic consequence; however, the bacteremia may also be associated with septic shock, decreased renal perfusion, and acute renal failure. Many of the patients with the most severe form of acute cholangitis, suppurative cholangitis, also develop multiple hepatic abscesses, and these patients have a high mortality.

Experimental and clinical studies by Dawson[59, 60] have shown that patients with obstructive jaundice have an increased chance of developing renal failure. Dawson proposed that circulating bile pigments sensitize the kidney to damage by ischemia. This contention is supported by experimental work in rats in which obstructive jaundice intensified the damage caused by 60 minutes of renal ischemia. However, Dawson was able to protect animals against ischemic damage by pretreating them with mannitol. In a retrospective study Dawson documented seven instances of acute renal failure among 103 patients with obstructive jaundice, and in six of the seven patients who developed acute renal failure, the preoperative bilirubin level was greater than 20 mg/dl. This incidence of renal failure in patients with jaundice most likely represents a decrease in renal blood flow associated with sepsis from cholangitis. In addition, the kidneys of these jaundiced patients may be more vulnerable to renal shut down because of the presence of retained bile pigments. Prompt treatment of the septic shock seen with acute cholangitis should decrease the incidence of acute renal failure. As pointed out in the section on treatment, this includes volume replacement, antibiotics, steroids, and frequently an ionotrophic agent such as dopamine. Since dopamine is a renal artery vasodilator as well, this drug can be particularly helpful. Avoidance of nephrotoxic antibiotics may also be important.

In patients with acute suppurative cholangitis, the infection may extend into the liver with the development of multiple liver abscesses. Initially, there are small collections of polymorphonuclear cells that are near the termination of the bile canaliculi. These areas may enlarge into true abscesses (Fig 25–4). Prior to the introduction of antibiotics, pylephlebitis secondary to appendicitis was the leading cause of pyogenic hepatic abscess.[61] However, several reports[61–64] in recent years have indicated that the relative incidence of intrahepatic abscesses secondary to cholangitis has been increasing. Cholangitis was the most frequent cause of hepatic abscess in a review of 130 cases reported by Sherman and Robbins[65] in 1960. An analysis of 10 studies published since 1960, including 417 instances of pyogenic hepatic abscess, revealed that 41% were due to cholangitis, while only 24% were transmitted via the portal vein.[62] Among 80 patients with pyogenic hepatic abscess seen at The Johns Hopkins Hospital between 1952 and 1972, 41 (51%) had a biliary etiology.[62] Among these 41 patients, 23 had benign biliary tract disease, and 21 of these patients had stones in the common bile duct. The remaining 18 patients had malignant extrahepatic obstruction, and 13 of these patients had adenocarcinoma of the head of the pancreas (Table 25–8). Most of these latter patients had undergone some form of biliary-intestinal bypass prior to the development of intrahepatic abscesses. In this series, malignant extrahepatic obstruction was more common in the later years of this study, and these patients accounted for 47%, or eight of 17 patients, seen during the last four years of the study. Two other recent reports[63, 66] have noted a 13%–15% incidence of pyogenic hepatic abscess secondary to malignant extrahepatic obstruction.

When intrahepatic abscesses develop, mortality is directly related to the multiplicity of abscesses. In the Hopkins series[62] the mortality rate was 31% among the 32 patients with a solitary abscess, and 88% among the 48 patients with multiple abscesses. In this series, 88% of the abscesses of biliary origin were multiple; therefore, these patients had a high mortality. Twenty of the 23 patients with benign biliary tract obstruction, and 17 of the 18 patients with malignant extrahepatic obstruction who developed intrahepatic abscesses died. In contrast, only two of 24 (8%) of those patients with solitary abscesses treated with antibiotics and surgical drainage died (Table 25–9).

As would be expected, the bacteriology of patients with liver abscesses of biliary origin is similar to the organisms grown from the bile in patients with cholangitis. In the series of patients with hepatic abscesses from Hopkins,[62] E. coli, Klebsiella and streptococcal species were the organisms most commonly isolated. However, a significant number of anaerobic organisms were also cultured directly from the abscesses or from the blood in these patients. In the Hopkins series anaerobes were grown in 27% of the patients, and the percentage of patients with anaerobic organisms isolated increased significantly from 16% during the first ten years of the study to 36% in the second ten years. Anaerobes were grown directly from the liver abscess in 25% of the patients cultured, whereas anaerobes were found in only 10% of the blood cultures and in only 7% of the bile cultures. These differences may be a reflection of culturing techniques, but they also may be an indication of the preferential ability of anaerobes to grow in liver parenchyma. As mentioned earlier, bile salts inhibit the growth of some anaerobic organisms.[32, 33]

In those patients with cholangitis who present with shock, lethargy, and mental depression, and in those patients who do not respond rapidly to nonoperative therapy, in addition to considering acute suppurative cholangitis, the possibility of liver abscesses must also be entertained. In addition to prompt surgical decompression of the biliary tree, consideration should be given to adding an antibiotic with anaerobe coverage, and possibly to the direct infusion of antibiotics via an umbilical vein catheter, as proposed by Piccone.[67] The mortality without prompt surgery approaches 100% in patients with multiple liver abscesses. Even with prompt surgical management and antibiotic coverage, the mortality is from 50% to 70%.[62]

TABLE 25–8.—ETIOLOGY OF PYOGENIC HEPATIC ABSCESS— THE JOHNS HOPKINS HOSPITAL*

ORIGIN	NO. OF PATIENTS	%
Biliary		
Benign		
Choledocholithiasis	21	
Cholecystojejunostomy	1	
Benign stricture	1	
Malignant		
Adenocarcinoma of pancreas	13	
Adenocarcinoma bile ducts, gallbladder, duodenum	4	
Metastatic carcinoma of cervix	1	
Total	41	51
Cryptogenic	16	20
Portal vein route	11	14
Direct extension	8	10
Trauma	3	4
Hepatic artery route	1	1

*Twenty-five patients with generalized sepsis and microscopic abscesses in several organs were excluded.

TABLE 25–9.—MORTALITY IN PYOGENIC HEPATIC ABSCESS—THE JOHNS HOPKINS HOSPITAL

	NO. OF PATIENTS	NO. OF DEATHS	MORTALITY, %
No. of abscesses			
Solitary abscess	32	10	31
Multiple abscesses	48	42	88
Total	80	52	65
Biliary etiology			
Benign	23	20	87
Malignant	18	17	94
Total	41	37	90
Adequate treatment*			
Solitary abscess	24	2	8
Multiple abscesses	17	12	71
Total	41	14	59

*Antibiotics plus abscess and, when indicated, biliary drainage.

ACUTE "TOXIC" CHOLANGITIS

Suppurative cholangitis refers to gross purulence, or pus, in the biliary tree. Charcot in his initial description of cholangitis was actually referring to acute suppurative cholangitis. In his account of hepatic fever,[1] he described it as being secondary to ". . . pus or purulent mucous mixed in stagnant bile." The first case of acute cholangitis treated by surgical decompression in 1903 by Rogers[2] was also in a patient with acute suppurative cholangitis. Acute suppurative cholangitis represents one end of a spectrum of acute bacterial cholangitis. Most instances of acute cholangitis are associated with partial biliary tree obstruction and infected bile. In acute suppurative cholangitis, the bile becomes grossly purulent, and the biliary tree fills with pus. With acute suppurative cholangitis the biliary tract obstruction is frequently complete. This variety of cholangitis fortunately is not common. Among the 78 patients with acute cholangitis admitted to The Johns Hopkins Hospital between 1952 and 1974, 11 (14%) proved to have acute suppurative cholangitis.[3] This is approximately one patient seen at a large, busy, urban hospital every two years. Two separate reviews compiled in 1970[22] and 1971[12] revealed fewer than 100 patients with acute suppurative cholangitis in the English-speaking literature.

Reynolds and Dargan[68] in 1959 added CNS depression and shock to Charcot's triad and suggested that this pentad was characteristic of a virulent form of acute suppurative cholangitis that they termed acute obstructive cholangitis. The authors felt that acute suppurative cholangitis in the absence of CNS depression and shock was probably secondary to a partially obstructed biliary tree containing pus. Acute obstructive cholangitis, they felt, occurred when the biliary tract obstruction became complete. For the sake of this discussion, we will not differentiate between acute suppurative cholangitis and acute obstructive cholangitis. Since the actual degree of biliary tract obstruction often cannot accurately be determined, the diagnosis of acute obstructive cholangitis rests purely on clinical grounds. It should be pointed out, however, that not all patients with acute suppurative or obstructive cholangitis have pus in their bile ducts at surgery. We would suggest, therefore, that a better term for these patients with the most severe forms of biliary sepsis might be acute "toxic" cholangitis.

Presentation and Diagnosis

A comprehensive review of acute "toxic" cholangitis was published by Pitt and Longmire in 1980.[69] These authors analyzed 303 patients with acute toxic cholangitis reported in the literature. They compared 112 patients who presented with shock to 191 reported patients who were not hypotensive. Fifty-two percent of the 303 patients were older than 70 years, and the subgroup who presented with shock was only slightly older than those who did not. More than 70% of each subgroup had a history of biliary tract disease. Likewise, these two groups differed very little in their clinical presentation. For the entire series, 88% had chills and fever, 93% were jaundiced, and 83% had right upper quadrant pain. However, patients presenting with shock were more likely to have a WBC count greater than 20,000/cu mm. The cause of biliary obstruction was stones in 84% of patients presenting with shock. Choledocholithiasis was also the cause of chol-

angitis in 75% of the nonhypotensive patients.

Thus, the presentation of patients with acute toxic cholangitis is similar to that of patients with acute nontoxic cholangitis. Their early identification on clinical grounds is important, however, since immediate surgery is essential for survival. An interesting study was carried out by Andrew and Johnson[22] in an attempt to identify patients presenting with acute toxic cholangitis. The authors compared 39 patients presenting to their hospital with classic Charcot's triad secondary to choledocholithiasis to 17 patients from their institution who were found to have acute toxic cholangitis. Mean age was similar in both groups. Prior common bile duct surgery, including biliary-intestinal anastomoses and sphincteroplasties, was more common in the group of patients with acute toxic cholangitis. Chills and fever on admission were actually seen more frequently in the patients with nontoxic cholangitis. The incidence of jaundice and right upper quadrant pain was similar in both groups. Septic shock, a temperature of 104°F or greater, and rebound tenderness were seen in a much higher proportion of patients with suppurative cholangitis. The mean WBC count in patients with acute toxic cholangitis was 22,000/cu mm and in nonsuppurative cholangitis 14,000/cu mm. The average serum bilirubin was 9 mg/dl in the patients with "toxic" cholangitis and 6 mg/dl in the patients with nontoxic cholangitis. Positive blood cultures were obtained in 43% of the patients with toxic cholangitis and in only 8% with nontoxic cholangitis. A similar analysis by Boey and Way[11] suggested that patients with toxic cholangitis were more likely to present with shock, a fever greater than 39°C, and a bilirubin greater than 4 mg/dl. Andrew and Johnson also collected 86 patients with acute toxic cholangitis from the literature. Fifty-eight percent were found to have a leukocytosis greater than 20,000/cu mm, and the average serum bilirubin was 10.2 mg/dl. Both of these figures are significantly greater than one usually encounters in patients with nontoxic acute cholangitis. Interestingly, Andrew and Johnson found that in the 86 patients collected from the literature, 69% developed liver abscesses.

The presentation of acute toxic cholangitis is similar to that of acute nontoxic bacterial cholangitis, differing only in degree of severity. Prior common duct surgery appears to be more common, a marked leukocytosis, significant hyperbilirubinemia and positive blood cultures more frequent, temperature over 104°F with a picture of septic shock seen in a high percentage, and rebound tenderness more frequently encountered. All of these findings obviously will alert the clinician to the fact that he is dealing with a markedly ill patient who has a high chance of having pus in his common duct. It is important to make this differentiation since the initial management of this infrequent form of cholangitis may differ from nontoxic cholangitis.

Treatment and Outcome

The treatment of acute toxic cholangitis is surgical drainage. Since the clinical presentation in most instances will be secondary to systemic sepsis, an initial effort should be made prior to surgery to control the systemic infection with IV antibiotics. If the patient is not in shock at the time of presentation, one may have as much as 12 to 24 hours for this initial preparation. However, if a patient is in septic shock and does not respond to initial fluid replacement and antibiotic administration, an emergency operation for ductal decompression might need to be carried out within hours of admission. In selected cases percutaneous transhepatic drainage may be an appropriate temporizing measure in these patients.

The bacteriology of acute toxic cholangitis is similar to that of nontoxic cholangitis. Therefore, an antibiotic regimen with coverage against gram-negative aerobes, enterococcus, and *B. fragilis* is necessary for these most severely ill patients. The usual supportive means for managing septic shock should also be initiated immediately. A central venous pressure catheter is mandatory and, in many instances, a Swan-Ganz catheter will be helpful. Initial treatment of the hypotension, which generally is secondary to peripheral vasodilatation, should be carefully monitored volumes of crystalloids and colloids. Most patients will not be anemic, but if a low hemoglobin is present, whole blood should be administered. If the patient does not respond with elevated arterial pressure prior to elevated central venous or pulmonary wedge pressure, therapy with an ionotropic drug such as dopamine should be started. Large doses of steroids are also generally administered for septic shock. Hypoglycemia has been documented in patients with acute toxic cholangitis, and may be in part responsible for the CNS depression seen. Therefore, blood glucose should be monitored and IV glucose administered. A Foley catheter is required for hourly monitoring of urinary output. A minimum of 30 ml of urine per hour is desired to insure that the cardiac output and renal blood flow are adequate. Most patients will require a nasogastric tube for gastric decompression. Since some of these patients may have chronic liver disease secondary to long-standing biliary tract problems, coagulation studies should be obtained and vitamin K administered if the prothrombin time is prolonged.

If there is an initial period of improvement, surgery may be delayed to await a more stable condition. One can only be suspicious of the diagnosis of suppurative cholangitis at this time, since the diagnosis can only be made by finding gross pus in the bile ducts at the time of surgery. If an initial improvement is seen, surgery may be delayed for 12 to 24 hours until optimal resuscitation has occurred. If the patient does not respond initially, surgical exploration should be carried out within hours of admission. At the time of surgery, a distended common duct will be encountered. Upon performing a choledochotomy, pus under pressure will be found. With gross purulence in the common duct, minimal biliary tract manipulation should be carried out. Any stones evident in the immediate vicinity of the choledochotomy should be removed. In addition, using very gentle irrigation, the biliary tree should be irrigated, possibly with an antibiotic solution. One should be extremely careful not to elevate the pressure in the biliary tree by irrigation, as this may facilitate further egress of bacteria from the biliary tree into the bloodstream. Once this has been performed, a T tube should be inserted and the operation terminated. No attempt should be made to completely rid the biliary tree of calculi or to perform operative cholangiography. If the patient's condition allows, a cholecystectomy should be performed. Under no circumstances should a cholecystostomy be used as a means of duct decompression. This has proved to be totally inadequate as a means of decompressing a common duct in the face of suppurative cholangitis and carries an extremely high mortality.[4, 70] In addition, the liver should be carefully palpated to ascertain whether liver abscesses are present. In the face of a benign or malignant biliary stricture, one has to be certain that the T tube or stent is placed above the point of obstruction. In most instances, no treatment should be carried out for the stricture at the time of exploration for toxic cholangitis. Following emergency duct decompression, secondary biliary tract procedures can be carried out weeks or months later under elective conditions.

Acute toxic cholangitis carries a high mortality. In the review compiled by Pitt and Longmire,[69] there were 29 deaths among the 191 patients (15%) who presented with toxic cholangitis in the absence of septic shock. Thirteen of the patients were not operated on, and six (46%) died. One hundred seventy-eight underwent surgery for biliary decompression, and 16 of these patients died (9%). Mortality was even higher among the 112 patients presenting with toxic cholangitis in septic shock. Thirty-four patients were not operated on, and all 34 died. Seventy-eight patients underwent surgical decompression with 26 not surviving (37%). Thus, 60 of the 112 patients (55%) presenting with acute toxic cholangitis in shock failed to survive. In the collective review of 86 patients by Andrew and Johnson,[22] all patients who did not have surgery died, and the mortality in those patients undergoing ductal decompression was in the range of 50%. The authors felt, on the basis of their review, that the most important factor leading to demise in acute toxic cholangitis was the failure to establish the correct diagnosis and to perform surgical decompression of the biliary tree as an emergency. Thus, if one is to manage the rare patient with acute toxic cholangitis successfully, a high index of suspicion is necessary. If a patient with a clinical picture of cholangitis presents and fails to respond to initial therapy, immediate surgery should be undertaken.

REFERENCES

1. Charcot J.M.: Lecons sur les maladies du fore des voices biliares et des veins. Paris, Faculte de Medecine de Paris. Recueillies et publiees par Bourneville et Sevestre, 1877.
2. Rogers L.: Biliary abscesses of the liver with operation. *Br. Med. J.* 2:706, 1903.
3. Saharia P.C., Cameron J.L.: Clinical management of cholangitis. *Surg. Gynecol. Obstet.* 142:369, 1976.
4. Saik R.P., Greenburg A.G., Farris J.M., et al.: Spectrum of cholangitis. *Am. J. Surg.* 130:143, 1975.
5. Saharia P.C., Zuidema G.D., Cameron J.L.: Primary common duct stones. *Ann. Surg.* 185:598, 1977.
6. Pitt H.A., Postier R.G., Cameron J.L.: Bacteremia after tube cholangiography. *Ann. Surg.* 191:30, 1980.
7. Flemma R.J., Flint L.M., Osterhout S., et al.: Bacteriologic studies of biliary tract infection. *Ann. Surg.* 166:563, 1967.
8. Davis J.L., Milligan F.D., Cameron J.L.: Septic complications following endoscopic retrograde cholangiopancreatography. *Surg. Gynecol. Obstet.* 140:365, 1975.
9. Burhenne H.J.: Complications of nonoperative extraction of retained common duct stone. *Am. J. Surg.* 131:260, 1976.
10. Pitt H.A., Postier R.G., Cameron J.L.: Consequences of preoperative cholangitis and its treatment on the outcome of surgery for choledocholithiasis. *Surgery* 94:447, 1983.
11. Boey J.H., Way L.W.: Acute cholangitis. *Ann. Surg.* 191:264, 1980.
12. Longmire W.P. Jr.: Suppurative cholangitis, in Hardy J.M. (ed.): *Critical Surgical Illness.* Philadelphia, W.B. Saunders Co., 1971, pp. 397–424.
13. Rosenthal L., Shaffer E.R., Lisboner R., et al.: Diagnosis of hepatobiliary disease by ^{99m}Tc HIDA cholescintigraphy. *Radiology* 126:467, 1978.

14. Okuda K., Tanikawa K., Emara T., et al.: Nonsurgical percutaneous transhepatic cholangiography—diagnostic significance in medical problems of the liver. *Am. J. Dig. Dis.* 19:21, 1974.
15. Bilbao M.K., Dotter C.T., Lee T.G., et al.: Complications of endoscopic retrograde cholangiopancreatography (ERCP): A study of 10,000 cases. *Gastroenterology* 70:314, 1976.
16. Cotton P.B.: Cannulation of the papilla of Vater by endoscopic and retrograde cholangiopancreatography (ERCP). *Gut* 13:1014, 1972.
17. Zimmon D.S., Fulkenstein D.G., Riccobono C., et al.: Complications of endoscopic retrograde cholangiopancreatography: Analysis of 300 consecutive cases. *Gastroenterology* 69:303, 1975.
18. Kasagai T., Kuno N., Kizu M.: Manometric endoscopic retrograde pancreatocholangiography. *Am. J. Dig. Dis.* 19:485, 1974.
19. Nakayama T., Ikeda A., Okuda K.: Percutaneous transhepatic drainage of the biliary tract: Technique and results in 104 cases. *Gastroenterology* 74:554, 1978.
20. Kadir S., Baassiri A., Barth K.H., et al.: Percutaneous biliary drainage in the management of biliary sepsis. *A.J.R.* 138:25, 1982.
21. Raine P.A.M., Gunn A.A.: Acute cholecystitis. *Br. J. Surg.* 62:697, 1975.
22. Andrew D.J., Johnson S.E.: Acute suppurative cholangitis, a medical and surgical emergency. *Am. J. Gastroenterol.* 54:141, 1970.
23. Fukunaga F.H.: Gallbladder bacteriology, histology, and gallstones. *Arch. Surg.* 106:169, 1973.
24. Edlund Y.A., Mollstedt B.O., Ouchterlong O.: Bacteriological investigation of the biliary system and liver in biliary tract disease correlated to clinical data and microstructure of the gallbladder and liver. *Acta Chir. Scand.* 116:461, 1959.
25. Keighley M.R.B., Flinn R., Alexander-Williams J.: Multivariate analysis of clinical and operative findings associated with biliary sepsis. *Br. J. Surg.* 63:528, 1976.
26. Pitt H.A., Postier R.G., Cameron J.L.: Biliary bacteria: Significance and alterations after antibiotic therapy. *Arch. Surg.* 117:445, 1982.
27. O'Connor M.J., Schwartz M.L., McQuarrie D.G., et al.: Cholangitis due to malignant obstruction to biliary outflow. *Ann. Surg.* 193:341, 1981.
28. Keighley M.R.B., Lister D.M., Jacobs S.I., et al.: Hazards of surgical treatment due to microorganisms in the bile. *Surgery* 75:578, 1974.
29. Mason G.R.: Bacteriology and antibiotic selection in biliary tract surgery. *Arch. Surg.* 97:533, 1968.
30. Chetlin S.H., Elliott D.W.: Biliary bacteremia. *Arch. Surg.* 102:303, 1971.
31. Gorbach S.L., Plant A.G., Nahas L., et al.: Studies of intestinal microflora: II. Micro-organisms of the small intestine and their relations to oral and fecal flora. *Gastroenterology* 53:856, 1967.
32. Binder H.J., Filburn B., Flock M.: Bile acid inhibition of intestinal anaerobic organisms. *Am. J. Clin. Nutr.* 28:119, 1975.
33. Williams R.C., Showalter R., Kern F. Jr.: *In vivo* effect of bile salts and cholestyramine on intestinal anaerobic bacteria. *Gastroenterology* 69:483, 1975.
34. Nielsen N.L., Justensen T.: Anaerobic and aerobic bacteriological studies in biliary tract disease. *Scand. J. Gastroenterol.* 11:437, 1976.
35. England D.M., Rosenblatt J.E.: Anaerobes in human biliary tracts. *J. Clin. Microbiol.* 6:494, 1977.
36. Shimada K., Inamatsu T., Yamashiro M.: Anaerobic bacteria in biliary disease in elderly patients. *J. Infect. Dis.* 135:850, 1977.
37. Bergen T., Dobloug I., Liavag I.: Bacterial isolates in cholecystitis and cholelithiasis. *Scand. J. Gastroenterol.* 14:625, 1979.
38. Jackaman F.R., Hilson G.R.F., Marlow L.S.: Bile bacteria in patients with benign bile duct stricture. *Br. J. Surg.* 67:329, 1980.
39. Taylor F.W.: Blood-culture studies of the portal vein. *Arch. Surg.* 72:889, 1956.
40. Orloff M.J., Peskins G.W., Ellis H.L.: A bacteriological study of human portal blood. *Ann. Surg.* 148:738, 1956.
41. Dineen P.: The importance of the route of infection in experimental biliary tract obstruction. *Surg. Gynecol. Obstet.* 119:1001, 1964.
42. Schatten W.E., Desprez J.D., Holden W.D.: A bacteriologic study of portal vein blood in man. *Arch. Surg.* 71:404, 1955.
43. Brooke B.N., Slaney G.: Portal bacteremia in ulcerative colitis. *Lancet* 1:1206, 1958.
44. Ong G.B.: A study of recurrent pyogenic cholangitis. *Arch. Surg.* 84:63, 1962.
45. Scott A.J., Khan G.A.: Origin of bacteria in bile duct bile. *Lancet* 2:790, 1967.
46. Mixer H.W., Rigler L.G., Gonzales-Oddone M.V.: Experimental studies on biliary regurgitation during cholangiography. *Gastroenterology* 9:64, 1947.
47. Edlund Y., Hanzon V.: Demonstration of the close relationship between bile capillaries and sinusoid walls. *Acta Anat. (Basel)* 17:105, 1953.
48. Rouiller C.: Les canalicules biliares: Etude au microscope electronique. *Acta Anat. (Basel)* 26:94, 1956.
49. Hampton J.C.: An electron microscope study of the hepatic uptake and excretion of microscopic particles injected into the blood stream and into the bile duct. *Acta Anat. (Basel)* 32:262, 1958.
50. Hultborn A., Jacobsson B., Rosengren B.: Cholangiovenous reflux during cholangiography. *Acta Chir. Scand.* 123:111, 1962.
51. Jacobsson B., Kjellander J., Rosengren B.: Cholangiovenous reflux. *Acta Chir. Scand.* 123:316, 1962.
52. Huang T., Bass J.A., Williams R.D.: The significance of biliary pressures in cholangitis. *Arch. Surg.* 98:629, 1969.
53. Mallet-Guy P.: Value of preoperative manometric and roentgenographic examination in the diagnosis of pathologic changes and functional disturbances of the biliary tract. *Surg. Gynecol. Obstet.* 94:385, 1952.
54. Williams R.D., Fish J.C., Williams D.D.: The significance of biliary pressure. *Arch. Surg.* 95:374, 1974.
55. Hopton D., White T.T.: An evaluation of manometric operative cholangiography in 100 patients with biliary disease. *Surg. Gynecol. Obstet.* 133:949, 1971.
56. Keighley M.R.B., Baddeley R.M., Burdon D.W., et al.: A controlled trial of parenteral prophylactic gentamicin therapy in biliary surgery. *Br. J. Surg.* 62:215, 1975.
57. Keighley M.R.B., Drysdale R.B., Quoraishi A.H., et al.: Antibiotics in biliary disease: The relative importance of antibiotic concentrations in the bile and serum. *Gut* 17:495, 1976.
58. Keighley M.R.B., Drysdale R.B., Quoraishi A.H.: Antibiotic treatment of biliary sepsis. *Surg. Clin. North Am.* 55:1379, 1975.
59. Dawson J.L.: Postoperative renal function in obstructive jaundice: Effect of mannitol diuresis. *Br. Med. J.* 1:82, 1965.
60. Dawson J.L.: Acute postoperative renal failure in obstructive jaundice. *Ann. R. Coll. Surg. Engl.* 42:163, 1968.
61. Ochsner A., DeBakey M., Murray S.: Pyogenic abscess of the liver: II. An analysis of 47 cases with review of the literature. *Am. J. Surg.* 40:292, 1938.
62. Pitt H.A., Zuidema G.D.: Factors influencing mortality in the treatment of pyogenic hepatic abscess. *Surg. Gynecol. Obstet.* 140:228, 1975.
63. Lazarchick J., deSouza e Silva N.A., Nichols D.R., et al.: Pyogenic liver abscess. *Mayo Clin. Proc.* 48:349, 1973.
64. Rubin R.H., Swartz M.N., Malt R.: Hepatic abscess: Changing clinical, bacteriologic, and therapeutic aspects. *Am. J. Med.* 57:601, 1974.
65. Sherman J.D., Robbins S.: Changing trends in the causistics of hepatic abscess. *Am. J. Med.* 28:943, 1960.
66. Joseph W.L., Kahn A.M., Longmire W.P. Jr.: Pyogenic liver abscess: Changing patterns in approach. *Am. J. Surg.* 115:63, 1968.
67. Piccone V.A.: Discussion of: Pyogenic liver abscess: Changing patterns in approach. *Am. J. Surg.* 115:63, 1968.
68. Reynolds B.M., Dargan E.L.: Acute obstructive cholangitis: A distinct clinical syndrome. *Ann. Surg.* 150:299, 1959.
69. Pitt H.A., Longmire W.P. Jr.: Suppurative cholangitis, in Hardy J.M. (ed.): *Critical Surgical Illness,* ed. 2. Philadelphia, W.B. Saunders Co., 1980, pp. 380–408.
70. Glenn F., Moody F.C.: Acute obstructive suppurative cholangitis. *Surg. Gynecol. Obstet.* 113:265, 1961.

PART V

Liver Disease and Portal Hypertension

26

The Liver
Malignant and Benign Tumors, Nonparasitic Cysts, Parasitic Cysts, Abscess, Liver Anatomy, Technique of Liver Resection

R. Scott Jones, M.D.

MALIGNANT LIVER TUMORS

Primary Tumors

Primary liver cancers can arise from hepatocytes or from epithelium of the intrahepatic bile ducts. Hepatocellular carcinoma constitutes about 90%–95% of primary liver cancers, while cholangiocarcinomas add about 5% of the total. Other malignancies such as sarcoma or mesenchymal tumors can occur. Hepatocellular carcinoma takes a quarter of a million lives annually worldwide. There is marked geographic variability in death rates from hepatoma, with high incidence in Africa and the Orient and relatively low incidence elsewhere. In Mozambique, for example, 99/100,000 people die of hepatoma each year. In the United States, however, the annual primary liver cancer death rate for 1975 was 3.7/100,000. There is a geographic variation within the United States for the annual death rate from primary liver cancer, with significantly higher mortality in the west south central states (4.6/100,000). Males have two to four times greater death rates from hepatoma than females. A statistically significant (45%) increase (2.5–3.6/100,000) in the age-adjusted death rate for hepatoma in non-white males occurred between 1958 and 1975 in the United States.[1]

Possible etiologies of primary liver cancer include hepatitis B virus (HBV), alcohol, cirrhosis, aflatoxins, organochlorine pesticides, and cigarette smoking.[2] The relative risks for several of these factors in Los Angeles included cigarette smoking, 2.6; alcohol, 4.2; hepatitis, 13.1; and blood transfusion, 7.0.[3, 4] Although not proved beyond doubt, a causal relation between hepatitis B virus and hepatocellular cancer is nearly certain.[2, 4–6] Evidence supporting the hypothesis that persistent infection with HBV causes the development of primary hepatocellular carcinoma includes the following:

1. Primary hepatocellular carcinoma is common in regions of the world where hepatitis B virus carriers are prevalent and is less common where hepatitis B virus carriers are not prevalent.

2. Ninety percent or more of patients with primary hepatocellular cancer who live in hepatitis B virus-endemic areas have HBsAg or high titers of antibody against virus core antigen in their blood.

3. Eighty percent of primary hepatocellular cancer arises in patients having cirrhosis, chronic active hepatitis, or both.

4. Hepatitis B virus protein is demonstrable in hepatic tissues of primary hepatocellular cancer patients.

5. Hepatitis B virus infection precedes primary hepatocellular cancer.

6. When hepatitis B virus is endemic, many chronic carriers acquire it from the mother.

7. Hepatitis B virus-DNA is not only present in primary hepatocellular cancer tissues but is also integrated into liver cell genomes.

8. There are other instances in nature in which viruses may cause liver tumors, as in woodchucks, Chinese ducks, and ground squirrels.

Understanding the relationship between hepatitis B virus and liver cancer is obviously important from the fundamental standpoint, because investigating the mechanisms by which the virus causes cancer will permit new insights into the issue of carcinogenesis. In addition, this understanding may permit development of strategies to reduce the occurrence of hepatocellular cancer. For example, the development of the hepatitis B vaccine can predictably reduce the numbers of people at risk for developing hepatocellular cancer. Personal sanitation and health practices in endemic areas of hepatitis B virus might reduce hepatitis and hence primary liver cancer. There is evidence for transmission of hepatitis B virus by certain insects such as bedbugs and mosquitoes; therefore, programs to eradicate these vectors may reduce hepatitis.[7]

Signs and Symptoms

Although hepatoma can develop in persons without liver disease, most liver cancers develop in persons with chronic liver disease. The symptoms include abdominal pain, weight loss, anorexia, fever. Patients can notice an abdominal mass or an increase in liver size. Physical examination may confirm fever and reveal jaundice, an abdominal mass, or findings of ascites in advanced cases.[8, 9]

When hepatoma develops without known preexistent liver disease, abdominal pain or an abdominal mass are commonly the findings. Infrequently, spontaneous intra-abdominal hemorrhage can be the first indication of primary liver cancer.

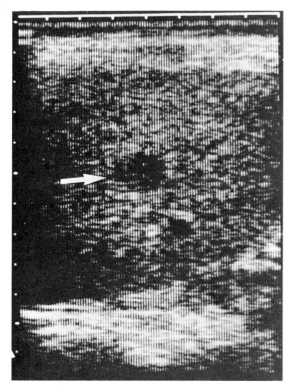

Fig 26–1.—Ultrasound examination disclosed a 1.2 × 1.6 cm hepatoma. (From Shinagawa T., et al.: *Gastroenterology* 86:495–502, 1984. Reprinted with permission of Elsevier Science Publishing Co., Inc. ©1984 by the Am. Gastroenterological Assoc.)

The best means of detecting primary liver cancers remains a controversial subject.[9, 10–16] A recent study conducted in Japan revealed that ultrasound examination found 72.5% of the tumors which developed in a group of patients undergoing follow-up evaluation of liver disease (Fig 26–1). In this

group of patients with hepatocellular cancers < 5 cm in diameter, ultrasound detected 92.2%, CT 73.2%, isotope scan 50.0%, and angiography 86.0% of the tumors. In this group of patients, the α-fetoprotein in the blood was normal in 25.5% and > 200 ng/ml in only 3.3% of the patients. These workers emphasized the utility of ultrasound in the detection of primary liver cancers in high-risk populations because of its utility, convenience, economy, and avoidance of radiation. It is interesting that they kept an ultrasound unit in the follow-up clinic.[9] Other workers suggested that arteriography was best for detecting minute hepatomas and indispensable for tumors < 2 cm. They suggested that α-fetoprotein values and ultrasound should be used for screening. Hepatomas usually appear as very vascular tumors during arteriography (Fig 26–2).[16]

The hepatoma having been detected, its identity can be confirmed by ultrasound-directed needle aspiration. Needle puncture should be avoided unless hemangioma has been confidently excluded.

Treatment

Surgical removal, when it can be applied, is the best treatment for hepatoma. For a patient to be treated surgically, the tumor should be confined to one hepatic lobe, there should be no evidence of metastatic disease in the lung or elsewhere, liver "function" should be normal or near normal, and the patient's general condition should be judged good enough to withstand a large surgical procedure. CT scanning should aid in evaluating resectability by delineating the size and position of the tumor and by revealing lesions in the contralateral liver lobe or in hilar or retroperitoneal nodes (Fig 26–3). In most cases, resectability will best be determined during laparotomy. Some authorities believe that cirrhosis is a contraindication to extensive liver resection, although small hepatomas in cirrhotics can be resected safely.[17] The need for arteriography is also controversial; it is not an absolutely necessary preoperative study, but the following helpful information can

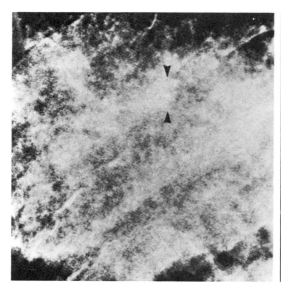

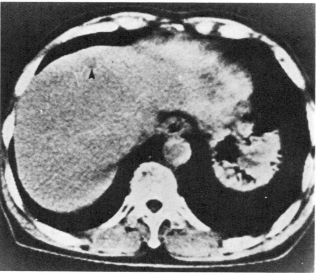

Fig 26–2.—**Left,** the capillary phase of this hepatic angiogram revealed a 1.6 × 1.6 cm hypervascular hepatoma. **Right,** this postcontrast CT scan confirmed the tumor detected by arteriogram. (From Takashima et al.: *Radiology* 145:635–638, 1982.)

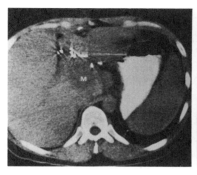
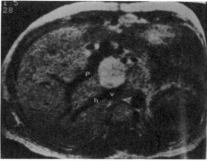

Fig 26–3.—Left, CT scan with contrast. A low-density mass *(M)* was a hepatoma in the caudate lobe. **Right,** NMR spin echo confirmed the presence of the hepatoma and demonstrated the relationships of the portal vein *(P)*, inferior vena cava *(V)*, and hepatic vein *(H)* to the tumor. (From Moss et al.: *Radiology* 150:141–147, 1984.)

be obtained in the arteriography suite: (1) the size, number, and location of tumors, particularly small tumors; (2) the relationship of the arteries to the tumor; (3) the anatomical relationship of the hepatic arteries including relations of bifurcation to the hepatic hilum and the presence of congenital anomalies; (4) hepatic venograms can delineate the relationships between the hepatic veins and tumors in the superior portion of the liver; and (5) inferior venacavograms can delineate the relationships between the vena cava and dorsally located tumors. Although this information is important in planning major hepatic resection, it can all be obtained during careful evaluation at laparotomy.

Most patients with hepatocellular cancer have advanced disease at the time the diagnosis is made, and resectability rates vary from 7%–40% of those with the disease. Generally, lobectomy or extended lobectomy is used to remove hepatomas (Figs 26–4 and 26–5). Limited resection can be employed for selected cirrhotic patients with primary liver tumor.[17] The operative mortality rate for resection of primary liver cancer varies from 4.3% to 24%. The survival rates (including actuarial analysis) of patients surviving operation at 1, 2, 3, and 5 years are, respectively, 35%–85%, 24%–59.5%, 20%–55.7%, and 14%–46%.[18–21]

A better perspective on the lethality of primary liver cancer comes from the recent review by Okuda and co-workers.[8] Of 600 consecutive Japanese patients with primary hepatocellular carcinoma, 98 (16.3%) had tumor resected, 169 (28.2%) underwent no treatment, and 333 (55.5%) were treated nonsurgically. The median survival time for surgically treated pa-

tients was 19.6 months (compared to 2.8 months for comparably staged, nonsurgically treated patients). The median survival time of untreated patients was 1.6 months.

One recommended chemotherapeutic regimen for primary liver cancer includes fluorouracil, cyclophosphamide, and vincristine, followed by doxorubicin (Adriamycin) if necessary. More recently, the four drugs have been administered simultaneously. Fluorouracil and mitomycin C have been employed.[18] There is, as yet, no convincing evidence for the efficacy of these regimens.

Other maneuvers such as hepatic artery ligation, radiation therapy, and the administration of BCG vaccine have been employed without demonstrable benefit in the treatment of primary liver cancer.

Metastatic Tumors

The vast majority of malignant liver tumors in the United States are metastatic from other sites. Although most human malignancies can spread to the liver, the most common source of liver metastases is intra-abdominal cancer, particularly cancers of the colon, pancreas, and stomach. The reasons for the liver's attraction for metastases are not completely understood, but must include its abundant and dual blood supply, its position in the splanchnic circulation draining the abdominal viscera, and its sinusoidal architecture. Because colorectal

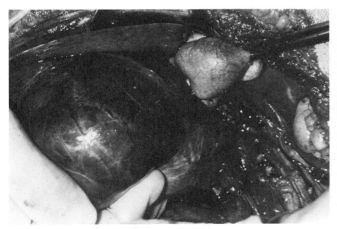

Fig 26–4.—Intraoperative photograph showing a large hepatoma in the right lobe.

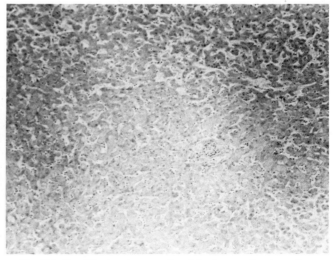

Fig 26–5.—Photomicrograph of features of a hepatoma. Note the absence of bile ducts.

cancers are the most common causes of hepatic metastases, their behavior will be emphasized.

Prognosis

The detection of hepatic metastases from most visceral cancers predicts that the patient will live only a few months. One report noted a median survival time of 75 days from the date of the diagnosis of liver metastases from colonic, pancreatic, and gastric primaries. Patients with colon primaries exhibited a median survival of 146 days following detection of the hepatic metastasis.[22] A recent analysis of 175 patients with liver metastases from colorectal cancer revealed a median survival of 6.7 months, although one patient lived 67 months. Many of the patients in that study had received treatment. A multifactorial analysis of 22 parameters from that material revealed seven statistically significant risk factors predicting earlier death: (1) elevated alkaline phosphatase; (2) elevated serum bilirubin; (3) location of metastases (bilobar vs. unilobar); (4) number of lymph nodes with cancer from primary; (5) decreased serum albumin; (6) whether the primary had been resected; and (7) chemotherapy administration.[23]

Detection of Liver Metastases

Among patients who develop metastases subsequent to surgical treatment of colorectal primary cancers, about half will be asymptomatic, and the other half will have signs and symptoms such as a palpable abdominal mass, abdominal pain, or discomfort or fever.[24]

Patients may undergo evaluation for liver metastases during treatment of the primary cancer (synchronous metastases) or subsequent to treatment of the primary cancer (metachronous metastases). The intraoperative inspection and palpation of the liver can detect metastases with an accuracy of 89%–95%. It is probable but unproved that intraoperative thin-needle aspiration and intraoperative ultrasound could increase the accuracy of intraoperative evaluation of hepatic metastases, particularly those located deep within hepatic parenchyma.

Blood tests or imaging studies are used for nonoperative detection of liver metastases. The accuracy of CEA, GGTP, SGPT, LDH, alkaline phosphatase, SGOT, LAP, and 5'nucleotidase in detecting liver metastases ranged from 53% to 65%, with no significant differences between tests. In patients with colorectal primaries, the CEA provided 86% sensitivity, 60% specificity, and 79% accuracy. When imaging techniques to detect liver metastases were evaluated prospectively, there was no significant difference between liver scintiscan, ultrasound, or CT. The sensitivities were 61%–79%, the specificities 81%–94%, and the accuracies 80%–84%. The use of contrast medium did not significantly influence the effectiveness of CT scan. Lesions 3 cm or greater in diameter were readily detected by each imaging study, while smaller lesions were usually missed. The choice of an imaging test to *screen* patients for liver metastases depends on availability, local expertise, cost, morbidity, and length of examining time and radiation exposure (Fig 26–6).[25]

Another imaging technique that promises to become helpful in evaluating patients with metastatic cancer, particularly metastatic colon cancer, is screening to detect localized radiolabeled antibody.[26–30] Radiolabeled antibodies to carcinoembryonic antigen detected a localized metastatic cancer in 18 patients in 48 hours, while all controls were negative. More recently, a radiolabeled fragment of an anticolorectal carcinoma monoclonal antibody detected metastatic lesions ranging from 1.5 to 8 cm.

Treatment

Having detected liver metastases, one must consider the following choices: (1) no treatment; (2) chemotherapy; (3) immunotherapy; (4) hyperthermia; (5) radiation; (6) hepatic artery ligation; and (7) surgical resection.

Patients with advanced liver metastases, particularly those with ascites, impaired liver function, and wasting, should get only palliative treatment, pain relief, and supportive care.

Currently the information available is insufficient to recommend immunotherapy, hyperthermia, or radiation therapy as therapies for general application to patients with liver metastases.

Studies of the treatment of liver metastases from colorectal cancer provide the bulk of the information concerning chemotherapy. There is currently no evidence that confidently supports chemotherapy as a treatment for metastatic liver cancer. Grage and co-workers[31] investigated the route of administration of chemotherapy for patients with liver metastases and concluded from a prospective randomized trial comparing intra-arterial to systemic infusion of fluorouracil that there was no significant difference in responses between

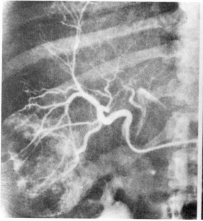
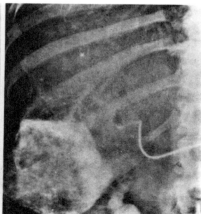

Fig 26–6.—Right hepatic arteriogram of a hypervascular liver metastasis. The tumor appears denser during the arterial hepatogram when the portal flow "washes" the contrast agent from the normal parenchyma. (From Chuang: *Radiology* 148:633–639, 1983.)

treatment and control groups. Since that study, an implant-able pump became available to permit chronic continuous in-fusion of drugs into the hepatic circulation, usually the he-patic artery.[32] Using this device to infuse FUDR (fluorouracil, deoxyriboside, or floxuridine) in the treatment of colorectal metastases, one study observed a median survival time of 26 months compared to a median survival time of eight months in a group of historic control patients.[33, 34] Another similar un-controlled study observed a median survival time of 25 months and provided the opinion that "no patients died solely of uncontrolled liver tumor . . ."[35]

Another study of long-term hepatic arterial infusion of FUDR observed no significant improvement in survival using unrandomized controls. Furthermore, significant toxicity oc-curred in the treated patients.[36]

There remains no conclusive evidence for the efficacy of chemotherapeutic treatment of liver metastases.

Because liver tumors derive their blood supply from the hepatic artery and because liver tumors become smaller fol-lowing hepatic artery ligation, hepatic artery ligation has been used to treat metastatic liver cancer. A recent report de-scribed 97 patients treated by hepatic artery ligation. No in-formation currently available allows evaluation of the efficacy of hepatic artery ligation in treating metastatic liver cancer.[37]

There is a role for hepatic artery ligation in patients with unresectable metastatic carcinoid tumors with associated car-cinoid syndrome. Hepatic artery ligation can relieve at least temporarily and provide significant palliation for the disabling symptoms of the carcinoid syndrome in patients with unre-sectable hepatic metastatic carcinoid tumors.[38]

Surgical Treatment

SYNCHRONOUS METASTASES.—When a small, peripher-ally located lesion can be removed by local excision, wedge resection, or segmental resection, and the lesion is accessible through the incision being employed, it should be removed at the time of the colon resection. Otherwise, the resection of the primary tumors should be completed, and the patient should be reevaluated for removal of the metastasis after com-plete recovery from operation.

METACHRONOUS METASTASES.—Good general health, normal liver function, metastases from colon or rectal pri-mary, a solitary unilobar lesion, and no preoperative or intra-operative evidence of other than a solitary lesion describes an ideal candidate for surgical resection of liver metastases. Technical factors such as size and location of the lesion should dictate the choice of operation. Small, peripheral lesions should be removed by wedge or local excision, while large, central lesions require lobectomy.

The operative mortality rate for surgical excision of liver metastases varies between 0% and 20%. Common causes of operative and postoperative death include hemorrhage, liver failure, GI hemorrhage, and infection. The five-year survival rate for the resection of hepatic metastases when heteroge-neous primary sites are included varies between 20% and 56.4%, because these reports include patients with endocrine tumors that may favorably influence survival. Recent publi-cations concerning resection of liver metastases from colon and rectal primaries report five-year survival rates of 18% to 29%.[18, 21, 24, 39–45]

It is impossible to know yet whether resection for meta-static cancer lengthens survival. Because there are no pro-spective randomized controlled studies, the results of hepatic resection must be compared to historic controls. It is gener-ally believed that the five-year survival of patients with un-treated hepatic metastases from colorectal cancer approaches zero.

Should hepatic resection for metastases be recommended? If the patient has been fully informed about the risks and the benefits, surgical resection of metastatic lesions should be car-ried out in selected patients.[46]

BENIGN LIVER TUMORS

Hepatic Adenoma

A hepatic adenoma is a tumor arising in the liver composed of liver cells with nuclear variation no greater than that of normal liver and which specifically lacks bile ducts or duc-tules. Ninety-one percent of hepatic adenomas occur in women, and most affected patients are in the third to fourth decades of life (20–40 years old). Prior to 1960, hepatic ad-enomas were rare lesions because, between 1940 and 1960, only eight cases had been described in the literature. Be-tween 1960 and 1977, 36 liver cell adenomas were reported. It is interesting that all adenomas reported prior to 1960 were solitary, while one fourth of those described since 1960 were multiple. Although literature reports may not reflect the true incidence of disease, it is highly probable that hepatic ade-noma increased in frequency after 1960, because reports from some institutions included no cases prior to 1960 and several cases subsequent to that time. Because oral contraceptives were introduced into general use in 1960, it is possible that these agents may influence the etiology and pathogenesis of hepatic adenoma. It is clear that some women with docu-mented adenomas have never taken oral contraceptives; how-ever, 89% of patients with hepatic adenomas have a clear and definite history of taking oral contraceptives. Furthermore, oral contraceptive preparations containing mestranol rather than ethynyl estradiol seem to be more closely related to the development of adenoma.[47–50]

Clinical Findings

About half of the patients with hepatic adenoma experi-enced abdominal pain. The pain can be chronic or intermit-tent, but is more commonly due either to hemorrhage or ne-crosis within the tumor or to tumor rupture with hemoperitoneum. In one report, 8/9 women with acute onset of pain due to hemorrhage into tumor or hemoperitoneum were taking birth control pills. Some cases are detected be-cause of a palpable abdominal mass. Thirty to forty percent of hepatic adenomas can be detected incidentally during medical examination, operation, or autopsy. Hepatomegaly or an up-per abdominal mass is a common physical finding in the dis-ease. Approximately 10% of patients will exhibit severe ab-dominal tenderness and shock owing to acute intraperitoneal rupture of the tumor and hemorrhage. Laboratory tests are usually normal, unless there has been hemorrhage associated with the tumor to produce elevated serum transaminase, al-kaline phosphatase, anemia, and leukocytosis.[49]

Imaging studies including isotope liver scan, ultrasound,

CT, and arteriography are all effective in detecting adenomas, particularly the larger ones. Arteriography reveals hypervascular liver tumors containing hypovascular regions, presumably due to hemorrhage or necrosis. Adenomas exhibit centripetal blood flow with numerous small arteries delineating the tumor. There is usually not an intense late stain in adenomas during arteriography (Fig 26–7).[49, 51]

Pathology

Almost half of the hepatic adenomas removed surgically at one institution were greater than 10 cm in diameter. The tumors are circumscribed and contain numerous surface vessels. There is frequently evidence of hemorrhage into the tumor (Fig 26–8). Generally well-differentiated hepatocytes without obvious arrangement compose the tumor without the presence of ducts or ductules. About 10% of specimens revealed foci of hepatocellular carcinoma.[49, 52]

Approach

Obviously, those patients experiencing acute hemorrhage should be operated on to remove the lesion. Generally, other patients believed to have hepatic adenomas should be treated surgically because of the risk of bleeding, the risk of cancer, and the uncertainty of the diagnosis. In many cases, it may

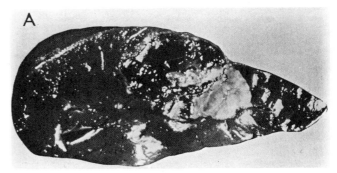

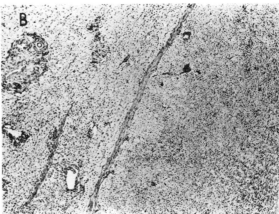

Fig 26–8.—A, a large hepatic adenoma with necrosis and hemorrhage. **B,** the tumor consists of hepatocyte devoid of ducts. Note normal liver to the left of the thin, fibrous capsule. (From Kerlin et al.: *Gastroenterology* 84:994–1002, 1983. Reprinted by permission of Elsevier Publishing Co., Inc. ©1983 by the Am. Gastroenterological Assoc.)

be impossible to discriminate among adenoma, hepatoma, and metastatic cancer. This evaluation should be done by laparotomy rather than needle biopsy because of the risk of hemorrhage and possible difficulty in interpreting small biopsy samples. After the diagnosis is established and the tumor removed, the patient should avoid taking birth control pills.[49] Some reports suggest regression of hepatic adenomas when birth control pills are discontinued.[48, 50, 53]

Focal Nodular Hyperplasia

Focal nodular hyperplasia is defined as one or more grossly visible, localized nodules in an otherwise normal liver, a predominance of normal hepatic cells mixed with some bile ducts or multiple ductules, and fibrous septae in the nodules, which usually radiate from a central stellate fibrous area. Twenty-four cases of focal nodular hyperplasia were reported in the English language literature between 1940 and 1960; they included 11 children and 13 adults (10 women and 3 men). Between 1960 and 1977, 37 cases of focal nodular hyperplasia have been described. This disease predominantly affects young women regardless of contraceptive hormone administration. These lesions may be evenly distributed between liver lobes; in about one eighth of the cases, the lesions are multiple. Prior to 1960, there were no reports of patients with focal nodular hyperplasia who experienced life-threatening

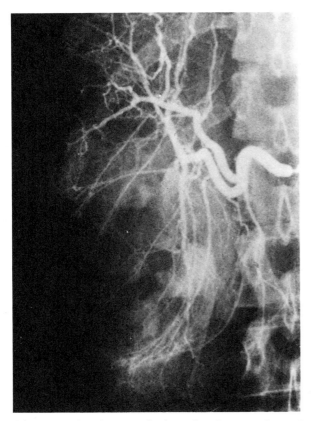

Fig 26–7.—Arteriogram of a hepatic adenoma shows that multiple vessels stretched around the tumor provide blood supply from the periphery. The avascular area was due to hemorrhage. (From Fechner, et al.: *Am. J. Surg. Pathol.* 1:217–224, 1977.)

hemorrhage; however, since 1960, several patients with intra-abdominal hemorrhage have been described. This suggests, but does not prove, that, while oral contraceptives probably do not cause focal nodular hyperplasia, they may increase the likelihood of bleeding complications from the lesions already present. At the moment, however, there is no convincing evidence that contraceptive hormones play an etiologic role in focal nodular hyperplasia.[47, 49, 51]

In one study, 88% of focal nodular hyperplasia occurred in women, predominantly young women. Fifty-eight percent of those affected had taken birth control pills. About 90% of lesions of focal nodular hyperplasia are discovered incidentally at autopsy, at laparotomy, or during a medical examination. About 10% of patients are symptomatic, having chronic or intermittent abdominal pain. Acute presentation of symptoms is unlikely in focal nodular hyperplasia. The majority of patients with focal nodular hyperplasia will exhibit normal physical examination, while 17% will have hepatomegaly, an abdominal mass, or abdominal tenderness.

Isotope scan, ultrasound, and CT scan frequently disclose focal nodular hyperplasia, but are not completely reliable. Arteriography is 100% sensitive in detecting focal nodular hyperplasia; however, its specificity is far lower. Arteriography usually discloses a single feeding artery, which is enlarged, tortuous, and untapered. Centrifugal filling of vessels is the rule. Focal nodular hyperplasia is sharply delineated and stained intensely in the late phase during arteriography (Fig 26–9).[49, 51]

Pathology

Most lesions in focal nodular hyperplasia are less than 10 cm in diameter. A cut-section gross inspection reveals stellate fibrous scars producing nodularity. A central scar may be present. Microscopically fibrous bands containing numerous bile ducts with numerous lymphocytes in and around the bands are usual. Normal-appearing hepatocytes may be arranged in cords about sinusoids (Fig 26–10).[49]

Management

Focal nodular hyperplasia is usually asymptomatic, carries a low risk for hemorrhage (in absence of birth control pills), and is not associated with malignancy. If a patient is found to have focal nodular hyperplasia, contraceptive pills should be interdicted. If the diagnosis of focal nodular hyperplasia could be established, the lesion could be left undisturbed. Unfor-

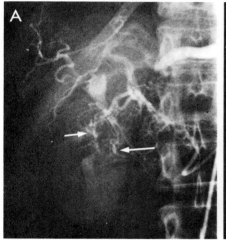
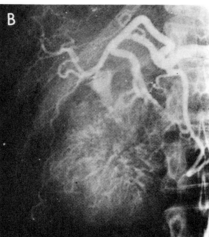
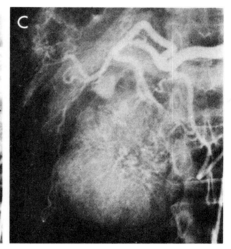
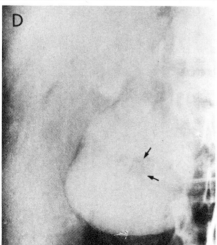

Fig 26–9.—Arteriogram from a case of focal nodular hyperplasia. **A,** the early arterial phase shows two arteries entering the center of the lesion. **B,** arterial branches radiate from the center toward the periphery. **C,** later phase delineating the mass filling by vessels within the lesion. **D,** later phase continued to delineate the lesion. The pale areas *(arrows)* may reveal a central fibrous zone. (From Fechner, et al.: *Am. J. Surg. Pathol.* 1:217–224, 1977.)

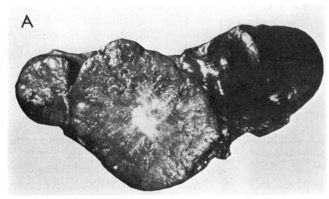

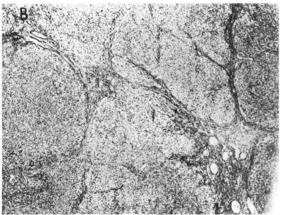

Fig 26–10.—Focal nodular hyperplasia. **A,** a large nodular lesion with a central scar. **B,** note fibrous bands with bile ducts and inflammatory cells. (From Kerlin et al.: *Gastroenterology* 84:994–1002, 1983. Reprinted by permission of Elsevier Publishing Co., Inc. ©1983 by the Am. Gastroenterological Assoc.)

tunately, it is not possible to establish the diagnosis accurately. Small, focal nodular hyperplasia lesions can be biopsied and treated simultaneously by wedge excision. Larger lesions can be defined by incisional biopsy and left intact if the diagnosis proves to be focal nodular hyperplasia.[49]

Hemangioma

Cavernous hemangiomas are the most common liver tumors, detected in about 2% of the livers examined during autopsy. Hemangiomas can vary from a few millimeters to many centimeters in diameter. Large, blood-filled endothelium-lined sinus, separated by fibrous septae, characterizes the microscopic appearance of hepatic hemangiomas.[54]

Many hepatic hemangiomas are detected incidentally during surgical operations or during radiologic evaluation for other conditions. Fewer than half of the patients with hepatic hemangiomas will be symptomatic. The usual symptoms are discomfort, a full feeling, and upper abdominal pain. Some patients (about 12%) will have fever. The most common physical finding is hepatomegaly or liver mass.[55] Although spontaneous hemorrhage from a hemangioma can occur, it is very infrequent. Trastek and co-workers[55] observed the course of 36 patients having hemangioma 4 cm in diameter; during an average period of 5.5 years, no patient died, no tumor bled,

and no patient experienced increased discomfort.

Liver isotope scan, ultrasound, and CT scan each can disclose hepatic hemangiomas, but angiography remains the most accurate diagnostic tool.[56] The numerous vascular spaces during the arterial phase and the "cotton-wool" appearance in the late phase are characteristic of hemangiomas (Figs 26–11 and 26–12). Scintigraphy with technetium Tc 99m-labeled erythrocytes may also accurately delineate and identify hepatic hemangiomas. Percutaneous needle biopsy of undefined liver masses should be avoided, because biopsy of hemangiomas can cause massive hemorrhage.

When liver hemangiomas cause persistent, bothersome symptoms such as pain and fever, when the tumor is deemed anatomically resectable, and when the patient's general health is good, surgical removal is appropriate and can be recommended. If, on the other hand, the patient is asymptomatic, operation can be safely delayed or avoided, provided the diagnostic studies are pathognomonic for cavernous hemangioma. Mortality rates for operation are low, and long-term follow-up is excellent after resection of hepatic hemangioma.

CYSTIC LIVER DISEASE

Nonparasitic Cysts

Liver cysts occur infrequently. They probably occur because of a developmental anomaly in which intralobular bile ducts fail during embryologic development to connect with interlobular bile ducts. Hepatic cysts are usually lined with cuboidal epithelium and usually do not communicate with bile ducts.[57, 58] There are several classifications of liver cysts, but the one employed here will include (1) adult fibropolycystic disease, (2) childhood fibropolycystic disease, (3) hepatic fibrosis, and (4) solitary nonparasitic cyst.

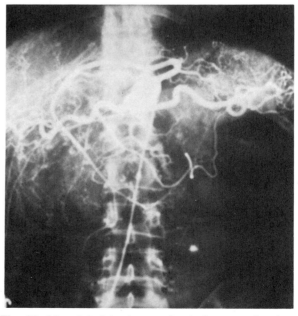

Fig 26–11.—Arterial phase of arteriogram showing a hemangioma.

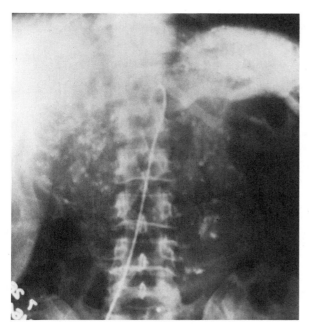

Fig 26–12.—Venous phase of angiogram showing a hemangioma with numerous vascular spaces and the "cotton-wool" appearance.

Adult Fibropolycystic Disease

Adult fibropolycystic disease is an inherited disorder transmitted as an autosomal dominant and is usually detected in adulthood. The patients usually have concomitant polycystic renal disease, which can impair renal function. The patients are usually asymptomatic and have normal liver function. In some cases the liver cysts can produce upper abdominal pain, discomfort, or pressure. There can be cystic disease of other organs, including spleen, pancreas, ovary, and lungs. About half of the patients with polycystic liver disease have polycystic kidneys, but the reverse is not true. Polycystic liver disease does not alter the life span, and the prognosis is determined solely by the extent and severity of the kidney disease.[59]

Infantile Fibropolycystic Disease

Infantile fibropolycystic disease is transmitted as an autosomal recessive trait, and the disease is usually evident in infancy, frequently at birth. Survival is determined by the severity of the renal disease. Patients with mild or minimal renal disease will live until childhood. The surviving patients develop progressive hepatic fibrosis, and some develop portal hypertension, esophageal varices, and variceal bleeding. Liver function tests in these patients may be normal. The variceal bleeding can be managed by surgical decompression of the varices.[59]

Congenital Hepatic Fibrosis

Congenital hepatic fibrosis may occur sporadically or may be due to autosomal recessive transmission. In this disease, bands of fibrous tissue containing cystic spaces and duct epithelial cells join the portal tracts. The patients almost always develop portal hypertension, which may become evident in infancy or adulthood. Liver function tests usually remain normal. If the patients develop recurrent bleeding from esophagogastric varices, they usually respond well to surgical decompression of the varices.[59, 60–62]

Solitary Nonparasitic Cysts

Solitary nonparasitic cysts are generally regarded as rare lesions. They may be detected incidentally at autopsy or operation. With the recent widespread application of hepatic imaging tests, solitary liver cysts are being detected with increasing regularity. Most patients with liver cysts are asymptomatic and have normal liver function. When symptoms occur, they are usually upper abdominal pain, discomfort, fullness, and, although only rarely, jaundice.[63]

Liver cysts are best detected and evaluated by ultrasound examination (Fig 26–13). The differential diagnosis will include parasitic cyst, abscess, and neoplasm, but it is usually not difficult to establish the diagnosis.

Treatment

The majority of patients with liver cysts require no treatment. If patients with polycystic liver disease develop severe pain, they should be treated surgically.[64] There is frequently a honeycomb appearance in the affected portion of the liver. This condition is best treated by the so-called fenestration procedure, in which the superficial cysts are unroofed followed by breaking the walls or septa into the adjacent and more deeply seated cysts. This permits drainage or communication of all cystic spaces with the peritoneal cavity.[65] Although liver resection is usually unnecessary, it may occasionally be needed.[66] When jaundice has occurred in polycystic liver disease, it has been ascribed to pressure or tension from the cysts causing mechanical bile duct obstruction.[67]

Solitary liver cysts are often superficial. They should be treated by unroofing and removal of as much of the cyst lining as possible.[68] One must use caution, because the cyst wall may be contiguous with ducts or vessels. Major hepatic resection is rarely necessary for solitary liver cysts.[66] When solitary cysts are associated with jaundice, careful cholangiography is mandatory, and the jaundice should not be ascribed to cyst pressure. There seems to be an increased association between solitary liver cysts and benign tumors of the bile ducts.[69] Although needle aspiration has been advocated for the treatment of liver cysts, recurrence following aspiration was 100% (Fig 26–14).[70, 71]

Parasitic Cysts

Hydatid Disease

Hydatid cysts, the most common parasitic cyst of the liver, are caused by the cestode *Echinococcus granulosus*. Hydatid disease is prevalent in South America, the Far East, Southern and Eastern Europe, and Australia. This disease is rare in the United States, but may occur in Alaska and the mid-South.[72]

Echinococcus granulosus is disseminated when the offal of infested sheep or swine is fed to dogs. The dogs' feces contaminate the ground or water around dwellings, and humans ingest the ova. After ingestion, the ova unencyst, pass

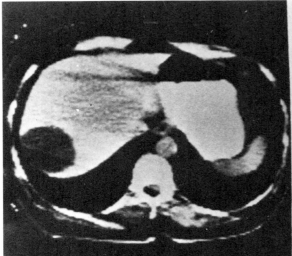
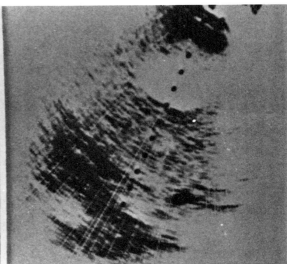

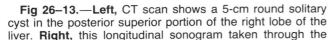

Fig 26–13.—Left, CT scan shows a 5-cm round solitary cyst in the posterior superior portion of the right lobe of the liver. **Right,** this longitudinal sonogram taken through the right lobe of the liver shows the cyst wall. (From Roemer, et al.: *A.J.R.* 136:1065–1070, 1981.)

through the intestinal epithelium into the portal blood, and pass to the liver. Although other organs, including lung, can be involved, the liver is the most common. Sixty to seventy percent of cysts arise in the right lobe, about 20% arise in the left lobe, and in 20%–30% both lobes are diseased. *Echinococcus* cyst of the liver is a chronic disease that affects both sexes equally and may occur at any age. The cyst may be asymptomatic for long periods and may be detected incidentally. Some patients may experience upper abdominal discomfort or detect a mass. Approximately one third of the patients will experience complications, in a decreasing order of frequency: (1) rupture into the bile ducts, (2) abscess, (3) intraperitoneal rupture, or (4) hepatic bronchial fistula. Rupture of an *Echinococcus* cyst into a bile duct causes colicky abdominal pain, jaundice, and fever.[73, 74] Plain films of the abdomen may reveal calcification in the cyst wall. Ultrasound is probably the best test for the diagnosis and delineation of *Echinococcus* cyst.[75, 76] One author stated that the ultrasound finding of the cyst with demonstrable daughter cysts was pathognomonic (Fig 26–15).[77] CT scans will delineate *Echinococcus* cysts with 98% accuracy; false negatives occur in patients with fatty livers (Figs 26–16 and 26–17).[78]

Immunologic testing may be employed. In one study the intradermal skin tests (Casoni test) were 69.4% positive in proved cases; however, authorities in Australia recommended that the Casoni test be abandoned. Immunoelectrophoresis is probably the test of choice.[77, 79]

Echinococcus cysts require surgical treatment. Several authors recommend evacuation of the cyst and the application of a scolecidal agent (either 0.5% silver nitrate or 1% cetrimide). Formalin should not be used because it can cause bile duct sclerosis or death.[80] Kune et al.[77] recommended filling the cavity with saline solution and closing the cavity and the abdomen without drainage. When cysts rupture into the bile ducts, common duct exploration and choledochostomy should be performed. There is controversy concerning treatment of *Echinococcus* cyst.[81–83] Some recommend excision of the cyst while others employ hepatic lobectomy. Resection must un-

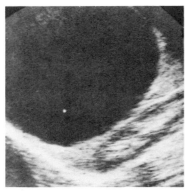
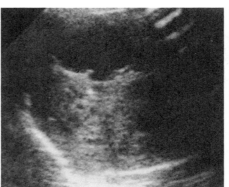
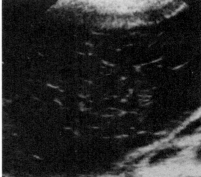

Fig 26–14.—Sonograms of a large solitary hepatic cyst. **Left,** large simple cyst. **Middle,** sonogram performed immediately following needle aspiration of 2,000 ml clear fluid. **Right,** sagittal sonogram performed one week following operation showing the recurrent cyst, which was treated surgically. (From Saini, et al.: *A.J.R.* 141:559–560, 1983.)

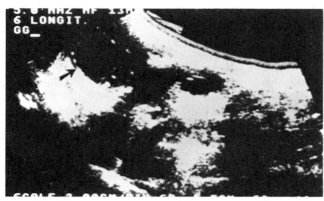

Fig 26–15.—This longitudinal hepatic sonogram shows an echinococcus cyst. *Arrow,* a daughter cyst. (From Kune, et al.: *Med. J. Aust.* 2:385–388, 1983.)

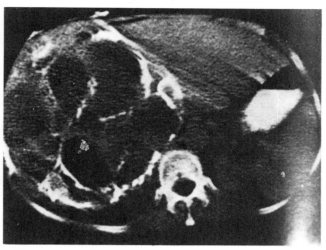

Fig 26–17.—CT scan reveals a calcified hydatid cyst. (From de Diego Choliz, et al.: *A.J.R.* 139:699–702, 1982.)

doubtedly be required infrequently. Dugalic et al.[82] recommend evacuation of the cyst contents, sterilization, excision of the cyst wall, and postoperative drainage of the cyst cavity. The cyst fluid is antigenic, and intra-abdominal leakage of fluid may cause anaphylactic shock.

LIVER ABSCESS
Pyogenic Abscesses

John Bright described pyogenic abscesses in 1836. Since then, the pathogenesis, diagnostic methods, and treatments of the disease have changed considerably. Despite improved methods for diagnosis and treatment, liver abscess remains difficult to diagnose and treat successfully.[84, 85] Fortunately, liver abscesses occur relatively infrequently in the United States, where the incidence is about 16 cases per 100,000 hospital admissions.[86, 87]

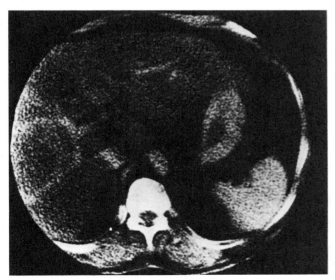

Fig 26–16.—CT scan showing a large hydatid cyst in the right hepatic lobe. The interior septae delineate daughter cysts. (From de Diego Choliz, et al.: *A.J.R.* 139:699–702, 1982.)

Etiology

Several conditions may cause liver abscesses; benign or malignant biliary diseases recently constitute the commonest etiology, contributing about half the cases. Cryptogenic abscesses, those with no well-defined etiology, may compose as much as 20% of pyogenic liver abscesses. About 14% of liver abscesses develop by portal vein bacteremia due to infection in one or more abdominal organs. The remaining 15% of liver abscesses are due to direct extension of infection into the liver from adjacent organs, direct inoculation by trauma, and hematogenous spread from a distant site via the hepatic artery.[86, 87]

In the earlier part of this century, intra-abdominal infection, particularly appendicitis with portal bacteremia, constituted the leading cause of liver abscesses; more recently, the sequelae of biliary disease have become the leading offenders.[86]

Bacteriology

The organisms recovered from liver abscesses vary greatly, probably because of antibiotic administration prior to culture, variation in culture technique, and various methods employed for culture, particularly for anaerobic organisms. *Escherichia coli, Klebsiella,* streptococcal species, and staphylococcal species commonly are cultured from liver abscesses. Recent work suggests that anaerobic organisms such as *Fusobacterium, Clostridium,* or *Bacteroides* may cause 20%–45% of all pyogenic hepatic abscesses. In a prospective study of 16 patients with liver abscess, all had positive cultures. *Streptococcus milleri* was isolated from 13 of the cases; in ten of the cases, it was the only organism recovered. Other organisms isolated during that study included *Fusobacterium, Bacteroides, Peptococcus,* and *E. coli.*

Anaerobes more commonly are cultured from solitary abscesses and are usually associated with lower mortality rates. Mortality of 29%, 50%, and 78% are associated with anaerobic organisms, mixed flora, and aerobic organisms, respectively.

Blood cultures may be positive in about half of the patients with liver abscesses. The growth of anaerobic or microaerophilic organisms in blood cultures should arouse suspicion for liver abscess.

Solitary lesions occur in about half the patients with liver abscesses, and approximately 60% of solitary abscesses occur in the right lobe. Most abscesses of biliary origin are multiple.[84, 88–93]

Diagnosis

Most patients with liver abscesses will be examined or will present with an illness of less than two weeks' duration, but a third of patients will have been sick a month or longer. The symptoms of liver abscess include fever, chills, malaise, anorexia, weight loss, abdominal pain or abdominal discomfort, and nausea and vomiting. The usual physical findings of liver abscess are enlarged, tender liver or tender abdominal mass, fever, jaundice, and pleural effusion. Leukocytosis and increased alkaline phosphatase, SGOT, and SGPT occur in 80% of patients, while two thirds exhibit elevated serum bilirubin, low serum albumin, and anemia. Half the patients with liver abscesses have abnormal chest x-rays; the abnormalities include elevated diaphragm, pleural effusion, basilar atelectasis or pneumonia, and an air-fluid level below the diaphragm. Liver isotope scan, ultrasound examination, and CT scan all can localize liver abscesses accurately (Fig 26–18).[86–88]

The diagnosis of liver abscess can be extremely difficult. One study reported that one third of liver abscesses went undiagnosed.[85] It is probable that the increased use of liver imaging studies in patients with unexplained fever will aid in detecting and diagnosing liver abscesses.

Treatment

Because of several reports of mortality approaching 100% in patients treated for liver abscess without surgical drainage, the traditional treatment for the disease includes antibiotic administration and prompt surgical drainage.[86, 87, 94–96] In the preantibiotic era, the extraserosal approach to drain liver abscesses was emphasized to avoid spilling pus into the peritoneal cavity. Before antibiotics, the transabdominal approach caused a mortality approaching 90%. After the introduction of antibiotics, however, the mortality fell markedly with the use of the transperitoneal approach. The transabdominal approach has the advantage of permitting evaluation of other intraabdominal pathology and allowing more complete evaluation of the liver, particularly for multiple abscesses. Antibiotic therapy must be started as soon as the diagnosis of liver abscess is made.

A review of hepatic abscesses treated by surgical drainage between 1954 and 1980 revealed an overall mortality of 57%. The mortality for patients with solitary abscesses was 24% compared to a mortality rate of 76% for patients with multiple abscesses.[89] It is interesting that in 1953 McFadzean and co-workers[97] from Hong Kong reported treating 15 patients with liver abscesses by needle aspiration plus antibiotics. All of their patients recovered. Since that time, there have appeared reports of patients treated successfully with antibiotics and needle aspiration.[93, 98–101] Dietrick[99] recently reported a large group of patients (109) treated for liver abscess by percutaneous needle aspiration and antibiotics. The mortality was 2.8% and the morbidity was 17.4%. In an unrandomized group of patients (83) from the same hospital treated with surgical drainage plus antibiotics, there were mortality and morbidity rates of 12.1% and 51.8%, respectively.

These excellent results have to be considered in any discussion of the treatment of pyogenic liver abscess. Successful CT-guided percutaneous catheterization of liver abscesses has been reported from many medical centers.[98, 102–107] In most cases, drainage can be affected with catheter drainage, but in some cases, surgical drainage becomes necessary. Scheinfeld et al.[108] added five cases of successful percutaneous drainage and reviewed the literature on that procedure. They found a mortality of 1.5% and compared that figure with reports of surgical drainage having mortality of 30%, 40%, and 65%.

Maher and co-workers[101] reported five patients treated successfully for pyogenic liver abscess with antibiotics and supportive care without abscess drainage. Reynolds[109] subsequently added nine cases, of which two required surgical therapy. The following guidelines were recommended:

1. Patients with acute surgical abdomen or bile duct obstruction should be operated on for treatment of the primary pathology and drainage of the abscess.

2. Patients with proved or presumed pyogenic hepatic abscess without coexisting surgical disease may be treated by antibiotics alone.

3. Percutaneous aspiration of the abscess may be employed to decompress the cavity and yield material for culture.

4. Multiple small abscesses cannot be successfully drained surgically and should be treated with antibiotics.

It therefore appears that the established surgical dictum of treating liver abscesses by surgical drainage is being challenged by reports of antibiotics alone, antibiotics plus needle aspiration, and antibiotics plus catheter drainage. It is currently impossible to determine whether case selection, chance, or other factors determine the suggested difference in mortality between surgical and nonsurgical therapy of liver abscesses. If either needle aspiration or percutaneous catheter drainage plus antibiotics continue to yield 97.2%–98.5% sur-

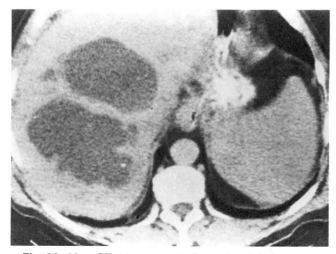

Fig 26–18.—CT scan reveals large loculated pyogenic abscess in right hepatic lobe. (From Bernardino, et al.: *J. Comput. Asst. Tomogr.* 8:38–41, 1984.)

vival with additional use, it will be a welcomed improvement for this difficult clinical problem.

Amebic Abscesses

Although amebiasis and its agent *Entamoeba histolytica* occur throughout the world, the highest prevalence occurs in tropical and subtropical zones. During the past 40 years, the prevalence of amebiasis in the United States decreased from 10% to 4% of the population. Generally, the cases occur in lower socioeconomic areas and in mental institutions. With increased tourism and especially with increased immigration into the United States from endemic areas, it is probable that the incidence of amebiasis and its complications will increase. This is already occurring in metropolitan areas and particularly in Southern California.[110, 111]

Amebic abscess of the liver occurs in 3%–9% of patients with amebiasis and is the most common extraintestinal complication of the disease. Amebic liver abscess develops most commonly in men aged 20–50 years.

Entamoeba histolytica occurs in two forms: trophozoites and cysts. The trophozoites are 10–20 nm in diameter and are motile. The cysts are similar in size. Infection occurs by ingestion of cysts because they are resistant to gastric juice, chlorine, and drying. The detection of cysts or trophozoites in the stool does not necessarily reflect active disease. In any event, when intestinal infection occurs, amebas may be carried to the liver in the portal vein.

Clinical Features

The common symptoms of amebic liver abscess include malaise, abdominal pain, fever, and weight loss developing over several days to a month. Some patients can have cough, pleuritic pain, and dyspnea. Rarely, ruptured abscesses can cause the syndrome of acute surgical abdomen and shock. Amebas may be isolated from the stools of 16%–33% of patients with amebic liver disease.

The common physical findings are fever, epigastric or right upper quadrant abdominal tenderness, and hepatomegaly. Often there will be abnormalities to auscultation or percussion over the right lung base.

In half the cases, a chest x-ray film will demonstrate either right lower lobe atelectasis, pleural effusion, an elevated diaphragm, or some combination of these. Ultrasound or isotope scan effectively delineates most lesions. Leukocytosis, anemia, and abnormalities of serum bilirubin, LDH, SGOT, SGPT, and alkaline phosphatase occur.

Serologic tests are very important to the diagnosis of liver abscess. The indirect hemagglutinin will be positive in 90%–100% of patients with amebic liver abscess. The gel diffusion precipitin test will be positive in 85%–95% of cases of amebic liver abscess. In one series, these tests were positive in all patients tested who had the disease.[112]

Therapy

Medical therapy is the cornerstone of the treatment of amebic liver abscess. Metronidazole, 750 mg three times daily, is effective therapy for more than 90% of patients. The duration of therapy required is not certain, but 10–20 days are recommended. Metronidazole is effective against the intestinal as well as the extraintestinal parasites. Other agents effective against extraintestinal *E. histolytica* are chloroquine and emetine. When they are used, an intraluminal amebicide, Diodoquin, should be used.

Most patients respond to the administration of metronidazole, and, if prompt response occurs, drug therapy alone is sufficient. If the patient fails to respond in five days, needle aspiration of the abscess should be performed.

Most amebic liver abscesses occur in the right lobe anteriorly and superiorly, while 4%–18% occupy the left lobe. Because left lobe abscesses frequently rupture into the peritoneal cavity, the pericardial sac, or the left pleural space, needle aspiration should accompany drug therapy for the left lobe lesions.

When metronidazole plus selective needle aspiration is employed to treat amebic liver abscesses, the mortality at one institution was 5.7%.

Complications

Four to seven percent of patients with amebic liver abscess experience complications, usually involving the thorax and including pulmonary abscess, bronchobiliary fistula, and empyema. In the past, bacterial superinfection of amebic liver abscess was common, but that complication is rare today.

SURGICAL RESECTIONS

Anatomy

The adult liver, weighing 1,200–1,600 gm, is the largest organ in the peritoneal cavity and occupies most of the upper abdomen, including the right hypochondriac, the epigastric, and some of the left hypochondriac regions (Fig 26–19). Although the liver is an intraperitoneal structure, it is closely related to the diaphragm, so that the upper portion of the right lobe may be located at the level of the fourth right intercostal space. Most of the liver, therefore, is normally enclosed by the thoracic cage. A portion of the medial segment of the left lobe occupying the epigastrium will not be covered by the thoracic cage, but the remainder of the left lobe will. The liver is roughly pyramidal, with the base of the pyramid located to the right and the apex to the left. Most of the liver is covered by peritoneum with the exception of the gallbladder fossa and the base area related to the diaphragm, the right kidney, the right adrenal gland, and the inferior vena cava. Although the liver is probably held in place by intra-abdominal pressure, there are several ligaments of surgical importance formed by the peritoneal reflection onto the liver about the base area. The transverse peritoneal reflection from the diaphragm onto the liver is the *coronary ligament*. As the coronary ligament passes to the right, its anterior and posterior leaves fuse to form the *right triangular ligament*. The fusion of the leaves of the coronary ligament on the left forms the *left triangular ligament* which attaches the left hepatic lobes to the diaphragm. Another peritoneal reflection, the falciform ligament, arises perpendicularly from the coronary ligament and passes inferiorly between the liver and the anterior abdominal wall from the diaphragm to the umbilicus. The dorsal edge of the falciform ligament contains the ligamentum teres hepaticus passing between the umbilicus and the left branch of the portal vein. Dorsally, the fossa of the umbilical vein is continuous with the fossa of the ductus venosus. To-

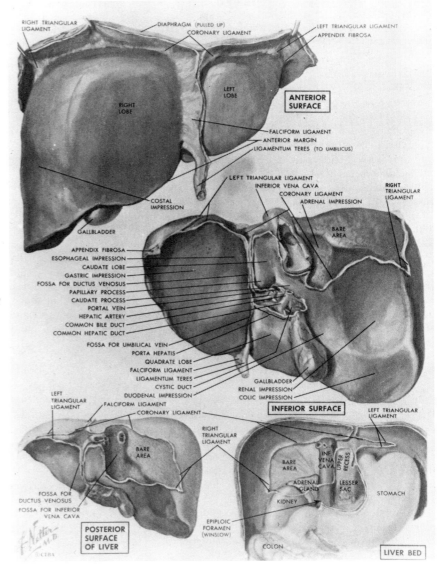

Fig 26–19.—Topography of the liver. (From Netter collection, *Digestive System,* vol. 3, part III, Section XV, plate 4. Copyright 1969, CIBA Pharmaceutical Co., Div. of CIBA-GEIGY Corp. Reprinted with permission from *The CIBA Collection of Medical Illustrations*; illustrated by Frank H. Netter, M.D. All rights reserved.)

pographically, the falciform ligament divides the liver into a right and a left lobe. From the dorsal perspective, the *caudate lobe* is bounded by the fossa for the ductus venosus and the inferior vena cava. The *quadrate lobe* is bounded by the *porta hepatis,* the gallbladder, and the fossa of the umbilical vein. The porta hepatis contains the common hepatic duct, hepatic artery, the portal vein, lymphatics, and nerves.

Hepatic Artery

The hepatic artery, which supplies approximately 25% of the liver's blood supply, commonly arises from the celiac axis and passes through the hepatoduodenal ligament, forming the right margin of the lesser omentum. The hepatic artery courses cephalad, lying to the left of the common bile duct and anteromedial to the portal vein. The hepatic artery gives off right gastric and gastroduodenal branches to become the common hepatic artery. The common hepatic artery divides at varying sites to provide the right and left hepatic arteries.

The right hepatic artery usually, but not always, courses dorsal to the common hepatic duct to give the cystic artery before entering the hepatic parenchyma. The left hepatic artery may give a "middle hepatic artery" before entering the hepatic parenchyma. There are numerous (40%) variations in the origin and branches of the hepatic artery. Some of the variations of the right hepatic artery include the common hepatic artery arising from the superior mesenteric artery, the right hepatic artery arising from the superior mesenteric artery, an accessory right hepatic artery arising from the superior mesenteric artery, a left hepatic artery arising from the left gastric artery, and an accessory left hepatic artery arising from the left gastric artery.

The Portal Vein

The portal vein provides approximately 75% of the liver's blood supply and arises between the head and neck of the pancreas and the body of the second lumbar vertebra by the union of the superior mesenteric vein and the splenic vein. The portal vein has no valves and receives the coronary vein and the pyloric vein. The portal vein is about 7–8 cm long and passes toward the liver in the hepatoduodenal ligament dorsal to the common bile duct and the common hepatic duct. Before reaching the liver, the portal vein divides into its right and left branches. The right portal vein is short and often branches before entering the hepatic parenchyma. The left branch of the portal vein is somewhat larger, 2–3.5 cm, and courses transversely across the base of the caudate lobe to enter the umbilical fissure to give segmental branches.

The Lymphatics of the Liver

The hepatic lymph derived from the spaces of Disse enters the lymphatics around the intrahepatic branches of the portal vein. The bile ducts also possess lymphatics. These lymphatics drain into the hepatic lymph nodes about the common bile duct and the portal vein. The lymphatics continue to the celiac nodes and subsequently to the cisterna chyli. Some hepatic lymphatics pass along the tributaries of the hepatic veins to pass through the vena caval diaphragmatic hiatus to enter lymph nodes about the inferior vena cava.

The Bile Ducts

The intrahepatic distribution of the bile ducts closely follows the hepatic arterioles and the portal venules in the portal triads. The small ducts unite to form segmental ducts which join to form the lobar ducts. The right hepatic duct formed by the union of the anterior and posterior segmental ducts near the hilus is about 0.9 cm long. The confluence of the ducts from segments II, III, and IV forms the left hepatic duct, which courses from left to right over the base of the quadrate lobe superior to the left branch of the portal vein but covered with hilar peritoneum. The extrahepatic left hepatic duct can be 2–3 cm long. The left and right lobar ducts join in the transverse fissure to form the common hepatic duct, which is very variable in length but averages 2.5 cm. There are many variations in the anatomy of the extrahepatic bile ducts.

Hepatic Veins

The venous drainage begins in the central vein of the hepatic lobules. The veins unite to form larger and larger veins. The principal venous drainage of the liver flows through the right hepatic vein, the middle hepatic vein, and the left hepatic vein. The right hepatic vein, the largest of the three, drains the posterior segment of the right lobe and a portion of the anterior segment of the right lobe. The middle hepatic vein drains a portion of the anterior segment of the right lobe and the superior part of the medial segment of the left lobe. The left hepatic vein drains the entire left lateral segment and a portion of the medial segment of the left lobe. The right hepatic vein usually empties directly into the inferior vena cava. The middle hepatic vein most frequently joins the left hepatic vein before the latter joins the inferior vena cava. Two or more veins drain directly from the caudate lobe into the left side of the inferior vena cava. Several (two to three) veins pass directly into the inferior vena cava from the posterior segment of the right lobe.[113]

Surgical Anatomy

For purposes of surgical approaches, the liver may be divided into right and left lobes by a plane or fissure extending from the gallbladder fossa anteriorly and inferiorly to the fossa of the inferior vena cava posteriorly and superiorly (Fig 26–20). Although not detectable by surface markings, this fissure clearly divides the liver into right and left lobes. The right lobe may be divided further into anterior and posterior segments. The left lobe of the liver consists of medial and lateral segments which can be delineated by the plane of the falciform ligament.[114]

Segmental Anatomy

Another system of nomenclature introduced by Couinaud divides the liver into eight segments (I–VIII), each lobe being composed of four segments. Segments I–IV compose the left lobe, while segments V–VIII form the right lobe (Fig 26–21).[115] In addition, Gupta and co-workers[116] studied the venous drainage of 95 human livers and observed five hepatovenous segments in every specimen: left, middle, right, paracaval, and caudate.

Hilar Dissection

Hilar dissection is necessary for either lobar resection. The hepatic artery is identified medial to the common bile duct and it is dissected out until its branches are clearly delineated. One must be aware of the common anomalies, particularly if preoperative angiography was not performed. The common hepatic duct should be identified and dissected proximally to the lobar duct confluence, and the duct of the lobe to be removed should be encircled with a ligature. The portal vein lies dorsal to the bile ducts and arteries. Dissection of the portal vein is usually easier to begin on its right side. No

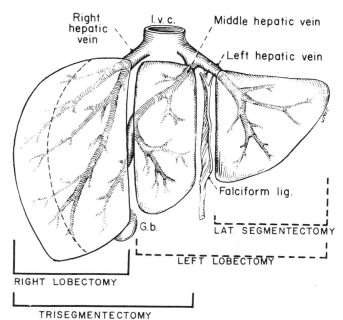

Fig 26–20.—Surgical anatomy of the liver. (Starzl, et al.: *Surg. Gynecol. Obstet.* 141:429–437, 1975.)

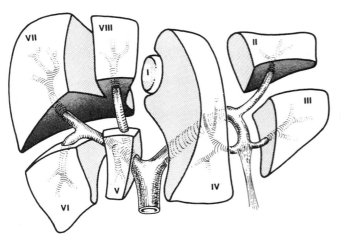

Fig 26–21.—Segmental anatomy of the liver according to Couinaud. (From Blumgart and Kelley: *Br. J. Surg.* 71:257–261, 1984. Reprinted by permission of Butterworth & Co., Ltd.)

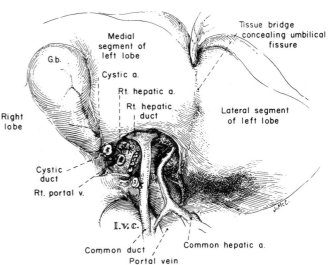

Fig 26–22.—Hilar dissection for right lobectomy or trisegmentectomy. (From Starzl, et al.: *Surg. Gynecol. Obstet.* 141:429–437, 1975.)

vein usually enters the portal vein between its bifurcation and the pancreas, except on the left side. The right portal vein is often short, and a more secure cuff sometimes can be obtained by dissecting out its major branches. The left portal vein is somewhat longer and can be exposed between its origin and the umbilical fissure.

Division of Hepatic Parenchyma

There are several techniques available for dividing the liver parenchyma, including finger fracture, electrocoagulation, laser, and an ultrasonic scalpel. The only techniques with which we are familiar are electrocoagulation and finger fracture. In any case, the intrahepatic vessels and ducts should be identified, if possible, and either be ligated or clipped.

Right Lobectomy

A right subcostal incision with extension to the left subcostal area as necessary usually provides satisfactory exposure for a right hepatic lobectomy. A right intercostal extension into the right thorax plus division of the diaphragm may be necessary. The right lobe may be mobilized by dividing the right triangular and coronary ligaments and retracting the lobe medially to assess resectability of the lesion.

Upon completion of the hilar dissection after ligation and division of the right hepatic artery, the right hepatic duct, and the right portal vein, the right lobe becomes discolored to permit delineation of the lobes. The line of resection lies between the gallbladder fossa anteriorly and the inferior vena cava posteriorly. The right lobe should be retracted anteriorly and medially to expose the inferior vena cava. The three to four hepatic veins draining into the cava should be carefully ligated and divided. The hepatic parenchyma along the line of demarcation should then be divided. Care should be taken in the area of the middle hepatic vein, which should remain intact after division of its anterolateral tributary. As the parenchymal dissection proceeds, the right hepatic vein should be identified. By securing the right hepatic vein after parenchymal division, a longer stump can be obtained, and it seems

easier to dissect the right hepatic vein in that way. After removing the specimen, small bleeding points may be controlled. A chest tube is inserted, if necessary, and soft, closed-system drains are placed adjacent to the cut surface of the liver.

Extended Right Lobectomy

Starzl described the trisegmentectomy for lesions of the right lobe which extend into the medial segment of the left lobe. Hilar dissection is performed as for a right lobectomy. The artery to the medial segment of the left lobe should be ligated and divided. The parenchymal dissection should pass near the falciform ligament. The middle hepatic vein will be ligated and divided with great care to preserve the left he-

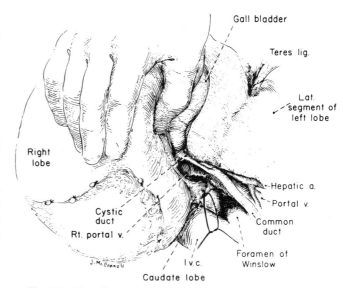

Fig 26–23.—Posterior approach to the bifurcation of the portal vein. (From Starzl, et al.: *Surg. Gynecol. Obstet.* 141:429–437, 1975.)

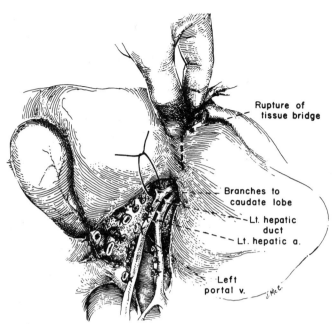

Fig 26–24.—Mobilization of the left branches of the portal triad for right trisegmentectomy. (From Starzl, et al.: *Surg. Gynecol. Obstet.* 141:429–437, 1975.)

patic vein. The right hepatic vein is handled as described previously (Figs 26–22 to 26–27).

Left Lobectomy

An abdominal midline incision provides good exposure for a left hepatic lobectomy. The left lobe should be mobilized

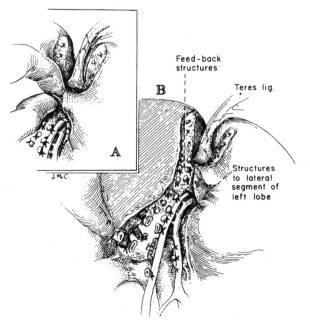

Fig 26–25.—Right trisegmentectomy: mobilization of structures between umbilical fissure and medial segment of left lobe. (From Starzl, et al.: *Surg. Gynecol. Obstet.* 141:429–437, 1975.)

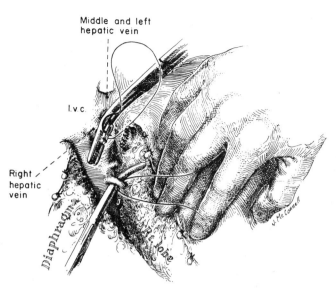

Fig 26–26.—Division of the right hepatic vein. (From Starzl, et al.: *Surg. Gynecol. Obstet.* 141:429–437, 1975.)

by dividing the left triangular ligament. Hilar dissection then permits ligation and division of the left hepatic artery, the left hepatic duct, and then the left portal vein. The discoloration of the left lobe delineates the dissection plane extending from the gallbladder fossa anteriorly to the inferior vena cava dorsally. Parenchymal dissection allows identification of the middle hepatic vein draining the medial segment of the left lobe and subsequently the left hepatic vein which is clamped, divided, and oversewn or ligated. After removal of the specimen, hemostasis can be completed, and a soft, closed-system drain should be placed adjacent to the cut surface of the liver.

Left Lateral Segmentectomy

Removal of the liver tissue left of the umbilical fissure consists of a left lateral segmentectomy. The left lateral segment can be mobilized by division of the falciform and left trian-

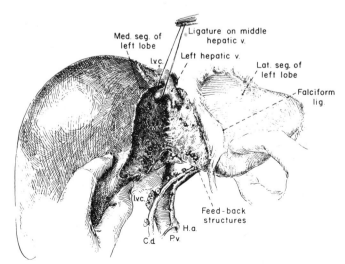

Fig 26–27.—Liver transsection nearly complete of right trisegmentectomy. (From Starzl, et al.: *Surg. Gynecol. Obstet.* 141:429–437, 1975.)

gular ligaments. Since hilar dissection is unnecessary, parenchymal division may then be carried out. Dissection should stay to the left of the umbilical fissure.

Regeneration

The liver possesses a remarkable capacity to regenerate. Humans may tolerate removal of 80% of hepatic parenchyma. In many cases of human liver resection, the disease, such as a tumor, may have slowly destroyed most of the lobe being removed, and regeneration of the remaining lobe may have occurred before lobectomy. In any event, regeneration is an important process, and some patients may require supportive care until adequate regeneration occurs.

REFERENCES

1. Sandler D.P., Sandler R.S., Horney L.F.: Primary liver cancer mortality in the United States. *J. Chronic Dis.* 36:227, 1983.
2. Lam K.C., Yu M.C., Leung J.W., et al.: Hepatitis B virus and cigarette smoking: Risk factors for hepatocellular carcinoma in Hong Kong. *Cancer Res.* 42:5246, 1982.
3. Resnick R.H., Stone K., Antonioli D.: Primary hepatocellular carcinoma following non-A, non-B post-transfusion hepatitis. *Dig. Dis. Sci.* 28:908, 1983.
4. Yu M.C., Mack T., Hanisch R., et al.: Hepatitis, alcohol consumption, cigarette smoking, and hepatocellular carcinoma in Los Angeles. *Cancer Res.* 43:6077, 1983.
5. Blumberg B.S., London W.T.: Hepatitis B virus: Pathogenesis and prevention of primary cancer of the liver. *Cancer* 50 (suppl. 11):2657, 1982.
6. Blumberg B.S., London W.T.: Primary hepatocellular carcinoma and hepatitis B virus. *Curr. Probl. Cancer* 6:1, 1982.
7. Arthur M.J., Wright R., Hall A.J.: Hepatitis B, hepatocellular carcinoma, and strategies for prevention. *Lancet* 1:607, 1984.
8. Okuda K., Obata H., Nakajima Y., et al.: Prognosis of primary hepatocellular carcinoma. *Hepatology* 4:35, 1984.
9. Shinagawa T., Ohto M., Kimura K., et al.: Diagnosis and clinical features of small hepatocellular carcinoma with emphasis on the utility of real-time ultrasonography: A study in 51 patients. *Gastroenterology* 86:495–502, 1984.
10. Aisen A.M., Martel W., Glazer G.M., et al.: Hepatic imaging: Positron emission tomography, digital angiography, and nuclear magnetic resonance imaging. *Hepatology* 3:1024, 1983.
11. Arias I.M.: Nuclear magnetic resonance and the future of hepatology. *Hepatology* 3:763, 1983.
12. Bernardino M.E., Lewis E.: Imaging hepatic neoplasms. *Cancer* 50:2666, 1982.
13. Chuang V.P.: Hepatic tumor angiography: A subject review. *Radiology* 148:633, 1983.
14. Lunderquist A., Owman T.: Preoperative diagnosis and evaluation of hepatic tumor resectability. *Gastrointest. Radiol.* 8:227, 1983.
15. Moss A.A., Goldberg H.I., Stark D.B., et al.: Hepatic tumors: Magnetic resonance and CT appearance. *Radiology* 150:141, 1984.
16. Takashima T., Matsui O., Suzuki M., et al.: Diagnosis and screening of small hepatocellular carcinomas: Comparison of radionuclide imaging, ultrasound, computed tomography, hepatic angiography, and alpha 1-fetoprotein assay. *Radiology* 145:635–638, 1982.
17. Kanematsu T., Takenaka K., Matsumata T., et al.: Limited hepatic resection effective for selected cirrhotic patients with primary liver cancer. *Ann. Surg.* 199:51, 1984.
18. Iwatsuki S., Shaw B.W. Jr., Starzl T.W.: Experience with 150 liver resections. *Ann. Surg.* 197:247, 1983.
19. Longmire W.P. Jr., Trout H., Greenfield J., et al.: Elective hepatic surgery. *Ann. Surg.* 179:712, 1974.
20. Ryan W.H., Hummel B.W., McClelland R.N.: Reduction in the morbidity and mortality of major hepatic resection: Experience with 52 patients. *Am. J. Surg.* 144:740, 1982.
21. Thompson H.H., Tompkins R.K., Longmire W.P. Jr.: Major hepatic resection: A 25-year experience. *Ann. Surg.* 197:375, 1983.
22. Jaffe B.M., Donegan W.L., Watson F., et al.: Factors influencing survival in patients with untreated hepatic metastases. *Surg. Gynecol. Obstet.* 127:1, 1968.
23. Lahr C.J., Soong S.J., Cloud G., et al.: A multifactorial analysis of prognostic factors in patients with liver metastases from colorectal carcinoma. *J. Clin. Oncol.* 1:720, 1983.
24. Kortz W.J., Meyers W.C., Hanks J.B., et al.: Hepatic resection for metastatic cancer. *Ann. Surg.* 199:182, 1984.
25. Kemeny M.M., Sugarbaker P.H., Smith T.J., et al.: A prospective analysis of laboratory tests and imaging studies to detect hepatic lesions. *Ann. Surg.* 195:163, 1982.
26. Goldenberg D.M., DeLand F., Kin E., et al.: Use of radiolabeled antibodies to carcinoembryonic antigen for the detection and localization of diverse cancers by external photoscanning. *N. Engl. J. Med.* 298:1384, 1978.
27. Harlyn M., Steplewski Z., Herlyn D., et al.: Colorectal carcinoma-specific antigen: Detection by means of monoclonal antibodies. *Proc. Natl. Acad. Sci. U.S.A.* 76:1438, 1979.
28. Mach J.P., Buchegger F., Forni M., et al.: Use of radiolabeled monoclonal anti-CEA antibodies for the detection of human carcinomas by external photoscanning and tomoscintigraphy. *Immunol. Today* 2:239, 1981.
29. Moldofsky P.J., Powe J., Mulhern C.B., et al.: Metastatic colon carcinoma detected with radiolabeled F(ab')2 monoclonal antibody fragments. *Radiology* 149:549, 1983.
30. Order S.E.: The history and progress of serologic immunotherapy and radiodiagnosis. *Radiology* 118:219, 1976.
31. Grage T.B., Vassilopoulos P.P., Shingleton W.W., et al.: Results of a prospective study of hepatic artery infusion with 5-fluorouracil versus intravenous 5-fluorouracil in patients with hepatic metastases from colorectal cancer: A Central Oncology Group study. *Surgery* 86:550, 1979.
32. Fortner J.G., Silva J.S., Cox E.B., et al.: Multivariate analysis of a personal series of 247 patients with liver metastases from colorectal cancer II: Treatment by intrahepatic chemotherapy. *Ann. Surg.* 199:317, 1984.
33. Balch C.M., Urist M.M., Soong S.-J., et al.: A prospective phase II clinical trial of continuous FUDR regional chemotherapy for colorectal metastases to the liver using a totally implantable drug infusion pump. *Am. Surg.* 198:567, 1983.
34. Bedikian A.Y., Chen T.T., Malahy M.A., et al.: Prognostic factors influencing survival of patients with advanced colorectal cancer: Hepatic artery infusion versus systemic intravenous chemotherapy for liver metastases. *J. Clin. Oncol.* 2:174, 1984.
35. Niederhuber J.E., Enswinger W., Gyves J., et al.: Regional chemotherapy of colorectal cancer metastases to the liver. *Cancer* 53:1336, 1984.
36. Weiss G.R., Garnick M.B., Osteen R.T., et al.: Long-term hepatic arterial infusion of 5-fluorodeoxyuridine for liver metastases using an implantable infusion pump. *J. Clin. Oncol.* 1:337, 1983.
37. Petrelli N.J., Barcewicz P.A., Evans J.T., et al.: Hepatic artery ligation for liver metastases in colorectal carcinoma. *Cancer* 53:1247, 1984.
38. Martin J.K. Jr., Moertel C.G., Adson M.A., et al.: Surgical treatment of functioning metastatic carcinoid tumor. *Arch. Surg.* 118:537, 1983.
39. Fortner J.G., Silva J.S., Golbey R.B., et al.: Multivariate analysis of a personal series of 249 consecutive patients with liver metastases from colorectal cancer I: Treatment by hepatic resection. *Ann. Surg.* 199:306, 1984.
40. Lim C.N., McPherson T.A.: Surgery as an alternative to chemotherapy for hepatic metastases from colorectal cancer. *Can. J. Surg.* 26:458, 1983.
41. Logan S.E., Meier S.J., Ramming K.P., et al.: Hepatic resection of metastatic colorectal carcinoma: A ten-year experience. *Arch. Surg.* 117:25, 1982.
42. Morrow C.E., Grage T.B., Sutherland D.E., et al.: Hepatic resection for secondary neoplasms. *Surgery* 92:610, 1982.
43. Nims T.A.: Hepatic trisegmentectomy for metastatic colo-

rectal cancer. *J. Surg. Oncol.* 24:154, 1983.

44. Nims T.A.: Resection of the liver for metastatic cancer. *Surg. Gynecol. Obstet.* 158:46, 1984.

45. Taylor B., Langer B., Falk R.E., et al.: Role of resection in the management of metastases to the liver. *Can J. Surg.* 26:215, 1983.

46. Adson M.A.: Hepatic metastases in perspective. *A.J.R.* 140:695, 1983.

47. Fechner R.E.: Benign hepatic lesions and orally administered contraceptives. *Human Pathol.* 8:255, 1977.

48. Henderson B.E., Preston-Martin S., Edmondson H.A., et al.: Hepatocellular carcinoma and oral contraceptives. *Br. J. Cancer* 48:437, 1983.

49. Kerlin P., Davis G.L., McGill D.B., et al.: Hepatic adenoma and focal nodular hyperplasia: Clinical, pathologic, and radiologic features. *Gastroenterology* 84:994, 1983.

50. Kolb A.: Benign liver tumors and oral contraceptives. *Acta Chir. Scand.* 148:89, 1982.

51. Fechner R.E., Roehm J.O.F.: Angiographic and pathologic correlation of hepatic focal nodular hyperplasia. *Am. J. Surg. Pathol.* 1:217, 1977.

52. Vecchio F.M., Fabiano A., Ghirlanda G., et al.: Fibrolamellar carcinoma of the liver: The malignant counterpart of focal nodular hyperplasia with oncocytic change. *Am. J. Clin. Pathol.* 81:521, 1984.

53. Edmondson H., Reynolds T.B., Henderson B., et al.: Regression of liver cell adenomas associated with oral contraceptives. *Ann. Intern. Med.* 86:180, 1977.

54. Ehren H., Majour G.H., Isaacs H. Jr.: Benign liver tumors in infancy and childhood. *Am. J. Surg.* 145:325, 1983.

55. Trastek V.F., van Heerden J.A., Sheedy P.F. II, et al.: Cavernous hemangiomas of the liver: Resect or observe? *Am. J. Surg.* 145:49, 1983.

56. Onodera H., Ohta K., Oikawa M., et al.: Correlation of the real-time ultrasonographic appearance of hepatic hemangioma with angiography. *J.C.U.* 11:421, 1983.

57. Longmire W.P. Jr., Mondiale S.A., Gordon H.E.: Congenital cystic disease of the liver and biliary system. *Ann. Surg.* 174:711, 1971.

58. Singh T., Jayaram G., Prakash P., et al.: Cystic disease of the liver. *J. Indian Med. Assoc.* 78:200, 1982.

59. Sherlock S.: *Diseases of the Liver and Biliary System*, ed. 6. London, Blackwell Scientific Publications, 1981.

60. Alvarez F., Bernard O., Brunelle F., et al.: Congenital hepatic fibrosis in children. *J. Pediatr.* 99:370, 1981.

61. McGonigle R.J., Mowat A.P., Bewick M., et al.: Congenital hepatic fibrosis and polycystic kidney disease: Role of porto-caval shunting and transplantation in 3 patients. *Q. J. Med.* 50:269, 1981.

62. Tazelaar H.D., Payne J.A., Patel N.S.: Congenital hepatic fibrosis and asymptomatic familial adult-type polycystic kidney disease in a 19-year-old woman. *Gastroenterology* 86:757, 1984.

63. Santman F.W., Thijs L.G., van den Veen E.A., et al.: Intermittent jaundice: A rare complication of nonparasitic liver cyst. *Gastroenterology* 72:325, 1977.

64. Henson S.W., Gray H.K., Dockerty M.B.: Benign tumors of the liver: III: Solitary cysts. *Surg. Gynecol. Obstet.* 103:607, 1956.

65. Lin T.Y., Chen C.C., Wang S.M.: Treatment of nonparasitic cystic disease of the liver. *Ann. Surg.* 168:921, 1968.

66. Armitage N.C., Blumgart L.H.: Partial resection and fenestration in the treatment of polycystic liver disease. *Br. J. Surg.* 71:242, 1984.

67. Wittig J.H., Burns R., Longmire W.P. Jr.: Jaundice associated with polycystic liver disease. *Am. J. Surg.* 136:383, 1978.

68. Hyde G.L., Bertram R.L., Schwartz R.W.: Solitary nonparasitic hepatic cysts. *South. Med. J.* 74:1357, 1981.

69. Austin E.H., Mitchell G.E., Oliphant M., et al.: Solitary hepatic cyst and benign bile duct polyp: A heretofore unheralded association. *Surgery* 89:359, 1981.

70. Roemer C.E., Ferrucci J.T. Jr., Mueller P.R., et al.: Hepatic cysts: Diagnosis and therapy by sonographic needle aspiration. *A.J.R.* 136:1065, 1981.

71. Saini S., Mueller P.R., Ferrucci J.T., Jr., et al.: Percutaneous aspiration of hepatic cysts does not provide definitive therapy. *A.J.R.* 141:559, 1983.

72. Daly J.J., McDaniel R.C., Husted G.S., et al.: Unilocular hydatid cyst disease in the mid-South. *J.A.M.A.* 251:932, 1984.

73. Ertan A., Sahin B., Kandilci U., et al.: The mechanism of cholestasis from hepatic hydatid cysts. *J. Clin. Gastroenterol.* 5:437, 1983.

74. Papadimitriou J., Tsiftsis D., Tountas C.: Hydatid cyst of the liver ruptured into the biliary tract. *Curr. Surg.* 40:339, 1983.

75. Fulton A.J., Picker R.H., Cooper R.A.: Ultrasonic appearance of hydatid cysts of the liver. *Aust. Radiol.* 26:64, 1982.

76. Hadidi A.: Sonography of hepatic echinococcal cysts. *Gastrointest. Radiol.* 7:349, 1982.

77. Kune G.A., Jones T., Sali A.: Hydatid disease in Australia: Prevention, clinical presentation, and treatment. *Med. J. Aust.* 2:385, 1983.

78. de Diego Choliz J., Lecumberri Olaverri F.J., Franquet Casas T., et al.: Computed tomography in hepatic echinococcosis. *A.J.R.* 139:699, 1982.

79. Varela-Diaz V.M., Coltorti E.A., de Zavaleta O., et al.: Immunodiagnosis of human hydatid disease: Application and contribution to a control program in Argentina. *Am. J. Trop. Med. Hyg.* 32:1079, 1983.

80. Aggarwal A.R.: Formalin toxicity in hydatid liver disease. *Anaesthesia* 38:662, 1983.

81. Belli L., de Favero E., Marni A., et al.: Resection versus pericystectomy in the treatment of hydatidosis of the liver. *Am. J. Surg.* 145:239, 1983.

82. Dugalic D., Djukic V., Milicevic M., et al.: Operative procedures in the management of liver hydatidoses. *World J. Surg.* 6:115, 1982.

83. Langer J.C., Rose D.B., Keystone J.S., et al.: Diagnosis and management of hydatid disease of the liver. *Ann. Surg.* 199:412, 1984.

84. Chattopadhyay B.: Pyogenic liver abscess. *J. Infect.* 6:5, 1983.

85. Northover J.M., Jones B.J.M., Dawson J.C., et al.: Difficulties in the diagnosis and management of pyogenic liver abscess. *Br. J. Surg.* 69:48, 1982.

86. Pitt H.A., Zuidema G.D.: Factors influencing mortality in the treatment of pyogenic hepatic abscess. *Surg. Gynecol. Obstet.* 140:228, 1975.

87. Rubin R.H., Swartz M.N., Malt R.: Hepatic abscess: Changes in clinical, bacteriologic, and therapeutic aspects. *Am. J. Med.* 57:601, 1974.

88. Heyman A.D.: Clinical aspects of grave pyogenic abscesses of the liver. *Surg. Gynecol. Obstet.* 149:203, 1979.

89. McDonald A.P., Howard R.J.: Pyogenic liver abscess. *World J. Surg.* 4:369, 1980.

90. Moore-Gillon J.C., Kykyn S.S., Phillips I.: Microbiology of pyogenic liver abscesses. *Br. Med. J.* 283:819, 1981.

91. Perera M.R., Kirk A., Noone P.: Presentation, diagnosis, and management of liver abscesses. *Lancet* 2:629, 1980.

92. Sabbaj J., Suttel V.L., Finegold S.M.: Anaerobic pyogenic liver abscess. *Ann. Intern. Med.* 77:629, 1972.

93. Stenson W.F., Eckert T.: Pyogenic liver abscess. *Arch. Intern. Med.* 143:126, 1983.

94. Altemeier W.A., Schowengerdt C.G., Whiteley D.H.: Abscesses of the liver: Surgical considerations. *Arch. Surg.* 101:258, 1970.

95. Joseph W.L., Kahn A.M., Longmire W.P. Jr.: Pyogenic liver abscesses: Changing patterns in approach. *Am. J. Surg.* 115:63, 1968.

96. Satiani B., Davidson E.D.: Hepatic abscesses: Improvement in mortality with early diagnosis and treatment. *Am. J. Surg.* 135:647, 1978.

97. McFadzean A.J.S., Chang K.P.S., Wong C.C.: Solitary pyogenic abscesses of the liver treated by closed aspiration and antibiotics: Report of 14 consecutive cases with recovery. *Br. J. Surg.* 41:141, 1953.

98. Berger L.A., Osborne D.R.: Treatment of pyogenic liver abscesses by percutaneous needle aspiration. *Lancet* 1:132, 1982.

99. Dietrick R.B.: Experience with liver abscess. *Am. J. Surg.* 147:288, 1984.

100. Herbert D.A., Rothman J., Simmons F., et al.: Pyogenic abscesses: Successful nonsurgical therapy. *Lancet* 1:134, 1928.

101. Maher J.A., Reynolds T.B., Yellin A.E.: Successful medical treatment of pyogenic liver abscesses. *Gastroenterology* 77:618, 1979.

102. Bernardino M.E., Berkman W.A., Plemmons M., et al.: Percutaneous drainage of multiseptated hepatic abscess. *J. Comput. Assist. Tomogr.* 8:38, 1984.

103. Gerzof S.G., Robbins A.H., Johnson W.C., et al.: Percutaneous catheter drainage of abdominal abscesses: A five-year experience. *N. Engl. J. Med.* 305:653, 1981.

104. Greenwood L.H., Collins T.L., Yrizarry J.M.: Percutaneous management of multiple liver abscesses. *A.J.R.* 139:390, 1982.

105. Johnson W.C., Gerzof S.G., Robbins A.H., et al.: Treatment of abdominal abscesses: Comparative evaluation of operative drainage versus percutaneous catheter drainage guided by CT or ultrasound. *Ann. Surg.* 194:510, 1981.

106. Mandel S.R., Boyd D., Jaques P.F., et al.: Drainage of hepatic, intraabdominal, and mediastinal abscesses guided by computerized axial tomography: Successful alternative to open drainage. *Am. J. Surg.* 145:120, 1983.

107. Martin E.C., Karlson K.B., Fankuchen E., et al.: Percutaneous

108. Scheinfeld A.M., Steiner A.E., Rivkin L.B., et al.: Transcutaneous drainage of abscesses of the liver guided by computed tomography scan. *Surg. Gynecol. Obstet.* 155:662, 1982.

109. Reynolds T.B.: Medical treatment of pyogenic liver abscesses. *Ann. Intern. Med.* 96:373, 1982.

110. Abuabara S.F., Barrett J.A., Jau T., et al.: Amebic liver abscess. *Arch. Surg.* 117:239, 1982.

111. Basile J.A., Klein S.R., Worthen N.J., et al.: Amebic liver abscess: The surgeon's role in management. *Am. J. Surg.* 146:67, 1983.

112. Peters R.S., Gitlin N., Libke R.D.: Amebic liver abscess. *Annu. Rev. Med.* 32:161, 1981.

113. Netter F.H.: *The CIBA Collection of Medical Illustrations*, vol. 3. *Digestive System, part III: Liver, Biliary Tract, and Pancreas.* New York, CIBA, 1957.

114. Kennedy P.A., Madding G.F.: Surgical anatomy of the liver. *Surg. Clin. North Am.* 57:233, 1977.

115. Couinaud C.: Controlled hepatectomies and exposure of the intrahepatic bile ducts. Paris 1981.

116. Gupta S.C., Gupta C.D., Gupta S.B.: Hepatovenous segments in the human liver. *J. Anat.* 133:1, 1981.

drainage in the management of hepatic abscesses. *Surg. Clin. North Am.* 61:157, 1981.

27

Trauma to the Liver

ALEXANDER J. WALT, M.B., CH.B., M.S..

NOT UNEXPECTEDLY, liver injuries are common, since the liver is soft and easily compressed. The liver is also the largest of the solid intra-abdominal organs, extending superiorly to the fourth intercostal space on expiration. Until the past decade, surgeons were misled in their treatment of liver injuries by concepts derived from obsolete data that discouraged alternative approaches, such as generous mobilization of the liver for exposure, hepatic artery ligation (HAL), and temporary gauze packing. More recently, the natural history of hepatic trauma has been clarified by new technology capable of delineating the hepatic parenchyma noninvasively. At the same time, critical reinterpretation of operative findings has resulted in the definition of well-defined subsets of injury demanding specific and different surgical approaches. Finally, the extrapolation of conclusions derived from military experience to the civilian environment is now recognized to be invalid in many respects.

The current approach to liver injury is characterized by increased conservatism with regard to major resection but a much more aggressive attitude toward intraparenchyma' control of bleeding (Tables 27–1 and 27–2). Maximal achievable resuscitation is established before any major surgical attempt is launched. Thereafter, an ordered surgical sequence is adopted with the recognition that a variety of valid options may need to be applied in any individual case depending on the topography and extent of the hepatic wound.

Reports in the recent literature and records of 1,635 patients with liver injury operated on in the Wayne State University Affiliated Hospitals between 1961–76 and 1980–83 constitute the basis of this review of current practice.

TYPES AND OUTCOMES OF LIVER INJURIES

Major trauma centers in the United States continue to report large series of cases: 1,592 from Detroit Receiving Hospital[1]; 1,590 from Ben Taub Hospital between 1939 and 1974[2]; 811 from Parkland Hospital, Dallas, between 1962 and 1971[3]; 546 from Charity Hospital, New Orleans, between 1964 and 1976[4]; and 1,124 from the San Francisco General Hospital between 1966 and 1980.[5] The mortality has plateaued between 10% and 20% in most series, although figures as low as 2.9% have been reported.[6] This wide variation in mortality may not necessarily reflect either excellence or in-

eptitude. Instead, the mortality rate may be a function of the time elapsed between injury and the appearance of the patient in the hospital emergency department, the quality of resuscitation provided by the emergency medical services at the scene of the injury and en route to hospital, the age and preinjury health of the patient, the level of expertise of the receiving team in the emergency department, the types of injury in the series, the multiplicity of visceral damage, and the degree and duration of shock. Paradoxically, poor results may appear to emanate from excellent trauma centers which receive rapidly delivered but moribund and essentially unsalvageable patients, who in the past would have been "dead on arrival,"[7] and good results from institutions where relatively minor injuries predominate.

In attempting to compare experience and results, it is necessary to compare subsets of patients with comparable anatomical and physiologic disruption. To this end, several classification systems have been proposed, of which the following from Denver General Hospital is practical and reflective of the percentage of patients likely to be found in each of the five categories (Table 27–3). It is important to note, however, that the distribution of categories may change substantially in different environments, with a shift toward the more serious groups 3, 4, and 5, where blunt injuries and higher-velocity missiles cause a high percentage of the injuries. Such categorizations are useful for purposes of comparison, but even then should be applied with considerable caution as the usual categorization applies only to the liver injury and does not take into account the number and variety of concomitant visceral injuries, either intra- or extra-abdominal. For example, a relatively minor liver injury incidental to major extrahepatic damage is categorized as low-grade. This phenomenon is reflected in Flint and Polk's series,[8] where 16.2% of grade II injuries died in contrast to 11.4% in grade III.

Death is due to the liver injury per se in about 40% of patients; in the other 60%, death is due to extrahepatic injury, most often hemorrhage from large adjacent vessels, such as the inferior vena cava (IVC) and abdominal aorta and its branches, or injury to the brain or chest.

Associated injuries are present in about 75% of patients. In the Wayne State University series, the organs involved in descending order of frequency were thoracic (lung, chest wall, diaphragm, and heart), stomach, colon, kidney, long bone fractures, small bowel, gallbladder, pancreas, duodenum, and

TABLE 27–1.—Liver Injuries: A 1978 Survey

INSTITUTION	ANNUAL NO. OF PATIENTS (Approximate)	HEPATIC ARTERY LIGATION*	LOBECTOMY*	IVC CANNULATION*† (1972–76)
Baylor	130	0/1590	2.5%	15 (7)
Dallas	110	3 (Hemobilia) in 5 yr	2 (1.8%)	4 (0)
Southern Illinois (Carbondale)	100	0	3–4 (3.5%)	3 (1)
Wayne State University	100	14/968	25/968 (2.6%)	8 (0)
SUNY (Downstate)	75	10 (Approx.)	0	0
Emory University	70	7/429	7/429 (1.6%)	0
LSU	70	Seldom	4 (5.7%)	2 (0)
UCSF	70	± 5%	± 4/yr (5.7%)	± 5/yr (10%)
Louisville	60	59/189 (31.2%)	3/189 (1.6%)	—
Colorado	40	"Extremely rarely"	Not available	9 (2)

*Figures derived either from published series, work in progress, or thoughtful estimates.
†Number of survivors in parentheses.
With permission of *American Journal of Surgery,* from Walt A.J.: The mythology of hepatic trauma or Babel revisited. 135:12–18, 1978.

spleen. When the liver alone is involved, the mortality is below 5%. When one additional organ is injured, the mortality rate rises to about 15%, but when more than four organs are injured, the mortality is over 60%. About 70% die of hemorrhage, 20% of subsequent sepsis in the lungs or abdomen, and about 10% of direct cerebral or cardiopulmonary injury.

In the past three years, 72% of those in our series who died did so in the first 24 hours, about half on the operating room table before definitive treatment could be accomplished. Of the patients who survived 24 hours, the commonest cause of death was sepsis, either in the abdomen (intrahepatic, perihepatic, or interloop abscess) or in the lungs. Consequently, all efforts should be directed toward combating the threats of hemorrhage and sepsis from the moment the patient is first seen.

The types of injury vary in different communities. The average age of our 1,635 patients was 32 years (range 13–93), and 80% were between 13 and 40 years of age. (No children were present in this series). In the urban Wayne State University series, the more recent distribution is presented in Table 27–4.

A few caveats are important. While the mortality of stab wounds is usually less than 1%, the outcome is worse in patients on whom long knives are used, injuring extrahepatic

structures, in those with cirrhosis in whom retraction of vessels may not occur, and in patients with a coagulopathy. All wounds below the right fourth intercostal space should be viewed as potentially damaging to the liver, since the diaphragm extends at least to this level on expiration. In addition, wounds of the left chest may cross to involve the liver.

In gunshot wounds, the mortality is usually 15%–20% and in shotgun wounds about 20%–25%, although more favorable results are reported. While the trajectory is important, only limited deductions may be safely made about the course of the track. The entry and exit points and the site of any retained missile are noted, but bizarre paths may be described, depending on the position of the patient at the time of injury and possible deflections of a bullet that is spent or that has bounced off bone or been shattered in any way. The kinetic energy of the injuring instrument helps to determine the degree of hepatic damage. For example, the local injury is directly influenced by the muzzle velocity of the weapon, which varies widely, e.g., 970 ft per second in the .38 revolver to 2,160 ft per second in the .303 hunting rifle.[9] Small-caliber, low-velocity bullets tend to produce a small track or trough of tissue, with so little surrounding necrosis that formal debridement of the parenchyma is not necessary. In contrast, high-

TABLE 27–2.—Liver Injuries: A 1984 Survey

INSTITUTION	NO. LIVER INJURIES PER YEAR	BLUNT TRAUMA	HEPATO-TOMY	HEPATIC ARTERY LIGATION	HEPATIC LOBEC-TOMY	VENA CAVAL SHUNT	LIVER PACKING	OVERALL MORBIDITY	PERIHE-PATIC ABSCESS	OVERALL MORTALITY	EXSAN-GUINA-TION
Harborview	208	67	20	3	3	1	10	12	4	5	4
Ben Taub General	194	14	9	2	2	1	6	13	4	16	13
San Francisco General	90	40	5	2	8	1	4	38	5	9	5
Louisville	68	41	24	1	4	1	4	14	3	7	4
Detroit Receiving	63	9	. . .	2	3	1	3	13	8	14	7
Denver General	61	32	10	2	4	1	2	28	4	10	6
Bellevue (NYU)	50	12	38	<1	<1	<1	0	5	5	5	5
St. Paul-Ramsey	36	42	. . .	2	7	0	4	45	1	26	15
Average	96	32	18	2	4	1	4	21	4	11	7

With kind permission of Moore E.E.: *Am. J. Surg.* 148:712–716, 1984.

TABLE 27–3.—A Classification of Civilian Hepatic Trauma

CLASS	LIVER INJURY	FREQUENCY (%)
I	Capsular avulsion	15
	Parenchymal fracture < 1 cm deep	
II	Parenchymal fracture 1–3 cm deep	55
	Subcapsular hematoma < 10 cm diameter	
	Peripheral penetrating wound	
III	Parenchymal fracture > 3 cm deep	25
	Subcapsular hematoma > 10 cm diameter	
	Central penetrating wound	
IV	Lobar tissue destruction	3
	Massive central hematoma	
V	Retrohepatic vena cava injury	2
	Extensive bilobar disruption	

With kind permission of Moore E.E.: *Am. J. Surg.* 148:712–716, 1984.

velocity missiles produce extensive damage, with poorly vascularized residual segments of tissue, large detached sequestra, and extensive vascular and biliary disruption. Shotgun wounds may produce widespread destruction, depending on the distance of the liver from the point of discharge, and sepsis when foreign material is introduced.

Blunt injuries produce a wide variety of injuries and a mortality of about 15%–30%. With the most severely compressive forces, the patient fails to survive because other organs such as the heart, thoracic aorta, diaphragm, and trachea also are ruptured. In more focused but severe blows, parenchymal damage is most often concentrated in the posterosuperior aspect of the right lobe. The resulting lesion is often stellate, ragged, and difficult to expose because of its posterior position. Following falls from heights in particular, but also after other blunt injury, the surface of the liver may be visually deceptive, showing little more than a slight purplish discoloration, a small crack, or a subcapsular hematoma, even though the parenchyma within may be pulpified, and the site of an enlarging hematoma that is sometimes difficult to appreciate by palpation. Preoperative ultrasonography, CT scan, or scintigraphy is invaluable in these situations if the clinical state of the patient permits.

In patients who survive major central compressions over the spinal column, the liver may suffer a fracture analogous to that of the body of the pancreas in blunt trauma. In such cases, the middle hepatic vein is likely to be lacerated intra-parenchymally and may be associated with a large intrahepatic hematoma.

Children might warrant special consideration in that contained hematomas seem relatively more common than in adults.[10] Children are also more likely to demonstrate a linear crack of the posterosuperior aspect of the right lobe extending into the right hepatic vein, the inferior vena cava, or both, associated with a torn right triangular ligament. When the tears are partial and temporarily tamponaded by the weight of the liver and the residual ligaments, bleeding may initially be very gradual.

Among miscellaneous factors predisposing to liver disease are cirrhosis, pregnancy, and sickle cell anemia (in which apparently spontaneous rupture may occur), peliosis, and vascular tumors. To this group may be added iatrogenic hepatic injury by closed chest massage and vascular damage in the course of needle biopsy, percutaneous transhepatic cholangiography (PTC), or the passage of a transhepatic stent. In any of these, exsanguinating intraperitoneal hemorrhage may occur, or, alternatively, when Glisson's capsule remains relatively intact, a large, expanding and subsequently exploding intrahepatic hematoma may develop.

ANATOMY SPECIALLY RELEVANT TO LIVER TRAUMA

Since the right lobe constitutes about 70% of the parenchyma of the liver, injuries predominate in this less accessible region. The most threatening bleeding is likely to originate from the posterosuperior surface and the area of confluence of the hepatic veins and IVC. Thirty percent of the blood supply but about 50% of the oxygenation is supplied by the hepatic arteries; 70% of the blood supply but only 50% of the oxygenation by the portal vein. In any marked reduction of hepatic artery blood flow, compensation is provided by increased extraction of oxygen from the portal blood and by the opening of collaterals over the first 4 to 24 hours. About 20–26 pairs of small collaterals have been demonstrated, of which the inferior phrenic are often the largest. Since several of these vessels pass through various attachments of the liver, it is desirable to keep these intact when technically feasible. However, incision of the triangular and falciform ligaments and separation of the bare area of the diaphragm is a fundamental step in delivering the liver as a midline organ, and many collaterals are unavoidably sacrificed. When the triangular ligaments are incised, great care must be taken not to continue the incision medially to the point of injuring the IVC.

The hepatic artery often has an anomalous distribution, of which the most important surgical variants are the origin of the right hepatic artery from the superior mesenteric artery in about 17% of humans and the left hepatic artery from the left gastric artery in about 15%.[11] Death of hepatic hemorrhage is more often due to venous disruption, and the closer the lesion to the large hepatic veins, the more precarious the situation. Because the bulk of the right hepatic lobe influences the site of disruption, laceration of the right hepatic vein is the most commonly encountered life-threatening venous injury in blunt and decelerating trauma. Exposure of the area of this vein is always difficult, and direct repair in adults is rarely possible. Direct exposure is made much easier by

TABLE 27–4.—Mortality of Liver Injuries (1974–76 and 1980–83): Wayne State University*

AGENT	NO. OF PATIENTS (1974–76)	DEATHS, No. (%)	NO. OF PATIENTS (1980–83)	DEATHS, No. (%)
Gunshot wound	186	28 (15.1)	110	19 (17.3)
Stabs	91	1 (1.1)	93	4 (4.3)
Blunt	40	8 (20.0)	22	6 (27.3)
Shotgun	13	3 (23.1)	5	1 (20.0)
Iatrogenic	1	0	1	0
Total	331	40 (12.1)	231	30 (13.0)

*Note: Mortality in 1961–68 was 10.5% (46/436); in 1969–73, 14.6% (93/637).

median sternotomy (or right thoracotomy) and incision of the diaphragm through the central tendon. The duel between surgeon and the right hepatic vein is most often engaged in as part of a hepatic lobectomy. The right hepatic vein averages about 1.7 cm in internal diameter, is about 2 cm long (with many variations), and is free of tributaries in its terminal 1 cm in only about 60% of patients,[12] accounting for some of the difficulty in obtaining formal extrahepatic ligation in many patients. Access is obtained by dislocation of the liver toward the midline and anteriorly. This maneuver is usually more difficult during trauma than in the elective situation because of the associated parenchymal injury and continuing blood loss if direct pressure is lost.

The left hepatic vein is smaller than the right and is readily accessible by incision of the left triangular ligament. In 75% of humans, the left hepatic vein is joined by the middle hepatic vein to form a common junction less than 1 cm from the IVC, but in 10% this junction is more than 1 cm distant. In the remaining 15%, the middle hepatic vein enters the IVC as a separate entity between the right and left hepatic veins.

A variable number of small veins drain directly from the liver into the IVC along the length of the posterior surface of the liver. When torn, these may bleed vigorously and on occasion catastrophically. In about 50% of humans, a large supplementary right hepatic vein, up to 1.8 cm in diameter, drains the posteroinferior surface of the right lobe. The size of this vein is inversely related to the size of the main right hepatic vein.

PREOPERATIVE MANAGEMENT

Liver injuries may be occult, and the patient will occasionally deny any injury because of inebriation or desire to protect a known, feared or loved assailant. About 30% of patients with subsequently proved hepatic injury are normotensive on arrival at the hospital. A small percentage of these—even with no initial abdominal symptoms, such as tenderness, pain, ileus, or distention—deteriorate suddenly due to hemorrhage from the liver, simulating the picture of a ruptured ectopic pregnancy. Potential predictors of impending disaster are few and limited to a careful history of the nature of the impact and observation of skin ecchymoses, seat-belt bruises, tire marks, and entry and exit wounds. Peritoneal lavage (PL) is invaluable in questionable cases such as the patient who is unconsciousness or obtunded by alcohol or drugs. A negative PL makes the presence of a liver injury highly unlikely, although not impossible, while a positive return indicates the presence of bleeding but obviously does not localize the site.

In stable patients with torso injuries in whom clinical signs are vague, ultrasonography, CT, or scintigraphy is indicated. The incidence of an unsuspected subcapsular hematoma or intrahepatic hematoma is greater than was appreciated in the past. If CT scan is contemplated, PL should be delayed so as not to obscure the estimate of the volume of blood in the peritoneal cavity. In patients in whom a contained intrahepatic lesion is demonstrated and in whom no other indication for laparotomy is thought to exist, watchful waiting is justified, especially in children.

A high suspicion of liver injury is entertained in the presence of a history of direct impact by a steering wheel, fender, boot, or other firm object; localized signs in the upper abdomen such as guarding and tenderness; evidence of contusions of the skin; the presence of fractured ribs on the right; or an appropriately placed wound. PL is unnecessary in most such cases, and laparotomy is indicated after resuscitation has been completed.

In many patients, the presence of an intrahepatic injury is obvious from the start. In these patients, the fundamental objective is to operate on the patient when the resuscitation curve is at its apogee. Premature operation on a patient in shock may be no less fatal than an inadvisedly delayed operation based on overoptimistic misinterpretation of the patient's clinical response. In our most recent series, 39% of patients with a systolic blood pressure (BP) below 90 mm Hg on admission subsequently died in contrast to 1.5% in those with a BP above this level. Similarly, Carmona et al.[5] reported initial shock in 38 of the 40 patients who died.

Massive transfusion of blood may be unavoidable.[13] Fifty-six of 231 recent patients (24.2%) required more than 10 units of blood. The need for a massive transfusion is obviously a reflection of an injury in the grade III–V categories. Early operation, timed to minimize the period of shock and the likelihood of coagulopathy and hypothermia, is mandatory. Autotransfusion may be helpful but may also contribute to the development of disseminated intravascular coagulation. The need for massive transfusion does not preclude a reasonable chance of salvage, however, and 27 of 56 such patients lived. Paradoxically, 17 of 30 (56.6%) requiring more than 20 units of blood survived in contrast to only five of 14 who were given 10–14 units, an expression of the number who die intraoperatively fairly rapidly.

Deep and persistent shock in the face of vigorous volume replacement is always ominous and is the ultimate indicator of the need for immediate operation. Consequently, the operating room is the most appropriate place for the conduction of any intense resuscitation. An attempt is made to restore intravascular volume by the rapid IV administration of Ringer's lactate through large-caliber cannulas or needles until cross-matched blood is available. If a subclavian line is inserted rather than a cannula by a cutdown, pneumothorax must be kept in mind as a possible complication if little or no response occurs. Ankle veins are avoided only if injuries to the IVC, hepatic, or pelvic veins are strongly suspected. Adequate ventilation is ensured, and the status of the CNS, chest, long bones, and kidneys is assessed to the extent possible. Seriously injured patients are not moved to a radiology suite for fear of severe complications ensuing there at a time and place where they would be less likely to be recognized and more likely to be poorly treated. If an indicated IVP is not feasible in the emergency department, it may be done later in the operating room by a bolus infusion of Renografin, provided the patient is not in substantial shock. Rh-negative or type-specific blood infusion is started if the response to crystalloid is inadequate and fully cross-matched blood is not yet available.

Optimal resuscitation is always desirable to combat the negative effects of any subsequent serious blood loss being grafted onto a background of acidosis, hypovolemia, hypoxemia, and hypotension. In certain well-defined circumstances, when further delay threatens to precipitate an irreversible situation, operation must be done even though the patient is in a suboptimal state. Ominous factors are (a) failure of shock to respond to fluid and blood replacement, (b) an initial response followed by sudden deterioration, (c) shock in the presence of a tightly tamponaded abdomen. Operation should be preceded by prophylactic antibiotics—we prefer cefazolin, gentamycin, and clindamycin—when concomitant intestinal spillage is suspected. In all patients with one or more fractured ribs, before general anesthesia is induced, a large chest tube is placed in the fifth intercostal space in the anterior axillary line to obviate an intraoperative tension pneumothorax. A nasogastric tube is passed and care taken to guard against aspiration.

In the special subgroup with a systolic BP persistently less than 60 mm Hg despite fluid administration and an abdominal tamponade, consideration should be given to a preliminary left thoracotomy and temporary clamping of the thoracic aorta above the diaphragm before the abdomen is opened.[14] Such action serves to increase the blood pressure and cardiac and cerebral perfusion, and to decrease subsequent blood loss at laparotomy. It has often been observed that rapid, irreversible collapse occurs in patients in this subgroup if special precautions are not taken to obtain immediate aortic control. An alternative to thoracotomy is the immediate occlusion of the abdominal aorta just below the diaphragm through the lesser omentum by fingers, sponge stick, vascular clamp, or aortic compressor, as is done with a leaking aortic abdominal aneurysm. The best approach remains controversial, but awareness of the problem does much to salvage some patients in this small select subgroup.

PRINCIPLES OF MANAGEMENT IN THE OPERATING ROOM

Resuscitation of patients with serious liver injury is best done in the operating room. Since death and morbidity are most likely to stem from hemorrhage, sepsis, or poor ventilation, these potential hazards are combated from the start. Volume replacement, assisted ventilation, and antibiotic coverage are provided. Large infusions of fluids and blood rapidly lead to core hypothermia, so the patient is placed on a heating blanket (which, in fact, contributes little), and provision is made to warm all the administered blood, crystalloids, and anesthetic gases. Vascular instruments, the autotransfusor, and adequate provision for suction should be available.

The skin is prepared from the neck to the pelvis. A midline incision is made from the xiphoid to the umbilicus. This incision is rapid, relatively bloodless, and most versatile, as it can be extended cephalad to split the sternum to gain access to the pericardium, heart, hepatic veins, and IVC, or caudally to expose the pelvis. In special cases, the incision may be led into one or other thoracic cavity depending on the anatomy of the associated injuries.

Large gauze packs are immediately placed over the liver, and pressure is exerted manually or by retractors to gain temporary local hemostasis. Clots and blood are rapidly evacuated and the situation is assessed. If aortic pulsation is weak, the aorta is occluded below the diaphragm, blood is given rapidly, and all efforts are directed to reducing or eliminating shock. A frequent error is a failure to spend five or ten minutes or whatever time is necessary to restore volume, reduce acidosis, and improve oxygenation before the liver injury is approached, with further loss of substantial quantities of blood. During this relative respite, a search is made for other injuries. Attention is directed immediately to any bleeding from extrahepatic vessels or solid viscera such as the spleen. Leaking intestinal content from lacerated bowel is controlled by a series of Babcock forceps. Contamination of the peritoneal cavity is reduced by irrigation with warm saline which has the benefit of reducing the significant hypothermia that is present in most severely injured patients. Bleeding from injured vessels is stopped by whatever means necessary. Splenectomy may be unavoidable, and protracted attempts to salvage the injured spleen in these adverse physiologic circumstances should be resisted.

With BP restored to a level above 90 mm Hg if possible, the packs are removed from the liver and the situation is reassessed. In some patients, bleeding will have ceased and will not recur; in others, bleeding continues or recurs as the blood pressure rises. The technique adopted to achieve hemostasis varies with the site and extent of the lesion.

If bleeding from the liver is considerable and persistent, further preliminary steps are taken. The vessels in the portal triad may be occluded by a soft clamp or a vascular clamp (Pringle's maneuver), but aortic occlusion should be used sparingly to avoid renal damage. If the bleeding now stops appreciably, the source can be assumed to be arterial or from intrahepatic portal veins. The clamp is then reapplied more selectively in an attempt to pinpoint the feeding vessel and to obviate the iatrogenic near-total hepatic ischemia. However, bleeding that continues after the portal triad is clamped may be assumed to arise from an anomalous hepatic artery or from a hepatic vein, especially when the lesion is in the posterior aspect of the liver. Frequently, inferior vena cava and hepatic vein injuries are associated with a very large retroperitoneal hematoma, which in fact reflects local containment of the bleeding and provides the explanation of the patient's survival to that point.

The Pringle maneuver is strictly a temporizing measure, and, in fact, none of Pringle's original eight cases survived.[15] Since the description in 1908, speculation has continued concerning the safe period of occlusion. Although long accepted as 15 minutes, many surgeons have had successful results with occlusion of the portal triad for prolonged periods.[16] Pachter et al.[17] reported no untoward results in 30 patients in whom the portal triad was occluded for more than 20 minutes, in 17 patients where this was done for > 30 minutes and in 3 patients for > 60 minutes. These patients received a preliminary IV bolus of methylprednisolone succinate (30–40 mg/kg) and subsequent hepatic hypothermia with iced saline aimed at keeping the intraparenchymal temperature below 32°C. As yet, no scientific basis for the efficacy of these additional adjuvants has been established and the immunosuppressive properties of the steroids in worrisome. Today, most surgeons accept the relative safety of ischemia times in excess of 30 minutes even in the shocked patient but feel that occlusion should be as selective and as short as possible. Temporary occlusion of the portal triad may also be valuable in reducing blood loss while gaining exposure of an injured area, as an adjunct to aortic compression, and in those desperate cases in whom placement of an intracaval shunt is unavoidable.

PRINCIPLES OF LOCAL CONTROL

In practice, a majority of hepatic injuries have stopped bleeding spontaneously by the time of laparotomy. In our 968 patients treated between 1968 and 1976, this was the case in 50.8%[18]; of the most recent 231 patients treated between 1980 and 1983, 65.1% had stopped. If a liver laceration or track is not bleeding and the patient is normotensive, no local treatment is necessary. However, in lesions conveniently situated, most surgeons tend to insert a few interrupted 2–0 chromic catgut sutures using a swedged-on, blunt-nosed liver needle as is done in oozing liver wounds or following formal elective liver wedge biopsy. Review of our data suggests that about 55% of liver injuries have stopped bleeding at the time of laparotomy, about 20% have the bleeding easily controlled by relatively simple suturing, about 10% require complex techniques of local control and 10% pose the need for large resections, arterial ligation, packing or caval cannulation (Table 27–5).

Certain caveats in the local management of the liver wound merit respect. Actively bleeding, deep stab wounds or lacerations should not be closed blindly because continuing or subsequent bleeding may create an intrahepatic hematoma that gradually builds up internal pressure over hours or days until the liver explodes, with consequent massive intraperitoneal hemorrhage. To obtain exposure, if necessary, the wound in the liver should be deliberately extended by an incision into normal tissue, with care taken to suture-ligate or Hemoclip deeper vessels and biliary radicles in the parenchyma as these appear in the course of finger fracture or blunt dissection with a knife handle. The fundamental principle of hemostasis of the liver is no different from elsewhere in the body—every attempt is made to visualize the bleeding vessels and to occlude them accurately and permanently. Unfortunately, hepatotomy, while easily accomplished for relatively superficial fissures or tracks, presents an extremely difficult technical problem when the missile or fissure passes through the depths of

the liver. In this circumstance, pursuit of the principle involves the deliberate incision of a considerable area of hepatic tissue and may appear excessively aggressive as a primary approach and therefore unjustified. Bleeding may stop completely with sustained firm manual pressure even in these wounds, in which case nothing more need be done beyond drainage of the area.

When bleeding continues from a deep track, the correct decision is much more difficult. Several alternatives are available: (A) Sustained bimanual pressure should be patiently applied, as bleeding may eventually stop. (B) The two ends of the track may be closed to produce a tamponading pressure. This is successful on occasion but is also risky, because a steadily expanding, unrecognized hematoma may develop with subsequent rupture and exsanguination. (C) A series of interrupted catgut sutures may be blindly inserted in the hope that the bleeding site will be occluded. Although the placement of sutures is likely to be inaccurate, this pragmatic technique is preferable to the closure of the two ends and, when technically feasible, is often successful. (D) The feeding hepatic artery may be ligated when preliminary temporary occlusion has demonstrated substantial hemostasis. (E) The walls may be tamponaded by the pressure exerted by multiple 1-in. Penrose drains pulled through the length of the track by a catheter and then left in situ with the ends of the drains brought through the abdominal wall. Bluett et al[6] have successfully used this in nine cases. (F) The liver may be mobilized to gain access to the region of the hemorrhage, after which segmental resection is performed. In a patient with multiple injuries who has been in shock for a long time and who has received many units of blood, this can be a formidable procedure fraught with many complications. (G) Hepatic lobectomy may be unavoidable. (H) The area may be compressed by gauze packs left in place for 2–3 days.

In the classic stellate injury of blunt trauma of the right lobe or following explosive destruction by high-velocity missiles, debridement of liver tissue is vital in addition to control of the often massive hemorrhage. The important principle in these patients is the use of the Pringle maneuver and local compression by packs until the blood volume and pressure have been improved, acidosis reduced, and the incision enlarged to provide optimal exposure. The liver is then mobilized by incision of the triangular and falciform ligaments and partially delivered out of the abdomen. Care is taken not to injure the hepatic vein-IVC confluence and the veins passing between the posterior aspect of the liver and the IVC. The temptation to inspect the lacerated area intermittently must be resisted, since each inspection tends to result in the loss of up the 200–300 ml of blood without benefit to the patient or surgeon. In addition, attempted inspection with inadequate exposure resulting in traction on the injured area may cause further tearing of the cracks in the liver or may lead to air embolism, when a differential pressure exists between the abdomen and the thoracic cavity. If the blood pressure suddenly falls in the absence of proportionate blood loss, the following possibilities should be considered: (1) obstruction of the vena caval return by the rotated liver or tamponading packs: (2) an unanticipated pneumothorax; or (3) air embolism.

With the bleeding area under direct vision, resectional de-

TABLE 27–5.—METHODS OF TREATMENT OF LIVER INJURIES (1968–76) IN 968 PATIENTS AND (1980–83) IN 231 PATIENTS

PROCEDURE	1968–76 (%)	1980–83 (%)
Laparotomy alone	50.8	66.0
Suture	37.9	15.6
Debridement	4.8	3.5
Hemihepatectomy	2.6	3.5
Hepatic artery ligation	1.4	1.3
Inferior vena cava cannulation	0.8	1.3
Packs	0.3	3.0
Death on table or details unavailable	1.4	5.2
Total	100	100

bridement may be performed. Large amounts of liver may be resected without observance of segmental boundaries, although the middle hepatic vein should always be protected. Determination of the optimal line of debridement is sometimes difficult. While viable tissue should line the cavity, insistence on brisk bleeding as the arbiter of viability may lead to unnecessary excision and prolongation of the operation. Hemostasis and bilostasis are obtained over the residual surfaces and a pedicle of omentum may be brought up over this area. In large resections, when oozing continues, ligation of the hepatic artery close to the liver may be advisable as an added safeguard.

When deep, troughlike resections are completed in central wounds, the use of a large rolled wad of viable omentum sewn into the area as a pack has its advocates.[19] The potential advantages claimed for this maneuver are obliteration of dead space, tamponading pressure, and the introduction of tissue rich in macrophages, which are helpful in combating infection. An omental pack should not be tied so tightly as to function as a plug that permits blood to collect under pressure beneath it. Alternatively, when the central resection leaves a deep, wedge-shaped defect, dead space may be obliterated by deep figure-of-8 chromic catgut sutures which approximate the walls of the cavity. The preliminary placement of a series of sutures parallel to the walls on each side may assist in preventing the tearing out of the figure-of-8 sutures.

Various hemostatic agents, notably Gelfoam and microcrystalline collagen, have been promoted as being of value. Application of these hemostatic adjuncts should be used only as a last-ditch measure, in part because their efficacy in such cases is questionable but mostly because they predispose to sepsis.[20]

In selected injuries thoracotomy should be seriously considered.[5] Thoracotomy was performed on 40 of our most recent 231 patients (17.3%), sometimes before celiotomy to obtain control of intrathoracic bleeding or to occlude the thoracic aorta in the presence of abdominal tamponade, sometimes to ensure adequate exposure of a fractured liver or retrohepatic bleeding, and occasionally to treat postoperative complications such as empyema or biliary fistula. Of those patients requiring thoracotomy, 17 (42.9%) survived.

HEPATIC ARTERY LIGATION (HAL)

Until the early 1970s, both packing and ligation of the hepatic artery to obtain hemostasis were regarded as the refuge of the incompetent or timid. The origins of these misconceptions are instructive. The virtual ban on HAL stemmed from the poor results obtained when HAL was used mainly in patients with liver failure, terminal cancer, or severe sepsis. Unwarranted extrapolation of the predictably dismal results to healthy young patients with acute traumatic lesions obscured the value of HAL. Similarly, condemnation of packing of civilian liver wounds rose from the poor experience of surgeons using this technique in World War II, when soldiers with multiple wounds treated after long delays, with comparatively poor resuscitation and no antibiotic coverage, developed intra-abdominal sepsis.

In a series of laboratory and clinical reports, Mays et al.[21] showed that HAL could be performed with an acceptable risk-benefit ratio in hepatic injuries. The initial enthusiasm which led to use of this technique in 31.1% of 178 cases has decreased; HAL is now advocated in only about 2%–4% of patients.[22] Used in appropriate anatomical circumstances, HAL undoubtedly stops or substantially slows bleeding from most intrahepatic arterial branches. Inevitably, HAL also produces hepatic ischemia, which is clearly visible as a line of demarcation. Sequelae are few after HAL ligation in those patients in whom shock is short and transient, all avascular liver tissue is debrided, no collections of blood form, and no spillage of intestinal content occurs. In these patients, collaterals appear in 6–24 hours, and the dearterialized parenchyma is soon oxygenated. In 20% of patients, however, in whom these favorable conditions are not present, the hypoxic liver constitutes a good culture medium, and sepsis occurs postoperatively. HAL is a seductively easy approach to hepatic hemostasis. The exchange of delayed sepsis for hemostasis is often not to the patient's advantage, and the overall mortality rate is inordinately high when HAL is used excessively. Furthermore, about 10%–20% of patients rebleed later. HAL should therefore be used only when assiduous attempts to obtain local control have failed. HAL is a tentative substitute for major resection but not for a determined attempt at local debridement and hemostasis.

If HAL is adopted, ligation should be performed as close to the liver as possible. In transverse cracks involving both lobes, the common hepatic artery is ligated. Packing may be added selectively, since refilling through large intact collaterals can be anticipated. Anecdotal data suggest that ligation of the hepatic artery proper should be avoided. If the common hepatic artery or right hepatic artery is ligated, the gallbladder should be removed. Not infrequently, cholecystectomy may be necessary anyway to gain access to the hepatic fissure or track in the vicinity of the gallbladder bed.

DRAINS

Most isolated liver injuries do not require drains. Fisher and co-workers[23] reported a nonrandomized series of 254 patients in whom an increased number of complications were noted in those who had drainage. This observation led to widespread reassessment of drainage policies, but most surgeons still drain major liver injuries in which resectional debridement, segmentectomy, or lobectomy have been done or when uneasiness about hemostasis remains. Penrose drains, with or without supplementary suction drains of the Jackson-Pratt variety, are favored. Excision of the 12th rib to provide the posterior site of exit of drains has been popular over the years, but many surgeons now fashion the site of exit from within the abdomen just beyond and lateral to the tip of the 12th rib of a size to admit one or two fingers. The Penrose drains are shortened and removed within 3–7 days, and the suction drains are left in place only as long as they produce material. Care is taken to avoid placing the drains across bowel that might later be eroded, especially if ileus occurs. Whatever method is adopted, it is important to pay meticulous attention to the skin and dressings around the drains, as well as to the drains themselves, to reduce the chance of the operative site's being colonized from outside. Drainage of the Penrose drains into a colostomy bag is useful.

The addition of T-tube drainage to the common bile duct (CBD) in moderate to severe injuries was widely accepted until the early 1970s, when a prospective randomized study proved that this was neither necessary nor desirable.[24] Increased complications occurred with T-tube use, such as jaundice, sepsis, ductal injury, and acute erosive gastritis. Use of a T tube in hepatic injury has now been abandoned except when the extrahepatic biliary tree has been injured and requires drainage or stenting in its own right.

INJURY TO THE HEPATIC VEIN—IVC COMPLEX (HV-IVC)

Patients with this injury remain the most difficult individuals to save. Injuries to the HV-IVC complex may be blunt or penetrating, and in most cases, the injury is such that the patient dies at the scene of the accident or soon after. The vascular lesion is seldom isolated in blunt injury in adults but is more likely to be so in children.[10] Obvious factors in any potential salvage are the number and variety of concomitant injuries and the degree of shock and blood loss. Iatrogenic causes of death in the treatment of these patients are: (1) failure to recognize the presence of the lesion while the bleeding is still contained retroperitoneally and surgical intervention may be lifesaving; (2) deliberate but ill-advised opening of a stable, nonexpanding hepatic hematoma in which the weight of the liver has successfully tamponaded the low-pressure venous system, resulting in loss of hemostatic control; (3) the launching of a surgical attack on the area when the patient is still in shock and deep metabolic acidosis rather than the application of local pressure until the patient's general condition has improved and adequate blood, exposure, instruments, and help are available; (4) intermittent inspection of the lesion resulting in further considerable blood loss; and (5) failure to consider adequately the possible alternative of packing.

The results of vena caval shunts in the literature are extremely poor, and it can be surmised that countless failures go unreported. In the Wayne State University series, all 14 patients with IVC cannulation have died. At the Ben Taub Hospital, where in 1977 eight of 15 patients survived,[18] subsequent poor experience led to the virtual abandonment of IVC cannulation. The best recent results of atriocaval shunts (ACS) have been reported from San Francisco Hospital, where four of 18 patients survived.[25] It is highly significant, however, that all four survivors were young and victims of penetrating rather than blunt injury. Furthermore, all had lesions that were primarily parenchymal and were operated on before gross physiologic deterioration had occurred by an experienced team. No surviving patient ever had a recorded BP of less than 70 mm Hg.

In the uncommon patient in whom the retroperitoneal hematoma is not quite contained and in whom packing is not appropriate, an IVC shunt may be needed. This decision should be made as early as possible when the patient is relatively stable, since substantial further bleeding may be anticipated during the insertion of the shunt. Three main techniques are available: (1) After a median sternotomy, an ACS with holes cut in the tube to allow passage of blood into the atrium may be inserted through the right atrium to the infrarenal area; tapes are tied around the IVC above and below

the liver.[26] (2) A large Foley catheter may be inserted through a purse-string suture placed just below the renal veins and positioned so as to ensure egress of renal blood and tamponading of the IVC wound by the balloon when inflated. (3) A special vena caval shunt tube (Bard) may be inserted through the saphenofemoral junction with the inflated balloon positioned opposite the hepatic veins.[27] As part of all of these shunt procedures, occlusion of the portal triad is added, and temporary occlusion of the abdominal aorta may be necessary.

The current clear trend away from the use of IVC cannulas is epitomized in recent publications from two previous proponents of this method who report satisfactory and presumably improved results from judicious packing.[28, 29] Some patients with more or less isolated right hepatic vein and IVC injuries may be saved by direct vascular repair without the use of an IVC cannula. This is much less often achieved in adults than in young children who, following blunt trauma, may be stable for many hours with a limited linear fracture of the right posterosuperior segment of the right lobe leading into a tear of the right hepatic vein or IVC or both. With time, the contained bleeding breaks through the right triangular ligament in the peritoneal cavity, and the child deteriorates suddenly. The anatomy of children permits easy exposure through a median sternotomy and vertical split of the diaphragm so that a partially occluding vascular clamp may be applied to the IVC, facilitating venous repair, with or without hepatic resection as necessary.

PLACE OF LOBECTOMY

About 2%–4% of all hepatic injuries require formal lobectomy. Not unexpectedly, given the fact that this procedure is reserved for a very severely injured group in whom less aggressive hepatic procedures are not feasible, the mortality in the United States remains about 35%–60%. Five of 13 (37.5%) of our most recent lobectomy patients died during a period when our overall mortality was 13.2%. While Balasegaram and Joisny[30] reported performing 94 major hepatic resections (including 29 extended hemihepatectomies with only three deaths (in a series of 443 patients, with a mortality for major resections of only 10.3%, the overall mortality in his entire series was 15.3%. This dichotomy of an unparalleled survival after lobectomy but a fairly high overall mortality is presumably a function of selection and pattern of injury, supported by the fact that only 24 of the 91 (26.3%) resected patients had associated injuries in contrast to the 80% or more in most comparable series.

In contradistinction to elective lobectomy, lobectomy for trauma is usually conducted on a depleted patient with several other injuries. Nevertheless, lobectomy is indicated when the lobe is shattered or obviously devitalized or when bleeding cannot be stemmed by any other method, as occurs with some hepatic venous injuries. The surgical principles employed are similar to those in elective lobectomy—temporary occlusion of the portal triad; ligation of the appropriate hepatic artery, portal vein, and bile duct; demarcation of the ischemic liver along a line between the gallbladder bed and the inferior vena cava; electrocoagulation of the superficial surface of the liver surface, followed by finger-fracture or blunt knife handle dissection of the parenchyma; suture-ligation or Hemoclipping of intraparenchymal vessels or biliary radicles to the right of the middle hepatic vein; ligation of the veins running between the posterior surface of the rotated liver and the IVC, and, finally, ligation of the right hepatic vein, usually within the hepatic parenchyma. In lesions of the lateral aspect of the lobe, bleeding may be reduced after mobilization of the ligament by the use of a special liver clamp such as the Storm-Longmire clamp or a broad Penrose drain slung around the lobe like a tourniquet. Omentum may be loosely tacked to the resected surface, and the subdiaphragmatic dead space should be well drained.

THE CURRENT STATUS OF PACKING

The packing of liver wounds was virtually outlawed in World War II because of the high mortality and morbidity that resulted. The alternative subsequently adopted was lobectomy which, although appealing to surgical machismo, resulted in a number of avoidable deaths. In retrospect, the poor results of packing are seen to have been the results of poorly selected packing. Walt,[18] Feliciano et al.,[28] Carmona et al.,[29] Calne et al.[31] have all in recent years made a case for the judicious use of this technique. Six of our last seven patients (one died of a head injury) have survived; Carmona et al.[29] has reported on 17 severely injured patients (average of 31 units of blood required) with a mortality of 12%. Packing may succeed where numerous other techniques, including debridement-resection, HAL, and even IVC cannulation, have failed. Packing is of special value when coagulopathy has supervened, in large transverse cracks of the liver, contained or nearly contained retro- or perihepatic hematomas, persistently bleeding hepatic surfaces or cavities, and in the hypothermic, shocked patient unable to withstand a prolonged operation. Above all, packing is useful in the blunt hepatic injury encountered in any hospital where facilities or experience are not available for major hepatic surgery. In such cases, the pack is inserted and the patient transferred to an appropriate center when stable.

The technique of packing includes insertion of large gauze packs against the liver surface(s) of all the bleeding areas to produce compression. Care is taken not to occlude the IVC and to ensure adequate ventilation in view of the unavoidable pressure on the diaphragm. The abdomen is closed without external drainage, and the packs are left in place for 1–3 days depending on the patient's progress. The packs are then removed in the operating room using general anesthesia, with all preparations made to do whatever may be necessary, including debridement, resection, or IVC cannulation and wide drainage of the area. In practice, recurrent bleeding is very uncommon beyond an occasional small artery which may need to be Hemoclipped or ligated. While antibiotics are given to patients in whom the pack is inserted, our experience, unlike that of some others, has been that intra-abdominal infection develops in about 40% of these patients. The tradeoff, however, when measured against uncontrollable hemorrhage remains very profitable.

SPECIAL DILEMMAS

Liver function tests are not reliable indicators of the presence, extent, or degree of resolution of hepatic injury. Serum enzyme levels may be normal early on or even later in the face of extensive damage. Newer technology including ultrasonography,[32] scintigraphy,[33] CT scanning,[34] arteriography and interventional radiologic procedures[35] have provided previously unappreciated insights into the natural history of liver injuries. These data have led to a wider range of options in the timing and variety of treatment, but insufficient experience has been acquired to permit dogmatism. Nevertheless, definite trends are discernible.

Isotopic delineation of the injured liver has long had advocates, but most institutions have not been able to provide around-the-clock service. Some surgeons have found results of scintigraphy to be unreliable or confusing, although it seems probable that many of these views are rooted in inexperience and insecurity. With the advent of technetium analogues of iminodiacetic acid (IDA), hepatobiliary injuries may be clearly delineated when of significant extent in a cooperative patient, and excellent results have been reported.

Ultrasonography, while inexpensive, requires a cooperative patient and an abdomen that permits accurate scanning. These factors are seldom available in a patient with acute multiple injuries. Ultrasonography has its greatest value as a noninvasive procedure to track the resolution of any intrahepatic filling defect and may be complementary to cholescintigraphy if bile leakage is suspected.

Arteriography, once advocated for the acute phase of injury, has its main value today in detecting an unidentified source of intrahepatic bleeding such as occurs in hemobilia or in postoperative hemorrhage. Of equal value, the arteriographic catheter provides access for embolization by Gelfoam pledgets or steel coils of the source of hemobilia, which may be an intrahepatic pseudoaneurysm, arteriovenous fistula, or lacerated vessel. The call for angiographic occlusion of such lesions more often occurs in patients who have already undergone one operation, and this technique obviates a difficult reoperation. Arteriography and embolization are not often required but are logical in selected patients in whom an intrahepatic source of bleeding has been demonstrated and in whom no extrahepatic lesion requiring operation is suspected. Sclafani et al.[35] demonstrated the versatility and benefits of embolization in patients with liver injury.

The advent of CT scanning as a relatively routine procedure has confirmed previous observations that liver injuries are often clinically occult. The San Francisco General Hospital group studied the potential of the CT body scanner in hemodynamically stable patients with blunt injury. Twenty-four patients with demonstrated hepatic injury (6% of all liver injuries in that period) were observed without laparotomy.[36] All were characterized by being younger than 40 years of age and clinically stable, having less than an estimated 250 ml of blood in the peritoneal cavity, and displaying an intrahepatic or subcapsular hematoma or both on CT scan. No complications of this expectant treatment were noted over a follow-up period of up to nine months. Similar conservative management has been described by Ritchie and Fonkalsrud,[37] Cheatham et al.,[38] and Athey et al.[39] Karp et al.[40] followed up 17 selected CT-proved lesions in children, of whom only one needed subsequent elective operation. Serial CT scans showed that healing occurred within about four months after a sequence of absorption and remodeling of the area of injury. This new and accurate knowledge acquired by noninvasive techniques poses fresh clinical dilemmas as the limits of conservative therapy are explored.

Potential pitfalls in nonoperative management have been analyzed by Geis et al.[41] Sixty-five of 283 (23% of patients with severe blunt torso injury) sustained hepatic injury; of these 65 patients, 49 required early operation, but in 16 (15.4%) stable intrahepatic hematomas were initially observed. Six of the 16 needed an operation over the next four weeks for sepsis or expansion of the hematoma. Operation is essential if the liver becomes palpable, pain persists or increases, the hemoglobin falls, signs of bleeding occur, serial scans show increase in the size of the lesion, or sepsis supervenes. If a localized abscess is suspected, percutaneous drainage of the lesion by percutaneously inserted catheters may be tried. *Serratia marcescens* appears disproportionately to be the infecting organism in hepatic hematomas, which may be a result of the prophylactic antibiotics usually given. Based on these data, when nonoperative treatment is selected, the patient must be watched very closely in the hospital for at least two weeks. Serial ultrasonography should be performed every few days at the start and then every two weeks or so, until the lesion is healed. During this period, the patient should avoid any physical exercise that may precipitate bleeding and should be warned to report urgently if any indication of bleeding such as weakness, pallor, hematemesis, or melena occurs at any time then or in the future.

Olsen[42] found that seven of 320 patients (2.2%) with acute hepatic injury developed central parenchymal complications that subsequently required reoperation. His review of a total of 21 such cases revealed that 11 presented with abscesses, 6 with sterile hematomas and 4 with hemobilia, 2 of whom had related biliary calculi. Some lesions were iatrogenic due to poor technique, others reflected the natural history of intrahepatic hematomas.

The entity of persistent posttraumatic hepatic cysts noted on serial scan is increasingly reported.[43] While some remain asymptomatic and may resolve spontaneously, the potential for subsequent bleeding or infection exists, and catheter drainage by the radiologist is probably advisable in established asymptomatic cases and certainly in persistent or symptomatic lesions.

COMPLICATIONS

All patients with hepatic injury inevitably suffer disruption of intraparenchymal arteries, veins, biliary radicles, and hepatic tissue to varying degrees. The final lesion is the result of these factors and may present as a subcapsular hematoma, intrahepatic hematoma, cyst or abscess, an arteriobiliary fistula, an ateriovenous fistula, or an intraperitoneal hemorrhage. Liver tissue has an unparalleled regenerative capacity, and even if 80% of the liver is resected, full replacement occurs within a few months. Most minor arterial and venous bleeding stops spontaneously, but major rebleeding may occur due to technical error, secondary sepsis, or arteriobiliary connections. Arteriography has demonstrated that acute arteriovenous fistulization is common in penetrating and blunt injuries and may in fact be almost inescapable in view of the intimate anatomical juxtaposition of the arteries and veins. Fortunately, the overwhelming majority of fistulas in the liver close spontaneously, even when initially large, and sometimes within a week.

Hemobilia

Delayed bleeding into the biliary system may occur following blunt trauma or percutaneous transhepatic cholangiography.[44, 45] Hemobilia is uncommon and is known to have occurred in only four of our 1,635 patients (0.002%); one of the four died. About 50% of patients present within one month and virtually all within a year. The clinical manifestations reflect the volume of blood loss. Some patients complain of pain in the right upper quadrant, but others present in shock with hematemesis or melena. Bleeding may be massive from the start or may occur in small amounts over a number of weeks, presumably due in part to intermittent dissolution of clot by bile. The patient may or may not be jaundiced and have abnormal liver function tests. In the presence of intrahepatic infection, fever may be a feature. Today, arteriography should be performed immediately if hemobilia is suspected. Because most lesions are essentially small pseudoaneurysms, they can be embolized successfully. If local sepsis follows, the cavity may be drained by a percutaneous catheter. Alternatively, if the cavity is large or if selected embolization fails, operation is necessary with unroofing of the cavity, ligation of the responsible vessel, and possibly ligation of the feeding hepatic artery. The cavity is left open and drained.

In children, spontaneous resolution of hemobilia with expectant treatment has been reported.[46] Most such lesions are small and situated in the peripheral areas of the liver. If this plan is adopted, the onus is very much on the surgeon.

Biliary Fistulas

Biliary fistulas are fortunately uncommon but take many forms. Given the ubiquity of biliary radicles within the liver and the size of the biliary structures in the hilum and porta hepatis, it is surprising that symptomatic biliary leaks do not occur more often. The importance to be attached to the leak is a function of its volume. In large hepatic injuries, some surgeons have advocated routine intraoperative retrograde cholangiography through a needle inserted into the gallbladder or common bile duct, but this is seldom necessary.

Postoperatively, ^{99m}Tc IDA scintigraphy has the advantage of potentially demonstrating the site and size of any biliary leak and has confirmed that small leaks, which are not infrequent, usually seal spontaneously. Larger leaks that occur through a drain site or the main wound usually cease within 1–6 weeks and are often best tracked by a fistulogram, which gives the most direct and accurate delineation. Bile that collects or becomes infected must be drained by a percutaneous catheter or operatively. Injury to an extrahepatic duct will usually need repair, but reasonably large intraparenchymal leaks may heal spontaneously.

Biliary-pleural fistulas occur in about 0.2% of liver injuries and must be drained through a thoracostomy tube.[47] If drainage does not cease spontaneously, the source in the liver must be identified and debrided or excised and the hole in the diaphragm repaired. Decortication may be necessary.

Biliary-bronchial fistulas[48] are very rare but are dangerous, since bile may suddenly flood the bronchial tree and drown the patient. The presence of bile in sputum serves as a clear warning, mandating an immediate search for the source. The fistula may not appear for several months after the trauma. Operation may be difficult because the origin may be surrounded by pleural adhesions, necrotic tissue, and obliterated tissue planes. A lower lobectomy may be unavoidable.

Traumatic Hepatic, Arteriovenous Fistula, and Pseudoaneurysms

Rarely, traumatic arteriovenous fistulas, so common in the acute phase, fail to obliterate spontaneously. In a review of 15 patients, Missavage et al.[49] classified three groups—the first recognized within a few weeks of trauma and manifested by hemorrhage or an epigastric bruit; the second with small fistulas and few symptoms; and the third, more chronic, characterized by portal hypertension, esophageal varices, and in two of three patients marked upper GI bleeding. Treatment may be successfully carried out by embolization, but in larger lesions a direct surgical attack may be necessary.

POSTOPERATIVE COMPLICATIONS

Approximately 40% of patients who survive hepatic trauma develop postoperative complications.[5] The spectrum and intensity of these complications tend to mirror the initial pathology and may be found intra- or extra-abdominally. Fever is common, and, while most often due to atelectasis or poor ventilation, potential sources abound.

The lungs are the commonest site of complications, characterized mainly by atelectasis, contusion, aspiration, or the adult respiratory distress syndrome of sepsis (ARDS). ARDS should be anticipated in patients who have been in shock or who have peritoneal contamination, massive transfusions, a major resection, or an overt abscess. Ventilation and arterial blood gases should be carefully monitored in those with major liver injury, and the endotracheal tube should not be removed until adequate spontaneous ventilation has been established. In blunt injury, allowance should be made for initially occult pulmonary contusion.

Of the abdominal complications, sepsis is the most frequent. The detection of a causative abscess may not be easy despite the availability of the many scanning techniques available today. While an intra- or peri-hepatic abscess is often anticipated and relatively easy to detect, the development of an interloop or pelvic abscess may be associated with vague symptoms and signs. Noninvasive scanning of all types is much less reliable when loculated pus is present in the central abdomen, and exploratory laparotomy (or so-called "second look" operation) may be unavoidable in patients who continue to show the picture of sepsis. In ARDS from an occult intra-abdominal collection of pus, such laparotomies have a positive yield of about 50%. The cost-benefit ratio of such explorations is difficult to determine as negative explorations sometimes compound the problems of ileus and respiratory dysfunction. Although such reexplorations occasionally produce intestinal fistulas, exploration can be lifesaving, and, consequently, the decision remains one of clinical judgment.

The abdominal wound may require special attention. In the presence of contamination, the skin and subcutaneous tissues are left open, to be closed at 4–7 days by secondary suture if the wound is clean. In shotgun wounds, when so much tissue is destroyed that the muscles cannot be approximated, eventual closure may be obtained by the initial use of Teflon mesh or parachute silk covered with moistened gauze sponges held in place by retention sutures. Care of this wound may necessitate light general anesthesia three or four times a week for debridement and replacement of fresh dressings, but even patients with exposed livers may gradually have successful wound closure.

Nutrition has a vital influence on wound healing. For patients in whom it can be predicted clinically that all intake is unlikely for a week or more, some favor the insertion of jejunal catheter at the primary operation. Since this procedure itself has potential complications in these circumstances, most surgeons favor IV total parenteral nutrition early. Postoperative fever is common in serious hepatic injuries; the potential of the hyperalimentation catheter to act as the source of infection and hence of the pyrexia may pose a clinical problem.

In the 10%–20% of patients with liver injuries who require more than 10 units of blood, coagulopathies are common. Intraoperative oozing may be due to the "washout" effect of the massive transfusion or to disseminated intravascular coagulation or mismatched blood. An acidosis below pH 7.2 and hypothermia below 32° C may add to the oozing. Precautions should be taken against all these eventualities, and a vigorous hematologic investigation conducted whenever oozing is present. Blood not older than 24 hours if possible should be used, with a unit of fresh frozen plasma given after each 6 units of blood to add component factors, platelet concentrates after each 10 units of blood or when the platelet count falls below 20,000/cu mm, and calcium chloride (1 gm IV) after each 5 units of blood. In the stable, non-oozing case, it is not necessary to treat temporarily deranged laboratory data such as a prolonged prothrombin time or partial thromboplastin time. Oliguria is avoided preoperatively and intraoperatively if possible. If oliguria ensues postoperatively, analysis of laboratory data and the response to volume replacement, often guided by information derived from a pulmonary artery balloon catheter, will determine the nature of the phenomenon and therefore its treatment. Polyuria may be due to intraoperative overloading, high-output renal failure, or sepsis causing an obligatory increase in urinary output. It is important that the latter be recognized so that fluid administration is not inappropriately restricted, with a resulting conversion, sometimes rapid, to intravascular volume contractions, renal damage, and oliguria.[50]

In sepsis, especially when added to shock, the stomach may be the target organ with consequent acute erosive gastritis. While the mucosal lesions may not be totally avoided by administration of hourly antacids to achieve a gastric pH greater than 5.0, with or without concomitant cimetidine, clinical bleeding of any serious degree is virtually eliminated.

CONCLUSIONS

As hepatic trauma has been critically studied over the past decade, a more rational approach has evolved that fits a variety of options to the broad spectrum of anatomical damage encountered. Some old fears have been dispelled, and aggressive conservatism has tended to replace illogical aggression. Since the mortality rate is now determined mainly by the occurrence of uncontrolled hemorrhage from the superior and posterior aspects of the liver, only modest further progress can be anticipated in the salvage of this group of patients, especially since they usually have serious concomitant injuries. Currently, the use of noninvasive techniques to delineate the presence, extent, and prognosis and possibility of spontaneous healing is attracting considerable attention as surgeons seek to reduce avoidable operations. It should be recognized, however, that this quest demands a high degree of clinical and technological sophistication and that misjudgment may carry considerable penalties for both patient and surgeon.

REFERENCES

1. Walt A.J., Bender J.S.: Injuries of the liver, in Schwartz S., Ellis H. (eds.): *Maingot's Abdominal Operations.* East Norwalk, Conn., Appleton-Century-Crofts, 1984, pp. 1577–1590.
2. DeFore W.W., Mattox K.L., Jordan G.L., et al.: Management of 1590 consecutive cases of liver trauma. *Arch Surg.* 111:493–497, 1976.
3. Trunkey D.D., Shires G.T., McClelland R.: Management of liver trauma in 811 consecutive patients. *Ann Surg.* 179:722–728, 1974.
4. Levin A., Gover P., Nance F.C., et al.: Surgical restraint in the management of hepatic injury: A review of Charity Hospital experience. *J. Trauma* 18:399–404, 1978.
5. Carmona R.H., Lim R.C., Clark G.C.: Morbidity and mortality in hepatic trauma—a 5 year study. *Am. J. Surg.* 144:88–94, 1982.
6. Bluett M.K., Woltering E., Adkins R.B.: Management of penetrating hepatic trauma. *Am. Surg.* 50:132–142, 1984.
7. Moore E.F.: Critical decisions in the management of hepatic trauma. *Am. J. Surg.* 148:712–716, 1984.
8. Flint L.M., Polk H.C.: Selective hepatic artery ligation: Limitations and failure. *J. Trauma* 19:319–323, 1979.
9. Mays E.T.: Hepatic trauma. *Curr. Probl. Surg.* Vol 5–73, 1976.
10. Coln D., Crighton J., Schorn L.: Successful management of hepatic vein injury from blunt trauma in children. *Am. J. Surg.* 140:858–860, 1980.
11. Michels N.: Newer anatomy of liver-variant blood supply and collateral circulation. *J.A.M.A.* 172:125–132, 1960.
12. Nakamura S., Tsuzuki T.: Surgical anatomy of the hepatic veins and the inferior vena cava. *Surg. Gynecol. Obstet.* 152:43–50, 1981.
13. Clagett G.P., Olsen W.R.: Coagulopathies causing hemorrhage in severe liver injury. *Ann. Surg.* 187:369–374, 1978.
14. Ledgerwood A.M., Kazmers M., Lucas C.E.: The role of thoracic aortic occlusion for massive hemoperitoneum. *J. Trauma* 16:610–615, 1976.
15. Pringle J.H.: Notes on the arrest of hepatic hemorrhage due to trauma. *Ann. Surg.* 48:541–549, 1908.
16. Huguet C., Nordlinger B., Bloch P., et al.: Tolerance of the human liver to prolonged normothermic ischemia. *Arch. Surg.* 113:1448–1451, 1978.
17. Pachter H.L., Spencer F.C., Hofstetter S.R., et al.: Experience with the finger fracture technique to achieve intra-hepatic hemostasis in 75 patients with severe liver injuries of the liver. *Ann. Surg.* 197:771–778, 1983.
18. Walt A.J.: The mythology of hepatic trauma or Babel revisited. *Am. J. Surg.* 135:12–18, 1978.
19. Stone H.H., Lamb J.M.: Use of pedicled omentum as an autogenous pack for control of hemorrhage in major injuries of the liver. *Surg. Gynecol. Obstet.* 141:92–94, 1975.
20. Scher K.S., Coil J.A.: Effects of oxidized cellulose and microfibrillar collagen on infection. *Surgery* 91:301–311, 1982.
21. Mays E.T., Conti S., Fallahzedeh H., et al.: Hepatic artery ligation. *Surgery* 86:536–543, 1979.
22. Flint L.M., Mays E.T., Aaron W.S., et al.: Selectivity in the management of hepatic trauma. *Ann. Surg.* 185:613–618, 1977.
23. Fischer R.P., O'Farrell K.A., Perry J.F.: The value of peritoneal drains in the treatment of liver injuries. *J. Trauma* 18:393–398, 1978.
24. Lucas C.E., Walt A.J.: Analysis of randomized biliary drainage for liver trauma in 189 patients. *J. Trauma* 12:925–930, 1972.
25. Kudsk K.A., Sheldon G.F., Lim R.C.: Atrial-caval shunting (ACS) after trauma. *J. Trauma* 22:81–85, 1982.
26. Schrock T., Blaisdell W., Mathewson C. Jr.: Management of blunt trauma to the liver and hepatic veins. *Arch. Surg.* 96:698–704, 1968.
27. Pilcher D.B., Harmon P.K., Moore E.E.: Retrohepatic vena cava balloon shunt introduced via the saphenofemoral junction. *J. Trauma* 17:837–841, 1977.
28. Feliciano D.V., Mattox K.L., Jordon G.L.: Intra-abdominal packing for control of hepatic hemorrhage: a reappraisal. *J. Trauma* 21:285–290, 1981.
29. Carmona R.H., Peck D.Z., Lim R.C. Jr.: The role of packing and planned reoperation in severe hepatic trauma. *J. Trauma* 24:779–784, 1984.
30. Balasegaram M.B., Joisny S.: Hepatic resection in trauma, in Shires G.T., (ed.): *Advances in Surgery.* Chicago, Year Book Medical Publishers, 1984, pp. 129–170.
31. Calne R.Y., Wells F.C., Forty J.: Twenty-six cases of liver trauma. *Br. J. Surg.* 69:365–368, 1982.
32. Uthoff L.B., Wyffels P.L., Adams C.S., et al.: A prospective study comparing nuclear scintigraphy and computerized axial tomography in the initial evaluation of the trauma patient. *Ann. Surg.* 198:611–616, 1983.
33. Weissman H.S., Byun K.J., Freeman L.M.: IDA scintigraphy in the evaluation of hepatobiliary trauma. *Semin. Nucl. Med.* 13:199–212, 1983.
34. Moon K.L., Federle M.P.: Computed tomography in hepatic trauma. *Am. J. R.* 141:309–314, 1983.
35. Sclafani S.J.A., Shaftan G.W., McAuley J., et al.: Interventional radiology in the management of hepatic trauma. *J. Trauma* 24:256–262, 1984.
36. Crass R.A., Myer A.A., Lim R.C., et al.: Selective non-operative management of blunt liver injury using abdominal CT. *Arch. Surg.* 120(5):550–554, 1985.
37. Richie J.P., Fonkalsrud E.W.: Subcapsular hematomas of the liver: nonoperative management. *Arch. Surg.* 104:781–784, 1972.
38. Cheatham J.E., Smith E.I., Tunell W.P., et al.: Nonoperative management of subcapsular hematomas of the liver. *Am. J. Surg.* 140:852–857, 1980.
39. Athey G.N., Rahman S.U.: Hepatic haematoma following blunt injury: Non-operative management. *Injury* 13:302–306, 1982.
40. Karp M.P., Cooney D.R., Pros G.A., et al.: The nonoperative management of pediatric hepatic trauma. *J. Pediatr. Surg.* 18:512–518, 1983.
41. Geis W.P., Schulz K.A., Giacchino J.L.: The fate of unruptured intrahepatic hematomas. *Surgery* 90:689–697, 1981.
42. Olsen W.R.: Late complications of central liver injuries. *Surgery* 92:733–743, 1982.
43. Sugimoto T., Yoshioka T., Sawada Y., et al.: Post-traumatic cyst of the liver found on CT scan—a new concept. *J. Trauma* 22:797–800, 1982.
44. Sandblom P., Mirkovitch V.: Hemobilia: Some silent features and their causes. *Surg. Clin. North Am.* 57:397–408, 1977.
45. Goodnight J.E., Blaisdell F.W.: Hemobilia. *Surg. Clin. North Am.* 61:973–979, 1981.
46. Lockwood T.E., Schorn L., Coln D.: Nonoperative management of hemobilia. *Ann. Surg.* 185:335–340, 1977.
47. Franklin D.C., Mathai J.: Biliary pleural fistula: A complication of hepatic trauma. *J. Trauma* 20:256–258, 1980.
48. Boyd D.P.: Bronchobiliary fistulas. *Ann. Thorac. Surg.* 24:481–487, 1977.
49. Missavage A.E., Jones A.M., Walt A.J., et al.: Traumatic hepatic arterio-venous fistula. *J. Trauma.* 24:355–358, 1984.
50. Lucas C.E.: The renal response to acute injury and sepsis. *Surg. Clin. North Am.* 56:953–975, 1976.

28

Portal Hypertension

LAYTON F. RIKKERS, M.D.

HISTORY OF SURGERY FOR PORTAL HYPERTENSION

The history of portal hypertension surgery has recently been discussed by Donovan and Covey[1] and by Warren.[2] The early history (1877–1912) was marked by original descriptions of surgical techniques, discovery of the physiologic consequences of portal diversion, and limited application of the techniques to patients with portal hypertension. The modern era (since 1945) has consisted of reintroduction of portal-systemic shunting as treatment for portal hypertension, wide application of shunt and nonshunt procedures throughout the world, and evaluation of some of the operations in randomized, controlled trials.

The first portacaval shunt was performed in a dog in 1877 by Nicolai Eck, a young military surgeon in St. Petersburg, Russia. Despite the fact that seven of eight shunted dogs died within the first week, and the lone survivor ran away before shunt patency could be documented, Eck concluded that complete portal diversion was compatible with survival and was an appropriate therapy for patients with ascites.

In 1893 Pavlov brilliantly described the physiologic consequences of complete portal diversion. His careful observations of 20 surviving dogs with Eck fistulas resulted in elucidation of portasystemic encephalopathy or "meat intoxication." His autopsy studies disclosed that dogs with encephalopathy had widely patent portacaval anastomoses and atrophic livers; unaffected dogs had thrombosed or narrowed shunts with collateral portal blood flow to the liver. Pavlov concluded that intestinally absorbed nitrogenous compounds, which bypass the liver, caused encephalopathy.

In 1903 Vidal performed the first human portacaval shunt. Because his patient developed symptoms of encephalopathy during a brief survival period, Vidal concluded that complete portal diversion was too radical a therapy for patients with portal hypertension. Because of Pavlov and Vidal's observations that total portal diversion could have devastating physiologic effects, the few other early attempts at portal decompression emphasized partial rather than total shunting of portal flow. Villard and Tavernier (1910) utilized an anastomosis between a superior mesenteric venous branch and the ovarian vein, and Rosenstein (1912) performed the first side-to-side portacaval shunt. Neither of these pioneering efforts were entirely successful.

The modern era of portal hypertension surgery began in 1945 when Whipple, Blakemore, and Lord reported their initial experience with portacaval and splenorenal shunts in patients with portal hypertension. These investigators reintroduced portal-systemic shunting because no other available therapies were effective for treatment of variceal hemorrhage and because they had recently devised improved methods for blood vessel anastomosis. In addition, contemporary laboratory studies had shown that the Eck fistula in dogs was compatible with prolonged survival. It is a remarkable achievement that all ten patients in this first shunt series survived the operation and were discharged from the hospital. After this initially successful experience, portal-systemic shunt therapy became widely disseminated. Several hundred end-to-side portacaval, side-to-side portacaval, and splenorenal shunts were done in many medical centers throughout the world, with the consensus being that these operations were the most effective means of preventing recurrent variceal hemorrhage.

It was not until the 1960s however, when the portacaval shunt was evaluated in randomized, controlled trials. Because of discouraging results from these studies, the emphasis in the 1970s and 1980s has been on development and testing of procedures which both prevent variceal hemorrhage and maintain portal perfusion of the liver. In 1967 Warren introduced the distal splenorenal shunt as a means of selectively decompressing esophagogastric varices while preserving portal blood flow to the liver. Multiple nonshunt operations, which interrupt collateral pathways to varices or obliterate varices have also been described. Finally, although first introduced in 1939, endoscopic variceal sclerosis has recently been resurrected and is presently competing with shunt and nonshunt operations for its role in the long-term management of patients with variceal hemorrhage.

ETIOLOGY AND PATHOPHYSIOLOGY OF PORTAL HYPERTENSION

With few exceptions, portal hypertension is initiated by increased vascular resistance within the portal venous system or liver. The elevated portal pressure is a stimulus to portal-systemic collateralization which develops wherever the splanchnic venous and systemic venous systems are in close apposition. Common pathways for collateral flow include the left and right gastric veins to the azygous vein (esophageal and gastric varices), umbilical vein to the epigastric veins (caput medusae), and superior hemorrhoidal vein to middle and inferior hemorrhoidal veins (hemorrhoids). Recent studies in experimental animals with portal hypertension secondary to either cirrhosis or portal vein ligation suggest that, when the collateral network is fully developed, vascular resistance returns to normal. Portal hypertension is then maintained by an increased inflow to the portal venous system.[3] Although the cause of the hyperdynamic splanchnic circulation is not known, in many cases it is associated with a hyperdynamic systemic circulation.

Despite the importance of increased portal flow in the pathogenesis of portal hypertension, etiologic classifications of portal hypertension have generally been based on the site of increased vascular resistance. The most common cause of prehepatic portal hypertension is portal vein thrombosis, which accounts for approximately 50% of portal hypertension cases in the pediatric population. Although neonatal omphalitis is occasionally the cause of portal vein thrombosis, in most cases the etiology is not known. Because hepatic vascular resistance is normal in patients with extrahepatic venous thrombosis, hepatopedal (to the liver) portal collaterals develop and maintain some portal blood flow to the liver. Typically, normal hepatic function is maintained, and these patients tolerate variceal hemorrhage well. An easily resolved variety of extrahepatic venous thrombosis is isolated splenic vein thrombosis, often secondary to chronic pancreatitis. Elevated pressures are confined to the gastrosplenic component of the splanchnic venous circulation and return to normal following surgical removal of the spleen.

Intrahepatic portal hypertension can be subclassified into presinusoidal, sinusoidal, and postsinusoidal types. However, this subclassification is an oversimplification as many liver diseases are associated with elevated resistance at more than one of these levels. Relatively pure presinusoidal portal hypertension is seen in schistosomiasis, sarcoidosis, congenital hepatic fibrosis, and arsenic toxicity. In all of these diseases, hepatocellular integrity remains intact, and liver function is generally well preserved.

Schistosomiasis is the most common cause of portal hypertension world-wide; however, in this country, cirrhosis is responsible for over 90% of cases of portal hypertension. All types of cirrhosis are caused by chronic hepatocellular necrosis and subsequent fibrosis and hepatic regeneration, resulting in distortion of the liver's architecture. In addition, collagen is deposited in the space of Disse, interfering with oxygen and nutrient exchange and leading to an elevated sinusoidal resistance. Alcohol is the responsible toxin in approximately 70% of cases. Alcoholic cirrhosis is characterized by elevated sinusoidal and postsinusoidal resistances, and most types of nonalcoholic cirrhosis such as chronic active hepatitis, cryptogenic cirrhosis, and primary biliary cirrhosis are also accompanied by an increased presinusoidal resistance. In approximately 5% of patients with cirrhosis, hepatic resistance becomes so elevated that portal venous blood no longer perfuses the liver, and a fraction of hepatic arterial flow drains via the portal vein (spontaneous reversal of portal flow).

Isolated postsinusoidal obstruction as a cause of portal hypertension is rare. Hepatic vein thrombosis (Budd-Chiari syndrome) occasionally develops in patients with a hypercoagulable state or idiopathically. When the thrombus involves all of the major hepatic veins, the only remaining outflow tracts for the liver are the small veins draining the caudate lobe and the portal vein. Hepatic congestion, which may eventually lead to hepatocellular failure, and intractable ascites result.

Finally, portal hypertension may occasionally develop secondary to enhanced portal blood flow alone. Both arterial venous fistulas in the splanchic vascular bed and massive splenomegaly have resulted in portal hypertension. Although increased flow probably initiates portal hypertension in these circumstances, liver biopsy usually reveals sclerosis of hepatic portal venules compatible with a secondary elevation of vascular resistance.

VARICEAL HEMORRHAGE

Variceal hemorrhage is the most life-threatening complication of portal hypertension. Reported mortality rates range from 22% to 84%[4] and are influenced by two main factors: hepatic functional reserve of the patient population under investigation and the time from onset of hemorrhage until patients are entered into the study. Since the greatest risk for mortality occurs immediately after the onset of hemorrhage, studies that do not consider this period report lower mortality than those that assess survival from the time of admission to the hospital.[5]

Only one third to one half of patients with portal hypertension and varices ever bleed from the varices. However, once bleeding occurs, the likelihood of a second episode of variceal hemorrhage exceeds 70%. The second episode of bleeding usually occurs within six weeks of the first, and the risk of recurrent hemorrhage diminishes thereafter.[5] There have been no reliable predictors as to which patients with varices will subsequently bleed. Therefore, prophylactic measures (before the first episode of hemorrhage has occurred) have had no beneficial impact on survival. However, it has recently been shown that patients with large varices are more likely to bleed than patients with small varices.[6] Both the size of varices and the risk of hemorrhage are independent of portal pressure.

The exact cause of variceal hemorrhage remains uncertain. Although gastroesophageal reflux would appear to be a possible factor, esophagitis is no more common in patients who bleed from varices than those who do not. It is more likely that intravariceal hydrostatic pressure leads to erosion of the overlying epithelium, resulting in hemorrhage.

Although varices may develop at any location within the gastrointestinal tract, the site of hemorrhage in over 90% of patients is within 2 cm of the gastroesophageal junction. This may be a particularly susceptible location for hemorrhage because the mucosal lining is often very thin (sometimes only one cell layer thick) at this anatomical site in patients with portal hypertension. Occasionally, variceal hemorrhage may occur in the esophagus or stomach at a site more remote from the gastroesophageal junction or even more rarely in the distal ileum, proximal colon, or rectosigmoid colon. Patients with an ileostomy and portal hypertension are particularly prone to hemorrhage from ileal varices. Likewise, dense adhesions between a segment of the GI tract and abdominal wall may provide a pathway for portal-systemic collateralization and a potential site for variceal hemorrhage.

DIAGNOSIS OF ACUTE VARICEAL HEMORRHAGE

The key to diagnosis of the acute variceal bleeder is upper GI endoscopy, either in the emergency department or soon after admission to the intensive care unit. Hemodynamic stabilization, a brief history and physical examination, initiation of essential laboratory tests, and gastric lavage should be done prior to endoscopy. A history of previously diagnosed chronic liver disease, alcoholism, or hepatitis make varices suspect as the cause of bleeding. Likewise, massive upper GI hemorrhage in a patient without abdominal pain is characteristic of variceal bleeding. Signs helpful in establishing a diagnosis of chronic liver disease include ascites, jaundice, asterixis, spider angiomas, palmar erythema, dilated abdominal wall veins, and splenomegaly.

Important laboratory tests include typing and cross-matching for at least four units of blood, hematocrit, platelet count, prothrombin time, partial thromboplastin time, electrolytes, BUN, and glucose. A complete chemistry profile, including conventional liver function tests, and serology for viral hepatitis can be obtained later.

Gastric lavage with a large bore nasogastric tube evacuates blood from the stomach ensuring accurate diagnostic endoscopy. It also determines whether the upper GI tract is the site of hemorrhage if the patient presents with melena or hematochezia rather than hematemesis and may contribute to cessation of hemorrhage in some patients. Although iced saline has traditionally been used as the lavage fluid, saline at room temperature is probably just as effective, if not more.

Although early studies suggested that lesions other than varices may be the cause of bleeding in as many as 50% of patients with varices and upper GI hemorrhage, more recent investigations indicate that patients with varices usually bleed from varices. In one study, varices were responsible for hemorrhage in 90% of patients.[7] The diagnosis of variceal hemorrhage can be established at the time of endoscopy by either observing a bleeding varix (approximately 30% of patients) or by detecting moderate to large-sized varices and no other lesions in a patient who has recently experienced a major upper GI hemorrhage (> 2 units), but who is not actively bleeding at the time of endoscopy.

Alcoholic cirrhotics are particularly prone to the other common causes of upper GI bleeding (duodenal ulcer, gastric ulcer, Mallory-Weiss tear, and erosive gastritis). The most frequently observed pathologic entity coexisiting with varices is gastritis. However, portal hypertension may be an important factor in the pathogenesis of gastritis, and portal decompression is sometimes the only effective treatment for controlling hemorrhage in these patients. In addition, the clinical course of patients with hemorrhagic gastritis and nonbleeding varices is similar to that of patients with bleeding varices and no gastritis.[8]

Although rarely indicated, a carefully performed barium swallow is also a sensitive means of detecting esophagogastric varices. The distinct disadvantage of this technique is that it does not determine whether the varices are the source of hemorrhage. Therefore, barium studies are never used in the acute situation. When the diagnosis is in doubt or other pathology is suspected, a barium study may be helpful prior to elective surgery.

ASSESSMENT OF PORTAL HEMODYNAMICS

Measurement of Portal Venous Pressure

The most common technique used to estimate portal venous pressure is measurement of hepatic venous wedge pressure, which closely correlates with portal vein pressure in patients with cirrhosis. Since the level of portal venous pressure does not predict which patients will bleed from varices, the only clinical usefulness of this measurement is in diagnosis. Patients with sinusoidal and postsinusoidal portal hypertension have an elevated hepatic venous wedge pressure while patients with presinusoidal portal hypertension have a normal pressure. Hepatic venous wedge pressure and free hepatic vein pressure are usually measured in two hepatic veins during hepatic angiography in the radiology suite. Corrected sinusoidal pressure is defined as hepatic venous wedge pressure minus free hepatic vein pressure and portal hypertension is defined as a pressure greater than 5 mm Hg. However, it is rare for variceal hemorrhage to occur when the corrected sinusoidal pressure is less than 12 mm Hg.[6] Prior to termination of the pressure studies, inferior vena caval pressure below the liver should also be measured to assess inferior vena caval hypertension (> 20 mm Hg) secondary to compression of the inferior vena cava by the caudate lobe. If this condition exists, an intra-abdominal portal-systemic shunting procedure is unlikely to be successful.

Portal pressure can also be directly measured by percutaneous transhepatic puncture of an intrahepatic portal venous radical, cannulation of the umbilical vein under local anesthesia, and splenoportography. These invasive methods of pressure measurement more accurately reflect portal pressure in some types of nonalcoholic cirrhosis and in all cases of presinusoidal portal hypertension.

Visualization of the Portal Venous System

Selective visceral angiography is the most frequently used method for opacification of the portal venous system and for qualitative estimation of hepatic portal perfusion.[9] Selective injections into superior mesenteric artery and splenic artery or celiac axis are followed by serial films well into the venous phase. Portal blood flow to the liver is estimated from the venous phase of the superior mesenteric angiogram and graded as follows: grade 1, normal hepatic portal perfusion; grade 2, intrahepatic portal venous radicles visualized; grade 3, portal vein only opacified; grade 4, portal vein not visualized (Fig 28–1).

Lack of portal vein opacification after superior mesenteric arterial injection is suggestive of either portal vein thrombosis or spontaneous reversal of portal flow. The latter diagnosis can usually be confirmed by observing portal venous opacifi-

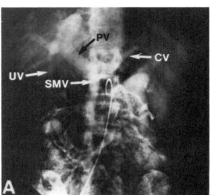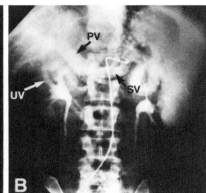

Fig 28–1.—Venous phases of selective superior mesenteric **(A)** and splenic **(B)** angiograms. The hepatic portal perfusion grade is 2. PV = portal vein; SMV = superior mesenteric vein; CV = coronary vein; UV = umbilical vein; SV = splenic vein.

cation during the venous phase of a selective hepatic arterial injection. The venous phase of the splenic arteriogram provides information about the size and position of the splenic vein and results in visualization of the coronary (left gastric) vein in approximately 70% of patients. When splenic collaterals such as an enlarged left gastroepiploic vein are opacified rather than the splenic vein, the likely diagnosis is splenic vein thrombosis, which may also cause variceal hemorrhage. When the left renal vein is to be used in the proposed surgical procedure, renal venography completes the angiographic study.

The portal venous system can also be visualized by the more invasive techniques of transhepatic portal venography, umbilical venography, and splenoportography. These techniques provide better splanchnic venous opacification, especially of collateral vessels, and a direct means of measuring portal venous pressure. However, these techniques are associated with a greater risk of complications than selective visceral angiography.

MANAGEMENT OF ACUTE VARICEAL HEMORRHAGE

Since most patients who present with acute variceal hemorrhage have cirrhosis and often one or more associated complications such as encephalopathy, ascites, coagulopathy, or malnutrition, they are at particularly high risk for emergency surgery. Therefore, initial management is directed toward nonoperative control of hemorrhage and overall metabolic support of the patient.

General Measures

Restoration of circulating blood volume and correction of coagulopathies are of prime importance. An isotonic crystalloid solution is rapidly infused through large-bore IV cannulas in both arms until blood is available. Blood pressure and urine output are carefully monitored by an arterial line and Foley catheter, respectively. If urine output is insufficient (<25 ml/hour) despite apparently adequate circulating volume, a Swan-Ganz pulmonary artery catheter should be inserted. If the prothrombin time is prolonged more than three seconds, fresh frozen plasma should be a component of the volume replacement. Platelet packs are administered only if the platelet count is persistently below 40,000–50,000/mm³.

If hypokalemic metabolic alkalosis is present, potassium chloride is infused IV until the situation is corrected. Alkalosis is deleterious for hypovolemic patients with chronic liver disease, because it causes a shift of the oxyhemoglobin curve to the left and facilitates transport of ammonia across the blood-brain barrier.

The combination of hypovolemia, with its adverse effects on hepatic metabolic function, and the presence of a large quantity of blood in the GI tract render cirrhotic patients who bleed from varices particularly susceptible to portal-systemic encephalopathy. In addition to restoration of adequate hepatic perfusion, blood should be removed from the GI tract by gastric lavage and administration of a cathartic through the nasogastric tube. If disorientation or asterixis develops, lactulose or neomycin should also be given.

When hemorrhage has been controlled, attention should be directed to restoration or maintenance of nutritional status. In most patients, only modest protein restriction (40–60 gm/day) is required. Salt intake should be limited to 1–2 gm/day to avoid development or worsening of ascites and edema. The recently introduced specialized nutritional solutions, which have a high concentration of branched-chain amino acids, have yet to be proved more efficacious than standard and much less expensive enteral and parenteral formulations.

Pharmacologic Therapy

Because they reduce splanchnic blood flow and thereby lower portal pressure, vasopressin, glypressin (an analogue of vasopressin), and somatostatin are all potentially effective in the management of acute variceal hemorrhage. Vasopressin is most commonly used and controls active variceal hemorrhage in approximately 50% of patients. In addition to its splanchnic vasoconstrictive properties, vasopressin adversely affects systemic hemodynamic parameters, including decreased cardiac output, increased blood pressure, bradycardia, and coronary vasoconstriction. Therefore, this drug should not be used in variceal bleeders with coronary artery disease. Simultaneous administration of nitroglycerin or nitroprusside may negate the adverse systemic hemodynamic effects of vasopressin infusion.

Vasopressin is most conveniently administered via a peripheral vein with an initial dose of 0.4 units/minute. Although selective superior mesenteric arterial infusion of vasopressin has been advocated, controlled trials have demonstrated that the peripheral IV route is just as effective, with fewer complications.[10] If vasopressin infusion at 0.4 units/

minute fails to control hemorrhage, the dose may be increased in 0.2 units/minute increments to a maximum of 1.0 units/minute. All patients receiving vasopressin should be carefully monitored in a critical care unit.

Although glypressin and somatostatin may be associated with fewer side effects than vasopressin, clinical experience with these alternatives has been limited. Whether or not they will be as or more effective than vasopressin has yet to be determined. Although propranolol has been used to prevent recurrent variceal hemorrhage following the acute bleeding episode, this drug has not been tested in patients with active variceal hemorrhage.

Balloon Tamponade

The most commonly used device for mechanical compression of bleeding esophagogastric varices is the Sengstaken-Blakemore tube (Fig 28–2). The advantages of balloon tamponade include rapid and sure control of hemorrhage in over 75% of patients and availability of the tube in most hospitals. However, use of the Sengstaken-Blakemore tube is controversial, because it has been associated with high morbidity and mortality in some centers, and because balloon deflation is followed by recurrence of variceal bleeding in 20%–50% of patients.[11] Lethal complications of balloon tamponade have included esophageal perforation secondary to intraesophageal inflation of the gastric balloon, ischemic necrosis of the esophagus due to prolonged overinflation of the esophageal balloon, upward migration of the esophageal balloon and subsequent asphyxiation after inadvertent deflation of the gastric balloon, and aspiration. These complications can be avoided by attaching a nasogastric tube to the Sengstaken-Blakemore tube above the esophageal balloon prior to insertion, by utilizing this device only in a critical care unit with personnel trained in its application, and by adhering to a strict protocol (Table 28–1). Because of the high frequency of recurrent bleeding following balloon deflation, more definitive therapy (surgery or endoscopic variceal sclerosis) should be planned for patients requiring balloon tamponade.

Percutaneous Transhepatic Embolization of Varices

Some interventional radiologists participate in the management of acute variceal bleeders by embolization of the coronary vein and short gastric veins after gaining entry to the portal venous system via a percutaneous, transhepatic approach. Although initial control of hemorrhage by this technique has been quite good (50%–85% of patients), rebleeding rates have been high (mean, 50%).[11] The only controlled trial comparing this technique to conventional medical therapy failed to show prolongation of survival following transhepatic embolization.[12] In addition, complications associated with this method have resulted in significant rates of morbidity and mortality in most series. Intra-abdominal hemorrhage, portal vein thrombosis, and failure to enter the portal vein are particularly frequent complications. Since portal vein thrombosis and obliteration of the short gastric veins limit future selection of portal-systemic shunt operations, all patients undergoing transhepatic embolization for acute control of variceal hemorrhage should have angiography prior to shunt surgery. In summary, percutaneous, transhepatic obliteration of varices has provided consistently good results in only a few centers that have radiologists who are experts in the application of this technique.

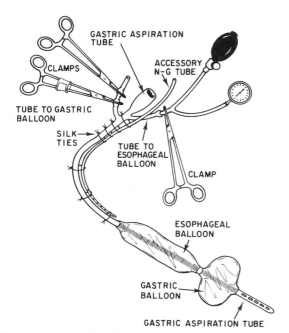

Fig 28–2.—Modified Sengstaken-Blakemore tube. An accessory nasogastric tube is attached for suctioning of secretions, which accumulate above the esophageal balloon.

TABLE 28–1.—PROTOCOL FOR USE OF THE MODIFIED SENGSTAKEN-BLAKEMORE TUBE*

A. Prior to insertion
  1. Always use new tube.
  2. Check balloons for leaks.
  3. Attach No. 18 salem sump tube above esophageal balloon.
  4. Evacuate stomach with Ewald tube.
  5. Insert through nose.
  6. Use ring forceps through mouth to facilitate passage if necessary.
B. After insertion
  1. Apply low, intermittent suction to stomach tube.
  2. Apply constant suction to salem sump.
  3. Inflate gastric balloon with 25-ml increments of air to 100 ml, observing the patient for pain.
  4. Snug gastric balloon to gastroesophageal junction and affix to nose, under slight tension, with soft rubber pad.
  5. Add 150 ml of air to gastric balloon.
  6. Place 2 clamps (1 taped closed) on tube to gastric balloon.
  7. Inflate esophageal balloon to 24–45 mm Hg, clamp, and check every 1 hour.
  8. Perform heavily penetrated upper abdomen-lower chest x-ray (portable) to confirm balloon positions.
  9. Determine serial hematocrits every 4–6 hours (gastric tube may occlude and fail to detect recurrent hemorrhage).
  10. Tape scissors to head of bed so tube can be transected and rapidly removed if patient develops respiratory distress.
  11. Deflate esophageal and gastric balloons after 24 hours.
  12. Remove tube in additional 24 hours if no recurrent hemorrhage.

*From Rikkers L.F.[4]

Endoscopic Variceal Sclerosis

Although first reported in 1939, endoscopic variceal sclerosis fell into disfavor after the introduction of portal-systemic shunt operations in the mid-1940s. Because of dissatisfaction with emergency surgical treatment of patients with acutely bleeding esophageal varices, a marked resurgence of interest in endoscopic sclerotherapy has occurred during the past decade.

Despite the greater than 100 recent publications regarding a variety of techniques of endoscopic sclerotherapy, no single method has emerged as superior.[11] A variety of endoscopes (rigid or flexible), anesthetics (local or general), methods of injection (intravariceal or paravariceal), sclerosants (sodium morrhuate, ethanolamine oleate, or sodium tetradecyl sulfate), and accessories (sheaths, balloons, or none) have been used. Although no controlled studies have compared the various techniques, most have reported temporary control of acutely bleeding esophageal varices in greater than 85% of patients. In contrast, sclerotherapy of bleeding gastric varices has been generally unsuccessful.

Complications directly attributable to endoscopic sclerotherapy have occurred in 2%–10% of patients in most reports.[11] Fever, retrosternal chest pain, and esophageal ulceration are common but relatively minor complications. Aspiration pneumonitis, worsening of variceal hemorrhage, and esophageal perforation are life-threatening complications, which are responsible for the 1%–3% of deaths reported in most sclerotherapy series.[11]

Because of no proved advantages for rigid esophagoscopy, which requires general anesthesia, accessories such as endoscopic sheaths and balloons, and the more difficult technique of paravariceal injection, most sclerotherapists in this country perform free hand intravariceal injections through flexible endoscopes in awake patients. The most frequently used sclerosants are sodium morrhuate (2.5%–5% solution) and sodium tetradecyl sulfate (0.5%–1.5% solution) often in combination with hypertonic dextrose (25%–70% solution). Higher concentrations of sclerosant have resulted in more frequent esophageal ulceration, stenosis, and perforation. Since effective sclerosis is difficult to achieve in the massively bleeding patient, temporary control of hemorrhage by vasopressin infusion or balloon tamponade should be achieved prior to sclerotherapy. If balloon tamponade is used or sclerosis must be done during fairly brisk bleeding, the airway should be controlled with a nasotracheal tube to prevent aspiration. Uncooperative patients may require paralysis with pancuronium bromide or general anesthesia. If the patient is unstable, only the bleeding varix is injected. In less emergent situations all varices are injected both at the gastroesophageal junction and 5 cm proximal to it. Fifteen to twenty milliliters of sclerosant is usually required for an initial treatment. A repeated sclerotherapy session is scheduled for two to four days following the initial one.

In the few controlled studies done thus far, endoscopic sclerotherapy has been superior to balloon tamponade[13] and inferior to emergency portacaval shunt[14] in controlling acute bleeding episodes. However, no short-term differences in survival have been detected in any of the trials.

Emergency Surgery

Orloff et al.[15] are among the few remaining advocates of routine emergency portal-systemic shunting for all patients with acute variceal hemorrhage. During the past two decades they have accumulated a series of 180 unselected, consecutive patients who have undergone emergency portacaval shunts for actively bleeding varices. This approach has resulted in an operative mortality of 42% and a five-year actuarial survival of 38%. Orloff and associates maintain that nonoperative methods for treating bleeding varices are generally ineffective and that, if emergency surgery is to be eventually required, the best time for intervention is soon after admission, before extensive blood loss and further deterioration of the patient's condition have occurred.

However, most portal hypertension surgeons selectively use emergency shunts for the minority of patients who fail conservative attempts at controlling variceal hemorrhage. This philosophy allows time for complete patient evaluation and improvement in hepatic function and nutritional status in most patients prior to surgical intervention. Since operative mortality rates are directly related to hepatic functional reserve at the time of surgery, this approach benefits the majority of patients who can be brought to elective surgery. Those patients (approximately 10%–20% of the total population) who fail all attempts at conservative management of the acute hemorrhage are generally higher operative risks when emergency surgery is eventually performed than they would have been immediately following admission. However, a policy of routine emergency surgery benefits only this small group to the detriment of the majority of patients, who can await elective surgery after improvement in hepatic functional status.

Nonshunt emergency operations directly obliterate varices or interrupt collateral venous pathways to the stomach and esophagus. The early prototype of these operations is transthoracic ligation of varices, which is associated with a high operative mortality, and, because recurrent bleeding is frequent in the late postoperative interval, a subsequent shunt operation is usually required. More recently, transection and reanastomosis of the distal esophagus with the EEA stapler through a gastrotomy incision, sometimes combined with ligation of the coronary vein, has gained popularity.[16] The major advantage of this procedure is the brief operating time required. Disadvantages are that the transection may be done above the variceal bleeding site, which is frequently at or just below the gastroesophageal junction, and that, even if initially successful, recurrent variceal hemorrhage is common in survivors. In addition, since endoscopic variceal sclerosis will be attempted in most institutions prior to an emergency surgical procedure, the stapled esophageal anastomosis may be more prone to leakage than usual.

Treatment Plan for Acute Variceal Hemorrhage

The simplest and safest initial treatment for the patient with actively bleeding esophagogastric varices is peripheral venous vasopression infusion (Fig 28–3). If hemorrhage persists despite increasing the dose of vasopressin, or is massive and requires immediate control to prevent shock, the most

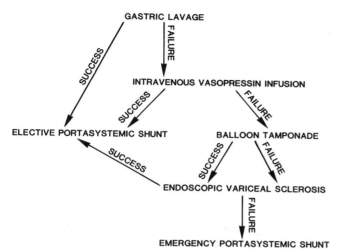

Fig 28–3.—Treatment algorithm for acute variceal hemorrhage. (From Rikkers L.F.: Portal hypertension, in Goldsmith H.S. [ed.]: *Practice of Surgery.* Philadelphia, Harper and Row, 1981, pp. 1–37.

reliable nonoperative measure is balloon tamponade. If bleeding is persistent but only mild or moderate, an acceptable alternative is endoscopic sclerotherapy without prior balloon tamponade.

Since recurrent hemorrhage is frequent following balloon deflation, further therapy should be planned for patients requiring the Sengstaken-Blakemore tube. If the patient is in a hospital without an experienced sclerotherapist or portal hypertension surgeon, the bleeding-free interval during balloon tamponade provides an opportunity for transfer of the patient to an institution with personnel experienced in the management of variceal hemorrhage. If hepatic function has recently deteriorated secondary to the bleeding episode or an alcoholic binge, endoscopic sclerotherapy should be done immediately after removal of the Sengstaken-Blakemore tube. Elective surgery should only be considered when hepatic function and nutritional status are optimal. Long-term definitive sclerotherapy is an alternative treatment, especially for patients who remain at high risk for surgery. If hepatic function is well preserved and there is no evidence of ongoing active liver disease, visceral angiography, followed by the most appropriate portal-systemic shunting procedure for that individual patient (see later section), should be completed while hemorrhage is controlled by balloon tamponade.

When variceal bleeding continues despite all nonoperative measures, emergency surgery without prior angiography is indicated. In this situation, the surgeon should select the operation with which he is most familiar and which he can perform most expeditiously and effectively. For most surgeons the end-to-side portocaval shunt best fits these criteria.

PREVENTION OF RECURRENT VARICEAL HEMORRHAGE

Since greater than 70% of patients who bleed from esophagogastric varices are destined to bleed again, the major objective of the long-term management of these patients

should be prevention of future bleeding episodes. If a portal-systemic shunt was done to treat the initial hemorrhage, this objective will already have been attained. However, in most centers emergency shunt operations are not routinely utilized, and cessation of hemorrhage is achieved by conservative measures. For these patients the options available for long-term control of variceal hemorrhage are propranolol, endoscopic sclerotherapy, portal-systemic shunt operations, and nonshunt operations.

Propranolol

Propranolol has recently been introduced by Lebrec and co-workers[17] as a simple, noninvasive means of preventing recurrent variceal hemorrhage. In a controlled trial of patients with alcoholic cirrhosis and either bleeding varices or hemorrhagic gastritis, propranolol administered in a dose sufficient to decrease the heart rate by 25% resulted in significant reduction of hepatic venous wedge pressure and frequency of recurrent hemorrhage. In addition, survival was prolonged in comparison to patients receiving placebo. However, these results should be interpreted considering that only good-risk patients were included, individuals with hemorrhagic gastritis and nonbleeding varices were also treated, and control patients were eliminated from survival analysis when they developed recurrent hemorrhage (inclusion of these patients negates the observed difference in survival). Although they also noted a significant decrease of hepatic venous wedge pressure secondary to propranolol treatment, Burroughs and coauthors[18] found that this drug did not prevent recurrent variceal hemorrhage or prolong survival in a controlled trial of unselected alcoholic and nonalcoholic cirrhotics who had experienced bleeding from esophageal varices. They concluded that the efficacy of propranolol in the long-term management of variceal hemorrhage has yet to be established and that its use for this purpose should be confined to carefully controlled trials. Studies comparing propranolol to medical treatment, endoscopic sclerotherapy, and portal-systemic shunt operations are presently in progress.

Endoscopic Variceal Sclerosis

After the reintroduction of endoscopic variceal sclerosis in the early 1970s, this technique was mainly used to control hemorrhage in patients who were not suitable candidates for shunt surgery because of advanced liver disease or diffuse splanchnic venous thrombosis and to control acute variceal hemorrhage prior to elective surgery.[19] However, as the method has gained popularity, it has increasingly been applied as a definitive, long-term treatment for prevention of recurrent bleeding in all categories of patients with esophageal variceal hemorrhage. Variceal sclerosis has not proved efficacious for patients who have bled from gastric varices.

Randomized controlled trials comparing endoscopic sclerotherapy to medical treatment have demonstrated that sclerotherapy repeated at intervals for three to six months decreases the frequency of recurrent hemorrhage.[20, 21] However, in these studies approximately 50% of patients rebled and, even though the majority of bleeding episodes occurred during the first year, the frequency of recurrent hemorrhage increased as the duration of follow-up lengthened. Although the bleeding episodes tend to be less severe than prior to sclerotherapy in some patients, others develop intractable hemorrhagic gastritis or bleeding gastric varices. The only remaining treatment options for these patients are surgical portal decompression or extensive devascularization of the proximal stomach and distal esophagus. Varices are completely eradicated in many of the long-term survivors, but sequential endoscopies are necessary because varices can recur and again cause life-threatening hemorrhage.

In one of the two trials comparing endoscopic sclerotherapy to conservative medical treatment, sclerotherapy resulted in significant prolongation of survival. However, this treatment modality needs to be compared in controlled trials to other long-term methods of preventing recurrent variceal hemorrhage, such as surgical portal decompression, nonshunt operations, and propranolol. In addition to frequency of recurrent bleeding and survival, other important factors including quality of survival, quantitative hepatic function, and cost need to be examined. Although some studies addressing these issues are presently in progress, results are not yet available.

Portal-Systemic Shunt Operations

All portal-systemic shunt procedures can be classified as either selective or nonselective, depending on whether they do or do not preserve portal blood flow to the liver (Figs 28–4 and 28–5). In addition to preserving hepatic portal perfusion, selective shunts maintain an elevated portal venous pressure, whereas nonselective shunts totally decompress the portal venous system. The advantages of preserving portal flow to the liver are that hepatotrophic hormones, such as insulin, are directly delivered to the liver following their secretion into the splanchnic venous effluent and that intestinally absorbed cerebral toxins are extracted and metabolized by the liver

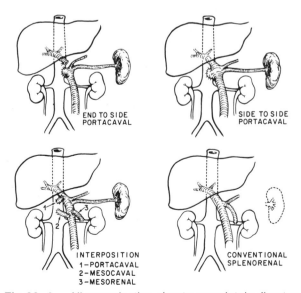

Fig 28–4.—All nonselective shunts completely divert portal blood flow away from the liver. Whereas the end-to-side portacaval shunt decompresses only the splanchnic venous system, the other procedures (side-to-side portal-systemic shunts) decompress the hepatic sinusoids as well.

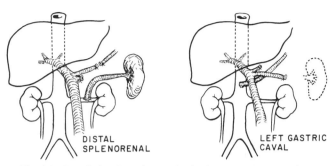

Fig 28–5.—Selective shunts both decompress esophago-gastric varices and maintain hepatic portal perfusion. The distal splenorenal shunt decompresses varices through the short gastric veins, spleen, and splenic vein to the left renal vein; the left gastric caval shunt directly decompresses varices via the coronary vein.

rather than entering the systemic circulation. Maintenance of intestinal venous hypertension may also be advantageous as there is evidence that total decompression of the hypertensive portal venous system results in enhanced absorption of passively absorbed substances such as ammonia, which may precipitate the syndrome of encephalopathy.[22] The distal splenorenal shunt and the left gastric-vena caval shunt are the only shunts, which consistently maintain hepatic portal perfusion and are, therefore, classified as selective shunts.

The nonselective shunt group can be divided into the following subgroups: (1) end-to-side portacaval shunt, (2) several varieties of side-to-side portal-systemic shunts which join splanchnic and systemic venous systems in a side-to-side fashion, and (3) end-to-side portacaval shunt with arterialization of the hepatic end of the divided portal vein. Each of these subgroups is hemodynamically distinct. Although all nonselective shunts decompress the entire splanchnic venous system, they have differing effects on intrahepatic hemodynamics. After an end-to-side portacaval shunt, the liver is entirely dependent on the hepatic artery for its blood supply. Depending on the hepatic vascular resistance, sinusoidal pressure may be decreased, remain the same, or be increased following this procedure.

Although the initial purpose of side-to-side portal-systemic shunts was to preserve portal blood flow to the liver, most evidence suggests that whenever a side-to-side portal-systemic anastomosis is of sufficient caliber to remain patent, portal flow is totally diverted from the liver. However, since the anastomosis remains in communication with the intrahepatic portal circulation, hepatic sinusoidal hypertension is relieved by these procedures. Because the liver is a major site of ascites formation, side-to-side portal-systemic shunts are effective in resolving intractable ascites as well as preventing recurrent variceal hemorrhage. In addition to patients with ascites and variceal hemorrhage, indications for side-to-side shunts are complete hepatic venous outflow obstruction (Budd-Chiari syndrome) and the occasional patient with advanced portal hypertension and spontaneous reversal of portal venous blood flow.

The objective of the end-to-side portacaval shunt with hepatic arterialization is to replace the lost portal venous component of hepatic flood flow with arterial blood. The hemodynamic consequence to the liver is that arterial rather than portal venous pressure is transmitted to the intrahepatic portal venous network.

Nonselective Shunts

END-TO-SIDE PORTACAVAL SHUNT.—Following its introduction into clinical practice in 1945, the end-to-side portacaval shunt was found to be the first consistently effective method for controlling variceal hemorrhage. In fact, recurrent hemorrhage was so infrequent following this procedure that its adverse side effects of encephalopathy and hepatic failure were largely ignored. Therefore, several large series were accumulated before the overall effectiveness of the end-to-side portacaval shunt was tested in appropriately designed trials.

Several randomized, controlled studies comparing the end-to-side portacaval shunt to medical management both for patients with varices and no prior hemorrhage (prophylactic) and for prevention of future bleeding episodes in patients who had previously experienced variceal hemorrhage (therapeutic) have been completed.[23] None of the prophylactic portacaval shunt trials have shown an advantage in survival for the surgically managed patients. Rather, only one third of the medically treated patients developed variceal hemorrhage and, though shunted patients did not bleed, they developed debilitating postoperative encephalopathy more frequently and died of hepatic failure more often.

The four controlled trials[24-27] comparing the therapeutic portacaval shunt to medical treatment are summarized in Table 28–2. Although all three American trials showed enhanced survival in the shunt group, in no single trial was the difference between treatment groups statistically significant. However, when the results of the VA Cooperative and BILG trials are combined, the shunted patients live significantly longer. Again, recurrent GI hemorrhage occurred infrequently in shunted patients, but was a common cause of morbidity and mortality in the medically treated groups. Although the frequency of encephalopathy was similar in shunted and medically treated patients in three of the studies, spontaneous, severe encephalopathy was mainly confined to the shunt groups. Encephalopathy in medically treated patients generally occurred only during recurrent variceal hemorrhage.

Although the results of these trials are often quoted to support both surgical and nonsurgical treatment of patients with bleeding esophageal varices, the limitations of the trials are seldom considered. Since the patient population consisted mainly of alcoholic cirrhotics and the only operation tested was the portacaval shunt, the results do not necessarily apply to patients with nonalcoholic liver disease and to newer shunt procedures, especially those that preserve hepatic portal perfusion. In addition, each trial contained a crossover bias in favor of the medically treated patients who underwent an end-to-side portacaval shunt when they developed intractable variceal hemorrhage. Despite these limitations, some cautious conclusions can be derived from the results of these studies: (1) end-to-side portacaval shunts effectively prevent variceal hemorrhage, (2) although not conclusively proved by these trials, end-to-side portacaval shunts probably prolong survival of alcoholic cirrhotics who bleed from varices, and (3) severe, spontaneous encephalopathy occurs more frequently in shunted than in medically treated patients.

SIDE-TO-SIDE PORTACAVAL SHUNT.—The side-to-side portacaval shunt was originally designed both to decompress varices and preserve hepatic portal perfusion. However, multiple studies have demonstrated that total portal diversion occurs following this procedure. In most patients who have had a side-to-side portacaval shunt, the hepatic limb of the portal vein functions as an outflow tract for the liver, and a fraction of the arterial perfusion of the liver is drained via the portal vein rather than the hepatic veins. Therefore, nutrient hepatic blood flow may be decreased to a greater degree following a side-to-side portacaval shunt or other similar side-to-side portasystemic shunts than after the end-to-side portacaval shunt. However, in the only controlled comparison of the two types of portacaval shunts, no differences were noted in either the survival rate or frequency of postoperative encephalopathy.[24] Because this procedure effectively decompresses the liver as well as the splanchnic venous system, it is more reliable than the end-to-side portacaval shunt for relief of intractable ascites in patients who bleed from esophageal varices. The major disadvantage of the procedure is that it is more difficult to construct than the end-to-side portacaval shunt. More extensive mobilization of the portal vein and inferior vena cava are required, and resection of an enlarged caudate lobe may be necessary to appose these two veins. Although the side-to-side portacaval shunt has been used in the past for cirrhotic patients with intractable ascites and no prior variceal hemorrhage, it is no longer indicated for this purpose. Rather, a peritoneovenous shunt is just as effective and is associated with considerably less morbidity and mortality than the side-to-side portacaval shunt.

TABLE 28–2.—RANDOMIZED STUDIES OF THE THERAPEUTIC PORTACAVAL SHUNT*

STUDY (FOLLOW-UP)		NO. OF CASES	SURVIVAL (%)	RECURRENCE OF BLEEDING (%)	ENCEPHALOPATHY (%)
VA Cooperative[24] (5-year follow-up)	Shunt	78	57	9	32
	Medical	77	36	65	43
BILG[23] (5-year follow-up)	Shunt	25	65	9	48
	Medical	25	48	70	52
USC[26] (12-year follow-up)	Shunt	45	24	0	35
	Medical	44	16	98	0
France[25] (3-year follow-up)	Shunt	40	47	8	40
	Medical	49	56	72	44

*From Rikkers L.F.[22]

INTERPOSITION SHUNTS.—Although either autogenous vein or synthetic grafts can be placed in the portacaval, mesocaval, mesorenal, and splenorenal positions, the most frequently utilized procedure has been the interposition mesocaval shunt using a large-bore (16–22 mm) Dacron graft. This operation was popularized by Drapanas and coauthors,[28] who reported a low surgical mortality, infrequent postoperative encephalopathy (11%), a five-year survival rate of 70%, and preservation of hepatic portal perfusion in 44% of patients. However, subsequent experience with this operation has not been nearly as encouraging. A controlled trial of the interposition mesocaval shunt vs. the side-to-side portacaval shunt failed to show any significant differences between these procedures with respect to survival or encephalopathy.[29] In addition, multiple investigators have found that large-bore interposition shunts completely divert portal flow and are hemodynamically indistinct from the side-to-side portacaval shunt. It is likely that the preservation of hepatic portal perfusion found by Drapanas et al. represented a misinterpretation of the postoperative angiographic studies.

When a side-to-side portal-systemic shunt is indicated, there are major advantages of the interposition procedures: they are technically easier to construct than a side-to-side portacaval shunt or conventional splenorenal shunt, and, if intractable postoperative encephalopathy ensues, they can be reversed by simple ligation. In the occasional patient with bleeding esophageal varices and dense adhesions in the upper abdomen, an interposition mesocaval shunt may be the only decompressive operation which can be safely achieved. When a side-to-side portacaval shunt cannot be done because an enlarged caudate lobe makes direct apposition of the portal vein and inferior vena cava impossible, an interposition portacaval shunt is preferable to excision of a large segment of liver. In addition to complete diversion of portal flow, synthetic interposition shunts have a high graft occlusion rate that approaches 50% at five years' follow-up.[30] Other potential disadvantages of synthetic grafts include compression of or erosion into the adjacent structures, such as the duodenum, and the development of graft infection. Thus far, these complications have been infrequent.

Recently, experience has been gained with small-diameter polytetrafluoroethylene grafts (10 mm) placed in the portacaval position. Early postoperative studies have suggested that hepatic portal perfusion may be preserved in approximately 40% of patients and that early shunt occlusion rates are surprisingly low.[31] Patients with preservation of hepatic portal perfusion have had infrequent postoperative encephalopathy. However, considering the experience with large-diameter interposition grafts, it is likely that shunt thrombosis and recurrent variceal hemorrhage will become significant problems when later postoperative evaluations are completed.

CONVENTIONAL SPLENORENAL SHUNT.—During the early years of portal hypertension surgery, the conventional splenorenal shunt was promoted by Linton et al.[32] as superior to the portacaval shunt for decompression of the portal venous system. Early noncontrolled studies of this procedure suggested that it was followed by a lower frequency of encephalopathy but a higher incidence of recurrent variceal hemorrhage than after the portacaval shunt. Subsequent studies utilizing postoperative angiography have suggested that these findings are due to a high thrombosis rate of the conventional splenorenal shunt. In most patients, shunt thrombosis occurs in the early postoperative interval, resulting in susceptibility to future variceal hemorrhage but preservation of hepatic portal perfusion and infrequent encephalopathy. Since the small proximal end of the splenic vein is used for shunt construction, it is not surprising that this shunt has a higher rate of thrombosis than the distal splenorenal shunt, which utilizes the larger distal end of the splenic vein. When a conventional splenorenal shunt of sufficient caliber to remain patent is constructed, it most likely eventually functions as a peripheral side-to-side portasystemic shunt and completely diverts the portal flow. More recent comparisons of the conventional splenorenal shunt and portacaval shunt have generally failed to show any clinical differences between these procedures.[33]

Since splenectomy is a component of the conventional splenorenal shunt procedure, one advantage of this operation is that it reliably relieves hypersplenism. However, clinically significant hypersplenism (platelet count consistently <30,000/mm³) rarely accompanies portal hypertension (three of 140 patients in the author's experience). Since severe hypersplenism is rare and splenic venous decompression after a shunt procedure generally results in an elevation of the platelet count, splenectomy is rarely indicated in this population of patients.

OTHER SIDE-TO-SIDE PORTAL-SYSTEMIC SHUNTS.—Several other infrequently used side-to-side portal-systemic shunts have been described. The portarenal and double-barrel portacaval shunts are nearly identical to the side-to-side portacaval shunt. The caval mesenteric shunt, which is constructed by anastomosis of the divided inferior vena cava to the side of the superior mesenteric vein, has mainly been used in pediatric portal hypertension. In general, the caval mesenteric shunt has provided better protection against future variceal hemorrhage than the conventional splenorenal shunt and makeshift shunts in children with extrahepatic portal hypertension.[34] Although postoperative hemodynamic studies have not been reported, it is likely that the caval mesenteric shunt functions as a completely diverting side-to-side portasystemic shunt. Because inferior vena caval interruption is often followed by severe leg edema in adults, this procedure has generally been confined to the pediatric population. Since the introduction of the interposition mesocaval shunt, the caval mesenteric shunt has been infrequently utilized.

END-TO-SIDE PORTACAVAL SHUNT WITH HEPATIC ARTERIALIZATION.—One means of maintaining total hepatic blood flow following an end-to-side portacaval shunt is arterialization of the hepatic stump of the portal vein. The arterial-portal vein fistula should be constructed with a small-caliber artery because the intrahepatic portal venous network poorly tolerates arterial pressure. Thus, the gastroepiploic artery, splenic artery, and a saphenous vein graft from the infrarenal aorta have all been used. The most carefully documented series of patients with portacaval shunt and hepatic arterialization was recently reported from Brussels.[35] The 62 patients undergoing this procedure were all carefully evaluated by intraoperative hemodynamic studies to determine if they had hepatopedal portal flow. After construction of an end-to-side portacaval shunt, an autogenous saphenous vein graft was interposed between the infrarenal aorta and the hepatic stump of the portal vein. Hepatic sinusoidal pressure was carefully monitored intraoperatively, and, if arterialization resulted in an increase in this pressure, the saphenous vein graft was banded. Utilizing this technique, measured pre- and post-shunt total hepatic blood flows were similar. Despite careful monitoring of sinusoidal pressure intraoperatively, six patients developed massive and intractable ascites in the early postoperative period and underwent a second operation for ligation or banding of the saphenous vein graft. Early postoperative angiograms showed graft patency in 84% of patients. The operation resulted in a five-year actuarial survival of 48% and a 20% incidence of chronic encephalopathy. The authors of this report correctly concluded that this operation cannot be meaningfully compared with end-to-side portacaval shunt without arterialization until a prospective controlled trial is completed. Such a trial is presently in progress in their institution. Theoretical objections to hepatic arterialization are that it does not restore portal hepatotrophic factors to the liver and that arterial pressure transmitted to the intrahepatic portal venous system may result in intractable ascites, hepatic necrosis, and accelerated hepatic failure.

Selective Portal-Systemic Shunts

DISTAL SPLENORENAL SHUNT.—The first method of selectively decompressing the gastrosplenic venous circuit was described by Warren and co-workers in 1967.[36] The distal splenorenal shunt procedure consists of anastomosis of the distal end of the splenic vein to the side of the left renal vein and disconnection of the superior mesenteric-portal venous component of the splanchnic venous system from the gastrosplenic component by interruption of the coronary vein, left gastroepiploic vein, and any other prominent collateral channels connecting these two venous beds. Portal-systemic collateralization is discouraged by ligation of the umbilical vein. Warren et al. originally listed three main objectives of this operation: (1) selective transsplenic decompression of esophagogastric varices, (2) preservation of hepatic portal perfusion, and (3) maintenance of portal venous hypertension.

During the early experience with this operation, candidates for the distal splenorenal shunt came from a group of patients with relatively good hepatic function, no preoperative ascites, evidence of hepatopedal portal blood flow on preoperative angiography, and an elective surgical setting. After experience with 348 patients who underwent the distal splenorenal shunt at Emory University, Warren et al. liberalized their criteria for this procedure.[30] They currently perform the distal splenorenal shunt in patients of all Child's classes, in the emergency setting, in patients with preoperative ascites, and in individuals with no evidence of hepatopedal portal flow on preoperative angiography. In fact, they state: "our sole indication for nonselective shunt is in the emergent situation where other non-surgical methods have failed or are not available."[30]

In this author's opinion, other than anatomical limitations (splenic vein <8 mm, prior splenectomy), the major contraindication to a distal splenorenal shunt is difficult-to-control as-

cites that develops prior to surgery. In contrast, the development of transient ascites during resuscitation from variceal hemorrhage is not a contraindication to this procedure. Intractable preoperative ascites is a good predictor of severe postoperative ascites, which may be a major cause of morbidity and even mortality following the distal splenorenal shunt.[37] Patients with minimal or absent hepatic portal perfusion on preoperative angiography, but without significant ascites, are reasonable candidates for the distal splenorenal shunt. Ligation of portal-systemic collaterals, an important component of the procedure, may restore hepatic portal perfusion in some of these patients. In addition, maintenance of intestinal venous hypertension, even in the absence of portal blood flow to the liver, may have a beneficial influence by inhibiting intestinal absorption of purported cerebral toxins, such as ammonia.[22]

Since the Warren group's original description, several investigators have modified the distal splenorenal shunt operation. Most modifications have consisted of less aggressive disconnection of the two components of the splanchnic venous system. However, failure to ligate the coronary vein and other collaterals converts the selective splenorenal shunt into a remote side-to-side portal-systemic shunt. Therefore, Warren et al. recently reemphasized the necessity for extensive devascularization, including ligation of the coronary vein at its junction with the portal vein as well as at the gastroesophageal junction, interruption of the umbilical vein as close to the liver as possible, obliteration of the full length of the gastroepiploic vein, and ligation of all other collaterals connecting the gastrosplenic and portal-superior mesenteric venous circuits.

Recently, Henderson and Warren[38] reviewed both the North American experience with the distal splenorenal shunt and the six randomized, controlled trials that have compared this procedure to nonselective shunts. Table 28–3 has been modified from their report by adding this author's own experience with the distal splenorenal shunt in Salt Lake City.[37] Operative mortality following the distal splenorenal shunt has been approximately 6%, with long-term survival ranging 50%–75%. These figures compare very favorably with any reported nonselective shunt experience. In addition, when the large Atlanta and Miami experiences with this operation are examined more closely, patients with nonalcoholic cirrhosis survive significantly longer than those with alcoholic cirrhosis. In all of the reports, frequency of postoperative encephalopathy has been less than 20%. Henderson and Warren[38] report that the frequency of ascites following the distal splenorenal shunt in their own series has been 56%. However, they also state that the majority of these patients can be managed by medical therapy alone and that peritoneovenous shunts have been necessary in only six patients. In the author's Salt Lake City experience, ascites severe enough to prolong significantly postoperative hospitalization developed in 28% of patients following the distal splenorenal shunt.[37] In addition, ascites was believed to be a major contributor to death in six patients. In the combined series, shunt patency rates have exceeded 90%, with recurrent hemorrhage developing in fewer than 7% of patients.

Table 28–4 summarizes the six controlled trials that have compared the distal splenorenal shunt with nonselective

TABLE 28–3.—The North American Experience with the Distal Splenorenal Shunt (Nonrandomized Studies)*

STUDY	NO. OF PATIENTS	ETIOLOGY		CHILD'S CLASS			OPERATIVE MORTALITY, No. (%)	SURVIVAL 3–5 yr. (%)	ENCEPHALOPATHY (%)
		Alcoholic	Non-alcoholic	A	B	C			
Atlanta	348	195	153	299	49		14(4)	58	4
Miami	91	52	39	Undefined			1(1)	57	—
Toronto	32	22	10	Undefined			5(16)	75	7
Los Angeles	17	6	11	7	7	3	2(12)	75	8
Columbus, Ohio	50	28	22	12	32	6	5(10)	70	10
Portland, Oregon	15	8	7	9	4	2	2(13)	75	20
Charlottesville	19	14	5	16	2	1	2(11)	—	—
Boston	22	22	0	Undefined			2(9)	47	15
St. Louis	15	12	3	7	7	1	1(7)	57	8
Salt Lake City	75	48	27	37	31	7	5(7)	45	12
Total	684	407	277				39(6)	50–75	≈10

*Modified from Henderson et al.[38]

shunts. Nonselective shunts utilized include the end-to-side portacaval shunt, the interposition shunt, and the conventional splenorenal shunt. In these trials, operative mortality and late mortality were similar in distal splenorenal and nonselective shunt populations. However, 83% of the patients entered into these studies had alcoholic cirrhosis. In consideration of the noncontrolled data of Warren et al.[30] and Zeppa et al.,[39] which showed better survival of nonalcoholic than alcoholic patients following the distal splenorenal shunt, it is possible that different survival results might be achieved if selective and nonselective shunts were compared in patients with nonalcoholic liver disease. With the exception of one of the six trials, encephalopathy occurred less frequently following the distal splenorenal shunt than after nonselective shunts. The overall incidence of encephalopathy after distal splenorenal and nonselective shunts was 14% and 36%, respectively.

A major controversy regarding the distal splenorenal shunt is whether this operation preserves hepatic portal perfusion in the late postoperative interval. Loss of portal blood flow to the liver in the early postoperative period is usually due to either complete portal vein thrombosis, which complicates the course of 5%–10% of patients, or failure to ligate major collaterals joining the portal-mesenteric and gastrosplenic components of the splanchnic venous circulation. However, even when these complications do not occur, progressive portal-systemic collateralization results in gradual diminution of hepatic portal perfusion in many patients. Patients with nonalcoholic cirrhosis are more likely than patients with alcoholic cirrhosis to maintain portal blood flow to the liver in the late postoperative period.[40] This may account for the significantly better long-term survival observed in some series for nonalcoholic cirrhotics.

Left gastric-vena caval shunt.—Experience with the left gastric-vena caval shunt has mainly been confined to

TABLE 28–4.—Results of the Six Prospective Randomized Studies Comparing Distal Splenorenal Shunt (DSRS) with Total Shunts*

SHUNT	POPULATION		OPERATIVE MORTALITY†	LATE MORTALITY‡	ENCEPHALOPATHY	SHUNT OCCLUSION
	Alcoholic	Non-alcoholic				
DSRS						
1	18	8	3/26	13/26	3/26	2/26
2	13	0	1/13	5/13	—	0/12
3	21	6	5/27	8/27	3/22	2/18
4	21	3	2/24	6/24	6/19	3/19
5	22	1	1/23	4/23	1/22	1/22
6	19	0	2/19	5/19	2/17	—
Total	114	18	14/132	41/132	15/103	8/97
Total shunt						
1	22	7	3/29	16/29	15/26	6/29
2	14	—	1/14	4/14	—	2/14
3	16	12	0/28	9/28	14/28	0/28
4	26	3	6/29	12/29	5/22	2/23
5	14	5	0/19	0/19	2/19	1/19
6	16	0	4/16	6/16	3/12	—
Total	108	27	14/135	47/135	39/107	11/113

*From Henderson et al.[38]
†In-hospital or 30-day mortality.
‡Wide variability between studies from 6 months to 10 years.

Japan. Selective decompression of esophagogastric varices is achieved by direct anastomosis of the coronary vein to the inferior vena cava or by interposing a graft between these two vessels. Inokuchi and associates[41] performed this procedure in 117 patients who had either nonalcoholic cirrhosis or noncirrhotic portal hypertension. Two thirds of these patients had previously bled from varices, and a prophylactic operation was done in the remaining third. Results have been excellent in this highly selected group of patients with a five-year survival rate of 78%, infrequent postoperative encephalopathy, and recurrent variceal hemorrhage in 10% of patients. The shunt has been patent in 90% of patients undergoing either postoperative angiography or autopsy. Although no large series of alcoholic cirrhotics undergoing this procedure has yet been reported, it may be technically more difficult in this population because the coronary vein is often of relatively small diameter and the retroperitoneum is frequently edematous and thickened.

Nonshunt Operations

The most effective nonshunt operations have been those in which the major objective has been extensive disconnection of the high pressure portal bed from esophagogastric varices. Procedures which attempt to decrease splanchnic inflow, such as splenic artery ligation and splenectomy, and operations which promote portal-systemic collateralization, such as subcutaneous transposition of the omentum or spleen, have generally been considerably less effective. The setting in which splenectomy alone reliably prevents future variceal hemorrhage is isolated splenic vein thrombosis without generalized portal hypertension. In such patients, high venous pressures are confined to the gastrosplenic component of the splanchnic circulation and removal of the spleen results in return of these pressures to normal. Splenic vein thrombosis is most frequently caused by chronic pancreatitis and can be diagnosed preoperatively if visceral angiography is a routine part of the work-up for patients who bleed from esophageal varices. The typical angiographic findings are nonvisualization of the splenic vein and the presence of a prominent left gastroepiploic venous collateral.

The nonshunt operation described by Sugiura and Futagawa[42] is the most extensive esophagogastric devascularization procedure that has been developed (Fig 28–6). The Sugiura procedure consists of splenectomy, proximal gastric devascularization, selective vagotomy, and pyloroplasty through an abdominal incision, and esophageal devascularization to the inferior pulmonary vein and esophageal transection and reanastomosis through a thoracotomy. The dissection is done close to the stomach and the esophageal wall so that the paraesophageal collateral pathways are maintained. Sugiura theorizes that maintenance of a paraesophageal collateral pathway prevents reformation of intraesophageal varices. The results of this operation in 276 patients with nonalcoholic liver disease have been excellent with an operative mortality of 4.3%, a seven-year survival of 83%, and recurrent variceal hemorrhage in less than 2% of patients.

A large series of Sugiura operations has yet to be reported in patients with alcoholic cirrhosis. However, esophagogastric devascularization procedures, as the one described by Johnson and co-workers,[43] have generally been complicated by

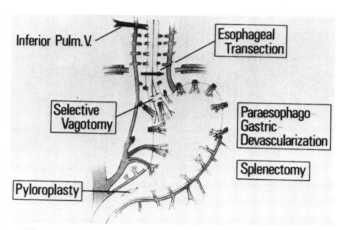

Fig 28–6.—Illustration of esophageal transection with paraesophagogastric devascularization (Sugiura procedure). (From Sugiura J., Futagawa S.: Further evaluation of the Sugiura procedure in the treatment of esophageal varices. *Arch. Surg.* 112:1317, 1977.)

frequent recurrent variceal hemorrhage in this patient population. The major differences of the Sugiura procedure from these earlier operations are preservation of the paraesophageal collateral pathways and transection of the esophagus. Whether these added features of the Sugiura procedure will make it more effective for control of recurrent variceal hemorrhage in American alcoholic cirrhotics remains to be proved. It is likely, however, that the combined thoracic and abdominal approaches will result in a high operative mortality in poor-risk patients. A less effective alternative for such patients is transabdominal esophageal transection and reanastomosis using the EEA stapling instrument together with ligation of the coronary vein.[16]

Selection of Therapy

Hemorrhage from esophagogastric varices is only one of many life-threatening complications that may develop in patients with chronic liver disease. Therefore, effective medical or surgical treatment of this isolated problem does not always result in prolongation of survival in large trials. Patients with alcoholic cirrhosis, who make up the highest percentage of most study groups, are particularly prone to relentless progression of their disease despite therapeutic intervention. Although survival of individuals with nonalcoholic cirrhosis and noncirrhotic portal hypertension may be influenced more favorably by the various treatment options for variceal hemorrhage, controlled trials confined to these disease categories have yet to be performed. Despite the conflicting and inconclusive data available, most authorities believe that active intervention of some type is indicated once an individual has bled from varices. Without treatment, the likelihood of recurrent hemorrhage approaches 100%, and the risk of death following each episode of bleeding ranges 20%–40%.

The only noninvasive therapy proposed has been propranolol. However, experience with this drug as treatment for variceal hemorrhage is limited, and available results are conflicting.[17, 18] Therefore, propranolol should only be used for patients who have been entered into controlled trials designed to determine its efficacy.

Although endoscopic sclerotherapy seems to be effective for acute control of variceal hemorrhage, its role in the long-term management of this problem has not yet been determined. Hopefully, ongoing trials comparing variceal sclerosis to surgical treatment will define patient subgroups for which one or the other of these therapies is more beneficial. For the present, it is reasonable to use chronic endoscopic sclerotherapy for patients who remain at high risk for surgery despite prolonged medical management and nutritional support.

Extensive experience has been gained with various surgical procedures for the long-term management of patients with variceal hemorrhage. Because patients with bleeding varices present with a wide spectrum of diseases, splanchnic hemodynamic alterations, and complications secondary to their underlying disease and portal hypertension, it is the belief of this author that no single operation is applicable to all situations. Rather, after careful preoperative evaluation, the operative procedure should be selected based on the specific clinical circumstances, the portal hemodynamic status, and the particular experience and skills of the surgeon involved. The surgical options include the end-to-side portacaval shunt, a side-to-side portal-systemic shunt, the selective distal splenorenal shunt, and one of the nonshunt operations. Since there has been minimal world-wide experience with the end-to-side portacaval shunt combined with hepatic arterialization and the left gastric-vena caval shunt, these procedures will not be discussed.

Two important clinical factors should influence selection of the operative approach: urgency of surgery, and the presence or absence of ascites. As previously mentioned, when surgical intervention is required during active, uncontrolled variceal hemorrhage, the two most important factors to consider are the reliability of the selected procedure for controlling acute hemorrhage and operative time. In this setting, the preference of this author is the end-to-side portacaval shunt, which can usually be performed expeditiously and is rarely complicated by recurrent hemorrhage in the early postoperative interval. If the surgeon is inexperienced, and all nonoperative treatments have failed, the only operative option not associated with an excessive mortality rate is transabdominal esophageal transection and reanastomosis with the EEA stapler and coronary vein ligation.[16] Since this procedure tends to be associated with a high frequency of recurrent hemorrhage in the late postoperative interval, a more definitive operation may be desirable when the patient has been stabilized. Contrarily, when the surgeon is experienced in management of these patients, and hemorrhage has been temporarily controlled by balloon tamponade, the distal splenorenal shunt is an effective emergency procedure, provided the patient meets the criteria for this operation.

Ascites frequently develops following fluid resuscitation from a major variceal hemorrhage. If the ascites responds to dietary salt restriction and/or diuretic therapy, the operation that would otherwise be appropriate for that patient should be selected. Ascites responsive to medical treatment should not be a deterrent to performing the distal splenorenal shunt. However, when ascites is intractable to prolonged medical management, a side-to-side portal-systemic shunt should be done, because it is the only procedure that relieves both hepatic sinusoidal and intestinal venous hypertension. It is debatable whether a direct vein-to-vein anastomosis is preferable to an interposition graft. Although the direct anastomosis is more likely to remain patent during the late postoperative interval, the interposition shunt is more easily reversed if severe encephalopathy develops.

Portal hemodynamic status, as judged from preoperative visceral angiography, is another important factor in shunt selection. When the venous phase of the superior mesenteric arterial injection shows hepatopedal portal flow, it is important to preserve this flow with distal splenorenal shunt unless the patient has a history of difficult to manage ascites. This procedure may also benefit patients with minimal or absent portal flow to the liver because it may restore hepatic portal perfusion and because it does maintain intestinal venous hypertension.[22] In our experience, approximately 65% of patients who bleed from varices are good candidates for the distal splenorenal shunt. If preoperative angiography reveals spontaneous reversal of portal blood flow, a distal splenorenal shunt may result in intractable postoperative ascites. Therefore, when this hemodynamic situation is present, a side-to-side portal-systemic shunt should be done.

When portal decompression is impossible because of diffuse splanchnic venous thrombosis, nonshunt operations and endoscopic sclerotherapy are the only therapeutic alternatives. Patients with variceal hemorrhage secondary to isolated portal vein thrombosis, however, are candidates for portal-systemic shunting procedures. Since these individuals usually have substantial hepatic portal perfusion through hepatopedal portal collaterals, a distal splenorenal shunt is preferred to a nonselective procedure. Other indications for a nonshunt operation are clinically significant hypersplenism (platelet count persistently less than 30,000/mm³ or leukocyte count less than 1,500/mm³) and patients with good hepatic portal perfusion but incompatible anatomy for a distal splenorenal shunt. Severe hypersplenism is uncommon in patients with cirrhosis and in this author's experience occurs in fewer than 2% of patients who bleed from esophageal varices. Patients who have undergone prior splenectomy or in whom the splenic vein is less than 7–8 mm in diameter are not candidates for a distal splenorenal shunt. If preoperative angiography reveals good hepatic portal perfusion, a nonshunt operation or endoscopic sclerotherapy may be preferable to a totally diverting shunt, which is frequently followed by encephalopathy.

Timing of Surgery

Since nonoperative methods successfully control acute variceal hemorrhage in 80% or more of patients, emergency surgery is infrequently required. An operation should be planned for an individual patient when risks of early postoperative morbidity and mortality are lowest. The two factors that have correlated best with early survival following shunt surgery are Child's classification and histologic activity of disease on liver biopsy. Child's classification consists of two biochemical indices, serum albumin and bilirubin, and three clinical parameters: ascites, encephalopathy, and nutrition. Several systems have been used to combine these parameters and grade individual patients as Child's A, B, or C.[4] In most series, operative mortality rates for A, B, and C risk patients are in the range of 0%–5%, 10%–15%, and greater than 25%, respectively. It has been demonstrated that Child's class can be considerably improved in many patients when an interval of medical management precedes surgery.[44] Although an individual may be admitted with decompensated cirrhosis secondary to hemorrhagic shock and/or recent alcoholism, it is often possible to improve hepatic functional status to Child's A or B when elective surgery is done weeks or months later. If the acute bleeding episode has had little impact on liver function, surgery can be scheduled as soon as the preoperative evaluation is complete.

Whether liver biopsy should routinely precede surgery is debatable. Although the degree of acute hyaline necrosis detectable on liver biopsy in patients with alcoholic liver disease has been a useful predictor of operative outcome in some series,[45] others[46] have found no correlation between liver histology and operative mortality rates. We currently obtain liver biopsies on patients with suspected alcoholic hepatitis or active chronic liver disease secondary to other causes, when coagulation parameters and ascites status permit.

ASCITES

Ascites frequently complicates portal hypertension, especially when the elevated vascular resistance is at the hepatic sinusoidal and/or postsinusoidal level. Ascites in patients with pure presinusoidal portal hypertension is much less common. Although the pathogenesis of ascites in portal hypertension is not completely understood, the most important factor seems to be altered hemodynamics in the hepatic and splanchnic circulations. Elevated hepatic sinusoidal pressure leads to transudation of protein-rich fluid into the liver's interstitium through porous sinusoidal endothelium. When the liver's capacity for transport of this excess fluid through the lymphatic system is exceeded, ascites results. A less important contributor to ascites formation is the splanchnic vascular bed. As ascites accumulates, circulating volume is depleted, and secondary mechanisms, such as aldosterone secretion and redistribution of blood flow within the kidney, are triggered to restore plasma volume. Subsequent expansion of plasma volume then results in further ascites formation.

The onset of ascites in patients with cirrhosis often portends a poor prognosis. In many patients the onset of ascites precedes hemorrhage from esophagogastric varices and ascites is necessary for the development of the life-threatening complication of spontaneous bacterial peritonitis. In addition, the hepatorenal syndrome, which is also associated with a high mortality rate, almost exclusively develops in patients with tense ascites.

Ascites can be effectively managed in 95% of patients by standard medical treatment. The most important elements of medical management are dietary salt restriction (20–30 mEq/day) and diuretic therapy. Water intake should also be restricted if hyponatremia is present. Because secondary hyperaldosteronism occurs in most patients with ascites, spironolactone is a rational first-line diuretic. The dose of spironolactone may be gradually increased within the range of 100–400 mg/day until a therapeutic effect is noted. Dietary salt restriction in combination with spironolactone therapy will re-

sult in an effective diuresis in approximately two thirds of patients. When salt restriction plus high doses of spironolactone fails to initiate a diuresis, either hydrochlorothiazide or furosemide should be added to the regimen. However, these diuretics are more frequently associated with electrolyte disturbances, azotemia, encephalopathy, and the hepatorenal syndrome; therefore, therapy should be carefully monitored including frequent estimations of serum electrolytes, BUN, and creatinine. Whatever drug therapy is used, weight loss should not exceed 2 lb/day, or prerenal azotemia may result from contraction of the intravascular volume.

The best surgical alternative for the fewer than 5% of patients with medically intractable ascites is the peritoneovenous shunt. Since LeVeen et al.[47] first popularized the peritoneovenous shunt in 1974, several devices have been marketed, but no studies have convincingly shown significant advantages of one over the others. All of these shunts function as a megalymphatic and return the ascitic fluid to the central venous system. The beneficial physiologic effects of the operation include increased cardiac output, renal blood flow, GFR, urinary volume and sodium excretion; and decreased plasma renin activity and plasma aldosterone concentration.

Although the peritoneovenous shunt results in resolution of ascites in many of the patients in whom it is used, no trial has yet shown that it prolongs survival. In addition, mortality and morbidity rates following this procedure are significant. One study reported a complication rate of 74% and an operative mortality of 24% following insertion of the peritoneovenous shunt for chronic intractable ascites.[48] Common complications include sepsis, shunt malfunction, and disseminated intravascular coagulation. This last complication is particularly likely to occur when the shunt is inserted in the early postoperative period following a portal-systemic shunt procedure. Because of the significant morbidity and mortality rates following this operation, it should be reserved for patients who are truly intractable to medical treatment of their ascites.

REFERENCES

1. Donovan A.J., Covey P.C.: Early history of the portacaval shunt in humans. *Surg. Gynecol. Obstet.* 147:423, 1978.
2. Warren W.D.: Presidential address: Reflections on the early development of portacaval shunts. *Ann. Surg.* 191:519, 1980.
3. Groszmann R.J., Atterbury C.E.: The pathophysiology of portal hypertension: A basis for classification. *Semin. Liver Dis.* 2:177, 1982.
4. Rikkers L.F.: Portal hypertension, in Goldsmith H.S. (ed.): *Practice of Surgery.* Philadelphia, Harper and Row, 1981, pp. 1–37.
5. Smith J.L., Graham D.Y.: Variceal hemorrhage: A critical evaluation of survival analysis. *Gastroenterology* 82:968, 1982.
6. Lebrec D., Defleury P., Rueff B., et al.: Portal hypertension, size of esophageal varices, and risk of gastrointestinal bleeding in alcoholic cirrhosis. *Gastroenterology* 79:1139, 1980.
7. Dave P., Romeu J., Messer J.: Upper gastrointestinal bleeding in patients with portal hypertension: A reappraisal. *J. Clin. Gastroenterol.* 5:113, 1983.
8. Sarfeh I.J., Tabok C., Eugene J., et al.: Clinical significance of erosive gastritis in patients with alcoholic liver disease and upper gastrointestinal hemorrhage. *Ann. Surg.* 194:149, 1981.
9. Nordlinger B.M., Nordlinger D.F., Fulenwider J.T., et al.: Angiography in portal hypertension: Clinical significance in surgery. *Am. J. Surg.* 139:132, 1980.
10. Chojkier M., Groszmann R.J., Atterbury C.E., et al.: A controlled comparison of continuous intraarterial and intravenous in-

fusions of vasopressin in hemorrhage from esophageal varices. *Gastroenterology* 77:540, 1979.

11. Joffe S.N.: Nonshunting procedures for control of variceal bleeding. *Semin. Liver Dis.* 3:235, 1983.
12. Smith-Laing G., Scott J., Long R.G., et al.: Role of percutaneous transhepatic obliteration of varices in the management of hemorrhage from gastroesophageal varices. *Gastroenterology* 80:1031, 1981.
13. Barsoum M.S., Bolous F.I., El-Rooby A.A., et al.: Tamponade and injection sclerotherapy in the management of bleeding oesophageal varices. *Br. J. Surg.* 69:76, 1982.
14. Cello J.P., Grendell J.H., Crass R.A., et al.: Randomized trial of endoscopic sclerotherapy vs. portacaval shunt in Child class C cirrhotics with massive variceal hemorrhage. *Gastroenterology* 86:1043, 1984.
15. Orloff M.J., Bell R.H. Jr., Hyde P.V., et al.: Long-term results of emergency portacaval shunt for bleeding esophageal varices in unselected patients with alcoholic cirrhosis. *Ann. Surg.* 192:325, 1980.
16. Wanamaker S.R., Cooperman M., Carey L.C.: Use of the EEA stapling instrument for control of bleeding esophageal varices. *Surgery* 94:620, 1983.
17. Lebrec D., Poynard T., Bernau J., et al.: A randomized controlled study of propranolol for prevention of recurrent gastrointestinal bleeding in patients with cirrhosis: A final report. *Hepatology* 4:355, 1984.
18. Burroughs A.K., Jenkins W.J., Sherlock S., et al.: Controlled trial of propranolol for the prevention of recurrent variceal hemorrhage in patients with cirrhosis. *N. Engl. J. Med.* 309:1539, 1983.
19. Johnston G.W., Rodgers H.W.: A review of 15 years' experience in the use of sclerotherapy in the control of acute haemorrhage from oesophageal varices. *Br. J. Surg.* 60:797, 1973.
20. MacDougall B.R.D., Westaby D., Theodossi A., et al.: Increased long-term survival in variceal haemorrhage using injection sclerotherapy: Results of a controlled trial. *Lancet* 1:124, 1982.
21. Terblanche J., Bornman P.C., Kahn D., et al.: Failure of repeated injection sclerotherapy to improve long-term survival after oesophageal variceal bleeding: A five-year prospective controlled clinical trial. *Lancet* 2:1328, 1983.
22. Rikkers L.F.: Portal hemodynamics, intestinal absorption, and postshunt encephalopathy. *Surgery* 94:126, 1983.
23. Rikkers L.F.: Operations for management of esophageal variceal hemorrhage (Medical Progress). *West. J. Med.* 136:107, 1982.
24. Resnick R.H., Iber F.L., Ishihara A.M., et al.: A controlled study of the therapeutic portacaval shunt. *Gastroenterology* 67:843, 1974.
25. Jackson F.C., Perrin E.B., Felix R., et al.: A clinical investigation of the portacaval shunt: V. Survival analysis of the therapeutic operation. *Ann. Surg.* 174:672, 1971.
26. Rueff B., Prandi D., Degos F., et al.: A controlled study of therapeutic portacaval shunt in alcoholic cirrhosis. *Lancet* 1:655, 1976.
27. Reynolds T.B., Donovan A.J., Mikkelsen W.P., et al.: Results of a 12-year randomized trial of portacaval shunt in patients with alcoholic liver disease and bleeding varices. *Gastroenterology* 80:1005, 1981.
28. Drapanas T., Lo Cicero J. III, Dowling J.B.: Hemodynamics of the interposition mesocaval shunt. *Ann. Surg.* 181:523, 1975.
29. Stipa S., Ziparo V., Anza' M., et al.: A randomized controlled trial of mesentericocaval shunt with autologous jugular vein. *Surg. Gynecol. Obstet.* 153:353, 1981.
30. Warren W.D., Millikan W.J. Jr., Henderson J.M., et al.: Ten years portal hypertensive surgery at Emory. *Ann. Surg.* 195:530, 1982.
31. Sarfeh I.J., Rypins E.B., Convoy R.M., et al.: Portacaval H-graft: Relationships of shunt diameter, portal flow patterns and encephalopathy. *Ann. Surg.* 197:422, 1983.
32. Linton R.R., Ellis D.S., Geary J.E.: Critical comparative analysis of early and late results of splenorenal and direct portacaval shunts performed in 169 patients with portal cirrhosis. *Ann. Surg.* 154:446, 1961.
33. Malt R.A., Szczerban J., Malt R.B.: Risks in therapeutic portacaval and splenorenal shunts. *Ann. Surg.* 184:279, 1976.
34. Voorhees A.B. Jr., Price J.B. Jr.: Extrahepatic portal hypertension: A retrospective analysis of 127 cases and associated clinical implications. *Arch. Surg.* 108:338, 1974.
35. Otte J.B., Reynaert M., De Hemptinne B., et al.: Arterialization of the portal vein in conjunction with a therapeutic portacaval shunt: Hemodynamic investigations and results in 75 patients. *Ann. Surg.* 196:656, 1982.
36. Warren W.D., Zeppa R., Fomon J.J.: Selective trans-splenic decompression of gastroesophageal varices by distal splenorenal shunt. *Ann. Surg.* 166:437, 1967.
37. Rikkers L.F., Soper N.J., Cormier R.A.: Selective operative approach for variceal hemorrhage. *Am. J. Surg.* 147:89, 1984.
38. Henderson J.M., Warren W.D.: Current status of the distal splenorenal shunt. *Semin. Liver Dis.* 3:251, 1983.
39. Zeppa R., Hensley G.T., Levi J.U., et al.: The comparative survival of alcoholics versus nonalcoholics after distal splenorenal shunt. *Ann. Surg.* 187:510, 1978.
40. Henderson J.M., Millikan W.J. Jr., Wright-Bacon L., et al.: Hemodynamic differences between alcoholic and nonalcoholic cirrhotics following distal splenorenal shunt—effect on survival? *Ann. Surg.* 198:325, 1983.
41. Inokuchi K., Kobayashi M., Ogawa Y., et al.: Results of left gastric vena caval shunt for esophageal varices: Analysis of one hundred clinical cases. *Surgery* 78:628, 1975.
42. Sugiura M., Futagawa S.: Further evaluation of the Sugiura procedure in the treatment of esophageal varices. *Arch. Surg.* 112:1317, 1977.
43. Johnson G., Dart C.H. Jr., Peters R.M., et al.: Hemodynamic changes with cirrhosis of the liver: Control of arteriovenous shunts during operation for esophageal varices. *Ann. Surg.* 163:692, 1966.
44. Holman J.M., Rikkers L.F.: Success of medical and surgical management of acute variceal hemorrhage. *Am. J. Surg.* 140:816, 1980.
45. Mikkelsen W.P.: Therapeutic portacaval shunt: Preliminary data on controlled trial and morbid effects of acute hyaline necrosis. *Arch. Surg.* 108:302, 1974.
46. Kanel G.C., Kaplan M.M., Zawacki J.K., et al.: Survival in patients with postnecrosis cirrhosis and Laennec's cirrhosis undergoing therapeutic portacaval shunt. *Gastroenterology* 73:769, 1977.
47. LeVeen H.H., Christoudias G., Ip M., et al.: Peritoneovenous shunting for ascites. *Ann. Surg.* 180:580, 1974.
48. Greig P.D., Langer B., Blendis L.M., et al.: Complications after peritoneovenous shunting for ascites. *Am. J. Surg.* 139:125, 1980.

29

Transplantation of the Liver*

BYERS W. SHAW, JR., M.D.
ROBERT D. GORDON, M.D.
SHUNZABURO IWATSUKI, M.D.
THOMAS E. STARZL, M.D.

INTRODUCTION

Within the past three to four years perhaps no other surgical endeavor has attracted more renewed attention, both from the lay and medical communities, than that of transplantation of solid organs. To discover the single most important cause for this sudden burst of interest, one need look no further than the introduction of the new immunosuppressant, cyclosporine. This claim in no way denies that many other important advances have been made in the field over the past 20–25 years. Several renal transplant centers were already obtaining outstanding graft and patient survival rates well before cyclosporine came along.[1, 2] No doubt judicious use of new knowledge regarding the value of tissue matching in the DR histocompatibility loci, and the discovery that deliberate blood transfusion protocols in kidney recipients could enhance graft survival, as well as careful management and selection of recipients all contributed to improvements in results. The assertion over the importance of cyclosporine also should do nothing to diminish the importance of certain other improvements, both technical and conceptual, made in the fields of heart, heart-lung, liver, and pancreas transplantation, where several groups continued to struggle for the kind of advances without which cyclosporine would have had a lesser impact.[3–5]

The importance of the arrival on the scene of a new, more effective immunosuppressive agent cannot be properly interpreted without an understanding of the larger history of the field of transplantation. This will become particularly evident in the early part of this chapter on hepatic transplantation. That cyclosporine is far from a "magic bullet" for the prevention of rejection will also become evident as we discuss the various difficulties and shortcomings encountered with its use.

The recent literature is replete with articles about liver transplantation, many of which can serve as comprehensive reviews of the subject.[6–9] In addition, virtually every major textbook of surgery or transplantation written within the past ten years contains a chapter or section concerning hepatic transplantation. The major purpose of the present chapter, then, is to serve not just as a general review of the subject, but also to share with the interested reader some of the issues currently facing physicians who are actively involved in offering liver transplantation as an effective approach to the treatment of a large variety of disorders of the liver.

COSTS AND BENEFITS OF THERAPY

Assessing the various costs involved in providing a form of therapy can be a formidable job. Furthermore, any form of therapy with which those costs run high naturally raises concern over whether the benefits accrued justify the costs. On the other hand, these questions are seldom posed by those physicians who may have devoted a lifetime toward developing and refining the particular therapeutic modality under scrutiny. Until recently, transplantation of the liver was such a rarely performed procedure, being done in the United States on a continual basis at only one center and at an average rate of fewer than 20 cases annually, that these issues seldom attracted much attention outside the relatively small brotherhood of health care personnel intimately involved with these procedures. But the improvement in results attending the introduction of cyclosporine in late 1979 and early 1980, as will be further emphasized throughout this chapter, stimulated such a renewal of interest in the procedure that major medical centers throughout the country, prodded by the professional and lay communities alike, began to look into the various cost-benefit ratios of providing liver transplantation as a service.

By the time the first symptoms of the national liver transplant fever had become undeniable in late 1982, the key question repetitively raising its head was "Who pays?" Although several major health insurance companies had decided in favor of covering the steep costs of the procedures for their policyholders, a far greater number denied any such obligations by maintaining that the procedure was still experimental. The various state welfare agencies were equally disparate in answering the question of payment.

In an effort to address some of these issues as well as oth-

*Supported by Research Grants from the Veterans Administration and Project Grant No. AM-29961 from the National Institutes of Health, Bethesda, Maryland.

ers, the National Institutes of Health convened a consensus conference in Washington, D.C., during June of 1983. The various opinions, facts, and data presented by the wide-ranging group of specialists invited to speak at the conference, as well as a consensus statement, have been published.[10] When interpreting some of this information, one must keep in mind both the speculative as well as the ephemeral quality of its accuracy. Nevertheless, the most important single conclusion of the conference was quite simply that liver transplantation is a viable therapeutic modality for a variety of disorders. Although one express intention of the conference was to steer clear of any opinions about who should pay, or for that matter how much should be paid or to how many or which centers, the official statement quite clearly removes the label "experimental" from hepatic transplantation therapy.

Formal debate of the question of payment is beyond the scope of this chapter. No doubt in the years to come, as liver transplant services begin to sprout in medical centers around the world, the issues involved will become more popular topics for discussion in a wide variety of venues (Fig 29–1).

Accurate information is available, however, regarding some of the costs involved with the procedure. These are illustrated in Table 29–1 for 31 adult patients selected at random from 1984 and for the total 55 pediatric patients transplanted during the 1983–84 fiscal year in Pittsburgh. The mean costs for all patients have a tremendous standard deviation because of the wide range of costs. The median figures give a more realistic accounting of "average" costs. Costs were lower for children overall than for adults. The median cost for all patients ($75,691) is virtually identical to the median costs for all children ($75,927) and for all adults ($75,691). The lowest costs were for pediatric patients who only required one graft,

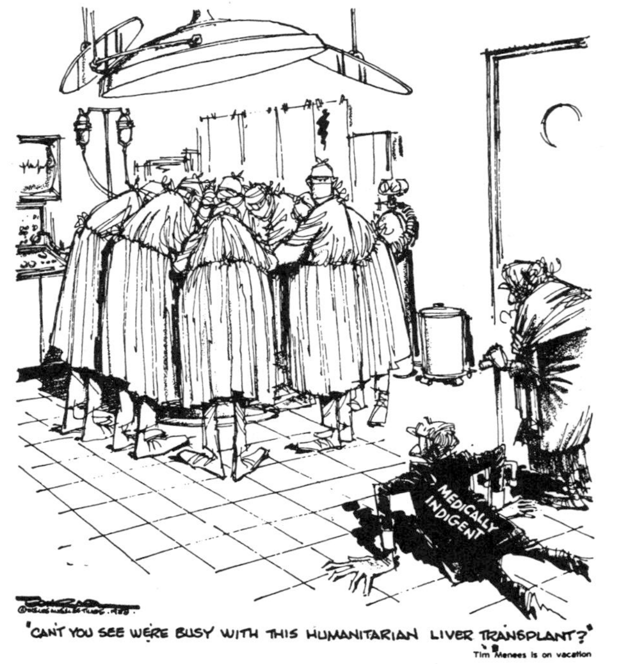

and highest for those 11 children who needed two or more livers.

One must keep in mind that these figures are being generated by a surgical service that, though the most experienced in the world, is constantly pushing the acceptable limits of patient candidacy for the procedure. If the number of high-risk patients could be minimized, either by earlier consideration for transplantation or by designation into other tracts of therapy, these costs could no doubt be lowered significantly. More will be said about the question of candidacy later in this chapter.

Attempting to compare these costs with alternative methods of care is, in most cases, a moot point, since no such alternatives exist. In these instances one must compare the costs of liver transplantation with the costs of death. Although the analysis begins to stretch beyond the intended scope of this chapter, a look at the numbers in terms of how many patients survived the treatment and how many are restored to a productive life is worth accounting.

Table 29–2 shows that in the precyclosporine era, of the 25 patients surviving five years or more and still living, 20 are employed full time, attending school, or involved in managing households. Although cyclosporine therapy has not been available for more than four years, Table 29–2 also shows similar information about 81 adult patients surviving six months or more after transplantation under the new drug. Of the 7 patients in the cyclosporine era who are disabled, 4 require recurring hospitalization for continued physical rehabilitation and 2 for adjuvant tumor therapy. Virtually all children are either back in school or otherwise doing well.[11]

HISTORICAL PERSPECTIVE

The transplantation of vascularized, solid organs was a logical extension of the development of the techniques for vascular anastomoses. Carrel[12] has been credited with showing that blood vessels could be sewn together with a reasonable expectation that blood would continue to flow through them for extended periods of time. Ullman in 1902 demonstrated that the removal of a kidney from one animal and revascularization in another was a technical feasibility.[13] Other early experiments revealed that autotransplants could be done successfully, but that even by using the same surgical techniques, allotransplants failed. This led Carrel in 1910[14] to claim that "the physiologic disturbance could not be considered as brought about by surgical factors. The changes undergone by the organ would be due to the influence of the host, that is the biological factors." Thus, with these technical successes, Carrel also demonstrated an observance if not an understanding of the phenomenon of tissue rejection. The early history of organ transplantation can be broken down into that dealing with advances in surgical methodology and that involving developments in immunology.

Early Experimental Techniques

The early work with *heterotopic* liver transplantation in dogs, reported first by Welch[15] and subsequently by others[16–18] was done without immunosuppression. These organs were destroyed after several days, apparently as a result of rejec-

"CAN'T YOU SEE WE'RE BUSY WITH THIS HUMANITARIAN LIVER TRANSPLANT?"
Tim Menees is on vacation

Fig 29–1.—By permission of the Los Angeles Times Syndicate, 1983.

TABLE 29–1.—TOTAL HOSPITAL COSTS ($), FISCAL 1983–84*

	ADULTS, ALL (n = 31)	CHILDREN, 1 GRAFT (n = 44)	CHILDREN, MULTIPLE (n = 11)	ALL CHILDREN (n = 55)	ALL PATIENTS (n = 86)
Mean	$111,062	$ 83,459	$196,998	$106,167	$107,931
SD	$ 91,213	$ 60,006	$ 97,321	$ 82,689	$ 85,891
Median	$ 75,691	$ 69,659	$164,762	$ 75,927	$ 75,691
Range	$ 45,339–$477,766	$ 30,937–$430,956	$ 93,209–$391,753		

*Costs include 31 adults and 55 children undergoing liver transplantation in Pittsburgh.

tion. Nevertheless, the observation that they produced bile, at least for an initial period, and appeared normal in color and texture was encouraging.

But the real test for the methodology for removal of a liver from one animal and revascularization into another took place when, in the late 1950s, Moore et al.[19] at Peter Bent Brigham Hospital and Starzl et al.,[20] then at Northwestern University (Evanston, Il.), developed their techniques for *orthotopic* transplantation in dogs. Survival following *orthotopic* replacement of an unpaired, vital organ requires, by definition, that a certain high level of organ function be obtained. In these early experiments on unmodified canine recipients, the death rate was exorbitantly high. Despite these discouraging results, Starzl and associates persisted in their efforts to improve the surgical technique, the methods of organ preservation, and the management of anesthesia. By 1965, they could report that 22 of 23 unmodified dogs survived at least two days following surgery, with 19 surviving at least six days. These animals served as one of the control groups in a series of elegant experiments which were presented in a landmark paper at the 26th annual meeting of the Society of University Surgeons in 1965.[21]

These studies demonstrated not only the course and nature of rejection of liver grafts in dogs, but also proved that, just as with renal allografts, rejection could be modified successfully with immunosuppression. In the same paper, Starzl and co-workers only casually mentioned the improvements in techniques responsible for the virtual elimination of perioperative mortality in these animals, an accomplishment which they modestly attributed to having gained "considerable experience." The paper belies the kind of herculean effort required from Starzl and colleagues to develop a whole new technology, perhaps the most complex and demanding in the field of surgery, technology that was necessary simply to get animals to survive long enough to approach the next great hurdle, that of tissue rejection. Without belaboring the point

TABLE 29–2.—REHABILITATION FOLLOWING LIVER TRANSPLANTATION

	PRECYCLOSPORINE THERAPY	CYCLOSPORINE THERAPY
Working	4	34
Housewife	6	34
School	10	4
Lost job, but able	5	2
Disabled	0	7
Total	25	81

suffice it to say that what the Starzl group describes as "gaining considerable experience" was responsible for their developing most of the techniques used today in the clinical transplantation of the liver. This will become more evident as we enter the discussion of operative techniques.

Early Experimental Immunology

The early observation that unmodified canine liver recipients would eventually succumb to rejection of their livers in a way not dissimilar to that seen with renal allografts was less surprising than the observation that sometimes the liver grafts failed to obey these so-called normal rules. Starzl et al. reported occasional long-term survival in unmodified dogs in 1961.[22] Later, Garnier et al.[23] observed even greater acceptance of liver grafts in unmodified pigs. These results were in contrast to those seen with random skin or kidney grafts, both of which were promptly rejected in all unmodified dogs or pigs. In 1969, Calne et al.[24] went on to show that unmodified pigs who failed to reject their liver allografts were subsequently rendered hyporeactive to skin or kidney grafts from the same donor. Although a similar immunosuppressive effect of liver grafts were not found in dogs by Starzl et al.,[21] or in primates by Myburgh et al.,[25] Zimmermann et al.[26] demonstrated an identical phenomenon in rats.

Early theories proposed to explain the apparent "privileged status" of liver grafts as well as the immunosuppressive effects in some animals were largely speculative.[3] One thought was that since the liver is such a large organ, the large antigenic mass simply overwhelmed the immune system of the recipient. Another theory was that since the liver comprises a large part of the reticuloendothelial system, a grafted organ replaced a large part of the machinery necessary for the organism to mount an immune response. A third proposal held that the transplanted liver released soluble factors into the serum which helped to block its own rejection.

Subsequent work with the rat model by the group at Cambridge has resulted in an increased understanding of the possible mechanisms for this so-called privileged status.[27] These authors conclude that the fate of liver grafts is primarily determined by immune response genes of the recipient. Accordingly, so-called high responders reject livers as readily as they do other organ grafts, whereas low responders not only fail to reject livers, but also appear to develop profound systemic tolerance to donor specific antigens. They have shown that this specific tolerance is accompanied by deletion of specific clones of cells normally responsible for reaction to the specific donor antigens, while those clones responsive to other antigens are retained. In addition, they found powerful and specific immunosuppressive molecules in the sera of liver grafted rats. They have found no evidence for the development of populations of either donor specific or nonspecific suppressor cells in these tolerant rats.

The direct impact of these studies on clinical liver transplantation is undetermined since, as yet, no similar mechanisms have been delineated in humans. On the other hand, working with the canine model, Starzl and colleagues were eventually able to obtain prolonged survival using immunosuppression with azathioprine[3, 21, 28] and antilymphocyte serum or its globulin derivative (ALG).[3, 29–32] These early successes using immunosuppressive agents to treat rejection of the liver in animals, combined with the massive experience accumulated with the operative technique led to the first human trials of hepatic transplantation.

Early Clinical Trials

On March 1, 1963, Starzl and associates[33] performed the first transplantation of the liver in a human. But that winter day in Denver is more important to the field as the day on which the Starzl team finally broke the ice than as the date on which liver transplantation became a clinical reality. This first attempt was the logical next step in the progression of the intensive research efforts started in the Denver and Boston dog laboratories over four years earlier. Nevertheless, the first patient, a 3-year-old boy with biliary atresia, died of uncontrollable hemorrhage on the operating table. Over the next ten months, four more attempts in Denver and one each in Boston and Paris were also unsuccessful (Table 29–3), halting further clinical trials for three more years. Starzl's sixth attempt in November 1966 and seventh in May 1967 also failed to provide prolonged survival. The first patient to obtain extended survival was a 1½ year-old girl who had transplantation on July 23, 1967, as treatment of primary hepatocellular carcinoma. She died 13 months later of diffuse metastases.

In May 1968 in the United Kingdom, Calne of the University Hospital at Cambridge and Williams of King's College in London embarked upon their series which, together with the Denver series of Starzl, account for the overwhelming majority of cases performed in the world during the subsequent decade. During that interval, however, single cases or small series of liver transplants in humans were also reported from Boston,[34, 35] Los Angeles,[36] Montreal,[37] Bonn,[38, 39] San

Paulo,[40] Calgary,[41] New York City,[42] Richmond,[43] Minneapolis,[44] Manchester,[45] and Oslo.[46] The importance of these early trials and the experience that they generated with the use of a variety of regimens of immunosuppression, originally developed for treatment of kidney recipients (Table 29–4), cannot be overestimated.

Yet by the end of 1978, little progress had been made toward significantly improving survival following hepatic transplantation. The best patient survival reported during this decade was a 50% one-year rate reported by Starzl for his so-called series II patients, a group of 30 patients who had transplantation between 1976 and 1978. However, the subsequent 26 patients were the subject of a paper entitled "Decline in Survival Following Liver Transplantation," published in 1980.[47] Of these 26 cases, only six (23%) survived beyond the first year following transplantation (Fig 29–2). Of particular note, most of the techniques of the operative procedure, of anesthesia management and postoperative care, as well as those of organ preservation, had been developed to a point where rejection or over immunosuppression in an attempt to control it were the major causes of death in a majority of patients during that era. Clearly the field lay open and fertile for the introduction of a new, more potent, and it was hoped, more specific immunosuppressant.

The Beginning of the Cyclosporine Era

An editorial in the July 11, 1981, issue of the *British Medical Journal* declared: "Liver transplantation has come of age: It gives a chance of excellent rehabilitation for patients with no other treatment available and the operation is probably less costly than prolonged care of a patient dying of liver disease in the hospital." The journal was responding to the reports from both Denver and Cambridge of marked improvements in survival of liver recipients following the introduction of the then new immunosuppressive agent, cyclosporin A.[48–52] In particular, Starzl's initial report of 71% one-year survival was startling and compared quite notably with previous results (Fig 29–3).

The ultimate impact upon the whole field of liver transplantation of these early reports has been a rebirth of enthusiasm for the procedure of epidemic proportions. At the end of 1980, after 17 years of clinical transplantation of the liver, the total number of cases performed in the world was probably fewer than 350. Most of these had been done at two centers

TABLE 29–3.—THE FIRST TRIALS OF ORTHOTOPIC LIVER TRANSPLANTATION

NO.	LOCATION	AGE/DISEASE	SURVIVAL DAYS	MAIN CAUSE OF DEATH
1	Denver	3/Extrahepatic biliary atresia	0	Hemorrhage
2	Denver	48/Hepatocellular cancer, cirrhosis	22	Pulmonary emboli, sepsis
3	Denver	68/Duct cell carcinoma	7½	Sepsis, pulmonary emboli, GI bleeding
4	Denver	52/Hepatocellular cancer, cirrhosis	6½	Pulmonary emboli, hepatic failure, pulmonary edema
5	Boston	58/Metastatic colon carcinoma	11	Pneumonitis, liver abscesses, hepatic failure
6	Denver	29/Hepatocellular cancer, cirrhosis	23	Sepsis, bile peritonitis, hepatic failure
7	Paris	75/Metastatic colon carcinoma	0	Hemorrhage
8	Denver	29/Hepatocellular cancer	7	Hepatic failure, sepsis
9	Denver	1/Biliary atresia	10	Hepatic failure, sepsis
10	Denver	1½/Hepatocellular cancer	400	Carcinomatosis

TABLE 29–4.—CLINICAL IMMUNOSUPPRESSIVE DRUG REGIMENS DEVELOPED
WITH KIDNEY TRANSPLANTATION

AGENTS	YEAR DESCRIBED AND REPORTED	PLACE	USED FOR LIVER TRANSPLANTATION
Azathioprine	1962	Boston	No
Azathioprine-steroids	1963	Denver, Boston, Richmond, Edinburgh	Yes
Thoracic duct drainage as adjunct	1963	Stockholm	Yes
ALG as adjunct	1966	Denver	Yes
Cyclophosphamide substitute for azathioprine	1970	Denver	Yes
Total lymphoid irradiation	1979	Palo Alto, Minneapolis	No
Cyclosporin-A alone	1978–79	Cambridge	Yes
Cyclosporin-A-steroids	1980	Denver	Yes
Azathioprine-steroids-adjuvant OKT*3	1981	Boston	No
Cyclosporine-steroids-adjuvant OKT*3	1984	Pittsburgh	Yes

(Denver and Cambridge), with steadily increasing involvement by two other institutions (Hanover[53] and Gronigen[54]). In four years following the introduction of cyclosporine, the world total will soon exceed 800 cases, and the number of centers around the world planning active involvement in the field is expanding on a weekly basis. Figure 29–4 shows the location of institutions participating in the middle of 1984, along with the number of cases at each center up to that time. The annual rate of cases in Pittsburgh has swollen stepwise from 30 in 1981 to over 175 in 1984. The coming years will no doubt witness the emergence of other centers able to take an active role and share the burden of providing liver transplantation to the increasing population of potential recipients.

THE LIVER DONOR

Several surveys have revealed that approximately 1%–1.5% of all in hospital deaths that occur annually in the United States are the result of irreversible brain damage.[55–58] Thus, the potential pool of donors has been estimated to be between 10,000 and 20,000 annually. Yet fewer than 3,000 donors per year provide organs for transplantation. The criteria which define a satisfactory kidney donor have become fairly standardized.[59] For the most part, many of these kidney donors would also be satisfactory donors for livers as well as hearts, pancreases, and other extrarenal organs. Yet probably fewer than 25% of kidney donors are actually utilized as extrarenal organ donors. The reasons for this under utilization of organ donors has been related largely to the lack of knowledge in both the medical and nonmedical communities about the tremendous increase in demand for extrarenal organs following the improvement in results with these transplants which attended the introduction of cyclosporine. The demand for donor livers at the end of 1984 remained concentrated in only a few centers across the country, with the University of Pittsburgh program continuing to utilize the vast majority of available organs. The high volume of liver transplant operations performed at Pittsburgh has been dependent on the referral of donors to Pittsburgh by a large number of other medical centers all across the country, most of which are not involved,

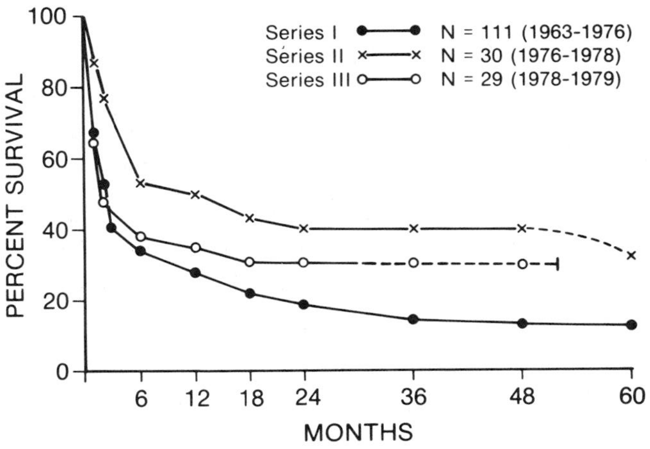

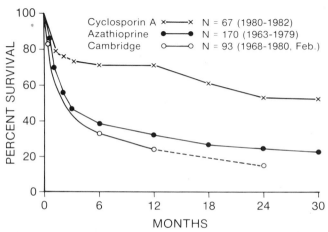

Fig 29–2.—Survival of patients given liver transplants in Denver under prednisone and azathioprine immunosuppression. (By permission of Hepatology.[6])

Fig 29–3.—Survival curves from initial reports of results of liver transplantation using cyclosporin-A and prednisone. (By permission of Hepatology.[6])

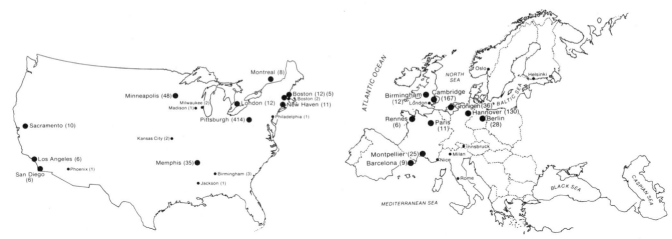

Fig 29–4.—Locations of active liver transplant centers in the United States and Europe as of July 1984. (By permission of Transplant Proceedings.[7])

as yet, in liver transplantation. But, as more medical centers enter the arena of liver transplantation, increasing the local availability of donor organs will become critical to meeting the needs of these transplant programs. This, in turn, will require continuing efforts on the part of transplant programs at making both the public and the rest of the medical community more aware of these needs so that fewer donor organs are wasted.

The techniques for procurement of multiple organs from a single donor have been described in many previous publications.[60–64] These methods have been designed to minimize or eliminate damage done to the various organs by warm ischemia. The basic principles of liver procurement are outlined herein. More detailed descriptions are available elsewhere.[60–64]

Donor Maintenance

Organ donors are heart beating cadavers. Prior to the declaration of death, the care of a brain-injured patient is the sole responsibility of the patient's primary physician(s) and should not be altered in any way which might be detrimental to the patient just because that patient is viewed as a possible organ donor. On the contrary, the functional quality of transplanted donor organs depends, to some degree, on how successful the primary physician(s) has (have) been in maintaining the normal physiology of the patient. Once a patient has been declared dead as the result of the complete and irreversible cessation of all brain function and permission for organ donation has been granted by the appropriate next of kin, usually the care of that cadaver is turned over to the transplant organ procurement agency.

At this point, the task of the procurement officer in charge of the donor is to assess the overall status of the donor in terms of its state of hydration, its cardiodynamic stability and ultimately, the level of end organ function. Any overt abnormalities are corrected, and an attempt is made to maintain a steady urine output of 2 ml/kg/hour or more. Diabetes insipidus, if present, is treated with judicious use of vasopressin, and fluid losses are replaced with a solution of extracellular composition (such as lactated Ringer's solution). Care must be exercised to avoid overhydration as well, especially if consideration is being given to procurement of the heart and lungs.

A central venous or pulmonary artery catheter is usually required for this purpose.

Hypoxia and hypotension are the two greatest dangers to the donor liver. Yet the liver is unique in its capacity to regenerate following injury. How extensive a period of hypoxia or hypotension a liver will tolerate and still provide satisfactory function in the recipient following transplantation is difficult to determine. A donor with a prolonged history of arterial hypoxia as evidenced by serial blood gas determinations warrants careful examination of the liver function tests. Likewise, a history of multiple or repeated cardiac arrests, of prolonged hypotension requiring the use of high doses of pressor agents for longer than brief periods of instability may have caused unacceptable degrees of hepatic injury. On the other hand, low doses of dopamine or inotropic agents may prove useful for maintaining good renal function and enhancing cardiac output.

The major point of this discussion is that in making the decision about whether to use a particular donor liver, one must take into account a number of variables. As an isolated set of values, liver function tests, whether entirely normal or grossly abnormal, are not particularly useful. Large elevations in serum transaminase levels as the result of a brief period of hypotension or of a recent episode of cardiopulmonary resuscitation often do not indicate an hepatic injury significant enough to preclude transplantation of the organ. On the other hand, a donor with extensive hepatic necrosis and massive fluid shifts may exhibit grossly normal serum transaminase levels. Serum bilirubin may be elevated secondary to the transfusion of blood, although usually with a higher than normal indirect fraction. A prolonged prothrombin or partial thromboplastin time should alert one to the possibility of the development in the donor of disseminated intravascular coagulation (DIC). Donor DIC may develop as the result of massive brain or other tissue necrosis secondary to multiple trauma or may indicate overt sepsis. In either case, an uncorrectable or unexplained coagulopathy should be considered a relative contraindication to liver donation, particularly if other evidence points to the presence of a significant hepatic injury.

Ultimately, responsibility for the decision about whether to use a particular liver for transplantation is borne by the surgeon performing the transplant. In making that decision, the surgeon may also take into account the condition of the recipient as well as the size, age, and blood type of the donor in terms of the relative frequency with which such a donor becomes available. For example, small pediatric donors are quite rare and the number of waiting candidates is large. The number of such patients who die waiting for the appropriate-sized donor is still greater than the number that receive transplants. Hence, when they become available, these donors are only infrequently deemed to be unsatisfactory.

Technique of Donor Hepatectomy

The heart-beating cadaver is placed on the operating table in a supine position. A heating blanket placed under the body is useful in maintaining donor core temperature above 34°C and thus avoiding premature development of cardiac arrythmias. An experienced anesthesiologist is invaluable in maintaining the integrity of donor cardiodynamic and pulmonary stability. An arterial catheter and a central venous or pulmonary artery catheter often has proved useful for the intraoperative management of the donor.

The donor abdomen is opened through a long midline incision combined with midline sternotomy. This provides excellent exposure to the abdominal viscera and allows for the option of removing the heart and/or lungs as well. In general, the liver procurement team performs the dissection of the hepatic hilum first. The hepatic arterial supply is identified and traced back to its origin from the aorta. The common bile duct is divided as close to the duodenum as possible, providing maximum length for anastomosis in the recipient. An incision is made in the gallbladder and bile flushed from the biliary tree with a bulb syringe. The portal vein is cleaned and the confluence of the splenic and superior mesenteric veins isolated. The latter is facilitated by dividing the pancreas between mass ligatures. A cannula for infusion of cold fluid is inserted into the portal vein via the splenic or mesenteric vein.

Once the hepatic hilar dissection has been completed, the nephrectomy team proceeds with isolation of the kidneys. We prefer *in situ* flush of the organs. Large-bore cannulas are inserted into the distal aorta and inferior vena cava at the level of the iliacs, the former for infusion of cold preservation solution into the arterial tree and the latter for drainage of blood and fluid from the venous system.

The so-called precooling step can be started at any time after the hepatic hilar dissection has been completed. The cannula in the distal vena cava is useful for draining off central venous volume as cold (4–10°C) lactated Ringer's solution is infused through the liver via the portal vein cannula. This is important to avoid central venous hypertension, which may cause swelling of the liver. The precooling step serves to cool the liver while it is still being perfused with oxygenated blood via the hepatic artery. In this way, warm ischemia is virtually eliminated. Infusion of cold lactated Ringer's is continued until donor core temperature falls to 28–30°C or until cardiac arrythmias develop. In practice, a stable donor will accept 3–5 L of portal infusion over approximately 45–60 minutes, with an attendant release via the vena caval cannula of 2–4 L.

The *in situ* flush of the aorta with preservation fluid (Collins or another fluid of intracellular composition) is started as soon as precooling is thought to be complete or at any time that cardiodynamic instability causes arterial perfusion pressures to become unsatisfactory. The aorta is clamped at the diaphragm, above the celiac axis, and the flush begun via the cannula in the distal aorta. At the same time, the vena caval cannula is opened and the fluid infusing through the portal vein is changed from lactated Ringer's to preservation solution for an additional liter of flush. The aorta is reclamped below the celiac axis after about 200–500 ml have been infused through the artery. While the kidneys continue to be flushed, the aorta is divided between the celiac axis and renal arteries and the liver is removed. The suprahepatic vena cava is divided at the base of the atrium and a small cuff of diaphragm left on the specimen. The hepatic ligaments are rapidly divided, the infrahepatic vena cava divided just above the renal vein and the liver lifted out of the abdomen. The organ is placed in plastic bags, packed in an ice slush solution and transported to the recipient hospital.

Liver Preservation

The average time interval at Pittsburgh between devascularization of a liver in the donor and revascularization in the recipient is 4½ hours, with a range of from 60 minutes in locally procured organs to over 12 hours in those flown in from the West Coast. In general, an effort is made to limit the cold ischemia time to less than 6–8 hours. This usually means starting the recipient procedure approximately two to three hours before the arrival of the donor organ at the recipient operating room. The timing is varied according to the anticipated degree of difficulty of the recipient hepatectomy.

Much research is currently being devoted to improving the methods of hepatic preservation. These efforts have centered around three main areas.

One involves attempts at cytoprotection and is founded on the principle that the major injury to the liver caused by hypotension or hypoxia in the donor or by the period of cold ischemia can be minimized by treatment of the liver or the donor with so-called cytoprotective agents. Different authors have proposed the use of calcium channel blockers,[65–67] somatostatin,[68] coenzyme Q,[69–71] and various prostaglandins.[72–75]

Protection may also be afforded to cells by a new method of cold storage called vitrification. This technique is being studied by the MRC Medical Cryobiology Group in Cambridge.[76] It involves very slow cooling of tissue under conditions of high atmospheric pressure with the intent being to avoid crystallization of tissue water while at the same time lowering tissue temperatures well below the freezing level, thus effectively arresting tissue metabolism.

A second area involves developing various methods of perfusion of the liver. Cold perfusion of the liver has been attempted by several authors.[77, 78] The extensive experiments of Brettschneider et al. showed that these methods of cold perfusion, even if combined with oxygenation of the perfusate, allowed no significant prolongation of preservation times beyond those allowed by simple cold storage. The extensive experience with cold perfusion for preservation of the kidney has demonstrated that these methods yield no clear advantage over simple cold storage, as witnessed by the general lack of agreement among kidney transplant centers about the preferred technique.[79, 80] The situation might change, however, if cold perfusion were to prove to be the preferred method for continual delivery of a cytoprotective agent.

The use of a warm, oxygenated perfusate may eventually prove a superior method for preservation of the liver. Rather than cool the liver to minimize its metabolic demands during a period of requisite ischemia, perhaps a better approach would involve eliminating the ischemic period altogether and providing the liver with everything that it needs during the time interval that it is between donor and recipient. Removal of the liver and placement of the organ into an extracorporeal circuit which employs a blood pump, oxygenator, and heat exchanger is combined with the administration into the circuit of appropriate metabolic substrate (glucose and amino acids) and the occasional use of a dialysis membrane. An even simpler solution may involve removal of the organs to be preserved en bloc with placement into a preservation box. Such a circuit might include the heart and lungs, liver, small bowel, pancreas, and kidneys. Critical to these techniques will be minimizing blood loss from leaks and hemolysis, avoiding thrombosis or the development of coagulopathies, and eliminating contamination with bacteria, fungi or other infectious agents which could lead to sepsis in the recipient.

The only method now of assessing the quality of a liver graft after it has been procured is to revascularize it in the recipient and then wait to see if it provides function adequate to support life. As discussed later in this chapter, although inadequate function of a grafted liver is the least common of the three major reasons for retransplantation, it is nevertheless the most devastating. Eliminating primary nonfunction as a cause of failure of a liver graft would result in decreasing the overall retransplantation rate by 25%.[81] Clearly, one can begin to understand the importance of developing ex vivo methods for measuring the degree of damage sustained by a liver either in the donor, at the time of procurement or during the subsequent period of cold storage. Histologic examination by either light or electron microscopic techniques has been inadequate for this purpose.

THE LIVER RECIPIENT

Indications for Liver Transplantation

The list of diseases leading to liver failure which can be corrected by hepatic transplantation reads like a textbook of hepatology. Table 29–5 shows the major diagnoses of 244 patients transplanted under cyclosporine therapy from March 1, 1980, to June 30, 1984, a period which allows for a minimum follow-up, at the time of this writing, of six months. The most frequent indication for liver replacement in adults is postnecrotic cirrhosis, usually following chronic active hepatitis. In children, if one includes with biliary atresia other congenital disorders of intrahepatic bile ductule formation, one can account for over 60% of patients 18 years old or younger who undergo liver transplantation.

A comparison of the indications for transplantation before and after the introduction of cyclosporine therapy reveals some important differences. Among adults, alcoholic cirrhosis and hepatic malignancies have become much more common. The list of metabolic disorders for which liver transplantation is indicated also has become more diverse. The reasons for these changes will become more evident later in this chapter,

TABLE 29–5.—INDICATIONS FOR 244 PRIMARY LIVER TRANSPLANTS PERFORMED BETWEEN MARCH 1, 1980, AND JUNE 30, 1984

INDICATION	ADULT	PEDIATRIC	TOTAL	%
Acute hepatic necrosis	3	0	3	1.2
Biliary atresia	0	56	56	23.0
Budd-Chiari syndrome	5	1	6	2.5
Cirrhosis	46	10	56	23.0
Familial cholestasis	0	7	7	2.9
Inborn errors of metabolism	11	23	34	13.9
Neonatal hepatitis	0	3	3	1.2
Primary biliary cirrhosis	36	0	36	14.8
Primary liver tumors	13	0	13	5.3
Secondary biliary cirrhosis	5	1	6	2.5
Sclerosing cholangitis	19	1	20	8.2
Others	2	2	4	1.6
Total	140	104	244	100

but in general, the survival rate following liver transplantation now exceeds that for other forms of therapy for virtually all causes of liver failure and this has had a major impact upon the selection of recipients.

Figure 29–5 shows actuarial survival curves for adults and children. The actuarial survival rate for all patients combined is 68% at one year and remains at 60% after the third year. Children have a 76% one-year and a 74% five-year survival rate, compared to 62% and 50% for adults at the same milestones, respectively.

Post Necrotic Cirrhosis

Most of these patients have so-called non-A, non-B hepatitis of a chronic nature and have developed cirrhosis with all of its sequelae. The actuarial one-year survival rate in the overall group of patients in this category is 62% (Fig 29–6). The best results have been obtained in patients in whom nutritional depletion or prior immune depression with steroid therapy has not taken place. The one-year survival rate in 45 of these patients who are aged 39 years or younger is 66.5% (Fig 29–7). Only five of 11 patients over 40 years of age survived the first year. Three of these patients are alive at 6, 9, and 12 months. Three others lived beyond one year, but all later died within 2½ years of transplantation. On the other hand, in patients with disabling complications of cirrhosis, delaying transplantation in an attempt to temporize with other forms of therapy may seriously hinder long-term survival.

Five patients who had transplantation with cyclosporine therapy had positive sera tests for hepatitis B surface antigen and for E antigen. All were treated with various regimens of human antihepatitis B immune globulin, and attempts have been made actively to immunize all patients transplanted since vaccine (Heptavax-B, Merck, Sharp & Dohme) has become available. One patient became antibody positive and antigen negative for over six months. A second patient became antigen negative for a brief period following surgery. All patients eventually reverted to their original hepatitis serology (positive for surface antigen and negative for antibody). Three of these patients died at 5, 14, and 14½ months, respectively, after transplantation. One of these three died with entirely normal liver function; the other two of septic complications attending the development of recurrent liver failure, both his-

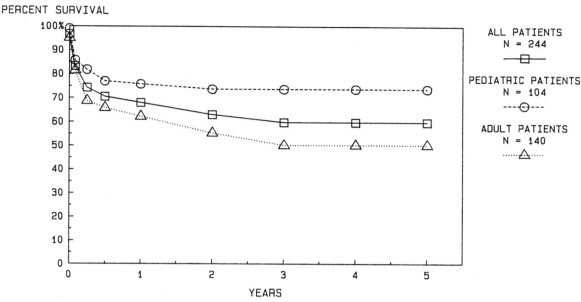

Fig 29–5.—Actuarial survival for 244 liver transplants done between March 1, 1980, and June 30, 1984.

topathologic evidence of recurrent hepatitis. The other two patients are presently alive one and three years after transplantation. The latter patient, although remaining antigen negative for over six months, eventually became antigen positive and has recently recovered from an episode of acute hepatitis. This limited experience suggests that hepatitis B positive patients remain at high risk for developing recurrent disease in the transplanted organ. Further attempts to transplant these patients must be accompanied by renewed efforts at eradicating the virus and preventing recurrent infection.

Because of the lack of serum markers for non-A, non-B hepatitis, the incidence of recurrent disease among patients who have had transplants for this entity is not known. Only

two of these patients developed episodes of what appears to have been acute hepatitis, and both have recovered fully. Overall, the results in these patients are quite good, and they remain a group for which transplantation should be considered early.

Primary Biliary Cirrhosis (PBC)

Virtually all of these patients are women in their fifth or sixth decade who have had documented disease for ten to 20 years or more. Many are deeply jaundiced with bilirubin levels in the 20 to 30 mg/dl range and have ascites, portal hypertension and severe bone disease. Recurrent bleeding from esophageal varices, repeated episodes of encephalopathy, or a

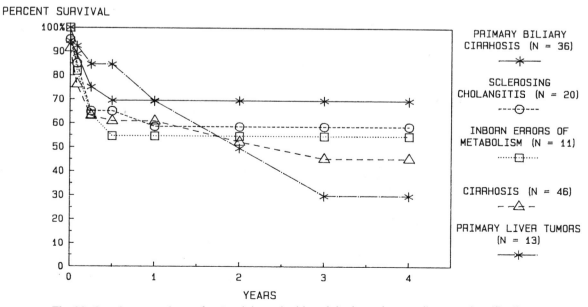

Fig 29–6.—A comparison of actuarial survival in adults based upon disease classification.

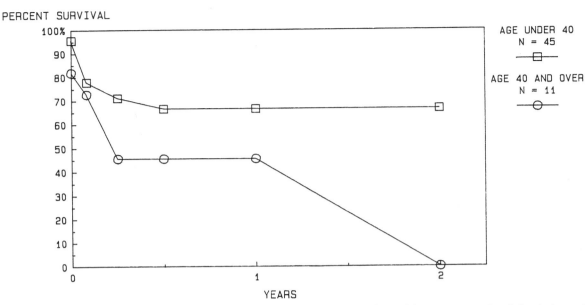

Fig 29–7.—A comparison of actuarial survival of 56 patients transplanted for post-necrotic cirrhosis based upon age.

sudden and relentless rise in bilirubin above 10 mg/dl are the most frequent reasons for referring these patients for transplantation. Although liver replacement can be a relatively easy operative procedure in many of these patients, advanced age, advanced liver disease, or a history of previous abdominal surgery are all factors which not only can markedly increase the operative risks but also may complicate recovery following transplantation.

The actuarial survival rate in these patients is 69.4% at one and five years (see Fig 29–6). Because of severe, preexisting osteoporosis, complicated by immunosuppressive therapy, ten of these 36 patients developed vertebral body compression fractures of a severity which required them to be hospitalized in rehabilitation centers following discharge from the hospital.

The question of recurrence of PBC in the transplanted liver has been raised before.[82] In virtually all of these patients, the antimitochondrial antibody titers remain positive following transplantation. In addition, the histologic appearance of chronic rejection of an hepatic allograft is extremely difficult to distinguish from primary biliary cirrhosis. The authors have seen chronic rejection in this group of patients, but do not believe they have seen recurrent PBC.

Sclerosing Cholangitis

Until recently, patients with sclerosing cholangitis (SC) had not obtained survival rates following liver transplantation as high as those for other diseases. The major reason has been that the vast majority of these patients have had multiple operative procedures designed to treat extrahepatic bile duct obstruction. The presence of extensive, dense adhesions in the face of portal hypertension can lead to inordinate blood loss during the transplant operation. Furthermore, preexisting infection in obstructed bile ducts greatly increases the risk of developing sepsis following surgery. Finally, in the past, because of the temptation for surgeons to treat the disease with repeated sundry procedures, many of these patients were referred for transplantation long after becoming moribund from advanced hepatic failure.

A recent analysis of survival statistics reveals that 13 of the overall group of 21 (62%) SC patients transplanted in Pittsburgh are still alive from six to 36 months following transplantation, with only one death occurring after six months. (The actuarial survival curve is shown in Figure 29–6.)

In making the diagnosis of sclerosing cholangitis, one must be wary of the possibility that the patient has a duct cell tumor. The absence of a history of ulcerative colitis or initial presentation of the disease in an older patient should increase the suspicion that malignancy may be the primary diagnosis. In addition, some evidence suggests that a long history of SC may predispose to development of duct cell tumor.

The treatment of colitis in these patients requires careful individualization. Patients with a significant risk for developing colonic malignancy by virtue of having a long history (greater than ten years) of active colitis are theoretically at even greater risk during immunosuppression therapy following transplantation. Whenever possible, if liver transplantation is a consideration for a patient, total proctocolectomy should be delayed until after the transplant. The presence of intra-abdominal adhesions and/or an ileostomy significantly increase the operative risk and may complicate recovery. If colitis is active following liver transplantation, definitive surgical therapy should be contemplated three to six months later when recovery is complete. The risk for recurrence of SC in the transplanted liver in patients with or without active colitis is not known, but no such cases have been reported thus far.

Malignancies

When discussing the results of liver transplantation for malignancies, one needs to distinguish between primary and metastatic lesions and between incidental and diffuse primary lesions. The initial determination must be that tumor is confined strictly to the liver and the assumption, therefore, is that a cure can be affected by total hepatectomy.

Until recently, the only reports involving metastatic lesion came from Calne at Cambridge. All five of their patients died from recurrent tumor within one year of transplantation, and their conclusion has been that metastatic malignancy should not be an indication for transplantation of the liver.[83] On the other hand, Huber and associates from Innsbruck, Basel, and Seattle reported the successful treatment of a 43-year-old woman with hepatic metastases from breast carcinoma by liver replacement combined with toxic doses of cyclophosphamide and irradiation followed by reconstitution with stored autologous bone marrow.[84] The patient is alive and free of tumor over two years later.[(personal communication, 1985)] This novel approach, though still experimental, nevertheless belies exciting possibilities for the future.

Primary hepatocellular tumors are found in association with diseases that also cause cirrhosis and liver failure. In the combined Denver and Pittsburgh series under cyclosporine immunosuppression, three patients with chronic active hepatitis, four with hereditary tyrosinemia, one with α_1-antitrypsin deficiency and one with sea blue histiocyte syndrome had such associated hepatomas. In all but one of these patients, the existence of the tumor was either known or strongly suspected prior to the transplant operation. In all of these cases, resection was not an alternative because of the presence of hepatic failure or extensive cirrhosis from other causes. A resection had been attempted in one patient with hereditary tyrosinemia with subsequent development of deep hepatic failure being the cause for referral of the patient for transplantation. Among the nine patients who survived, with follow-up of from ten months to 3½ years (eight of whom are still alive), none has developed recurrent tumor.

Primary hepatic malignancies with diffuse involvement of the liver have been the major cause for liver transplantation in a total of 32 patients (exclusive of those with cirrhosis or hereditary tyrosinemia), treated with transplantation from March 1963 to September 1983. Table 29–6 lists the tumor types for both groups of patients.

Twenty of these patients were treated before the introduction of cyclosporine, 12 of whom survived long enough to observe them for evidence of recurrent tumor. Seven of these patients died between two and 11 months, four more between 13 and 54 months following transplantation. Metastatic disease was present in all 11 and was a major factor in the death of seven of these patients. One patient who had transplantation for a sarcoma of undetermined cell type and who had miliary abdominal metastases at the time of transplantation is

TABLE 29–6.—PRIMARY LIVER TUMORS

TYPE OF LESION	BEFORE CYCLOSPORINE	AFTER CYCLOSPORINE
Hepatoma	12 (0)*	6 (5)*
Fibrolamellar	1 (0)	5 (4)
Klatskin's	5 (0)	2 (0)
Cholangiocarcinoma	1 (0)	2 (0)
Sarcomas	2 (1)	3 (1)

*Number in parentheses, currently alive after one year.

alive eight years later with no evidence of active growth of residual tumor.

An actuarial survival curve is shown in Figure 29–6 for the 12 patients with tumors treated in the cyclosporine era. Eight survived at least one year and five are still alive between 1½ and 3½ years postoperatively. Two of the five long-term survivors have known metastatic disease, one of whom has had a positive response to chemotherapy.

The fibrolamellar type hepatoma has been described as a particularly slow growing variant of hepatoma.[85, 86] Our experience suggests that these tumors represent a group of patients for whom transplantation may offer both reliable palliation and a reasonable chance for cure. This variant was originally described in 1956 by Edmondson,[87] and further elucidated by Peters in 1975.[88] Five patients in the cyclosporine era have been identified as having this type of tumor. Three patients are alive and tumor free, one over three years and the other two over one year after transplantation. One of the remaining two died after 2½ years and the other is alive after 31 months, having undergone chemotherapy for treatment of pulmonary metastases. This patient is remarkable for having originally undergone a right trisegmentectomy for her tumor in 1977, with transplantation having been undertaken 4½ years later for recurrence of tumor in the residual liver.

Three patients in the cyclosporine group had epithelioid hemangioendothelial sarcomas. Two died, one of sepsis at 79 days, the other of metastatic disease after 16 months. A total of seven patients had cholangiocarcinomas, five of which were Klatskin's tumors. All three Klatskin's tumor patients from the precyclosporine era died, one at two months with no evidence of metastatic tumor and two of metastatic disease at 24 and 54 months. One of two patients with Klatskin's tumors treated under cyclosporine survived the perioperative period, eventually succumbing to metastatic disease after 8½ months. The two other patients with non-Klatskin's cholangiocarcinomas died at 12 and 20 months of metastatic tumor.

This experience is similar to that reported from other centers. Wight reported 24 patients with primary hepatoma, 20 of whom did not have cirrhosis and therefore, presumably had tumors which were unresectable by virtue of their extensive involvement of the liver.[83] Five of these patients obtained survival for two years or more, two of whom then died of disseminated tumor, three of whom lived five years or more without evidence of recurrence. Of all 120 cases in the Cambridge-Kings College series, 26 survived for six months or more, and although 15 (58%) of these died as the direct result of tumor recurrence, Wight concludes that transplantation improved the quality of life in these patients therefore providing worthwhile palliation.

Since in our experience, with the exception of about 50% of patients with fibrolamellar hepatomas, virtually all hepatic malignancies have recurred, many in less than one year and often with such an aggressive behavior that death occurred very rapidly after the appearance of the recurrence, further attempts to treat tumor patients with malignancies are justifiable only if combined with other therapeutic modalities. More experience needs to be obtained in this arena to determine whether transplantation will become a satisfactory form of treatment for tumor patients.

Budd-Chiari Syndrome

Thrombosis of the hepatic veins has presented as an indication for liver transplantation in both the acute and chronic setting. Six of the seven patients in the authors' series were treated after the introduction of cyclosporine. The one patient from the precyclosporine period and three from the current series are still alive at 10 and 4½ years and 54, 9, and 8 months. One patient died of sepsis in less than one month after transplantation, but two others obtained long-term survival of 16 and 20 months. The latter of these two patients died following retransplantation for liver failure secondary to chronic rejection. The other died of recurrent Budd-Chiari syndrome when long-term coumadin therapy was discontinued in preparation for an elective surgical procedure.

The two most recently treated patients were women who presented with acute thrombosis of both the intrahepatic vena cava and the hepatic veins. One also had complete thrombosis of the portal vein, both renal veins, and both iliofemoral systems. These patients required extensive thrombectomies during the transplant procedure and both have now survived on chronic anticoagulation therapy with no recurrent thromboses.

Biliary Atresia and Related Disorders

These disorders account for over 60% of all children who have received liver transplants in the cyclosporine era at Pittsburgh and Denver (Fig 29–8). Biliary atresia per se is the diagnosis in fully 54% of children, making it the single most frequent diagnosis among all patients receiving liver transplantation in this series.

Most biliary atresia patients have had a Kasai procedure and many have had subsequent attempts at modification of the original procedure in order to obtain drainage of bile. For the most part, a single attempt at a Kasai procedure, even with an attempted revision does not pose an increased oper-

ative risk to the recipient at the time of liver transplantation. On the other hand, multiple reoperations for revision of jejunal limbs, creation of stomas, and other repeated attempts designed to obtain better drainage may seriously complicate removal of the recipient liver.

Bylers disease, congenital biliary hypoplasia, and Alagille's syndrome are other disorders of bile ducts which lead to hepatic failure in childhood and require consideration for transplantation. Some of these patients may also have had attempts at correction through biliary drainage procedures, usually because of some confusion about the true diagnosis.

One- and five-year actuarial survival in this group is 76%. Twenty-six of the total 56 patients are alive one year or more, and 12 two years or more following transplantation. The major impediment to treating adequately all potential candidates with this disorder, as pointed out earlier, is the lack of availability of appropriate donors. Biliary atresia and related disorders are cured by liver replacement. Many patients who are accepted for transplantation die while waiting for a donor to become available.

Metabolic Disorders

Under cyclosporine therapy, a total of 34 patients with inborn errors of metabolism have been treated with liver transplantation, all for cirrhosis rather than solely for correction of the metabolic disorder (Table 29–7). Twenty three of the 34 patients were 18 years old or younger at the time of surgery.

The most common metabolic disorder treated by liver transplantation is α_1-antitrypsin (α_1-A) deficiency. Patients with Pi_{zz} phenotype can develop macronodular cirrhosis that is sometimes confused with post necrotic cirrhosis. Replacement of the liver results in restoration of serum α_1-A levels to normal and conversion to Pi phenotype.[89] Suitability for transplantation is somewhat dependent on the patient's pulmonary status in that severe obstructive airway disease may preclude survival following the procedure. In general, pa-

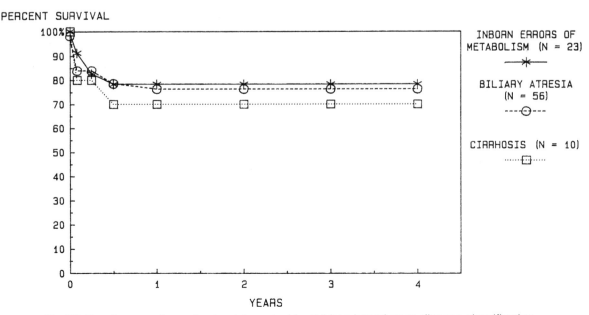

Fig 29–8.—A comparison of actuarial survival in children based upon disease classification.

TABLE 29–7.—INDICATIONS FOR 34 PRIMARY
LIVER TRANSPLANTS PERFORMED FOR INBORN
ERRORS OF METABOLISM

INDICATION	ADULT	PEDIATRIC	TOTAL
α_1-Antitrypsin deficiency	6	15	21
Wilson's disease	3	4	7
Tyrosinemia	1	3	4
Glycogen storage disease	0	1	1
Hemochromatosis	1	0	1
Total	11	23	34

tients with this disorder are excellent candidates for liver replacement. They usually have not had multiple previous abdominal procedures. Because transplantation cures the underlying disorder, they are generally referred for the procedure soon after they begin to manifest signs of significant liver failure, usually before serious physiologic deterioration and malnutrition have developed. Of the 21 patients with α_1-A, 15 were children, six adults. The actuarial one- and four-year survival rate is 67% (Fig 29–9).

Wilson's disease is the second most common diagnosis among the metabolic disorders. These patients suffer from markedly reduced copper excretion and decreased serum ceruloplasmin levels and experience increased copper deposition in liver and brain tissue. Medical treatment consists of strict adherence to low copper diets, oral potassium sulfide to reduce enteral absorption of copper, and, more recently, the use of D-penicillamine. Liver replacement corrects the disorder of copper metabolism and is indicated when hepatic involvement with the disease becomes significant. Patients may present for the first time in hepatic failure or in acute hemolytic crisis.[90] In the authors' series, seven patients have been transplanted with four surviving between six months and 13 years (Fig 29–9). In general, waiting for recovery from the acute hemolytic crisis and then planning for liver transplantation on a semi-elective basis is the preferred route.

Hereditary tyrosinemia is another hepatic based disorder of metabolism which is corrected by replacement with a normal liver. The accumulation of abnormal metabolites of tyrosine which are carcinogenic results in a high incidence of malignancies in patients who present with this disorder, although the major indication for transplantation is usually cirrhosis.[91] All four patients treated for tyrosinemia in this series after the introduction of cyclosporine are alive from seven to 37 months following transplantation.

The two other patients with metabolic disorders include a 17-year-old girl with type IV glycogen storage disease and a 41-year-old man with hemochromatosis. Both are alive at 35 and 12 months, respectively.

More recently, the authors had an opportunity to treat a 10-year-old girl with homozygous familial hypercholesterolemia (FH), who had developed cardiac failure and intractable angina despite three different attempts at coronary artery reconstruction. This patient underwent a combination heart and liver transplantation procedure. The patient underwent liver replacement solely to correct the underlying disorder, since the native liver was anatomically and otherwise outwardly normal. The procedure appears to have been a success since serum cholesterol levels were markedly reduced from over 1,000 mg/dl prior to transplantation down to less than 300 mg/dl following liver transplantation.[92] With the continuing improvement in the success rate with liver transplantation, the future will undoubtedly see an increasing role for the operation in the treatment of not only FH but for a growing list of other metabolic disorders which may prove to be hepatic based.[93] As an example, at Cambridge recently, a young man with severe complications of oxalosis was transplanted with no indication other than treatment of the metabolic defect.

Alcoholic Cirrhosis

Results of transplantation for patients with cirrhosis secondary to alcohol abuse are difficult to assess. Since the introduction of cyclosporine, only three patients have been treated

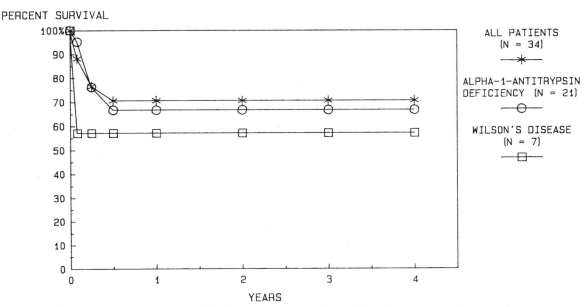

Fig 29–9.—Actuarial survival for 34 patients transplanted for inborn errors of metabolism.

and two are dead. Both of these must be considered technical failures, since they died on the operating table. One patient, a 52-year-old businessman, is alive and well, leading a productive life one year following surgery. Before the advent of cyclosporine, 15 alcoholics had transplants, four of whom lived over one year, three of whom are still alive. One patient returned to his former ways following surgery and 56 months later was found unconscious in a roadside ditch in Florida, eventually dying of pneumonitis. The most difficult issue in deciding to treat these patients with liver replacement will continue to be the satisfactory definition of reformation from alcoholism.

THE RECIPIENT OPERATION

Although the development of the surgical techniques necessary for the successful completion of an orthotopic transplantation of the liver began in the laboratory in the late 1950s, the operation in normal dogs often bears little resemblance to the operation in a cirrhotic human. The presence of severe portal hypertension, particularly in the face of adhesions resulting from previous surgical procedures or liver biopsies, can present a markedly different kind of challenge. Much of the inherent difficulty of the procedure lies in the recipient hepatectomy. Failure to carry off this initial step in reasonable safety can jeopardize all of the steps that must follow.

The recipient operation can be divided into three distinct phases, each with its own special problems. The first phase encompasses those steps necessary for the removal of the recipient liver. The second phase begins after the recipient liver has been removed and the new organ is being sewn into place: the so-called anhepatic phase. Restoring blood flow to the new liver in the recipient begins the third phase, a phase which also involves the sometimes arduous process of obtaining complete hemostasis.

The Recipient Hepatectomy

The abdomen is generally opened through bilateral subcostal incisions, with a vertical extension in the midline toward the xyphoid. Excision of the xyphoid provides for greater expansion of the midline wound. Alternatively, a Reynolds flap type of incision often provides adequate exposure. A self-retaining retractor which attaches to the operating table and can effectively spread the rib cage is an indispensable tool for maximizing exposure.

The recipient operation is begun early enough to allow the surgeon sufficient time to exercise meticulous care in removing the diseased liver. Liberal use of the electrocautery to make the incision and elsewhere in the dissection can help minimize blood loss, but is not a suitable substitute for careful surgical technique. Lymphatics and collateral blood vessels in the hepatic hilum are ligated and divided to expose the common bile duct, portal vein, and hepatic arterial supply. The supporting ligaments of the liver can be divided with the electrocautery, care being taken to ligate larger blood vessels to avoid bleeding later. The retrohepatic vena cava can be freed from the diaphragm superiorly down to a point just above the right renal vein. Alternatively, in adults, if exposure to the hepatic ligaments or the vena cava is limited, ei-

ther because of the extreme size of the liver or because retraction of the liver out of the hepatic fossa causes hemodynamic instability, the dissection behind the liver can be delayed until after the patient has been placed on venous bypass. In this case, hemostasis can be obtained readily after the native liver has been removed and before implanting the new liver.

Bleeding during this initial phase can also be minimized by aggressive treatment of preexisting coagulopathy with blood components. In Pittsburgh, the use of the thromboelastograph has allowed the anesthesiologists to constantly monitor the status of the patient's coagulation and to react accordingly.[94] This technique has proven more useful in the operating room than repeated measurements of conventional coagulation factors.

The Anhepatic Phase

Once dissection of the liver has been completed and the organ is ready to be removed, preparations are made for the anhepatic phase. In the past, this has always been the most critical phase, from a physiologic standpoint, for the recipient. Venous return from the inferior vena cava to the heart is completely interrupted. At the same time, both the portal and caval venous beds are completely obstructed. Patients tolerate this stage to varying degrees. Children in general fare much better than do adults. A venous bypass technique which does not require anticoagulation of the recipient was developed in the laboratory in Pittsburgh in late 1982[95] and has been used routinely in all adults undergoing liver transplantation since February 1983. The details of the technique and the improvements in results attending its routine use were the subjects of earlier reports.[96] In short, the method of venous bypass involves cannulating the divided portal vein and the femoral vein through a saphenous vein, cut down to provide decompression of the respective venous beds through a closed system which employs a centrifugal force pump to return blood to the superior vena cava by way of the axillary vein (Fig 29–10). Venous bypass results in the maintenance

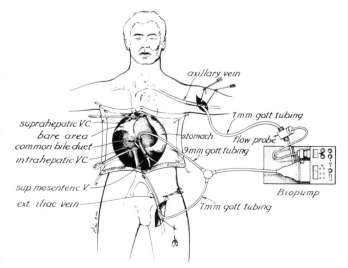

Fig 29–10.—Anatomy of venous bypass for anhepatic phase of orthotopic liver transplantation.

of normal physiology during the anhepatic phase, a virtual elimination of intraoperative mortality, a lower incidence of postoperative renal failure or GI bleeding, and lower blood loss during the transplant operation. The technique also markedly reduces the difficulty of those cases wherein exposure to retrohepatic structures is impossible or inadequate, by allowing one the option of extending the anhepatic phase in order to obtain hemostasis in the hepatic fossa after the native liver has been removed.

In children, the decision about whether to use bypass can usually be made after performing a test clamping of the inflow to the liver and the suprahepatic vena cava. Those who experience a marked fall in central venous or pulmonary arterial wedge pressure and a resultant decrease in cardiac output may require venous bypass. This can be accomplished in most children weighing more than 20 kg without the need for systemic anticoagulation, because flow rates in the bypass circuit will be adequate to prevent activation of clotting mechanisms. More recently, work has begun in the laboratory which no doubt will redefine the acceptable lower limits of flow rate so that venous bypass without systemic anticoagulation of the recipient may soon be an option for all high-risk children undergoing the procedure.

The native liver is excised by dividing the inflow vessels and the vena cava above and below the liver. The upper vena cava and hepatic veins are transected as distally as possible to maximize length of the upper cuff. The septa between these vessels can be cut or one or more of the hepatic vein ostia oversewn to tailor the diameter of the upper cuff to that of the donor upper cava (Fig 29–11). The lower cava is cut as long as possible as well, and excess length trimmed to fit the donor organ.

Once the liver has been removed, some time can be spent obtaining hemostasis in the hepatic bed. If bypass is employed, this time is well spent because decompression of the caval and portal beds prevents the kind of increasing venous congestion that would normally make such attempts futile.

The Revascularization and Hemostasis Phase

The sequencing of the vascular anastomoses requires careful judgment on the part of the operating surgeon. In general, the liver should be revascularized within 60 to 75 minutes after it has been removed from cold storage and brought up to the recipient. Usually all four anastomoses can be accomplished in that period, so that the liver receives its complete

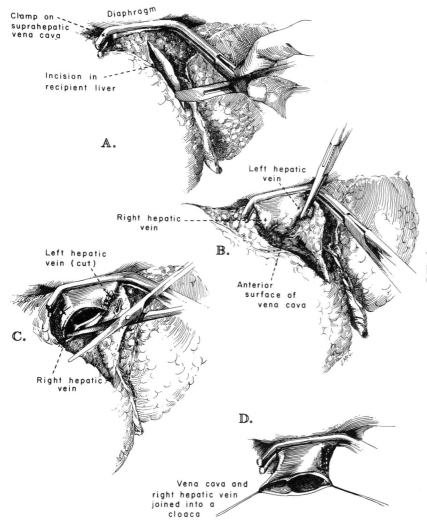

Clamp on suprahepatic vena cava

Diaphragm

Incision in recipient liver

A.

Left hepatic vein

Right hepatic vein

B.

Anterior surface of vena cava

Left hepatic vein (cut)

C.

Right hepatic vein

D.

Vena cava and right hepatic vein joined into a cloaca

Fig 29–11.—Development of upper vena caval cuff in recipient. (By permission of Surgery, Gynecology, and Obstetrics.[103])

blood supply all at once. Normally the upper vena caval anastomosis is followed by that of the lower cava. In adults on venous bypass, the arterial anastomosis can be done next, since the portal vein is decompressed. Following that, if clamping the portal vein side of the venous bypass (to remove the bypass cannula and perform the portal vein anastomosis), results in dimunition of bypass flow to less than 800–1,000 ml/minute, the arterial inflow to the liver can be restored, the caval clamps removed, and the patient removed from venous bypass before starting the portal vein anastomosis. Most often, however, clamping the portal vein cannula does not seriously jeopardize bypass flow. If one anticipates that the arterial anastomosis will be particularly difficult or that the inflow from the artery may be unreliable, the portal venous anastomosis should be done first. This is particularly the case in children or in any patient not benefiting from venous bypass. In these instances, the effort should be directed toward completing the portal vein anastomosis and releasing the obstructed caval and portal systems as rapidly as possible, and then completing the arterial anastomosis thereafter.

Before completing the lower vena caval anastomosis, the donor liver is flushed out with cold (4–10°C) lactated Ringer's solution through the cannula which was placed into the donor splenic vein during the procurement procedure. This precaution washes the preservation solution, high in potassium, out of the organ, at the same time evacuating air from the donor hepatic veins and vena cava, lessening the chance of hyperkalemic cardiac arrest or massive air embolism at the time that flow is released to the new liver.[97]

What usually proves to be the longest stage of the operation follows the revascularization of the new liver. The degree of difficulty in obtaining hemostasis at this point is largely dependent on how successful the team has been in controlling the bleeding during the performance of the recipient hepatectomy. But following revascularization of the donor liver in the recipient, a period of fibrinolysis often occurs. This period can be quite short, even clinically unnoticeable, but may sometimes last for several hours if it is not anticipated, looked for, and effectively treated. The thromboelastograph has proved to be particularly useful in this regard. The appearance of clot lysis is an indication to use cryoprecipitate and/or judicious use of ε-aminocaproic acid (Amicar). Ultimate control of bleeding requires persistence upon the parts of both the surgical team in managing so-called surgical bleeding and the anesthesia team in reversing coagulopathies. Closing the abdominal incision too early, with the attitude that improving hepatic function or some other feat of "Nature" will take care of the problem of persistent hemorrhage is a trap which the surgeon should avoid.

Bile duct reconstruction is delayed until after hemostasis has been completed. This allows thorough exposure to all hilar structures while looking for bleeding points and at the same time allows full manipulation and retraction of the liver without fear of disrupting the biliary anastomosis.

Biliary Reconstruction

If the liver recipient has a normal native bile duct, the preferred method of reconstruction is a duct-to-duct anastomosis over a T tube. With this method, the advantage of an intact sphincter of Oddi is preserved. In small pediatric patients or in any situation in which either recipient or donor bile duct is too small to allow the use of a T tube (the smallest normally available is an 8 F), a Roux-en-Y loop of jejunum is constructed and a choledochojejunostomy performed. In those patients in whom the bile duct is diseased (e.g., sclerosing cholangitis or biliary atresia and related disorders) or damaged (e.g., secondary biliary cirrhosis or previous bile duct surgery), a Roux-en-Y choledochojejunostomy is the method of reconstruction we prefer. The anastomosis is stented with an appropriately sized plastic (polyethylene) tube. We have had limited experience using the method of reconstruction employed by Calne[98] and have not found the technique to offer any advantage over conventional methods of reconstruction.

At the completion of the biliary anastomosis, a cholangiogram is obtained, either through the T tube or via a catheter in the cystic duct. Routine cholangiography confirms both patency and competency of the duct anastomosis and also serves to ensure proper positioning of the T tube or stent.

Auxiliary or Heterotopic Transplantation

The possibility of successfully treating some patients with a new liver without the need to remove the native organ has remained an intriguing possibility. But the world experience, as summarized by Fortner et al.,[99] has been rather discouraging, with only one of 50 cases reviewed obtaining unequivocal success. Houssin and associates[100] from Paris later reported a second success. The major problems have been the frequency of thrombosis of the venous outflow and ensuring satisfactory portal venous inflow. Optimal revascularization of a liver graft appears to require inflow from the native portal system, as demonstrated by previous work.[101, 102]

Nevertheless, if a satisfactory technical solution were forthcoming, heterotopic transplants would offer the best alternative for patients suffering from metabolic disorders with otherwise normal livers, patients with hepatic dysfunction of a temporary nature, or in patients at high risk for removal of their native liver secondary to a history of extensive surgery in the area or from portal vein thrombosis.

RETRANSPLANTATION

Until recently, few patients were offered a second transplant for treatment of a failing hepatic graft. Figure 29–12 shows the yearly rate of retransplantation and Figure 29–13 the survival following retransplantation before and after the introduction of cyclosporine. The 19% one-year survival rate for those given second grafts in the azathioprine era did little to justify its increased application. Since 1980, however, survival has begun to exceed 50%, and the rate of retransplantation has been between 20% and 25% annually.

Details of this group of patients given retransplantation were the subject of a previous report.[81] Rejection of the graft continues to represent the most common cause of graft failure leading to retransplantation, with technical failures (mostly arterial thromboses), and primary nonfunction of a graft being the other two major categories (Fig 29–14). Technical failures occurred with a frequency that was significantly greater in children than adults.

A total of nine patients in the Pittsburgh series have received three liver transplants, five of whom have obtained greater than one-year survival. As with secondary transplants, timing and the setting under which the retransplant occurs

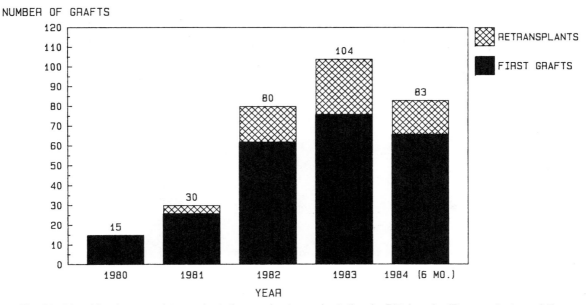

Fig 29–12.—Yearly rate of transplantation and retransplantation in Pittsburgh. (By permission of Transplant Proceedings.[81])

are major determinants of ultimate survival. When retransplantation is performed in an emergent setting and in the face of severe liver failure, the chances of success are much lower than in the more elective situation. Likewise, hepatic dysfunction as the result of failure to reverse rejection is an indication to consider retransplantation rather than to subject the recipient to the greater risks of increasing immunosuppression.

FUTURE PROSPECTS

Both 1983 and 1984 saw marked improvements in survival rates for liver recipients over those for 1982 (Fig 29–15). Aggressive retransplantation, more enlightened use of the new

drug cyclosporine and the routine use of venous bypass for adults are the major reasons for the better results.

Further improvements could be obtained through better selection of patients for the procedure. An examination of the group of adults transplanted using venous bypass revealed that bypass had a significant effect on 30-day survival in high-risk patients, but that these patients went through a period of increased mortality thereafter, so that their 90-day survival was similar to that of those patients transplanted without the use of bypass. High risk factors included recurrent episodes of severe encephalopathy, massive ascites, severe coagulopathy, recurrent episodes of massive GI hemorrhage, marked malnutrition and muscle wasting, renal failure, or a history of

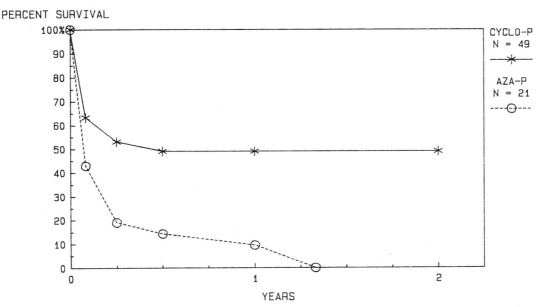

Fig 29–13.—A comparison of survival following hepatic retransplantation before and after cyclosporine. (By permission of Transplant Proceedings.[81])

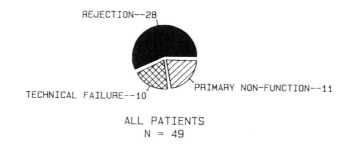

Fig 29–14.—Indications for hepatic retransplantation under cyclosporine and prednisone. (By permission of Transplant Proceedings.[81])

multiple previous abdominal surgeries. In another analysis, patients were assigned to one of three groups, solely dependent on their physical location at the time they were called to the operating room for the transplant. Six-week survival in those who were in the intensive care unit was 42% compared to 84% for those in the hospital, but on the ward, and 68% for those who were called in from home.

The survival curves in the Pittsburgh series have been obtained without any formal process of patient selection. Better results would follow the institution of even the most lenient process of selection. In general, when assigning priorities to recipients of a service as difficult to obtain in this country (and the world) as liver transplantation, careful consideration must

be given not just to which patient is the most ill, but also to the question of which patient will most likely be benefited by the procedure.

Suitability for survival of a liver transplant operation is often seriously jeopardized by the ravages of advanced hepatic failure. Unlike the field of kidney transplantation, transplantation of the liver has had to be developed without the benefit of a form of dialysis which would allow for stabilization and proper preparation of recipients prior to surgery. The development of an effective and practical technique of hepatic dialysis undoubtedly would markedly enhance survival for recipients currently classified as high risk for physiologic reasons.

The increasing participation in the field by a number of

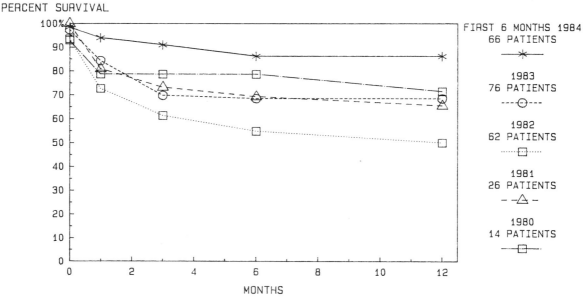

Fig 29–15.—Yearly actuarial survival curves since the introduction of cyclosporine.

new centers promises to provide both greater availability of the procedure as a service and greater diversity of results. Liver transplantation has become a high-profile news item, leading some institutions to view the procedure as one which might enhance their prestige. Other programs may view a liver transplantation service as a means of filling unoccupied hospital beds. But to be successful, a liver transplant program requires a tremendous commitment of resources, both financial and human. Provided that natural selection rather than governmental assignment is allowed to operate, the next few years will undoubtedly see the emergence of between 15 and 20 active centers from the initial milieu of institutions now starting up programs.

Major research efforts will center around improving immunosuppression. In the near future, a better cyclosporine (cyclosporin G) which is less nephrotoxic may be forthcoming. In addition, the use of antilymphocyte preparations, especially monoclonal antibodies, may prove to be useful additions to the armamentarium against rejection. On the other hand, the ultimate goal of inducement of donor specific tolerance still appears to be beyond the current horizon.

Developing better methods for liver preservation as well as for assessing viability of a liver graft before implantation are areas in which much research is needed. The future will also see multiple organ transplants (such as heart-liver transplants for familial hypercholesterolemia or liver-kidney grafts for polycystic disease) receiving greater application now that the initial trials with these procedures have begun.

The field of liver transplantation is in its infancy in terms of the potential for development that remains ahead. The first 20 years, largely as the result of the unflagging efforts of a few men, saw one of the most difficult of all surgical procedures refined to the point that it could be taught successfully to other surgeons. The availability, beginning in 1980, of a new and better immunosuppressant led to better control of what remains the greatest single source of failure: cell-mediated rejection of the liver allograft. The future offers physicians involved in the field the challenge of making the next chapter one of even greater success in the treatment and ultimate prevention of hepatic failure.

REFERENCES

1. Salvatierra O., Vincenti F., Amend W., et al.: Deliberate donor-specific blood transfusions prior to living related renal transplantation: a new approach. *Ann. Surg.* 192:543, 1980.
2. Persijn G.G., van Leeuwen A., Parlevliet J., et al.: Two major factors influencing kidney graft survival in Eurotransplant: HLA-DR matching and blood transfusion(s). *Transplant. Proc.* 13:150, 1981.
3. Starzl T.E. (with the assistance of Putnam C.W.): *Experience in Hepatic Transplantation.* Philadelphia, W.B. Saunders Co., 1969.
4. Oyer P.E., Stinson E.B., Reitz B.A., et al.: Cardiac transplantation: 1980. *Transplant. Proc.* 13:199, 1981.
5. Calne R.Y., Williams R., Lindop M., et al.: Improved survival after orthotopic liver grafting. *Br. Med. J.* 283:115, 1981.
6. Starzl T.E., Iwatsuki S., van Thiel D.H., et al.: Evolution of liver transplantation. *Hepatology* 2:614, 1982.
7. Starzl T.E., Iwatsuki S., Shaw B.W. Jr., Gordon R.D.: Orthotopic liver transplantation in 1984. *Transplant. Proc.* In press.
8. Starzl T.E., Iwatsuki S., Shaw B.W. Jr., et al.: Analysis of liver transplantation. *Hepatology* 4 (suppl. 1):47S, 1984.
9. Starzl T.E., Iwatsuki S., Shaw B.W. Jr., et al.: Consensus conference report on liver transplantation. *Dial. Transplant. Burn* 1:27, 1983.
10. *Hepatology* 4 (suppl. 1):1984.
11. Gartner J.C. Jr., Zitelli B.J., Malatack J.J., et al.: Orthotopic liver transplantation in children: 2 year experience with 47 patients. *Pediatrics* 74:140, 1984.
12. Carrel A.: La technique operatoire des anastomoses vasculaires et la transplantation des visceres. *Lyon Med.* 98:859, 1902.
13. Ullmann E.: Experimentelle nierentransplantation. *Wien. Klin. Wochenschr.* 15:281, 1902.
14. Carrel A.: Remote results of the replantation of the kidney and the spleen. *J. Exp. Med.* 12:146, 1910.
15. Welch C.S.: A note on transplantation of the whole liver in dogs. *Transplant. Bull.* 2:54, 1955.
16. Goodrich E.O., Welch H.F., Nelson J.A., et al.: Homotransplantation of the canine liver. *Surgery* 29:244, 1956.
17. Paronetto F., Horowitz R.E., Sicular A., et al.: Immunologic observations on homografts: I. The canine liver. *Transplantation* 3:303, 1965.
18. Sicular A., Dreiling D.A., Paronetto F., et al.: Studies of the rejection of the homotransplanted liver. *Surg. Forum* 14:202, 1963.
19. Moore F.D., Wheeler H.B., Demissianos H.V., et al.: Experimental whole-organ transplantation of the liver and of the spleen. *Ann. Surg.* 152:374, 1960.
20. Starzl T.E., Kaupp H.A., Brock D.R., et al.: Reconstructive problems in canine liver homotransplantation with special reference to the postoperative role of hepatic venous flow. *Surg. Gynecol. Obstet.* 111:135, 1960.
21. Starzl T.E., Marchioro T.L., Porter K.A., et al.: Factors determining short and long term survival after orthotopic liver homotransplantation in the dog. *Surgery* 58:131, 1965.
22. Starzl T.E., Kaupp H.A., Brock D.R., et al.: Studies on the rejection of the transplanted homologous dog liver. *Surg. Gynecol. Obstet.* 112:135, 1961.
23. Garnier H., Clot J.P., Bertrand M., et al.: Liver transplantation in the pig: surgical approach. *C.R. Seances Acad Sci. (Paris)* 260:5621, 1965.
24. Calne R.Y., Sells R.A., Pena J.R., et al.: Induction of immunological tolerance by porcine liver allografts. *Nature* 223:472, 1969.
25. Myburgh J.A., Abrahams C., Mendelsohn D., et al.: Colestatic phenomenon in hepatic allograft rejection in the primate. *Transplant. Proc.* 3:501, 1971.
26. Zimmermann F.A., Butcher G.W., Davies H.ff.S., et al.: Techniques for orthotopic liver transplantation in the rat and some studies of the immunologic responses to fully allogeneic liver grafts. *Transplant. Proc.* 11:571, 1979.
27. Roser B.J., Kamada N., Zimmerman F., et al.: Immunosuppressive effect of experimental liver allografts, in Calne R.Y. (ed.): *Liver Transplantation.* London, Grune & Stratton, 1983, pp. 35–54.
28. Mikaeloff P., Pichlmayr R., Rassat J.P., et al.: Orthotopic transplantation of the liver in the dog: II. Immunosuppressive treatment (Imuran and Actinomycin C). *Ann. Chir. Thorac. Cardiovasc.* 4:649, 1965.
29. Starzl T.E., Marchioro T.L., Faris T.D., et al.: Avenues of future research in homotransplantation of the liver: with particular reference to hepatic supportive procedures, antilymphocyte serum, and tissue typing. *Am. J. Surg.* 112:391, 1966.
30. Starzl T.E., Marchioro T.L., Porter K.A., et al.: The use of heterologous antilymphoid agents in canine renal and liver homotransplantation and human renal homotransplantation. *Surg. Gynecol. Obstet.* 124:301, 1967.
31. Mikaeloff P., Pichlmayr R., Rassat J.P., et al.: Orthotopic homotransplantation of the liver in the dog: Immunosuppressive treatment with antilymphocyte serum. *Presse Med.* 75:1967, 1967.
32. Birch A.G., Orr W.M., Duquella J.: Evaluation of horse antidog antilymphocyte globulin in the treatment of hepatic allografts. *Surg. Forum* 19:186, 1968.
33. Starzl T.E., Marchioro T.L., Von Kaulla K.N., et al.: Homotransplantation of the liver in humans. *Surg. Gynecol. Obstet.* 117:659, 1963.

34. Alper C.A., Johnson A.M., Birtch A.G., et al.: Human C'3: Evidence for the liver as the primary site of synthesis. *Science* 163:286, 1963.

35. Birtch A.G., Moore F.D.: Experiences in liver transplantation. *Transplant. Rev.* 2:90, 1969.

36. Fonkalsrud E.W., Stevens G.H., Joseph W.L., et al.: Orthotopic liver allotransplantation using an internal vascular shunt. *Surg. Gynecol. Obstet.* 127:1051, 1968.

37. Daloze P., Delvin E.E., Glorieux F.H., et al.: Replacement therapy for inherited enzyme deficiency: liver orthotopic transplantation in Niemann-Pick disease Type A. *Am. J. Med. Genet.* 1:221, 1977.

38. Lie T.S., Kauffer C., Siedek M., et al.: Prolonged ischemic tolerance time of the human liver with successful grafting. *M.M.W.* 116:1013, 1974.

39. Bechtelsheimer H., Gedigk P., Muller R., et al.: Pathologic anatomic observations after three allogeneic transplantations of the liver in adults. *Virchows Arch. (Pathol. Anat.)* 360:287, 1973.

40. Machado M.D., Moneiro da Cunha J.E., Margarido N.F., et al.: Hyperosmolar coma associated with clinical liver transplantation. *Int. Surg.* 61:368, 1976.

41. Abouna G.M., Preshaw R.M., Silva J.L.U., et al.: Liver transplantation in a patient with cholangiocarcinoma and ulcerative colitis. *Can. Med. Assoc. J.* 115:615, 1976.

42. Fortner J.G., Beattie E.J. Jr., Shiu M.H., et al.: Orthotopic and heterotopic liver homografts in man. *Ann. Surg.* 172:23, 1970.

43. Hume D.M., Wolf J.S., Lee H.M., et al.: Liver transplantation. *Transplant. Proc.* 4:781, 1972.

44. Lampe E.W., Simmons R.L., Najarian J.S., et al.: Hyper-glycemic nonketotic coma after liver transplantation. *Arch. Surg.* 105:774, 1973.

45. Orr W.M., Charlesworth D., Mallick N.P., et al.: Liver transplantation in man after an extended period of preservation by a simple technique. *Br. Med. J.* 4:28, 1969.

46. Aune S., Schistad G., Skulberg A., et al.: Human liver transplantation without azathioprine. *Surg. Gynecol. Obstet.* 135:727, 1972.

47. Starzl T.E., Koep L., Porter K.A., et al.: Decline in survival after liver transplantation. *Arch. Surg.* 115:815, 1980.

48. Calne R.Y., Rolles K., White D.J.G., et al.: Cyclosporin A initially as the only immunosuppressant in 34 patients of cadaveric organs; 32 kidneys, 2 pancreases, and 2 livers. *Lancet* 2:1033, 1979.

49. Calne R.Y., White D.J.G., Evans D.B., et al.: Cyclosporin A in cadaveric organ transplantation. *Br. Med. J.* 282:934, 1981.

50. Calne R.Y., Rolles K., White D.J.G., et al.: Cyclosporin A in clinical organ grafting. *Transplant. Proc.* 13:349, 1981.

51. Starzl T.E., Iwatsuki S., Klintmalm G., et al.: Liver transplantation 1980, with particular reference to cyclosporin A. *Transplant. Proc.* 13:281, 1981.

52. Starzl T.E., Klintmalm G.B.G., Weil R. III, et al.: Liver transplantation with the use of cyclosporin A and prednisone. *N. Engl. J. Med.* 305:266, 1981.

53. Brolsch C.H.E., Neuhaus P., Pichlmayr R.: Gegenwartiger Stand der Leber—Transplantation. *Z. Gastroenterologie* 20:117, 1982.

54. Gips C.H., Krom R.A., de Groot E.H., et al.: The fate of 30 patients for whom liver transplantation was considered during the period 1977 to 1979 included, and actually performed in 7 of them. *Ned. Tijdschr. Geneeskd.* 125:868, 1981.

55. Stuart F.: Need, supply and legal issues related to organ transplantation in the United States. *Transplant. Proc.* 16:87, 1984.

56. Bart K., Macon E.J., Humphries A.L. Jr., et al.: Cadaveric kidneys for transplantation: a paradox of shortage in the face of plenty. *Transplantation* 31:383, 1981.

57. Cooper K.: The potential supply of cadaveric kidneys for transplantation. *Trans. Am. Soc. Artif. Intern. Organs* 23:416, 1977.

58. Denny D.: Testimony on organ procurement and distribution for transplantation. Subcommittee on Investigations and Oversight of the Committee on Science and Technology, U.S. House of Representatives, 98th Congress. *Organ Transplants*. U.S. Government Printing Office: 134, 1983.

59. Denny D.: Organ procurement for transplantation in the United States, *Transplant. Today* 1:41, 1984.

60. Shaw B.W. Jr., Hakala T., Rosenthal J.T., et al.: Combination donor hepatectomy and nephrectomy and early functional results of allografts. *Surg. Gynecol. Obstet.* 155:321, 1982.

61. Shaw B.W. Jr., Rosenthal J.T., Griffith B.P., et al.: Techniques for combined procurement of hearts and kidneys with satisfactory early function of renal allografts. *Surg. Gynecol. Obstet.* 157:261, 1983.

62. Shaw B.W. Jr., Rosenthal J.T., Hardesty R.L., et al.: Early function of heart, liver and kidney allografts following combined procurement. *Transplant. Proc.* 16:238, 1984.

63. Rosenthal J.T., Shaw B.W. Jr., Hardesty R.L., et al.: Principles of multiple organ procurement from cadaveric donors. *Ann. Surg.* 198:617, 1983.

64. Starzl T.E., Hakala T., Shaw B.W. Jr., et al.: A flexible procedure for multiple cadaveric organ procurement. *Surg. Gynecol. Obstet.* 158:223, 1984.

65. Bersohn M.M., Shine K.I.: Verapamil protection of ischemic isolated rabbit heart: dependence on pretreatment. *J. Mol. Cell. Cardiol.* 15:659, 1983.

66. Ishigami M., Magnusson M.O., Stowe N.T., et al.: The salutary effect of verapamil and d-propranolol in ischemically damaged kidneys. *Transplant. Proc.* 16:40, 1984.

67. Papadimitriou M, Alexopoulos V., Vargemezis V., et al.: The effect of preventive administration of verapamil on acute ischemic renal failure in dogs. *Transplant. Proc.* 16:44, 1984.

68. Szabo S., Usadel K.H.: Cytoprotection—organoprotection by somatostatin: gastric and hepatic lesions. *Experientia* 38:254, 1982.

69. Marubayashi S., Dohi K., Ezaki H., et al.: Preservation of ischemic rat liver mitochondrial functions and liver viability with CoQ_{10}. *Surgery* 91:631, 1982.

70. Marubarashi S., Dohi K., Ezaki H., et al.: Preservation of ischemic liver cell—prevention of damage by coenzyme Q_{10}. *Transplant. Proc.* 15:1297, 1983.

71. Monden M., Toyoshima K., Gotoh M., et al.: Effect of coenzyme Q_{10} on cadaveric liver transplantation in dogs. *Transplant. Proc.* 16:138, 1984.

72. Monden M., Fortner J.G.: Twenty four and 48-hour canine liver preservation by simple hypothermia with prostacyclin. *Ann. Surg.* 196:38, 1982.

73. Ghuman S.S., Rush B.F. Jr. Machiedo G.W., et al.: Effect of prostaglandin on cell membrane permeability and hepatic high-energy stores following hemorrhagic shock. *J. Surg. Res.* 32:484, 1982.

74. Makowka L., Falk R.E., Cohen M.M., et al.: Protective effect of 16,16-dimethyl prostaglandin E_2 on acute ethanol induced inhibition of hepatic regeneration. *Surg. Forum* 33:183, 1982.

75. Miyazaki M., Makowka L., Falk R.E., et al.: Protection of thermochemotherapeutic-induced lethal acute hepatic necrosis in the rat by 16,16-dimethyl prostaglandin E_2. *J. Surg. Res.* 34:415, 1983.

76. Pegg D.E.: The future of organ preservation. *Transplant. Proc.* 16:147, 1984.

77. Brettschneider L., Kolff J., Smith G.V., et al.: An evaluation of perfusion and constituents in liver preservation. *Surg. Forum* 19:354, 1968.

78. Brettschneider L., Bell P., Martin A.J., et al.: Conservation of the liver. *Transplant Proc.* 1:132, 1969.

79. Spees E.K., Vaughn W.K., Mendez-Picon G., et al.: Preservation methods do not affect cadaver renal allograft outcome: The SEOPF prospective study 1977–1982. *Transplant. Proc.* 16:177, 1984.

80. van der Vliet J.A., Vroemen J.P.A.M., Cohen B., et al.: Comparison of cadaver kidney preservation methods in Eurotransplant. *Transplant. Proc.* 16:180, 1984.

81. Shaw B.W. Jr., Gordon R.D., Iwatsuki S., et al.: Hepatic retransplantation. *Transplant. Proc.* 17(suppl.) In press.

82. Neuberger J., Portmann B., Macdougall B.R., et al.: Recurrence of primary biliary cirrhosis after liver transplantation. *N. Engl. J. Med.* 306:1, 1982.

83. Wight D.G.D.: Pathology of liver transplantation (other than rejection), in Calne R.Y. (ed.): *Liver Transplantation*. London, Grune & Stratton, 1983, pp. 289–316.

84. Huber C., Niederwieser D., Schonitzer D., et al.: Liver trans-

plantation by high dose cyclophosphamide, total body irradiation and autologous bone marrow transplantation for treatment of metastatic breast cancer: A case report. *Transplantation* 37:311, 1984.

85. Craig J.R., Peters R.L., Edmondson H.A., et al.: Fibrolamellar carcinoma of the liver: a tumor of adolescents and young adults with distinctive clinicopathologic features. *Cancer* 46:372, 1980.

86. Berman M.M., Libbey N.P., Foster, J.H.: Hepatocellular carcinoma: polygonal cell type with fibrous stroma—an atypical variant with a favorable prognosis. *Cancer* 46:1448, 1980.

87. Edmondson H.A.: Differential diagnosis of tumors and tumor-like lesions of the liver in infancy and childhood. *Am. J. Dis. Child.* 91:168, 1956.

88. Peters R.L.: Pathology of hepatocellular carcinoma, in Okuda K., Peters R.L. (eds.): *Hepatocellular Carcinoma.* New York, John Wiley & Sons, 1975, pp. 107–168.

89. Hood J., Koep L., Peters R., et al.: Liver transplantation for advanced liver disease with alpha$_1$-antitrypsin deficiency. *N. Engl. J. Med.* 302:272, 1980.

90. Deiss A., Lynch R.E., Lee G.R., et al.: Long term therapy of Wilson's disease. *Ann. Intern. Med.* 75:57, 1971.

91. Starzl T.E., Zitelli B.J., Shaw B.W. Jr., et al.: Changing concepts: liver replacement for hereditary tyrosinemia and hepatoma. *J. Pediatr.* In press.

92. Starzl T.E., Bilheimer D.W., Bahnson H.T., et al.: Heart-liver transplantation in a patient with familial hypercholesterolemia. *Lancet* 1:1382, 1984.

93. National Institutes of Health Consensus Development Conference Statement: Liver Transplantation—June 20–23, 1983. *Hepatology* 4(supp. 1):107S, 1984.

94. De Nicola P.: *Thromboelastography.* Springfield, Ill., Charles C Thomas Publisher, 1957.

95. Denmark S.W., Shaw B.W. Jr., Griffith B.P., et al.: Veno-venous bypass without systemic anticoagulation in canine and human liver transplantation. *Surg. Forum* 34:380, 1983.

96. Shaw B.W. Jr., Martin D.J., Marquez J.M., et al.: Venous bypass in clinical liver transplantation. *Ann. Surg.* 200:524, 1984.

97. Starzl T.E., Schneck S.A., Mazzoni G., et al.: Acute neurological complications after liver transplantation with particular reference to intraoperative cerebral air embolus. *Ann. Surg.* 187:236, 1978.

98. Calne R.Y.: A new technique for biliary drainage in orthotopic liver transplantation utilizing the gall bladder as a pedicle graft conduit between the donor and recipient common bile ducts. *Ann. Surg.* 186:605, 1976.

99. Fortner J.G., Yeh S.D.J., Kim D.K., et al.: The case for and technique of heterotopic liver grafting. *Transplant. Proc.* 11:269, 1979.

100. Houssin D., Berthelot P., Franco D., et al.: Heterotopic liver transplantation in end-stage HBsAg positive cirrhosis. *Lancet* 1:990, 1980.

101. Marchioro T.L., Porter K.A., Dickinsin T.C., et al.: Physiologic requirements for auxiliary liver homotransplantation. *Surg. Gynecol. Obstet.* 121:17, 1965.

102. Starzl T.E., Terblanche J.: Hepatotrophic substances, in Popper H., Schaffner F., (eds.): *Progress in Liver Disease.* New York, Grune & Stratton, 1979, pp. 135–152.

103. Starzl T.E., Koep L.J., Weil R. III, et al.: Development of a suprahepatic recipient vena cava cuff for liver transplantation. *Surg. Gynecol. Obstet.* 149:76, 1979.

PART VI

Pancreatic Disease

30

Injuries to the Pancreas

ARTHUR J. DONOVAN, M.D.
ALBERT E. YELLIN, M.D.

INJURIES to the organs in the right upper quadrant may pose formidable challenges to the surgeon. The liver, duodenum, and pancreas are in relatively fixed positions that render them liable to the shear effects of blunt trauma. Resectional and reconstructive surgery to these organs is technically more difficult than that for the remainder of the GI tract, the spleen, or the genitourinary tract. The risk of serious postoperative complications is high, particularly if the injuries are not initially identified and properly treated. There may be concurrent injury to the major blood vessels in the area. These generalities are particularly applicable to injuries of the pancreas.

HISTORY

The first report of pancreatic injury due to blunt trauma is believed to be that of Travers in 1827.[1] A young woman was struck by the wheel of a stagecoach and died. At autopsy, she was found to have a completely transected pancreas. Only five injuries to the pancreas from penetrating trauma were reported by the Surgeon General during the American Civil War.[2]

Among the earliest discussion of rational therapy for pancreatic injury is that included in the remarkable address of Mikulicz-Redecki to the Congress of American Physicians and Surgeons in 1903.[3] This was the first article in *Annals of Surgery* for July of that year and was entitled "Surgery of the Pancreas." He regretted the "tardy development of surgery of the pancreas" and listed "three general reasons":

"First, the topographical relations of the organ should be considered."

The technical problems of exposure, the preferable routes by which the pancreas can be explored, the need for mobilization of the head to examine completely the organ, and the high incidence of often lethal injury to surrounding organs were all considered. He emphasized that because of the severity of associated injuries, the pancreatic injury may be overlooked:

Another factor that has prevented the advancement of pancreatic surgery is the difficulty in diagnosis. . . . Even today, assisted by a variety of diagnostic modalities that include peritoneal lavage, ultrasound, computerized axial tomography (CAT), and endoscopic retrograde cholangiopancreatography (ERCP), diagnosis of pancreatic injury remains difficult.

A third reason which has prevented the rapid development of pancreatic surgery is that the operation, so far as it includes the organ itself, is much more dangerous than an operation upon any other abdominal organ. . . . A danger much greater than that from hemorrhage—is that due to the special secretion of the gland leaking from the injured parenchyma in larger or smaller quantities . . . injuries of the pancreas . . . seriously affect the peritoneum and the neighboring tissues . . . it prepares a nutrient medium for bacterial invasion and makes infection extremely easy.

Mikulicz-Redecki did not believe that one could reliably prevent pancreatic secretions from leaking into the peritoneal cavity by turning the pancreas "inward" and by closing the gland with deep sutures. He advocated the use of sutures to control hemorrhage and placement of drains to the "exposed pancreas." Pseudocyst as a complication of pancreatic injury was clearly recognized. Early operation, thorough exploration of the pancreas, hemostasis, and generous drainage are the basic principles that we pursue today in the treatment of pancreatic injury. They were all advocated by Mikulicz-Redecki over 80 years ago.

Subsequent notable developments in treatment of pancreatic injury have been importantly related to attempts to negate the effects of disruption of the major pancreatic ducts. Although Garré in 1905 resutured the gland,[4] it remained for Newton in 1929 to attempt to reanastomose the pancreatic duct.[5] A pseudocyst developed. Doubilet and Mulholland[6] advocated duodenotomy and transampullary insertion of a small plastic catheter into the duct of Wirsung. This catheter was used as a stent and passed into the separated distal segment of the gland in an attempt to promote healing of the duct. Walton[7] in 1930 recommended distal pancreatectomy for disruption of the pancreas. In 1959 Letton and Wilson[8] established Roux-en-Y jejunal drainage of the distal segment in two cases of pancreatic transection. Jones and Shires[9] used a Roux-en-Y jejunal segment to drain both the head and the distal segment of the divided pancreas. Selected examples of these operations are depicted in Figure 30–1.

In this chapter the term "distal pancreas" will refer to that portion of the gland remote from the ampulla of Vater and "proximal pancreas" to that portion nearer to the ampulla of Vater. This is consistent with common usage, but is the direct opposite of the terminology employed with respect to the common bile duct that joins the pancreatic duct to enter the

WALTON - 1923   DOUBILET AND MULHOLLAND - 1963

LETTON - 1959   JONES AND SHIRES - 1965

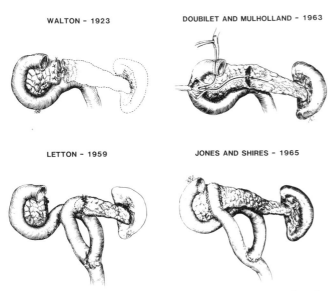

Fig 30–1.—Four suggested techniques for repair of major pancreatic injury. (From Fitzgibbons, T.J., Yellin A.E., Maruyama M.M., et al.: Management of the transected pancreas following distal pancreatectomy. *Surg. Gynecol. Obstet.* 154:225, 1982. Used by permission.)

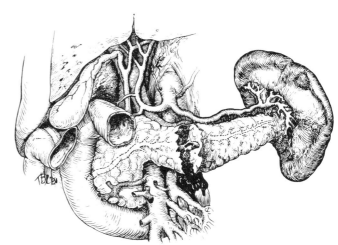

Fig 30–2.—A typical prevertebral fracture of the pancreas. (From Fitzgibbons T.J., Yellin A.E., Maruyama M.M., et al.: Management of the transected pancreas following distal pancreatectomy. *Surg. Gynecol. Obstet.* 154:225, 1982. Used by permission.)

duodenum at the ampulla of Vater. The distal common bile duct is generally accepted to be that portion nearest to the ampulla of Vater.

The incidence of pancreatic injuries has clearly increased during recent decades. Accidents involving vehicles traveling at high speed and the increasing violence of urban society are significant factors in this regard. Northrup estimated that the pancreas was injured in 2% of all abdominal injuries.[10]

NATURE OF PANCREATIC INJURY

Injury to the pancreas from blunt trauma occurs when there is a forceful blow in the upper abdomen that compresses the pancreas. The offending agent is most frequently the steering wheel of a car, but the handles of a bicycle or a motorcycle, or a rapidly moving free object, such as a surfboard or a human fist, or foot, may be the cause. In its retroperitoneal position, the pancreas may be only contused, or an overt disruption of pancreatic substance may result. Contusion may lead to capillary leakage, minor hemorrhage reflected as petechiae, and to pancreatic cellular disruption at the microscopic level. When the pancreas is compressed against the vertebral column by force applied in the epigastrium, a prevertebral fracture of the pancreas can occur. The fracture is usually just to the left of the superior mesenteric vessels. Small venous tributaries are torn, and a peripancreatic hematoma develops that obscures the fracture. Major vascular injury is unusual. The pancreatic fracture itself may be complete or incomplete. An incomplete fracture can involve the posterior portion of the gland with an intact anterior "capsule." Injury to the pancreatic ducts is most unlikely to result from blunt trauma in the absence of overt disruption of the pancreas. We have never encountered such a case. Figure 30–2 is an illustration of a prevertebral fracture of the pancreas.

When the force is applied from the right anterior or lateral aspect of the abdomen, the head of the pancreas may be crushed against the vertebral column. Synchronous injury to the head of the pancreas and a "blow out" injury of the duodenum may occur. If the force is extreme, the common bile duct can be avulsed from the liver or pancreas. Major vessels in the portahepatis or behind the pancreas may be torn.

Any penetrating wound that involves the upper abdomen can injure the pancreas. When the pancreas is injured owing to penetrating trauma, injury to adjacent organs is the rule rather than the exception. These organs are the stomach, transverse colon, duodenum, liver, small intestine, spleen, and kidney, as well as the major vessels around the pancreas, including the portal and superior mesenteric veins, splenic vein, aorta, superior mesenteric artery, and vena cava. Even a brief contemplation of the anatomical relations of the pancreas will establish that it is almost impossible for a knife or bullet to reach the pancreas without inflicting injury to another organ. On the contrary, the pancreas is often the only organ injured with blunt trauma. The likelihood of pancreatic injury from a posterior abdominal stab wound is very low— only two instances among 465 such cases.[11]

The critical determinant in injuries to the pancreas is the nature of the injury to the ducts. If only a contusion occurs, without a major leak of pancreatic exocrine secretions from the substance of the pancreas and into the peripancreatic tissues, only mild clinical manifestations of injury will occur, such as transient hyperamylasemia. When overt disruption of pancreas occurs, the possibility of duct injury exists. With a small laceration in the tail, only a minor duct may be opened. With a fracture owing to blunt trauma or a deep penetrating wound, a major duct may be divided. For purposes of these discussions, major duct is defined as the duct of Wirsung or Santorini. Varying degrees of peripancreatic inflammation can develop if duct injury exists and there is continuing leak of pancreatic secretions into the peripancreatic tissue. Proteolytic and lipolytic enzymes when activated cause tissue necrosis and invite subsequent hemorrhage. Bacterial invasion can follow with development of pancreatic abscess. Erosion into the GI tract can occur. A pancreatic pseudocyst may form, although it may not become apparent for several weeks. We have encountered cases of free communication between the duct system and the peritoneal cavity leading to "pancreatic ascites." If a major duct injury is treated surgically by external drainage, a pancreatic fistula may become established. An established fistula is defined as one that persists longer than two months without spontaneous closure. A fistula becomes established because the injured duct does not heal or heals with a stricture. Secretions from the distal pancreas continue to egress along the drains. Pancreatitis may develop in the inadequately drained distal pancreas. If the duct proximal to the injury is not obstructed, any fistula drainage from the proximal pancreas will ultimately cease as the exocrine secretions drain through the ampulla of Vater into the duodenum. The likelihood of development of these serious complications is unknown. With timely diagnosis and utilization of the appropriate treatments, discussed subsequently, their incidence should be very low to nonexistent.

Pancreatic injury that is associated with a duodenal injury is a particularly difficult problem that has been associated with a high incidence of regional complications. Among nine cases that we reported in 1966, there were 17 major regional complications of the injury itself and three deaths, or a 33% mortality.[12] The exact reason for this high morbidity has not been established. Leakage of pancreatic juice onto the external surface of a freshly sutured wound in a contused duodenum may lead to disruption of the suture line. A fistula that occurs at or distal to the ampulla of Vater has, in the past, been associated with a very high mortality, and the majority have not closed spontaneously.[13] The current widespread utilization of parenteral and enteral nutrition has had a favorable impact on the adverse consequences of such a sidewall duodenal fistula. When nutrition is maintained, the fistula may close.

Associated injuries to major vessels is common, particularly with penetrating injury of the pancreas. Such wounds, rather than the pancreatic injury, are often the major injury. Indeed, when pancreatic injury occurs concomitant with major vascular injury, mortality is most often the consequence of hemorrhage from the injury to the aorta, superior mesenteric artery, or vena cavae or portal venous system, and not the result of the pancreatic injury.

EVALUATION

Injuries of the pancreas owing to penetrating trauma are generally identified during surgical exploration of the abdomen undertaken for treatment of a stab or gunshot wound. The application of nonsurgical techniques to detect pancreatic injury is a major consideration in blunt trauma.

The typical patient with pancreatic injury from blunt trauma is admitted to the hospital with a complaint of mild upper abdominal pain, with slight to moderate upper abdominal tenderness, and with voluntary rigidity of the upper abdominal musculature. Occasionally, clear evidence of peritonitis with involuntary rigidity of abdominal musculature, absence of bowel sounds, and marked tenderness are present

on admission. Even with serious pancreatic injury, these latter findings more often evolve over the initial few hours of observation.

A pancreatic injury may first be suspected because of an elevation of the serum amylase. The serum amylase will be elevated in approximately 90% of patients with pancreatic injury caused by blunt trauma but in only about one half caused by penetrating trauma.[14] The absence of hyperamylasemia does not provide any ensurance that there is not major pancreatic injury. Conversely, the serum amylase may be modestly elevated without pancreatic injury in cases of duodenal perforation. Amylase-rich duodenal fluid leaks from the duodenum and is presumably absorbed through the peritoneum into the bloodstream, producing hyperamylasemia.

When the patient with hyperamylasemia is to undergo exploratory celiotomy because of other indications, the cause of hyperamylasemia will be established during the operation. Further preoperative investigation of hyperamylasemia is not indicated. Should the patient have only mild epigastric tenderness, if bowel sounds are present and muscle rigidity is absent, the question of whether hyperamylasemia could be due to duodenal perforation must be resolved. Retroperitoneal perforation of the duodenum can be reflected in minimal physical findings in the early hours after injury. A patient with retroperitoneal perforation of the duodenum may mistakenly be treated as a case of mild acute pancreatitis of insufficient severity to require surgery. Serious consequences of retroperitoneal perforation of the duodenum may develop before the injury is recognized. Therefore, our policy has been to perform an upper GI series with water-soluble contrast mediums in such cases to exclude a perforation of the duodenum masquerading as mild acute pancreatitis. A case of retroperitoneal perforation of the duodenum due to blunt trauma with initially minimal physical findings is depicted in Figure 30–3.

The provisional diagnosis in the patient with blunt abdominal trauma, hyperamylasemia, equivocal physical findings, and a negative gastroduodenogram will be pancreatic injury, and the question of indication for surgery will still exist. The patient can be observed over a period of hours to detect increasing abdominal tenderness, involuntary muscle rigidity, decreasing or absent bowel sounds, or "third spacing"—all suggestions of a progressive intra-abdominal process. Special diagnostic procedures can be performed in an attempt to resolve more rapidly the question of major pancreatic injury. Such studies may also provide intraoperative guidance to the surgeon.

We believe that peritoneal lavage has limited application in the attempt to detect pancreatic injury. The level of amylase in the peritoneal fluid may not be elevated with pancreatic trauma, reflecting the retroperitoneal location of the organ. Conversely, elevation of amylase in the fluid does not mean that there is a pancreatic injury of sufficient magnitude to require definitive surgical treatment.

It was hoped that the newer imaging techniques, such as ultrasound and CAT scan, would assist in evaluation of acute injury to retroperitoneal structures such as the pancreas, but they have proved disappointing. Ultrasound is often able to identify peripancreatic fluid collections, such as hematoma, but rarely can identify pancreatic disruption. The ileus that

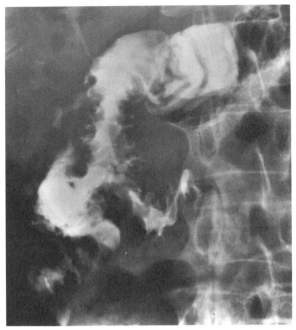

Fig 30–3.—This diatrizoate (Hypaque) gastroduodenogram was performed with water-soluble contrast medium in a 23-year-old man with blunt trauma to the upper abdomen. On admission examination he had moderate upper abdominal tenderness, bowel sounds, but no abdominal muscle rigidity. Temperature was 38°C and WBCs 13,000/cc. Serum amylase was 325 units (normal 75–140 U/L). Leak of contrast media from retroperitoneal perforation of the duodenum is apparent. (From Fitzgibbons T.J., Yellin A.E., Maruyama M.M., et al.: Management of the transected pancreas following distal pancreatectomy. *Surg. Gynecol. Obstet.* 154:225, 1982. Used by permission.)

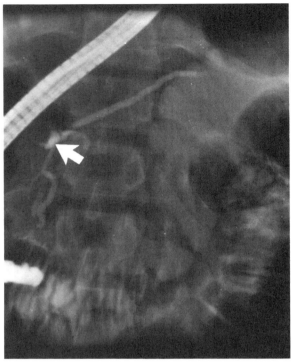

Fig 30–4.—This ERCP was performed in a patient who sustained blunt abdominal trauma and who on admission to the hospital had a bruise in the epigastrium. The physical examination revealed only mild epigastric tenderness. The serum amylase was 750 units (normal 75–140 U/L). Leak of contrast *(arrow)* from a prevertebral fracture of the pancreas is apparent in the ERCP performed within four hours of injury.

frequently accompanies abdominal trauma markedly reduces the efficacy of ultrasound. CAT scan has been evaluated in over 500 patients at the trauma unit of San Francisco General Hospital.[15] It was much less reliable in identifying pancreatic injury than injuries to the liver or spleen, where it is highly accurate. In most cases, the plane of laceration within the pancreas could not be detected. Secondary changes suggestive of pancreatic injury often are not evident until 12 hours postinjury.

The exact role of ERCP in the early evaluation of suspected pancreatic injury is not precisely established but in our experience it has been useful. A retrograde pancreatic ductogram may demonstrate an intact duct. This supports the diagnosis of pancreatic contusion. In the absence of progressive signs of peritoneal irritation and with a negative gastroduodenogram, nonoperative therapy can be pursued. More important, disruption of the duct system may be demonstrated, an indication for surgical exploration and a finding that may assist the surgeon's intraoperative planning. A prevertebral fracture of the pancreas with division of the duct of Wirsung as detected by preoperative ERCP is depicted in Figure 30–4. ERCP should be performed with infusion of dye into the pancreatic duct by gentle pressure, since forceful injection can provoke acute pancreatitis. If any diagnostic study reliably documents the presence of a major pancreatic injury, such as

laceration of the pancreatic duct or disruption of pancreatic substance, exploratory celiotomy is indicated, even in the absence of overt signs of peritonitis.

The principal problems in patients who are seen over variable periods following blunt abdominal trauma with late consequences of unrecognized or inappropriately treated pancreatic injury are those of pseudocyst, persistent pancreatitis, or pancreatic fistula. Pancreatic abscesses, pancreatic ascites or hemorrhage are less frequent. Ultrasound or CAT scan may disclose a pseudocyst or abscess. ERCP may reveal disruption of the ductal system with an abrupt cutoff or with a stricture. If the patient underwent initial surgical exploration with peripancreatic drainage and an established pancreatic fistula developed, injection of water-soluble contrast medium through the fistula tract may identify a communication with the distal fragment of the pancreas (Fig 30–5). These special imaging techniques alone or in combination will usually identify precisely the nature of the late consequences of unrecognized or inadequately treated pancreatic injury.

SURGERY

Exploration

In cases of abdominal trauma, the abdomen is best explored through a midline abdominal incision. Mikulicz-Redecki in 1903[3] stated with reference to pancreatic injury:

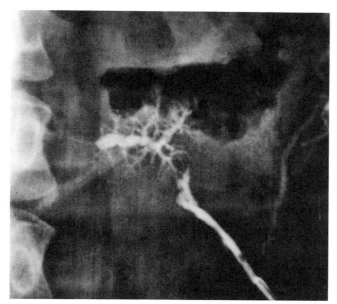

Fig 30–5.—Drains were placed to the side of a pancreatic injury six months before this fistulogram was performed with water-soluble contrast medium. The medium has entered the dilated duct system of a distal fragment of pancreas that is separated from the body of the gland.

With the uncertainty of diagnosis it is best to make the incision, as a rule, in the median above the umbilicus. This is also true for penetrating wounds which lie some distance from the midline. From this midline incision, one can best determine what changes are present in the peritoneal cavity, and can enlarge the incision above, below or to one side, as needed, exposing the pancreas according to the location of injury.

This advice remains timely and relevant.

The entire pancreas must be examined meticulously if pancreatic injury is suspected. A Kocher maneuver is performed to mobilize the head of the pancreas so its posterior aspect can be elevated and the region of the uncinate process can be scrutinized. The pancreas within the lesser peritoneal bursa must be exposed. In a thin patient, this can occasionally be accomplished by incising the gastrohepatic ligament. Usually the lesser peritoneal sac must be opened by dividing the gastrocolic ligament. An injury to the pancreas may be readily apparent when the lesser sac is explored, but usually with such injury there is a hematoma about the pancreas. This masking hematoma (Fig 30–6) must be evacuated to identify the pancreatic injury. Failure to evacuate a peripancreatic hematoma is the most common reason for a surgeon to overlook a major pancreatic injury.[16]

In searching for a prevertebral fracture of the pancreas, after any hematoma is evacuated, the loose areolar tissues along the superior and inferior margins of the pancreas should be incised. A finger may then be slipped behind the pancreas. On occasion, a dorsal fracture of the pancreas will be identified when the anterior pancreatic capsule is intact. The fracture is not apparent on visualization of the ventral surface of the gland.

A most difficult technical problem is controlling hemorrhage from and repairing the major vessels that lie behind the pancreas. The superior mesenteric artery and the portal ve-

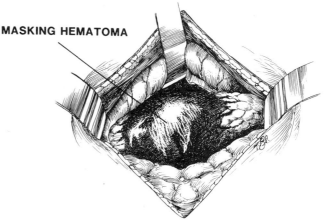

Fig 30–6.—Masking hematoma. The lesser peritoneal sac has been entered by dividing the gastrocolic ligament. A hematoma overlies the midportion of the pancreas and masks an underlying prevertebral fracture.

nous system can be manually compressed between the surgeon's left thumb, which is placed on the anterior aspect of the pancreas, and the index and middle fingers, inserted through the foramen of Winslow and onto the posterior aspect of these vessels (Fig 30–7). Exposure of the vessels posterior to the neck of the pancreas for proximal and distal control and for repair is a surgical challange. One method is to lift the pancreas off the vessels at the site of vascular injury and to transect it. Such a transection of the pancreas usually cannot be achieved speedily under any circumstances, particularly while attempting simultaneously to control the hemorrhage. A preferred approach is to control hemorrhage with pressure, as described above, or by direct pressure applied to the site of injury, and to expose the mesenteric vessels by mobilization of the spleen and the pancreas from their beds. These organs are elevated from left to right until the mesenteric vessels are reached. This approach is discussed in detail in the section of this chapter that concerns distal pancreatectomy.

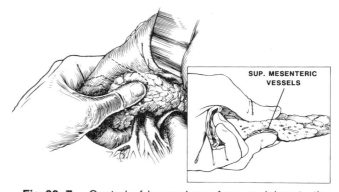

Fig 30–7.—Control of hemorrhage from an injury to the mesenteric vessels that lie behind the head and neck of the pancreas can often be achieved by insertion of the index and middle fingers through the foramen of Winslow, compressing the vessels between these fingers and the thumb, which is placed on the anterior aspect of the pancreas. These relationships are more precisely depicted in the inset *(lower right)*.

When the entire pancreas has been exposed, the surgeon must decide whether there is injury to a major duct, which may have been determined by a preoperative ERCP. This will importantly influence decisions as to surgical treatment. An overt disruption to the gland that clearly involves the duct of Wirsung may be obvious. When a duodenal injury is present through which the ampulla of Vater may be identified, a small polyethylene tube may be inserted and a pancreatic ductogram performed to establish the integrity of the major ducts. This can be particularly useful in a penetrating wound that involves both the duodenum and the head of the pancreas.

A suggestion has been made that in cases of traumatic pancreatitis with hyperamylasemia but not overt pancreatic disruption, the duodenum should be opened and the ampulla cannulated or the tail of the pancreas amputated to obtain a pancreatic ductogram.[17] We do not believe that the yield in identification of injury to a major duct can justify the potential morbidity of these procedures. As already stated, we have never encountered disruption of a major duct in the absence of overt disruption of pancreatic substance.

The most difficult questions arise when there is a penetrating wound into the pancreatic substance or when a fracture involves pancreatic substance but there is uncertainty as to whether the major ducts are injured. In the final analysis, the surgeon must decide the probability of major duct injury based on his experience. Our policy has been to assume injury to a major duct if the wound or fracture penetrates deeply into the substance of the pancreas.

SURGICAL OPTIONS

The optimal surgical procedure for a pancreatic injury avoids regional complications such as established pancreatic fistula, pseudocyst, abscess, hemorrhage, or pancreatitis, minimizes the possibility of pancreatic endocrine or exocrine insufficiency, and has an inherently low risk of mortality. The principal surgical procedures that have been recommended for pancreatic injury should be evaluated against these aforementioned goals.

EXTERNAL DRAINAGE.—Liberal drainage of the pancreas is a routine component of all operations for pancreatic injury. Soft Penrose drains are placed to the site of pancreatic injury and brought out of the abdomen through a stab wound in the flank. When the injury is a pancreatic contusion without disruption of pancreatic substance, leakage of pancreatic secretions is most unlikely, but these drains should permit its egress. A contusion of the pancreas treated by drainage is depicted in Figure 30–8. If there is any disruption of pancreatic substance, the placement of a soft sump drain is also recommended. If there is not an injury to a major duct, any pancreatic fistula that develops should be transient. If a major duct is injured, drainage with Penrose drains with or without sump suction but without a more definitive procedure may result in pancreatic fistula, pseudocyst, or chronic pancreatitis. The exact risk of these complications is unknown. Penrose drains should be quarantined in sterile plastic bags to minimize the danger of nosocomial infection. Several sump drains have been designed with a closed or filtered system that should reduce the risk of retrograde contamination. Sump

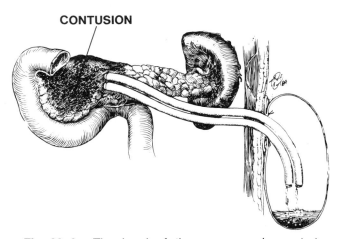

Fig 30–8.—The head of the pancreas demonstrates edema and petechial hemorrhage consequent to blunt trauma. Overt disruption of pancreatic substance has not occurred. Penrose drains have been placed to the head of the pancreas. A sterile wound bag is placed around these drains where they exit from the abdomen. The bag is intended to quarantine the drains and to reduce the likelihood of nosocomial infection.

drains, even of the soft type, are removed by the fifth day because of risk of erosion into a blood vessel or into the GI tract.

ENTERIC DRAINAGE TO THE SITE OF INJURY TO A MAJOR DUCT.—A Roux-en-Y loop of jejunum may be fashioned, as suggested by Jones and Shires,[9] and brought up to the pancreas at the site of a complete fracture. The end of the loop is closed. Both proximal and distal ends of the transected pancreas are implanted into the sides of the loop. When the pancreas is not totally transected but division of the duct of Wirsung is obvious, the remaining pancreas is divided to facilitate the procedure. This operation was recommended by Jones and Shires for a fracture well to the right of the midline when they believed that resection of the distal pancreas might lead to pancreatic endocrine or exocrine insufficiency or both. Drainage of both segments of the pancreas into a Roux-en-Y loop is a rather complex and time-consuming operation. Leakage from the site of anastomosis invites the development of a peripancreatic abscess and enteric or pancreatic fistula. Pancreaticoenterostomy is not recognized as a highly secure anastomosis. This operation should reduce the risk of pseudocyst and pancreatitis and ensure endocrine and exocrine function. In practice, anastomosis of the proximal pancreas to the jejunum to ensure pancreatic exocrine drainage is not necessary. A fistula from the proximal gland would be transient. Drainage into the duodenum through the ampulla of Vater will be reestablished in the natural course of events, unless there is obstruction in the duct of Wirsung in the proximal pancreas. Rather than anastomosis of both the proximal and distal pancreas to a Roux-en-Y loop, the pancreatic duct in the proximal segment may be ligated and the distal pancreas implanted into the Roux-en-Y loop. The proximal pancreas will drain through the ampulla of Vater. This operation was suggested by Letton and Wilson.[8] It should reduce the likelihood of established fistula and other regional pancreatic complications, as well as ensure endocrine and exocrine function. As in the case of a double Roux-en-Y anastomosis, there is the risk of a leak from the suture line. The operation is moderately complex, and its use must be balanced against the magnitude of associated injuries, the intraoperative condition of the patient, and the potential for development of endocrine and exocrine insufficiency should the distal pancreas be resected. We believe this risk to be low. These procedures are depicted graphically in Fig 30–1.

DIRECT REPAIR OF THE PANCREAS.—Suture of the pancreatic capsule[18] or reconstruction of the duct of Wirsung has been attempted in recent years.[19, 20] Suture of the capsule should be unnecessary if a major duct is not injured and would be unlikely to be effective in preventing pancreatic complications if a major duct is divided. Doubilet and Mulholland[6] recommended that the duodenum be opened for transampullary cannulation of the duct of Wirsung. A plastic tube was passed through the duct, out of the proximal segment, and into the duct in the distal separated segment. The operation was designed to permit drainage of the segments and to allow the duct to heal. Pellegrine and Stein[19] reported successful direct suture of the pancreatic duct. These procedures for repair of the pancreatic duct have not been widely adopted. To open the intact duodenum in a case of major pancreatic injury invites a postoperative duodenal fistula. The likelihood of long-term success of pancreatic duct repair is questionable—the duct is small, leakage at the site of repair with fistula or pseudocyst seems likely, and stricture with distal pancreatitis is a possibility.

DISTAL PANCREATECTOMY WITH OR WITHOUT SPLENECTOMY.—The pancreas distal to the site of injury can be resected as a definitive surgical procedure. The operation is easier if the spleen is removed and if the pancreatic injury is to the left of the superior mesenteric vessels. A resection to the left of the inferior mesenteric vein is defined as limited, between the inferior mesenteric vein and the superior mesenteric vessels as major, and a resection to the right of the superior mesenteric vessels as extended. The latter is comparable to a "95% pancreatectomy," as defined by Child and associates.[21] The uncinate process remains after this procedure. These types of resection are depicted in Figure 30–9.

Established pancreatic fistula, pseudocyst, hemorrhage, and persistent pancreatitis are essentially nonexistent complications following distal pancreatectomy for trauma. Transient pancreatic fistula is common, and left upper quadrant abscess may occur. Pancreatic endocrine and exocrine insufficiency are extremely rare. Transient hyperglycemis requiring insulin for control may occur in the early postoperative period after major or extended resection. This may reflect a delay in adaptation of residual islet cells and is undoubtedly accentuated by the usual tendency to postoperative glucose intolerance—the "diabetes of trauma".[22] Among 116 cases of distal pancreatic resection for trauma reported from Los Angeles County-University of Southern California Medical Center over the past 15 years, there has been only one instance of established postoperative diabetes.[14, 23] Twenty-seven of these resections were of the extended type. The islet cells are uniformly distributed throughout the pancreas. Of patients undergoing 95% pancreatectomy for chronic pancreatitis as re-

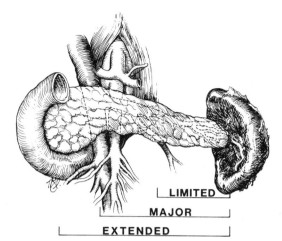

Fig 30–9.—Distal pancreatectomies are classified as *Limited* if to the left of the inferior mesenteric vein, *Major* if the division is between the superior mesenteric vessels and inferior mesenteric vein and *Extended* if transection is to the right of the superior mesenteric vessels.

ported by Child and associates,[21] diabetes was not inevitable among patients who were not diabetic preoperatively. This presumably is due to the function of the residual islet cells in the uncinate process. We have not identified an instance of pancreatic exocrine insufficiency among patients with distal pancreatectomy. The operation of distal pancreatectomy has the virtue of a very low to nonexistent incidence of exocrine or endocrine insufficiency and an inherently low mortality. The enteric suture lines of the Roux-en-Y loop used for pancreaticoenterostomy are avoided.

Biliary drainage may be a desirable adjunct in certain cases after pancreatic resection. These would be extended resections for blunt or penetrating trauma as well as major resections for blunt trauma. These are the instances in which mild pancreatitis in the residual pancreas is more likely to occur and in which transient obstruction of the common bile duct can develop. If the serum bilirubin rises postoperatively, obstruction of the biliary tract can be excluded as a diagnosis, and the biliary tract will be decompressed. In a small or normal-sized common duct, a cholecystostomy is preferred. With a duct greater than 1 cm in diameter, a T tube may be inserted in the common bile duct.

A rather protracted ileus is frequent following major pancreatic surgery. Additionally, if a transient pancreatic fistula develops, it may be desirable temporarily to avoid oral feedings. A gastrostomy will decompress the stomach and eliminate the need for nasogastric suction. A jejunostomy for enteral feeding will obviate the use of parenteral nutrition. Both gastrostomy and jejunostomy are desirable adjuncts to a major or extended distal pancreatectomy.

To initiate a distal pancreatectomy with splenectomy, the spleen is gently retracted anteriorly and to the right, and the peritoneal reflection posterior to the spleen and pancreas entered. The loose areolar tissue behind the pancreas is separated by blunt and sharp dissection, and the pancreas is mobilized from left to right and retracted anteriorly and toward the midline. When the splenic artery is identified, it is ligated, transfixed with a silk suture, and divided. The inferior mesenteric vein is divided. The vasa brevia may be divided at this time or later. Deferment may be preferable if the spleen and pancreas are being mobilized for exposure and control of hemorrhage from the region of the superior mesenteric vessels. As one approaches the confluence of the splenic vein and the superior mesenteric vein, care must be taken not to continue the mobilization to the point that a tear occurs in these veins at their junction. The splenic vein is isolated, ligated, transfixed, and divided. This approach to exposure of the superior mesenteric vessels is depicted in Figure 30–10.

When there is pancreatic disruption, the dissection is carried to the point of disruption, whether to the left or to the right of the superior mesenteric vessels. If the pancreatic transection is not complete, the remaining pancreatic substance is teased apart with the back side of a small, curved hemostat or with a small sucker. The pancreatic duct is identified. Magnifying loops may be of assistance. The injection of secretin IV may provoke a brisk flow from the severed pancreatic duct and aid in its identification. When the duct is identified, it is ligated with a fine monofilament nonabsorbable suture. A few small vessels may require ligation, but most of the bleeding from the transected surface of the pancreas can be controlled by electrocoagulation.

Several options exist for management of the stump of the pancreas. If the main duct has been identified and ligated and hemostasis ensured, it is not essential to perform further procedure on the pancreas. Traditionally, vertical mattress sutures have been placed in the transected pancreas to control bleeding from small vessels and to prevent leakage of pancreatic juice from small ducts, the latter effort usually unsuccessful. Some surgeons have wedged the pancreas in a fishmouth fashion prior to placement of these sutures. If sutures are placed, we recommend using absorbable suture. In recent years, it has become customary to occlude the pancreas with an automatic stapling device, using the TIA stapler with the 0.5-mm staples to compress the substance of the gland.[23]

Two soft Penrose drains are placed close to the transected surface of the pancreas. These are fixed to the loose areolar tissue in the pancreatic bed with chromic catgut sutures and are brought out through a generous stab wound in the flank, inferior to the costal margin. A soft sump is also placed in the pancreatic bed and brought out through a separate flank incision. Biliary drainage, gastrostomy, and jejunostomy are established for previously described indications. The gastrostomy is of the Stamm type, and the feeding jejunostomy is created with either a #6 French infant feeding tube or a #8 French rubber catheter. The jejunostomy tube is tunneled into place. Both the stomach and the jejunum are fixed with nonabsorbable sutures to the anterior parietes at the site of their exit through the abdominal wall. If the stomach does not reach the anterior abdominal wall conveniently and without tension, the tube is wrapped in omentum from the gastric wall to the parietal peritoneum (Fig 30–11). Figure 30–12 is a magnified view of the pancreas occluded by staples.

From the sump and from the site of the Penrose drains, drainage of fluid high in amylase content is the rule rather than the exception following distal pancreatectomy, irrespective of the management of the pancreatic stump. This fistula may not become apparent until the 7–10 days postoperatively. For that reason, although the sump is removed on the fourth or fifth day, the Penrose drains are left in place for at least ten days. In our experience, pancreatic fistulas following distal pancreatectomy have, without exception, closed spontaneously. An established fistula has been seen only in cases of injury to a major pancreatic duct treated by drainage alone.

We recently studied the incidence of regional complications

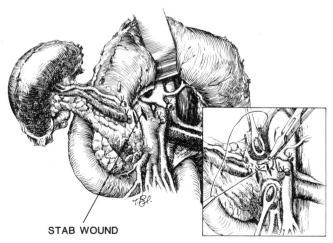

STAB WOUND

Fig 30–10.—The spleen and pancreas have been refracted from left to right to expose a stab wound of the superior mesenteric vein. The splenic artery and vein have been divided. The inset *(right)* depicts a vascular repair. Hemostasis during repair is more easily achieved by the use of proximal and distal compression by sponges than by mobilization of the vein. The latter maneuver may incur increasing hemorrhage. An injury of the posterior wall of the vein may be repaired through the anterior venotomy.

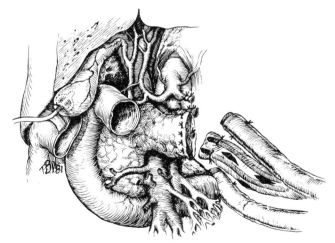

Fig 30–11.—A distal pancreatectomy with splenectomy. The pancreatic duct has been ligated with nonabsorbable suture and the cut surface of the pancreas compressed with absorbable sutures. The placement of a sump drain and Penrose drain as noted. A cholecystostomy has been performed, and a gastrostomy and feeding jejunostomy will also be performed. (From Fitzgibbons T.J., Yellin A.E., Maruyama M.M., et al.: Management of the transected pancreas following distal pancreatectomy. *Surg. Gynecol. Obstet.* 154:225, 1982. Used by permission.)

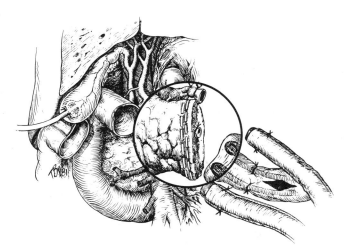

Fig 30–12.—A distal pancreatectomy has been performed and the cut surface of the pancreas has been occluded with the use of the stapler. The pancreatic duct has been separately ligated. (From Fitzgibbons T.J., Yellin A.E., Maruyama M.M., et al.: Management of the transected pancreas following distal pancreatectomy. *Surg. Gynecol. Obstet.* 154:225, 1982. Used by permission.)

in a nonrandomized series of 56 patients who underwent distal pancreatectomy for trauma. The pancreas was occluded by a stapler in 29 cases and with suture in 27 cases.[23] An abscess occurred in the left upper quadrant that required drainage in six of the 56 cases. A pancreatic fistula persisted at hospital discharge in seven cases, but each closed before two months and thus would not be defined as established. These regional complications were equally divided between the two groups—those closed with a stapler and those with suture of the pancreas. In the sutured group, the complications were more frequent in cases without ligation of the pancreatic duct, an observation not true of cases occluded with the stapler. The stapler was employed with more severe injuries. Six associated duodenal injuries occurred among cases stapled, and only one with suture closure of the pancreas. An extended resection was performed in ten cases in which the stapler was used compared with four cases in the sutured group. These results support the use of the stapler for occlusion of the pancreas. The results in these cases and those in a prior reported series of distal pancreatectomies are summarized in Table 30–1.

Resection of the spleen together with the pancreas facilitates the operation but sacrifice of the spleen is not without a price. The long-term effects of the asplenic state, including susceptibility to sepsis, are well recognized. The distal pancreas can be resected without the spleen and the operation should be considered in selected instances with a stable patient without major associated injury. This procedure is probably most easily performed by dissection of the pancreas from the right to the left in contradistinction to the technique of distal pancreatectomy with splenectomy. A Kocher clamp may be placed on the distal pancreas at the site of disruption and gentle traction applied inferiorly and to the left. This will expose and place slight tension on the small branches of the splenic artery and the splenic vein as they pass from superi-

TABLE 30–1.—DISTAL PANCREATECTOMY (116 CASES)*

DESCRIPTION	NO. OF CASES (%)
Type	
Blunt trauma	39 (34)
Stab wound	21 (18)
Gunshot	56 (48)
Extent of resection	
Limited	39 (34)
Major	50 (43)
Extended	27 (23)
Regional complications	
Diabetes	1 (.08)
Steatorrhea	0
Pancreatitis	2 (1.7)
Established fistula	0
Pseudocyst	1 (.08)
Secondary hemorrhage	2 (1.7)
Left upper quadrant abscess	13 (12)

*References 14 and 23.

orly downward and into the pancreas. Each is individually identified, ligated, and divided or occluded with a hemoclip. The dissection is somewhat tedious but not difficult. The management of the pancreatic stump and the use of drains are identical to the techniques described for distal pancreatectomy with splenectomy. A distal pancreatectomy without splenectomy is depicted in Figure 30–13.

DUODENAL "DIVERTICULIZATION".—Treatment of combined injuries of the duodenum and pancreas by closure of the duodenal wound and drainage of the pancreas has been followed by such frequent regional complications, including lateral duodenal fistula, that alternative operations have been recommended. A report from Los Angeles County-University of Southern California Medical Center in 1966 included nine cases of combined pancreaticoduodenal injury.[12] Three of the

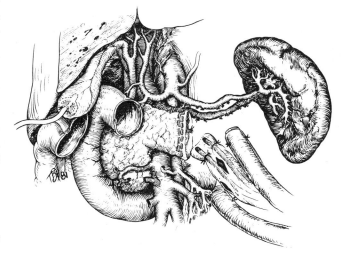

Fig 30–13.—A distal pancreatectomy in which the spleen has been preserved. Branches to the pancreas from the splenic artery and vein are individually identified and ligated. This operation is appropriate in a stable patient without major associated injuries.

nine patients underwent as a primary procedure an operation now known as duodenal diverticulization. This operation had previously been employed as a secondary procedure in patients who developed sidewall duodenal fistula after closure of complex duodenal wounds. Success in these latter cases led to its adoption as a primary procedure. Duodenal diverticulization as described consists of antrectomy, tube duodenostomy, closure of the duodenal wound, end-to-side gastrojejunostomy, vagotomy, and extensive drainage.[24] This operation shunts gastric contents away from the duodenum and converts the duodenum with the attached biliary and pancreatic ductal systems into a diverticulum. The vagotomy is performed to prevent late marginal ulceration.

The concept that diversion of gastric content from the duodenum would be beneficial in severe duodenal injury dates from at least 1904 when Summers[25] suggested that with duodenal trauma "one should . . . in addition to repairing the duodenal wound or wounds . . . occlude the pylorus by means of a purse string stitch . . . a gastroenterostomy must be made." Berg, in 1907,[26] treated lateral duodenal fistula with pyloric occlusion and gastroenterostomy and Colp[27] subsequently supported this concept. Welch and Edmunds[13] in 1960 recommended antrectomy, gastroenterostomy, and tube duodenostomy in patients with a duodenal fistula at or distal to the ampulla of Vater. The operation converted a side fistula with a high mortality and low rate of spontaneous closure into an end fistula with a lower mortality and a higher rate of spontaneous closure.

Diverticulization as primary therapy was employed rather extensively at the Los Angeles County-University of Southern California Medical Center as the primary operation for combined pancreaticoduodenal injury during the 1960s and early 1970s. The first report by Berne and associates[24] that was devoted to this procedure was published in 1968, and a series of 50 cases was reported in 1974.[28] The mortality among these 50 cases with diverticulization as a primary procedure was 16%. This was considerably lower then the previously reported mortality for these injuries. The incidence of regional complications was extraordinarily low. Seven duodenal fistulas occurred, and all closed spontaneously. The mortality was almost exclusively due to massive hemorrhage from associated vascular injury and from postoperative major organ failure. Diverticulization was combined with distal pancreatectomy in cases of major pancreatic duct injury.

In recent years, with the increasing use of feeding jejunostomy and with emphasis on the nutritional support of these patients, the consequences of sidewall duodenal fistulas have become less devastating. We are now more prone to close a duodenal wound, to establish drainage, and to initiate early enteral nutrition with a feeding jejunostomy in patients who a decade ago would have undergone a diverticulization procedure for the same severity of wound.

A few technical details of diverticulization deserve emphasis. The afferent limb of the gastrojejunostomy should be at least 18 in. long to discourage reflux to the site of the duodenal injury. The duodenal stump is best closed in a standard fashion. The duodenal wound is sutured. The tube used to decompress and drain the duodenum is a #12 or #14 French red rubber catheter, which is inserted into the duodenum with a Witzel technique. The likelihood of leakage around the tube and from the duodenum is lower when the tube is placed through a separate stab wound than through the duodenal stump. Penrose drains are placed lateral to the duodenum and egress through the right flank. Essential features of duodenal diverticulization combined with distal pancreatectomy are depicted in Figure 30–14.

Pyloric Exclusion

Pyloric exclusion has been recently recommended by Vaughan and associates[29] for more complex duodenal injuries that would include some combined pancreaticoduodenal injuries. The antrum is opened on its posterior aspect and the pylorus exposed and closed with a purse-string suture of catgut. An autostapler is an alternative technique to occlude the pylorus. A gastroenterostomy is established at the site of the antrotomy. This operation may incur a risk of gastrojejunal ulceration. If an absorbable suture is employed and is ultimately resorbed, GI continuity will be restored. If necessary, the gastroenterostomy can be taken down with restoration of normal anatomy. This operation achieves the goal of gastric diversion but has not been widely adopted, reflecting, to a degree, concern about the possibility of marginal ulceration.

Pancreaticoduodenectomy

Pancreaticoduodenectomy has been employed for selected cases of combined injury of the duodenum and the head of the pancreas.[30] Stricture of a choledochojejunostomy is more likely to occur when the anastomosis is made to a common duct that is not dilated. Most of the literature on pancreaticoduodenectomy consists of isolated case reports or reports of two or three cases that were successfully treated. Surgeons may report one or two successful cases but not one or two failures. Thus, the collective mortality from the literature is unrepresentative. The mortality for ten cases of pancreaticoduodenectomy for trauma at the Los Angeles County-University of Southern California Medical Center reported in 1975 was 60%.[30] The mortality for pancreaticoduodenectomy will

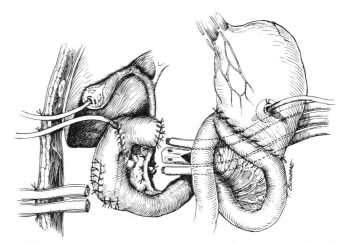

Fig 30–14.—The gastric antrum has been resected and a gastroenterostomy established. The duodenal wound has been closed and a tube duodenostomy established. A distal pancreatectomy has been combined with this diverticulization of the duodenum because of a fracture of the head of the pancreas.

be influenced by the magnitude of associated injury and the experience of the surgeon. Oreskovich and Carrico[31] recently reported ten cases of pancreaticoduodenectomy for trauma without a death.

RECOMMENDED SURGICAL PROCEDURES

The operations that we recommend for pancreatic injury are as follows.

CONTUSION.—The placement of Penrose drains at the site of injury is the only treatment indicated.

MINOR DISRUPTION OF THE PANCREATIC SUBSTANCE WITH PROVED OR PRESUMPTION OF INTACT MAJOR DUCTS.—Penrose drains are placed at the site of injury, as well as a soft sump of the Jackson-Pratt type.

MAJOR PANCREATIC DISRUPTION WITH PROVED OR PRESUMPTION OF MAJOR DUCT INJURY.—The preferred treatment for this lesion is a distal pancreatectomy, performed with splenectomy in cases of multiple injury or if the patient's intraoperative condition is unstable. With an injury in a stable patient without major associated injury, an attempt is made to preserve the spleen. The bed of the pancreas is drained extensively with soft Penrose drains and sump suction. If the resection is major or extended and or if injury is due to blunt trauma, the biliary tract is drained by a cholecystostomy. In injuries due to penetrating trauma, a cholecystostomy is performed for extended resections. A gastrostomy and a feeding jejunostomy are inserted in major or extended resections.

If the pancreatic injury due to either a penetrating wound or blunt trauma is considerably to the right of the superior mesenteric vessels, a distal pancreatectomy could, rarely, result in diabetes. When, in such cases, the duct of Wirsung is proved to be divided, the patient is stable, and other major injuries are not present, a Roux-en-Y loop of jejunum may be anastomosed to the distal pancreas at the site of transection and the duct in the proximal pancreas ligated. We do not have experience with this operation.

The more difficult question is when to insert drains rather than when to perform resectional or reconstructive surgery, even though injury to a major duct is thought likely or even proved to be present. A number of factors weigh in this judgment, to include the magnitude of associated injury, the location of the injury in the pancreas, and the general condition of the patient. A limited resection of the distal 3 cm of pancreas for treatment of a stab wound involves considerations vastly different from a resection or reconstructive surgery for a penetrating wound of the head of the pancreas. In a patient with major associated injuries and complicating other disease, drains to the head of the pancreas may be the better choice, despite risk of fistula, pseudocyst, and pancreatitis. The surgeon must remember that the mortality as opposed to morbidity related to the pancreatic wound, if adequately drained, is far more likely to be due to the associated injury than to the pancreatic injury. Discretion can be the better part of valor.

COMBINED PANCREATICODUODENAL INJURY.—The procedure of duodenal diverticulization is reserved for those patients with severe duodenal injury combined with a pan-

creatic injury. These are cases with a severity of duodenal injury that strongly suggest that a duodenal suture line would be in serious jeopardy. If the pancreatic injury includes an injury to a major duct, distal pancreatectomy is also performed. Pancreaticoduodenectomy should be reserved exclusively for those patients with devastating injury to the duodenum and pancreas in which the operation is a debridement of devitalized parts or is performed to control exsanguinating hemorrhage. These recommendations are summarized in Table 30–2.

COMPLICATIONS

Early

Abscess in the upper abdomen, particularly in the left upper quadrant, is a serious sequela of pancreatic injury. The abscess may develop in a case of unrecognized pancreatic injury or when a major injury to the pancreas does not receive definitive treatment. Unfortunately, it has also in our experience been the most common regional complication after definitive surgical treatment. Pancreaticoenterostomy to the site of disruption of a major duct does not eliminate the problem. Following distal pancreatectomy and splenectomy, the residual dead space may invite a collection of fluid that becomes infected. Leakage of pancreatic juice into the area that is not totally evacuated by drains is a risk factor for sepsis. Contamination from associated enteric injury is a consideration. Finally, the drains employed in an attempt to control leakage of pancreatic secretions may, although quarantined in a sterile drainage bag, act as an avenue for nosocomial infection. Despite this latter possibility, surgeons have not as yet been so venturesome as to omit drainage of an overt pancreatic disruption.

We prefer posterior drainage of pancreatic abscess through the bed of the resected left 12th rib, synchronous with anterior celiotomy to unroof any pockets of purulence and to guide placement of the drains.[32] Devitalized pancreas should be resected. If the spleen is intact, synchronous anterior celiotomy and posterior drainage establishes dependent drainage while avoiding injury to the spleen and splenic vessels.

Late

Established pancreatic fistula, pseudocyst, or chronic pancreatitis may occur in a patient in whom there has not been definitive treatment of a recognized injury to a major duct or in whom a major pancreatic injury was not identified. Chronic pancreatitis may evolve over a period of months, during which the patient has persistent smouldering pancreatitis or recurring exacerbation of clinical acute pancreatitis. A posttraumatic pseudocyst is treated as any pseudocyst of the pancreas. Occasionally, the distal pancreas, together with the pseudocyst, can be mobilized for resection. More often, internal drainage by cystojejunostomy is the treatment of choice. Our preference is for use of a Roux-en-Y loop. In a patient with a persistent external pancreatic fistula, a combination of a sinogram and ERCP will usually demonstrate the site of duct injury. Definitive treatment consists of surgical exploration, identification of the pancreas at the site of fistula and a distal pancreatectomy. The anastomosis of the fistula tract to a loop of jejunum is an undesirable alternative. With

TABLE 30–2.—GUIDELINES FOR PREFERRED TREATMENT OF PANCREATIC INJURY

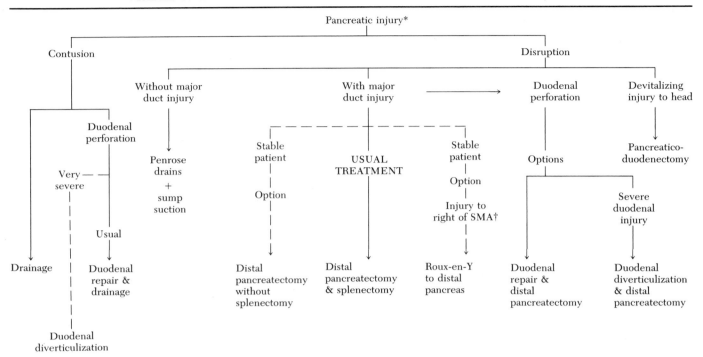

*Unstable condition of a patient might warrant abandoning preferred procedure for drainage of the pancreatic injury.
†Superior mesenteric artery

chronic pancreatitis distal to the duct injury, a resection is the preferred treatment. If dilatation of the duct of Wirsung has occurred, a Roux-en-Y loop may be fashioned and a pancreaticojejunostomy established.

MORTALITY

The mortality of pancreatic injury is dominantly the mortality of the associated vascular and, to a lesser extent, enteric injuries. When suture lines in the GI tract of ligatures on major vessels are bathed with activated pancreatic juice, the risk of enteric fistula and secondary hemorrhage will be increased.

The mortality among 116 cases of major pancreatic injury treated by distal pancreatectomy and reported in two series from the Los Angeles County-University of Southern California Medical Center has been 13%.[14, 23] The mortality for 60 cases reported in 1967 was 12% and that for 57 cases reported in 1983 was 14%. Although these rates are essentially the same, the causes of death among these two groups of patients were very different. In the first group, the majority of deaths were postoperative and due to major organ failure, often associated with sepsis. In the more recent group, the deaths were due to neurological injury or consequent to exsanguinating hemorrhage from vascular injury. Death occurred soon after arrival at the hospital. These altering circumstances probably reflect at least two factors. With evolution of prehospital care, including emergency medical services and efficient transportation, patients arrive at major trauma centers with a magnitude of injury to which they would have suc-

cumbed "in the field" 15–20 years ago. Concurrently, improved techniques of intensive care and postoperative support of major organ dysfunction have undoubtedly reduced postoperative mortality. Reduction of the mortality of major pancreatic injuries much below 15% will be most difficult, not because of the pancreatic injury, but because of the associated vascular injuries from which a higher salvage rate is unlikely.

REFERENCES

1. Travers B.: Rupture of the pancreas—hospital report of St. Thomas Hospital. *Lancet* 12:384, 1827.
2. Otis G.A.: *The Medical and Surgical History of the War of the Rebellion, Vol. II, Pt. II. Surgical History.* Washington D.C., U.S. Government Printing Office, 1876.
3. Mikulicz-Redecki J. von: Surgery of the pancreas. *Ann. Surg.* 38:1, 1903.
4. Garré C.: Totaler querris des pankreas durch nahtgeheilt. *Beitr. Klin. Chir.* 46:233, 1905.
5. Newton A.: A case of successful end to end suture of the pancreas. *Surg. Gynecol. Obstet.* 48:808, 1929.
6. Doubilet H., Mulholland J.H.: Some observations on the treatment of trauma to the pancreas. *Am. J. Surg.* 105:741, 1963.
7. Walton A.J.: *A Textbook of the Surgical Dyspepsias.* London, Edward Arnold & Co., 1923.
8. Letton A.H., Wilson J.P.: Traumatic severance of pancreas treated by Roux-y anastomosis. *Surg. Gynecol. Obstet.* 109:473, 1959.
9. Jones R.C., Shires G.T.: The management of pancreatic injuries. *Arch. Surg.* 90:502, 1965.
10. Northrup W.F. III, Simmons R.L.: Pancreatic trauma: A review. *Surgery* 71:27, 1972.
11. Peck J., Berne T.V.: Posterior abdominal stab wounds. *J. Trauma* 21:298, 1981.

12. Donovan A.J., Hagen W.E.: Traumatic perforation of the duodenum. *Am. J. Surg.* 111:341, 1966.
13. Welch C.E., Edmunds L.H.: Gastrointestinal fistulas. *Surg. Clin. North Am.* 42:1311, 1960.
14. Yellin A.E., Vecchione R.T., Donovan A.J.: Distal pancreatectomy for pancreatic trauma. *Am. J. Surg.* 124:135, 1972.
15. Federle M.P.: Computed tomography of blunt abdominal trauma. *Radiol. Clin. North Am.* 21:461, 1983.
16. Donovan A.J., Turrill F., Berne C.J.: Injuries of the pancreas from blunt trauma. *Surg. Clin. North Am.* 52:649, 1972.
17. Bach R.D., Frey C.F.: Diagnosis and treatment of pancreatic trauma. *Am. J. Surg.* 121:20, 1971.
18. Howell J.F., Burrus G.R., Jordan G.L. Jr.: Surgical management of pancreatic injuries. *J. Trauma* 1:32, 1961.
19. Pellegrine J.A., Stein I.J.: Complete severance of pancreas and its treatment with repair of main pancreatic duct of Wirsung. *Am. J. Surg.* 101:707, 1961.
20. Martin L.W., Henderson B.M., Welsh N.: Disruption of the head of the pancreas caused by blunt trauma in children: A report of two cases treated with primary repair of the pancreatic duct. *Surgery* 63:697, 1968.
21. Child C.G. III, Frey C.F., Fry W.J.: A reappraisal of removal of 95% of the distal portion of the pancreas. *Surg. Gynecol. Obstet.* 129:49, 1969.
22. Cahill G.F. Jr.: Body fuels and their metabolism. *Bull. Am. Coll. Surg.* 79:279, 1953.
23. Fitzgibbons T.J., Yellin A.E., Maruyama M.M., et al.: Management of the transected pancreas following distal pancreatectomy. *Surg. Gynecol. Obstet.* 154:225, 1982.
24. Berne C.J., Donovan A.J., Hagen W.E.: Combined duodenal pancreatic trauma: The role of end to side gastrojejunostomy. *Arch. Surg.* 96:712, 1968.
25. Summers J.E. Jr.: The treatment of posterior perforation of the fixed portions of the duodenum. *Ann. Surg.* 39:727, 1904.
26. Berg A.A.: Duodenal fistula: Its treatment by gastrojejunostomy and pelvic exclusion. *Ann. Surg.* 45:721, 1907.
27. Colp R.: External duodenal fistula. *Ann. Surg.* 78:725, 1923.
28. Berne C.J., Donovan A.J., White E.J., et al.: Duodenal "diverticulization" for duodenal and pancreatic injury. *Am. J. Surg.* 127:503, 1974.
29. Vaughan G.D. III, Frazier O.H., Graham D.Y., et al.: The use of pyloric exclusion in the management of severe duodenal injuries. *Am. J. Surg.* 134:785, 1977.
30. Yellin A.E., Rosoff L.: Pancreatoduodenectomy for combined pancreatoduodenal injuries. *Arch. Surg.* 110:1177, 1975.
31. Oreskovich M.R., Carrico C.J.: Pancreatoduodenectomy for trauma: A viable option? *Am. J. Surg.* 147:618, 1984.
32. Berne T.V., Donovan A.J.: Synchronous anterior celiotomy and posterior drainage of pancreatic abscess. *Arch. Surg.* 116:527, 1981.

31

The Diagnosis and Early Treatment of Acute Pancreatitis

JOHN H. C. RANSON, B.M., B.CH.

THE TERM "ACUTE PANCREATITIS" is used to describe a wide variety of pancreatic inflammatory conditions. It includes pancreatitis associated with etiologic factors as diverse as chronic alcohol abuse, gallstones, or the bite of the scorpion *Tityus trinitatis*. The spectrum of pathologic findings includes pancreatic edema and interstitial inflammation as well as frank pancreatic necrosis or hemorrhage. Finally, the clinical findings range from mild, self-limiting symptoms to a fulminant, rapidly lethal disease. It is hoped that better methods for the classification of pancreatic inflammatory disease will be developed in the future. Meanwhile, however, it is important to remember that multiple differing entities are grouped under this term, and the management of patients must be highly individualized.

The earliest reports of pancreatic inflammation were based on findings at autopsy. Aubert in 1579[1] and Tulpius in 1641[2] described the occurrence of pancreatic abscesses. Edouard Ancelet[3] in 1856 recognized that pancreatic suppuration was a consequence of pancreatitis. He also described the "very rare" occurrence of pancreatic gangrene, but he did not specifically relate this to pancreatitis.

Nicholas Senn,[4] a Milwaukee and Chicago surgeon, published a description of clinical and experimental studies of pancreatic diseases in 1886. In this monograph, he provides a description of acute pancreatitis and notes that this may lead to pancreatic suppuration, abscess or gangrene. Diffuse pancreatic hemorrhage was also described but was not related to pancreatic inflammation. Three years later, the Middleton-Goldsmith Lecture of Reginald Fitz[5] led to wider recognition of acute pancreatitis as a disease process. Fitz classified pancreatitis as suppurative, hemorrhagic, or gangrenous. He observed that the clinical course of suppurative pancreatitis was usually subacute or chronic, while that of hemorrhagic pancreatitis was hyperacute or apoplectiform. The course of gangrenous pancreatitis was described as "acute." The possibility that these pathologic findings represented different stages of the same process does not appear to have been considered. Pancreatic hemorrhage was retained as a separate entity, not necessarily associated with pancreatitis. The occurrence of fat necrosis was also described and related to underlying acute pancreatitis.

During the first quarter of this century, a confident diagnosis of acute pancreatitis was reached only at exploratory celiotomy or postmortem examination. Since a proportion of those who were diagnosed at celiotomy survived the acute illness, operative treatment was often recommended at this time. In 1925, Moynihan[6] wrote that although "there can be no doubt that recovery from acute pancreatitis, of all grades, except the most severe, is possible without operation . . . . [this occurrence] is so rare that no case should be left untreated." He recommended operative evacuation of any peripancreatic fluid, incision of the pancreatic capsule and external drainage.

The subsequent development of methods for the estimation of urinary and serum levels of amylase led to the more frequent nonoperative diagnosis of acute pancreatitis. It became clear that most patients could recover without surgical intervention and, in recent years, operative treatment has been considered only for those patients with the most severe pancreatitis or with associated cholelithiasis, or for the management of complications such as pancreatic abscess.

DIAGNOSIS

Clinical Presentation

The diagnosis of acute pancreatitis depends primarily on a careful evaluation of the patient's history and physical findings. Unfortunately, the clinical features vary widely and may closely mimic those of peptic ulcer, biliary lithiasis, intestinal obstruction, or other acute extrapancreatic illnesses. The first and dominant symptom is usually pain, which is characteristically located in the epigastrium (Table 31–1). It may radiate to the back and to both flanks. The onset of pain is rapid but less sudden than that of peritonitis secondary to perforated gastic or duodenal ulcer. The pain often begins after a heavy meal or during an alcoholic drinking binge. It is constant in character and may be extremely severe. Milder pain may be relieved somewhat by sitting forward or by lying curled on the right or left side. Occasionally, striking relief of pain follows the institution of nasogastric suction.

Nausea and vomiting are almost invariably present and are often a prominent early feature. The vomiting may be repeated but is usually not copious. The vomitus contains gas-

TABLE 31–1.—INCIDENCE
OF CLINICAL SYMPTOMS AND SIGNS
IN ACUTE PANCREATITIS*

SYMPTOM	% INCIDENCE
Abdominal pain	85–100
Radiation to back	50
Nausea, vomiting	54–92
Fever	12–80
Arterial hypotension	1–60
Palpable abdominal mass	6–20
Jaundice	8–20

*Adapted from Dürr.[7]

tric and duodenal contents, and, in contrast to patients with mechanical obstruction of the small intestine, it is not feculent. Many patients give a history of previous biliary disease or of alcohol abuse.

The physical findings also vary widely. The patient may be restless with a rapid pulse and respiratory rate. The blood pressure may be mildly elevated, normal, or decreased. The temperature is usually 99–100°F. Cyanosis may be present in severe cases. The abdomen is usually moderately distended and may exhibit a characteristic epigastric fullness. Tenderness is usually most marked over the epigastrium and upper abdomen. It may be diffuse, especially in more severe cases. Muscle spasm is frequent but true rigidity is unusual. Grey Turner's sign, which is a grey-green or purple discoloration of the flank, is present in about 1% of patients.

Laboratory Findings

AMYLASE.—Serum and urinary levels of amylase remain the most widely used laboratory measurements in the evaluation of possible pancreatitis. Although the lack of specificity of amylase levels is well known, initial serum amylase levels are elevated in 95% of patients with acute pancreatitis. In patients with acute abdominal pain due to other causes, it was found that only 5% had elevated initial amylase levels.[8]

Among patients with pancreatitis who have a normal serum amylase level reported, approximately 40% have hyperlipidemia with lactescent serum. The serum of such patients interferes with measurements of amylase levels.[9] Accordingly, in patients with lactescent serum and abdominal pain, pancreatitis must be considered strongly even if elevated serum amylase levels are not reported. True amylase levels may be demonstrated in these patients by repeat determinations after dilution of the serum.

In large groups of patients with acute abdominal conditions, approximately 20% have elevated serum amylase levels. Of these, approximately 75% have pancreatitis and, among the 25% with extrapancreatic disease, only about 50% had conditions which might be confused with acute pancreatitis.[10] The acute extrapancreatic abdominal conditions most commonly associated with elevated serum amylase levels are perforated peptic ulcer, acute biliary tract disease, intestinal obstruction, and mesenteric infarction.

In some patients, elevation of serum amylase levels are related to decreased urinary excretion. This possibility can be evaluated by measurement of the renal clearance of amylase. This is normally 1.2–5.8 ml/minute. In patients with acute

pancreatitis, the renal clearance of amylase is often increased. Because of variation in underlying renal function, this can be most easily estimated by determination of the ratio of amylase clearance to creatinine clearance according to the formula:

$$\frac{C_{Am}}{C_{Cr}} = \frac{\dfrac{(Amylase)_{urine}}{(Amylase)_{serum}}}{\dfrac{(Creatinine)_{urine}}{(Creatinine)_{serum}}}$$

The ratio of C_{Am}/C_{Cr} is normally 1%–4%. In patients with pancreatitis, the ratio may be increased, and it had been hoped that this measurement would improve the laboratory diagnosis of acute pancreatitis. Unfortunately, in most reported experiences, this calculation has not proved helpful in the routine evaluation of patients with possible pancreatitis.

Techniques are available for the separation of total serum amylase activity into three or more isoamylases. Such studies allow differentiation of patients with hyperamylasemia secondary to increased salivary gland amylase or macroamylasemia from those with increased pancreatic amylase. The role of such measurements in the routine evaluation of patients with possible acute pancreatitis is uncertain at present.[11, 12]

LIPASE.—Increased levels of lipase activity in blood and serum occur in patients with acute pancreatitis, and it has been reported that measurement of lipase levels may increase the specificity of the laboratory diagnosis of acute pancreatitis. In the past, measurement of lipase levels required a prolonged period of incubation and was not widely used. The recent development of rapid methods for the estimation of lipase activity has led to renewed interest in the value of this measurement. It is, unfortunately, clear that elevated levels of lipase can occur in patients with acute extrapancreatic intra-abdominal conditions which may mimic pancreatitis, such as acute cholecystitis or intestinal perforation or infarction.[13]

OTHER LABORATORY MEASUREMENTS.—Hyperglycemia and hypocalcemia are features of severe acute pancreatitis which may occasionally be of help in diagnosis. If patients with known diabetes mellitus are excluded, an initial blood glucose level above 300 mg/dl is uncommon in patients with acute extrapancreatic abdominal conditions. Hyperglycemia of this degree was present in 7% of our patients with acute pancreatitis. Similarly an initial serum calcium level below 8 mg/dl was observed in 9% of our patients with acute pancreatitis. This degree of hypocalcemia may occur in patients with perforated duodenal ulcer but has been rare in other acute intra-abdominal diseases.

Diagnostic Paracentesis

Diagnostic peritoneal lavage has proved valuable in the evaluation of abdominal trauma, and it has been suggested that this technique may also be helpful in the differential diagnosis of acute abdominal pain. Experimental studies have shown that lavage fluid returned from the peritoneal cavity of animals with acute pancreatitis differs significantly in amylase, lactic dehydrogenase, and proteolytic content from that of animals with mesenteric ischemia or perforated ulcer during the first five hours after induction of pathology.[14] Unfortunately, in clinical practice, the time at which patients are first seen following the onset of acute pancreatitis is variable, and no consistent pattern of findings in peritoneal lavage fluid has been observed. The amylase content may be normal in acute pancreatitis and elevated in patients with GI perforations. Observed peritoneal fluid WBC counts vary from 22 to 350 cells/cu mm, and the hematocrit may be as high as 24%. Occasionally, diagnostic paracentesis and peritoneal lavage may yield fluid which is not consistent with uncomplicated acute pancreatitis. Specifically, the presence of bile, fibers, or organisms on Gram smear suggest some other intra-abdominal process. In addition, lavage fluid obtained from patients with infarcted bowel often has a characteristic, musty ammoniacal odor that can be readily recognized. Overall, however, paracentesis and peritoneal lavage usually do not provide valuable positive evidence for a diagnosis of acute pancreatitis.

Radiology

Plain radiographic films of the chest and abdomen are a routine part of the evaluation of patients with acute abdominal pain and shows how one or more positive findings in approximately 80% of patients with acute pancreatitis. The most common findings are listed in Table 31–2. Best known is segmental dilatation or ileus of a loop of small bowel in the left upper abdominal quadrant, present in 42% of cases (Figure 31–1). Dilatation of the transverse colon with a relative paucity of gas in the descending colon has been termed "pseudo-obstruction" or "the colon cut-off sign" and is present in 22% of patients. Loss of psoas margins and other radiographic findings are observed less frequently. Duodenal ileus, with an air-filled duodenum outlining an enlarged pancreatic head, is the most specific plain radiographic finding of acute pancreatitis, but was present in only 11% of patients. Most radiographic findings on plain film studies are nonspecific but may prove valuable in the overall evaluation of suspected acute pancreatitis.

UPPER GI SERIES.—Perforations of the upper GI tract or intestinal obstruction or infarction are important extrapancreatic conditions which may closely mimic acute pancreatitis. A water-soluble contrast study of the esophagus, stomach, and small intestine, therefore, may be exceedingly valuable in the initial evaluation of patients with pancreatitis. Findings which support the diagnosis of acute pancreatitis may sometimes be observed. These include displacement of the stomach, duo-

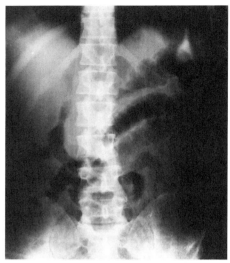

Fig 31–1.—Abdominal radiogram illustrating a dilated small-bowel loop in the left upper quadrant. Duodenal ileus with the air-filled duodenum outlining an enlarged pancreatic head is also shown. (From Ranson J.H.C.: Acute pancreatitis. *Curr. Probl. Surg.* Chicago, Year Book Medical Publishers, November, 1979, p. 14. Used by permission.)

denum, or proximal small bowel, and edema or irregularity of duodenal mucosa. In most patients, however, positive findings are absent, and this study is primarily valuable in excluding perforation or obstruction.

ANGIOGRAPHY.—Selective visceral angiography rarely shows significant abnormalities early in patients with acute pancreatitis. In those with severe pancreatitis, splenic vein obstruction may be observed, but this study is primarily of value in evaluating patients with possible pancreatitis in whom mesenteric infarction must be excluded.

CHOLANGIOGRAPHY.—In patients with known or suspected gallstones, the differentiation of acute pancreatitis from acute biliary tract disease associated with elevated serum amylase levels may be exceedingly difficult. In most patients, this differentiation may not be essential, since both conditions usually respond well to a period of nonoperative therapy. However, in patients who are severely ill or who are not responding to treatment, a precise diagnosis may be of critical importance. Ultrasonography may be helpful in the demonstration of gallbladder stones, but distention of the gallbladder and thickening of the gallbladder wall are observed in both acute cholecystitis and acute pancreatitis.

Attempts to visualize the biliary tree radiographically employing oral or IV contrast materials are rarely successful in this setting. Demonstration of the biliary tree by radionuclide scanning may demonstrate patency of the cystic duct, but delineation of the common duct is not adequate to exclude common duct stones. Furthermore, failure to visualize the gallbladder by this means has been observed in patients with acute pancreatitis in the absence of cholelithiasis.

Endoscopic retrograde cholangiopancreatography (ERCP) provides excellent visualization of the biliary tree, and it is clear that this study may be safely accomplished in many pa-

TABLE 31–2.—INCIDENCE (%) OF
RADIOGRAPHIC SIGNS SUGGESTING ACUTE
PANCREATITIS ON INITIAL CHEST AND ABDOMINAL
RADIOGRAPHS IN 73 PATIENTS WITH ACUTE
PANCREATITIS

RADIOGRAPHIC SIGN	% INCIDENCE
Segmental small-bowel ileus	41
Colonic dilatation	22
Obscure psoas margin	19
Increased epigastric soft tissue density	19
Increased gastrocolic separation	15
Gastric greater curvature distortion	14
Duodenal ileus	11
Pleural effusion	4
Pancreatic calcification	3
One or more of the above signs	79

tients with acute pancreatitis. In addition, it permits possible endoscopic sphincterotomy and stone extraction if calculous obstruction of the common bile duct is demonstrated. We have been reluctant to employ ERCP in patients with possible severe acute pancreatitis because of the potential for exacerbation of pancreatitis. In addition, introduction of nonsterile contrast material into a pancreas with areas of devitalized tissue may lead to pancreatic abscess formation.

In those patients with suspected acute pancreatitis in whom full visualization of the biliary tree is judged to be essential, we have preferred percutaneous transhepatic cholangiography (PTC) using the Chiba needle technique.[15] Clearly, this measure should not be used unless adequate information cannot be gained by safer, noninvasive measures, and the potential benefits of the information sought justify the potential morbidity. In patients with severe pancreatitis it may, however, be valuable in excluding obstructive cholangitis or gangrenous cholecystitis which require urgent surgical correction.

ULTRASONOGRAPHY.—Ultrasonography has an established role in the diagnosis of gallbladder disease and pancreatic cysts or masses. In patients with suspected acute pancreatitis, marked gaseous distention of the bowel often interferes with ultrasound studies, and, in studies of McKay et al.,[16] adequate imaging of the gallbladder and pancreas was achieved in only 70%–75% of cases. When the gallbladder was visualized, the presence or absence of gallstones could be determined with a high degree of accuracy. When satisfactory imaging of the pancreas was achieved, the gland was judged to appear normal in 41%, to show generalized enlargement in 33%, and to have localized swelling or a cyst in 26%. In this study, 64% of patients who had localized swelling or cystic collections developed subsequent pancreatic pseudocysts or abscess. Thus, while ultrasonography is of limited value in determining the presence or absence of pancreatitis, it is useful for evaluating the possibility of associated gallbladder stones, and it may help to identify those patients with an increased risk of late pancreatic complications.

COMPUTED TOMOGRAPHY.—Although more complex and expensive than ultrasonography, CT usually provides excellent images of the pancreas and peripancreatic retroperitoneum. The most frequent findings in patients with acute pancreatitis are diffuse pancreatic enlargement, obliteration of the peripancreatic fat planes, and inflammation of the left anterior pararenal space (Fig 31–2). Peripancreatic fluid collections may also be visualized.[17] Such positive findings on CT scan provide strong evidence for a diagnosis of acute pancreatitis. However, in our experience, early CT findings were interpreted as being normal in 16% of patients judged to have acute pancreatitis; a negative scan does not exclude this diagnosis. Later in the course of acute pancreatitis, both ultrasonography and CT may be extremely valuable for the diagnosis and localization of pancreatic cysts or infected abscesses.

Diagnostic Celiotomy

In most patients, a diagnosis of acute pancreatitis can usually be achieved on the basis of careful nonoperative evaluation. In a small proportion, however, celiotomy is required to exclude or treat acute extrapancreatic disease. It should be stressed, in this regard, that strong positive evidence of acute

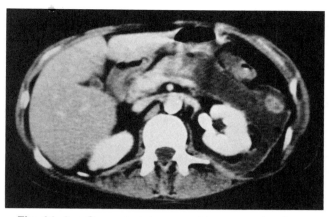

Fig 31–2.—Computed tomographic scan showing enlargement and disruption of the pancreas. Fluid is seen around the distal pancreas and in the left anterior pararenal space.

pancreatitis does not exclude the possibility of coexistent gangrenous cholecystitis, mesenteric infarction, or other pathology requiring urgent surgical correction.

When uncomplicated acute pancreatitis is found at diagnostic celiotomy, the choice of surgical procedure should be determined by specific therapeutic goals. Once surgical exploration has been undertaken, this choice is different from that of a decision for or against a specific surgical procedure compared to nonoperative therapy. There are little data available that compare different surgical procedures in patients undergoing early diagnostic celiotomy. Gliedman and co-workers[18] reported that simple closure of the abdomen without drainage was associated with 100% mortality in 48 patients. It has been our experience that if mild pancreatitis is found at early celiotomy, the patient's course is not ameliorated by any surgical measure. The placement of drains in the area of the pancreas in this group should be avoided, since this is associated with an increased incidence of late peripancreatic infection. If gallstones are present and pancreatitis is mild, definitive surgical correction of biliary disease can usually be undertaken safely to prevent recurrent pancreatitis.

In patients with severe acute pancreatitis who undergo early celiotomy, the choice of surgical procedure is less clear. In this group, it has been our experience that early definitive correction of associated biliary calculous disease is hazardous, and morbidity has been lower if biliary surgery was limited to cholecystostomy.[8] There is no evidence that cholecystostomy ameliorates the course of severe pancreatitis. It does, however, simplify the evaluation of fever and jaundice in patients with severe gallstone-associated disease.

Pancreatic drainage and pancreatic resection have both been recommended in patients with severe acute pancreatitis. It has been our experience that once celiotomy has been undertaken, the overall mortality has been the same whether the procedure was limited to placement of catheters for postoperative peritoneal lavage or more extensive procedures were undertaken. Kivilaakso et al.[19] compared celiotomy and placement of lavage catheters to early pancreatic resection in a controlled clinical trial. They found that morbidity tended to be lower in patients undergoing resection, but this difference did not achieve statistical significance. Since no clear benefit has been demonstrated from more extensive surgical measures, we continue to limit the operative procedure to placement of lavage catheters in most patients who are diagnosed at early celiotomy.

PROGNOSTIC ASSESSMENT

In most reports of acute pancreatitis, approximately 60%–75% of patients recover uneventfully with general supportive care. Between 25% and 40% of patients develop life-threatening complications, and 4%–26% (an average of 10%) die of the acute illness. Many special therapeutic measures have been proposed for patients who have life-threatening acute pancreatitis. Evaluation of the efficacy of these measures, however, has been uncertain because of difficulty in identifying the severity of the pancreatitis being treated.

Clinical Classification

Prognostic classification of patients with acute pancreatitis is usually made primarily on clinical findings. Marked abdominal tenderness, distention or muscle spasm, and the presence of peritoneal fluid or a palpable abdominal mass are all considered evidence of severe disease. In addition, hypotension, respiratory distress, or mental confusion may indicate a poor prognosis. Most of these factors are, however, difficult or impossible to quantify objectively and may, therefore, be subject to observer variation. Furthermore, in a prospective study, McMahon et al.[20] found that initial clinical assessment successfully identified only 39% of patients who proved to have severe disease. Thus, while a careful clinical assessment is clearly of the greatest importance for individual patients, it must be recognized that clinical findings alone are an unreliable prognostic guide and provide an unsound basis for evaluation of the efficacy of proposed therapies.

Pathologic Classification

A precise classification of acute pancreatitis based on pathologic examination of the gland would be of considerable interest. Unfortunately, only a small and unrepresentative group of patients with pancreatitis come to autopsy or celiotomy, and our knowledge of the gross and microscopic features of human acute pancreatitis is therefore fragmentary. The morbidity and mortality of patients with extensive pancreatic hemorrhage or necrosis is usually greater than that of patients with pancreatic edema alone. In a recent collective review of findings in 397 patients who came to autopsy examination, 76% had necrotizing or hemorrhagic pancreatitis.[7] However, 24% of patients who died had edematous or interstitial pancreatitis without evidence of necrosis. In patients who undergo celiotomy, it is customary to categorize the gross appearance of the pancreas as edematous, hemorrhagic, or necrotizing. Use of these terms is, however, highly subjective, and the same operative findings may be interpreted differently by different observers. From a pathologic standpoint, all patients who have gross fat necrosis have "necrotizing" pancreatitis. Many such patients do not, however, have a complicated clinical course. Surgeons use the term "necrotizing" when extensive peripancreatic necrosis is present. Use

of this term, therefore, involves a judgment as to the degree of necrosis.

Table 31–3 shows the relationship between the early operative findings and mortality in 52 patients in whom celiotomy was undertaken during the first five days of illness. "Hemorrhagic" pancreatitis was identified by gross and extensive retroperitoneal hemorrhagic exudate. In "edematous" pancreatitis, pancreatic inflammation was often associated with fat necrosis, but the general anatomical relationships were maintained. Frank liquefaction necrosis of the pancreas was identified during this early phase of disease in only one patient, who was grouped with a larger number of patients who had a pancreatic "phlegmon." In this group, pancreatic enlargement was marked, and anatomical landmarks were obscured by inflammatory masses. There was a clear relationship between the early operative findings and overall mortality. It must be stressed, however, that sharp distinctions between these groups did not exist, and categorization was often arbitrary. Furthermore, most patients with pancreatitis do not undergo operation or autopsy, and no pathologic classification is possible in this group.

Etiologic Association

The relationship between the etiology of pancreatitis and mortality in a group of 450 patients is shown in Table 31–4. It appears that pancreatitis occurring in postoperative patients is a far more lethal illness than that which occurs in other clinical settings. Unfortunately, differences in mortality in different etiologic groups are clearly related to diagnostic criteria. For example, in our data, gallstone-related pancreatitis is associated with a mortality approximately twice that of alcohol-associated disease. A diagnosis of gallstone-associated pancreatitis is often reached on the basis of abdominal pain, nausea and vomiting, and elevated serum amylase levels. However, in patients meeting these criteria, if early operation or autopsy is undertaken, approximately 60% have no gross evidence of significant pancreatic inflammation. Morbidity and mortality in this group is low. In our data, we have included only those patients who had gross operative or clinical findings of pancreatitis other than simple hyperamylasemia. If all patients with hyperamylasemia were included in this group, mortality would be lower. Similarly, in patients who have recently undergone surgery, the presence of abdominal pain, nausea, and elevated serum amylase levels is often attributed to the preceding operative procedure, unless other complications of pancreatitis arise. It is clear, therefore, that until better methods are available to establish the diagnosis of acute pancreatitis, etiologic associations are not a reliable prognostic criterion.

TABLE 31–3.—OPERATIVE APPEARANCE OF THE PANCREAS RELATED TO MORTALITY IN 52 PATIENTS WHO UNDERWENT CELIOTOMY ON DAYS 0–5

OPERATIVE FINDINGS	NO. OF PATIENTS	MORTALITY, %
Edema	25	4
Hemorrhage	14	86
Phlegmon	13	54

TABLE 31–4.—THE MORTALITY OF ACUTE
PANCREATITIS RELATED TO SEX, ETIOLOGIC
ASSOCIATIONS, AND HISTORY OF PREVIOUS
EPISODES IN 450 PATIENTS

	NO. OF PATIENTS	NO. DEAD	% DEAD
All patients	450	32	7.1
Etiology			
Alcohol	315	12	3.8
Biliary	74	5	6.8
Postoperative	23	10	43.5
Other	38	5	13.2
Previous episodes			
0	282	27	9.6
1	76	4	5.3
> 1	92	1	1.1
Men	351	22	6.3
Women	99	10	10.1

History of Previous Pancreatitis

Table 31–4 also shows that most deaths from acute pancreatitis occurred during the first or second episodes of acute illness. In our hospital population, most patients with recurring pancreatitis abuse alcohol. In this group, all of the respiratory, cardiovascular, and septic complications of other etiologic subgroups may occur during the first or second acute episodes. These complications are rare after the first two episodes. In gallstone-associated and postoperative pancreatitis, the third and subsequent acute episodes have also been mild in our experience, but we have observed only a few of these patients with more than one previous acute attack. By contrast, in patients with pancreatitis associated with hyperlipoproteinemia, each recurring episode appears to have the potential virulence of the initial illness.

Objective Prognostic Signs

In 1974, we carried out a statistical analysis of the relationship between 43 measurements made during the initial 48 hours of treatment of acute pancreatitis and overall morbidity in 100 patients.[21] As a result of this analysis, 11 early objective prognostic signs were identified. They are listed in Table 31–5. Fluid sequestration was estimated crudely by subtracting the total volume of nasogastric aspirate and urinary output from the volume of fluid administered IV during the overall initial 48-hour period. The change in hematocrit and in BUN was also calculated on the basis of the change between hour 0 and hour 48, without regard to intermediate measurements. The only measurements that have been deliberately excluded from prognostic consideration are blood glucose levels in patients with known diabetes mellitus. Each of the signs listed in Table 31–5 correlates on a statistical basis with an increased risk of death or major complications from acute pancreatitis. The relationship between the number of these signs and overall mortality in a series of 450 patients is shown in Figure 31–3. In approximately 80% of patients, fewer than three positive signs were present, and in this group overall mortality was 0.9%. In patients with three or four positive signs, mortality rose to 16%; in those with five or six positive signs, it was 40%; and in those with seven or more signs, mortality was 100%.

TABLE 31–5.—THE 11 EARLY
OBJECTIVE SIGNS USED TO CLASSIFY
THE SEVERITY OF PANCREATITIS

At admission or diagnosis
  Age over 55 years
  WBC count over 16,000/cu mm
  Blood glucose over 200 mg/dl
  Serum lactic dehydrogenase over 350 IU/L
  SGOT over 250 Sigma-Frankel units %
During initial 48 hours
  Hematocrit fall greater than 10 percentage points
  BUN rise more than 5 mg/dl
  Serum calcium level below 8 mg/dl
  Arterial Po_2 below 60 mm Hg
  Base deficit greater than 4 mEq/L
  Estimated fluid sequestration more than 6,000 ml

It should be stressed that the prognostic signs do not have any diagnostic value and should not be used to differentiate patients with pancreatitis from those with other causes of acute abdominal pain. Furthermore, not every patient with three, four, or even five positive signs has severe pancreatitis. The signs only identify a group of patients with an increased risk of life-threatening complications. Although most of our patients had pancreatitis associated with alcohol abuse, these 11 signs have been shown to achieve good prognostic separation in patients with biliary, postoperative, or other forms of acute pancreatitis.[22]

Imrie et al.[16] described a system of prognostic signs similar to that shown in Table 31–5. Other studies have found that serum methemalbumin and cAMP levels may have prognostic value.[22] In addition, Warshaw and Lee[23] found a relationship between serum ribonuclease levels and pancreatic necrosis. McMahon et al.[20] reported that the severity of pancreatitis may be estimated by the volume and color of peritoneal fluid obtained by early paracentesis of peritoneal lavage. The usefulness of this approach may be limited by the potential hazards of paracentesis. It is certainly to be hoped that simpler

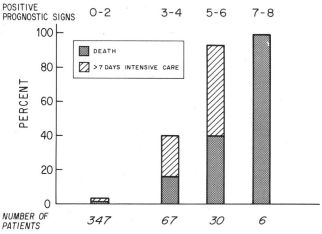

Fig 31–3.—The relationship between the number of positive early prognostic signs recorded and the percent mortality and morbidity in 450 patients with acute pancreatitis. (From Ranson J.H.C.: Acute pancreatitis. *Curr. Probl. Surg.* Chicago, Year Book Medical Publishers, November 1979, p. 33. Used by permission.)

and more precise methods of classifying pancreatitis will be developed in the future. Nonetheless, the existing prognostic signs do allow the early objective identification of a group of patients who have a high risk of life-threatening complications. It is hoped that the use of these signs will allow improved management for individual patients and a more rational evaluation of proposed treatments for acute pancreatitis.

EARLY TREATMENT

A wide variety of medical and surgical measures has been proposed for the early treatment of patients with acute pancreatitis. The primary objective of these measures may be broadly categorized as: (1) to limit the severity of pancreatic inflammation; (2) to ameliorate the course of disease by interrupting the pathogenesis of its complications; and (3) to support the patient and treat specific complications. Many of these measures are listed in Tables 31–6 and 31–7. In general, measures in the first two categories were recommended initially on the basis of our limited understanding of the pathogenesis of acute pancreatitis and its complications. With the possible exception of antacid administration to prevent acute gastroduodenal hemorrhage, none of the measures in these two categories has been clearly demonstrated to be of benefit in clinical pancreatitis.[7, 24] In recent years, some of these measures have been evaluated by controlled clinical trials. Unfortunately, interpretation of the results of many of these trials has been clouded by the wide variation which exists in the natural history of pancreatitis. This wide variation tends to result in no statistically demonstrable difference between treatment groups in unstratified clinical trials unless very large numbers of patients are included. For example, studies of the therapeutic efficacy of nasogastric suction which failed to show significant benefit included only 29 to 58 patients and

TABLE 31–6.—NONOPERATIVE MEASURES PROPOSED FOR THE TREATMENT OF ACUTE PANCREATITIS

To limit the severity of pancreatic inflammation
  Inhibition of pancreatic secretion
    Nasogastric suction
    Pharmacologic
      Anticholinergics, glucagon, fluourouracil,
        acetazolamide, cimetidine, propylthiouracil,
        calcitonin, somatostatin
    Hypothermia
    Pancreatic irradiation
  Inhibition of pancreatic enzymes
    Aprotinin, ε-aminocaproic acid, soybean trypsin inhibitor,
      insulin, snake antivenom
  Corticosteroids
To interrupt the pathogenesis of complications
  Antibiotics
  Antacids, cimetidine
  Heparin, fibrinolysin
  Low molecular weight dextran
  Vasopressin
To support the patient and treat complications
  Restoration and maintenance of intravascular volume
  Electrolyte replacement
  Respiratory support
  Analgesia
  Nutritional support
  Heparin

TABLE 31–7.—OPERATIVE MEASURES PROPOSED FOR THE TREATMENT OF ACUTE PANCREATITIS

To limit the severity of pancreatic inflammation
  Biliary operations
To interrupt the pathogenesis of complications
  Pancreatic drainage
  Pancreatic resection
  Thoracic duct drainage
  Peritoneal lavage
To support the patient and treat complications
  Feeding jejunostomy
  Drainage of abscesses or cysts

are probably too small for valid statistical interpretation. By contrast, aprotinin and glucagon have been convincingly shown to have no beneficial effect in trials which included 161 to 246 patients.[25, 26]

NONOPERATIVE MANAGEMENT

The treatment of all patients must include careful observation of their overall clinical condition together with their response to treatment. The possibility of an error in diagnosis must be closely evaluated.

Inhibition of Pancreatic Secretion

Nasogastric suction is usually introduced to reduce vomiting and abdominal distention. It has also been suggested that aspiration of gastric acid may decrease pancreatic exocrine secretion by reducing secretion release. As discussed above, small unstratified controlled studies of nasogastric suction have failed to demonstrate statistically significant amelioration of pancreatitis by this measure, and certainly many patients with mild disease recover without it.[7, 8] We continue, however, to recommend nasogastric suction for most patients because of the symptomatic improvement which often results and because of the decrease in evidence of pancreatic inflammation which occasionally ensues.

Whatever the role of nasogastric suction, experimental studies have demonstrated that gastric feedings during acute pancreatitis increase the severity of pancreatic inflammation.[8] It has been our repeated clinical experience that the resumption of oral feedings prior to resolution of pancreatitis is followed by reactivation of pancreatitis and further complications. Oral feedings should, therefore, be withheld until pain, tenderness, fever, and leukocytosis have resolved, and, in most patients, the serum amylase has returned to normal. When oral feedings are resumed, they should be low in fat content. In patients with severe pancreatitis, CT scans may show evidence of pancreatic inflammation long after clinical signs of pancreatitis have resolved. These radiographic findings may take weeks or months to resolve and, in most patients, the nutritional status can be safely maintained by low-fat oral feedings during this convalescent phase.

Inhibition of pancreatic exocrine secretion by a wide variety of pharmacologic agents, hypothermia, or pancreatic irradiation has been recommended on the basis of uncontrolled clinical experience or experimental studies. Of these, atropine, glucagon, cimetidine, and calcitonin have been found to be ineffective in controlled clinical trials.[27]

Inhibition of Pancreatic Enzymes

The concept that the severity of pancreatitis and its complications might be reduced by inhibition of pancreatic enzymes has been extensively investigated over the past 25 years. In particular, aprotinin, a polypeptide that inhibits trypsin and kallikrein, has been repeatedly studied in clinical trials and has been convincingly shown to be ineffective in reducing the morbidity of pancreatitis. Epsilon-amino caproic acid inhibits plasmin and trypsin. Insulin may decrease lipase activity, but both agents have been ineffective in controlled trials.[27, 28] Administration of corticosteroids has been recommended in the past because of their anti-inflammatory effects, but there is, at present, no clinical evidence to support their use.

Antibiotics

Three small, unstratified controlled clinical studies have failed to demonstrate any reduction in the morbidity of pancreatitis from the administration of ampicillin.[27] Many of the patients in these studies had mild alcoholic pancreatitis, and although there is no clear evidence of benefit, we continue to recommend broad-spectrum antibiotic administration, usually a cephalosporin, in patients with severe or gallstone-associated pancreatitis.

Antacids

Upper GI hemorrhage from acute ulceration is a frequent complication in patients with severe pancreatitis. The incidence of such bleeding can be sharply reduced by monitoring of gastric pH and administration of antacids to maintain a pH greater than 4.

Heparin and Fibrinolysin

Intravascular coagulation has been documented in the pancreas, lungs, and other tissues during acute pancreatitis. This has led to the suggestion that the administration of heparin or fibrinolysin might ameliorate the course of disease. Experimental evaluation of this suggestion has yielded conflicting results.[29] However, in clinical experience with ten patients receiving heparin during the first few days of acute pancreatitis, no benefit was observed, and marked retroperitoneal hemorrhage occurred in two instances. Thus, anticoagulants should, if possible, be avoided during the early phase of pancreatitis.

Although the early administration of heparin may be hazardous, serial studies of coagulation factors have demonstrated marked thrombocytosis and hyperfibrinogenemia during the second and third weeks of treatment in some patients with severe acute pancreatitis. In such patients, heparin administration may have a role in the prevention of pulmonary embolism.

Low Molecular Weight Dextran and Vasopressin

Modification of pancreatic blood flow by the administration of low molecular weight dextran or vasopressin has been reported to ameliorate the severity of experimental acute pancreatitis, but the clinical applicability of these findings is unknown.

Restoration and Maintenance of Intravascular Volume

The intravascular volume of the patient must be carefully restored, monitored, and maintained. In most patients this requires placement of a central venous catheter for monitoring of central venous pressures and the introduction of an indwelling urethral catheter for measurement of hourly urine output. In patients with marked fluid shifts or associated cardiopulmonary disease, monitoring of pulmonary arterial pressure by means of a Swan-Ganz catheter may be essential for appropriate IV fluid therapy.

In most patients, intravascular volume can be satisfactorily restored and maintained by the administration of crystalloid solutions. Measurements of serum albumin or of hematocrit may indicate the need for transfusion of plasma or blood. In patients who require the administration of colloid solutions, the use of fresh frozen plasma may theoretically be advantageous because of the natural proteinase inhibitors which are present.[30]

Electrolyte Replacement

Hypokalemia is frequent and potassium replacement is usually required. Intravenous replacement of calcium and magnesium have been advocated.[31] However, hypocalcemia is often related to hypoalbuminemia,[32] and since hypercalcemia has been implicated in the pathogenesis of pancreatitis, calcium administration should be carried out with caution.

Respiratory Support

Clinically occult respiratory insufficiency is a frequent early feature of acute pancreatitis, occurring in about 40% of patients.[33–35] It may occur in patients who do not have severe disease by the usual clinical criteria, and physical and radiographic examinations of the chest are usually normal at this time. Since early arterial hypoxemia may be lethal if undiagnosed or untreated, it is essential that arterial blood gas determinations be obtained at the time of diagnosis and at intervals of not more than 12 hours in every patient for the initial 48–72 hours of treatment.

In most patients, early hypoxemia improves as pancreatitis subsides, and the only management needed is close monitoring and administration of oxygen. Clinically obvious progressive respiratory insufficiency or pulmonary complications tend to occur in patients with severe or protracted pancreatitis and in those who undergo early laparotomy, and it should be anticipated in these groups. In patients with progressive pulmonary insufficiency, the severity of this complication may be ameliorated by restricting the volume of fluid administered IV and by increasing urinary output with diuretic drugs.[34] When needed, endotracheal intubation and mechanically assisted ventilation with positive end-expiratory pressure should be instituted early.

Analgesia

The pain associated with acute pancreatitis may be very severe, and it is traditional to administer meperidine rather than morphine, because spasm of the ampulla of Vater is associated with morphine. Splanchnic block or continuous epidural anesthesia has been recommended because they avoid ampullary spasm and may increase pancreatic blood flow. They are not, however, widely used.

Nutritional Support

Marked nutritional depletion occurs in patients with acute pancreatitis. In those with mild disease, low-fat oral feedings can usually be resumed within a few days. In those with severe pancreatitis, oral feedings may not be tolerated for prolonged periods, and nutritional support by IV alimentation should be instituted as soon as the patient's cardiovascular condition allows. The use of IV lipids as a source of nutrition has given rise to concern because of the association of hyperlipidemia with acute pancreatitis. In patients with hypertriglyceridemia, lipids should be avoided. In other patients, however, standard doses of Intralipid 10% IV Fat Emulsion appear to be well tolerated. They usually do not result in elevated triglyceride levels, and no exacerbation of pancreatitis has been documented.[36] When intestinal peristalsis returns, enteric feedings of a low-fat formula diet may be instituted by a fine catheter introduced into the jejunum under fluoroscopic control.

OPERATIVE MEASURES

In patients with acute pancreatitis, early celiotomy may be required to exclude or treat acute extrapancreatic disease. In addition, surgical intervention may be required for the management of complications such as pseudocyst or abscess. It has also been proposed that early operative measures may ameliorate the course of acute pancreatitis, and the procedures which have been suggested are listed in Table 31–7.

It is usually agreed that most patients with acute pancreatitis recover following nonoperative management, and most of the measures listed in Table 31–7 have been recommended for patients with "severe" disease. Much of the controversy surrounding the efficacy of these measures is related to difficulty in the identification and definition of "severe" pancreatitis. In many reports concerning the efficacy of operative therapy, the severity of pancreatitis is estimated by the operative appearance of pancreatic hemorrhage or necrosis. As discussed earlier in this chapter, these findings are subject to variable interpretation and cannot, in any event, be used to evaluate the relative efficacy of operative and nonoperative treatments. It is to be hoped that the use of objective criteria to estimate the risk of death or major complications of acute pancreatitis will clarify the role of the operative treatments described.

Biliary Operations

In patients with acute pancreatitis and gallstones, surgical intervention may be undertaken to exclude or treat associated gangrenous cholecystitis or obstructive cholangitis. It has also been proposed that early biliary operation may ameliorate the course of acute gallstone-associated pancreatitis. In general, operation has been recommended for patients with severe pancreatitis, and the procedures recommended have included cholecystostomy, external drainage of the common bile duct, and cholecystectomy.[8] More recently, Acosta and associates[36]

proposed that persistent calculus obstruction of the ampulla of Vater may be responsible for progression of pancreatic inflammation. They reviewed 132 patients judged to have acute gallstone pancreatitis with symptoms of less than 48 hours' duration. In 86 patients treated prior to 1972, a nonoperative early approach was followed, and the mortality during that period was 16%. Between 1972 and 1975, 46 patients were managed by early definitive biliary surgery. In this group, a gallstone was found to be impacted in the ampulla of Vater in 72% of cases, and overall mortality fell to 2%.[37] Acosta et al. therefore recommended cholecystostomy, common bile duct exploration, and, when indicated, transduodenal sphincterotomy, when surgery could be accomplished within 48 hours of the onset of symptoms.

Stone et al.[38] evaluated the role of early biliary surgery in patients with gallstone-associated pancreatitis by a controlled clinical trial. Thirty-six patients with gallstones, abdominal pain, and elevated amylase levels were assigned to operation within 73 hours of hospital admission. This group underwent cholecystectomy, transduodenal sphincteroplasty, and pancreatic duct septotomy. Thirty-four similar patients received conventional nonoperative therapy and were scheduled for the same operative procedure three months later. In patients who underwent early operation, a rapid clinical improvement was commonly recorded. One of these patients died (2.9%), and the average hospital stay of the survivors was 13.5 days. In patients managed nonoperatively, there were no deaths during this admission, and the average hospital stay was 10.7 days. These findings do not suggest that early biliary surgery ameliorated the pancreatitis. However, among 29 patients who returned for delayed elective biliary surgery, there were two postoperative deaths (6.8%), and the average duration of the second hospital stay was 12.1 days. It is not clear why the morbidity and mortality of elective biliary surgery was so high in this study, but the authors concluded that, in patients with gallstone-associated pancreatitis, early definitive biliary operation is safe and reduces the overall morbidity of the disease by obviating a second hospital admission for correction of biliary disease.

Evaluation of the efficacy of early biliary surgery in ameliorating acute pancreatitis has been confused by difficulty in determining the diagnosis and estimating the severity of pancreatitis. Up to 75% of patients with acute abdominal pain, gallstones, and elevated amylase levels have no gross evidence of significant acute pancreatitis at early operation or autopsy. In such patients, early definitive treatment of biliary disease may usually be undertaken safely, with prompt subsidence of biliary symptoms. Among patients who have clear evidence of pancreatitis, approximately 80% have mild disease, and in this group early biliary surgery can often be undertaken safely, but, as indicated by the Stone study, does not clearly ameliorate the course of the acute illness. Twenty percent of patients have severe pancreatitis, and in our experience early intra-abdominal surgery has been associated with a substantially higher morbidity and mortality than early nonoperative treatment in this group.

Our experience with the management of 133 episodes of acute pancreatitis associated with cholelithiasis is summarized in Figure 31–4. These data include only patients who had clear operative or clinical evidence of acute pancreatitis and

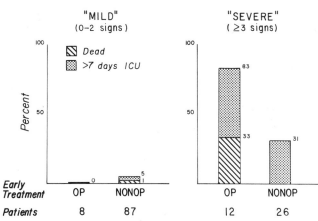

Fig 31–4.—Morbidity and mortality of 133 episodes of acute gallstone pancreatitis. Patients undergoing intra-abdominal surgery during the initial 48 hours *(OP)* are compared with those managed nonoperatively during this period *(NONOP)*. "Severity" of pancreatitis is classified by early objective prognostic signs. (From Ranson J.H.C.: The surgical treatment of acute pancreatitis. *Bull. N.Y. Acad. Med.* 58:604, 1982. Used by permission.)

exclude those with elevated serum amylase levels alone. Ninety-five episodes of acute pancreatitis were designated as "mild" on the basis of the presence of fewer than three positive prognostic signs. In this group, there was only one death, which occurred from respiratory failure in a patient who underwent definitive biliary surgery on the fourth hospital day, while clinical evidence of pancreatitis was still present. Twenty-nine percent of the whole group of patients was considered to have "severe" pancreatitis on the basis of early prognostic signs. There were four deaths (33%) in the group of 12 patients who underwent intra-abdominal surgery, usually consisting of cholecystectomy and common bile duct exploration, during the first 48 hours after diagnosis. By contrast, 26 of these patients were managed initially by nonoperative means with no deaths, although 31% developed complications which required at least seven days of intensive care.

Prior to 1972, we followed a policy of early biliary surgery in patients considered to have severe, gallstone-associated pancreatitis. Mortality during that period was high, and it is striking that, since returning to a nonoperative early approach, there has been a dramatic reduction in morbidity and mortality.[8] It is, therefore, our current practice to manage gallstone pancreatitis by nonoperative measures if gangrenous cholecystitis or obstructive cholangitis can be excluded.

Encouraging results have recently been described following endoscopic sphincterotomy in patients judged to have gallstone pancreatitis.[39, 40] Because it is difficult or impossible to differentiate by nonoperative means obstructive cholangitis with minimal pancreatitis from severe pancreatitis with gallstones, these results are hard to interpret. We have been reluctant to carry out endoscopic sphincterotomy in patients with severe pancreatitis because of the potential hazards of further pancreatic injury and of introducing unsterile contrast material into a devitalized gland. This technique may, however, prove a valuable approach in the rare patient in whom

pancreatitis will not resolve until ampullary obstruction is relieved.

Although early biliary surgery has not in our experience been effective in reducing the morbidity of acute pancreatitis, correction of cholelithiasis is needed to prevent recurrent episodes of pancreatic inflammation. In the past, a four- to six-week period of convalescence has often been recommended after acute pancreatitis before the elective biliary procedure. During this period, the patient is exposed to the risk of recurrent pancreatitis, and in most patients correction of cholelithiasis can be safely undertaken as soon as evidence of acute pancreatic inflammation has subsided. In the relatively small group of patients with severe pancreatitis, it may be advisable to allow the pancreatic inflammatory mass to resolve over a period of several weeks before undertaking biliary surgery.

Gallstone-associated pancreatitis may occasionally occur during pregnancy. In this setting, pancreatitis clearly poses a risk not only to the life of the mother but also to that of the fetus. These risks are related to the severity of the underlying pancreatitis, and there is no evidence that termination of pregnancy will reduce the maternal risk. Early management of pancreatitis should be by nonoperative means. After pancreatitis has subsided, operative correction of associated cholelithiasis has been recommended during the second trimester in patients who develop pancreatitis during the first or second trimesters. In the third trimester, biliary surgery may often be postponed until after delivery, but management must depend on the clinical course and estimates of the maturity of the fetus.[41]

Pancreatic Drainage

Early operative drainage of the pancreas was often recommended for severe acute pancreatitis in the first 30 years of this century, and has received renewed attention recently.[42, 43] Our own evaluation of this approach was by a small controlled clinical trial in patients considered to have "severe" pancreatitis. Wide sump drainage of the pancreas combined with cholecystostomy, gastrostomy, and jejunostomy (Fig 31–5) were carried out within 48 hours of hospital-

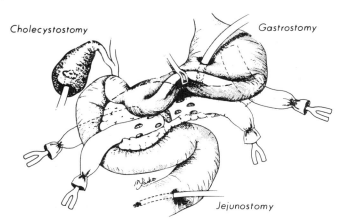

Fig 31–5.—Diagrammatic representation of early pancreatic drainage procedure evaluated in a small controlled trial. (From Ranson J.H.C.: Acute pancreatitis. *Curr. Probl. Surg.* Chicago, Year Book Medical Publishers, November, 1979, p. 49. Used by permission.)

ization in patients assigned to early surgery and compared to standard nonoperative treatment. Only ten patients were included in this study, but the frequency of intra-abdominal sepsis and the severity of respiratory complications were dramatically increased in those patients who underwent early surgery. All ten patients survived, but the mean period of intensive care rose from 10.3 days for unoperated patients to 27.8 days in the operative group. Furthermore, it was striking that the most marked increases in morbidity following early surgery were observed in patients with the most severe acute pancreatitis.[21]

Pancreatic Resection

In 1963, Watts[44] described survival of a patient with pancreatitis who had been treated by total pancreatectomy approximately 48 hours after the onset of symptoms. Since that report, there has been extensive interest in the possibility that early removal of part or all of the pancreas may decrease the devastating systemic and local sequelae of severe acute pancreatitis. Experimental studies have not demonstrated a reduction in mortality over that achieved with supportive treatment, unless resection is undertaken within 30 minutes of the induction of disease.[8] In clinical reports of resection, pancreatitis is described as "necrotizing" or "hemorrhagic," but the severity of disease is usually not estimated by objective criteria.[45] In a collective review of 129 patients treated by primary pancreatic resection, Edelmann and Boutelier[46] found an overall survival of 61%. Mortality rose from 29% in those treated by resection of necrotic tissue alone to 67% in those who underwent total pancreatectomy.[47]

Some years ago, we carried out distal subtotal pancreatic resection within 48 hours of diagnosis in five patients with severe acute pancreatitis. All had extensive retroperitoneal hemorrhage or frank liquefaction necrosis of the gland itself. The average number of positive prognostic signs was five (range, three to eight). Unfortunately, the subsequent clinical course of these patients was similar to that of other patients with pancreatitis of comparable severity. It was marked by respiratory failure, intra-abdominal sepsis, and eventual death in all cases.

In a recent controlled clinical study,[19] celiotomy and pancreatic resection was compared with celiotomy and placement of catheters for postoperative peritoneal lavage. Four of 18 resected patients died (22%) compared to 8 of 17 patients treated by lavage (47%). Although this difference did not achieve statistical significance, it raises the possibility that, in patients who are subjected to early celiotomy, resection may be superior to placement of lavage catheters alone. Unfortunately, in this study all patients underwent celiotomy, so that no conclusions can be reached concerning the relative merits of operative measures compared to nonoperative treatment. The severity of pancreatitis in this study was estimated by objective prognostic signs. The patients in the two treatment groups had an average of 3.7 and 3.9 positive signs, suggesting that possible inclusion of patients with a low statistical risk of life-threatening complications.

Our overall clinical experience has been that early intra-abdominal surgery does not ameliorate the course of acute pancreatitis in any group identified. In patients with mild pancreatitis, early celiotomy may be tolerated without diffi-

culty, but the frequency of respiratory and septic complications is increased. In patients with "severe" pancreatitis, defined by the presence of three or more positive prognostic signs, celiotomy has been associated with clearly increased mortality (Fig 31–6).

Thoracic Duct Drainage

Since pancreatic enzymes may reach the bloodstream by lymphatic channels, it has been proposed that diversion of thoracic duct lymph by construction of a thoracic duct fistula may benefit patients with acute pancreatitis. Controlled clinical trials have not been reported, but experimental studies have suggested that relative thoracic duct obstruction may obviate the potential advantages of this procedure.[47]

Peritoneal Lavage

In 1965, Wall[48] reported marked clinical improvement in three patients with acute pancreatitis when peritoneal dialysis was instituted to treat associated renal failure. Subsequent experimental and clinical studies by several other authors[49–52] indicated that peritoneal lavage may be a valuable treatment in acute pancreatitis.

INDICATIONS AND TECHNIQUES OF PERITONEAL LAVAGE.—We have considered any patients who were experiencing their first or second episode of acute pancreatitis and had three or more positive prognostic signs to be candidates for peritoneal lavage.[53] Because bowel distention is common in patients with severe pancreatitis, we have attempted to minimize the risk of visceral injury by introducing lavage catheters through an open incision, about 4–5 cm long, with direct visualization of the peritoneum. Catheters are placed in the midline below the umbilicus using sterile technique and local infiltration of anesthesia. In patients with previous abdominal incisions, an area remote from these incisions is selected. We currently use a soft, noncollapsible silastic drain

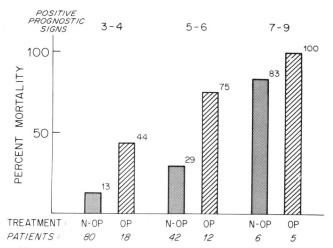

Fig 31–6.—Overall mortality following early (day 0–7) intra-abdominal surgery (OP) compared to that following early nonoperative management (NONOP) in 163 patients with severe acute pancreatitis defined by early objective prognostic signs. (From Ranson J.H.C.: The surgical treatment of acute pancreatitis. *N.Y. Bull. Acad. Med.* 58:607, 1982. Used by permission.)

as our peritoneal lavage catheter. The abdominal incision is closed tightly about the catheter. The lavage fluid is an approximately isotonic electrolyte solution containing 15 gm/L of dextrose (Dianeal). Potassium, 4 mEq/L, heparin, 500 USP/L, and ampicillin, 125 mg are usually added to each liter of lavage fluid. In general, 2 L of the fluid is allowed to run into the peritoneal cavity over about 15 minutes, to remain intraperitoneally for about 30 minutes, and then drained out by gravity over 15 minutes. The cycle is usually repeated hourly, employing 48 L of lavage fluid during each 24 hours. Lavage has been instituted within 48 hours of diagnosis in all patients. It has been discontinued after 48 hours to seven days, depending on the patient's course.

In addition to the risk of visceral injury during catheter placement, there are two important hazards of peritoneal lavage. First, respiratory insufficiency is a frequent feature of severe pancreatitis. The addition of 2 L of fluid to the peritoneal cavity may cause a significant decrease in pulmonary ventilation. Therefore, respiratory function must be closely monitored throughout lavage, including regular arterial blood gas measurements. It is sometimes necessary to reduce the volume and timing of the lavage cycle to avoid undue respiratory distress. Second, the tonicity of the lavage fluid is maintained with glucose. Since impaired glucose tolerance is a feature of severe pancreatitis, serum glucose levels must be measured regularly and insulin administered as needed. With these precautions, lavage has been free of complications in our experience.

THERAPEUTIC EFFICACY OF PERITONEAL LAVAGE.— Our initial evaluation of peritoneal lavage was by a controlled trial in ten patients with three or more positive prognostic signs.[54] We compared peritoneal lavage with conventional nonoperative management. No patient in this study underwent operation within the first seven days of treatment, and it was found that lavage reduced the mean period of intensive care from 17.4 days to 8.4 days. The only death in that small study occurred in a nonlavaged patient. Following this early trial, peritoneal lavage has been used more widely in patients with acute pancreatitis associated with three or more positive early prognostic signs. Striking clinical improvement has usually been noted shortly after the institution of lavage.

Figure 31–7 shows the early (day 0–10) mortality in patients managed with peritoneal lavage compared to those managed without peritoneal lavage. These data include patients who underwent early celiotomy as well as those who were managed nonoperatively for the initial period. In 110 nonlavaged patients, early mortality was 15%. In this group, approximately 40% of all deaths occurred during the first ten days of treatment, primarily from cardiovascular and respiratory failure. By contrast, there were only two early deaths (4%) in 48 similar patients managed with peritoneal lavage. In one of these patients, lavage was carried out for a short period, followed by celiotomy because of failure to respond. Nonocclusive mesenteric infarction affecting his entire bowel was found, in addition to extensive hemorrhagic pancreatitis.

The therapeutic efficacy of peritoneal lavage has generally been attributed to removal of toxic material in the peritoneal exudate of acute pancreatitis. Since hemodialysis has not been associated with significant improvement, it is probable that

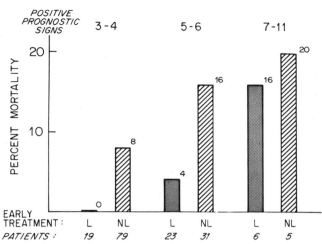

Fig 31–7.—Early (day 0–10) mortality in patients with three or more positive prognostic signs managed with peritoneal lavage (L) or without lavage (NL). Those in whom lavage catheters were introduced at laparotomy are included, as are those who underwent other surgical procedures. (From Ranson J.H.C.: The surgical treatment of acute pancreatitis. *Bull. N.Y. Acad. Med.* 58:608, 1982. Used by permission.)

the efficacy of lavage is not due to improvement in fluid and electrolyte balance or to removal of dialysable substances from the blood. Studies of the peritoneal exudate formed during acute pancreatitis have shown that this exudate contains amylase, lipase, phospholipase A, trypsinogen, prostaglandin-like activity, and kinin-forming enzymes. In addition, the peritoneal exudate has been shown to produce systemic hypotension, histamine release, and increased vascular permeability.[54] Whatever the factor or factors responsible for the toxic effects of the peritoneal exudate in acute pancreatitis, it is clear that its removal, however incomplete, by peritoneal lavage is associated with a decreased early mortality from severe acute pancreatitis.

Unfortunately, the overall hospital mortality has not been greatly altered by the use of peritoneal lavage. In patients managed nonoperatively for the first seven days of treatment, shown in Fig 31–8, there is some slight improvement in mortality in each group. This improvement is, however, disappointingly small. Virtually all deaths in patients managed by peritoneal lavage have been due to late peripancreatic sepsis. We have examined the possibility that lavage might be associated with an increased risk of sepsis and found that this was not the case.[53] Clearly, however, early peritoneal lavage does not prevent the late sequelae of peripancreatic necrosis; specifically, infected pancreatic abscess.

Three subsequent randomized control studies of peritoneal lavage have been reported.[55–57] In Stone and Fabian's study,[55] 85% of 34 patients managed with lavage showed "decided improvement in overall condition" at the end of 24 hours. This contrasted with similar improvement in only 36% of 36 patients managed without peritoneal lavage. In an unstated proportion of patients in these two groups, severe pancreatitis was diagnosed at celiotomy. Evaluation of the overall efficacy of lavage in this study is clouded by the fact that 17 patients

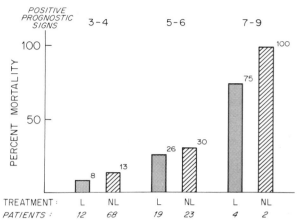

Fig 31–8.—Overall hospital mortality in 128 patients with severe pancreatitis whose early (day 0–7) management did not include laparotomy. Those treated by peritoneal lavage *(L)* are compared to those managed by conventional nonoperative measures *(NL)*. (From Ranson J.H.C.: The surgical treatment of acute pancreatitis. *Bull. N.Y. Acad. Med.* 58:609, 1982. Used by permission.)

TABLE 31–8.—SUMMARY OF CURRENT MANAGEMENT OF ACUTE PANCREATITIS

All patients
　Diagnostic evalution: clinical, radiographic, serum amylase
　Nasogastric suction: in moderate or severe disease
　Monitoring and maintenance of intravascular volume
　Analgesia
　Respiratory monitoring and support
　Antibiotics in severe or gallstone disease
　Early celiotomy only for diagnosis
　Prognostic assessment
"Severe" pancreatitis
　Peritoneal lavage
　Nutritional support
　Late heparin after 14 days if hypercoagulable
　Suspect and treat pancreatic sepsis

in the nonlavaged group who did not improve were subsequently transferred to the peritoneal lavage group. Nonetheless, of a total of 51 patients who did receive early peritoneal lavage, there were eight deaths (15.6%). By contrast, in the 19 patients who were managed without lavage, there were six deaths (31.6%).

In the studies reported by Mayer et al.[56] and by Ishe et al.,[57] all patients were managed without formal early laparotomy, and there was no significant difference in overall mortality between the lavage and nonlavage groups. The time of death, however, tended to be later in patients managed by early peritoneal lavage.

Since peritoneal lavage does not appear to reduce the overall mortality of severe acute pancreatitis, its use may be questioned. As indicated above, we have found that it is a valuable adjunct to the management of the early cardiovascular and respiratory complications of severe pancreatitis and continue to recommend it for this specific purpose. Clearly, improved methods are still needed for the prevention and more effective treatment of pancreatic abscesses.

CONCLUSIONS

The diagnosis of acute pancreatitis can usually be reached on the basis of a careful clinical, laboratory, and radiographic assessment of the patient. Unfortunately, there is no objective test that reliably establishes the presence or absence of acute pancreatitis in all patients, and celiotomy is occasionally required to exclude or treat acute extrapancreatic disease.

The clinical spectrum of acute pancreatitis is broad, and objective prognostic assessment of individual patients helps the selection of appropriate management for individual patients and permits more rational evaluation of proposed therapeutic regimens.

At present, no treatment has been clearly demonstrated to limit the severity of pancreatic inflammation or reduce complications. Management, therefore, remains primarily suppor-

tive. Although the treatment of patients must be individualized, the general approach which we currently follow is summarized in Table 31–8. Overall mortality with this regimen is 4%–6%, and deaths are primarily related to the septic sequelae of extensive peripancreatic necrosis.

REFERENCES

1. Aubert J.: *Progymnasmata* (1579), quoted by J. Browne in *Adenochoiradelogia, or An Exact Anatomical Treatise of the Glandules*. London, S. Lowndes, 1684, pp. 142–143.
2. Tulpius (1641), quoted by Mayo A.W., Moynihan B.G.A., in *Diseases of the Pancreas and Their Surgical Treatment*. Philadelphia, W.B. Saunders Co., 1903, pp. 58–134.
3. Ancelet E.: *L'anatomie Pathologique du Pancreas*. Paris, Rignoux, 1856, pp. 21–24.
4. Senn N.: *The Surgery of the Pancreas*. Philadelphia, W.J. Dornan, 1886, pp. 71–107.
5. Fitz R.H.: Acute pancreatitis. *Boston Med. Surg.* 120:181–229, 1889.
6. Moynihan B.: Acute pancreatitis. *Ann. Surg.* 81:132, 1925.
7. Dürr G.H.-K.: Acute pancreatitis, in Howat H.T., Sarles H. (eds.): *The Exocrine Pancreas*. London, W.B. Saunders Co., 1979, pp. 352–401.
8. Ranson J.H.C.: Acute pancreatitis. *Curr. Probl. Surg.* 16:1, 1979.
9. Warshaw A.L., Bellini C.A., Lesser P.B.: Inhibition of serum and urine amylase activity in pancreatitis with hyperlipidemia. *Ann. Surg.* 182:72, 1975.
10. Stefanini P., Ermini M., Carboni, M.: Diagnosis and management of acute pancreatitis. *Am. J. Surg.* 110:866, 1965.
11. Levitt M.D.: Clinical use of amylase clearance and isoamylase measurements. *Mayo Clin. Proc.* 54:428, 1979.
12. Collins R.E.C., Frost S.J., Spittlehouse K.E.: The P₃iso-enzyme of serum amylase in the management of patients with acute pancreatitis. *Br. J. Surg.* 69:373, 1982.
13. Banks P.A.: *Pancreatitis*. New York, Plenum Medical Book Co., 1979, pp. 75–76.
14. Machiedo G.W., Brown C.S., Lavigne J.E., et al.: Use of peritoneal lavage in the diagnosis of experimental acute pancreatitis. *Surg. Gynecol. Obstet.* 140:889, 1975.
15. Coppa G.F., LeFleur R., Ranson J.H.C.: The role of Chiba-needle cholangiography in the diagnosis of possible acute pancreatitis with cholelithiasis. *Ann. Surg.* 193:393, 1981.
16. McKay A.J., Imrie C.W., O'Neill J., et al.: Is an early ultrasound scan of value in acute pancreatitis? *Br. J. Surg.* 69:369, 1982.
17. Jeffrey R.B., Federle M.P., Cello J.P., et al.: Early computed tomographic scanning in acute severe pancreatitis. *Surg. Gynecol. Obstet.* 154:170, 1982.
18. Gliedman M.L., Bolooki H., Rosen R.G.: Acute pancreatitis. *Curr. Probl. Surg.* 17, 1970.
19. Kivilaakso E., Lempinen M., Mäkeläinen A., et al.: Pancreatic

resection versus peritoneal lavation for acute fulminant pancreatitis. *Ann. Surg.* 199:426, 1984.

20. McMahon M.J., Playforth M.J., Pickford I.R.: A comparative study of methods for the prediction of severity of attacks of acute pancreatitis. *Br. J. Surg.* 67:22, 1980.

21. Ranson J.H.C., Rifkind K.M., Roses D.F., et al.: Prognostic signs and the role of operative management in acute pancreatitis. *Surg. Gynecol. Obstet.* 139:69, 1974.

22. Ranson J.H.C.: Etiological and prognostic factors in human acute pancreatitis. *Am. J. Gastroenterol.* 77:633, 1982.

23. Warshaw A.L., Lee K.-H.: Serum ribonuclease elevation and pancreatic necrosis in acute pancreatitis. *Surgery* 86:227, 1979.

24. Regan P.T.: Medical treatment of acute pancreatitis. *Mayo Clin. Proc.* 54:432, 1979.

25. Imrie C.W., Benjamin I.S., Ferguson J.C., et al.: A single-centre double-blind trial of Trasylol therapy in primary acute pancreatitis. *Br. J. Surg.* 65:337, 1978.

26. Welbourne R.B., Armitage P., Gilmore O.J.A., et al.: Death from acute pancreatitis. *Lancet* 2:632, 1977.

27. Creutzfeldt W., Lankisch P.G.: Intensive medical treatment of severe acute pancreatitis. *World J. Surg.* 5:341, 1981.

28. Svenson J.-O.: Role of intravenously infused insulin in treatment of acute pancreatitis. *Scand. J. Gastroenterol.* 10:487, 1975.

29. Ranson J.H.C., Lackner H.: Coagulopathies, in Bradley E.L. (ed.): *Complications of Pancreatitis.* Philadelphia, W.B. Saunders Co., 1982, pp. 154–175.

30. Cushchieri A., Wood R.A.B., Cumming J.R.G., et al.: Treatment of acute pancreatitis with fresh frozen plasma. *Br. J. Surg.* 70:710, 1983.

31. Wills M.R.: Hypocalcemia and hypomagnesaemia in acute pancreatitis. *Br. J. Surg.* 53:174, 1966.

32. Imrie C.W., Allam B.F., Ferguson J.C.: Hypocalcemia of acute pancreatitis: The effect of hypoalbuminaemia. *Curr. Med. Res. Opinion* 4;101, 1976.

33. Imrie C.W., Ferguson J.C., Murphy D., et al.: Arterial hypoxia in acute pancreatitis. *Br. J. Surg.* 64:185, 1977.

34. Ranson J.H.C., Turner J.W., Roses D.F., et al.: Respiratory complications in acute pancreatitis. *Ann. Surg.* 179:557, 1974.

35. Lankisch P.G., Rahlf G., Koop H.: Pulmonary complications in fatal acute hemorrhagic pancreatitis. *Dig. Dis. Sci.* 28:111, 1983.

36. Acosta J.M., Pellegrini C.A., Skinner D.B.: Etiology and pathogenesis of acute biliary pancreatitis. *Surgery* 88:118, 1980.

37. Acosta J.M., Rossi R., Galli O.M.R., et al.: Early surgery for acute gallstone pancreatitis. *Surgery* 83:367, 1978.

38. Stone H.H., Fabian T.C., Dunlop W.E.: Gallstone pancreatitis. *Ann. Surg.* 199:165, 1984.

39. Rosseland A.R., Solhaug J.H.: Early or delayed endoscopic papillotomy (EPT) in gallstone pancreatitis. *Ann. Surg.* 199:165, 1984.

40. Safrany L., Cotton P.B.: A preliminary report: Urgent duodenoscopic sphincterotomy for acute gallstone pancreatitis. *Surgery* 89:424, 1981.

41. McKay A.J., O'Neill J., Imrie C.W.: Pancreatitis, pregnancy and gallstones. *Br. J. Obstet. Gynaecol.* 87:47, 1980.

42. Warshaw A.L., Imbembo A.L., Civetta J.M., et al.: Surgical intervention in acute necrotizing pancreatitis. *Am. J. Surg.* 127:484, 1974.

43. Waterman N.G., Walsky R., Kasdan M.L., et al.: The treatment of acute hemorrhagic pancreatitis by sump drainage. *Surg. Gynecol. Obstet.* 126:963, 1968.

44. Watts G.T.: Total pancreatectomy for fulminant pancreatitis. *Lancet* 2:384, 1963.

45. Alexandre J.-H., Guerrieri M.T.: Role of total pancreatectomy in the treatment of necrotizing pancreatitis. *World J. Surg.* 5:369, 1981.

46. Edelmann G., Boutelier P.: Le traitement des pancreatites aigues necrosantes par l'ablation chirurgicale precoce des portions necrosees. *Chirurgie* 100:155, 1974.

47. Schiller W.R., Duprez A., Iams W.B., et al.: Experimental pancreatitis—treatment by colloid replacement and adrenocorticosteroid therapy combined with thoracic duct drainage. *Arch. Surg.* 98:698, 1969.

48. Wall A.J.: Peritoneal dialysis in the treatment of severe acute pancreatitis. *Med. J. Aust.* 2:281, 1965.

49. Bolooki H., Gliedman M.L.: Peritoneal dialysis in treatment of acute pancreatitis. *Surgery* 64:466, 1968.

50. Rogers R.E., Carey L.C.: Peritoneal lavage in experimental pancreatitis in dogs. *Am. J. Surg.* 111:792, 1966.

51. Rosato E.F., Chu W.H., Mullen J.L., et al.: Peritoneal lavage treatment of experimental pancreatitis. *J. Surg. Res.* 12:138, 1972.

52. Rosato E.F., Mullis W.F., Rosato F.E.: Peritoneal lavage therapy in hemorrhagic pancreatitis. *Surgery* 74:106, 1973.

53. Ranson J.H.C., Spencer F.C.: The role of peritoneal lavage in severe acute pancreatitis. *Ann. Surg.* 187:565, 1978.

54. Ranson J.H.C., Rifkind K.M., Turner J.W.: Prognostic signs and nonoperative peritoneal lavage in acute pancreatitis. *Surg. Gynecol. Obstet.* 143:209, 1976.

55. Stone H.H., Fabian T.C.: Peritoneal dialysis in the treatment of acute alcoholic pancreatitis. *Surg. Gynecol. Obstet.* 150:878, 1980.

56. Mayer A.D., McMahon M.J., Corfield A.P.: A randomized trial of peritoneal lavage for the treatment of severe acute pancreatitis (abstract). *Gastroenterology* 86:1178, 1984.

57. Ishe I., Evander A., Gustafson I.: A controlled randomized study on the value of peritoneal lavage in acute pancreatitis, in Hollender L.F. (ed.): *Controversies in Acute Pancreatitis.* Berlin, Springer-Verlag, 1982, pp. 200–202.

32

Treatment of the Complications of Acute Pancreatitis

ANDREW L. WARSHAW, M.D.
JIN GONGLIANG, M.D.

ACUTE PANCREATITIS is most often a self-limited disease without severe manifestations or associated irreversible organ injury, but its many potential complications can be spectacular when they occur. Since Fitz's classic description[1] of "hemorrhagic, suppurative, and gangrenous pancreatitis" in 1889, there has been a tendency to think that pancreatitis occurs in various "forms" (cf. edematous and hemorrhagic), and is attended by a list of possible complications, any of which just might develop at one time or another. In our experience that way of viewing pancreatitis is perhaps suitable to a pathologist like Fitz, but fails to convey the clinical reality that pancreatitis occurs not so much in different varieties as in a spectrum of severity, from mild to fulminant, from simple edema and inflammation to regional necrosis and enzymatic digestion. The specific clinical complications, rather than being a haphazard potpourri of catastrophes, occur for particular reasons at particular times.* Awareness of this order of events can greatly simplify at least part of the management of severe acute pancreatitis by focusing surveillance. By knowing what *ought* to happen at any given time, the aware clinician can often interpret diagnostic tests more precisely than diagnosticians (such as radiologists), who recognize an abnormality but who cannot distinguish the appearances of competing diagnoses such as pancreatic phlegmon, necrosis, early pseudocyst, or abscess, without clinical data.

TIMING OF COMPLICATIONS

It is our thesis that acute pancreatitis evolves through three phases: early, middle, and late.

The *early phase,* lasting one to four days and the only one that the majority of patients pass through, is a period of completely reversible pathophysiology. The inflammation, fluid shifts, cardiovascular dysfunction, pulmonary failure and metabolic aberrations may be life-threatening or even lethal, but all of these phenomena can resolve by endogenous control mechanisms or perhaps with exogenous specific treatment, leaving no sequela.

The *middle phase,* beginning about day 4 and lasting one to five weeks, is the time during which prolonged pancreatic swelling (phlegmon) occurs, with or without areas of necrosis. The tissue injury is believed to be a direct consequence of ischemia[2] from circulatory deficits during the early phase. Infarction and gangrene of the pancreas (Fig 32–1) and its surroundings are the results. Activated pancreatic enzymes may extend the area of damage by eroding contiguous tissues and penetrating into new locations and viscera.

The *late phase* of pancreatitis rarely begins before day 10 and is characterized by infection of the necrotic tissues produced in the middle phase. The pancreas is normally resistant to infection. In contrast to the rare local foci of infection caused by septic emboli or the widespread miliary abscesses secondary to high-grade bacteremia, pancreatic abscesses after pancreatitis have as their prerequisite a culture medium to nurture bacterial growth. For that reason pancreatic abscesses will not occur until at least enough time has passed to allow substantial tissue necrosis. Secondary infection of the dead tissues may occur soon, not for several weeks, or not at all (allowing for resorption and healing).

The problems of the early phase and their management have been treated in chapter 31. This section will discuss the middle and late phase complications of pancreatitis.

MIDDLE PHASE COMPLICATIONS

Phlegmon

The earliest and simplest manifestation of the middle phase is the pancreatic phlegmon or swelling, predominantly due to inflammation and edema, but possibly containing areas of local infarction. These masses will be detectable on ultrasound or CT scan in 30%–60% of cases, and may vary from minimal enlargement of the gland to massive involvement of the upper abdomen all the way to the perirenal spaces and out into the mesenteric roots (Fig 32–2). The higher rates are generally reported from CT studies, in part because there is no problem of technical failure due to obscuring intestinal gas, as is the case with ultrasonography. A mass is palpable in 15%–20% of patients. Patients with a phlegmon may be asymptomatic, but commonly have at least some degree of pancreatic

---

*For more extensive references and discussion of this concept, see Warshaw A.L., Richter J.M.: A practical guide to pancreatitis. *Current Problems in Surgery* 21:1–104, 1984.

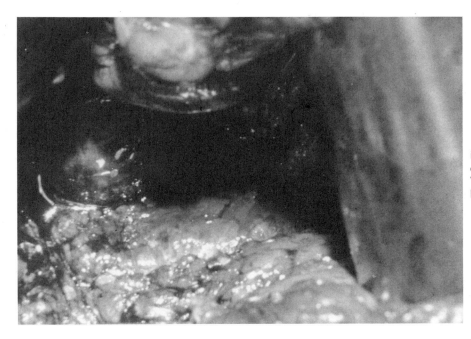

Fig 32–1.—Total pancreatic infarction, eight days after the onset of acute pancreatitis. (From Warshaw A.L., Richter J.M.[34] Used by permission.)

pain, low-grade fever, and anorexia along with hyperamylasemia.

The mass effect of the phlegmon may compress and partially obstruct the common bile duct (Fig 32–3), stomach and duodenum (Fig 32–4), or transverse colon. Localized ileus of the bowel segments adjacent to the phlegmon, presumably a reaction to inflammation or irritation by loosed pancreatic enzymes, may contribute to functional obstruction of the gut, particularly of the duodenum. Whereas clinically significant gastric outlet obstruction does occasionally require surgical intervention, rarely if ever is it necessary to bypass or decompress the bile duct or the colon because of a phlegmon unless an additional complication such as visceral infarction supervenes.[3]

Mucosal hemorrhage from gut segments adjacent to the phlegmon is relatively common. The cause is usually erosive gastritis (hemorrhagic gastritis, stress ulcers), perhaps no different from the hemorrhagic gastritis seen in many other acute illnesses (Fig 32–5). However, the fact that similar mucosal erosions and bleeding also occur in the duodenum and transverse colon in this disease suggests that a local factor related to the pancreas (ischemia, enzymes, vasoactive substances?) may act on adjacent bowel segments to produce the ulcers directly.

Treatment of a pancreatic phlegmon consists of the same expectant measures used to treat the underlying pancreatitis. There is no drug of proved effectiveness. It is probably beneficial to withhold oral feedings until fever and hyperamylasemia have abated and the mass is clearly diminishing in size. Fasting may also reduce the likelihood of progression of regional necrosis and abscess formation.[4] Nasogastric suction does not appear to be necessary at this stage unless there is

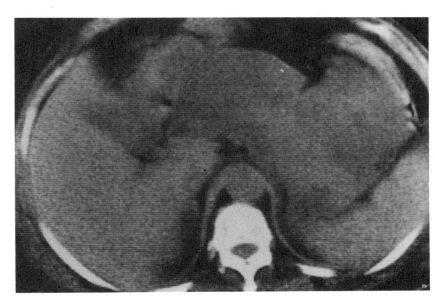

Fig 32–2.—CT scan in acute pancreatitis. There is a huge pancreatic phlegmon, with swelling extending across the upper abdomen to the perirenal tissues.

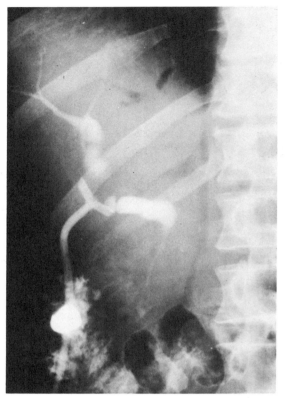

Fig 32–3.—Cholangiogram showing compression and narrowing of the lower segment of the common bile duct as it passes through the swollen pancreatic head. A T tube had been placed in the common duct at exploration for pancreatitis.

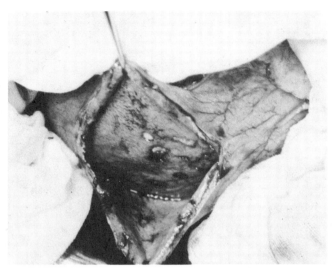

Fig 32–5.—Multiple gastric erosions seen through an anterior gastrotomy. The patient had an acutely inflamed pancreas and acute pseudocyst in the lesser sac behind the stomach.

evidence of inadequate gastric emptying. Periodic evaluation of the phlegmon with CT scanning, perhaps once a week, is suggested to detect areas of liquefaction necrosis for possible debridement before they become superinfected.

Mucosal ulceration is best treated by prevention, which is possible within the stomach by routine prophylactic alkalinization and/or H_2-blockade with cimetidine or ranitidine. Because the mechanism of colonic ulceration is not understood, there is no known preventive measure. The treatment of uncontrolled mucosal hemorrhage at any level of the GI tract may respond to selective intra-arterial infusion of pitressin or embolization.

Obstruction of the lower segment of the bile duct within the swollen pancreas may cause hyperbilirubinemia, usually less than 6 mg/dl,[5] but never needs to be treated directly by operation or intubation. The biliary stenosis always subsides spontaneously unless there is also a preexisting chronic fibrotic stricture caused by chronic pancreatitis. Clinically significant bacterial cholangitis has not been reported in the absence of common duct stones, instrumentation, or chronic stricture.

Gastric outlet obstruction, usually due to duodenal inflammation, atony and compression, also resolves in most cases but may take four weeks or more (Fig 32–6).[3] After a reasonable period of observation, variable with the circumstances, a gastrojejunostomy should be considered.

Colonic distortion and narrowing related to compression by the pancreatic mass or local inflammatory reaction rarely produces clinical signs of obstruction, even though radiographic studies show local narrowing and some proximal colonic dilatation (Fig 32–7). Spontaneous resolution is the rule and surgical resection or diverting colostomy is rarely if ever needed or justifiable, unless there is evidence for colonic perforation.

Regional Necrosis

Infarction may consume small foci or the entire pancreas (see Fig 32–1). Appearances are frequently deceiving, however, and much of the involved tissue is likely to be only

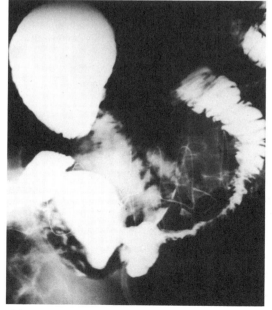

Fig 32–4.—Barium study of the stomach and duodenum in a patient with acute pancreatitis. There is compression and partial obstruction by the pancreatic phlegmon.

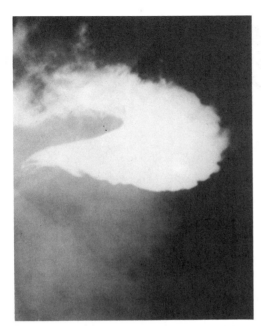

Fig 32–6.—Complete gastric outlet obstruction associated with a pancreatic phlegmon. After four weeks a gastrojejunostomy was performed.

peripancreatic fat. Histologically verifiable tissue death seems not to occur until at least several days after the onset of the attack. Small volumes of necrotic tissues can probably be reabsorbed and healed if digestion by liberated pancreatic enzymes does not compound and propagate the injury. Contiguous or connected organs may be recruited into the region of necrosis by thrombosis of their arteries.

Pancreatic and peripancreatic necrosis may be difficult to recognize. If large areas are involved, the patient may be sick with pain, tachycardia, fever, and leukocytosis. Often, how-

ever, the symptoms and signs are subtle or absent. Elevation of the serum amylase does not happen with reliability. Ultrasound or CT scans can demonstrate areas of irregular lucency, now being recognized as consistent with liquefaction necrosis (Fig 32–8),[6] but even the CT scan is relatively insensitive and not as specific as would be desired. A sizable volume of necrotic tissue, probably a few centimeters in diameter, is necessary for detection by CT. Even so, the finding appears relatively late and may be difficult to distinguish from edema. The first sure evidence of regional necrosis may only come later when signs of infection appear. Because pancreatic ribonuclease is released from dead pancreatic cells into the bloodstream (Fig 32–9), measurement of polycytidine-specific serum RNase has been suggested as a sensitive means of monitoring for pancreatic necrosis,[7] and investigation of this test continues.

Although comparative studies do not exist, it appears that if there is sufficient pancreatic necrosis to be recognized as such, morbidity and mortality are reduced by excising it. Untreated, these patients are at high risk of developing abscesses, hemorrhage, and visceral infarction. The mortality after debridement operations is generally reported in the range of 20%–40%.[8] We have had one death among 18 such patients in the last four years.

Any patient with evidence of pancreatic necrosis attended by fever and leukocytosis should certainly be operated upon promptly to forestall further complications. It may be safe to follow and observe patients who are asymptomatic, but only so long as they remain asymptomatic and the lesion is shown to resolve. Because premature feeding is thought to increase the likelihood of an abscess, it is prudent not to feed such patients until resolution occurs, but to maintain their nutrition by parenteral feedings. The use of Intralipid in this setting is somewhat controversial. We recommend avoiding it because of possible injury to the inflamed pancreas by breakdown of triglycerides to toxic free fatty acids.[9]

The specific treatment of pancreatic necrosis is debridement. By this is meant excision of dead tissue—"necrosectomy" according to European surgeons—rather than anatom-

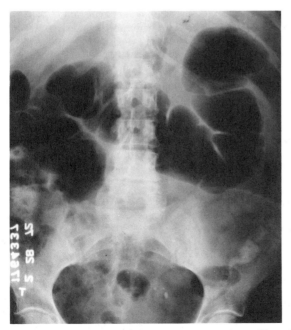

Fig 32–7.—Distention of the transverse colon with cutoff at the splenic flexure in acute pancreatitis.

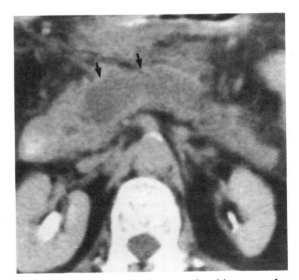

Fig 32–8.—CT scan of a pancreatic phlegmon. *Arrows,* irregular lucent area of liquifaction necrosis. (From Warshaw A.L., Richter J.M.[34] Used by permission.)

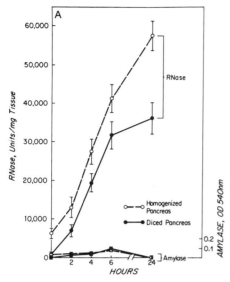

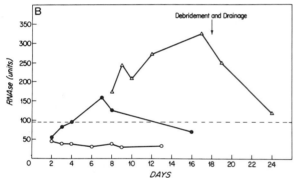

Fig 32–9.—Release of RNase from ischemic pancreas. **Top,** comparison of RNase and amylase appearing in the medium during anoxic incubation of rat pancreas slices (reprinted from *Surgery* 95:537, 1984). **Bottom,** serum levels of RNase in three patients: only the patient with persistently elevated RNase levels required operation for debridement of necrotic tissues. (Reprinted from *Surgery* 86:227, 1979.)

ical pancreatic resection (Fig 32–10). It may be necessary to incise the pancreatic surface to uncover the necrotic core (Fig 32–11). As much of the dead tissue as possible is removed by a combination of blunt and sharp dissection. At the time these operations are usually done, the dead tissue generally has the consistency of wet blotting paper and swamp muck. The plane of dissection is kept through devitalized tissues to minimize bleeding and injury to viable structures. Multiple soft rubber drains and sumps are left in the cavity upon completion, and are allowed to remain for at least a week or until there is no further significant drainage.

Complications after pancreatic debridement include hemorrhage from eroded blood vessels in the cavity, appearance of a bowel or biliary fistula from visceral injury by the pancreatitis or by the surgeon, extension of the necrotizing process to new areas (or inadequate debridement of existing areas), infection of residual dead tissues, and persistence of a pancreatic fistula. Reoperation to deal with these problems is an

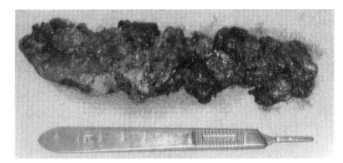

Fig 32–10.—Necrotic pancreatic tissues debrided from the patient described in Figure 32–9.

inescapable reality and obligation for the surgeon who must treat pancreatitis. These problems will be discussed in more detail in following sections.

Pancreatic Fistula

Pancreaticocutaneous fistulas are always an aftermath of surgery upon the pancreas, never of the pancreatitis alone. They manifest as continuing drainage of pancreatic secretions, with or without purulent slough, usually out through an established drain site. Not being considered here are those communications that develop between a necrotic pancreas and necrotic adjacent areas of bowel—they are included among bowel injuries, which are the predominant factor in treatment.

A pancreatic fistula is common after extensive debridement of the pancreas or external drainage of a pseudocyst. Leakage of pancreatic secretions from the disrupted parenchyma and perhaps from a major duct usually begins several days (or longer) after operation, as the pancreas resumes functioning. The fluid is initially a characteristic turbid tan-grey, comprising pancreatic juices, dead tissue particles, and pus. Flecks of fresh blood or intermittent bursts of hemorrhage are common. Later, the drainage may become simply clear pancreatic secretions. The daily volume can reach 1,500 ml depending on the location of the leak, and it increases with oral feeding.

Ninety percent of the fistulas will close spontaneously with time and healing. The time required will range from a few days to several months. Some fistulas will close temporarily, only to resume draining a few days or weeks later. If the abdominal wall was healed solidly in the interim, a new pseudocyst will form. When a fistula persists indefinitely, the drainage is usually from the distal pancreatic remnant which has been separated from the proximal gland by necrosis and loss of a segment of intervening duct.

It is believed that a fistula will heal more rapidly if the flow through it is minimized. Because oral feeding stimulates pancreatic secretion, common sense suggests a course of fasting and parenteral nutrition. Clear liquids, elemental diets, or even a low-fat diet may be used as the patient stabilizes and the waiting period lengthens.

Drains should be left in the fistula tract, at least through the abdominal wall, until the drainage has ceased. Otherwise the fistula efflux may collect within the abdomen and produce recurrent pain and fever due to a pseudocyst or abscess. Man-

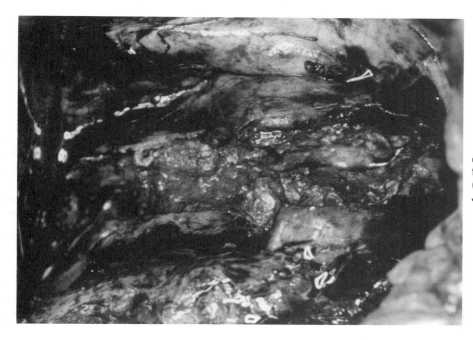

Fig 32–11.—Necrotic pancreatic core, apparent only after incision of the pancreatic capsule and surface. (From Warshaw A.L., Richter J.M.[34] Used by permission.)

agement of the skin around the fistula is not difficult—the pancreatic enzymes are usually not activated and generally do not excoriate. Karaya or Stomahesive wafers can be used to protect the skin around the fistula when necessary.

If the fistula shows no intention to close, its origin should be defined by contrast sinography or endoscopic pancreatography (Fig 32–12). A non-healing fistula is usually the result of obligate drainage from an isolated distal pancreatic segment.

Definitive surgical treatment of persistent pancreatic fistula consists either of excising the isolated distal segment which is the source (Fig 32–13), or laying on a Roux-en-Y loop of jejunum to channel the fistula back onto the GI tract. Excision is preferable for distal fistulas when the mobilization of the pancreatic tail is not excessively difficult. The Roux loop should be used with proximal fistulas and when inflammation has obliterated the surgical planes distal pancreatectomy is dangerous. By the time that the operation is performed, the pancreas around the fistula will have become firm and fibrotic and will hold the sutures for the anastomosis securely.

Acute Pseudocysts

While it is common practice to view all pancreatic pseudocysts in the same way, there is good reason for dispensing with that monolithic view.[10, 11] Most pseudocysts are found in patients with chronic pancreatitis who have not had an identifiable recent acute attack and who are not acutely ill at presentation (most present because of pain). Chronic pseudocysts usually are within the pancreatic parenchyma or capsule, communicate with the pancreatic duct system, often with a stenosis of the duct proximal to the cysts, and rarely undergo spontaneous regression. These pseudocysts are thick-walled at the time of discovery, and most are suitable for internal drainage by anastomosis to the stomach, jejunum, or duodenum.

In contrast, so-called acute pseudocysts (also termed acute pancreatic fluid collections) are pools of exudate and escaped pancreatic secretions, often in the lesser sac (Fig 32–14). They are the consequence either of a necrotizing injury and slough of tissue or of inflammatory reaction to severe acute pancreatitis. These patients have been and often continue to be acutely ill, and are characteristically febrile, tachycardic, and in need of IV volume support. Many of them in essence have ongoing necrotizing pancreatitis, and perhaps 25% will die[10] because of sepsis arising in the necrotic tissues, hemor-

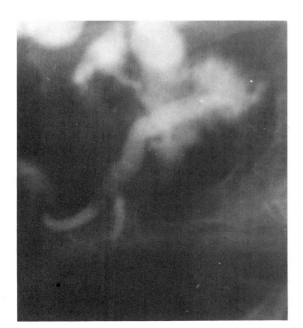

Fig 32–12.—Retrograde pancreatogram showing a leak from the duct in the body of the pancreas following necrotizing pancreatitis.

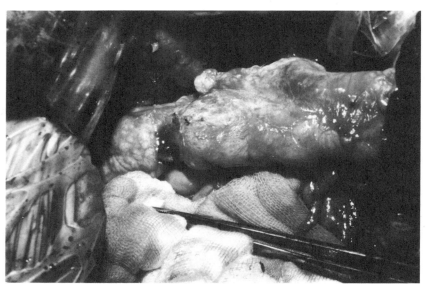

Fig 32–13.—Defect in the body of the pancreas at the origin of a pancreatic fistula.

rhage from eroded blood vessels, visceral infarction and perforation, and the combined effects of unrestrained enzymatic destruction of the region. Acute pseudocysts have been estimated to occur in 25%–30% of patients with acute pancreatitis.[12]

Paradoxically, it is likely that most of the pseudocysts reported to have resolved spontaneously have been of the acute type. If the pancreatitis abates, a race ensues between the body's efforts to reabsorb the fluid collection and its simultaneous efforts to encapsulate it. The factors which tilt the outcome in one direction or the other are not well understood but probably depend in part on whether or not there is continued leakage of pancreatic secretions. Occasionally a pseudocyst will rupture into an adjacent structure (duodenum or colon; stomach, esophagus, bile duct (Fig 32–15) and portal

vein have also been reported). The resulting communication can allow uneventful drainage and healing of the pseudocyst (Fig 32–16), but often there is accompanying major hemorrhage which can be lethal. Rupture of the cyst into the peritoneal cavity can manifest either as an acute abdominal catastrophe with peritonitis or, more likely, as chronic amylase-rich ascites. When the rupture is retroperitoneal, the fluid may dissect cephalad above the diaphragm and into the pleural space to produce a chronic amylase-rich pleural effusion or pericardial effusion.

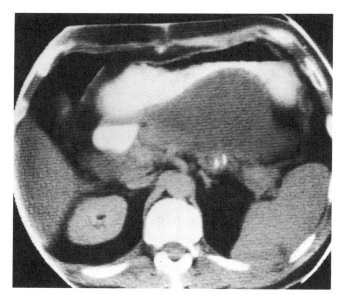

Fig 32–14.—CT scan showing an acute pseudocyst in the lesser sac behind the pancreas. Subsequent studies showed spontaneous resolution of this collection.

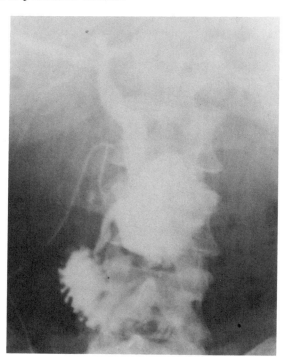

Fig 32–15.—Cholangiogram showing filling of a pseudocyst which had eroded into the common bile duct. The pseudocyst was treated by draining it into a Roux-en-Y jejunal loop.

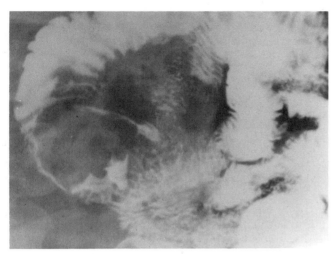

Fig 32–16.—Upper GI series showing a barium-filled sinus tract into the pancreatic head, the remains of a pseudocyst which spontaneously ruptured and decompressed into the duodenum.

TREATMENT.—Safe guidelines for the management of acute pseudocysts have not been worked out to universal agreement, in part because of the failure to distinguish between potentially dangerous pseudocysts representing escaped pancreatic secretions and less threatening (harmless?) inflammatory effusions. The former is the product of a major structural injury in necrotizing pancreatitis. The latter represents an exudate in response to inflammation and has no communication with the duct system. The amylase content will be astronomically high in the escaped pancreatic secretions but equal to or even less than serum levels in the exudate. Percutaneous aspiration to obtain a fluid sample for amylase determination may prove to be singularly valuable in making that distinction and thereby in facilitating judgments about the need for drainage, but there is little experience with this approach to date. So-called amylase-poor pseudocysts[13] may not need drainage at all, or, if persistent, may only require percutaneous aspiration since they should have no reason or means to refill from the pancreas.

The natural history of an acute pseudocyst can end with spontaneous resolution or with evolution into unforewarned disaster.[12, 14] The observation period is therefore a time of indeterminate hazard. The patient should remain in the hospital during this time. Oral feedings should be restricted to clear liquids at most and nutritional support given by parenteral means until the cyst has essentially resolved. If he remains toxic (febrile, tachycardic, in need of IV volume support) surgical drainage should not be delayed. Only if his condition stabilizes and he appears well should a waiting period be allowed to continue. It has been estimated that 25%–50% of acute pseudocysts will resolve.[11, 12, 14]

The size of the pseudocyst should be monitored by ultrasound or CT scans, perhaps weekly. The CT scan has the advantage of being able to detect associated areas of liquefaction necrosis in and around the pancreas, which may determine the need for surgical debridement. As long as the patient remains stable or improves, observation is tolerable in

the hopes of spontaneous resolution. The need for operation will be precipitated by increasing size of the pseudocyst, persistence past four to six weeks, and, of course, a new complication such as bleeding, infection, rupture, or visceral perforation.[14] Larger pseudocysts (> 6 cm) are said to be far less likely to resolve spontaneously. In addition to the hope for spontaneous resolution, a purpose of the observation period is to allow the wall of the acute pseudocyst time to "mature" and thicken with enough fibrous tissue to hold sutures, thereby allowing internal drainage by anastomosis to the upper GI tract rather than external drainage. Current practice holds that the necessary waiting period is four to six weeks, but we have seen pseudocysts mature within two weeks in some cases. Because amylase stagnant in a mature pseudocyst undergoes characteristic physical changes which are detectable by electrophoresis, it has been suggested that the finding of "old amylase" in the bloodstream may be an index of pseudocyst maturity and readiness for internal drainage (Fig 32–17).[15] The waiting period may have to be abandoned if the patients shows continuing signs of pancreatitis, and in that case external drainage will be necessary.

The definitive treatment of an acute pseudocyst is drainage *and debridement.* Nonoperative percutaneous drainage by catheter placement under ultrasound or CT guidance has been used in a few cases,[16] but its effectiveness is limited by the possible presence of substantial amounts of necrotic tissues in need of removal. It may be reasonable in some cases to try nonoperative percutaneous drainage first, to see how

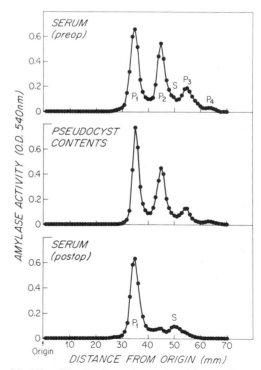

Fig 32–17.—Electrophoresis study of isoamylases in the serum and pseudocyst contents of a patient with a mature pseudocyst. The P_2 isoamylase is an altered or "aged" form found in the pseudocyst. It is easily detected in the serum preoperatively but disappears after drainage of the pseudocyst. (Reprinted from *Gastroenterology* 79:1246, 1980.)

effective it will be. In most cases, however, surgical means will be needed, especially if there is duodenal or bile duct obstruction by the pseudocyst.[17]

Exploration through an anterior midline incision gives the simplest widest exposure of the entire pancreatic lesion. Obvious collections in areas of destroyed tissue must be opened and drained. The planes around the pancreas should be carefully opened where there is induration even if no collection is obvious: an incredible amount of devitalized tissue and fluid can be hidden in the retroperitoneum. The safest avascular approaches include a Kocher maneuver to explore behind the pancreatic head and an incision along the inferior margin of the pancreas to the left of the ligament of Treitz (either above or below the mesocolon) to explore behind the body and tail. Soft rubber drains and swamps are left in all explored areas. Anastomosis of an acute pseudocyst to the stomach or jejunum is not feasible or safe. The drains are removed only after drainage has ceased. Recurrence after external drainage has been reported to be 25%,[18] but that figure probably applies to externally drained chronic pseudocysts, not acute pseudocysts.[11]

When the pseudocyst is found at operation to have a thick fibrous wall, internal drainage by anastomosis to the stomach or intestine is preferable to external drainage. It does not seem to matter whether stomach, duodenum, or a Roux-en-Y loop of jejunum is used. We choose whatever of those is closest to the cyst or adherent to it. If the pseudocyst is adherent to the posterior wall of the stomach, a transgastric approach is used. If not, a Roux loop of jejunum is safest. The chance of recurrence of the pseudocyst after internal drainage should be less than 5%.[18]

Pancreatic Hemorrhage

Hemorrhage from necrotizing pancreatitis occurs as a consequence of several possible mechanisms[19]: (A) regional necrosis involving the contained small or large vascular structures; (B) enzymatic injury to blood vessel walls by elastase and other proteolytic enzymes, causing formation of pseudoaneurysms (Fig 32–18), some of which rupture. The splenic,

gastroduodenal, and colic branches of the superior mesenteric artery are the most common sites of major hemorrhage; (C) bleeding from the walls of pseudocysts and abscesses, either as ooze from the granulation tissue or erosion of an exposed vessel on the wall of the cavity. Depending on the size of the vessel and whether it is an artery or vein, bleeding may be slow and subclinical, or exsanguinating. The blood loss may be contained by the cavity, dissect through retroperitoneal planes, burst into a viscus, or empty into the intestine via the pancreatic duct or bile duct to present as GI bleeding.

Pancreatic bleeding, as contrasted with "hemorrhagic pancreatitis," is a phenomenon of the middle phase of necrotizing pancreatitis and parallels the development of tissue death in the second and third week of a severe attack, or even later. Bleeding from these mechanisms also poses a continuing threat after surgical debridement and drainage of necrotic areas, as the injury continues to extend inexorably further. Its incidence is hard to ascertain, but it and overwhelming sepsis are the two most important causes of death after the first week of pancreatitis.

Control of massive hemorrhage is the first imperative. Surgical exploration and ligation of the bleeding vessels is recommended but often difficult to accomplish.[19] In our experience, isolation of the bleeding points can be inexact and hazardous, with further bleeding and fistulas following. We have found that initial stabilization can often be attained by angiographic identification, embolization, and occlusion of the arterial source of hemorrhage (Fig 32–19). This maneuver can only be considered a temporary means of control, inasmuch as the necrotic and infected tissues which are underlying must still be debrided and drained. However, with the bleeding stopped, the subsequent operation can be planned and executed under far more controlled circumstances and at lower risk. Five of our last ten patients treated in this manner have survived, in contrast to 100% mortality among the previous group treated by surgery alone. Others have reported individual experiences that are similar.[20, 21] Immediate laparotomy to stop the bleeding is necessary when the hemorrhage is so rapid as not to allow time for an attempt at angiographic

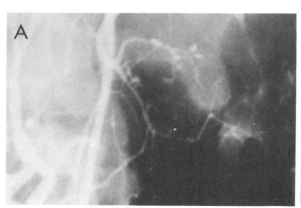
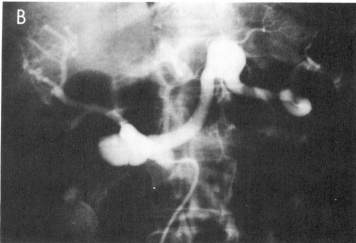

Fig 32–18.—Arteriograms in two patients after necrotizing pancreatitis showing **(A)** multiple small pseudoaneurysms and **(B)** two large pseudoaneurysms.

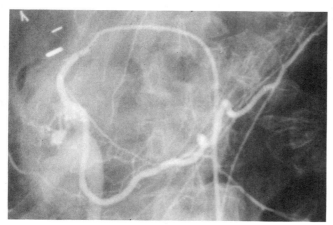

Fig 32–19.—Arteriogram showing extravasation from a branch of the gastroduodenal artery seven days after onset of necrotizing pancreatitis in a 74-year-old woman. The bleeding was controlled by transcatheter embolization. Subsequently the necrotic tissues were debrided, and she survived. (From Warshaw A.L., Richter J.M.[34] Used by permission.)

control or when angiographic means have failed.

At surgery, identification of the exact source of bleeding and access to it can be exceedingly difficult. The vessel is often at the far and deep end of a cavity whose entrance is hemmed in by bowel or major mesenteric vessels. The walls of the cavity may ooze large volumes of blood in addition to specific holes in major vessels. Where possible, suture ligatures are preferable for localized bleeding points, especially when arterial, but packs may be needed for diffuse or venous bleeding. We prefer to place sump catheters beside the packs to provide egress for pancreatic secretions and blood. If the cavity to be packed is relatively small, multiple stuffed latex drains can be used in place of gauze packs and subsequently removed without necessitating another laparotomy under an anesthesia. Ligation of feeding vessels in a clean area outside the debrided cavity adds insurance against rebleeding but is rarely feasible.

There has been revival of interest in open packing of large necrotizing pancreatitis cavities, particularly if infected.[22, 23] The cavity is debrided and packed with multiple large gauze pads, which are replaced on a planned basis every few days. Initially these replacements are combined with further debridement using anesthesia, but later the exchanges can be done in bed on the ward. It has been reported that the problems of major rebleeding, which can be expected to occur in more than one third of patients treated by either means, are nearly eliminated.

Major Vascular Thrombosis

Vessels injured by the adjacent inflammatory process and enzymatic injury may thrombose rather than leak blood. Because of collateral flow, many of these events do not have sequellae. Venous thrombosis rarely is apparent, except that acute *splenic* vein thrombosis can lead to splenic rupture, hypersplenism, or gastric varices.[24] Thrombosis of local pancreatic arteries can add to the loss of pancreatic tissues. However, it is thrombosis of major visceral arteries that produces dramatic, catastrophic new chapters in the story.

The superior mesenteric artery, and especially its colic branches, are at highest risk, along with the gastroduodenal, and splenic arteries. Occlusion of the latter two may go unnoticed, but occlusion of the middle colic or right colic arteries frequently leads to infarction of segments of the colon, probably because the thrombosis extends peripherally to segmental branches near or at the bowel wall. Similar processes involving the jejunal branches can destroy the small intestine,[25] and thrombosis of the gastroduodenal artery at terminal branches can cause slough of the duodenum. Lesser consequences of visceral artery thrombosis include bleeding from mucosal slough without transmural necrosis and strictures developing later in ischemic segments (Fig 32–20).

Early detection of bowel necrosis before perforation may be difficult. The signs attributable to the intestinal ischemic injury are frequently masked by or mistaken for ongoing pancreatic inflammation. Consequently, the first recognition of bowel infarction may only come with unequivocal peritonitis. One early sign not to be ignored is the appearance of rectal bleeding. The mucosa being the bowel coat most susceptible to ischemia, bleeding from areas of mucosal slough will occur days before perforation from full-thickness bowel infarction. The blood usually appears fresh and red, rather than as melena, and there is a tendency to underestimate its importance and to dismiss it as hemorrhoidal. Theoretically, angiographic study of patients who develop rectal bleeding, even in small

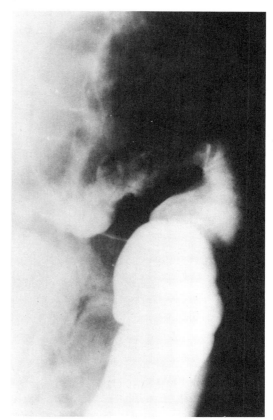

Fig 32–20.—Barium enema showing a colonic stricture at the splenic flexure after acute pancreatitis.

amounts, could distinguish those patients with important arterial thrombosis and help to select the ones for whom pre-emptive bowel resection is less risky than waiting for perforation and pertonitis.

Once bowel infarction occurs, it presents with increasing signs of inflammation, including pain, tenderness, fever and leukocytosis. There may be localized perforation which gives rise to an abscess (Fig 32–21), or free perforation into the peritoneal cavity (Fig 32–22) with generalized peritonitis. Major gastrointestinal hemorrhage from the viable margins of the bowel can occur.[18, 26] Fistulas from the bowel lumen into an adjacent cavity of necrotic tissue (duodenopancreatic, colomesenteric) may develop before surgical intervention, and are even more likely after drains have been left in a paravisceral cavity. The latter phenomenon is heralded by the appearance of feculent or bilious drainage material.

The *treatment* of small- or large-bowel injury after pancreatitis almost always requires eventual resection of the damaged segment. The hole is otherwise too extensive to close spontaneously, even with adequate drainage. Because of the environment of bacterial and enzymatic inflammation in which the injury has occurred and because the thrombosis of mesenteric vessels may extend, primary resection and reanastomosis carries a high risk of breakdown of the anastomosis, sepsis, and refistulization. It is far safer to bring out the bowel ends as stomas and to delay the reanastomosis to a much later time when it can be accomplished in a clean, quiet field. The

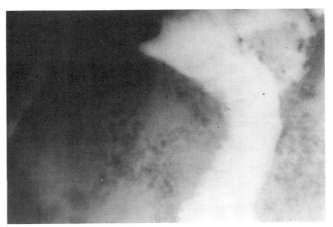

Fig 32–22.—Barium leaking from the colon into the free peritoneal cavity after necrosis of the left colon 14 days after onset of pancreatitis. (From Warshaw A.L., Richter J.M.[34] Used by permission.)

initial operation should nonetheless accomplish resection of the destroyed bowel segment when possible—simple drainage of the perforation usually fails to control associated sepsis. At the very least, if primary resection is considered too hazardous, a proximal diversion of the bowel contents via a double-barreled stoma is necessary. The resection and reanastomosis can be accomplished in one or two subsequent stages. If it is the duodenal wall that has been destroyed, extensive drainage of the right upper quadrant may suffice,[27] but isolation of the duodenum by stapling the pylorus and T-tube drainage of the common duct may be helpful. Ultimately a pancreaticoduodenectomy may well be required. Primary pancreaticoduodenectomy for acute pancreatitis carries a mortality of approximately 60% in experienced hands.[28]

Bile Duct Necrosis

The lower common bile duct, which traverses the head of the pancreas, is at special risk of perforation in severe necrotizing pancreatitis. Such disruption of the bile duct cannot be repaired, and either a persistent fistula or stricture occurs if inadequately treated. The initial treatment is by adequate drainage and by placement of a T tube. A needle-catheter or tube jejunostomy can be useful to refeed the bile lost through the fistula. Ligation of the duct above the pancreas may be helpful, but rerouting of bile flow to the jejunum should be reserved for a later time because of the high risk of anastomotic breakdown in the setting of necrotizing pancreatitis. Biliary reconstruction with a Roux-en-Y jejunal loop is to be preferred, but a cholecystojejunostomy may suffice in some cases (Fig 32–23).

LATE PHASE COMPLICATIONS
Pancreatic Abscess

The main event of the late phase is infection. For infection to occur, there must be a culture medium in which the invading bacteria can grow. As noted earlier, viable pancreas is resistant to infection, but devitalized tissues, including those in an acute pseudocyst, welcome and support microbes. The

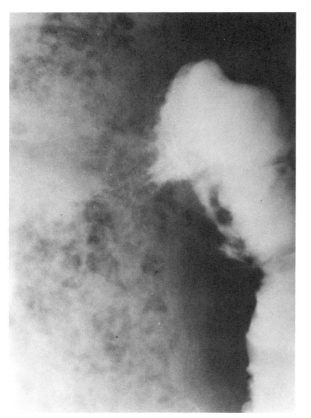

Fig 32–21.—Barium enema showing leak of barium from the splenic flexure of the colon into retroperitoneal necrotic tissues.

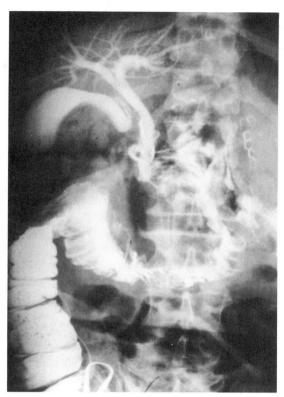

Fig 32–23.—Cholecystogram in a patient whose intra-pancreatic common bile duct had sloughed in necrotizing pancreatitis. The resulting bile leak was treated by ligation of the bile duct and cholecystojejunostomy. This study shows the appearance after the anastomosis and outlines the swollen pancreatic head.

components giving rise to a pancreatic abscess require at least seven to ten days to develop, and the signs of infection may not become obvious until the third week or even later.[29, 30] Pancreatic abscesses follow acute pancreatitis in approximately 4% of cases.[29]

The origin of the bacteria in a pancreatic abscess is not known for certain. Although hematogenous and lymphatic seeding has been suggested, it seems most likely that they migrate transmurally from the lumen of the adjacent colon. Earlier reports found that many pancreatic abscesses were caused by gram-positive cocci, staphylococci and streptococci, but the prevailing current experience is that gram-negative coliforms clearly predominate.[30] Many of the abscesses have more than one bacterial component. Bacteroides and other anaerobes have not been frequent. *Candida albicans* is also being recognized, probably most often as an opportunistic replacement in patients receiving broad-spectrum antibiotics, but also as a primary agent.[31]

Like acute pseudocysts, pancreatic abscesses seem to occur in two clinical forms. In the first, the attack of pancreatitis is severe and ongoing. The secondary infection of the damaged tissues adds a further insult to the continuing unbridled enzymatic injury. These patients remain acutely ill and deteriorate obviously during the second and third weeks. The signs of infection are intermingled with and indistinguishable from

the signs of ongoing pancreatitis. If an operation is performed at seven to 14 days, the findings are those of edema, necrosis, and extensive permeation of the retroperitoneal tissues with pancreatic juices and exudate. Although these tissues are laden with bacteria, there are not well-defined gross pockets of pus, abscesses in the common conception. In the second form, the pancreatitis runs its course and ends, leaving behind a substantial nidus of devitalized tissue. Eventually, sometime in the succeeding weeks, this tissue becomes infected. Typically, such patients appear to have recovered from their attack either completely or largely. Some may actually have been discharged from the hospital, only to reappear with a fever as long as six weeks after the original attack of pancreatitis began. In general, these patients appear much less "toxic" than those of the first type, the difference probably being due in large part to the presence or absence of continuing pancreatitis. Not surprisingly, major additional complications and death are more likely to occur among patients of the first type. We estimate that the mortality of the type I pancreatic abscess has been in excess of 50%, whereas 5% or fewer of the type II patients die of their disease.

With no known exceptions, inadequately treated pancreatic abscesses of either type are lethal. In addition to the general effects of sepsis in producing shock, respiratory failure (ARDS), acute renal failure, and hemorrhagic gastritis, pancreatic abscesses increase the likelihood of retroperitoneal hemorrhage, vascular injury to the bowel, and fistulas that were the threats of the middle phase. Probably because of the activated proteolytic enzymes contained in the abscesses, they have a proclivity for extending the area of necrosis and penetrating out along retroperitoneal planes, into the bowel mesentery, and up into the mediastinum. They may rupture into the bowel, pleural space, or bronchial tree.[18] Pancreatic abscesses have been drained via the neck and via the scrotum (see Fig 32–27).

DIAGNOSIS.—of a pancreatic abscess depends, before any laboratory or radiologic tests, on an understanding of the natural history of pancreatitis and on a high index of suspicion. Any patient who remains or becomes febrile after ten days must be suspected of harboring an abscess. In this situation, ultrasound and CT scanning have become the only diagnostic tests of importance, superseding all other laboratory and radiographic techniques (Fig 32–24). Both are sensitive in detecting fluid collections and in demonstrating the gas bubbles that are virtually pathognomonic of infection (Fig 32–25). Even without gas, any collection in a febrile patient must be considered for drainage in preference to waiting for clinical complications (Fig 32–26). When there is doubt, percutaneous needle aspiration of the fluid collection can be performed under ultrasound or CT guidance to obtain a sample for analysis and culture.[16] Infected collections must be drained, while sterile fluid pockets might be watched.

TREATMENT.—Antibiotics have a role in limiting the septicemia from pancreatic abscesses, but antibiotics alone cannot effect a cure. If the contents of the abscess have not been sampled and cultured, the coverage by the antibiotics should be broad enough to include gram-negative coliforms (particularly *E. coli*) and gram-positive cocci. Gentamicin and a ceph-

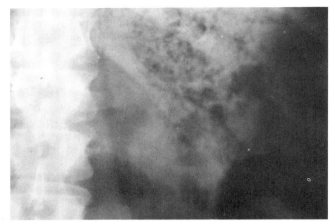

Fig 32–24.—Plain x-ray of the abdomen in a patient with a pancreatic abscess, showing the classic mottling of the "soap-bubble sign." This sign appears in only 20% of cases and therefore must not be awaited or relied on.

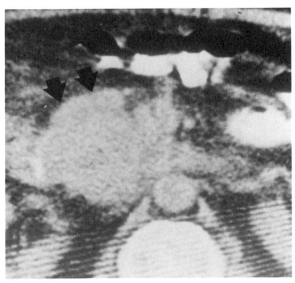

Fig 32–26.—CT scan in patient with a proved pancreatic abscess. The head of the gland contains an obvious large swelling but no gas.

alosporin or cefoxitin alone are reasonable first choices until information from cultures is available.

Patients suspected of having a pancreatic abscess should routinely be treated by prophylactic alkalinization of the stomach. If bleeding from gastric erosions occurs, it may be temporarily controlled by selective intra-arterial infusion of vasopressin (Pitressin), but the hemorrhagic gastritis itself is a further indication of the urgent need for control of the underlying sepsis.

Percutaneous catheter drainage under radiographic guidance has been suggested for draining pancreatic abscesses, much as the technique has been used successfully in definitive treatment of other types of intra-abdominal abscesses.[32] However, in contrast to the 90% success rate for those others, the success rate for pancreatic abscesses is closer to 60%. The greater number of failures is probably due to the associated solid debris of necrotic tissues, which cannot be effectively

evacuated by the small catheters, to the associated continuing enzymatic injury, and to the loculations and multiplicity of abscesses in this disease (nearly 30% will have more than one abscess). Percutaneous catheter drainage may still have a role in some patients as a first maneuver to reduce the ill effects of high-grade sepsis in an unstable patient—to improve his condition in preparation for definitive drainage. We have also used percutaneous drainage to good advantage as an adjunct for draining small residual and recurrent abscesses after surgical drainage, when reoperation may be deemed excessively difficult or hazardous.

The definitive treatment of pancreatic abscesses is surgical debridement and drainage (Fig 32–27). Our preference is for transabdominal exploration via a midline incision to give the

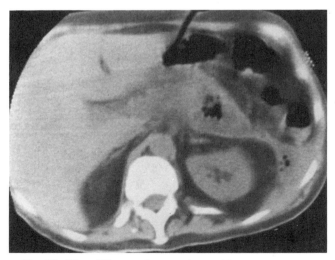

Fig 32–25.—CT scan in a patient with a pancreatic abscess, showing gas bubbles in the swollen pancreas and in the perirenal space. (From Warshaw A.L., Richter J.M.[34] Used by permission.)

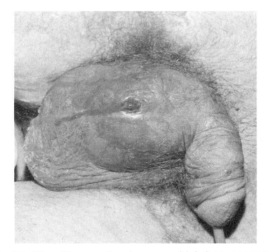

Fig 32–27.—Pancreatic abscess which has necessitated debridement down the gutter behind the right colon, out along the inguinal canal, and drainage through the scrotum. (Reprinted from *Surg. Clin. North Am.* 54:621, 1974.)

widest exposure. Flank incisions are too limiting, both in the search for additional loculations and in the event of hemorrhage from the depths of a cavity. Indurated areas must be viewed with suspicion and penetrated, great care being required to avoid injuring the bowel. It may be helpful to enter the abscess cavity from below the transverse mesocolon, dissecting up through it to the peripancreatic space. This route is safest to the left of the ligament of Treitz, where there is no retroperitoneal duodenum and no important blood vessel in the mesentery. The exploration and debridement must be thorough enough to ensure that all loculations, extensions, and separate abscesses have been emptied. We prefer to insert a combination of soft, stuffed rubber drains and soft rubber sumps (or Jackson-Pratt type suction catheters), to pack the cavity as well as to aspirate it.

In up to 30% of cases, further abscesses requiring drainage become apparent after the first operation. It is necessary to be as aggressive in pursuing adequate drainage of these later abscesses as it was for the first one. As mentioned earlier, percutaneous placement of a drainage catheter may substitute for reoperation in some cases.

The sumps and drains should be removed slowly, beginning a week after the operation and progressing as the drainage allows. In the event of a pancreatic fistula, the drains should remain until it closes.

Bowel Necrosis and Fistula

It is not unusual to discover at exploration that the abscess has destroyed the wall of the colon, stomach, or even duodenum. In a recent study of 45 patients with pancreatic abscesses treated at the Massachusetts General Hospital, there were four perforations of the colon, two of the duodenum, and one of the stomach.[30] As discussed earlier in the section on bowel injuries of the second phase, it is not sufficient simply to drain the area of the damaged bowel. Resection of the involved segment along with end stomas is preferable when possible. A proximal diverting stoma is highly advisable for colon injuries which cannot be resected.

Appearance of bowel contents via the drains at any point in

the postoperative period may indicate the development of an enterocutaneous fistula, even if none was found at the operation. The origin of the fistula can be defined by fistulography (Fig 32–28). Reoperation will almost always be necessary to resect the damaged bowel, because the hole is too big to heal itself, but the reoperation can be delayed if the condition of the patient is stable. Complicating conditions which force earlier reoperation include sepsis and bleeding from the fistula tract.[26] The latter is particularly common with gastrocutaneous fistulas, perhaps because of the additional problem of acid digestion of the fistula tract. We have treated three such, in all of which bleeding forced a gastric resection earlier than planned. Spontaneous healing of enteric fistulas caused by pancreatic abscesses is very exceptional and has not occurred in our personal experience.

In spite of aggressive surgical treatment, most series have continued to report mortality from pancreatic abscesses of 30%–50% or even higher.[29, 33] Most of the deaths are related to the adverse effects of the associated pancreatitis, complicating injuries to other viscera, and bleeding. In our own recent experience, we have found a surprising improvement over the past few years.[30] Between 1974 and 1978, 10 of 26 patients (38%) died. In striking contrast, during the subsequent five years only one of 19 (5%) died. This, the best survival record reported so far, may be the product of earlier diagnosis by the use of ultrasound and CT scans, a policy of early and aggressive surgical drainage and debridement, and a ready willingness to reoperate for further drainage.

PERSISTING PANCREATITIS

A few patients continue for months to have signs of pancreatic inflammation or develop acute recurrences immediately on feeding. Even long periods of TPN do not succeed in effecting a termination to the persistent attack. These patients represent a mixture of problems, including unrecognized microabscesses in the pancreas, nonhealing duodenal wall injury, underlying congenital lesions,[34] and, most important, duct injuries produced during the original attack but

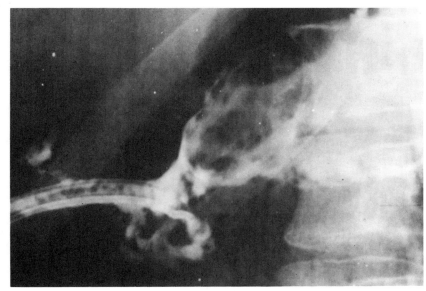

Fig 32–28.—Injection of contrast medium into the drains left in a pancreatic abscess, showing a fistula into the colon.

now acting to propagate it by obstructing pancreatic secretion. The spectrum of their symptoms ranges from pain to full-blown acute pancreatitis. Laboratory findings may be normal, but many will have pancreatic swelling on examination by CT scan.

Since the group of patients under consideration do not have an abscess, pseudocyst, or area of necrotic tissue to target for drainage or debridement, the persistence of their problems is puzzling and frustrating. ERCP may demonstrate a duct anomaly or injury which points to a solution.

Treatment of persisting pancreatitis is, almost by definition, difficult. Once nonsurgical options have been exhausted, surgical solutions may become unavoidable. We have on a few occasions had success with transduodenal sphincteroplasty of the sphincter of Oddi and the orifice of the duct of Wirsung when these appeared to be stenotic. If a stenosis or obstruction is found farther out along the main pancreatic duct, distal pancreatectomy may be of benefit. In six patients, we have resorted to a Whipple operation for persisting pancreatitis.[34] The head of the gland appeared to be the principal location of the swelling and inflammation in five of these, and only the pancreatic head was resected. In one patient, the pancreas was uniformly involved from head to tail and the entire gland was removed. The pylorus-preserving (Longmire) method of pancreaticoduodenectomy was used in two, and a mucosa-to-mucosa pancreaticojejunal anastomosis was constructed in four of five candidates. Although the technical aspects of pancreaticoduodenectomy are particularly difficult when the pancreas is acutely inflamed, all six patients survived without complication and were discharged from the hospital within two weeks after operation. Their preoperative hospitalization had ranged from six weeks to three months.

LATE RESIDUALS OF ACUTE PANCREATITIS

Pancreatic Duct Obstruction

Even in those patients who have recurrent attacks of acute pancreatitis, there ordinarily is not evolution to chronic pancreatitis. That is, the gland heals each time, unless the damage has been great enough to cause permanent scarring. If, however, there has been segmental necrosis involving the pancreatic duct, the loss of the segment leaves the distal fragment of pancreas with nowhere to drain. The partially or completely distal fragment either atrophies and becomes asymptomatic or it retains function and becomes a focus of recurrent pain and attacks of pancreatitis.[35, 36] This phenomenon has been described as "upstream pancreatitis."[36] It has been recognized most commonly after drainage of pseudocysts or debridement of necrotic tissues in the region of the midpancreas, both being indications of regional injury to the gland.

The diagnosis of upstream pancreatitis is most easily made by ERCP, preferably carried out during a quiescent interval between acute attacks. The pancreatogram shows a block (or less commonly a high-grade stenosis) in the pancreatic duct at the point of injury and scar (Fig 32–29). When the point of obstruction is within a few centimeters of the sphincter, the foreshortened appearance of the duct of Wirsung may be mistaken for the congenital anomaly pancreas divisum.[35]

At operation, the proximal portion of the pancreas may have a normal texture and size, but the obstructed distal segment is fibrotic, indurated, and generally swollen. The transition is abrupt and obvious. There may even be a gap between the two parts, the location once occupied by a pseudocyst or necrotic pancreas (see Fig 32–13).

The most effective treatment for this condition is distal pancreatectomy. The operation is easy and safe, removes useless damaged tissue, and leaves essentially normal pancreas.

Pancreatic Insufficiency

Pancreatic insufficiency after acute pancreatitis is quite exceptional. Hyperglycemia during the attack suggests inadequate insulin production at that time, but blood glucose and insulin levels almost always return to normal without the need for insulin therapy. Even after necrotizing pancreatitis requiring extensive debridement, there is enough pancreatic tissue left in most patients to allow recovery and compensa-

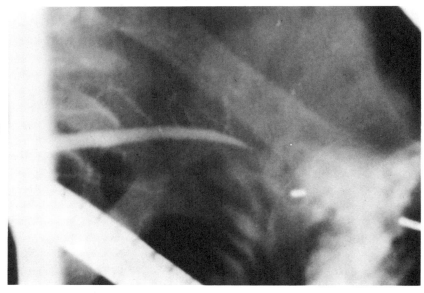

Fig 32–29.—Retrograde pancreatogram in a patient who had previously undergone debridement after necrotizing pancreatitis. It shows tapering and obstruction of the pancreatic duct in the body of the gland. The patient suffered recurrent attacks of pancreatitis, which were cured by excising the pancreatic tail distal to the demonstrated block.

tory hyperplasia. Diabetes rarely persists. We have not seen exocrine insufficiency requiring oral pancreatic enzyme supplements as a consequence of acute pancreatitis unless the pancreas has been formally resected.

REFERENCES

1. Fitz R.H.: Acute pancreatitis: A consideration of pancreatic hemorrhage, hemorrhagic, suppurative, and gangrenous pancreatitis and of disseminated fat necrosis. *Boston Med. Surg. J.* 120:181, 1889.
2. Warshaw A.L., O'Hara P.J.: Susceptibility of the pancreas to ischemic injury in shock. *Ann. Surg.* 188:197, 1978.
3. Bradley E.L. III.: Enteropathies, in: Bradley E.L. (ed.): *Complications of pancreatitis, medical and surgical management.* Philadelphia, W.B. Saunders Co., 1982, p. 265.
4. Ranson J.H.C., Spencer F.C.: Prevention, diagnosis, and treatment of pancreatic abscess. *Surgery* 82:99, 1977.
5. Bradley E.L., Salam A.A.: Hyperbilirubinemia in inflammatory pancreatic disease: Natural history and management. *Ann. Surg.* 188:626, 1978.
6. White M., Wittenberg J., Mueller P.R., et al.: Pancreatic necrosis: computed tomographic manifestations. *Radiology* (submitted for publication).
7. Warshaw A.L., Lee K.-H.: Serum ribonuclease elevations and pancreatic necrosis in acute pancreatitis. *Surgery* 86:227, 1979.
8. Kivilaakso E., Fraki O., Nikki P.: Resection of the pancreas for acute fulminant pancreatitis. *Surg. Gynecol. Obstet.* 152:493, 1981.
9. Saharia P., Margolis S., Zuidema G.D., et al.: Acute pancreatitis with hyperlipemia: Studies with an isolated perfused canine pancreas. *Surgery* 82:60, 1977.
10. Crass R.A., Way L.W.: Acute and chronic pancreatic pseudocysts are different. *Am. J. Surg.* 142:660, 1981.
11. McConnell D.B., Gregory J.R., Sasaki T.M.: Pancreatic pseudocyst. *Am. J. Surg.* 143:599, 1982.
12. Bradley E.L. III, Gonzalez A.C., Clements J.L. Jr.: Acute pancreatic pseudocysts: Incidence and implications. *Ann. Surg.* 184:734, 1976.
13. Weaver D.W., Bouwman D.L., Walt A.J., et al.: "Amylase-poor" pancreatic pseudocysts: A new entity? *Surg. Gastroenterol.* 1:341, 1982.
14. Bradley E.L., Clements J.L., Gonzalez A.C.: The natural history of pancreatic pseudocysts: A unified concept of management. *Am. J. Surg.* 137:135, 1979.
15. Warshaw A.L., Lee K.-H.: Aging changes of pancreatic isoamylases and the appearance of "old amylase" in the serum of patients with pancreatic pseudocysts. *Gastroenterology* 79:1246, 1980.
16. Gerzof S.G., Johnson W.C., Robbins A.H., et al.: Percutaneous drainage of infected pancreatic pseudocysts. *Arch. Surg.* 119:888, 1984.
17. Warshaw A.L., Rattner D.W.: Facts and fallacies of common bile duct obstruction by pancreatic pseudocysts. *Ann. Surg.* 192:33, 1980.
18. Warshaw A.L.: Inflammatory masses following acute pancreatitis: Phlegmon, pseudocyst, and abscess. *Surg. Clin. North Am.* 54:621, 1974.
19. Stroud W.H., Cullom J.W., Anderson M.C.: Hemorrhagic complications of severe pancreatitis. *Surgery* 90:657, 1981.
20. Stabile B.E., Wilson S.E., Debas H.T.: Reduced mortality from bleeding pseudocysts and pseudo-aneurysms caused by pancreatitis. *Arch. Surg.* 118:45, 1983.
21. Huizenga W.K.J., Kalideen J.M., Bryer J.V., et al.: Control of major hemorrhage associated with pancreatic pseudocysts by transcatheter arterial embolization. *Br. J. Surg.* 71:133, 1984.
22. Stone H.H., Strom P.R., Mullins R.J.: Pancreatic abscess management by subtotal resection and packing. *World J. Surg.* 8:340, 1984.
23. Bradley E.L. III, Fulenwider J.T.: Open treatment of pancreatic abscesses. *Surg. Gynecol. Obstet.* In press.
24. Sitzmann J.V., Imbembo A.L.: Splenic complications of a pancreatic pseudocyst. *Am. J. Surg.* 147:191, 1984.
25. Collins J.J. Jr., Peterson L.M., Wilson R.E.: Small intestinal infarction as a complication of pancreatitis. *Ann. Surg.* 167:433, 1968.
26. Poole G.V., Wallenhaupt S.L.: Massive rectal bleeding from colonic fistula in pancreatitis. *Arch. Surg.* 119:732, 1984.
27. Storm F.K., Wilson S.E.: Survival of patients with duodenal fistulas from necrotizing pancreatitis. *World J. Surg.* 1:105, 1977.
28. Alexandre J.H., Guerrieri M.T.: Role of total pancreatectomy in the treatment of necrotizing pancreatitis. *World J. Surg.* 5:369, 1981.
29. Warshaw A.L.: Pancreatic abscesses. *N. Engl. J. Med.* 287:1234, 1972.
30. Warshaw A.L., Jin G.: Improved survival of patients with pancreatic abscesses. *Ann. Surg.* In press.
31. Richter J.M., Jacoby G.A., Schapiro R.H., et al.: Pancreatic abscess due to *Candida albicans*. *Ann. Intern. Med.* 97:221, 1982.
32. Gerzof S.G., Robbins A.H., Johnson W.C., et al.: Percutaneous catheter drainage of abdominal abscesses: A five-year experience. *N. Engl. J. Med.* 305:653, 1981.
33. Aranha G.V., Prinz R.A., Greenlee H.B.: Pancreatic abscess: An unresolved surgical problem. *Am. J. Surg.* 144:534, 1982.
34. Warshaw A.L., Richter J.M.: A practical guide to pancreatitis. *Curr. Probl. Surg.* 21:1984.
35. Warshaw A.L., Cambria R.C.: False pancreas divisum: Acquired pancreatic duct obstruction simulating the congenital anomaly. *Ann. Surg.* 200:595, 1984.
36. Laugier R., Camatte R., Sarles H.: Chronic obstructive pancreatitis after healing of a necrotic pseudocyst. *Am. J. Surg.* 146:551, 1983.

33

Chronic Pancreatitis

HERBERT B. GREENLEE, M.D.

ALTHOUGH the gross anatomical features of chronic pancreatitis had been reported as early as 1799 by Baille, a more precise characterization of chronic pancreatitis and its complications was presented by Mayo-Robson in 1904 in a series of Hunterian lectures.[1] The Symposium of Aetiology and Pathology of Pancreatitis held in Marseilles in 1963 was helpful in defining the distinctions between acute and chronic pancreatitis. The futher separation of the chronic disease into relapsing chronic pancreatitis and chronic pancreatitis based on the presence of pain-free periods in the former has not been particularly useful, however, in determining prognosis and therapy. It is useful, nonetheless, to classify pancreatitis based on the presumed etiology of the disease. In acute pancreatitis and recurrent acute pancreatitis, associated biliary tract disease is identified consistently as the major etiologic factor. In contrast, the vast majority of patients with chronic pancreatitis are suffering from alcoholism.[2, 3] The evidence that alcohol use is a significant etiologic factor is overwhelming. Confirmed alcoholics are 20 to 50 times more likely to suffer from some type of pancreatitis than the general population.[4] Although the exact mechanism whereby chronic alcoholism results in pancreatitis is unknown, Sarles and Sahel[5] demonstrated early changes in the pancreas consisting of precipitation of enzymatic protein with resulting obstruction of the pancreatic ducts. Further, it is now clear that there is an increased output of calcium in pancreatic juice in patients with chronic pancreatitis.[6] The incorporation of calcium into precipitated protein plugs is a plausible explanation of intraductal pancreatic calcification frequently seen in advanced chronic pancreatitis.

The mortality of acute pancreatitis has been reported from several medical centers[7-9] and ranges from 7% to 20%. The risk of mortality for the initial episode of acute pancreatitis is considerably higher than that for recurrent bouts. In patients with chronic pancreatitis, the likelihood of surviving an individual episode is better than for acute pancreatitis. In fact, follow-up studies of patients with chronic pancreatitis suggest that relatively few patients die as a direct result of their disease.[10, 11] Rather, the ravages of chronic alcoholism and its related diseases primarily account for the high death rate seen in the follow-up studies of patients with alcoholic pancreatitis.[12]

This presentation will focus on the role of surgery for chronic pancreatitis and its complications. The available alternatives for the management of these problems will be discussed and a rationale for treatment recommended based on this author's experience and perspective.

MANAGEMENT OF CHRONIC INCAPACITATING ABDOMINAL PAIN

The goal of operative therapy for chronic pancreatitis is to relieve abdominal pain while preserving as much exocrine and endocrine function as possible. A variety of complications of pancreatic inflammatory disease is responsible for pain emanating from the pancreas. In chronic pancreatitis, those seen most frequently include distention of a pancreatic duct behind a stricture and/or pancreatic calculi, pseudocyst, and/or involvement of the nerves supplying the pancreas by scarring and inflammation. The parasympathetic nerve supply to the pancreas is involved primarily in the control of pancreatic secretions. Mediation of pain, on the other hand, is primarily by sympathetic nerve fibers. The pain of chronic pancreatitis is usually located in the upper midabdomen with radiation to the back. The pain may be continuous in some patients or have periodic fluctuations in others. Typically, there is exacerbation of the pain after eating. In fact, weight loss frequently occurs as the result of a self-imposed diet owing to the fear of pain secondary to eating.

A variety of operations has been tried to control the pain of chronic pancreatitis.[13-16] Diversion of bile to prevent reflux into the pancreatic duct, peptic ulcer surgery to lower the acid entering the duodenum and put the "pancreas at rest" by reducing hormonal stimulation of the pancreas, and sphincterotomy and sphincteroplasty have proved to be uniformly unsuccessful in relieving the disabling symptom of pain secondary to chronic pancreatitis. There is, however, a subset of patients with stenosing papillitis and recurrent pancreatitis identified by Nardi et al.[17] who are benefited by sphincteroplasty. Direct operations on the pancreas which have been most successful in controlling the pain of chronic pancreatitis are drainage procedures to relieve obstruction of the pancreatic ducts or resection of part or all of the diseased pancreas. Proponents of ductal drainage believe that the pain of chronic pancreatitis is due, in large part, to obstruction and distention of the major pancreatic ducts. Drainage of these obstructed ducts with a pancreaticojejunostomy is relatively safe and simple, and it preserves as much exocrine and endocrine function as possible.[12, 18–24] Proponents of pancreatic resection counter that not all patients have major ductal obstruction with dilatation[25] and that extended removal of the diseased organ reliably eliminates the source of the abdominal pain.[26–32] During recent years, considerable agreement has evolved as to a reasonable approach for those patients with incapacitating abdominal and back pain due to chronic pancreatitis. In patients with a dilated pancreatic ductal system (> 8 mm diameter) demonstrated by endoscopic retrograde cholangiopancreatography (ERCP), an adequate pancreaticojejunostomy will relieve pain in most patients with little or no impairment of exocrine and/or endocrine function secondary to the operative procedure. The hypothesis that pancreatic function would be improved or preserved by pancreatic ductal decompression, however, has been disproved by follow-up study and observation of these patients.[12, 22, 33] Pancreatic resections are best reserved for those patients with no demonstrable dilation of the major pancreatic ducts and evidence of substantial existing impairment of exocrine and endocrine pancreatic function, severe involvement of the gland limited primarily to the body and tail, or a failed drainage procedure. Although operative mortality rates are similar for both operations, early postoperative morbidity is higher following major resections of the pancreas, and the incidence of insulin dependent diabetes is significantly increased.[34] Management of diabetes is particularly precarious in this population group, many of whom continue to use excessive amounts of alcohol. A third alternative involving left or bilateral splanchnicectomy with or without partial ganglionectomy has been used intermittently for the treatment of the pain of pancreatitis, particularly in those patients with chronic pancreatitis who have a small, hard pancreas with obstructed ducts.[35, 36] Varying periods of pain relief may be obtained by these nerve-cutting procedures in contrast to alcohol injections of the coeliac ganglia, which have provided only transient relief of pain. Further use and study of coeliac ganglionectomy is warranted to determine its role in the management of pain due to chronic pancreatitis, particularly after failed pancreatic ductal drainage operations and in patients with unobstructed, nondilated pancreatic ducts.

Diagnosis

A spectrum of diagnostic tests is available for the patient with the presumed diagnosis of chronic pancreatitis. The simplest test for islet cell function is the two-hour postprandial blood glucose and the glucose tolerance test. Forty percent of our patients were diabetic as defined by these parameters prior to operation.[12] Exocrine function is measured most accurately by duodenal intubation and measurement of bicarbonate and enzyme concentrations with hormonal stimulation. Steatorrhea was severe enough in 20% of our patients to require pancreatic enzyme replacement prior to pancreatic duct drainage.[12]

Structural abnormalities of the pancreas are best defined by sonography and CT scanning. These methods have largely replaced the traditional contrast roentgenograms of the GI system to detect pancreatic enlargement and pseudocyst formation. Ultrasound and CT scans are helpful in the identification of dilation of the ducts in the biliary tract and the pancreas as

well as in the recognition of previously undetected pancreatic calcification. ERCP remains the key test for ascertaining the structural anatomy of the pancreatic ducts and the presence of an associated biliary structure. The presence of strictures and dilations ("chain-of-lakes") in the pancreatic ductal system provides guidance in identifying those patients in whom pancreatic duct drainage can be expected to be of benefit (Fig 33–1). The sensitivity of ultrasound in detecting pseudocysts renders ERCP unnecessary in most of these patients, although in long-standing pancreatitis, the additional identification of dilated ducts by ERCP may persuade the surgeon to combine drainage of the pseudocysts and pancreatic duct decompression at the same operation.

Frequently overlooked in the diagnostic studies for chronic pancreatitis is the presence of partial or nearly complete common bile duct obstruction. An elevated bilirubin or alkaline phosphatase level suggests the presence of an associated biliary stricture. Identification of the biliary stenosis may be accomplished by ERCP if dye can be injected successfully so as to outline the stricture with proximal dilation. Frequently, a better picture of the anatomy is obtained by percutaneous transhepatic or operative cholangiography.

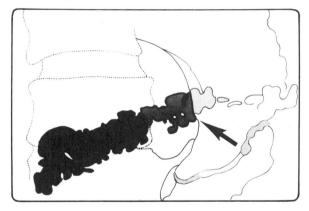

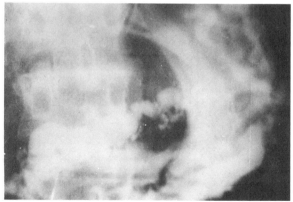

Fig 33–1.—The instillation of contrast material into the pancreatic duct during ERCP in this patient with alcoholic pancreatitis demonstrates sites of multiple strictures with dilation of the duct ("chain-of-lakes"). Incidentally noted is considerable reflux of dye into the stomach *(arrow).* (Reprinted with permission from Greenlee H.B.: The role of surgery for chronic pancreatitis and its complications, *Surg. Annu.* 15:283–305, 1983.)

Evolution of Pancreatic Ductal
Drainage Procedures

Assuming that obstruction of the pancreatic duct is a major factor in the production of pain associated with chronic pancreatitis in many patients, pancreatic duct decompression is a logical maneuver. The belief that the site of obstruction was at the sphincter of Oddi suggested sphincterotomy as an initial approach to this problem.[14] Disappointment with the results of this procedure prompted attempts at more direct ductal decompression. DuVal[37] first employed this concept by retrograde drainage of the duct of Wirsung to a defunctionalized loop of jejunum anastomosed to the distal process (Fig 33–2). The belief that caudal pancreaticojejunostomy would effectively drain the pancreatic ductal system was based on the mistaken presumption that a single structure of the duct of Wirsung near the ampulla was responsible for the pathophysiologic picture of chronic pancreatitis in most instances. Puestow and Gillesby[38] subsequently showed that multiple strictures and dilations (the "chain-of-lakes" phenomenon) frequently occurred in the ductal system in chronic pancreatitis. To achieve better drainage of the pancreatic ductal system, they recommended a longitudinal opening of the pancreatic duct from the site of pancreatic transection in the tail to a point just to the right of the mesenteric vessels (Fig 33–3). A splenectomy and excision of the tail of the pancreas are tech-

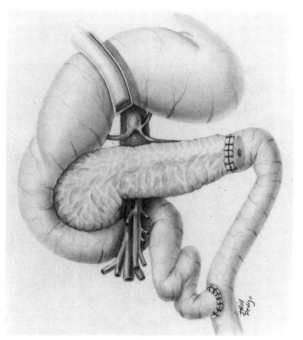

Fig 33–2.—The concept of pancreatic duct decompression by retrograde drainage into a Roux-en-Y loop of jejunum (caudal pancreaticojejunostomy) was introduced by DuVal. Frequently, pancreatic duct decompression was ineffective because of multiple sites of ductal obstruction in the body and head of the pancreas. (Reprinted with permission from Greenlee H.B.: The role of surgery for chronic pancreatitis and its complications, in Nyhus L.M. (ed.): *Surg. Annu.* Norwalk, Connecticut, Appleton-Century-Crofts, 1983, pp. 283–305.)

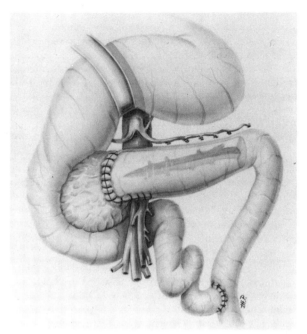

Fig 33–3.—Unroofing of the pancreatic duct after resection of the tail of the pancreas, as described by Puestow and Gillesby, recognized the problem of multiple strictures within the pancreatic duct. This method of longitudinal pancreaticojejunostomy achieves better pancreatic duct decompression. (Reprinted with permission from Greenlee H.B.: The role of surgery for chronic pancreatitis and its complications, in Nyhus L.M. (ed.): *Surg. Annu.* Norwalk, Connecticut, Appleton-Century-Crofts, 1983, pp. 283–305.)

nical requirements for this operation as they are for the DuVal procedure. Side-to-side pancreaticojejunostomy is a refinement of the Puestow procedure first suggested by Partington and Rochelle[39] and requires neither splenectomy nor resection of the tail of the pancreas (Fig 33–4). We favor this method as the procedure of choice in chronic pancreatitis. Less dissection is required to perform this operation. Since the greatest concentration of islet cells is in the tail of the pancreas,[40] preservation of this tissue is desired in patients in whom diabetes may develop during the course of their disease. The pancreas need not be implanted into the jejunum, so the restriction imposed by the mesenteric vessels at the body of the pancreas is eliminated. This permits the pancreatic duct to the right of the mesenteric vessels to be unroofed to a point close to the duodenum and ampulla. More effective drainage of the ductal system in the head of the pancreas and uncinate process is thus achieved.

Technique of Side-to-Side
Pancreaticojejunostomy

Step-by-step details of this operation (see Fig 33–4) with diagrams have been published.[41] A brief narrative description of the key technical aspects is included here. Preoperative preparation is similar to that for any other major intra-abdominal procedure. Nutritional status must be carefully evaluated, as these patients are frequently malnourished due to limited intake related to the exacerbation of abdominal pain after eat-

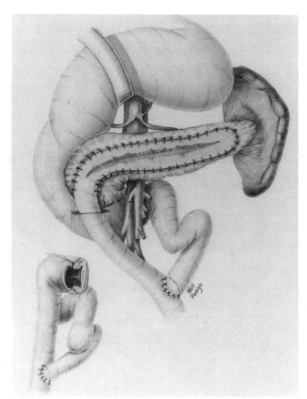

Fig 33–4.—A modification of the Puestow procedure suggested by Partington permits wide drainage of the pancreatic duct from the tail to the head of the pancreas without resection of the tail or splenectomy. This method of side-to-side pancreaticojejunostomy must now be considered the procedure of choice for pancreatic duct drainage in chronic pancreatitis. (Reprinted with permission from Greenlee H.B.: The role of surgery for chronic pancreatitis and its complications, in Nyhus L.M. (ed.): *Surg. Annu.* Norwalk, Connecticut, Appleton-Century-Crofts, 1983, pp. 283–305.)

ing. A period of preoperative parenteral nutrition is appropriate if the serum albumin is below 3.0 gm/dl. As most of these patients are alcoholics, evaluation of liver function and derangements of coagulation parameters is important in determining operative risk.

A transverse upper abdominal incision is favored, although any incision that gives adequate exposure to the upper abdomen is satisfactory. The lesser omental bursa is entered by wide incision of the gastrocolic ligament and greater omentum. The posterior wall of the stomach is often adherent to the anterior surface of the pancreas from long-standing pancreatic inflammation. These adhesions must be divided by sharp dissection, staying close to the surface of the pancreas. It is important to expose the entire anterior surface of the pancreas from the splenic hilum to the duodenum. When this has been accomplished, the stomach can be retracted superiorly, providing good exposure for the unroofing of the pancreatic duct. The location of the pancreatic duct may frequently be determined by palpating the fluctuation of fluid under pressure through the anterior surface of the pancreas. This can be confirmed by needle aspiration. If these maneu-

vers are unsuccessful, an oblique incision to the expected course of the duct in the body of the pancreas is performed. Once the duct is identified, the overlying pancreas is incised so that the duct is unroofed to within 1 to 2 cm of the spenic hilum and also to within the same distance from the duodenum and the ampulla of Vater. The duct of Wirsung curves inferiorly in the head of the pancreas as the unroofing proceeds from the initial entrance into the duct in the body of the pancreas. It is crucial to open widely this area of the duct in the head of the pancreas and in the uncinate process. Failure to accomplish this is a common reason for failure of pancreatic ductal decompression procedures. Pancreatic duct stones are encountered in many patients. Those that are accessible are removed, but the success of the operation has little to do with complete removal of the stones, as wide drainage has been established. Bleeding along the cut edge of the pancreas can be controlled in a variety of ways including electrocautery probe or suture ligature. Due to the fibrotic nature of the gland in chronic pancreatitis, significant bleeding is unusual. An exception to this rule occurs in the head of the pancreas, where branches of the pancreatic duodenal arterial arcade are divided frequently with brisk bleeding ensuing. Biopsy of the pancreas is always obtained to rule out the possibility of pancreatic cancer.

Attention is now turned to the preparation of the jejunal limb for Roux-en-Y drainage of the pancreas. The jejunum is divided 30–40 cm distal to the ligament of Treitz. The distal segment is closed and brought through a window in the avascular portion of the transverse mesocolon to the right of the middle colic vessels. The jejunal loop is placed parallel to the opened pancreatic duct so that the closed end of the jejunum lies adjacent to the tail of the pancreas and the splenic hilum. A row of interrupted nonabsorbable sutures is then placed between the jejunum and the tough fibrous capsule of the pancreas just inferior to the opened pancreatic duct. The jejunum is then opened along a course parallel to the opened pancreatic duct. The anastomosis is completed by interrupted sutures joining the jejunum to the pancreas just superior to the unroofed pancreatic duct. I do not believe it is necessary to perform a mucosa-to-mucosa anastomosis. Drains are not routinely used, as this is a low-flow, low-pressure anastomosis securely held to the fibrotic capsule of the pancreas.

Gastrointestinal continuity is reestablished by a jejunojejunostomy approximately 40 cm distal to the pancreaticojejunostomy. Postoperative care is similar to that for any other upper abdominal case involving a small-bowel anastomosis. Nasogastric suction is continued until flatus is passed, and diet is advanced as tolerated.

If the patient fails to achieve relief of abdominal pain or develops recurrence of pain during the follow-up period, the effectiveness of the pancreaticojejunostomy in decompressing the pancreatic duct can be evaluated by a repeated ERCP. Figure 33–5 demonstrates prompt dispersal of the dye into the Roux-en-Y jejunal limb. This type of information concerning the adequacy of pancreatic duct decompression will provide the surgeon the necessary data base to determine whether revision of the pancreaticojejunostomy can be expected to be effective in controlling the pain or whether other measures, such as resection, nerve blocks, or interruption, will be necessary.

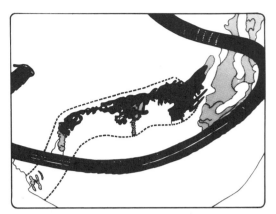
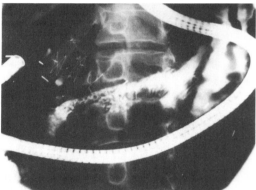

Fig 33–5.—Evaluation of the effectiveness of pancreatic duct drainage following pancreaticojejunostomy is accomplished by injection of contrast material into the pancreatic duct during ERCP. Immediate filling of the Roux-en-Y jejunal limb, as demonstrated here, confirms excellent pancreatic duct decompression. (Reprinted with permission from Greenlee H.B.: The role of surgery for chronic pancreatitis and its complications, in Nyhus L.M. (ed.): *Surg. Annu.* Norwalk, Connecticut, Appleton-Century-Crofts, 1983, pp. 283–305.)

RESULTS AFTER PANCREATICOJEJUNOSTOMY

The following conclusions are based on 100 consecutive patients who underwent surgical treatment of chronic pancreatitis to relieve intractable abdominal pain and to interrupt a cycle of repeated hospital admissions or narcotic dependence or both.[12] Although cholelithiasis was documented in 32 of these patients, alcoholism was considered to be the primary cause of the chronic pancreatitis that required pancreatic duct drainage in an attempt to relieve abdominal pain. A variety of operations had been undertaken before ductal drainage in 30 patients. These included cholecystectomy or common duct exploration or both in 18 patients, exploratory laparotomy in 12, drainage of pseudocysts in 9, gastric operations in 6, sphincterotomy in 4, and splanchnicectomy in 1 patient. Seven patients had two or more operations. Associated diseases such as cholelithiasis and duodenal ulcer may require surgical treatment based on the morbidity secondary to these conditions. It is important to understand, however, that the pathophysiologic changes of chronic pancreatitis and abdominal pain will almost certainly persist in the alcoholic and eventually require a direct operation on the pancreas.

Postoperative Complications

The operative mortality in this series was 3.8%, but there were no in-hospital deaths in the last 50 patients. For the most part, the postoperative complications that occurred in 21 patients were managed without prolonged morbidity. These included pneumonia in 6; wound infection in 6; GI hemorrhage in 3 patients from gastritis or acute stress ulcers, plus massive bleeding in 1 patient from the jejunal side of the pancreaticojejunostomy which required reoperation; subphrenic abscess in 2; wound seroma in two; and stroke, parotiditis, and small-bowel obstruction in 1 patient each. Of particular interest are three patients who died of metastatic carcinoma of the pancreas within one year of the operation. In each instance, biopsy of the pancreas had been obtained at the time of pancreatic duct drainage, and the operating surgeon did not suspect the presence of carcinoma. Recognition of occult carcinoma in a pancreas displaying the typical findings of chronic pancreatitis remains an unsolved problem.

Relief of Pain

The primary goal is to achieve relief of the disabling abdominal and back pain. Eighty-seven percent of the patients were available for follow-up evaluation as to the effectiveness of pain relief; postoperative deaths, patients with misdiagnosed carcinoma, and patients lost to follow-up were excluded. Table 33–1 presents the incidence of pain relief following three methods of pancreatic duct drainage; caudal pancreaticojejunostomy (DuVal), longitudinal pancreaticojejunostomy (Puestow and Gillesby), and side-to-side pancreaticojejunostomy (Partington and Rochelle). It is clear that the incidence of pain relief correlates with the more extensive pancreatic duct drainage achieved by side-to-side pancreaticojejunostomy: greater than 80% of the patients reported good to excellent results. An added benefit of this method of pancreatic duct decompression is that splenectomy and resection of the tail of the pancreas are not necessary.

Metabolic Consequences

The optimistic concept that pancreatic duct decompression would improve or stabilize pancreatic exocrine and endocrine function has not been supported by follow-up studies.[12, 33] Although the operative procedure does not appear to add to this problem, the destructive process in the pancreatic islets and acinar cells initiated by chronic alcoholism continues during the years after operation. Figures 33–6 and 33–7 summarize the progressive deterioration of endocrine and exocrine function during long-term follow-up. Eventually, 28% of our patients developed insulin-dependent diabetes, and one third required oral pancreatic enzyme replacement therapy for clinically significant steatorrhea.

Carcinoma and Chronic Pancreatitis

There appears little question that chronic pancreatitis predisposes to the development of malignant tumors of the pancreas. In three of the 100 patients in our series, carcinoma was not detected at the time of pancreatic duct drainage in

TABLE 33–1.—RESULTS OF PANCREATICOJEJUNOSTOMY

TYPE OF PANCREATIC DUCT DRAINAGE	COMPLETE RELIEF (%)	SUBSTANTIAL RELIEF (%)	MINIMAL TO NO RELIEF (%)	OPERATIVE MORTALITY	UNSUSPECTED CARCINOMA	LOST TO FOLLOW-UP
Side-to-side	21/50(42)	20/50(40)	9/50(18)	1/53	1/53	1/53
Longitudinal	10/36(28)	18/36(50)	8/36(22)	2/43	1/43	4/43
Caudal	1/5 (20)	1/5 (20)	3/5 (60)	1/8	1/8	1/8

(Reprinted with permission. Prinz R.A., Greenlee H.B.: Pancreatic duct drainage in 100 patients with chronic pancreatitis. *Ann. Surg.* 194:313, 1981.)

spite of pancreatic biopsy. Death from metastatic pancreatic carcinoma occurred within one year of operation. Temporary relief of pain occurred in each of these three patients. Two other patients were found to have carcinoma of the pancreas at autopsy or operation six and ten years, respectively, after pancreaticojejunostomy for chronic pancreatitis.

Continued Alcoholism and Late Outcome

Continued alcoholism proved to be a major factor both in relation to continued pain relief and late mortality due to alcohol-associated diseases. The period of follow-up study ranged from one to 25 years (average, 7.9 years). Forty-six of the 87 patients subsequently died seven months to 20 years after operation (average survival period, 6.1 years). The major causes of death were those frequently attributed to alcoholism and smoking: cardiovascular disease (24%), cirrhosis or chronic alcoholism (17%), pneumonia or pulmonary tuberculosis (15%), and carcinoma (15%), including oropharyngeal cancer in four patients and lung cancer in two patients. Death directly or indirectly related to chronic pancreatitis occurred only in two patients who developed carcinoma of the pancreas

during the follow-up period and in four patients who developed uncontrolled diabetes. In three of these patients, brittle diabetes occurred after pancreatic resection for failed drainage operations. The successful management of diabetes in the alcoholic is a difficult problem. Figure 33–8 shows an illustration of the influence of continued alcoholism on survival.

Successful pain relief is improved somewhat if the patient can be convinced to abstain from alcohol. Of the 23 of 87 patients who stopped all alcohol intake after operation, 21 continued free of significant pain. On the other hand, 14 of the 16 patients who continued to drink received no pain relief from the ductal drainage.

Failure of Pain Relief

In the reported experience for drainage operations, there remains a hardcore of 15%–30% of patients who fail to obtain pain relief after operation. The key diagnostic test to evaluate the effectiveness of pancreatic duct decompression following pancreaticojejunostomy is to determine whether there is immediate filling of the Roux-en-Y jejunal limb after injection of contrast material into the pancreatic duct during ERCP (see Fig 33–5). If all or a portion of the pancreatic ductal system is inadequately drained, revision of the pancreaticojejunostomy may help. Other alternatives including resection, nerve blocks or celiac ganglionectomy, or general supportive care, including analgesics, must be considered if ERCP demonstrates adequate pancreatic duct drainage.

It is tempting to theorize that certain as yet undetermined factors determine the successful amelioration of abdominal

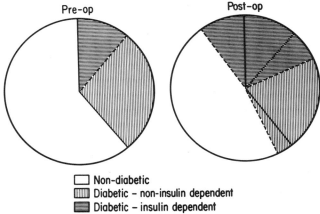

Pre-op   Post-op

☐ Non-diabetic
▥ Diabetic – non-insulin dependent
▧ Diabetic – insulin dependent

Fig 33–6.—Thirty-four of 87 patients available for follow-up study were diabetic as defined by an elevated fasting blood glucose level prior to pancreaticojejunostomy, but only ten of these required insulin. Six patients with preoperative diabetes required insulin after operation. Diabetes also developed in 11 of the 53 nondiabetic patients, eight of whom 11 required insulin. Only 28% of our patients are insulin-dependent diabetics. *Open area:* nondiabetic; *vertical stripes:* diabetic—noninsulin dependent; *horizontal stripes:* diabetic-insulin dependent. (Reprinted with permission from Prinz R.A., Greenlee H.B.: Pancreatic duct drainage in 100 patients with chronic pancreatitis. *Ann. Surg.* 194:313, 1981.)

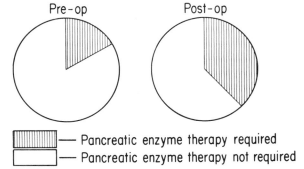

Pre-op   Post-op

▥ — Pancreatic enzyme therapy required
☐ — Pancreatic enzyme therapy not required

Fig 33–7.—Seventeen of 87 patients required treatment with pancreatic enzymes before pancreatic duct drainage. Twelve more patients required exocrine replacement therapy after operation. *Vertical stripes:* pancreatic enzyme therapy required: *open area:* pancreatic enzyme therapy not required. (Reprinted with permission from Prinz R.A., Greenlee H.B.: Pancreatic duct drainage in 100 patients with chronic pancreatitis. *Ann. Surg.* 194:313, 1981.)

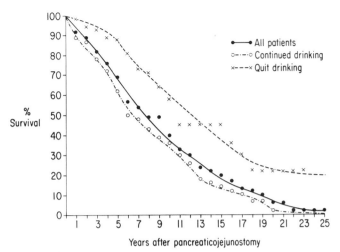

Fig 33–8.—Continued alcoholism is a crucial factor determining patient outcome. The survival rate of patients who abstain from alcohol is substantially better than that of those patients who continue to drink. ●———●: all patients; ○————○: continued drinking; x———x: quit drinking. (Reprinted with permission from Prinz R.A., Greenlee H.B.: Pancreatic duct drainage in 100 patients with chronic pancreatitis. *Ann. Surg.* 194:313, 1981.)

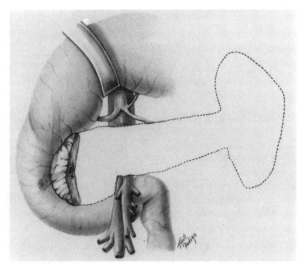

Fig 33–9.—A 60%–95% pancreatectomy is an acceptable alternative for the patient with refractory abdominal pain due to chronic pancreatitis if: (1) the pancreatic ducts are not dilated, and (2) the disease is concentrated in the body and tail of the pancreas. (Reprinted with permission from Greenlee H.B.: The role of surgery for chronic pancreatitis and its complications, in Nyhus L.M. (ed.): *Surg. Annu.* Norwalk, Connecticut, Appleton-Century-Crofts, 1983, pp. 283–305.)

pain. This reflects incomplete understanding of the mechanism of pain in all cases of pancreatitis. The simplistic explanation that pancreatic duct dilation is the sole reason for pain secondary to chronic pancreatitis does not explain adequately the documented observation of ductal dilation without pain[42] and the equally documented observation of incapacitating abdominal pain with normal pancreatic ducts on ERCP.[25] There may well be some common factors responsible for poor results after both drainage or resection related to narcotic addiction, continued alcoholism, or some currently unrecognized pathophysiologic changes in the pancreas or sympathetic innervation of the pancreas.

RESECTION FOR CHRONIC PANCREATITIS

A unique and extensive experience with resection therapy for the treatment of chronic pancreatitis has been achieved at the University of Michigan.[26, 34, 43] The concept of near-total pancreatectomy (80%–95%) was introduced there by Child and associates in 1959 based on the hypothesis that both the pain and complications associated with this disease would be eliminated by removing most of the pancreas. Due to the limited number of these patients seen in any one medical center, they elected to concentrate their attention on resectional therapy and to leave to others the task of evaluating other methods of surgical therapy.

In performing near-total pancreatectomy, an attempt is made to remove as much pancreas as possible without injury to the common bile duct (Fig 33–9). In many instances, it is necessary to leave more than 5% of the pancreas in situ because of the anatomy of the pancreaticoduodenal sweep and distortions caused by disease. Excessive alcohol intake was the major etiologic factor in the University of Michigan series, similar to that found in other reported series discussing the surgi-

cal management of chronic pancreatitis. Their low postoperative mortality of 3% is admirable for this major operation, frequently performed in malnourished patients. A significant number of early postoperative complications occurred, including pneumonia in one fifth of the patients and subphrenic abscess in one sixth of the series. Pancreatic fistula requiring long-term drainage from the pancreatic stump with associated abscess was the most troublesome of these complications. To minimize the frequency of these complications, they have advocated three technical maneuvers: ligation of the pancreatic duct individually with nonabsorbable suture; inversion of the pancreatic stump with Lembert sutures when feasible; and bringing the pancreatic drains directly anterior through the abdominal wall, rather than attempting lateral dependent drainage, to provide a shorter drainage tract should a pancreatic fistula develop. They speculate that splenectomy, performed as a part of near-total pancreatectomy, may have been a contributing factor in the difficulty of controlling sepsis. Based on sufficiently detailed information available on 55 patients, the incidence of insulin-dependent diabetes increased from 9% preoperatively to 67% following near-total pancreatectomy.[34] Insulin requirements tended to parallel the extent of the resection: patients undergoing conservative pancreatectomies frequently required no insulin. The need for insulin tended to increase with time, an observation previously noted following drainage operations and undoubtedly related to the continuing destructive process in the remaining pancreas. Success in relieving pain was comparable to that achieved with drainage procedures; one half of the patients were eventually pain free and another one fourth experienced only mild pain. Late mortality is high and parallels that reported from other institutions, regardless of the type of surgery performed. Common causes of death include complications of continued alco-holism, cardiovascular disease, cancer, and complications of diabetes. Other authors have reported roughly similar results with left subtotal pancreatectomies,[44–46] although selection of patients in these series was usually based on the extent of the disease and the absence of dilated pancreatic ducts.

Another approach using pancreaticoduodenectomy to achieve major resections of diseased pancreas in chronic pancreatitis has been utilized in some centers.[47–51] The reasons for selecting this extensive procedure for benign disease of the pancreas vary, but indications center on the presence of intractable pain in patients with the preponderance of the inflammatory disease located in the head of the pancreas and the absence of dilated pancreatic ducts. Associated biliary and/or duodenal obstruction plus exocrine and endocrine insufficency have been offered as additional indications for pancreaticoduodenectomy. Any evaluation of this type of extensive surgery for benign disease must first take into account its safety. In skilled and experienced hands, the operative mortality has been reported to range from 2% to 14.7%.[51] Particularly in the lower range, this risk is acceptable and compares favorably with other operations for chronic pancreatitis. The reported satisfactory results in surviving patients range from 50% to 93.3%, again an acceptable result. In particular, the relief of pain compares favorably with other modes of surgical therapy. For surgeons with extensive experience with pancreatic resection, there is an evolving consensus that long-term results appear to favor pancreaticoduodenectomy over left subtotal pancreatectomy.[28, 30, 48, 52–54] Late morbidity and mortality following pancreaticoduodenectomy, however, must be assessed in defining the proper role of this procedure in the management of pain secondary to chronic pancreatitis. Late deaths and complications related to continued alcoholism, diabetes, cancer, and cardiovascular disease occur in these patients at a rate similar to that seen after other methods of surgical control of chronic pancreatitis. Pancreaticoduodenectomy, however, may be followed by complications initiated by the procedure itself. Anastomotic ulcers may occur if vagotomy is not done. Alternatively, vagotomy may not be necessary if the antrum and pylorus are preserved and the line of transection is across the proximal duodenum.[55] Short-term results suggest improvement in the nutritional state of these patients without the complication of anastomotic ulcer when compared to follow-up studies after the traditional pancreaticoduodenectomy.[56] Strictures of the choledochojejunal anastomosis may be troublesome, reflecting the difficulty and hazard of working with a normal-sized rather than dilated duct. In patients undergoing total pancreatectomy, the presence of the apancreatic state has been correlated with a "failure to thrive" in the patient population.[32]

Pancreaticoduodenectomy remains an option for the surgical treatment of advanced chronic pancreatitis, but should be reserved for special situations. If a dilated pancreatic duct is present, the more conservative and equally effective side-to-side pancreaticojejunostomy is preferable. In the absence of pain, associated biliary stricture and/or duodenal stenosis can be managed effectively by the appropriate bypass. Pancreaticoduodenectomy may be utilized for those patients with major involvement of the pancreatic head, unrelenting pain, and a nondilated pancreatic duct.

The metabolic problems which develop after extended pancreatic resections have deterred many surgeons from recommending pancreatectomy with greater frequency. The management of insulin-dependent diabetes in this patient population is difficult. Refinements in autotransplantation of pancreatic islet cell tissue eventually may prevent the development of worsening of diabetes after pancreatectomy; but, at present, it has had limited success.[29, 57–60] Although cautious optimism is expressed by these investigators, the failure to achieve an insulin-independent status and to avert surgically induced diabetes mellitus in most patients leads to the general conclusion that further developments in islet cell autotransplantation are necessary before this technique is a practical adjunct to major resections of the pancreas for chronic pancreatitis.

NERVE PROCEDURES FOR CHRONIC PANCREATITIS

The transmission of pain from the pancreas is primarily through the sympathetic nerve fibers. Some information on the localization of pain secondary to lesions in the pancreas has been provided by the electrical stimulation of the pancreas during abdominal operations performed with local anesthesia.[61, 62] The site of stimulation correlated closely with the location of visceral sensation of pain—e.g., left-sided stimulation produced pain in the left side, and stimulation of the head of the pancreas produced right-sided pain. Stimulation of the central portion of the pancreas produced pain on both sides of the abdomen. Presumably the pain in chronic pancreatitis is related either to distention of the pancreatic duct behind a proximal obstruction or direct involvement of the sympathetic nerve fibers by the inflammatory process itself or both.

Inasmuch as the main goal of operative therapy for chronic pancreatitis is relief of abdominal pain, it is appropriate to consider nerve ablation procedures as a primary method or secondary alternative to manage this problem. Nerve injection or cutting procedures do not sacrifice additional pancreatic tissue in patients whose exocrine and endocrine function has already been compromised. Most of the sensory nerves to the pancreas pass through the celiac ganglia and splanchnic nerves. This has been confirmed by the injection of anesthetic agents or alcohol directly into the area of these ganglia anterior to the aorta and adjacent to the celiac axis, or by left or bilateral splanchnicectomy with or without partial ganglionectomy.[35, 63] These operations do not alter the long-term course of the disease but may relieve pain for varying periods. The relief of disabling pain from pancreatic cancer is more successful than control of pain secondary to chronic pancreatitis.[64] Only slightly over one half of patients with chronic pancreatitis received effective pain relief, and the mean pain-free interval was only two months. In contrast, almost 90% of cancer patients were relieved of pain, and most remained pain-free until death.

Transthoracic splanchnicectomy does not appear to help patients with pancreatic cysts or dilated pancreatic ducts and pancreatic duct calculi.[35] White[65] has reported long-term relief of pain using this technique in 12 of 20 patients with chronic pancreatitis of unknown origin who had a small, hard pancreas with unobstructed ducts. The more commonly used approach of celiac ganglionectomy has been described by White and Harrison.[66] Unfortunately, the celiac ganglia and splanchnic nerves are not easily accessible due to their location, in intimate association with the anterior surface of the aorta, superior mesenteric artery, and diaphragmatic crura. One approach is through the lesser omentum. The splenic artery is located superior to the pancreas and followed down posteriorly to the aorta until the two semilunar ganglia and splanchnic nerves are identified, adjacent to the celiac axis and between the crura of the diaphragm. A partial removal of the ganglia with a short segment of the splanchnic nerves is adequate for relief of pain. Unfortunately, this approach is complicated by the presence of many inflammatory nodes, and excessive bleeding results frequently. Another approach utilizes an extended Kocher maneuver that mobilizes the duodenum, pancreas, and portal triad anteriorly and permits retropancreatic exposure of the inferior vena cava and aorta. The right celiac ganglia is identified between the superior mesenteric artery and celiac axis and can be dissected free and partially resected. A third approach is through the bed of the left 12th rib. The splanchnic nerves can be identified emerging from behind the crura. The left celiac ganglion is located medial to the adrenal just superior to the renal vessels and around the celiac axis. Dissection with a nerve hook and control of bleeding with clips will permit removal of a significant portion of the ganglia and left splanchnic nerve.

Pancreaticojejunostomy for patients with dilated pancreatic ducts and resection in patients with normal or small pancreatic ducts remains the preferred approach to the control of pain due to chronic pancreatitis. Nerve ablation procedures, however, should be considered as alternatives to extensive pancreatic resections with their resulting disabilities and for failed drainage or resection operations. This approach deserves further study; it has been underutilized in most centers. Unfortunately, the initial good results in achieving pain relief after nerve interruption are frequently lost with time.

BILIARY STRICTURE AND CHRONIC PANCREATITIS

The fibrosis and inflammation that characterize chronic pancreatitis may cause obstructive jaundice by compressing the intrapancreatic portion of the common bile duct, resulting in a long, smooth stricture of the distal portion of the duct.[67, 68] Recognition of this complication of chronic pancreatitis is important, since it can lead to cholangitis, biliary cirrhosis, diagnostic confusion with pancreatic carcinoma, and persistence of pain following operations on the pancreas itself. It is possible to isolate those patients with chronic pancreatitis who have fixed obstruction of the distal common bile duct by the more frequent use of PTC and ERCP. The latter procedure permits delineation both of the pancreatic duct and the biliary tree prior to operation. These bile duct strictures have been reported to occur in 3%–27% of patients with chronic pancreatitis.[69] In our own experience, approximately 15% of patients with chronic pancreatitis were found to have associated obstruction of the biliary tree.[67]

In patients with chronic pancreatitis, the suspicion of associated common duct obstruction is based on a substantial elevation in the level of alkaline phosphatase and a mild hyperbilirubinemia (Tables 33–2 and 33–3). In our experience, elevation of the alkaline phosphatase level was the most common abnormal laboratory finding; in 75% of the patients, it exceeded three times the normal value. The total and direct bilirubin levels, on the other hand, were moderately elevated and were characterized by a rising and falling pattern. This disproportionate increase in the alkaline phosphatase level as compared with the bilirubin levels is compatible with benign obstruction of the distal common duct.[68, 70] The precise delineation of the anatomical abnormality in the common duct requires the use of invasive radiologic procedures. A long, smooth, gradual tapering of the distal common duct is characteristic of a benign stricture due to pancreatic fibrosis. The proximal dilated duct often appears as a "bent-knee" deformity superior to the pancreas (Fig 33–10). When successful, PTC and ERCP provide valuable preoperative information in planning the operation and eliminates the need for such time-consuming intraoperative manipulations as cholangiography and pancreatography. The identification of pancreatic duct abnormalities permits simultaneous pancreatic duct decompression by pancreaticojejunostomy in addition to bypass of the biliary stricture, a combination that we performed in ten of 51 patients.[68] Ultrasound examination of the pancreas is useful in detecting pseudocysts of the pancreas that may require simultaneous drainage. In patients with persistent nausea and vomiting, an upper GI tract roentgenographic series helps to identify incidental abnormalities in the stomach and duodenum or to rule out obstruction secondary to pancreatitis which may require surgical bypass.

The obstructed biliary tree proximal to the periductal fibrosis is in constant jeopardy of bacterial infection. Only three of our patients showed clinical signs of cholangitis, but of the 30 cultures of bile taken during surgery, 18 cultured a variety of gram-negative bacteria. This finding of contaminated bile in the absence of clinical evidence of cholangitis has been reported by others.[71] On the other hand, life-threatening cholangitis may be present, requiring urgent or emergency operation. Warshaw and associates[72] found that four of five patients with common duct obstruction from chronic pancreatitis had gram-negative enteric organisms in their bile at the time of surgery; in one of these, acute cholangitis and hepatic abscesses were found at operation. Gregg and co-workers[73] obtained positive cultures of bile at the time of ERCP in four of eight patients, and all four had symptomatic cholangitis.

Biliary cirrhosis is a complication of long-standing biliary obstruction that may be prevented by biliary tract decompression.[69, 71, 72, 74] We did not identify biliary cirrhosis in our series, but Laënnec's cirrhosis was diagnosed in six of 51

TABLE 33–2.—ABNORMAL SERUM TEST RESULTS IN PATIENTS WITH COMMON DUCT OBSTRUCTION FROM CHRONIC PANCREATITIS

TEST	NORMAL	MEAN ± SEM	RANGE
Total bilirubin, mg/dl	<1.2	5.8 ± 0.7	0.6–23.6
Direct bilirubin, mg/dl	<0.5	4.4 ± 0.6	0.3–18.8
Amylase, IU	<200	228.6 ± 35.7	55–2,300
Alkaline phosphatase, IU	30–85	655.3 ± 105.2	56–3,810
Serum transaminase, IU	0–50	120.6 ± 9.5	20–818

TABLE 33–3.—DIAGNOSTIC RADIOLOGIC TESTS

TEST*	NO. OF PATIENTS	ABNORMAL COMMON DUCT	ABNORMAL PANCREATIC DUCT	UNSUCCESSFUL TEST
PTC	23	23	None	None
ERCP	17	9	10	3
IOC	17	17	None	None
IVC	2	1	None	1

*PTC indicates percutaneous transhepatic cholangiography; ERCP, endoscopic retrograde cholangiopancreatography; IOC, intraoperative cholangiogram; and IVC, intravenous cholangiogram. (Reprinted with permission. Aranha G.V., Prinz, R.A., Freeark R.J., et al.: The spectrum of biliary tract obstruction from chronic pancreatitis. *Arch. Surg.* 119:595, 1984.)

patients.[68] It is unclear whether hepatic deterioration is hastened by common duct obstruction in the presence of preexisting alcoholic cirrhosis.

Determining whether biliary obstruction is due to chronic pancreatitis or underlying malignancy can be a very challenging clinical problem. Although there is no absolute way of resolving this difficulty in all cases, Wapnick and associates[75] have defined several parameters which make a diagnosis of inflammatory disease of the pancreas more likely than cancer. In their experience, patients with chronic pancreatitis were significantly younger than patients with carcinoma (average age, 47 vs. 62). The total serum bilirubin was much higher typically in patients with carcinoma, 18.5 ± 2.1 mg/dl compared with 5.6 ± 1.5 mg/dl in chronic pancreatitis. Perhaps more important than the absolute level of bilirubin was the pattern of elevation. In patients with malignancy, bilirubin

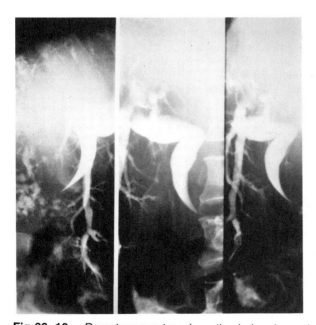

Fig 33–10.—Percutaneous transhepatic cholangiography showing long, smooth, concentric narrowing of distal common duct with "bent-knee" deformity as seen in obstruction from pancreatitis. (Reprinted with permission from Aranha G.V., Prinz R.A., Freeark R.J., et al.: The spectrum of biliary tract obstruction from chronic pancreatitis. *Arch. Surg.* 119:595, 1984.)

rose relentlessly until the biliary tree was decompressed. In contrast, bilirubin levels in chronic pancreatitis tended to wax and wane. Newton and colleagues[76] suggested that in patients with biliary obstruction due to pancreatitis, abdominal and back pain usually antedated the onset of jaundice, which tended to wax and wane. In contrast, patients with carcinoma experienced no pain, or only a brief interval, before a progressive and relentless increase in the bilirubin level developed. These historical observations and laboratory findings combined with the radiographic appearance of the common duct will differentiate most cases of benign obstruction from malignancy. In carcinoma, cholangiograms demonstrate an abrupt cutoff at the common duct in contrast to the long, smooth, tapering obstruction seen in chronic pancreatitis. In spite of a thorough history, laboratory and radiographic investigation, and operative evaluation, an occasional patient with the typical findings of chronic pancreatitis will have an underlying malignancy. Three of 100 patients undergoing pancreaticojejunostomy for presumed chronic pancreatitis died within one year, of metastatic pancreatic cancer, in spite of pancreatic biopsy at the time of the initial operation in our series.[12]

The cause of pain in patients with chronic pancreatitis is multifactorial. In my opinion, it is mainly related to the diseased pancreatic gland with lesser contributions secondary to the involvement of the biliary and GI tracts. In patients with biliary obstruction and chronic pancreatitis, biliary decompression alone may not be sufficient to relieve abdominal pain.[45] Identification of patients with associated pancreatic and duodenal abnormalities is necessary if complete relief of the patient's symptoms is to be achieved.[67, 68, 77] In addition to biliary decompression in our patients, lateral pancreaticojejunostomy was necessary in ten patients, as well as drainage of pseudocysts in six patients and gastrojejunostomy in six patients. On the other hand, unrecognized biliary obstruction may be responsible for persistent or recurrent pain after drainage of the pancreatic duct for chronic pancreatitis. Warshaw and co-workers[72] reported two patients with chronic pancreatitis in whom pain relief was achieved only after drainage of the common duct. It is apparent that the origin of the symptom complex of pain in chronic pancreatitis frequently is difficult to identify in many patients. This underlines the importance of investigating associated anatomical abnormalities that are present and correcting all of them, preferably at the initial operation.

Choledochoduodenostomy or Roux-en-Y choledochojejunostomy are the preferred methods of biliary bypass for those patients.[67, 68, 74, 78–80] When possible, choledochoduodenostomy is preferable because it does not divert bile from the duodenum, it is easier to construct, and it leaves the jejunum free to be used for associated procedures that may be required on the stomach and pancreas (Fig 33–11). Several technical reasons, such as nonmobility of the duodenum or duodenal stricture secondary to pancreatic inflammation, may render this choice difficult or unsatisfactory. In these instances, Roux-en-Y choledochojejunostomy is a satisfactory alternative (Fig 33–12). If necessary, pancreatic duct decompression and gastroenterostomy can be accomplished utilizing the same Roux-en-Y jejunal loop. Sphincteroplasty has been unsuccessful in relieving common duct obstruction

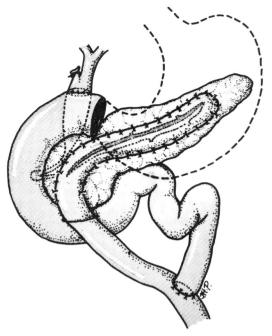

Fig 33–11.—Choledochoduodenostomy is an effective method of biliary bypass for distal common bile duct stricture due to chronic pancreatitis. This permits a Roux-en-Y jejunal loop to be used for pancreatic duct drainage, if necessary.

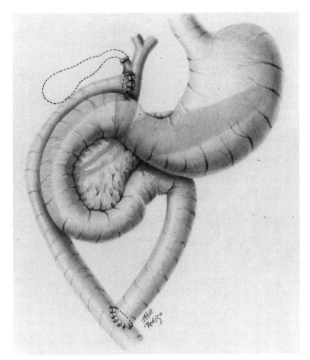

Fig 33–12.—Relief of biliary obstruction secondary to chronic pancreatitis may be achieved by choledochojejunostomy to a Roux-en-Y jejunal limb. (Reprinted with permission from Greenlee H.B.: The role of surgery for chronic pancreatitis and its complications, in Nyhus L.M. (ed.): *Surg. Annu.* Norwalk, Connecticut, Appleton-Century-Crofts, 1983, pp. 283–305.)

from pancreatitis in most series due to the length of the distal common duct stricture proximal to the sphincter.[68, 74, 78] A cholecystenteric anastomoses to bypass common duct stenosis is also associated with a high incidence of failure due to the unpredictability of the long term patency of the cystic duct. Is is reserved for those patients in whom direct access to the common duct is extremely difficult and cystic duct patency has been established. Common bile duct exploration and T-tube drainage is doomed to failure except, perhaps, as a temporary measure in an occasional patient.

The resolution of common bile duct stenosis following pancreatic duct drainage is controversial. Wisloff and coworkers[81] have concluded that stenosis of the common bile duct is a frequent complication of chronic pancreatitis and that biliary enteric bypass is unnecessary in most patients with such complications. They noted that 50% of their patients who were icteric at the time of the initial investigation had spontaneous resolution of jaundice. Only a few of their patients, however, were subjected to long-term follow-up, and the waxing and waning of elevated bilirubin levels is characteristic of such patients. Our own experience has led us to conclude that the vast majority of these strictures are fixed by surrounding fibrotic pancreas, and little, if any, change results from pancreatic duct decompression or prolonged medical management.[67, 68] On the other hand, partial or complete obstruction of the common bile duct may be secondary to a pseudocyst in the head of the pancreas.[82, 83] The presence of a pseudocyst in this location, however, does not necessarily mean that the pseudocyst is solely responsible for obstruction

of the biliary system. After drainage of the pseudocyst, it is imperative that operative cholangiography be performed to demonstrate the presence or absence of underlying periductal fibrotic compression of the common duct by chronic pancreatitis.[79] Should significant stenosis still be present, it is wishful thinking to expect that the jaundice will clear as a result of pseudocyst drainage alone.

The above discussion forms the basis we use for the management of patients with biliary obstruction and chronic pancreatitis. In a patient with chronic pancreatitis and abdominal pain who has an elevated alkaline phosphatase, distal common duct stenosis is suspected. The anatomical defect is best demonstrated by either PTC or ERCP. The latter procedure permits the demonstration of associated pancreatic duct abnormalities. Surgical decompression of the obstructed bile duct is necessary to prevent the complications of biliary cirrhosis and cholangitis. Identification of associated problems, including pancreatic duct obstruction and dilatation, pseudocysts, and duodenal obstruction, is important because they can be corrected during the same operation. This increases the likelihood of relieving abdominal pain and/or nausea and vomiting that may be due to these factors rather than to the obstructed biliary tract. When possible, the preferred operation for distal biliary stricture is choledochoduodenostomy, since it can be constructed easily and leaves the jejunum free to be used for concomitant procedures on the pancreas or stomach.

GASTROINTESTINAL COMPLICATIONS

Due to their close anatomical relationship to the pancreas, the stomach and duodenum may be affected by diseases involving the pancreas. Considerable attention has been devoted to involvement of the upper GI tract by carcinoma of the pancreas,[84] but relatively little has been given to gastric and duodenal involvement from inflammatory pancreatic disease. The incidence of fixed gastric outlet and duodenal obstruction from all aspects of pancreatic inflammatory disease is small. In our hospital,[85] 16 patients were identified during a ten-year period among 1,911 patients who were discharged with a diagnosis of pancreatitis, an incidence of 0.8%. The cause of obstruction was chronic pancreatitis in 10 patients, pseudocysts in 5 patients, and pancreatic abscess in 1 patient. In contrast, of those patients with severe chronic pancreatitis requiring pancreatic duct drainage, approximately 10% have required simultaneous or subsequent relief of duodenal obstruction. Thus, in the setting of chronic pancreatitis, upper GI tract obstruction should be suspected in a patient with persistent nausea and vomiting.

The diagnosis is confirmed by barium examination of the stomach and duodenum and by endoscopy. A long, constricting lesion of the duodenum is most frequently seen when the obstruction is caused by pancreatitis (Fig 33–13). Carcinoma of the head of the pancreas tends to involve the medial wall of the C-loop of the duodenum. Endoscopically, a cone-shaped, smooth obstruction of the duodenum suggests obstruction from pancreatitis. In contrast, with carcinoma the endoscopist is likely to encounter friable duodenal mucosa due to duodenal invasion by the malignancy.

There is considerable disagreement regarding how long upper GI tract obstruction from pancreatitis should be treated medically. Bradley and Clements[86] pointed out that 25% of the patients admitted to their hospital had functional duodenal obstruction. The mean interval from the time of diagnosis to surgery in our patients was 30 days.[85] A three- to four-week interval permits the associated inflammation and edema of the duodenal wall secondary to pancreatitis to subside.[86, 87] Patients who continue to manifest symptoms of upper GI tract obstruction beyond this period and who have had past similar episodes should be suspected of having fixed obstruction unlikely to respond to conservative measures. A trial of hyperalimentation for several weeks may be carried out in indeterminate cases.

The operative treatment selected depends on the underlying pathologic condition. In two of our patients, obstruction was relieved by lysis of fixed inflammatory adhesions around the duodenum. If the obstruction is due to external pressure from a pseudocyst, drainage of the cyst may suffice.[88] Our results suggest that gastroenterostomy is sufficient to relieve duodenal obstruction. A vagotomy is added if the patient has a previous history of peptic ulcer disease. If abdominal pain as well as duodenal obstruction is a significant part of the clinical picture, additional diagnostic measures are instituted to determine concomitant biliary or pancreatic duct obstruction. If these conditions are recognized preoperatively and relieved surgically at the time of operation, pain will be relieved in the majority of the cases (Fig 33–14).

The possibility of carcinoma of the pancreas masquerading as a benign duodenal obstruction must always be considered. Although carcinoma of the pancreas may appear as a duodenal obstruction without causing jaundice, patients usually are found to have widespread metastatic disease at the time of surgical exploraton.[89] In such cases, the use of ultrasound,

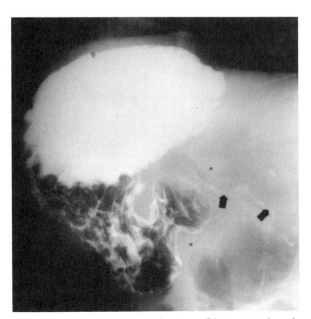

Fig 33–13.—Lateral view of upper GI tract series demonstrating long constricting lesion *(arrows)* of duodenum from pancreatitis. (Reprinted with permission from Aranha G.V., Prinz R.A., Greenlee H.B., et al.: Gastric outlet and duodenal obstruction from inflammatory pancreatic disease. *Arch. Surg.* 119:833, 1984.)

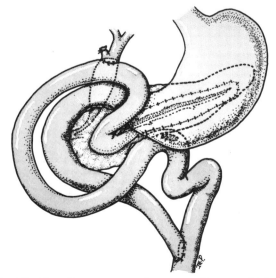

Fig 33–14.—If necessary, the same Roux-en-Y jejunal loop may be used for pancreatic duct drainage, biliary bypass for distal bile duct stricture, and gastroenterostomy for duodenal stenosis when these complications occur secondary to chronic pancreatitis.

ERCP with cytology, CT scans, and angiography are helpful in differentiating carcinoma from pancreatitis,[90] plus evaluation of operation including biopsy.

The above discussion has focused on the area of the GI tract most frequently involved by chronic pancreatitis—i.e., the distal stomach and duodenum. It would be remiss not to indicate that a functional or anatomical obstruction may result at other sites contiguous to the pancreas, including the duodenojejunal junction and the transverse colon, particularly at the splenic flexure. The obstruction may be secondary to an inflamed pancreas or the inflammatory reaction about an associated pseudocyst. Therapy is aimed at treatment of the underlying problem; for example, drainage of the pseudocyst. Appropriate bypass procedures may be necessary if the primary lesion cannot be corrected.

PANCREATIC ASCITES AND PANCREATIC PLEURAL EFFUSIONS

In chronic pancreatitis, the accumulation of pancreatic fluid in the peritoneal cavity is most frequently caused by leakage of a pancreatic pseudocyst or disruption of the main pancreatic duct.[91] Peritoneal fluid may accumulate with other diseases of the pancreas. In acute pancreatitis, ascites may occur secondary to chemical peritonitis. In abdominal carcinomatosis from pancreatic carcinoma, ascites often results from peritoneal metastases. The term "pancreatic ascites" in this discussion is reserved for those patients with chronic pancreatitis who develop massive ascites from an internal pancreatic fistula to the peritoneal cavity due to a disruption of the main pancreatic duct or a leaking pseudocyst. The accumulation of a chronic massive pleural effusion is a closely related entity secondary to the retroperitoneal tracking of an internal pancreatic fistula to the mediastinum and pleural space. Although the clinical presentation of chronic pancreatic pleural effusion may differ considerably from that of pancreatic ascites, their etiologies are identical. In fact, both conditions may occur in the same patient.

The exact incidence of pancreatic ascites is unknown. Sankaran and Walt[92] identified 26 patients with 31 episodes of pancreatic ascites during a 17-year period. During this time, 15% of all patients treated for pseudocysts at that hospital had associated pancreatic ascites. The recognition of chronic pleural effusions of pancreatic origin has been more recent. Cameron and associates,[93] in a series of 34 patients with pancreatic ascites and/or pleural effusions, identified 12 (35%) who had a pleural effusion alone or in conjunction with ascites. The recognition of these fluid collections of pancreatic origin in the peritoneal cavity or pleural space will increase with greater clinical awareness.

Several theories have been proposed as possible mechanisms for pancreatic ascites. Blocked intraperitoneal lymphatics was suggested by Schmidt and Whitehead.[94] Gambill and co-workers[95] suggested that ascites was secondary to subacute peritoneal inflammation from the presence of pancreatic enzymes. It is now clear that pancreatic ascites results from the leakage of pancreatic secretions from a ductal disruption or incompletely formed pseudocyst.[93] In the presence of acute pancreatitis, the inflammatory reaction will usually seal off any leak with the resulting formation of a pseudocyst. In the

absence of acute inflammation, this leak may persist and result in chronic collections of fluid of pancreatic origin in the peritoneal cavity and/or pleural space. The location of the duct disruption has some bearing on the direction of the internal pancreatic fistula. Anterior disruptions usually track into the peritoneal cavity, whereas posterior disruptions into the retroperitoneum will track along the path of least resistance, often through the esophageal and/or aoritc hiatus up into the mediastinum. The pancreatic secretions may be contained in the mediastinum or rupture into one or both pleural cavities and present as pleural effusions. Acute peritonitis or acute pleuritis does not develop, since the pancreatic enzymes have not been activated by the duodenal contents. The patient experiences little or no pain. A chronic peritoneal or pleural exudative reaction does occur, however—possibly secondary to the high albumin content of the fluid. It is important to distinguish these chronic massive pleural effusions from the small, usually left-sided, pleural effusions that occur in response to attacks of acute pancreatitis. These latter effusions are sympathetic in origin and will usually resolve spontaneously.

Most patients presenting with pancreatic ascites have a history of excessive alcohol intake. The usual admitting diagnosis is alcoholic cirrhosis with ascites. Frequently there is little historical evidence of inflammatory disease of the pancreas. On physical examination, tense ascites is the predominant feature. The abdomen is usually nontender in contrast to patients with acute pancreatitis. The patients appear chronically rather than acutely ill. For those patients with chronic massive pleural effusions, the clinical presentation is even more misleading. Their symptoms are primarily respiratory in origin, with minimal, if any, complaints referable to the abdomen. The usual admission diagnosis relates to pulmonary parenchymal or pleural disease. The differentiation of internal pancreatic fistula as the source of these fluid collections from other conditions can be easily and rapidly accomplished by the simple biochemical analysis of the fluid. The amylase in the fluid is always markedly elevated, usually in the thousands.[93] The albumin content of the fluid is usually greater than 3 gm/dl. The serum amylase level is almost always elevated, probably resulting from absorption of amylase from the fluid rather than as a result of active pancreatic inflammation.

Once the diagnosis of pancreatic internal fistula with ascites and/or pleural effusion has been confirmed, most physicians choose an initial period of nonoperative management.[96] The basis of this treatment regimen is to "put the pancreas at rest" by decreasing pancreatic secretion and to keep ascitic or pleural fluid to a minimum. This is accomplished by nothing by mouth and/or nasogastric tube suction plus the use of atropine and acetazolamide (Diamox). Daily paracentesis and/or thoracentesis or chest tube drainage is used to keep the peritoneal or pleural cavities free of fluid. These measures are performed in the hope that the fistula will seal by peritoneal or pleural approximation. As many as 50% of patients may avoid surgery with this management.[96] Hyperalimentation and the maintenance and improvement in nutrition is extremely important, not only as an adjunct in the initial conservative management, but as preparation for operation should it be necessary.

Surgery is indicated if nonoperative therapy is unsuccessful over a period of two weeks. The choice of operative treatment must be based on an adequate knowledge of the pathologic anatomy—e.g., presence of a pseudocyst or demonstration of a pancreatic ductal leak. Preferably, this information is obtained preoperatively by ERCP, since identification of the source of the pancreatic internal fistula at operation may be difficult and unnecessarily prolong the length of the operation.[97] If a direct leak from the pancreatic duct is present and no pseudocysts are present, an anastomosis between the site of ductal rupture and a Roux-en-Y jejunal loop is the preferred treatment. In a collected series, only 10% of patients were found to have a free duct rupture.[96] Most patients will have small pseudocysts. If the cyst is small and located in the tail, distal pancreatectomy is the preferred treatment. If pancreatography has demonstrated proximal obstructive duct disease, the pancreatic remnant should be drained by a pancreaticojejunostomy utilizing a Roux-en-Y jejunal loop rather than simply oversewing the pancreatic remnant. If the pseudocyst is large or located in the head of the gland, internal drainage by a cystogastrostomy or cystojejunostomy is indicated. These principles of operative treatment hold regardless of whether the internal pancreatic fistula has resulted in pancreatic ascites or pancreatic pleural effusion.

Although the overall mortality for these patients ranges from 15% to 20%, and recurrent ascites occurs in 16% based on an analysis of collected series,[96] it is evident that the results are improving now that a standardized therapeutic approach is evolving in the management of these patients. The key elements in achieving an increasing success rate is the more liberal use of parenteral nutrition as an adjunct in both the nonoperative and operative management and the skillful use of ERCP in identification of the precise location of the internal pancreatic fistula, so that the proper choice of operative correction may be selected for those patients requiring surgery.

PSEUDOCYST

Pseudocyst formation as a complication of acute pancreatitis has been discussed elsewhere in this book. Pseudocyst formation in chronic pancreatitis will be reviewed briefly here, with emphasis on diagnosis and management. The exact mechanism of pseudocyst formation varies, but two main processes are probably involved. In one, an attack of acute pancreatitis results in extravasation of pancreatic juice, which becomes walled off, a fibrous capsule developing after some weeks. The second mechanism occurs in a patient with chronic pancreatitis and ductal obstruction. The pseudocyst probably begins as a retention cyst, which gradually outgrows its epithelial lining as it enlarges.[98] This latter presentation typically occurs as an established entity without an antecedent acute illness in a patient with chronic pancreatitis. Serial ultrasonic examinations in these patients indicate that these pseudocysts do not resolve spontaneously,[99] and further, the cyst wall is usually mature at the time of presentation, so that surgical drainage may be accomplished soon after diagnosis.

Ultrasound is the key diagnostic test for the initial demonstration and follow-up study of pseudocysts. The sophistication of this technique permits identification of multiple pseudocysts, suggests ancillary problems such as biliary tract

obstruction with bile duct dilation, and may even suggest pancreatic duct dilation ("chain-of-lakes"). CT scan is reserved for patients in whom the presence and cystic nature of the lesion is in question. Angiography is not necessary unless resection is contemplated. In these situations, it is obtained for delineation of the vascular anatomy, providing help in the technical conduct of the operation. The use of ERCP in the diagnostic evaluation of the pseudocysts remains controversial. It is contraindicated after an attack of acute pancreatitis with pseudocyst formation because of the risk of a flare-up in the pancreatitis or infection of the pseudocyst contents. We reserve ERCP for patients with documented chronic pancreatitis and pseudocyst formation in whom associated pancreatic duct obstruction and dilation are suspected. In these patients, consideration is given to draining the pancreatic duct as well as the pseudocyst into a Roux-en-Y jejunal limb (Fig 33–15). This conclusion has been based on the observation that approximately one half of our patients who required additional operations on the pancreatic duct remote from a pseudocyst operation were for persistent abdominal pain related to pancreatic duct obstruction and dilation.[100] When ERCP is performed in patients with a pseudocyst, antibiotic coverage is given and operation is scheduled, usually within the next 24 hours.

Three methods of surgical drainage of pseudocysts include resection and internal and external drainage. The main criteria for selecting the type of drainage are the anatomical presentation of the cyst and the characteristics of the wall. At our institution, we prefer internal drainage of a pancreatic pseudocyst into the stomach (Fig 33–16), duodenum, or a Roux-

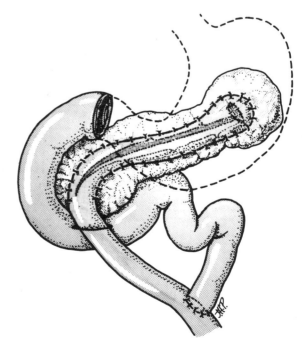

Fig 33–15.—Drainage of a pseudocyst in the tail of the pancreas is combined with pancreatic duct drainage by the same Roux-en-Y jejunal limb in this diagram demonstrating the feasibility of combining pseudocyst and pancreatic duct drainage when the latter exhibits multiple strictures and dilations.

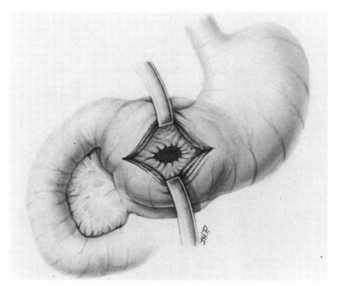

Fig 33–16.—Cystogastrostomy is an excellent method of internal drainage for pancreatic pseudocysts posterior to the stomach in which the anterior cyst wall has become adherent to the posterior wall of the stomach. (Reprinted with permission from Greenlee H.B.: The role of surgery for chronic pancreatitis and its complications, in Nyhus L.M. (ed.): *Surg. Annu.* Norwalk, Connecticut, Appleton-Century-Crofts, 1983, pp. 283–305.)

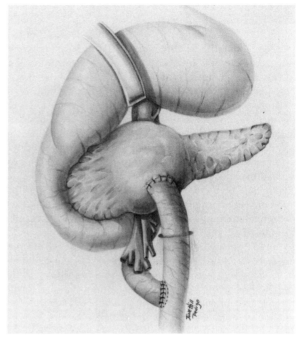

Fig 33–17.—Internal drainage of a pancreatic pseudocyst into a Roux-en-Y loop of jejunum is. the preferred method of treatment, particularly if the cyst wall is not adherent to the stomach or duodenum, precluding drainage into these organs. (Reprinted with permission from Greenlee H.B.: The role of surgery for chronic pancreatitis and its complications, in Nyhus L.M. (ed.): *Surg. Annu.* Norwalk, Connecticut, Appleton-Century-Crofts, 1983, pp. 283–305.)

en-Y loop of jejunum (Fig 33–17) whenever possible.[100] The choice between these sites of drainage is based primarily on the anatomical location of the cyst, rather than favoring one recipient viscus over another based on a physiologic advantage. External drainage resulted in recurrent cysts in one third of our patients. We reserve this method of treatment for those patients with infected cysts and clinical signs of sepsis or those with flimsy and immature cyst walls that cannot be drained internally for technical reasons. This latter finding is unusual in patients whose pseudocysts develop in the chronic pancreatitis setting. Resection effectively eradicates the pseudocyst (Fig 33–18). This approach however, requires resecting the contiguous pancreas, which, from a practical point of view, limits resection to pseudocysts situated in the body and tail of the pancreas. In our experience, resection is associated with higher morbidity and mortality, which offsets any potential advantage of this method in preventing recurrent cyst formation.

SUMMARY

Chronic alcoholism is the etiologic factor initiating most instances of chronic pancreatitis and its complications. Impairment of exocrine and endocrine function parallels the severity of the chronic pancreatitis. Ultrasound and CT scans are the most accurate tests for the identification of gross anatomical changes in the pancreas, but ERCP is critical for the evaluation of pancreatic ductal anatomy.

Severe, persistent abdominal and back pain requiring narcotics is significantly relieved in approximately 80% of patients receiving pancreatic duct drainage operations. Pan-

creatic resection utilizing left subtotal pancreatectomy or pancreaticoduodenectomy is an acceptable alternative if pancreatic ductal dilation is absent. A high incidence of insulin-dependent diabetes remains the main drawback of pancreatic resection, a problem often difficult to manage in the alcoholic. Further progress in islet cell autotransplantation must occur before this technique is practical as an adjunct to major resections of the pancreas for chronic pancreatitis. Nerve ablation procedures as alternatives to extensive pancreatic resections and for failed drainage operations deserve further study and use. Unfortunately, the initial good results in achieving pain relief after nerve interruption are frequently lost with time.

Strictures secondary to chronic pancreatitis involving the biliary tract and contiguous GI tract require an individual approach based on the site and cause of the problem. Fixed obstruction resulting from fibrosis secondary to long-standing chronic pancreatitis is effectively treated by a bypass procedure. If a pseudocyst is present and compressing these structures, drainage of the pseudocyst may relieve the obstruction.

Pancreatic ascites and pancreatic pleural effusions result from an internal pancreatic fistula due to a disruption of the pancreatic duct or a leaking pseudocyst. A standardized therapeutic approach involving a period of medical management, in which the pancreas is "put at rest," followed by surgery for the failures has resulted in a significant lowering of mortality for these complications. Hyperalimentation to maintain and improve nutrition is an important adjunct, not only in the

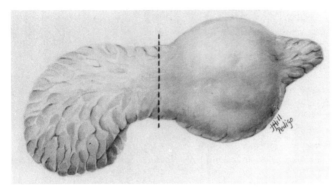

Fig 33–18.—Pancreatic pseudocysts located in the body and tail of the pancreas may be managed by distal pancreatectomy. This method effectively eradicates the pseudocyst but is frequently associated with a higher morbidity and mortality because of the surrounding inflammatory reaction or involvement with contiguous abdominal organs. (Reprinted with permission from Greenlee H.B.: The role of surgery for chronic pancreatitis and its complications, in Nyhus L.M. (ed.): *Surg. Annu.* Norwalk, Connecticut, Appleton-Century-Crofts, 1983, pp. 283–305.)

initial conservative management but also as preparation for operation should it necessary. The preoperative use of ERCP to identify the precise location of the internal pancreatic fistula has proved to be a significant advance in the operative management of these patients.

Internal drainage of pancreatic pseudocysts is favored whenever possible. If the contents of the pseudocyst are infected or the cyst walls are immature, external drainage is indicated. Resection of the pseudocyst and the contiguous pancreas effectively treats the pseudocyst, but at the price of higher morbidity and mortality. The role of percutaneous aspiration of pseudocyts has not yet been adequately tested.

REFERENCES

1. Mayo-Robson A.W.: The pathology and surgery of certain diseases of the pancreas: Inflammatory affections of the pancreas. *Lancet* 1:845, 1904.
2. Sarles H., Sales J.C., Camatte R., et al.: Observations on 205 confirmed cases of acute pancreatitis, recurring pancreatitis and chronic pancreatitis. *Gut* 6:545, 1965.
3. White T.T.: Inflammatory diseases of the pancreas. *Adv. Surg.* 9:247, 1975.
4. Sarles H.: Alcohol and the pancreas. *Adv. Exp. Med. Biol.* 856:429, 1977.
5. Sarles H., Sahel J.: Pathology of chronic calcifying pancreatitis. *Am. J. Gastroenterol.* 66:117, 1976.
6. Clain J.E., Barbezat G.O., Marks I.N.: Exocrine pancreatic enzyme and calcium secretion in health and pancreatitis. *Gut* 22:355, 1981.
7. Aldrete J.S., Jiminez H., Halpern N.B.: Evaluation and treatment of acute and chronic pancreatitis. *Ann. Surg.* 191:664, 1980.
8. Jacobs M.L., Daggett W.M., Civetta J.M., et al.: Acute pancreatitis: Analysis of factors influencing survival. *Ann. Surg.* 185:43, 1977.
9. Satiani B., Stone H.H.: Predictability of present outcome and future recurrence in acute pancreatitis. *Arch. Surg.* 114:711, 1979.
10. Levrat M., Descos L., Molinier B., et al.: Evolution au long

course des pancréatites chroniques (A propos de 113 observations). *Arch. Fr. Mal Appar. Dig.* 59:5, 1970.
11. Read G., Braganza J.M., Howat H.T.: Pancreatitis: A retrospective study. *Gut* 17:945, 1976.
12. Prinz R.A., Greenlee H.B.: Pancreatic duct drainage in 100 patients with chronic pancreatitis. *Ann. Surg.* 194:313, 1981.
13. Bowers R.G.: Choledocojejunostomy: Its ability to control chronic recurring pancreatitis. *Ann. Surg.* 142:682, 1955.
14. Doubilet H., Mulholland J.H.: Eight year study of pancreatitis and sphincterotomy. *J.A.M.A.* 160:521, 1956.
15. Mallet-Guy P.: Surgical treatment of chronic relapsing pancreatitis. *Arch. Surg.* 70:609, 1955.
16. Priestley J.T., Taylor L.M., Rogers J.D.: Surgical treatment of chronic relapsing pancreatitis. *Surgery* 37:317, 1955.
17. Nardi G.L., Michelassi F., Zannini P.: Transduodenal sphincteroplasy. 5–25 year follow-up of 89 patients. *Ann. Surg.* 198:453, 1983.
18. Prinz R.A., Kaufman B.H., Folk F.A., et al.: Pancreaticojejunostomy for chronic pancreatitis: Two to 21 year follow-up. *Arch. Surg.* 113:520, 1978.
19. Greenlee H.B.: The role of surgery for chronic pancreatitis and its complications. *Surg. Annu.* 15:283–305, 1983.
20. Potts J.R. III, Moody F.G.: Surgical therapy for chronic pancreatitis: Selecting the appropriate approach. *Am. J. Surg.* 142:654, 1981.
21. Sato T., Noto N., Matsuno S., et al.: Follow up results of surgical treatment for chronic pancreatitis: Present status in Japan. *Am. J. Surg.* 142:317, 1981.
22. Warshaw A.L., Popp J.W. Jr., Schapiro R.H.: Long-term patency, pancreatic function and pain relief after lateral pancreaticojejunostomy for chronic pancreatitis. *Gastroenterology* 79:289, 1980.
23. Proctor H.J., Mendes O.C., Thomas C.G. Jr., et al.: Surgery for chronic pancreatitis: Drainage versus resection. *Ann. Surg.* 189:664, 1979.
24. Jordan G.L. Jr., Strug B.S., Crowder W.E.: Current status of pancreaticojejunostomy in the management of chronic pancreatitis. *Am. J. Surg.* 133:46, 1977.
25. Grodsinsky C., Schuman B.M., Block M.A.: Absence of pancreatic duct dilation in chronic pancreatitis: Surgical significance. *Arch. Surg.* 112:444, 1977.
26. Frey C.F., Child C.G. III, Fry W.: Pancreatectomy for chronic pancreatitis. *Ann. Surg.* 184:403, 1976.
27. Cohen J.R., Kuchta N., Geller N., et al.: Pancreaticoduodenectomy for benign disease. *Ann. Surg.* 197:68, 1983.
28. Taylor R.H., Bagley F.H., Braasch J.W., et al.: Ductal drainage or resection for chronic pancreatitis. *Am. J. Surg.* 141:28, 1981.
29. Najarian J.S., Sutherland D.E., Baumgartner D., et al.: Total or near total pancreatectomy and islet autotransplantation for treatment of chronic pancreatitis. *Ann. Surg.* 192:526, 1980.
30. Traverso L.W., Tompkins R.K., Urrea P.T., et al.: Surgical treatment of chronic pancreatitis: Twenty-two years experience. *Ann. Surg.* 190:312, 1979.
31. Adson M.A.: Surgical treatment of pancreatitis: Review of a series. *Mayo Clin. Proc.* 54:443, 1979.
32. Braasch J.W., Vito L., Nugent F.W.: Total pancreatectomy of end-stage chronic pancreatitis. *Ann. Surg.* 188:317, 1978.
33. Bradley E.L. III, Nasrallah S.M.: Fat absorption after longitudinal pancreaticojejunostomy. *Surgery* 95:640, 1984.
34. Turcotte J.G., Eckhauser F.E.: Near total pancreatectomy for chronic pancreatitis, in Dent T.L. (ed.): *Pancreatic Disease: Diagnosis and Therapy.* New York, Grune & Stratton, 1981, pp. 353–360.
35. Mallet-Guy P., Feroldi J.: Bases pathologiques, experimentales et cliniques de la splanchnicectomie gauche dans le traitement des pancréatities chroniques récidivantes. *Presse Med.* 61:99, 1953.
36. White T.T., Lawinski M., Stacher G., et al.: Treatment of pancreatitis by left splanchniectomy and celiac ganglionectomy: Analysis of 146 cases. *Am. J. Surg.* 112:195, 1966.
37. DuVal M.K. Jr.: Caudal pancreatico-jejunostomy for chronic relapsing pancreatitis. *Ann. Surg.* 140:775, 1954.

38. Puestow C.B., Gillesby W.J.: Retrograde surgical drainage of pancreas for chronic relapsing pancreatitis. *Arch. Surg.* 76:898, 1958.

39. Partington P.F., Rochelle R.E.L.: Modified Puestow procedure for retrograde drainage of the pancreatic duct. *Ann. Surg.* 152:1037, 1960.

40. Wittingen J., Frey C.F.: Islet concentration in the head, body, tail and uncinate process of the pancreas. *Ann. Surg.* 179:412–414, 1974.

41. Greenlee H.B.: Pancreaticojejunostomy (Roux-en-Y) for chronic pancreatitis, in Nyhus, L.M., Baker R.J. (eds.): *Mastery of Surgery*. Boston, Little, Brown & Co., 774–779, 1984.

42. Bornman P.C., Marks I.N. Girdwood A.H., et al.: Is pancreatic duct obstruction or stricture a major cause of pain in calcific pancreatitis? *Br. J. Surg.* 67:425, 1980.

43. Child C.G., III, Frey C.F., Fry W.J.: A reappraisal of removal of ninety-five percent of the distal portion of the pancreas. *Surg. Gynecol. Obstet.* 129:49, 1969.

44. White T,T., Hart M.J.: Pancreaticojejunostomy versus resection in the treatment of chronic pancreatitis. *Am. J. Surg.* 138:129, 1979.

45. Way L.W., Gadacz T., Goldman L.: Surgical treatment of chronic pancreatitis. *Am. J. Surg.* 127:202, 1974.

46. Trapnell J.E.: Chronic relapsing pancreatitis: A review of 64 cases. *Br. J. Surg.* 66:471, 1979.

47. Warren K.W.: Surgical management of chronic relapsing pancreatitis. *Am. J. Surg.* 117:24, 1969.

48. Leger L., Lenriot J.P., Lamaigre G.: Five to twenty year follow-up after surgery for chronic pancreatitis in 148 patients. *Ann. Surg.* 180:185, 1974.

49. Clot J.P., Chigot J.P., Richer R., et al.: Attitude thérapeutique face à une pancréatite chronique autonome: A propos de 147 cas. *Ann. Chir.* 32:733, 1978.

50. Guillemin G., Berard P., Bigay D., et al.: 103 Duodéno-pancréactomies cephaliques pour panréatite chronique: Reflexions sur une expérience de 20 ans. *Chirurgie* 105:147, 1979.

51. Moreaux J.: Long-term follow up study of 50 patients with pancreaticoduodenectomy for chronic pancreatitis. *World J. Surg.* 8:346, 1984.

52. Gall F.P., Mühe E., Gebhart C.: Results of partial and total pancreaticoduodenectomy in 117 patients with chronic pancreatitis. *World J. Surg.* 5:269, 1981.

53. Sarles J.C., Nacchiero M., Garani F., et al.: Surgical treatment of chronic pancreatitis: Report of 134 cases treated by resection or drainage. *Am. J. Surg.* 144:317, 1982.

54. White T.T., Slavotinek A.H.: Results of surgical treatment of chronic pancreatitis: Report of 142 cases. *Ann. Surg.* 189:217, 1979.

55. Traverso L.W., Longmire W.P. Jr.: Preservation of the pylorus in pancreaticoduodectomy: A follow-up evaluation. *Ann. Surg.* 192:306, 1980.

56. Newman K.D., Braasch J.W., Rossi R.L., et al.: Pyloric and gastric preservation with pancreaticoduodenectomy. *Am. J. Surg.* 145:152, 1983.

57. Toledo Persyra L.H.: Islet cell autotransplantation after subtotal pancreatectomy. *Arch. Surg.* 118:851, 1983.

58. Grodsinsky C., Malcolm S., Goldman J., et al.: Islet cell autotransplantation after pancreatectomy for chronic pancreatitis: Its limitations. *Arch. Surg.* 116:511, 1981.

59. Cameron J.L., Mehigan D.G., Broe P.J., et al.: Distal pancreatectomy and islet autotransplantation for chronic pancreatitis. *Ann. Surg.* 193:312, 1981.

60. Traverso L.W., Abou-Zamzam A.M., Longmire W.P. Jr.: Human pancreatic cell autotransplantation following total pancreatectomy. *Ann. Surg.* 193:191, 1981.

61. Bliss W.R., Burch B., Martin M.M., et al.: Localization of referred pancreatic pain induced by electric stimulation. *Gastroenterology* 16:317, 1950.

62. Ray B.S., Neill C.L.: Abdominal visceral sensation in man. *Ann. Surg.* 126:709, 1947.

63. Flanigan D.P., Kraft R.O.: Continuing experience with palliative chemical splanchnicectomy. *Arch. Surg.* 113, 509, 1978.

64. Leung J.W., Bowen-Wright M., Aveling W., et al.: Coeliac plexus block for pain in pancreatic cancer and chronic pancreatitis. *Br. J. Surg.* 70:730, 1983.

65. White T.T.: Pain, in Bradley E.L. III (ed.): *Complications of Pancreatitis: Medical and Surgical Management*. Philadelphia, W.B. Saunders Co., 1981, pp. 203–222.

66. White T.T., Harrison R.C.: *Reoperative Gastrointestinal Surgery*. ed. 2nd. Boston, Little, Brown & Co., 1979, pp. 228–232.

67. Prinz R.A., Aranha G.V., Greenlee H.B., et al.: Common duct obstruction in patients with intractable pain of chronic pancreatitis. *Am. Surg.* 48:373, 1982.

68. Aranha G.V., Prinz R.A., Freeark R.J., et al.: The spectrum of biliary tract obstruction from chronic pancreatitis. *Arch. Surg.* 119:595, 1984.

69. Scott J., Summerfield J.A., Elias E., et al.: Chronic pancreatitis: A cause of cholestasis. *Gut* 18:196, 1977.

70. Gremillion D.E. Jr., Johnson L.F., Cammerer R.C., et al.: Biliary obstruction: A complication of chronic pancreatitis diagnosed by endoscopic retrograde cholangiopancreatography (ERCP). *Dig. Dis. Sci.* 24:145, 1979.

71. Littenberg G., Afroudakis A., Kaplowitz N.: Common bile duct stenosis from chronic pancreatitis: A clinical and pathological spectrum. *Medicine* 58:385, 1979.

72. Warshaw A.L., Schapiro R.H., Ferrucci J.T. Jr., et al.: Persistent obstructive jaundice, cholangitis, and biliary cirrhosis due to common bile duct stenosis in chronic pancreatitis. *Gastroenterology* 70:562, 1976.

73. Gregg J.A., Carr-Locke D.L., Gallagher M.M.: Importance of common bile duct stricture associated with chronic pancreatitis. *Am. J. Surg.* 141:199, 1981.

74. Yadegar J., Williams R.A., Passaro E. Jr., et al.: Common duct stricture from chronic pancreatitis. *Arch. Surg.* 115:582, 1980.

75. Wapnick S., Hadas N., Purow E., et al.: Mass in the head of the pancreas in cholestatic jaundice: Carcinoma or pancreatitis? *Ann. Surg.* 190:587, 1979.

76. Newton B.B., Rittenburg M.S., Anderson M.C.: Extrahepatic biliary obstruction associated with pancreatitis. *Ann. Surg.* 197:645, 1983.

77. Creaghe S.B., Roseman D.M., Saik R.P.: Biliary obstruction in chronic pancreatitis: Indications for surgical intervention. *Am. Surg.* 47:243, 1981.

78. Schulte W.J., LaPorta A.J., Condon R.E., et al.: Chronic pancreatitis: A cause of biliary stricture. *Surgery* 82:303, 1977.

79. Bradley E.L. III, Salam A.A.: Hyperbilirubinemia in inflammatory pancreatic disease: Natural history and management. *Ann. Surg.* 188:626, 1978.

80. Gadacz T.R., Lillemoe K., Zinner M., et al.: Common bile duct complications of pancreatitis: Evaluation and treatment. *Surgery* 93:235, 1983.

81. Wisloff F., Jakobsen J., Osnes M.: Stenosis of the common bile duct in chronic pancreatitis. *Br. J. Surg.* 69:52, 1982.

82. Grace R.R., Jordan P.H. Jr.: Unresolved problems of pancreatic pseudocysts. *Ann. Surg.* 184:16, 1976.

83. Karatzas G.M.: Pancreatic pseudocysts. *Br. J. Surg.* 63:55, 1976.

84. Sarr M.G., Gladen H.E., Beart R.W. Jr., et al.: Role of gastroenterostomy in patients with unresectable carcinoma of the pancreas. *Surg. Gynecol. Obstet.* 152:597, 1981.

85. Aranha G.V., Prinz R.A., Greenlee H.B., et al.: Gastric outlet and duodenal obstruction from inflammatory pancreatic disease. *Arch. Surg.* 119:833, 1984.

86. Bradley E.L. III, Clements J.L. Jr.: Idiopathic duodenal obstruction: An unappreciated complication of pancreatitis. *Ann. Surg.* 193:638, 1981.

87. Makrauer F.L., Antonioli D.A., Banks P.A.: Duodenal stenosis in chronic pancreatitis: Clincopathological correlations. *Dig. Dis. Sci.* 27:525, 1982.

88. Rheingold O.J., Walker J.A., Barkin J.S.: Gastric outlet obstruction due to a pancreatic pseudocyst. *Am. J. Gastroenterol.* 69:92, 1978.

89. Lindenauer S.M., Reuter S.R., Joseph R.R.: Carcinoma of the head of the pancreas presenting as duodenal obstruction without jaundice. *Am. J. Surg.* 115:705, 1968.

90. Moosa A.R., Levin B.: The diagnosis of "early" pancreatic can-

cer: The University of Chicago experience. *Cancer* 47:1688, 1981.

91. Cameron J.L., Anderson R.P., Zuidema G.D.: Pancreatic ascites. *Surg. Gynecol. Obstet.* 125:328, 1967.

92. Sankaran S., Walt A.J.: Pancreatic ascites: Recognition and management. *Arch. Surg.* 111:430, 1976.

93. Cameron J.L., Kieffer R.S., Anderson W.J., et al.: Internal pancreatic fistulas: Pancreatic ascites and pleural effusions. *Ann. Surg.* 184:587, 1976.

94. Schmidt E.H., Whitehead R.P.: Recurrent ascites as an unusual complication of chronic pancreatitis. *J.A.M.A.* 180:533, 1962.

95. Gambill E.E., Walters W., Scanlon P.W.: Chronic relapsing pancreatitis with extensive subacute peritonitis and chronic recurrent massive "chylous" ascites. *Am. J. Med.* 28:668, 1960.

96. Broe P.J., Cameron J.L.: Pancreatic ascites and pancreatic pleural effusions, in *Complications of Pancreatitis: Medical and Surgical Management*. Philadelphia, W.B. Saunders Co., 1982, pp. 245–264.

97. Sankaran S., Sugawa C., Walt A.J.: Value of endoscopic retrograde pancreatography in pancreatic ascites. *Surg. Gynecol. Obstet.* 148:185, 1979.

98. Bradley E.L. III: Pancreatic pseudocysts, in Bradley E.L. III (ed.): *Complications of Pancreatitis: Medical and Surgical Management*. Philadelphia, W.B. Saunders Co., 1982, pp. 124–153.

99. Aranha G.V., Prinz R.A., Esguerra A.C., et al.: The nature and course of cystic pancreatic lesions diagnosed by ultrasound. *Arch. Surg.* 118:486, 1983.

100. Aranha G.V., Prinz R.A., Freeark R.J., et al.: Evaluation of therapeutic options for pancreatic pseudocysts. *Arch. Surg.* 117:717, 1982.

34

Recurrent Acute Pancreatitis

LARRY C. CAREY, M.D., F.A.C.S.

RECURRENT ACUTE PANCREATITIS is a controversial diagnosis. While it was identified in the classification of pancreatitis established in 1963 in Marseilles, it was excluded from the Cambridge classification in 1983 and the more recent Marseilles conference in 1984. Perhaps it is appropriate to include recurrent acute pancreatitis under the general heading of acute pancreatitis, but experience indicates that the recurrent form of the illness may warrant special consideration.

In most patients, the cause is established before, during, or shortly after the attack takes place. The cause of alcoholic pancreatitis is often known to be present before the first attack. If gallstones are at fault, ultrasound may establish their presence during the attack. Hyperlipidemia or hypercalcemia may be confirmed after the initial attack has subsided. However, once a single attack of pancreatitis of obscure etiology occurs, there is a 30%–70% chance that it will recur,[1-4] presumably because the cause is unrecognized. When the illness does recur, commonly recognized etiologic factors such as alcohol abuse and gallstones are usually again investigated. If they are not found, then the disease must be considered to be "idiopathic," and attacks may be expected to continue to recur.

At the outset, a definition is in order. The uncertainty of the diagnosis of acute pancreatitis continues to create controversy. It seems that, in general, abdominal pain compatible with pancreatitis and an elevation in amylase must be accepted as the benchmarks of the diagnosis.

If this definition is used, the majority of errors will be made in overdiagnosing pancreatitis, although in a few instances, the diagnosis will not be made. Spechler et al.[5] in an evaluation of patients with clinical evidence of acute pancreatitis found the amylase level to be misleading in 32%. Increased accuracy in diagnosis promises to result from new imaging techniques such as CT scan and ultrasound, but the quest continues for improved clinical laboratory accuracy since no test has yet proved superior to the traditional measurement of blood amylase with or without lipase. There is hope that accuracy may be improved by isoenzyme measurements of amylase. What role nuclear magnetic resonance (NMR) will play in the diagnosis of pancreatic disease remains speculative.

With the problems related to diagnosis recognized, recurrent acute pancreatitis can be simply defined as acute pancreatitis that occurs over and over. The condition differs from chronic pancreatitis in that it does not as a rule result in permanent functional or histologic abnormality in the gland. Pancreatic insufficiency develops occasionally after a single episode of severe acute pancreatitis, but it appears that once recovery is complete, the gland is not chronically inflamed or fibrotic as it is in chronic alcoholic pancreatitis. There are exceptions, but in the nonalcoholic patient they are unusual.

Recurrent acute pancreatitis causes distress for the patient as well as the physician. From the patient's perspective, life is clouded by the constant threat of another attack. There is little clue as to what precipitates the events, and the patient has no idea how to protect himself. His life may be disrupted at any time without warning. The attacks vary in severity from a few hours of mild to moderate abdominal pain to incapacitating pain requiring hospitalization, IV fluids, and narcotics. Even when an attack is of sufficient intensity to require care by a physician, the diagnosis may remain obscure, and until an amylase determination is done the diagnosis of pancreatitis is in question. Ultrasound is less accurate. When the acute attack has subsided and when there has been at least one previous attack, an orderly diagnostic program should be instituted. Since most acute recurrent pancreatitis in the United States is related to alcohol consumption or the presence of gallstones, these two possible etiologic factors should be pursued first.

ETIOLOGY AND TREATMENT

Alcoholism

When attacks of pancreatitis recur, the cause must be sought and then treatment may be planned. The first step in establishing a cause is to secure an accurate and detailed history. An essential component of that history is directed at quantifying the patient's alcohol consumption. Unfortunately, the minimum amount of alcohol required to cause pancreatitis has not been identified.

In studies by Sarles,[6] 150–175 gm of pure alcohol was the average amount of alcohol consumed by patients with pancreatitis. This translates into 10 shots of 100 proof whiskey, 1.5 L of wine, or 3 L of beer. While these figures are averages for patients with pancreatitis, the disease may follow the consumption of much smaller amounts of alcohol. As little as 20 gm may precipitate an attack. From a practical consideration, modest social drinking rarely results in alcohol-induced pancreatitis. Nevertheless, total abstinence from alcohol is advisable in a patient who has had an attack of pancreatitis related to the consumption of alcohol. If no further attacks occur, it is reasonable to assume alcohol to be the inciting factor, and continued abstinence is required. It is worth restating the fact that while the initial attacks of pancreatitis may be clinically isolated events, the morphology of the pancreas is permanently altered and histologically the gland resembles one affected by chronic pancreatitis. If alcohol consumption ceases, the disease may be arrested, but the gland will remain abnormal.

It is tempting to speculate on the relationship of alcohol to pancreatic disease. Most alcoholics develop neither cirrhosis nor pancreatitis. Those who suffer pancreatitis usually do not get cirrhosis and vice versa. Sarles[7] suggested that precipitation of protein in the pancreas is an initial step in causing alcoholic pancreatitis. Others[8-10] have found antigenic similarity in patients with alcohol-induced pancreatitis. This finding strengthens the suspicion that perhaps this subgroup of people is more susceptible than the population at large to the toxic effects of alcohol.

When alcohol has been eliminated as the cause of the illness, an exhaustive search must be initiated, since there is a significant chance that another cause will be found that can be corrected and the recurrent attacks will cease without permanent damage to the pancreas.

Gallstones

While it is widely recognized that gallstones are related to pancreatitis, the mechanism remains poorly defined. Opie's[11] observation of an impacted gallstone in the ampulla of Vater in a patient with fatal pancreatitis added in some degree to confusion in the understanding of the relationship of biliary calculi to pancreatitis. It wasn't until more than five decades later that Acosta[12] examined the stool of patients recovering from pancreatitis and found gallstones. Until then, it was quite mysterious that patients operated upon in the period of convalescence after pancreatitis seldom had stones in their common bile ducts, much less impacted in the ampulla of Vater. Since the stones pass when a patient has recurrent attacks of pancreatitis, the chances are that gallstones are at fault. Opie's hypothesis that gallstones occlude a "common channel" at the ampulla of Vater allowing reflux of bile into the pancreas is probably not accurate. Bile will not flow into the pancreas under normal conditions, and it is extraordinarily rare to find bile staining of the pancreas in severe pancreatitis. When the entire flow of bile is diverted through the pancreatic duct in experimental animals, pancreatitis does not develop. Elliott[13] found that bile and pancreatic juice mixed together would flow into the pancreas at normal ductal pressures and produce severe experimental pancreatitis. McCutcheon[14] found no "common channel" in 7 of 10 patients with severe nonalcoholic pancreatitis and suggested reflux of duodenal content to be a possible factor. In experiments in our laboratories, we have been unable to cause reflux of duodenal contents into the pancreatic duct of dogs even at enormous pressure.[15] At this point, it is clear that gallstones are related to pancreatitis. It is also clear that stones in patients with acute pancreatitis pass through the duct into the duo-

denum. Beyond these facts, all else pertaining to gallstones and pancreatitis remains speculative.

The presence of gallstones in patients with acute recurrent pancreatitis is usually detected by ultrasonography during the acute attack or by oral cholecystography after the patient has recovered. Each of these procedures has a high degree of accuracy, but alone or in combination they will fail to confirm gallstones in an occasional (Fig 34–1) patient. Almost inevitably, those overlooked will be very small (Fig 34–2) multiple stones. Endoscopic retrograde cholangiopancreatography (ERCP) will detect stones that are not identified by more standard means in some patients.[16] Duodenal drainage of bile and inspection for pigment aggregates or microstones has proved useful.[17] In addition to demonstrating gallstones, ERCP has been useful in demonstrating other (Fig 34–3) causes of pancreatitis, including cancer, papillary stenosis, choledochal cysts, cystic fibrosis, and ductal obstruction from previous trauma or inflammation.[18]

When a complete and thorough search is made for a cause of pancreatitis and none is found, cholecystectomy should be performed. The patient should be informed that if stones are not found, attacks may recur. Although the capability to diagnose even tiny gallstones is very (Fig 34–4) good, it is not perfect. When patients are carefully screened, the majority who have unexplained recurrent pancreatitis will have gallstones and they will be cured by cholecystectomy.

The time to perform cholecystectomy has changed in recent years. It was formerly thought best to allow the patient to recover and go home for six weeks and then return for elec-

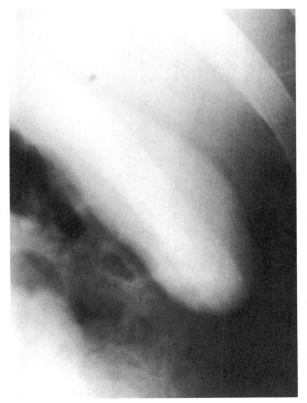

Fig 34–1.—Normal-appearing cholecytogram in patient with recurrent episodes of pancreatitis.

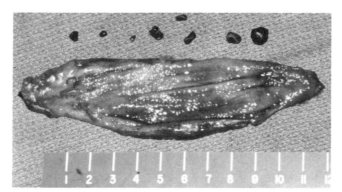

Fig 34–2.—The gallbladder and the stones found at the time of cholecystectomy of patient in Fig 34–1. No further pancreatitis has developed in this individual.

tive cholecystectomy.[19, 20] When this approach is used, many will have another attack of pancreatitis during this interval. A more aggressive approach has been suggested by some, who recommend operation in the first 48 hours accompanied by sphincteroplasty, in all or many cases for common duct stones.[20, 21] A less aggressive alternative permits resolution of the acute attack, a systematic diagnostic evaluation, and elective operation, usually within the first week of hospitalization. This approach is associated with few exacerbations. Most stones will have cleared the common duct or can be easily removed. Emergency operation is reserved for patients who are getting worse in the first 12 to 24 hours of nonsurgical treatment.

Choledochal Cyst

Most adults with choledochal cyst have cholangitis and symptoms of biliary tract disease. Most of the few reported instances of recurrent acute pancreatitis associated with choledochal cyst occur in adults. Babbitt[22] has suggested that an unusual anatomic relationship between the pancreatic duct and common bile duct could be etiologic in the development

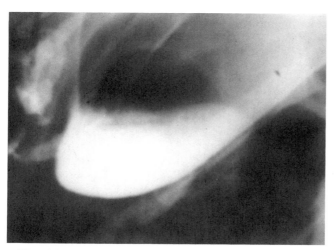

Fig 34–3.—A demonstration of the effectiveness of ERCP in demonstrating stones which may have been missed on other methods of gallbladder evaluation including oral cholecystography and ultrasonography.

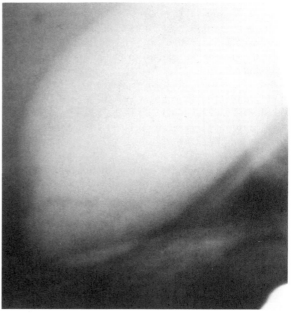

Fig 34–4.—Demonstrates a fine layer of gallstones in this oral cholecystogram. Of interest is the fact that this was the 23rd oral cholecystogram in this particular patient, all the previous ones having shown no stones in spite of recurrent episodes of pancreatitis.

of choledochal cyst. More recently, Todani and associates[23] from Japan reported an abnormal relationship with a long "common channel" and an abnormal angle between the common duct and pancreatic duct and supported the ideas of Babbitt. An earlier report by Okada[24] made similar observations. While speculations about the etiologic significance of choledochal cyst are interesting, an abnormal relationship between the cyst and the pancreatic duct appears to be common in adults with choledochal cysts.

My experience suggests two important matters. It is important to perform ERCP before operation to clearly delineate the relationship of the pancreatic and bile ducts. It is also important to resect the choledochal cyst and to remove that portion in the head of the pancreas down to the junction with the pancreatic duct. Particular care is required to avoid injury to the pancreatic duct. The diagnosis of choledochal cyst in an adult is best made with ultrasound and confirmed with ERCP. When the cyst is resected and the integrity of the pancreatic duct preserved, the recurrent pancreatitis is controlled.

Duodenal Diverticula

In general, duodenal diverticula do not cause major problems. They do, however, occasionally lead to recurrent pancreatitis. They do so when the diverticulum arises from the duodenum adjacent to the papilla of Vater. The narrow opening allows food to become inspissated, and with distention of the diverticulum, pancreatic duct compression occurs and pancreatitis ensues.

Pancreatitis may also occur when a duodenal diverticulum involves the papilla of Vater so that the common bile duct and pancreatic duct empty into the apex of the diverticulum. This condition may be synonymous with the lesion called by some choledococele. These problems are technically more difficult than periampullary diverticula or choledochal cysts. They require excision of the diverticulum and reimplantation of the papilla into the duodenum. This is best done by opening the papilla as one would do in a sphincteroplasty and implanting it into the side of the duodenum as a patch graft.

One must also be aware that duodenal diverticula are associated with an increased incidence of biliary tract disease. Gallstones have been reported in 13% to 31% of patients with a duodenal diverticulum.[25, 26] This high frequency may cause a dilemma in the treatment of a patient with a duodenal diverticulum and gallstones who is experiencing recurrent attacks of pancreatitis. In these cases, it is probably best to remove the gallbladder. When the gallstones have not been identified preoperatively, I would proceed with cholecystectomy. If gallstones are found upon opening the gallbladder or have been identified preoperatively, I would stop with cholecystectomy. If recurrent pancreatitis persists, then diverticulectomy is indicated. Operative cholangiography should be done. This is particularly important when ERCP cannot be done preoperatively. When the papilla of Vater is within the duodenal diverticulum, retrograde cannulation is extremely difficult. Operative or preoperative cholangiography is important because of the increased incidence of choledocholithiasis.[27]

As previously described, duodenal diverticula adjacent to the papilla of Vater are best managed by dissection from the head of the pancreas, inversion into the lumen of the duodenum and amputation. While tedious, this is not a particularly difficult operation for the experienced pancreatic surgeon. In these cases, I have found no need for sphincteroplasty or drainage procedure.

When the ampulla of Vater is within the diverticulum, the surgical treatment is more complex. The duodenal diverticulum is dissected from the head of the pancreas and great care must be taken to avoid injury to the pancreatic duct. The papilla of Vater is identified and this may be facilitated by passage of a small catheter from the cystic duct stump into the duodenum. The papilla is opened as in a sphincteroplasty and the opened duct anastomosed to the side of the duodenum. While I have not found it necessary, a T-tube in the duct with a long arm through the anastomosis can be used for the first 10 to 14 days. A few cases of intraluminal diverticula and pancreatitis have been reported[28] and are easily managed by simple excision of the diverticulum.

Papillary Stenosis

Few surgical conditions have caused so much controversy as papillary stenosis. Opinions vary from enthusiasm to incredulity. Even among the enthusiasts, there is no uniform agreement about symptoms, but most who accept the diagnosis of papillary stenosis agree that it may cause pancreatitis. The etiology of papillary stenosis is speculative, but trauma to the sphincter of Oddi seems the likeliest explanation. Zollinger[29] showed in 1938 that vigorous dilation of the sphincter of Oddi produced damage with possible ultimate scarring. Acosta[12] and Kelly[30] have both recovered gallstones in the stool of most patients with acute pancreatitis related to gallstones.

From these observations it is clear that gallstones pass through the bile ducts very often in people with acute pancreatitis associated with gallstones. Recognition that forcible dilation of the sphincter produces damage and clear evidence that gallstones pass through the sphincter establish a mechanism for papillary stenosis. It also seems reasonable that excessively vigorous common duct exploration may produce sphincteric damage with ultimate stenosis. Once stenosis has developed, the mechanism for recurrent pancreatitis is explained by partial pancreatic duct obstruction preventing the free flow of pancreatic juice.

The diagnosis of sphincteric stenosis may be difficult to establish. Jaundice is usually not present. The alkaline phosphatase may or may not be elevated and some degree of common duct dilation may be present. Tests that depend on increasing flow through the sphincter have lost favor. These include the Nardi test, which involves administration of morphine and prostigmine, and which has not withstood the scrutiny of prospective analysis. However, in Nardi's[31] large series of patients treated by sphincteroplasty, those with a positive test preoperatively showed better results. The same is generally true of tests involving the use of cholecystokinin. Endoscopic cholangiopancreatography has been helpful.

Geenen has found a relationship between symptoms and increased pressure in the common duct measured at endoscopy.[32] If papillary stenosis does indeed happen, it certainly is common. Sphincteroplasty of the common bile duct sphincter has been suggested as the treatment. In 1977, Moody[33] described an operation which he called septectomy that consisted of sphincteroplasty of both the common duct and pancreatic duct of Wirsung. An occasional patient who has had a common duct sphincteroplasty will continue to have pancreatitis until the pancreatic duct orifice is enlarged. Routine enlargement of the opening of both ducts seems appropriate.

Nardi[31] has been a major advocate of sphincteroplasty of both the common duct and duct of Wirsung for the treatment of recurrent pancreatitis. His results show 50% of the patients to be totally free of symptoms for 5 years. The early results were better, with 60% of patients reporting complete relief of symptoms. In my experience, sphincteroplasty of the common duct alone may lead to continued attacks of pancreatitis until the pancreatic duct orifice is opened.

The major problem in the use of sphincteroplasty in the treatment of recurrent pancreatitis is selection of patients. Most would agree that in the absence of ductal dilation, a thorough search must be made for an alternative cause of pancreatitis. Sphincteroplasty should be reserved for only those with no other known cause of pancreatitis or those with evidence of obstruction at the pancreatic duct orifice.

AFFERENT LOOP SYNDROME.—It is really surprising that afferent loop obstruction does not produce pancreatitis more often. Obstruction of the duodenum may be used to produce experimental pancreatitis.

Not only will afferent loop obstruction produce abdominal pain and hyperamylasemia but the large distended loop may be mistaken on CT scan for a pseudocyst, adding credibility to the diagnosis of acute pancreatitis. Generally, surgical decompression of the obstructed loop will solve the problem. On gross examination, the pancreas usually shows little or no evidence of acute inflammation.

Pancreas Divisum

In about 5% of people, the duct of Santorini drains most of the pancreatic parenchyma and is fused to the ventral duct of Wirsung.[34] Although this anatomic variation has been recognized for years, only because of the increasing skill of endoscopists has the condition been diagnosed more often recently (Fig 34–5). Since many people have pancreas divisum but do not have recurrent pancreatitis, other causes must be sought. Pancreas divisum should not be considered the primary cause of pancreatitis until the gallbladder has been removed, since treating gallstones with no manipulation of the ductal system may relieve recurrent attacks.

When all other causes of pancreatitis have been excluded, the patient with recurrent attacks may benefit from enlargement of the opening of the duct of Santorini. Warshaw's experience with this approach has been generally favorable.[34] In a series of 40 patients, he reported that those with stenosis fared better than those without. Stenosis was defined as a ductal orifice of 0.75 mm or less. He also found 12 of 15 with recurrent attacks of pancreatitis had good results with sphincteroplasty of the duct of Santorini, while all 5 with chronic pain were failures. There was no benefit to performing sphincteroplasty on both pancreatic ducts. Gregg et al.[35] found a high incidence of stenosis of the common duct orifice and suggested that enlargement of the duct of Santorini as well as the common bile duct should be done.

Cotton[36] reported discouraging results of sphincteroplasty of the Santorini orifice using both endoscopic and surgical means. In my initial experience in 6 cases, the early results were encouraging. Since then, an experience with 18 patients operated upon for well established recurrent pancreatitis has been disappointing. While the majority had cessation of recurrent attacks of pancreatitis, all continue to have abdominal

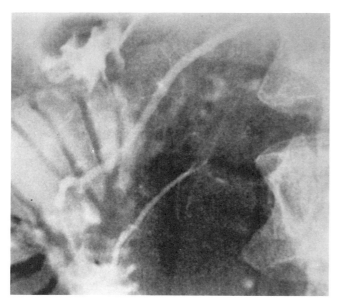

Fig 34–5.—Demonstrates pancreas divisum by use of retrograde pancreatography. The small duct at the inferior portion of the photograph drains a portion of the head and uncinate process of the gland and was the original ventral duct of the pancreas.

pain, and two have progressed to advanced chronic pancreatitis in the absence of alcohol ingestion. Best results have been obtained when another cause of pancreatitis such as gallstones or hyperparathyroidism can be identified.

A major problem has been the ability to establish pancreas divisum as the etiologic factor in recurrent pancreatitis. Warshaw has described a test involving real-time ultrasonographic assessment of the pancreatic duct with administration of secretin.[37] Ductal dilation is interpreted as evidence that the duct opening is inadequate. When correlated with surgical outcome, the test was useful in predicting success. At this point, I am very skeptical of the role of operative management of pancreas divisum and suspect that, in most cases, it is an anatomic variant of little clinical significance. The less common anomaly of annular pancreas is rarely associated with acute pancreatitis.[38]

Hyperparathyroidism

While not a frequent problem, hyperparathyroidism is related to and apparently etiologic in certain cases of recurrent acute pancreatitis. There have been reports of recurrent pancreatitis in normocalcemic patients with parathyroid adenoma.[39]

A note of caution is appropriate with respect to the time of evaluation of hyperparathyroidism. Since hypocalcemia may be associated with acute pancreatitis, it is important to evaluate calcium homeostasis after the acute phase of pancreatitis has abated. It is possible that hypercalcemia can be obscured during the acute attack. Hyperparathyroidism may cause recurrent acute pancreatitis, but it is uncertain whether in fact it is the hypercalcemia or the hyperparathyroidism which is at fault.

The relationship between pancreatitis and hyperparathyroidism has been recognized clinically for at least 40 years.[40] The mechanism is unclear but does not seem to be related to the magnitude of hypercalcemia. While hyperparathyroidism with little or no hypercalcemia is related to pancreatitis in some cases, hypercalcemia without hyperparathyroidism is also suspect.[41] We recently treated a patient whose normal serum calcium and phosphorus were documented but ionized serum calcium was elevated as was parathormone. Ultrasound examination showed a lesion suggesting a parathyroid adenoma and the tumor was excised. It is too early to know whether the recurrent pancreatitis will be relieved. Clearly, a patient with recurrent acute pancreatitis needs to be studied vigorously with regard to calcium homeostasis.

Hyperlipidemia

There is no question that hyperlipidemia is associated with acute recurrent pancreatitis.[42] Beyond that, almost nothing else about the relationship is certain. Types I, IV, and V are the hyperlipid states most often associated with pancreatic inflammation, with Type V the most common. Several unresolved issues cloud the understanding of the relationship. Many patients with hyperlipidemia and pancreatitis have other known causes of pancreatitis such as gallstones and alcoholism.

Many patients observed to have lipemic serum and acute pancreatitis do not have lipemic serum once the attack has subsided. The issue is further clouded by the fact that acute abdominal pain without pancreatitis occurs in hyperlipidemic states.[43] In addition, hyperlipidemia interferes with amylase determination, making the diagnosis of pancreatitis less certain.[44] In the face of all of these difficulties, it is still clear that certain of the hyperlipidemic states are related to pancreatitis. Cameron,[45] studying isolated perfused pancreas, found that an increase in the neutral fat content of the perfusate produced edema of the perfused gland with an increase in free fatty acid in the venous effluent. This ingenious experiment suggests that conversion of neutral fat to free fatty acid is the mechanism for pancreatitis in hyperlipidemia.

Zieve[46] suggested that hyperlipidemia and pancreatitis occurred only when there was fat infiltration of the liver. That does not appear to be the case. While the lactescent serum may clear spontaneously as the pancreatitis improves, experimental pancreatitis may induce lipemia. There is evidence that lowering the triglyceride level may reduce the frequency of attacks of pancreatitis.[47, 48] This is most often done by reducing fat in the diet, avoiding drugs and alcohol which may increase triglycerides, and occasionally in severe refractory cases by partial small bowel bypass to diminish fat absorption. Pancreatitis may be induced by intravenous fat infusion, and care should be used in administering intravenous fat, especially in alcoholics.[49]

Drug-Induced Pancreatitis

The issue of recurrent acute pancreatitis as a sequel to the ingestion of certain drugs is nearly as confusing as the relationship of pancreatitis to hyperlipidemia. Most studies of drug-induced pancreatitis exclude alcohol, since the relationship of alcohol to pancreatic inflammation is widely accepted even if poorly understood.

Recently two different authors have reviewed the problem in detail.[50, 51] Both have presented evidence that the relationship of certain drugs to pancreatitis seems clear enough to be accepted, while the relationship of other drugs is not clear. Unfortunately, the two authors do not agree. Thomas[50] suggests that in order for the relationship to be clearly accepted, the following criteria should be met. Pancreatitis should develop in patients taking the drug who do not have a history of or other obvious causes of pancreatitis. The pancreatitis should subside when the drug is stopped. If the drug is resumed, pancreatitis should recur. Obviously, the last step is not to be recommended. One of the problems that prevents the clear establishment of a relationship between drugs and pancreatitis is the fact that many of the suspected drugs are very commonly used. Furthermore, in certain of the diseases for which the drugs are used, pancreatitis may be suspected to be a part of the clinical presentation. Table 34–1 lists drugs that seem to be related to pancreatitis and Table 34–2 lists drugs suspected but not shown to be clearly related to pancreatitis.

While many drugs seem related to pancreatitis, very few mechanisms have been suggested. When a patient being treated with drugs develops pancreatitis, the drugs should be stopped if possible and a search made for an alternative cause of the pancreatitis, such as gallstones. If no cause is found, the medications least likely to be related to pancreatitis should be reintroduced one at a time. A drug of high probability as a causative factor should be exchanged for another

TABLE 34–1.—DRUGS WITH PROBABLE OR CERTAIN RELATIONSHIP TO PANCREATITIS

Azathioprine	Procainamide
Calcium	Mercaptopurine
Estrogen	Sulfonamides
Furosemide	Tetracycline
Methyldopa	Thiazides
Pentamidine	Vitamin D

drug if possible or introduced very cautiously. In addition to single drugs, there is some evidence that a combination of drugs may produce pancreatitis. Altman[52] reported an apparent relationship between pancreatitis and cytosine arabinoside and L-asparaginase. This appears to be one of the few chemotherapeutic agents or combination of agents that may produce pancreatitis. Certain medications such as estrogen also seem to trigger the pancreatitis in some patients.[53] Industrial toxins have also been incriminated. Both pentachlorophenol (PCP)[54] and anticholinesterase insecticides[55] have been shown to cause pancreatitis.[62, 63]

Cancer

Reviewing a large series of patients with pancreatic cancer, Gambill[56] found pancreatitis grossly or histologically in about 10%, but in only 3% was there clinical evidence of pancreatitis. Conversely, when cases of acute pancreatitis are reviewed, cancer is found in only 1 or 2%.[57] While it is uncommon, the possible relationship between acute recurrent pancreatitis and cancer should not be overlooked. In operations for cancer, rather severe induration in the distal pancreas is often noted, and the finding seems to be related to complete occlusion or high-grade stenosis of the main pancreatic duct. These patients are usually jaundiced and have a clinical history that suggests pancreatic cancer. ERCP shows the expected finding of compromise of the pancreatic duct in the head of the gland. In one case reported by Van Waes et al.[57] and in one unreported from my own experience, the cancer was in the body of the gland with no endoscopic evidence of ductal obstruction.

Cancer of the pancreas associated with clinical recurrent pancreatitis is very uncommon. It may occur in the absence of ductal obstruction and with normal ERCP. If ERCP and CT scan show no abnormality, the diagnosis will probably be made at laparotomy.

Trauma

While direct trauma to the pancreas may cause acute pancreatitis, its onset may be delayed sometimes for several years. We have encountered three patients who have had recurrent bouts of pancreatitis several months or years after an episode of blunt upper abdominal trauma. All other causes of pancreatitis were excluded. In each patient, ERCP showed a normal segment of pancreatic duct that ended (Fig 34–6) abruptly, usually at the vertebral column. At operation, the gland beyond the site of obstruction was atrophic and fibrotic (Fig 34–7). This distal segment may be managed by resection or internal drainage using a Roux-en-Y conduit. Resection is done unless surrounding inflammation is present. More lib-

TABLE 34–2.—DRUGS WITH POSSIBLE
RELATIONSHIP TO PANCREATITIS

Acetaminophen	Histamine
Amphetamines	Indomethacin
Anticoagulants	Isoniazid
Asparaginase	Meprobamate
Chlorthalidone	Methanol
Cholestyramine	Opiates
Cimetidine	Propoxyphene
Corticosteroids	Propylthiouracil
Cyproheptadome	Rifampin
Diazoxide	Salicylates
Ethacrynic acid	

eral use of intraoperative pancreatography as advocated by Berni et al. might avoid these early problems.[58]

Systemic Illnesses

A clear relationship between certain systemic illnesses and recurrent pancreatitis has been difficult to establish. In many instances, treatment of the primary disease may involve drugs that have been incriminated as a cause of pancreatitis. The treatment of systemic lupus erythematosus (SLE) with corticosteroids is an excellent example of this situation. As data have accumulated, however, it seems quite likely that patients with SLE have an increased incidence of recurrent pancreatitis unrelated to steroid medication. Reynolds et al.[59] in an excellent review of 20 patients with SLE and acute pancreatitis reported that all were in an active state of SLE with multiple organ involvement. Vasculitis with ischemic necrosis and autoimmune reactions have been suspected to incite pancreatitis in patients with SLE. Of practical importance is the institution, continuation, or increase in steroid dose to treat the SLE, since the pancreatitis does not seem to be related to the administration of steroids.

Because of improved management, cystic fibrosis is now

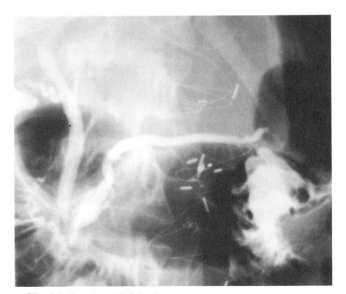

Fig 34–6.—An ERCP of a patient with a previous history of trauma and recurrent episodes of pancreatitis and abdominal pain. Note the cut-off at the end of the pancreatic duct.

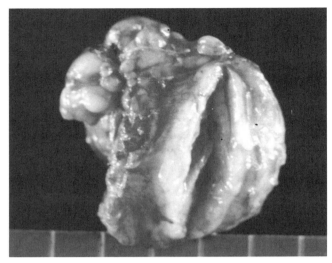

Fig 34–7.—The distal pancreas from the patient whose pancreaticogram is seen in Fig 34–6. Note the fibrosis and ductal dilatation of this segment of gland which had been separated from the main ductal system. We have called this condition "pancreatic sequestrum."

encountered more often in adults. Occasionally, acute pancreatitis may be the initial symptom in an adult with unrecognized cystic fibrosis.[60] Most adults with cystic fibrosis have some degree of pulmonary dysfunction, but it may be quite mild. Measurement of sweat chloride is the key to the diagnosis. Levels above 70 mg/L of sweat chloride are characteristic of cystic fibrosis.

A host of isolated reports of systemic illness including hepatitis, uremia, transplantation, cardiopulmonary bypass, and many others describe recurrent pancreatitis as a complication.

Heredity

Hereditary pancreatitis is rare. It is transmitted as a non-sex-linked autosomal dominant trait. Only about 250 patients and 25 families have been reported.[62, 63] Some authors have described an abnormal sphincter of Oddi and good response to sphincteroplasty. The majority of surgical procedures have been performed to relieve a greatly dilated duct, to resect a destroyed gland, or to treat complications such as pseudocyst. The diagnosis is made by exclusion plus a history of familial incidence. In one instance a 16-year-old boy was thought to have familial pancreatitis since his mother also had pancreatitis. Careful evaluation proved the boy to be an alcoholic and his mother to have had pancreatitis associated with gallstones. Familial pancreatitis certainly exists. It is so rare that a careful search for other causes should always be conducted.

Summary

It would be very satisfying to establish a unified concept of the pathophysiology of recurrent acute pancreatitis. At this moment, this remains an unattained goal. Although many factors are related, none is a clear cause. Alcoholism may prove to make the pancreas susceptible to a toxin owing to an inborn error of metabolism. Gallstones, pancreas divisum, papillary stenosis, cancer, and afferent loop syndrome may all have a combination obstruction-stimulation mechanism. The common channel theory remains as elusive as it was after Opie's original report.

Metabolic and endocrinologic disorders such as hyperlipidemia and hyperparathyroidism, drugs, systemic lupus erythematosus, and the hereditary form of the disease may prove to have a common pathway at the cellular level. Perhaps superoxides, mesotrypsins, prostaglandins, vasoactive peptides, and other cellular and subcellular compounds will eventually be disclosed.

For now, we are steadily reducing the percentage of patients with idiopathic recurrent pancreatitis and steadily improving our ability to find a cause or at least a relationship. We are also more able to prevent, stop, or reduce the frequency of the attacks.

Recurrent acute pancreatitis is a puzzling and often frustrating illness. A firm knowledge of the possible causes is necessary if help is to be given to those afflicted. By securing a careful history and following an appropriate diagnostic plan, a cause will be identified in most cases.

REFERENCES

1. Satiani B., Stone H.: Predictability of present outcome and future recurrence in acute pancreatitis. *Arch. Surg.* 114:711–716, 1979.
2. Trapnell J.E.: The natural history and prognosis of acute pancreatitis. *Ann. Roy. Coll. Surg. Engl.* 38:265–287, 1966.
3. Olsen H.: Pancreatitis: A prospective clinical evaluation of 100 cases and review of the literature. *Am. J. Dig. Dis.* 19:1077–1090, 1974.
4. Reid B.G., Kune G.A.: Natural history of acute pancreatitis: a long-term study. *Med. J. Aust.* 2:555–558, 1980.
5. Spechler S.J., Dalton J.W., Robbins A.H., et al.: Prevalence of normal serum amylase levels in patients with acute alcoholic pancreatitis. *Dig. Dis. Sci.* 28:865–869, 1983.
6. Sarles H., Figarella C., Clemente F.: The interaction of ethanol, dietary lipids, and proteins on the rat pancreas. *Digestion* 4:13–22, 1971.
7. Sarles H., Lebreuil G., Tasso F., et al.: A comparison of alcoholic pancreatitis in rat and man. *Gut* 12:377–388, 1971.
8. Dani R., Antunes L.J., Ribeiro J.E.F., et al.: Immunological participation in chronic calcifying pancreatitis. *Digestion* 11:333–337, 1974.
9. Gullo L., Tabacchi P.L., Corazza G.R., et al.: HLA-B13 and chronic calcific pancreatitis. *Dig. Dis. Sci.* 27:214–216, 1982.
10. Gosselin M., Fauchet R., Genetet B., et al.: Les antigenes HLA dans la pancreatite chronique alcoolique. *Gastroenterol. Clin. Biol.* 2:883–886, 1978.
11. Opie E.L.: The etiology of acute hemorrhagic pancreatitis: Pathological report and experimental study. *Bull. Johns Hopkins Hosp.* 12:182, 1901.
12. Acosta J.M., Ledesma C.L.: Gallstone migration as a cause of acute pancreatitis. *N. Engl. J. Med.* 290:484–487, 1974.
13. Elliott D.W., Williams R.D., Zollinger R.M.: Alterations in pancreatic resistance to bile in the pathogenesis of acute pancreatitis. *Ann. Surg.* 146:669–682, 1957.
14. McCutcheon A.D., Melb M.D.: Aetiological factors in pancreatitis. *Lancet* 2:710–712, 1962.
15. Myers J.C., Garzia F.M., Martin D.T., et al.: Pancreatic reflux of duodenal contents in experimental animals. (Unpublished).
16. Hamilton I., Bradley P., Lintott D.J., et al.: Endoscopic retrograde cholangiopancreatography in the investigation and management of patients after acute pancreatitis. *Br. J. Surg.* 69:504–506, 1982.
17. Goldstein F., Kucer F.T., Thornton J.J., et al.: Acute and relapsing pancreatitis caused by bile pigment aggregates and diagnosed by biliary drainage. *Am. J. Gastroenterol.* 74:225–230, 1980.
18. Blustein P.K., Gaskin K., Filler R., et al.: Endoscopic retrograde

cholangiopancreatography in pancreatitis in children and adolescents. *Pediatrics* 68:387–393, 1981.
19. Elfstrom J.: The timing of cholecystectomy in patients with gallstone pancreatitis. *Acta Chir. Scand.* 144:487–490, 1978.
20. Acosta J.M., Rossi R., Galli O.M.R., et al.: Early surgery for acute gallstone pancreatitis: Evaluation of a systematic approach. *Surgery* 83:367–370, 1978.
21. Stone H.H., Fabian T.C., Dunlop W.E.: Gallstone pancreatitis. *Ann. Surg.* 194:305–312, 1981.
22. Babbitt D.P.: Choledochal cyst: New etiological concept based on anomalous relationships of common bile duct and pancreatic bulb. *Ann. Radiol.* 12:231–240, 1969.
23. Todani T., Watanabe Y., Fujii T., et al.: Anomalous arrangement of the pancreatobiliary ductal system in patients with choledochal cyst. *Am. J. Surg.* 147:672–676, 1984.
24. Okada A., Oguchi Y., Kamata S., et al.: Common channel syndrome: Diagnosis with endoscopic retrograde cholangiopancreatography and surgical management. *Surgery* 93:634–642, 1983.
25. Chitambar A.: Duodenal diverticula. *Recent Adv. Surg.* 33:768, 1953.
26. Landor J.H., Fulkerson C.C.: Duodenal diverticula: Relationship to biliary tract disease. *Arch. Surg.* 93:192, 1966.
27. Leinkram C., Roberts-Thomson I.C., Kune G.A.: Juxtapapillary duodenal diverticula: Association with gallstones and pancreatitis. *Med. J. Aust.* 2:209–210, 1980.
28. Griffen M., Carey W.D., Hermann R., et al.: Recurrent acute pancreatitis and intussusception complicating an intraluminal duodenal diverticulum. *Gastroenterology* 81:345–348, 1981.
29. Zollinger R.M., Branch C.D., Bailey O.T.: Instrumental dilatation of the papilla of Vater. Experimental and clinical observations. *Surg. Gynecol. Obstet.* 66:100–104, 1938.
30. Kelly T.R.: Gallstone pancreatitis. *Arch. Surg.* 109:294–297, 1974.
31. Nardi G.L., Michelassi F., Zannini P.: Transduodenal sphincteroplasty: 5–25 year follow-up of 89 patients. *Ann. Surg.* 198:453–461, 1983.
32. Geenen J.E.: Sphincter of Oddi diagnosis and treatment. *Am. Soc. Gastrointest. Endoscopy*, New Orleans, La., May 1984.
33. Moody F.G., Berenson M.M., McCloskey D.: Transampullary septectomy for post-cholecystectomy pain. *Ann. Surg.* 186:415–419, 1977.
34. Warshaw A.L., Richter J.M., Schapiro R.H.: The cause and treatment of pancreatitis associated with pancreas divisum. *Ann. Surg.* 198:443–452, 1983.
35. Gregg J., Somomon J., Clark G.: Pancreas divisum and its association with choledochal sphincter stenosis. *Am. J. Surg.* 147:367–371, 1984.
36. Cotton P.B.: Congenital anomaly of pancreas divisum as cause of obstructive pain and pancreatitis. *Gut* 21:105–114, 1980.
37. Warshaw A.L., Simeone J., Schapiro R.H., et al.: Objective evaluation of ampullary stenosis with ultrasound and pancreatic stimulation. *Am. J. Surg.* (In press).
38. Chevillotte G., Sahel J., Raillat A., et al.: Annular pancreas: Report of one case associated with acute pancreatitis and diagnosed by endoscopic retrograde pancreatography. *Dig. Dis. Sci.* 29:75–77, 1984.
39. Ballon S., Cohen N., Strasberg Z.: Recurrent pancreatitis due to parathyroid adenoma in a normocalcemic patient. *Can. Med. Assoc. J.* 106:51–54, 1972.
40. Smith F.B., Cooke R.T.: Acute fatal hyperparathyroidism. *Lancet* 2:650–651, 1940.
41. Madison R.R.: Acute pancreatitis secondary to iatrogenic hypercalcemia: Implications of hyperalimentation. *Arch. Surg.* 108:213–215, 1974.
42. Greenberger N.J., Hatch F.T., Drummey G.D., et al.: Pancreatitis and hyperlipidemia: A study of serum lipid alterations in 25 patients with acute pancreatitis. *Medicine* 45:161–174, 1966.
43. Miller A., Lees R.S., McCluskey M.A., et al.: The natural history and surgical significance of hyperlipemic abdominal crisis. *Ann. Surg.* 190:401–408, 1979.
44. Lesser P.B., Warshaw A.L.: The diagnosis of pancreatitis masked by hyperlipemia. *Ann. Intern. Med.* 82:795–798, 1975.
45. Saharia P., Margolis S., Zuidema G.D., et al.: Acute pancreatitis

hyperlipidemia: Studies with an isolated perfused canine pancreas. *Surgery* 82:60–67, 1977.

46. Zieve L.: Relationship between acute pancreatitis and hyperlipemia. *Med. Clin. North. Am.* 52:1493–1500, 1968.

47. Hollister L.E., Kanter S.L.: Essential hyperlipemia treated with heparin and chlorpromazine. *Gastroenterology* 29:1069, 1955.

48. Klatskin G., Gordon M.: Relationship between relapsing pancreatitis and essential hyperlipemia. *Am. J. Med.* 12:3, 1952.

49. Buckspan R., Woltering E., Waterhouse G.: Pancreatitis induced by intravenous infusion of a fat emulsion in an alcoholic patient. *South. Med. J.* 77:251–252, 1984.

50. Thomas F.B.: Drug-induced pancreatitis: Fact versus fiction. *Drug. Ther. Hosp.* March:60–71, 1982.

51. Mallory A., Kern F.: Drug-induced pancreatitis: A critical review. *Gastroenterology* 78:813–820, 1980.

52. Altman A.J., Dinndorf P., Quinn J.J.: Acute pancreatitis in association with cytosine arabinoside therapy. *Cancer* 49:1384–1386, 1982.

53. Glueck C.J., Scheel D., Fishback J., et al.: Estrogen-induced pancreatitis in patients with previously covert familial Type V hyperlipoproteinemia. *Metabolism* 21:657–666, 1972.

54. Cooper R.G., Macaulay M.B.: Pentachlorophenol pancreatitis. *Lancet* 1:517, 1982.

55. Dressel T.D., Goodale R.L. Jr., Arneson M.A., et al.: Pancreatitis as a complication of anticholinesterase insecticide intoxication. *Ann. Surg.* 189:199–204, 1979.

56. Gambill E.E.: Pancreatitis associated with pancreatic carcinoma in a study of 26 cases. *Mayo Clin. Proc.* 46:174, 1971.

57. Van Waes L., Van Maele V., Demeulenaere L., et al.: Carcinoma of the pancreas presenting as relapsing pancreatitis. *Am. J. Gastroenterol.* 68:88–90, 1977.

58. Berni G.A., Bandyk D.F., Oreskovich M.R., et al.: Role of intraoperative pancreatography in patients with injury to the pancreas. *Am. J. Surg.* 143:602–605, 1982.

59. Reynolds J.C., Inman R.D., Kimberly R.P., et al.: Acute pancreatitis in systemic lupus erythematosus: Report of twenty cases and a review of the literature. *Medicine* 61:25–32, 1982.

60. Masaryk T.J., Achkar E.: Pancreatitis as initial presentation of cystic fibrosis in young adults: A report of two cases. *Dig. Dis. Sci.* 28:874–878, 1983.

61. Robechek P.J.: Hereditary chronic relapsing pancreatitis: A clue to pancreatitis in general. *Am. J. Surg.* 113:819–824, 1967.

62. Williams R.A., Caldwell B.F., Wilson S.E.: Idiopathic hereditary pancreatitis. *Arch. Surg.* 117:408–412, 1982.

35

Pancreatic Cancer

A. R. MOOSSA, M.D., F.R.C.S., F.A.C.S.
RICHARD DAVIES, M.D.

THIS CHAPTER deals primarily with adenocarcinoma of the exocrine pancreas. Rarer pancreatic malignancies such as cystadenomas, cystadenocarcinomas, apudomas, lymphomas, sarcomas, etc., will be covered in other chapters. There are two main reasons why pancreatic cancer is assuming increasing surgical importance. The first is that the incidence of this once rare disease is increasing and has tripled over the past 40 years. About 25,000 new cases of pancreatic cancer are currently seen each year in the United States.[1, 2] Most Western countries report a similar alarming rise. The second reason is that the disease remains highly lethal, with an estimated cure rate of only 2%–5%. Despite representing only 2%–3% of all cancers, this is the fourth commonest cause of cancer death in the United States. Males are affected about twice as commonly as females, with a peak incidence in both sexes of about 60 years. There is also an increased incidence among blacks compared to whites.

Surgeons must strive to develop a balanced attitude between therapeutic nihilism and unbridled enthusiasm while evaluating improved and multidisciplinary treatment options in dealing with this dismal disease. As more is learned about etiology, prevention, and earlier diagnosis, the future holds some hope; meanwhile surgeons will be called on to make decisions based on recent developments. While general guidelines are helpful and acceptable, the management of every patient must be individualized.

ETIOLOGY

The causal factors responsible for the development of pancreatic carcinoma have not been identified. Industrial pollutants have been cited as carcinogens that may be responsible in chemical, coke and metal, and glass plant workers. Alcohol ingestion is not thought to be a risk factor, but cigarette smoking is.[3, 4] The data concerning coffee drinking are at best speculative.[5] Diabetes appears to be an increased risk factor in women, who show a sixfold increase in pancreatic cancer, although diabetic men are not at increased risk.[1-4] A causal relationship between carcinoma of the exocrine pancreas and the disturbance in function of the endocrine pancreas cannot be clearly identified for two main reasons: (1) there is uncertainty regarding the exact duration of the in situ phase of human pancreatic cancer or of the hyperglycemia; and (2) at least some of the patients with hyperglycemia have a true hereditary diabetes mellitus or a hyperglycemia of the aged. It has been postulated that there may be two types of diabetes mellitus in pancreatic cancer patients: one in a group of individuals in whom a long-standing hereditary type of diabetes is present, with its possible increase risk of pancreatic cancer; the other is in a set of patients in whom the hyperglycemia is of shorter duration and is a direct result of the pancreatic cancer. The suggestive bimodality of duration of clinical diabetes mellitus (40% of patients with a duration greater than two years, and 50% with less than one year) is supportive of this hypothesis.[6]

The association of pancreatitis with pancreatic cancer is a rather confusing one because the word pancreatitis is often loosely used to connote different clinical or pathologic (macroscopic and microscopic) entities. The relationship can be summarized as follows:

1. Patients with the *very rare* type of hereditary pancreatitis have a *definite* increased incidence of pancreatic cancer.

2. There is *no* evidence that the acquired types of acute or chronic pancreatitis (of whatever etiology) are a risk factor in the development of pancreatic cancer.

3. An attack of acute pancreatitis may be the first clinical manifestation of a pancreatic cancer.

4. Every pancreatic tumor compresses and destroys normal acinar tissue and causes varying degrees of edema and ductal obstruction. Thus, an inflammatory reaction is always present and, on histologic examination, is labeled as "associated pancreatitis" in over 90% of cases.

SURGICAL PATHOLOGY

Since the pancreas is principally a glandular organ, most cancers are adenocarcinomas. Any physician treating pancreatic cancer has to be cognizant with all aspects of pathology to plan rational treatment. A review of over 500 patients from Memorial Hospital in New York has shown that only 14% of patients had disease limited to the pancreas, 21% had spread to the regional nodes, and 65% had advanced local disease with or without distant metastases.[7, 8] All series have shown a predilection for the head of the pancreas for carcinoma, 65%–75% located there; the remainder are found in the body and tail of the gland. The distal (body and tail) lesions present late

TABLE 35–1.—NONENDOCRINE CARCINOMA OF
THE PANCREAS (N = 508)

HISTOLOGIC TYPE	% OF PATIENTS
Ductal origin	
Duct cell adenocarcinoma	75
Giant cell carcinoma	4
Giant cell carcinoma (epulis with osteoid)	0.2
Adeno squamous carcinoma	4
Microadenocarcinoma	3
Mucinous ("colloid") carcinoma	2
Cystadenocarcinoma (mucinous)	1
Acinar cell origin	
Acinar cell adenocarcinoma	1
Undetermined cell type	
Pancreaticoblastoma	0.2
Papillary cystic tumor	0.2
Mixed cell type	
Acinar, duct, and islet cell carcinoma	0.2
Unclassified cell type	
Large cell	8
Small cell	1
Clear cell	0.2
Total	100

and therefore have a mean size of 10 cm compared with 5 cm for lesions in the head of the pancreas.

Table 35–1 summarizes the histologic types of pancreatic cancer. Ductal adenocarcinomas are of two types. Those arising from large end ducts contain mucin as opposed to those arising from the smaller ducts. It must also be noted that the vast majority of pancreatic adenocarcinomas are associated with a desmoplastic reaction, pancreatitis, and fibrosis. The surrounding pancreatitis and fibrosis make biopsy fraught with the possibility of sampling errors and must be borne in mind by the surgeon treating the disease.

Acinar cell pancreatic cancer is of interest despite its rarity, since these patients may present with constitutional symptoms of arthralgias and may develop inflammation of their subcutaneous fat with a severe panniculitis. An elevated serum lipase and an eosinophilia often accompany this syndrome.

It must also be emphasized that a mucinous cystadenocarcinoma may in fact masquerade as a pancreatic pseudocyst and despite its usually distal pancreatic location, long-term survivals of 30%–60% have been reported.[9] Newer imaging techniques have helped to identify these "cysts."

The issue of multicentricity is important although, as in other cancers, its clinical relevance is hard to define, since long-term survival with metachronous tumor development is unusual. It is generally estimated that about 25% of all pancreatic resection specimens with a pancreatic cancer will have evidence of multifocal disease.[7–9]

SURGICAL ANATOMY OF THE PANCREAS

The retroperitoneal location of the pancreas and its close proximity to vital vascular structures are the factors that limit its resectability and are also mainly responsible for the late presentation of pancreatic carcinoma. Were it not for clinical jaundice, most patients would fail to present until the onset of pain due to perineural involvement or of vomiting due to duodenal obstruction; both situations are usually indicative of incurability. A thorough knowledge of the anatomical relations of the pancreas is paramount in both the successful surgical treatment of pancreatic carcinoma as well as in planning effective ports for radiotherapy. Figure 35–1 summarizes the anatomical relationships. To describe it as the "seat of the soul" is not an exaggeration when one considers the proximity of the stomach, duodenum, liver, gallbladder, common bile duct, colon, transverse mesocolon, aorta, vena cava, superior and inferior mesenteric vessels, portal and splenic vessels, spleen, kidneys and adrenal glands. It is clear that the pancreas is situated at a complex anatomical crossroad where its central position provides lymphatic drainage radially along several major routes (splenic, hepatic, and superior mesenteric vessels). This makes it hard to design an adequate cancer operation that, in an orderly manner, removes the primary

Fig 35–1.—Oblique cross section of upper abdomen viewed from below. Section passes through the long axis of the pancreas at approximately the level indicated in the inset figure. The disposition and relations of structures shown approximate those seen on oblique/transverse ultrasonic scanning. (From Moossa A.R.: *Tumors of the Pancreas,* ed. 1. Baltimore, Williams and Wilkins, 1980. Reproduced by permission.)

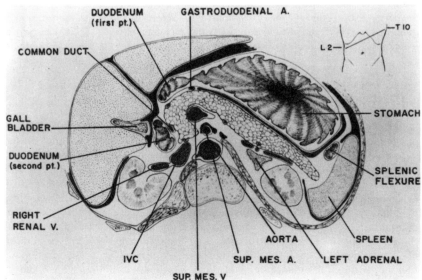

tumor en bloc with primary, secondary, and tertiary lymphatic nodal basins. Moreover, the intimate association of the pancreas with the major vessels of the epigastrium at once limits the extent of the procedure and dictates what must be removed. Thus, when a tumor spreads a short distance to involve the portal vein or superior mesenteric vessels, it usually becomes incurable. Similarly, if the gland is excised in radical fashion, the need to excise many of the vessels and lymph nodes that go with it makes removal of the duodenum, common bile duct, gallbladder, upper jejunum, a large segment of the stomach and the spleen necessary.

Vascular encroachment by tumor of the celiac axis, its major branches, the portal vein or the superior mesenteric vessels generally renders the pancreatic lesion unresectable for cure. Although resection of the pancreas with the involved major vessels has been described[10] convincing evidence that such extensive procedures result in long-term survival is not yet forthcoming.

The head of the pancreas and its uncinate process wrap themselves around the portal and superior mesenteric veins. The superior pancreaticoduodenal vein drains into the portal vein and the inferior pancreaticoduodenal vein into the superior mesenteric vein. Several unnamed short, smaller branches from the head of the pancreas and uncinate process also drain directly into the portal and superior mesenteric veins. There is a relatively avascular plane between the anterior surface of the portal and superior mesenteric veins immediately posterior to the neck of the pancreas without significant tributaries draining into the immediate anterior surface of these two large veins. This relative avascular portion enables the neck of the pancreas to be elevated and transected with minimal risk in a Whipple operation. It should be emphasized that, occasionally, the unexpected proximity of branches somewhat more anterior than usual may result in serious bleeding.

The distal common bile duct traverses the head of the pancreas; hence, the relatively early presentation of pancreatic carcinoma in those patients who become jaundiced because of an obstructing lesion involving the bile duct adjacent to its confluence with the pancreatic duct to form the ampulla of Vater. Lesions arising from pancreatic ductal epithelium more distally will reach a considerable size before involving the lower common bile duct. Obviously, lesions arising at the ampulla present earliest with jaundice and have correspondingly higher surgical resection and cure rates after surgical excision.

It is important to realize that the accessory pancreatic duct (Santorini's duct) may give rise to pancreatic cancer and if the duct opens into the duodenum through an accessory ampulla the main pancreatic duct (Wirsung's duct) will appear normal on ERCP and jaundice may be a relatively late presentation despite the tumor's origin from the uncinate process.

Because the duodenum and pancreas have a common blood supply most operations have been based on the resection of both organs. Lesser operations have been described for benign conditions of the pancreas. However, preservation of part of the duodenum as part of a pancreatic cancer operation will invariably result in local recurrence as it fails to achieve an adequate margin of resection.

Figure 35–2 summarizes the lymphatic pathways and nodal

LYMPHATIC DRAINAGE OF THE PANCREAS

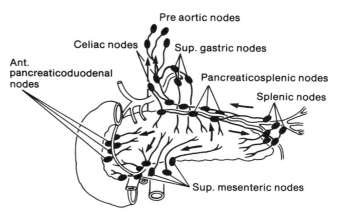

Fig 35–2.—Lymphatic drainage of the pancreas.

groups that drain the pancreas. This complicated network of drainage is one of the principal reasons for early dissemination of pancreatic cancer. An appreciation of lymphatics is important both for surgical extirpation and in planning radiation ports if the results of treatment are to be improved.

PATTERNS OF DISSEMINATION IN PANCREATIC CANCER

Although the natural history of pancreatic cancer may be capricious certain patterns emerge when large series are analyzed. The proximity and thinness of the posterior parietal peritoneum facilitate early peritoneal seeding once this structure is breached. In addition, a rich lymphatic network with multiple pathways for dissemination and the large numbers of venous tributaries draining the pancreas are largely responsible for the variety of patterns that may emerge in the dissemination of pancreatic cancer.[7–9]

Table 35–2 adapted from the autopsy study of Cubilla and Fitzgerald[7, 8] demonstrates that adjacent organs are invaded depending on their regional relationship to the primary cancer.

Table 35–3 demonstrates the variety of organs to which

TABLE 35–2.—DIRECT INVASION BY PANCREATIC CANCER IN 75 PATIENTS AT AUTOPSY (%)

ANATOMICAL SITE	PRIMARY SITE OF PANCREATIC CANCER		
	Head (36)	Body (25)	Tail (14)
Duodenum	67	24	0
Stomach	25	40	7
Spleen	0	12	36
Left adrenal gland	0	4	29
Transverse colon	3	12	14
Left kidney	0	4	7
Jejunum	3	4	7
Right ureter	3	0	0
Total, %	48	33	19

TABLE 35–3.—METASTATIC SITES IN PANCREATIC CANCER (%)

SITE	HEAD (N = 5,233)	BODY AND TAIL (N = 1,912)
Regional lymph nodes	75	76
Liver	65	71
Lungs	30	14
Peritoneum	22	38
Duodenum	19	5
Adrenal glands	13	24
Stomach	11	5
Gallbladder	9	0
Spleen	6	14
Kidney	6	5
Intestines	4	5
Mediastinal nodes	4	5
Other sites	19	28
No metastases	13	0

metastatic carcinoma of the pancreas disseminates, and, again, this tends to explain the poor results of local therapy for pancreatic cancer.

STAGING OF PANCREATIC CANCER

To make meaningful comparisons between the results of different treatment options for pancreatic cancer accurate staging is essential and has not received the rigorous attention that staging for other cancers has. This is due to the late stage of many pancreatic cancers at presentation and the dismal survival figures regardless of past therapy. With the recent small but definite improvement in survival figures and the use of multidisciplinary therapy, it is essential that all pancreatic cancers be accurately staged.

TABLE 35–4.—DEFINITIONS OF TNM CATEGORIES FOR CANCER OF THE PANCREAS, SURGICAL-EVALUATIVE ASSESSMENT

T: Primary tumor
- T1: No direct extension of the primary tumor beyond the pancreas
- T2: Limited direct extension (to duodenum, bile ducts, or stomach), still possibly permitting tumor resection
- T3: Further direct extension, incompatible with surgical resection
- Tx: Direct extension not assessed or not recorded

N: Regional lymph node involvement
- N0: Regional nodes not involved
- N1: Regional nodes involved
- Nx: Regional node involvement not assessed or not recorded

M: Distant metastasis
- M0: No distant metastasis
- M1: Distant metastatic involvement
- Mx: Distant metastatic involvement not assessed or not recorded

STAGE	TNM CATEGORY
I	T1 N0 M0
	T1 Nx M0
	T2 N0 M0
	T2 Nx M0
	Tx N0 M0
	Tx Nx M0
	T1,2, x N0, x M0
II	T3 N0 M0
	T3 Nx M0
	T3 N0, x M0
III	T1 N1 M0
	T2 N1 M0
	T3 N1 M0
	Tx N1 M0
	T-N1 M0
IV	T-N-M1
Stage unknown	T-N-Mx

Table 35–4 outlines the common pathologic staging used in the United States and compares it with the TNM system preferred by the American Joint Committee on Cancer (AJCC). The staging form preferred by the AJCC is reproduced (Fig 35–3).

CLINICAL PRESENTATION

Multiple studies have analyzed the presenting symptoms of pancreatic cancer.[10, 11] Most attest to the period of latency with only vague prodromal symptoms to warn the patient and physician of the impending obdurate neoplasm. Earlier diagnosis obviously might improve survival. Unfortunately, blanket screening in the absence of more concrete criteria for patients at substantially increased risk is not practicable or

PANCREAS (ICD-O 157)

Data Form for Cancer Staging

Patient identification
Name ______
Address ______
Hospital or clinic number ______
Age ____ Sex ____ Race ______

Institutional identification
Hospital or clinic ______
Address ______

Oncology Record

Anatomic site of cancer ______
Chronology of classification* [ ] Clinical-diagnostic (cTNM) [ ] Surgical-evaluative (sTNM)
Date of classification ______

Histologic type ______ Grade (G)† ______
[ ] Postsurgical resection–pathologic (pTNM)
[ ] Retreatment (rTNM) [ ] Autopsy (aTNM)

Definitions: TNM Classification

Primary Tumor (T)
[ ] TX Minimum requirements to assess the primary tumor cannot be met.
[ ] T1 No direct extension of the primary tumor beyond the pancreas
[ ] T2 Limited direct extension to duodenum, bile ducts, or stomach, still possibly permitting tumor resection
[ ] T3 Further direct extension (incompatible with surgical resection)

Nodal Involvement (N)
[ ] NX Minimum requirements to assess the regional nodes cannot be met.
[ ] N0 Regional nodes not involved
[ ] N1 Regional nodes involved

Distant Metastasis (M)
[ ] MX Minimum requirements to assess the presence of distant metastasis cannot be met.
[ ] M0 No (known) distant metastasis
[ ] M1 Distant metastasis present
Specify ______

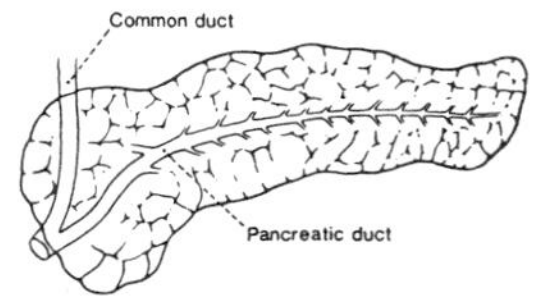

Indicate on diagram primary tumor and regional nodes involved.

Location in Pancreas

[ ] Head
[ ] Body
[ ] Tail
[ ] Diffuse
Size (largest diameter) ____ cm

*Use a separate form each time a case is staged.
†See reverse side for additional information

Nodes

Number positive ______
Location ______

Stage Grouping

[ ] Stage I T1, T2; N0, M0
[ ] Stage II T3, N0, M0
[ ] Stage III T1–T3, N1, M0
[ ] Stage IV T1–T3, N0–N1, M1

Other Site-Specific Information

Diagnostic Confirmation

History [ ] Pain Duration ______
[ ] Jaundice Duration ______
[ ] Weight loss Duration ______
[ ] Diabetes mellitus Duration ______
Physical findings [ ] Abdominal mass
[ ] Ascitic fluid
Roentgenogram [ ] Arteriography
[ ] CT scan
[ ] Endoscopic retrograde cholangiopancreatography (ERCP)
Ultrasound results ______

Cytology [ ] Duodenal fluid
[ ] ERCP
[ ] Needle
[ ] Ascitic fluid
Pathology [ ] From pancreas
[ ] Extrapancreatic
Type ______

Histopathology

[ ] Duct cell adenocarcinoma
[ ] Giant cell carcinoma (pleomorphic carcinoma)
[ ] Giant cell carcinoma (epulis type) with osteoid
[ ] Adenosquamous carcinoma
[ ] Microadenocarcinoma
[ ] Mucinous (colloid) carcinoma
[ ] Cystoadenocarcinoma
[ ] Acinar cell adenocarcinoma
[ ] Pancreatoblastoma
[ ] Papillary cystic tumor
[ ] Mixed type
[ ] Unclassified
Specify ______

Examination by ______ M.D.
Date ______

Postsurgical Resection Residual Tumor (R)

[ ] R0 No residual tumor
[ ] R1 Microscopic residual tumor
[ ] R2 Macroscopic residual tumor
Specify ______

Tumor Grade (G)

[ ] G1 Well differentiated
[ ] G2 Moderately well differentiated
[ ] G3–G4 Poorly to very poorly differentiated

Performance Status of Host (H)

Several systems for recording a patient's activity and symptoms are in use and are more or less equivalent as follows:

AJCC	Performance	ECOG Scale	Karnofsky Scale (%)
[ ] H0	Normal activity	0	90–100
[ ] H1	Symptomatic but ambulatory; cares for self	1	70–80
[ ] H2	Ambulatory more than 50% of time; occasionally needs assistance	2	50–60
[ ] H3	Ambulatory 50% or less of time; nursing care needed	3	30–40
[ ] H4	Bedridden; may need hospitalization	4	10–20

Fig 35–3.—Staging form for pancreatic cancer recommended by the American Joint Committee on Cancer.

economically feasible at this time. Until the relatively late symptoms or sign of icterus appear, the physician has to be vigilant and have a high index of suspicion, particularly in the patient with unexplained weight loss, lassitude, abdominal pain, anorexia, nausea, or vomiting. Obviously these symptoms may be due to pathologies other than pancreatic cancer. Without jaundice these findings may be overlooked[10–12] and, even when noted, the patient may be unwilling to undergo the extensive invasive diagnostic work-up necessary to establish the existence of an early pancreatic cancer.

The current state of the art in pancreatic cancer diagnosis can be summarized as follows: - if a large number of patients with minimal symptoms suggestive of possible pancreatic cancer are investigated under the best possible circumstances, a substantial percentage (40%–60%) will undergo "unnecessary" tests because they will turn out not to have the dreaded disease. Only about one third of all patients with pancreatic cancer will have a resectable lesion at the time of diagnosis. Only one third of these resectable lesions, i.e., one ninth of all pancreatic cancers, are "early" and potentially curable.[12] Thus, unless the surgeon can lower his mortality rate to well under 11%, he may do more harm than good. All early lesions are located in the head of the pancreas.

We have retrospectively defined an early pancreatic cancer as one which satisfies all the following criteria following a pancreaticoduodenal resection[12]:

1. Tumor less than 2 cm in diameter.

2. No histologic evidence of invasion of the pancreatic pseudocapsule.

3. Absence of lymph node invasion on careful histologic examination of all regional nodal basins.

4. No evidence of peritoneal seeding or distant metastasis at laparotomy.

PREOPERATIVE EVALUATION

Any surgical strategy must include adequate preoperative diagnosis, careful selection of patients who are deemed suitable for attempted pancreatic resection, documentation of informed consent from the patient and immediate relatives, and optimum preparation of the patient for a major operation.[12]

Four investigative tools (ultrasonography, computed tomography [CT], endoscopic retrograde cholangiopancreatography [ERCP], and angiography) are most useful in the evaluation of patients with suspected pancreatic cancer because they provide the surgeon with vital preoperative information and prevent time-consuming, often unrewarding diagnostic maneuvers in the operating room. Ultrasonography and/or CT will delineate localized masses, glandular enlargement, alteration in the contour of the gland, and biliary or pancreatic ductal dilatation. With modern CT scanners, enlargement of peripancreatic nodes or even major vascular invasion may sometimes be evident. Both techniques also may demonstrate the presence of hepatic metastases greater than 1 cm in diameter. ERCP is the test that is most likely to provide a definitive diagnosis of pancreatic cancer, especially when it is combined with cytologic examination of the aspirated pancreatic juice. However, it has become clear in recent years that this test is often overused, even when the diagnosis is obvious by noninvasive methods. This has resulted in a small

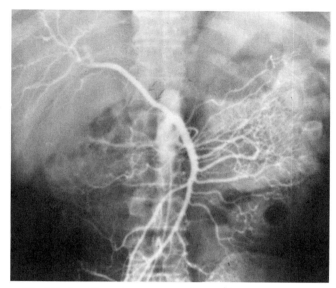

Fig 35–4.—Superior mesenteric arteriogram showing a common anatomic variant. The right hepatic artery originates from the superior mesenteric artery and can be damaged during pancreaticoduodenal resection.

but substantial percentage of patients developing septic cholangitis.

Angiography is advisable as the last preoperative investigation in those selected patients who are deemed to be candidates for a major pancreatic resection. It has a high predictive value for resectability of the tumor. Major arterial (hepatic, splenic, superior mesenteric) or venous (portal, superior mesenteric, or splenic) encasement is virtually pathognomonic of unresectability. The other major role of angiography is to outline important variations of the foregut vasculature, and this may be helpful to the surgeon in the planning of major pancreatic resections. It must be emphasized that a major anomaly of the foregut arteries is demonstrated in at least 25%–30% of angiography studies. Damage to the hepatic arterial blood supply, especially likely when it originates from the superior mesenteric artery and is not easily palpable behind and to the right of the common bile duct, will lead to fatal hepatic necrosis in the jaundiced patient (Fig 35–4).

CONTRAINDICATIONS TO LAPAROTOMY

The frail, elderly patient with multiple systemic disorders who is a high surgical risk should be spared a purely diagnostic laparotomy especially when surgical palliation is not desirable or feasible. This applies especially to lesions in the body and tail of the pancreas, which are virtually always unresectable. In such instances, the technique of percutaneous fine-needle aspiration, with ultrasonography or CT used for guidance, is a simple and effective way of obtaining material for cytologic examination. Caution, however, must be exercised in the interpretation of a cytologic smear, since it may sometimes be difficult to differentiate among a lymphoma, an islet cell carcinoma, and a ductal adenocarcinoma of the pancreas. Hence, the technique should not be applied to the relatively fit young patient in whom a definite histologic, as opposed to a cytologic, diagnosis is essential prior to the aggressive administration of chemotherapy or radiation therapy. The technique also should not be applied to small, potentially resectable cancers because of the high probability of sampling error and the theoretical risk of tumor seeding along the needle tracts.

"Percutaneous needling" for preoperative diagnosis is also another test which is overutilized in a haphazard fashion. It is unnecessary for the unresectable lesion when the patient needs surgical palliation. It is meddlesome for the small resectable tumor, both because of the likelihood of sampling error and because it can result in a traumatic pancreatitis leading to undue adherence of the portal vein. This can make subsequent resection technically difficult.

CONTRAINDICATIONS TO PANCREATIC RESECTION

Pancreatic resection for a ductal adenocarcinoma of the pancreas must not be attempted in the following circumstances:

1. When the patient's general condition is poor. Frail elderly (more than 70 years old) patients with multiple systemic disorders fall into this category.

2. When the patient has clinical, laparoscopic, or operative evidence of distant metastasis.

3. When the patient's life expectancy is estimated to be less than three years because of other concomitant diseases.

4. When the surgeon is inexperienced in this field or does not have adequate backup facilities and manpower in his institution.

A positive lymph node in the immediate vicinity of the pancreas or invasion into any adjacent organ to be removed as part of the pancreatoduodenal resection is not a contraindication to pancreatic resection. Unlike other rare tumors of the pancreas (cystadenocarcinoma, apudomas, etc.) which have a much better prognosis, an adenocarcinoma of the pancreas must never knowingly be resected for palliation, although this is all that may be achieved in most instances.

PREPARATION FOR OPERATION

In addition to careful selection and adequate preoperative evaluation, the patient with cancer of the pancreas must be carefully prepared for operation. This applies especially to the jaundiced patient with a lesion in the head of the pancreas who has a small chance of being cured. Particular attention must be paid to the state of hydration and nutrition, correction of blood deficits, and assessment of cardiopulmonary, renal, and hepatic function. Because starvation for long hours is mandatory prior to many tests, supplemental IV fluids must be given to ensure good hydration and a continuous diuresis. Renal failure to hypovolemia is a tremendous hazard in the jaundiced patient. It also occurs more frequently than is generally realized following injection of contrast material for angiography. In selected severely malnourished individuals a brief period of IV nutrition both before and after operation may be of additional benefit.

Anemia should be corrected by transfusion of packed RBCs as deemed necessary. Because hemorrhage is the single most common complication of pancreaticoduodenectomy, especially in jaundiced patients, a preoperative hematocrit of approximately 40% is advisable. All jaundiced patients should receive daily injections of vitamin K IM, preferably for five days prior to operation, whether the prothrombin index is normal or not. Six units of fresh frozen plasma, six units of platelets, and at least six units of blood should be made available in the operating room. All patients should have an adequate mechanical bowel preparation, which can be supplemented by an nonabsorbable antibiotics for approximately two days prior to operation. In addition, IV broad-spectrum antibiotic coverage should be given perioperatively to all patients who have biliary tract obstruction.

The question of preoperative percutaneous transhepatic biliary decompression became fashionable a few years ago based on theoretical considerations. Prior to the introduction of nonoperative techniques for external and internal biliary decompression, several surgeons, including Whipple, had proposed that severely jaundiced patients requiring pancreatoduodenectomy should undergo staged operations with preliminary decompression of the biliary tract at the initial laparotomy. In recent years, several nonoperative methods for biliary decompression, including percutaneous transhepatic biliary drainage (PTD), endoscopic or percutaneous insertion of an indwelling biliary endoprosthesis, with or without an endoscopic sphincterotomy, have been developed.

Over the past five years, PTD has been recommended routinely for palliation of patients with advanced malignant disease of all types causing biliary obstruction and for the preoperative preparation of the severely jaundiced patient. On theoretical grounds, we have also previously recommended preliminary percutaneous biliary decompression in three types of situations prior to a pancreatoduodenectomy for a lesion in the periampullary region[10]: (1) patients who have a highly elevated serum bilirubin (greater than 20 mg/100 ml); (2) those who have an intercurrent treatable illness; or (3) those who need a period of parenteral hyperalimentation prior to surgical exploration.

Our more recent experience is making us rather more cautious about this recommendation since a significant percentage of patients with temporary or permanent PTD have developed both early and late complications including recurrent catheter blockage, intractable sepsis, hemorrhage in the form of hemobilia, intrahepatic arteriovenous fistula, biliary ascites, pleural effusion, etc. The initial report from Japan claimed a 30-day hospital mortality of 6%–8% in patients prepared preoperatively by PTD compared to a 28% mortality among similar patients operated on without prior PTD. The control group was a historical series and both groups were evaluated retrospectively.[13] Another retrospective nonrandomized study from this country did not show any difference in operative mortality (16% among patients undergoing preoperative PTD and 25% in the control group). This difference was not statistically significant, but PTD seemed to have lowered the incidence of postoperative complications (28% vs. 56%, $P < 0.05$).[14]

Two prospective randomized studies, from South Africa and the United States, have failed to demonstrate any clear advantage of preoperative PTD in terms of both postoperative morbidity and mortality. Thus, it may well be that we have been too enthusiastic about the theoretical advantages of preoperative PTD. It is still possible that the length of preoperative drainage in all these studies has been too short (10 to 18 days) to reverse the multiple metabolic disturbances, coagulation defects, and immunologic abnormalities associated with obstructive jaundice.[15, 16]

SURGICAL CONSIDERATIONS

Surgical considerations are different for lesions in the head of the pancreas from those in the body and tail of the gland for several reasons. We have demonstrated, in prospective diagnostic studies, that a small but definite group of individuals with cancer of the head of the pancreas has a relatively early lesion with a possible chance of cure. The same subset of patients usually need surgical palliation to relieve obstruction jaundice and/or duodenal obstruction. No such palliation is needed for cancer of the body and tail of the pancreas, which are invariably seen at an advanced stage when distant metastases are evident.

During the period of preoperative evaluation and preparation, it is important for the surgeon (not his resident) to have a full discussion of all the possibilities and implications with the patient and his relatives. The natural history of pancreatic cancer, the certainty or uncertainty of the exact diagnosis, and the need for various operative procedures such as biopsy, resection of all types, or bypass, should be discussed in simple terms. The desirability of resecting a lesion in spite of a negative tissue diagnosis should be carefully outlined. Too many medicolegal problems have resulted simply because of failure of the surgeon to communicate properly and outline his plans prior to operation, with the patient and patient's relatives.[17]

OPERATIVE MANAGEMENT

The key words are access, exposure, and assistance.[18, 19] The abdominal incision must be exceedingly generous for full exploration of the pancreas. The type of incision depends on the patient's build. If the patient is tall and has an acute subcostal angle, a long midline incision starting at the xyphisternum and ending well below the umbilicus is appropriate. If the patient is broad and has a wide subcostal angle, an oblique sabre-type of incision along the long axis of the pancreas is recommended. Alternatively, some surgeons prefer a bilateral subcostal incision, starting in the right subcostal region and extending the incision if no obvious metastases in the liver and peritoneal cavity are encountered on initial exploration.

Exploration of the entire abdomen must be meticulous and thorough, using both inspection and palpation. Distant metastasis in the liver or omentum or peritoneal implants are obvious contraindications to resection. Two less obvious sites must also be evaluated:

1. Extension of tumor into the base of the transverse mesocolon and the root of the small-bowel mesentery must be visualized by elevating the transverse colon and tensing the transverse mesocolon. Obvious puckering in this area, just below the region where the superior mesenteric vessels pass beneath the neck of the pancreas, indicates tumor extension beyond the margin of resectability.

2. Obvious extension of tumor around the celiac axis is also indicative of unresectability.

If full exploration of the peritoneal cavity appears favorable for a resective procedure, two further maneuvers are essential to determine the resectability of a cancer of the head of the pancreas.

1. The hepatic flexure of the colon is mobilized by freeing its peritoneal attachments to the infrahepatic structures, including the right kidney, duodenum, and head of pancreas. The peritoneal reflection lateral to the second part of the duodenum is divided, and an extensive Kocher maneuver is attempted to elevate the duodenum and head of pancreas from the right kidney, the inferior vena cava, and both renal veins. If the tumor has invaded these gutter structures, resection is abandoned.

2. The greater omentum is detached from the transverse colon to open the lesser sac widely. The stomach and greater omentum are retracted superiorly and the transverse colon and mesocolon are retracted inferiorly to expose the anterior surface of the head, neck, and body of the pancreas. The middle colic vein is gently traced down to the inferior border of the pancreas and to its junction with the superior mesenteric vein. Careful palpation and elevation of the neck of the pancreas will reveal any tumor extension into the superior mesenteric vein. It is often necessary to feel the superior border of the neck of the pancreas at the same time to be certain that the neck of the pancreas is free from the anterior aspect of both the portal and superior mesenteric veins. This must be done from above, and ligation and division of the gastroduodenal artery facilitate this exposure. If either the portal or the superior mesenteric vein is invaded, the tumor is deemed unresectable.

The Need for Intraoperative Tissue Diagnosis

Many experts believe that any operation of the magnitude and risk of a major pancreatic resection must not be undertaken unless a positive microscopic diagnosis of malignancy has been established. With the currently available diagnostic aids discussed previously, a cytologic diagnosis is often obtained prior to operation, and virtually all doubtful cases are sorted out preoperatively. Thus, the dilemma of intraoperative differentiation between a cancer of the head of the pancreas and chronic pancreatitis, or an impacted stone at the ampulla, is greatly exaggerated in the present-day context of adequate preoperative evaluation. Occasionally, a doubtful situation arises, and this should have been discussed with the patient and his relatives preoperatively. The surgeon then must decide whether he should try to establish a diagnosis by frozen section histologic examination of intraoperative biopsy before attempting a resection. He must remember that truly representative biopsies of the pancreas are often difficult to obtain because of sampling error and because of the confusion between tumor and associated pancreatitis. The diagnosis by histologic examination of frozen-section biopsies is often time-consuming and can be traumatizing. A pancreatoduodenal resection has sometimes been performed simply because of the surgical trauma inflicted to this region. Thus, the patient must not be "biopsied to death," nor must an opportunity to resect a small tumor be missed by obsessive reliance on the establishment of an exact tissue diagnosis. Each surgeon is, quite rightly, influenced by his own philosophy, his experience and expertise, and his pathologist's experience in this field, as well as by the overall clinical picture.[20]

The standard technique of biopsying a mass in the head of the pancreas is to employ the Tru-cut (Travenol) needle inserted through the intact duodenum into the suspicious area after an adequate Kocher manuever. If an experienced cytopathologist is available, the skinny needle aspiration technique is much safer and equally accurate. Some surgeons have advocated the tedious, time-wasting task of biopsying lymph nodes adjacent or peripheral to a pancreatic mass for frozen section histologic examination. We disagree with this recommendation, because the presence of a positive regional node per se does not preclude a satisfactory outcome.[21] Several patients in many series have survived for substantial periods (greater than three years) following pancreatic resection for cancer which had metastasized to adjacent lymph nodes. Thus, in carefully selected cases, when all conditions are favorable and the issues and uncertainties have been explained to the patient and relatives, we proceed with a resection in the absence of a positive tissue diagnosis for cancer, so as not to miss the opportunity of curing an early small lesion.

ATTEMPTS AT CURE AND THE CHOICE OF A RESECTIVE PROCEDURE

Statistically, the only patients who have a chance of cure are those with a localized cancer in the head of the pancreas.[10, 17] In spite of some disagreement about the extent of resection, most surgeons agree that extirpation of a carcinoma of the head of the pancreas is advisable whenever possible. The reported salvage rate is low for two main reasons:

1. The postoperative mortality is too high. This can be blamed on faulty selection and inadequate preparation of the patient and on the surgeon's inexperience with the operation and its complications.

2. The very small percentage of patients with early lesions, because the vast majority of cancers are diagnosed late.

It is clear, however, that survival of patients with cancer of the head of pancreas has been appreciable only after some form of pancreatoduodenal resection as opposed to palliative bypass procedures. The technical details of these operations have been well described.[18, 19, 21, 22] There are currently four resective choices for a cancer in the head of the pancreas.

Pancreatoduodenectomy (Whipple's Operation)

This procedure entails en bloc removal of the duodenum, head, and neck of the pancreas; a variable portion of the distal stomach and of the upper jejunum, the gallbladder, and common bile duct; and, as far as possible, the regional lymphatic nodal basin. All surgeons agree that the operation is ideally suited to patients with resectable localized cancers of the ampulla, distal common bile duct, or duodenum. It is also applicable to benign tumors in the periampullary region that are too large or too deeply embedded to be ennucleated. Whether the operation is adequate for a ductal adenocarcinoma arising in the head of the pancreas is clearly still a debatable issue.

Total Pancreatoduodenectomy (Total Pancreatectomy)

This is an extension the Whipple operation and entails the additional removal of the body and tail of the pancreas, the spleen, and a more extensive regional lymphadenectomy. The pros and cons of a total pancreatoduodenectomy vs. a Whipple operation have been amply emphasized by numerous authors. The rationale for total pancreatoduodenectomy are as follows:

1. Eradication of multicentric disease.

2. Eradication of spread to distal pancreas by direct extension, intraductal seeding, and lymphatic permeation.

3. A better cancer operation is achieved and the operative technique is enhanced by en bloc tissue resection, avoiding confusion of a transection level, avoiding multiple frozen section examinations, and obviating a pancreatojejunal anastomosis.

4. A decrease in severity and frequency of complications, such as postoperative pancreatitis and leakage of pancreatojejunostomy.

5. An acceptable operative mortality of around 5% in the best of hands.

6. Manageable metabolic derangment provided the patient and relatives are properly educated.

7. High incidence of pancreatic endocrine and exocrine insufficiency following the standard Whipple procedure.

The arguments against total pancreatecomy are rather weak and include: (1) loss of endocrine function; (2) loss of exocrine function; and (3) increase risk of peptic ulcer disease, which is totally avoidable by either performing a substantial (60% or more) gastric resection or by adding a truncal vagotomy to the operation. To these reasons may be added the author's personal prejudice against partially resecting any gland harboring a lethal carcinoma. The fear of inducing diabetes mellitus by total pancreatecomy is irrational, because 34% of all our pancreatic cancer patients are insulin-dependent diabetics at the time of presentation. Another 47% have abnormal glucose tolerance as defined by the American Diabetic Association's age-adjusted criteria.

Regional Pancreatectomy

The concept of extended resection or super-radical pancreatectomy dates as far back as the early 1950s, when tangential clamping of the portal vein with partial resection of its wall, total resection of the vein with reanatomosis, or portacaval shunt, were tried in both animals and man. These procedures were uniformly attended by an increase in morbidity and mortality without a concomitant improvement in cure rate. In 1973 Fortner[24-25] reactivated the concept of a super-radical or regional approach to pancreatic cancer. He advocated resection of any or all of the three major vessels near the neck of the pancreas; namely, the portal vein, the superior mesenteric artery, and the celiac axis. The portal vein was usually reconstructed with end-to-end anastomosis, and the major arteries were reconstructed either by direct reimplantation into the aorta or by the insertion of a communicating graft. If only the portal vein is excised as part of the total pancreatoduodenectomy, the operation is labeled type 1, and if a major artery is resected with an appropriate reconstruction, the procedure is labeled type 2. Four years later, Fortner and associates updated his experience and introduced a concept of type O regional pancreatectomy in which none of the three vessels were resected. This is exactly the same operation as had been advocated by several authors; namely, a total pancreatectomy with regional lymphadenectomy. The objective data supporting such an extensive procedure with a prohibitive mortality and morbidity is still lacking.[24–26]

The Pylorus-Preserving Pancreatoduodenal Resection (Whipple or Total)

Traverso and Longmire[27] popularized this variation of the Whipple procedure or total pancreatectomy. The entire stomach, pylorus, and first part of the duodenum are preserved. The advantage of this operation is that the patient can eat normal-sized meals and does not develop dumping syndrome. Long-term survival data with the operation are not yet available. The procedure is clearly advantageous in cases of benign disease of the pancreas or selected localized tumors of the duodenum or ampulla of Vater. In the senior author's opinion, it is indefensible to apply the operation to cancer of the head of the pancreas or of the lower end of the common bile duct, since it may compromise the only chance of cure.

Evaluation of the published data in the literature to identify the most appropriate of these four operations is virtually impossible for several reasons: (1) Most of the series reported are retrospective, and accurate histologic diagnosis, staging, and postmortem data are often lacking.[10, 21] (2) Many surgeons report their results of "periampullary cancers" and include ampullary, duodenal, common bile duct, pancreatic cystic, and islet cell cancers; these lesions have a much better prognosis than carcinoma of the head of the pancreas.[10, 21, 28] (3) The number of surgeons involved in the operations and the experience and expertise are not clear from the reports. Very few surgeons have reported personal series. It is clear, however, that the results of small personal series are far better than those of large institutional ones. The value of experience and specialization in this area is documented by the acceptable low mortality (currently in the region of 5% or less) in experienced hands. Such results lend support to the concept of centralization to specialized centers where a small number of surgeons can perform more frequent resections and can reduce the mortality and morbidity of pancreatic surgery to an acceptable level.[10, 21, 23, 28] (4) Uncertainty of histologic diagnosis has been a frequent concomitant of most conservative (nonresectional) procedures. Between 1964 and 1968, only three of 19 reports reviewed indicated that a tissue diagnosis by biopsy and histology or by autopsy was obtained.[21] Most authorities agree that many cancers of the head of the pancreas cannot be easily distinguished from cancers originating in the ampulla, duodenum, or lower common bile duct until the entire resected specimen is examined in the pathology laboratory. If these more favorable tumors are treated by bypass procedures, the patients are then denied the 50% five-year survival that can be expected after an adequate resection.

The probability of a high mortality and morbidity for pancreatoduodenal resections which are reported in the literature are largely due to these inherent defects. Even in recent reports mortality rates of around 20% are quoted for the Whipple operation or total pancreatectomy.[28] Comparison of survival after various types of resections and bypass procedures are impossible, since there has, quite rightly, been a tendency to allocate patients to treatment group on the basis of multiple variable factors, such as age and fitness of the patient, stage of the disease, and the surgeons' personal preferences. The small number of patients who are operated on when the disease is still at the curative stage makes further analysis difficult. Statistical analysis of retrospective noncomparable, and sometimes incomprehensible data are processed and offered to give validity to some preconceived thesis.[21, 23, 28]

The main current controversy is whether a Whipple operation or a total pancreatectomy is the most appropriate operation for a carcinoma of the head of the pancreas. It has not been documented that the long-term results of the Whipple operation are different from those of total pancreatectomy, but the main issue is whether the series compared are in fact comparable. Jordan[29] performed a literature survey of 898 patients with adenocarcinoma of the head of the pancreas treated by a Whipple operation, and 203 patients who underwent a total pancreatectomy. After excluding the operative deaths, he found that the five-year survival to be 6.5% and 8.2%, respectively. Each group included patients who were alive at periods of less than five years, so the length of survival will probably increase with time in both groups.[29] Edis et al.[23] reviewed the Mayo Clinic experience of a 25-year period and compared 124 patients who had a Whipple operation with 38 who had a total pancreatectomy. The five-year survival was 8% for each group. Of the special note is that the operative mortality for total pancreatectomy remains high (17%–15%) during the whole period of study. The latest recommendation from the Mayo Clinic group is that the Whipple operation should be performed in the first instance in all patients who are not insulin-requiring diabetics. The operation is converted into a total pancreatectomy only if there is tumor at the pancreatic transection line on frozen-section histology or if a pancreatojejunal anastomosis is not technically feasible.

It is clear that either of the two currently popular operations (Whipple procedure or total pancreatectomy) can be performed with an acceptable risk in a center where there is adequate interest, experience, and expertise in pancreatic surgery as well as competence in the management of these patients preoperatively and postoperatively. In the senior author's personal experience with the first 74 resections for ductal adenocarcinoma of the pancreas (19 Whipple, 55 total), there appears to be marginal but not statistically significant difference in survival favoring total pancreatectomy. The mean survival following total pancreatectomy is 35 months compared to 29 months following a Whipple operation. The operative mortality does not appear to be different, one of 19 for Whipple operation and four of 55 for total pancreatectomy. Caution is advised in the interpretation of these apparently superb results, which must be carefully analyzed against the background of what happens to the relatively long survivors.

One of our five operative deaths had a very early cancer, and the death was directly related to operative and postoperative hemorrhage. Eight of our patients have survived for longer than five years, an additional 2 have survived 4 years, and 23 have survived over 3 years. Nine of these "long-term" survivors have died of unrelated problems such as myocardial infarction and cerebrovascular accidents; 4 have died of autopsy-proved primary lung cancer; 1 patient has died of an insulin overdose; and 5 patients have died of metastases from pancreatic cancer.

It is apparent that a small but definite percentage of patients who have cancer of the head of the pancreas is potentially salvageable and can have appreciable survival either after a Whipple operation or a total pancreatectomy, provided that the patient does not die of the operation or of its complications. It is also clear that patients with pancreatic cancer, even if it can be eradicated, are also at high risk of dying of other disorders, many of which are associated with cigarette smoking.

The Reconstruction Following Pancreatic Resections

Numerous variations in technique of reconstruction have been championed to reduce the postoperative mortality and morbidity and to provide a better functional result. The exact technical details vary and are mainly dependent on the surgeon's personal preferences rather than on sound surgical principles.[21, 30] Some important guidelines, however, should be followed:

1. The pancreatic remnant after a Whipple pancreatoduodenectomy should be reanastomosed to the jejunum. The senior author finds it difficult to defend simple ligation and/or injection of the pancreatic duct with drainage of the pancreatic stump to the exterior. We prefer the method described by Hunt of end-to-end pancreaticojejunostomy, which is done by simply plugging the pancreatic stump into the jejunum and holding it with interrupted 3–0 and 4–0 silk sutures on the outside. No attempt is made to obtain mucosa-to-mucosa approximation. This technique is ideal when the pancreatic duct is very small.[21] An alternative method, which is specially applicable when the pancreatic duct is dilated, is to perform an end-to-side pancreaticojejunostomy, using fine (5–0) nonabsorbable sutures to perform a mucosa-to-mucosa anastomosis between the pancreatic duct and the jejunal mucosa. The anastomosis is splinted with a small silastic catheter and reinforced by an outer layer of interrupted 3–0 or 4–0 silk sutures.[21]

2. The common hepatic duct, not the gallbladder, is used for biliary-jejunal anastomosis. The gallbladder, common bile duct, and porta hepatic nodes should have been removed en bloc with the specimen.

3. The time-honored principle that the alkaline fluid of the upper GI tract should enter the jejunum before the acid juice from the stomach to prevent marginal ulceration is entirely unproved. Hence, whether the biliary-enteric anastomosis is performed proximal or distal to the gastrojejunostomy is irrelevant. However, if less than 60% of the stomach is resected, a bilateral truncal vagotomy must be added to eliminate the risk of developing a stomal ulcer.

PALLIATION FOR CANCER OF THE HEAD OF THE PANCREAS

Palliation is defined as the relief, even temporarily, of any symptom or impending symptom due to a disease process without attempting to treat the disease itself. The emphasis of any palliative procedure is on improvement of the *quality* of life, the lessening of suffering, and, if possible, the return to some occupation even on a temporary basis. If the symptom relieved is associated with a life-threatening complication, i.e., cholangitis and liver failure due to obstructive jaundice or severe malnutrition due to duodenal obstruction, the duration of survival is also increased.[19]

The surgeon has an enormous responsibility to the patient and to the other physicians who are going to treat the patient subsequently. If the cancer is unresectable or metastatic it is *essential* that a tissue diagnosis by biopsy and frozen-section histology is made prior to leaving the operating room. This takes the matter out of the realm of doubt, an especially important point when the palliative procedure restores the patient to relatively good health for a relatively long period. In this situation, doubt is often raised about the true diagnosis. A known positive biopsy for ductal adenocarcinoma of the pancreas will then prevent an unnecessary second-look laparotomy.

Relief of Jaundice

Decompression of the biliary tract is recommended for several reasons. Most patients find the physical stigma of jaundice very distressing and the intractable pruritus intolerable, especially during the summer months. Suppurative cholangitis, progressive liver failure, and coagualopathy are secondary lethal complications which can be avoided.

The actual anatomical arrangement of the biliary bypass is not of great importance, provided that it does decompress the biliary tree adequately. It is highly surprising that mortality rates ranging from 6% to more than 50% have been reported following operative biliary decompression.

The use of the gallbladder for providing internal biliary drainage is quick, simple, and safe. The gallbladder is the biliary tract organ of choice when the cystic duct is widely patent and enters the common bile duct high in the biliary tree, well away from the tumor mass. The gallbladder must not be employed when the cystic duct is unusually long and narrow and enters the lower part of the common bile duct close to the tumor, or when there is evidence of cholangitis, or when the gallbladder itself is diseased. In such situations, the common hepatic duct should be used for exit of bile and the gallbladder should be removed.

Most authorities agree that the stomach or duodenum should not be used for the biliary-enteric bypass. A loop of jejunum brought up in antecolic fashion is the preferred method. The Roux-en-Y hepaticojejunostomy is very acceptable. An equally effective arrangement is to bring a loop of small bowel up to the dilated biliary tree and to add a side-to-side enteroenteroanastomosis some 12 in. below the biliary-enteric bypass so that small-bowel food content is prevented from regurgitating into the biliary tree.

Relief From Duodenal Obstruction

Overt duodenal obstruction is rare in cancer of the head of the pancreas, since many patients die before such a complication can develop. However, functional or partial duodenal obstruction is clinically evident in some 40%–60% of patients. Contrary to common belief, the second part of the duodenum is rarely the actual site of the obstruction. It is the mass that grows inferiorly toward the root of the mesentery that tends to produce duodenal obstruction in the third and fourth part of the duodenum and around the ligament of Treitz. Most authorities advocate a gastrojejunostomy to be used selectively based on preoperative and operative impressions of obstruction rather than because of fear of future difficulties. We believe that the gastrojejunostomy should be performed routinely, especially in the younger, more fit patient who is likely to survive a reasonable time and who is a candidate for agressive chemotherapy or radiation therapy. It is a tragedy to have to reoperate after four or five months of such therapy to relieve duodenal obstruction in these individuals, since the second laparotomy is obviously more hazardous. Whether a retrocolic or antecolic gastrojejunostomy is performed depends on the patient's anatomy and on the exact location of the tumor. It is important to place the anastomosis well to the left of the main tumor mass and to use the most dependent part of the stomach usually just posterior to the greater curvature. A gastrojejunostomy in the anterior wall of the stomach is mechanically unsatisfactory, since the stomach does not empty very well whether the patient is sitting up or lying down. A truncal vagotomy to prevent stomal ulceration is unnecessary in most instances. However, in the relatively young good-risk patient who is likely to have a prolonged survival, it is wise to add a quick, bilateral truncal vagotomy. Finally, the gastrojejunostomy should always be performed proximal to the biliary-enteric anastomosis.

Control of Pain

Epigastric and back pain are incapacitating, distressing symptoms of pancreatic cancer especially when it involves the body of the pancreas. Biliary and duodenal bypass procedures contribute nothing to the relief of pain. Intraoperative chemical splanchnicectomy at the time of laparotomy is the most expedient and easily performed procedure. Injection of either 6% phenol or 50% alcohol along both sides of the celiac axis is still the best of all the recommended methods. For a satisfactory splanchnicectomy an adequate volume of the chemical—about 25 ml—must be injected on each side of the celiac axis. Unfortunately, adequate relief of pain for a reasonable length of time is only achieved, in our hands, for approximately one third of the patients.[21]

A tense, distended, obstructed main pancreatic duct is believed by Cattel and Smith to contribute substantially to the pain.[21] Hence, they recommended decompression of the main pancreatic duct in these situations. The construction of yet another anastomosis in these debilitated patients should, however, be attempted with extreme caution. Rodney Smith advocated placing a large T tube through a small incision in the main pancreatic duct and bringing out the long limb of the T tube through both walls of the stomach and out of the

anterior abdominal wall, where it can be placed on low-grade continuous suction for a few days. After three to four weeks, the posterior wall of the stomach is sealed around the incision in the pancreas, and a direct pancreaticogastric fistula is formed. The T tube can then be removed.

Other more elaborate maneuvers, including stereotaxic thalamotomy and cordotomy, have been advised for the relief of pain but they have a very limited role in the management of the majority of patients with pancreatic cancer, since most do not live long enough to warrant such drastic interventions. Judicious use of narcotic drugs and other analgesics in various combinations is the best that we have to offer at the present time.[19]

NONOPERATIVE PALLIATION OF PANCREATIC CANCER

Percutaneous transhepatic external or internal-external drainage of the biliary system is a valuable alternative for palliating obstructive jaundice under the following circumstances[13-16, 19]:

1. The patient is unfit for or refuses operative internal biliary drainage.

2. The diagnosis of pancreatic carcinoma (using cytologic aspiration of duodenal-pancreatic juice or material obtained by direct percutaneous needle aspiration) and its spread beyond the confines of resectability are established beyond a reasonable doubt.

3. The potential of complications (subcutaneous infections, catheter blockage, recurrent biliary sepsis, bleeding), the inconveniences, and the discomfort inherent in using an external tube and a collecting device are fully appreciated by the patient and the family.

Endoscopic papillotomy with insertion of an internal biliary-duodenal catheter stent is an acceptable alternative, but more experience is necessary before its widespread use can be recommended. Its main disadvantage is that it is much more difficult to change a blocked catheter endoscopically than it is using the radiologic method.

Percutaneous injection of the celiac ganglia, using 50 ml of 50% alcohol after a diagnostic trial with tetracaine hydrochloride (Pontocaine), can be attempted for the relief of pancreatic pain. An increasingly popular alternative is the anterior approach to the celiac ganglia using CT scan for guidance. In our experience, significant and prolonged relief of pain is obtained in only the minority of patients.[19]

TREATMENT OF CANCER OF THE BODY AND TAIL OF THE PANCREAS

Surgical treatment of adenocarcinoma of the body and tail of the pancreas is even more depressing than that of a similar lesion in the head of the gland. As far as the senior author knows, the only long-term survivor from resection of a cancer of the body of the pancreas was reported in 1934 by Gordon-Taylor.[31] By the time the patient presents with symptoms, the disease is invariably at a very late or terminal stage. In our hands, no patient with cancer of the body and tail of the pancreas has survived longer than one year with or without a pancreatic resection. Longmire quotes an average of eight months, with range of 0–20 months.[32]

The two aims of a surgeon exploring cancer of the body and tail of the pancreas are (1) to establish a tissue diagnosis beyond doubt and (2) to relieve pain. If the tumor can be mobilized from the posterior parietes, the senior author prefers a palliative distal pancreatectomy and splenectomy. The margins of the pancreatic bed is then outlined with hemoclips to help in the designing of a radiation port postoperatively. If the tumor is too extensive to be resected locally and/or is widely metastatic, all that can be achieved is to obtain adequate tissue diagnosis. The injection of phenol or absolute alcohol around the celiac plexus should be performed as previously described. Occasionally, the duodenojejunal junction is obstructed by tumor invasion at the ligament of Treitz. A palliative gastrojejunostomy is advisable in such a situation.

The "tissue diagnosis at all costs" philosophy in patients with cancer of the body and tail of the pancreas has to be tempered and individualized. The frail, elderly patient should clearly be spared a purely diagnostic laparotomy; the percutaneous needle aspiration technique for cytologic diagnosis can be performed as previously discussed. On the other hand, the patient who is relatively fit and young should always be explored, since occasionally the surgeon and the patient will have the relatively pleasant surprise of finding an islet cell tumor or a lymphoma, which has a much better prognosis than a ductal adenocarcinoma of the pancreas.

POSTOPERATIVE COMPLICATIONS OF PANCREATIC RESECTION FOR CANCER

Intra-abdominal hemorrhage is the commonest operative and postoperative complication encountered during pancreaticoduodenal resection. Hemostasis must be meticulous during the operation and all divided vessels carefully ligated. In spite of this, blood may ooze at an alarming rate from all raw areas inside the abdomen during the first 24 hours following operation. Adequate replacement of blood and blood clotting factors during and after operation is essential. Reoperation is mandatory when the surgeon has reason to suspect a major bleeding site, when clot accumulation in the abdomen causes distention, or when a consumption coagulopathy is recognized. In the latter two situations, one never finds a discrete bleeding point at reoperation. The clots are gently evacuated and the whole abdomen irrigated prior to reclosure with drainage. A similar amount of bleeding may occur in the form of hemobilia following decompression of a dilated obstructed biliary tree. This invariably stops on its own. Hepatorenal failure and cardiopulmonary failure are the two commonest events leading to postoperative death after major pancreatoduodenal resections. Other complications which may also be fatal include intractable sepsis, mesenteric infarction, myocardial infarction, congestive heart failure, cerebrovascular accident, and, very rarely, pulmonary embolism. Anastomotic leakage and fistula formation should not occur, since they are highly preventable by careful and proper construction of the anastomoses. Nonfatal complications described include pneu-

monia, delayed gastric emptying, wound infection or dehiscence, cardiac arrhythmias, fecal fistula, and gastrojejunocolic fistula.[21]

LONG-TERM MANAGEMENT OF THE TOTAL PANCREATECTOMIZED PATIENT

The totally pancreatectomized patient has to be suitably educated and rehabilitated before he leaves hospital. He has to learn to eat multiple, small meals with a low-fat content and to take his enzyme supplements. NPH insulin (with or without some regular insulin) is given every morning, and the patient and a member of his relatives are taught how to administer the insulin and how to perform standard urine or blood assay monitoring for glucose. Most patients take two to three weeks to adjust to the new regimen. The patient and his relatives must be reminded repeatedly that his diabetes is different from the spontaneously occuring diabetes mellitus, in that hypoglycemia is the big danger, probably due to the absence of pancreatic glucagon. The hypoglycemic attacks can be easily avoided by increasing the food intake slightly and decreasing the insulin dose, especially when physical activity is resumed. Death may occur during a hypoglycemic attack; it is mandatory for the physician to reiterate this danger at each clinic visit. The patient should carry sugar with him at all times and also keep it at his bedside. It may even be beneficial for some patients to experience an early hypoglycemic attack (tachycardia, sweating, nervousness, confusion, etc.,) while he is still in the hospital to see that these symptoms are easily relieved by taking sugar. The patient must never miss evening meals because this is the time that hypoglycemia most often develops with long-acting insulin preparations. If the patient is selected properly, he can lead a relatively normal life following total pancreatoduodenectomy, provided that he is adequately educated and supported by his physician and relatives.

RADIATION THERAPY OF PANCREATIC CANCER

Postoperative photon or mixed-beam therapy in doses of 4,000–6,000 rad given as a split course over a period of six to eight weeks using fluorouracil (5-FU) as a radiosensitizer is currently the standard method of palliating locally unresectable pancreatic cancer.[33] It is most useful for the surgeon to outline the tumor mass with silver clips when performing the palliative bypasses. Treatment should be planned carefully, using CT tumor analysis data and treatment simulators in combination with ultrasound and the utilization of multiple field techniques. Median survival in the region of 12 months can be anticipated.

The advent of fast neutron therapy for curative radiation has until now not fulfilled the promised improvement in results. Despite the relatively high doses and consequent high morbidity, residual microscopic tumor has been demonstrated in most of the patients who underwent autopsy.

Considerable interest now centers on intraoperative radiation therapy of pancreatic cancer. Several trials of interstitial implantation of radioactive needles and seeds (198 AU, 125 I) followed by high-dose photon beam irradiation have yielded a significantly reduced local recurrence rate but not an unexpected increase in distant metastases. The morbidity and mortality from this highly traumatic procedure is appreciable, and local implantation of radioactive material has now been largely abandoned in most institutions.

The use of intraoperative beam radiation for patients with unresectable pancreatic cancer carcinoma is currently being tried in several centers.[34, 35] Intraoperative beam therapy (mainly of high-energy electrons) has several advantages over radioactive seed implantation: (1) larger tumors can be treated; (2) the dose delivered is more uniform; (3) the trauma to the peripancreatic tissues and the pancreas is less; (4) the radiation therapy field is broader so that high-dose volume can include 1- to 2-cm margin outside the gross tumor volume; and (5) the possibility of seeding cancer from implantation is eliminated. Preliminary data from the Massachusetts General Hospital shows a 16.5-month median survival with generally good palliation. There is also a possible added benefit from using a radiosensitizer such as misonidazole. If these observations are confirmed, the logical extension is to use intraoperative radiation following radical resection for cancer of the head of the pancreas. The preliminary data from Japan on 12 patients show that there is improvement in the one-year survival compared to pancreatoduodenectomy alone, but not in the two-year survival rate. Autopsy of three patients who underwent the combined therapy did not reveal any involvement of the lymph nodes in the irradiation field. However, there was involvement of the lymph nodes outside the field; namely, around the aorta just below the diaphragm and around the origin of the inferior mesenteric artery. Liver metastases continue to be a prominent cause of death.[35]

CHEMOTHERAPY OF PANCREATIC CANCER

There is no single drug available which is effective against adenocarcinoma of the exocrine pancreas. In spite of enormous time and effort invested in the design and evaluation of chemotherapeutic drugs, only two combinations of multiple agents have resulted in modest increments in response rates. Some prolongation of life has been reported using the FAM (5-FU, Adriamycindoxorubicin, mitomycin C) or SMF (streptozotocin, mitomycin C, 5-FU) regimens. The FAM regimen, however, has considerably less toxicity than the SMF.[36]

It is clear the chemotherapeutic management of patients with pancreatic cancer must be directed by clinical oncologists with experience and special interest in GI cancer to ensure optimal results. The importance of agressive nutritional, pharmacologic, and emotional support cannot be overemphasized. It is the senior author's opinion that these patients should not be treated outside of the rigid framework of a controlled trial. Only in this way can we improve our chemotherapeutic armamentarium against this lethal cancer.

CONCLUSIONS

We have previously emphasized that the early symptoms of pancreatic cancer are vague and nonspecific and are often ig-

nored both by the physician and patient. A normal physical examination and a normal routine blood and radiologic investigation do not exclude pancreatic cancer. The presence of common disorders such as gallstones, hiatal hernia, and diverticular disease of the colon does not preclude the concomitant presence of a pancreatic cancer. About 10%–15% of all patients presenting with pancreatic cancer are potentially curable at the time of presentation. All favorable lesions are located in the head of the pancreas. Whether a Whipple operation or a total pancreatectomy is performed, the operative mortality should not be greater that 5%. Intraoperative radiation therapy following a radical resection to eliminate minimal residual disease will probably improve the results of pancreatic resections. Regionalization or centralization of patients with these difficult problems to specialty centers is clearly of the utmost importance.

REFERENCES

1. Buncher C.R.: Epidemiology of pancreatic cancer, in Moossa A.R. (ed.): *Tumors of the Pancreas.* Baltimore, Williams & Wilkins Co., 1980, pp. 415–427.
2. Levin D.L., Connelly R.R.: Epidemiology, in Cohn I., Hastings P.R. (eds.): *Pancreatic Cancer.* Geneva, UICC, 1981, pp. 5–12.
3. Wynder E.L., Mabuchi K., Marachi N., et al.: Epidemiology of cancer of the pancreas. *Cancer* 31:641, 1973.
4. Gordis L.: Epidemiology of pancreatic cancer, in Lilienfeld A. (ed.) *Reviews of Cancer Epidemiology.* New York, Elsevier/North-Holland, 1980, pp. 84–110.
5. MacMahon B., Yen S., Trichopolos D., et al.: Coffee and cancer of the pancreas. *N. Engl. J. Med.* 384:630, 1981.
6. Moossa A.R., Lewis M.H., Bowie J.D.: Clinical features and diagnosis of pancreatic cancer, in Moossa A.R. (ed.): *Tumors of the Pancreas.* Baltimore, Williams & Wilkins Co., 1980, pp. 429–442.
7. Cubilla A.L., Fitzgerald P.J.: Surgical pathology of cancer of the ampulla—head of the pancreas region, in Fitzgerald P.J., Mornson A.B. (eds.): *The Pancreas.* Baltimore, Williams & Wilkins Co., 1980, pp. 67–81.
8. Cubilla A.L., Fitzgerald P.J.: Surgical pathology of tumors of the exocrine pancreas, in Moossa A.R. (ed.): *Tumors of the Pancreas.* Baltimore, Williams & Wilkins Co., 1980, pp. 159–193.
9. Moossa A.R., Dawson P.J.: The diagnosis of pancreatic cancer. *Pathobiol. Annu.* 11:299, 1981.
10. Moossa A.R.: Pancreatic cancer—approach to diagnosis, selection for surgery and choice of operation. *Cancer* 50:2689, 1982.
11. Braganza J.M., Howat H.T.: Cancer of the pancreas in the exocrine pancreas. *Clin. Gastroenterol.* 1:219, 1972.
12. Moossa A.R., Levin B.: The diagnosis of early pancreatic cancer. *Cancer* 47:1688, 1981.
13. Nakayama T., Ikeda A., Okuda K.: Percutaneous trans-hepatic drainage of the biliary tract: Technique and results in 104 cases. *Gastroenterology* 74:554, 1978.
14. Denning D.A., Ellison E.C., Casey L.C.: Preoperative percutaneous biliary decompression lowers operative morbidity in patients with obstructive jaundice. *Am. J. Surg.* 141:61, 1981.
15. Hatfield A.R., Tobias R., Terblanche J., et al.: Preoperative external biliary drainage in obstructive jaundice: A prospective controlled clinical trial. *Lancet* 2:899, 1982.
16. Pitt W.A.: Personal communication, 1982.
17. Moossa A.R.: Reoperation for pancreatic cancer. *Arch. Surg.* 114:502, 1979.
18. Moossa A.R.: Total pancreatectomy, in Dudley H., Pories W., Carter D. (eds.): *Operative Surgery,* ed. 4. London, Butterworths, 1983, pp. 773–782.
19. Moossa A.R.: Surgical treatment of pancreatic cancer—when to resect, how to palliate. *Surg. Rounds* September, pp. 38–50, 1982.

20. Moossa A.R., Altorki N.: Pancreatic biopsy. *Surg. Clin. North Am.* 63:1205, 1983.
21. Moossa A.R.: Surgical treatment of pancreatic cancer, in Moossa A.R. (ed.): *Tumors of the Pancreas.* Baltimore, Williams & Wilkins Co., 1980, p. 443.
22. Moossa A.R.: Total pancreatectomy, in Schwartz S.I., Ellis H. (eds.): *Maingot's Abdominal Operations,* ed. 8. Norwalk, Conn., Appleton-Century-Crofts, 1984, p. 2231.
23. Edis A.J., Kiernan P.D., Taylor W.F.: Attempted curative resection of ductal carcinoma of the pancreas: Review of the Mayo Clinic experience. *Mayo Clin. Proc.* 55:531, 1980.
24. Fortner J.G.: Regional resection of cancer of the pancreas: A new surgical approach. *Surgery* 73:307, 1973.
25. Fortner J.G.: Surgical principles for pancreatic cancer. *Surgery* 47:1712, 1981.
26. Moossa A.R.: Scott M.H., Lavelle-Jones M.: The place of total and extended total pancreatectomy in pancreatic cancer. *World J. Surg.* 8:895, 1984.
27. Traveso L.W., Longmire W.P. Jr.: Preservation of the pylorus in pancreatoduodenectomy. *Surg. Gynecol. Obstet.* 146:959, 1978.
28. Cooperman A.V., Hester F.B., Marboe G.A., et al.: Pancreatoduodenal resection and total pancreatectomy: An institutional review. *Surgery* 90:707, 1981.
29. Jordan G.L. Jr.: Surgical management of pancreatic cancer, in Stroehlein J.R., Romsdahl M.M. (eds.): *Gastrointestinal Cancer.* New York, Raven Press, 1981.
30. Brooks I.R. (ed.): *Surgery of the Pancreas.* Philadelphia, W.B. Saunders Co., 1983.
31. Gordon-Taylor G.: The radical surgery of cancer of the pancreas. *Ann. Surg.* 100:206, 1934.
32. Longmire W.P. Jr.: Cancer of the pancreas: Palliative operation, Whipple operation or total pancreatectomy? *World J. Surg.* 8:872, 1984.
33. Dobelbower R.R. Jr., Miligan A.J.: Treatment of pancreatic cancer by radiation therapy. *World J. Surg.* 8:906, 1984.
34. Shipley W.U., Wood W.C., Tepper J.E., et al.: Intraoperative electron beam irradiation for patients with unresectable pancreatic carcinoma. *Ann. Surg.* 200:289, 1984.
35. Hiroka T., Watanabe E., Michinaga M., et al.: Intraoperative irradiation combined with radical resection for cancer of the head of pancreas. *World J. Surg.* 8:766, 1984.
36. Harvey T.H., Schein P.S.: Chemotherapy of pancreatic carcinoma. *World J. Surg.* 8:935, 1984.

36

Pancreas Transplantation in Man

DAVID E.R. SUTHERLAND, M.D., PH.D.
DAVID KENDALL, B.A.
FREDERICK C. GOETZ, M.D.
JOHN S. NAJARIAN, M.D.

THE APPLICATION of pancreas transplantation for the treatment of diabetes mellitus has increased dramatically.[1] More pancreas transplants were performed during the two years from Jan. 1, 1982, to Dec. 31, 1983, than in the preceding 16 years,[2] following the first transplant performed by Kelly et al.[3] in 1966.

The evidence that the complications of diabetes are secondary to disordered metabolism is very convincing,[5] and many diabetologists are now making intense efforts to maintain nearly constant euglycemia in diabetic patients.[5] However, the new techniques of exogenous insulin delivery have risks, specifically hypoglycemia.[6] Pancreas transplantation is the most physiologic approach to maintain euglycemia in the treatment of diabetes. Clinical transplantation has had limited application because of immunologic and technical problems, but these problems are gradually being overcome, and the number of successful transplants has increased in recent years.

The American College of Surgeons/National Institutes of Health (ACS/NIH) Organ Transplant Registry recorded information on 57 pancreas transplants in 55 diabetic patients from Dec. 17, 1966, to June 30, 1977, when the Registry closed.[7] One primary and two secondary pancreas transplants performed in 1976 were not reported to the ACS/NIH Registry, but were reported to the new International Human Pancreas Transplant Registry.[8] The new Registry has received data on all known cases of pancreas transplantation since July 1, 1977.[1] The information on vascularized pancreas transplant cases reported to the Registry from Dec. 17, 1966, through June 30, 1984, is summarized in the following section. The experience at the University of Minnesota, where more than one fifth of the transplants have been performed,[9] are described in a subsequent section.

PANCREAS TRANSPLANT REGISTRY

Number of Pancreas Transplants and Overall Results

From Dec. 17, 1966, to June 30, 1984, 485 pancreas transplants were performed in 454 diabetic patients at 52 institu-

tions (Fig 36–1). Four hundred forty-five transplants were from cadaver donors (414 primary, 29 secondary, and 2 tertiary grafts), and 40 were from living related donors (all primary grafts). The 425 transplants performed since July 1, 1977, were placed in 400 patients (Table 36–1). Two patients in the new Registry, one from Stockholm and one from Lyon, had had previous transplants recorded by the ACS/NIH Registry.

The institutions with the largest and most recent experiences, Minnesota,[10, 11] Lyon,[12] Stockholm,[13] Munich,[14] Cambridge,[15] Zurich,[16] Detroit,[17] Wisconsin,[18] Birmingham,[19] and Cincinnati,[20] have published the details on all except their latest cases of pancreas transplantation. The reports published on pancreas transplants from most other institutions are referenced in an earlier comprehensive review article.[21]

One hundred twenty-nine patients currently (as of August 1984) are listed in the Registry as having functioning grafts. Of these, at least 60 have been insulin-independent for more than one year. Thirteen other grafts have functioned for more than one year and then either failed and the patients resumed exogenous insulin, or the recipients died with functioning grafts. The other 343 grafts ceased to function at less than one year because of either technical complications, rejection, or death of the recipients. All of the currently functioning grafts were transplanted since 1978.

The actuarial graft and patient survival rate curves, according to era, for all pancreas transplant cases are shown in Figures 36–2 and 36–3, respectively. The results have improved in recent years, and transplantation has definitely become safer. For 60 recipients of 56 grafts transplanted before July 1, 1977, the one-year actuarial graft survival rate was 3% and the patient survival rate was only 39%. In contrast, of the 192 patients who received 205 transplants from July 1, 1977, to Dec. 31, 1982, the one-year graft survival rate was 20% and the one-year patient survival rate was 72%. For 1983–84 (219 transplants in 207 recipients), the one-year graft survival rate was 38% and the patient survival rate was 77%.

Most recipients of successful pancreas transplants are normoglycemic. However, the metabolic test results can be quite variable.[22, 23] Examples of the types of test results in individual pancreas transplant recipients are illustrated from the University of Minnesota experience in a later section.

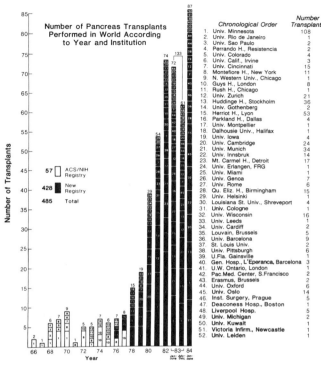

Fig 36–1.—Number of pancreas transplants by year and institution reported to the Registries between Dec. 17, 1966, and June 30, 1984. Each institution is assigned a number according to the chronological order in which it did its first transplant.

Pancreas Transplant Results According to Association With or Without Kidney Grafts

Most pancreas transplant recipients have had diabetic nephropathy and/or other far advanced complications of diabe-

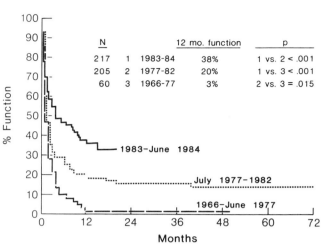

Fig 36–2.—Functional graft survival rates for all pancreas transplants reported to the Registries by year of transplantation through June 30, 1984.

tes. Kidney transplants were performed in 322 of the 400 recipients (80%) of 425 pancreas grafts transplanted since July 1, 1977.

The pancreas transplant success rates have been approximately the same in nonuremic, nonkidney transplant recipients and in kidney transplant recipients (Fig 36–4). There also were no significant differences in the functional survival rates of pancreas grafts transplanted either simultaneously with or after a kidney transplant. One-year actuarial graft survival rates were 31% in recipients of simultaneous kidney transplants, 26% in recipients of previous kidney transplants, and 24% for nonuremic, nonkidney transplant patients ($P > 0.2$). Both recipients of kidney grafts after a pancreas transplant lost pancreas graft function before the kidney transplant.

Patient survival rates have been lower in pancreas trans-

TABLE 36–1.—PANCREAS TRANSPLANT EXPERIENCE OF INDIVIDUAL INSTITUTIONS REPORTING > 10 CASES BETWEEN JULY 1, 1977, AND JUNE 30, 1984

INSTITUTION	NO. TX. (PTS.)	NO.	REPORTED TO BE FUNCTIONING,* MO. (Technique†)
Minnesota	94 (82)	27	57,61,73 (open peritoneal); 15,21,23,31,44 (duct-inj); 8,8,12,12,13,13,16,16,17,21, 25,31,34,36 (enteric)‡
Lyon	48 (46)	13	3,7,8,10,11,12,16,16,16,20,28,33,41 (duct-inj)
Stockholm	30 (27)	5	2,6,16,29,33 (enteric)
Munich	34 (33)	18	2,2,3,3,3,4,4,5,6,8,12,12,12,13,16,18,28,38 (duct-inj)
Cambridge	24 (23)	9	3,3,5,6,7,7,12,21 (enteric); 60 (duct-inj)
Zurich	17	4	3,9,40,49 (duct-inj)
Detroit	17	2	10,37 (duct-inj)
Wisconsin	16	8	2,2,3,4,4,8,13,17 (urinary)
Birmingham	15	5	3,5,29,35,39 (duct-inj)
Innsbruck	14 (13)	5	3,4,6,16,17
Cincinnati	14 (12)	4	5,8,24 (urinary); 32 (duct-inj)
Oslo	10	7	2,3,3,4,6,8,9
≤ 10 cases	92 (89)	22	2,3,3,5,5,8,9,10,10,16,21 (enteric); 4,5 (urinary); 2,3,4,6,6,14,18,44 (duct-inj)
Total	425 (400)	129	2–71 mo.

*Recipients insulin-independent, assuming continuous function of cases reported to be functioning between June 1984 and August 1984.
†For drainage or occlusion of exocrine secretion.
‡Duct-injection, enteric drainage.

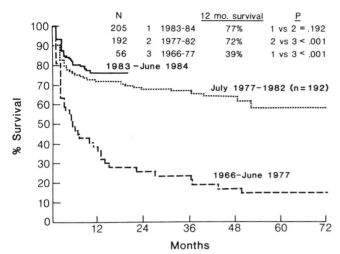

Fig 36–3.—Patient survival rates for all recipients of primary pancreas transplants reported to the Registries by year of transplantation through June 30, 1984.

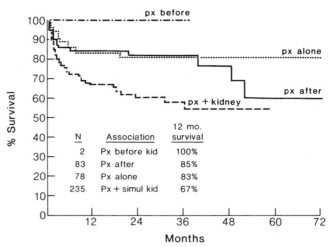

Fig 36–5.—Patient survival rates for recipients of primary pancreas transplants reported to the Registry from July 1, 1977, to June 30, 1984, according to association with or without kidney transplants.

plant recipients of simultaneous kidney grafts than in recipients of pancreas grafts alone or pancreas grafts after a successful kidney graft (Fig 36–5). Patient survival rates would be expected to be higher in recipients of pancreas transplants alone, since the nonuremic diabetic patients would be more likely to have less advanced complications than the uremic diabetic recipients, but the fact that patient survival rates are also higher in uremic diabetic patients who received a kidney transplant before pancreas transplant than in those receiving both grafts simultaneously suggests that a penalty is paid for synchronous as opposed to asynchronous grafting in uremic diabetic patients. This interpretation is supported by an analysis of pancreas graft and patient survival rates according to whether the recipients of pancreas transplants did or did not have end-stage diabetic nephropathy (ESDN). Although pancreas graft survival rates are approximately the same in the two categories of recipients (Fig 36–6), patient survival rates

were significantly higher in patients with than without ESDN (Fig 36–7).

There is no evidence that pancreas transplants have improved the outcome of kidney transplants in uremic diabetic patients. Kidney graft as well as patient survival rates in pancreas transplant recipients with ESDN[24] are lower than those reported for diabetic uremic recipients of kidney transplants alone.[25, 26] It thus appears that correction of uremia by kidney transplantation is more beneficial and more important than total endocrine replacement therapy in diabetic patients with renal failure.

Pancreas Transplant Results According to Surgical Technique

A variety of surgical techniques has been used for pancreas transplantation, attesting to the fact that a single totally satisfactory method has not yet been devised. The methods can

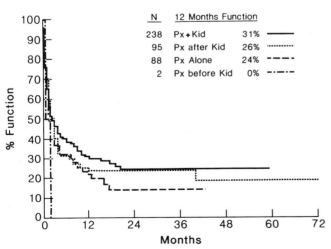

Fig 36–4.—Graft survival rates for all pancreas transplants reported to the Registry from July 1, 1977, to June 30, 1984, according to association with or without kidney transplants.

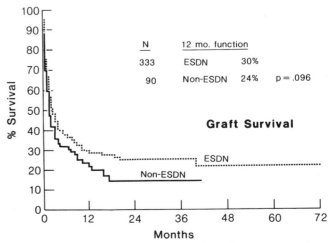

Fig 36–6.—Graft survival rates for all pancreas transplants reported to the Registry from July 1, 1977, to June 30, 1984, in recipients with or without end-stage diabetic nephropathy (ESDN).

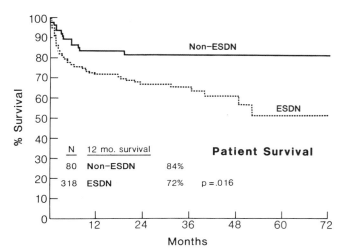

Fig 36–7.—Patient survival rates for recipients of primary pancreas transplants reported to the Registry from July 1, 1977, to June 30, 1984, according to the presence or absence of end-stage diabetic nephropathy *(ESDN).*

be classified according to the type of graft (whole organ or segmental) and technique used for duct management (occluded or drained into a hollow viscus). Whole organ grafts can be further divided into those that include all or part of the duodenum or papilla of Vater and those that do not. Duct-occluded grafts can be divided into those in which the duct is simply ligated or those in which the entire ductal system is obliterated by injection of a synthetic polymer. Duct drained grafts can be divided into those in which an anastomosis is made to either the urinary system (ureter or bladder) or the gut.

The first pancreas transplant performed was a segmental graft.[3] However, in the ACS/NIH Registry encompassing the period from 1966 to 1977,[7] 26 grafts, nearly half of those transplanted, were whole pancreaticoduodenal grafts. With this approach, the pancreas, duodenum, an aortic patch encompassing the celiac axis and superior mesenteric artery, and the portal vein are removed en bloc from the donor, and vascular anastomoses are made to the iliac vessels of the recipient.[27] In eight of the first 26 cases transplanted by this technique, a cutaneous duodenostomy was performed, while in 18 cases the duodenum was anastomosed to a Roux-en-Y limb of recipient jejunum. A high technical complication rate of pancreaticoduodenal transplantation led to a near abandonment of this approach by the mid-1970s, and, until recently,

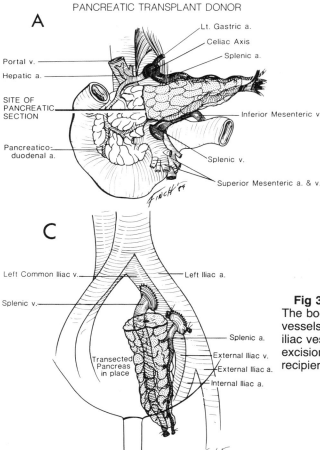

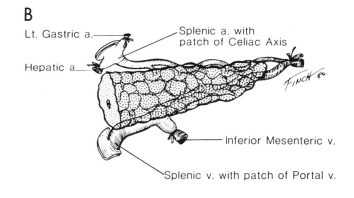

Fig 36–8.—Technique of segmental pancreas transplantation. The body and tail are transplanted with anastomoses of the splenic vessels (or portal vein and celiax axis of the donor pancreas to the iliac vessels of the recipient. **A,** donor anatomy. **B,** graft after excision from a cadaver donor. **C,** graft after implantation in the recipient.

LIGATION OF DISTAL SPLENIC ARTERY & VEIN
IN PANCREAS TRANSPLANT LIVING RELATED DONOR

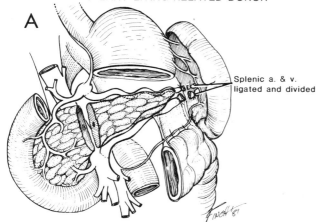

Splenic a. & v.
ligated and divided

SPLENIC ARTERIAL SUPPLY IN PANCREAS TRANSPLANT
LIVING RELATED DONOR

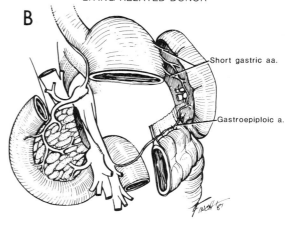

Short gastric aa.

Gastroepiploic a.

Fig 36–9.—A, technique of distal pancreatectomy in living related donor for segmental transplantation. **B,** collateral blood supply to the donor spleen is preserved. (From Sutherland D.E.R., et al.: Pancreas and islet transplantation in diabetic patients with long-term followup in selected cases, in Friedman E.A., L'Esperance F.A. (eds.): *Diabetic Renal Retinal Syndrome, Prevention and Management.* New York, Grune and Stratton, 1982, pp. 463–494. Used by permission.)

the segmental technique was used almost exclusively (Fig 36–8). With this approach, the body and tail (approximately 50%) of the pancreas are removed. The celiac axis (or splenic artery) and portal vein (or splenic vein) are used for vascular anastomoses, usually to the iliac vessels of the recipient. The recipient's splenic vessels have also been used for anastomoses, a technique that results in drainage of the graft venous effluence into the portal circulation.[28] Either a retroperitoneal or intraperitoneal approach can be used to expose the vessels of the recipient for graft placement. The technical details for removal of segmental pancreas grafts from cadaver donors, before[29, 30] or after circulatory arrest,[31] have been well described.

The segmental approach also allows for the use of living related donors for pancreas transplantation (Fig 36–9).[32] The splenic artery and vein can be ligated in the hilum of the spleen, and the spleen will survive on the collateral blood supply.[33] If the donors have normal glucose tolerance prior to hemipancreatectomy, the metabolism will remain normal postdonation.[33, 34]

In recent years, there has been a renewed interest in transplantation of the entire pancreas from cadaver donors, with or without the duodenum (Fig 36–10). The entire duodenum can be transplanted[35]; or the duodenum can be trimmed to just a bubble encompassing the portion that is most intimate with the pancreas[35]; or the pancreas can be meticulously freed from the duodenum so only the papilla of Vater is left attached[36]; or it can be completely separated so that both the common bile duct and pancreatic duct are divided before they enter into the duodenum.[36] Division of the duct before it en-

PANCREATIC TRANSPLANT DONOR

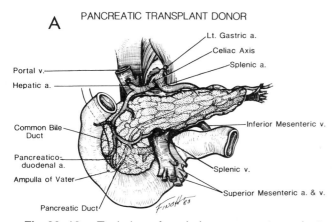

Lt. Gastric a.
Celiac Axis
Splenic a.
Portal v.
Hepatic a.
Common Bile Duct
Pancreatico-duodenal a.
Ampulla of Vater
Pancreatic Duct
Inferior Mesenteric v.
Splenic v.
Superior Mesenteric a. & v.

PANCREAS DONOR ORGAN

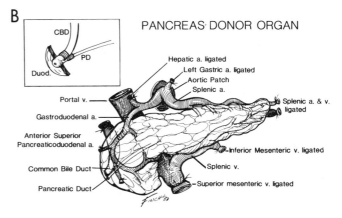

CBD
PD
Duod.
Hepatic a. ligated
Left Gastric a. ligated
Aortic Patch
Splenic a.
Portal v.
Gastroduodenal a.
Anterior Superior Pancreaticoduodenal a.
Common Bile Duct
Pancreatic Duct
Splenic a. & v. ligated
Inferior Mesenteric v. ligated
Splenic v.
Superior mesenteric v. ligated

Fig 36–10.—Technique for whole pancreas transplantation. **A,** pancreas anatomy in donor prior to excision. The duodenum can be excised en bloc with the pancreas graft for transplantation to the recipient, or **(B)** the pancreas can be entirely separated from the duodenum, or *(inset)* only the portion of the duodenum accompanying the papilla of Vater can be retained *(inset)*. (From Sutherland D.E.R., et al.: Maximization of islet mass and pancreas graft by near total or total organ excision without duodenum from cadaver donors. *Transplant. Proc.* 16:111, 1984.)

ters the duodenum obviates enteric contamination from the donor and has been used for duct management techniques that do not include drainage into a hollow viscus, while the preservation of the papilla of Vater has been exclusively with the viscus drainage techniques. Some surgeons have also left the spleen attached to the pancreas graft to increase the blood flow through the large splenic vessels, thus theoretically reducing the probability of vascular thrombosis.[35, 37]

The most important issue in pancreas transplantation is the provision made for the management of the exocrine secretions. Several methods of duct management have been used. Suppression of exocrine function and obstruction of residual secretions by polymer injection of the duct[30] has been the most widely used technique (Fig 36–11); 235 of 425 grafts transplanted since July 1, 1977, were duct-injected (55%). The complication rate for polymer injection remains relatively low, but fibrosis induced by the injected agent can involve the islets and may lead to graft failure.[38] Duct ligation was used in the first pancreas transplant case[3] and has been used sporadically since July 1, 1977 (11 cases, 3%). The pancreatic duct has also been left open to drain freely into the peritoneal cavity,[39] and the secretions are absorbed if the pancreatic enzymes are not activated (19 cases since July 1, 1977, 4%). Pancreaticoenterostomy[40] and pancreaticoductoureterostomy[29] were used in some of the earliest pancreas transplant cases. A variety of anastomotic techniques has been used, including direct insertion of the pancreatic duct into the bladder in recent cases.[18] Enteric drainage has been established most often by an intussusception technique for segmental grafts (Fig

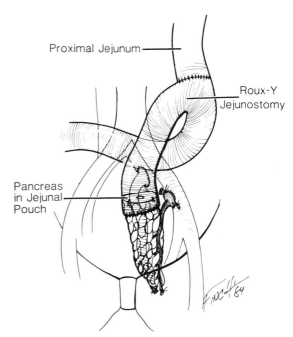

Fig 36–12.—Technique for drainage of the segmental pancreas graft exocrine secretion via a Roux-en-Y limb of recipient bowel. (From Sutherland D.E.R., Goetz F.C., Elick B.A., et al.: Pancreas and islet transplantation in diabetic patients with long-term following in selected cases, in Friedman E.A., L'Esperance F.A. (eds.): *Diabetic Renal Retinal Syndrome, Prevention and Management.* New York, Grune & Stratton, 1982, pp. 463–494.)

36–12) and by mucosal-to-mucosal anastomosis for whole pancreas[41] (Fig 36–13) or pancreaticoduodenal grafts.[35] Currently, pancreaticoenterostomy[13, 42, 43] and urinary drainage[18, 20, 44] are gaining in popularity (120 cases and 37 cases [19 ureter, 18 bladder] since July 1, 1977, 28% and 8%, respectively).

PANCREATIC DUCT JEJUNOSTOMY

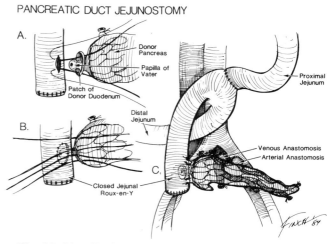

Fig 36–13.—Technique for enteric drainage of a whole pancreas graft with anastomosis of the papilla of Vater to a Roux-en-Y limb of recipient jejunum. (From Sutherland D.E.R., et al.: Pancreas transplantation, in Najarian J.S., Simmons R.L., (eds.): *Manual of Organ Transplantation.* New York, Springer-Verlag, 1984, p. 427.)

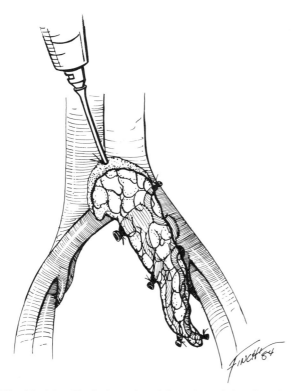

Fig 36–11.—Technique for obliteration of the ductal system by injection of a synthetic polymer immediately following revascularization of a whole pancreas transplant.

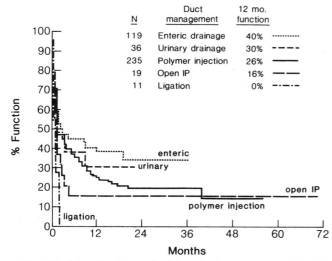

Fig 36–14.—Graft survival by duct management technique for all pancreas transplants reported to the Registry from July 1, 1977, to June 30, 1984, excluding three cases not classified due to immediate technical failure.

Except for duct ligation, all methods of duct management have been associated with long-term graft function (Fig 36–14). The one-year actuarial functional survival rates of pancreas grafts transplanted since July 1, 1977, were 40% with enteric drainage, 30% with urinary drainage, 26% with duct-injection, and 16% for intraperitoneal open duct; the differences are not statistically significant ($P > 0.1$). The methods of duct management associated with the highest patient survival rates have been ligation and enteric drainage, but again none of the differences is statistically significant (Fig 36–15).

Fifty of the transplants performed in the world between July 1, 1977, and Dec. 31, 1983, were whole-pancreas grafts (27 without and 23 with all or a portion of the duodenum). The other 376 were segmental (hemipancreas) grafts. Although the graft survival rates have been higher for whole-pancreas than for segmental grafts, the differences are not sta-

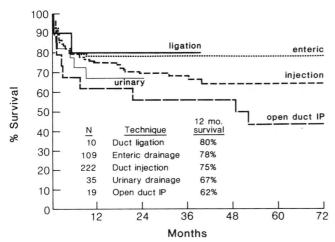

Fig 36–15.—Patient survival rates for recipients of primary pancreas transplants for cases reported to the Registry from July 1, 1977, to June 30, 1984, according to duct management technique.

tistically significant, except for those in which the duct was drained into the urinary system (Fig 36–16).

Pancreas Transplant Results According to Immunosuppression in the Recipients

Before June 30, 1977, azathioprine was used to treat all pancreas transplant recipients. Since July 1, 1977, cyclosporine has been the principal immunosuppressant in 217 recipients and azathioprine in 198 recipients of pancreas allografts. An actuarial analysis, according to immunosuppression (Fig 36–17), showed that the pancreas allograft functional survival rates were significantly higher in all patients treated with cyclosporine than with azathioprine (37% vs. 20% at one year). When technically successful transplants only were considered, the one-year pancreas allograft function rates in recipients given cyclosporine (n = 189) and azathioprine (n = 152) were 41% and 26%, respectively (Fig 36–18).

Pancreas Transplant Results According to Duration of Graft Preservation

Many of the pancreas grafts were transplanted immediately following removal from the donor. However, since July 1, 1977, the intervals between removal from the donor and transplantation to the recipient were reported on 225 grafts preserved by hypothermic storage in electrolyte solutions. An actuarial analysis showed a statistically higher functional survival rate for grafts preserved less than six hours than for those stored more than six hours (Fig 36–19). The longer storage times were associated with a higher percentage of early (less than three days) graft failures, but late losses were nearly equivalent. Thus, at one year the differences in graft survival rates were not substantial, 26% for the < 6-hour and 24% for the > 6-hour preservation groups. An earlier analysis had shown that the immediate function rates were similar for all storage times up to 24 hours.[45] The capacity to preserve pancreas grafts has greatly facilitated the logistical aspects of pancreas transplantation.[46]

PANCREAS TRANSPLANT EXPERIENCE AT THE UNIVERSITY OF MINNESOTA

Transplants of immediately vascularized pancreas grafts or of free grafts of islet tissue have been performed at the University of Minnesota since 1966.[27, 47] There have been two series each of pancreas and islet transplants. In neither of the islet transplant series (ten cases each) did any recipients become permanently insulin-independent.[48, 49]

The first series of pancreas transplants was from 1966 through 1973.[10] Only one recipient survived for greater than one year with a functioning pancreas graft.[50] The most recent series began in July 25, 1978,[39] and through June 30, 1984, included 94 pancreas transplants performed in 82 diabetic patients. The results in this series have been periodically reported.[9, 11, 34, 42, 51, 52]

Patient Population, Transplant Technique, and Immunosuppression

Of the 82 patients undergoing pancreas transplantation in the most recent University of Minnesota series, 43 had functioning renal grafts (42 allografts, one isograft) placed six

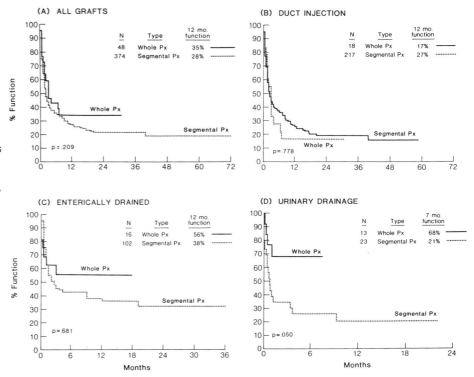

Fig 36–16.—Functional survival rate of whole pancreas vs. segmental pancreas grafts reported to the Registry from July 1, 1977, to June 30, 1984, for *(A)* all cases, *(B)* duct injected grafts, *(C)* enteric-drained grafts, and *(D)* urinary-drained grafts.

months to nine years previously for treatment of ESDN. Thirty-nine patients were nonuremic and had not received kidney grafts at the time of the pancreas transplant. Fifty-six of the 94 pancreas grafts came from cadaver donors (60%) and 38 came from living related donors (40%). Seventy-two grafts were segmental (all of those from living related and 32 from cadaver donors), while 22 were cadaveric grafts of the whole pancreas as previously described.[36, 41] Twenty-four grafts (11 cadaver, 13 related) failed for technical reasons (9 thrombosis, 7 infections, 3 inadequate preservation, 3 ascites, 2 bleeding). All of the pancreas grafts were placed intraperitoneally.

Four different techniques were used for management of the pancreatic duct (Table 36–2). Enteric drainage into a Roux-en-Y limb of recipient jejunum is now preferred.

We have previously described in detail the immunosuppressive protocols used in our patients.[9, 52–54] Twenty-three recipients of pancreas allografts were treated with azathioprine (AZA), prednisone, and antilymphocyte globulin (ALG); 7 were treated with AZA and prednisone only; 9 were treated with cyclosporine (CSA) (and usually prednisone) after an initial course of conventional (AZA, prednisone, ALG) immunosuppression; 36 were treated with CSA and prednisone begin-

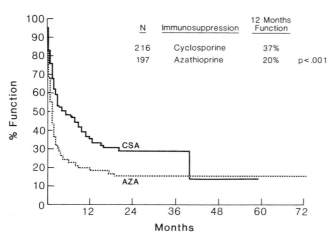

Fig 36–17.—Pancreas allograft functional survival rates according to principal immunosuppressant used in the recipients for all cases reported to the Registry between July 1, 1977, and June 30, 1984.

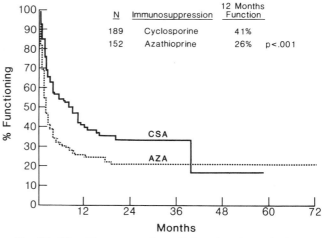

Fig 36–18.—Pancreas allograft functional survival rates according to principal immunosuppressant used in recipients of technically successful transplants only reported to the Registry between July 1, 1977, and June 30, 1984.

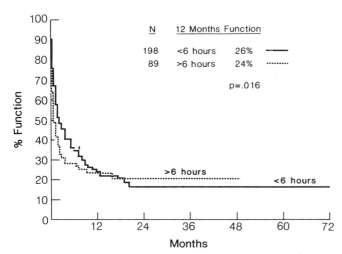

Fig 36–19.—Pancreas graft functional survival rates according to preservation time for transplants from cadaver donors reported to the Registry between July 1, 1977, and June 30, 1984. (From Sutherland D.E.R., Kendall D.M.: Clinical pancreas and islet transplant registry report. *Transplant. Proc.*[1])

ning immediately after transplantation; and 13 patients received a combination of CSA, AZA, and prednisone (triple therapy; see Table 36–2). Four patients were treated with CSA for the first three to six months posttransplant and were then switched to AZA. One of the converted patients had no change in grafts function and is currenty insulin-independent with a functioning graft at more than two years after transplantation. The other three switched patients experienced decline of graft function and resumed exogenous insulin two to six months after conversion. Fifteen grafts in the conventionally immunosuppressed patients failed for technical reasons, while seven grafts in the CSA group were lost to technical failure.

Current Status of Pancreas Transplant Recipients at the University of Minnesota

As of August 1984, 67 of 82 patients were alive (82%), and 27 had full function (22 cases, receive no exogenous insulin)

or partial function (5 cases, have C-peptide levels along baseline and are no longer ketosis prone but require supplemental insulin to maintain normoglycemia) of their pancreas grafts (33%). Twenty grafts have functioned for longer than one year, of which 18 are still functioning, the longest for 6.1 years. Sixteen of the 27 currently functioning grafts are from living related donors.[34]

In 36 instances the pancreas grafts functioned for one to 12 months before hyperglycemia recurred and the recipients had to resume permaenently exogenous insulin. Grafts biopsies were performed in 16 cases at the time of or a few months after loss of function and showed rejection in 13 instances.[54a] In three instances (including two isografts with insulitis) it appeared that specific β-cell destruction resulted in recurrence of diabetes independent of rejection,[42, 55, 56] most likely because of an autoimmune insulitis.[54, 55]

Hyperglycemia that occurred weeks or months after transplantation was presumptively diagnosed as rejection in 24 graft recipients (10 from related, 14 from cadaver donors). Rejection episodes were treated with either an increase in prednisone dose or with administration of antilymphocyte globulin.[9, 52, 53] Four recipients of related and three recipients of cadaver grafts reverted to euglycemia after antirejection treatment and are currently insulin-independent.

The results of oral glucose tolerance tests and metabolic profiles in most of the insulin-independent patients with functioning grafts are normal or nearly normal.[9, 11, 22, 34, 52] There is great variability, however, in the response of individual patients (Fig 36–20). The patient whose grafts has functioned the longest (now 73 months posttransplant) has normal glucose tolerance test results at 2, 3, and 4 years, while the results were abnormal at 1 and 5 years (Fig 36–20,C). That absolutely normal metabolic profiles and glucose tolerance test (both oral and IV) results occur in some pancreas transplant recipients (Fig 36–21) means that the denervated state of the graft or drainage of the venous effluent into the systemic circulation are not by themselves responsible for the abnormalities seen in other recipients.

All 38 related donors of segmental pancreas grafts are currently alive. Two donors (5%) required reoperation, one for a splenectomy and one to ligate the pancreatic duct at the line of transection. Glucose tolerance tests results changed in

TABLE 36–2.—OUTCOME AFTER PANCREAS TRANSPLANTATION IN 1978–84 MINNESOTA CASES ACCORDING
TO TECHNIQUE, DONOR SOURCE, AND IMMUNOSUPPRESSION

TECHNIQUE	NO. OF TXS (REL/CAD)	IM. SUP.* C/A/T	TECHNICAL FAILURES	LATE LOSS† OF FUNCTION	GRAFTS NO.	CURRENTLY FUNCTIONING‡ DURATION IN MOS
Duct ligated	3 (0/3)	0/3/0	3 (100%)	0 (0%)	0 (0%)	—
Open peritoneal	15 (5/10)	1/14/0	8 (53%)	4 (27%)	3 (20%)	57(A)ᶜ, 61(A)ʳ, 73(A)ᶜ
Enteric	37 (28/9)	15/9/11	10 (27%)	6 (16%)	19 (51%)	2(T)ʳ, 2(T)ᶜ, 3(T)ᶜ, 5(A)ʳ, 5(T)ᶜ, 8(T)ᶜ, 8(T)ʳ, 12(T)ᶜ, 12(T)ᶜ, 13(A)ʳ, 13(C)ʳ, 16(C)ʳ, 16(A)ʳ, 17(A)ʳ, 21(C)ʳ, 25(C)ʳ, 31(C)ʳ, 34(A)ʳ, 36(C)ʳ
Duct-injection	39 (5/34)	29/8/1	3 (8%)	28 (72%)	5 (13%)	15(T)ᶜ, 21(A)ʳ, 23(C)ᶜ, 31(C)ᶜ, 44(A)ʳ
Total	94 (38/56)	45/34/12	24 (26%)	38 (40%)	27 (37%)	2–73

*The patients received prednisone in addition to either cyclosporine (C), azathioprine (A), or triple therapy (T, combination of cyclosporine and azathioprine).

†Does not include 4 patients with technically successful transplants (2 duct-inj., 2 enterically drained) who died with functioning grafts. As of August 1984, 16/38 (42%) related and 11/56 (20%) cadaver grafts were fuctioning. Of technically successful allografts, 9/17 (53%) treated with azathioprine, 9/40 (23%) with cyclosporine, and 9/10 (90%) with triple therapy are functioning.

‡Immunosuppression in parenthesis (C, A, or T), and donor source cadaverᶜ or relatedʳ, as superscripts.

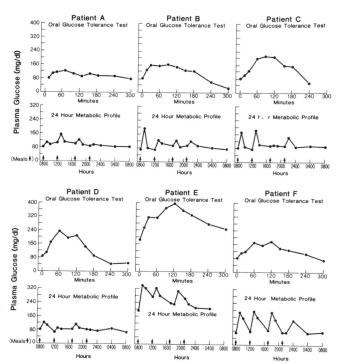

Fig 36–20.—Results of metabolic studies (glucose tolerance tests and 24-hour profiles) in the absence of exogenous insulin in six recipients of segmental pancreas transplants functioning at > 12 months, illustrating the variability in response of individual patients. **Patient A,** *12 months posttransplant,* has both a normal glucose tolerance test (GTT) results and a normal metabolic profile during a day of normal meals and activity. **Patient B,** *36 months posttransplant,* is normal except for a slight hypoglycemic trend at 4–5 hours during the GTT. **Patient C,** at *60 months posttransplant,* has an abnormal GTT with elevated 2 hour glucose value, but *is* euglycemic through a day of standard meals and activity. **Patient D,** *24 months posttransplant,* has abnormal GTT (with both hyperglycemia and hypoglycemia), but displays a normal 24 hour glucose profile. **Patient E,** *36 months posttransplant,* has highly abnormal GTT as well as fasting and postprandial hyperglycemia during a day of normal meals and activity. **Patient F,** *12 months posttransplant,* has a normal GTT but an abnormal profile with elevated postprandial glucose during 24-hour profile. (From Sutherland D.M., Kendall D.M., Goetz F.C., et al.: Pancreas transplantation in man. *Diabetes Annu.* In press.)

some donors postoperatively, but were physiologically significant in only one obese donor.[33]

Comments

The current protocol for pancreas transplantation at the University of Minnesota has been derived from lessons learned during 128 attempts at endocrine replacement therapy in 109 patients since 1966. The experience includes 12 pancreaticoduodenal, 20 islet, 23 whole, and 73 segmental pancreas transplants. At this time, we offer pancreas transplants to patients whose diabetic complications are, or poten-

tially will be, more serious than the possible side effects of long-term immunosuppression. Thirty-nine of the 82 patients who received transplants since 1978 were nonuremic, nonkidney transplant recipients (48%), including 21 of 30 (70%) in 1983 and the first half of 1984. Early nephropathy or progressive neuropathy or retinopathy were indications for pancreas transplantation in these patients. Fifteen of the 27 patients whose grafts are currently functioning (56%) had not received previous kidney grafts.

We have focused most of our efforts on simply achieving an acceptable pancreas graft functional survival rate with a low morbidity and mortality rate. At this time it is our preference to drain exocrine pancreas secretions into a hollow viscus, and enteric drainage is the most physiologic method.

The diagnosis of rejection can be particularly difficult, as noted by other groups.[57] Home monitoring of plasma glucose levels and early use of a graft biopsy have been the most useful indicators of rejection in our series.[9, 54]

We are following up the recipients closely for the effect of the procedure on secondary complications. Observations (unpublished) on kidney biopsies in two patients, followed up for longer than four years after successful pancreas transplantation, suggest that the progression of renal lesions can be prevented and that early lesions may actually regress. Certain aspects of our protocols, including the use of cyclosporine for recipient immunosuppression[53] and pancreaticoenterostomy[42] for management of exocrine function, are similar to those of other groups[13, 43, 58] applying pancreas transplantation to the treatment of diabetes.

However, our treatment of uremic diabetic patients differs from most groups performing pancreas transplantation. We do not place kidney and pancreas grafts simultaneously. Kidney transplantation alone will rehabilitate most uremic diabetics,[26, 59] and simultaneous pancreas and kidney grafting does not improve renal graft survival rates.[24] Thus, we delay pancreas transplantation until the renal graft is well established, and perform the procedure only in patients whose rehabilitation will be further enhanced by correction of diabetes.

Pancreas transplantation should, if possible, be accomplished much earlier in the course of the disease than has been the case for most recipients. Since generalized immunosuppression is required to prevent rejection, this approach cannot be taken unless the patients clearly have or are developing serious secondary complications.

In summary, of 94 pancreas transplants performed in 82 diabetic patients at the University of Minnesota since 1978, 27 patients currently (as of August 1984) have functioning pancreas grafts. Twenty patients have functioning grafts longer than one year posttransplant. Simultaneous advances in immunosuppressive therapy, in surgical technique, and in patient selection criteria have been associated with a progressive increase in the success rate of pancreas transplantation at our institution.[52]

DISCUSSION

Nearly one third of the pancreas transplants performed worldwide since 1966 were done in 1983 and the first half of 1984, emphasizing the renewed interest in pancreas trans-

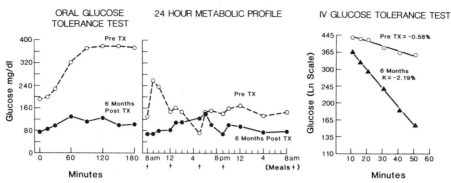

Fig 36–21.—Results of metabolic profiles and oral and IV glucose tolerance tests before and six months after a segmental pancreas transplant with enteric drainage of the pan- creatic duct and systemic drainage of the graft venous effluent. The results after transplantation are entirely normal.

plantation in recent years. The success rate is steadily improving, and long-term graft function with normal or near-normal glucose metabolism has been sustained in several patients. Ultimately, pancreas transplantation could have the same impact on the treatment of diabetes as kidney transplantation has had on the treatment of end-stage renal disease. Pancreas transplantation may also provide information answering many fundamental questions related to the nature of diabetes mellitus.[60]

Most pancreas graft recipients have had far advanced secondary complications of diabetes prior to transplantation. Ideally, pancreas transplantation should be performed early in the stages of the disease. There is some tendency in this direction, particularly in the recent Minnesota series.

Immunologic barriers have been the greatest hindrance to successful pancreas transplantation. The use of cyclosporine has been associated with an improvement in the results of pancreas transplantation (see Figs 36–16 and 36–17). However, the success rate is still much lower than that reported for kidney transplantation.[15] Cyclosporine is also a generalized immunosuppressive agent that has adverse side effects. Nevertheless, the use of cyclosporine has expanded the patient population that can be considered for pancreas transplantation.

Clinical attempts at islet allotransplantation have been unsuccessful.[1] The manipulations that can lead to a relatively high success rate in experimental animals models[61] may not be applicable in the clinical situation. Islet transplantation is not simpler for the transplant team. It is very difficult to procure a sufficient quantity of viable islet tissue from a single donor pancreas, and techniques to alter graft immunogenicity must be made practical. If the methods currently being used in animals are effective for human islet isolation and reduction of immunogenicity,[62] a rational basis for attempts at clinical islet transplantation will be established, but it is unlikely that clinical islet transplantation will be successful in the immediate future.

Pancreas transplants are being performed in diabetic patients subjected to rigorous selection criteria at this time. Because generalized immunosuppression is needed to prevent rejection, pancreas transplantation has been restricted to patients whose secondary complications of diabetes are, or pre-

dictably will be, more serious than the potential side effects of antirejection therapy. Patients who have had or who require a kidney transplant meet this criteria and are also obligated to immunosuppressive therapy. However, many nonuremic, nonkidney transplant patients also and such as those with preproliferative retinopathy have serious complications are thus at great risk for loss of vision.

When a specific immune response in humans can be abrogated, and when the risks of transplantation are minimal, the limiting factor will be the availability of donor pancreases. This problem is solveable. In the United States more than 5,000 kidney transplants are done each year.[63] The incidence of new cases of type I diabetes is approximately 10,000/year in the United States, and fewer than half of the patients with the disease develop serious complications.[64]

Thus, the current kidney transplant rate is the same as the yearly incidence of complication-prone type I diabetes. Only a small proportion of potential donors are currently used as a source of organs.[65] However, there is no inherent reason why donor procurement should be any more difficult for pancreas transplantation than for kidney transplantation. Measurement of joint stiffness[66] or of insulin-like growth factors[67] might identify diabetic patients who are at high risk to develop secondary complications. It should be possible also to identify diabetics who have impaired counter-regulatory mechanisms and who are at high risk for hypoglycemic reactions while on insulin pump or other intensified insulin therapy regimens.[6] Patients with these characteristics[6, 66, 67] are those most likely to benefit from a pancreas transplant. A sufficient number of pancreases from cadaver and related donors should be available for this select group.

In conclusion, pancreas transplantation is becoming increasingly effective for the treatment of human diabetes. Islet transplantation has been successful only in the laboratory. Until islet yield can be improved and methods to reduce immunogenicity can be made practical, pancreas transplantation is the only practical method of total endocrine replacement therapy that can succeed in diabetes. Pancreas transplantation has the potential to be applied on as large a scale as renal transplantation. Eventually, pancreas transplantation could be routinely performed at a stage sufficiently early to prevent the development of diabetic nephropathy and could supersede kidney transplantation in the management of complication-prone diabetic patients.

ADDENDUM

Two pancreas transplants, one performed at Institution No. 37 (whole organ preserved < 6 hours, transplanted after a previous kidney, with enteric drainage in an azathioprine treated recipient) in the last half of 1983 and one at Institution No. 40 (segmental grafts preserved > 6 hours, transplanted simultaneously with a kidney, and drained into the urinary system of a cyclosporine treated recipient), were reported to the Registry after Aug. 1, 1984, the date of this analysis, and were not included in the calculations for Figures 36–2 to 36–7 and 36–14 to 36–19. Since both failed within six weeks of transplantation for technical reasons, their exclusion does not alter the results reported.

ACKNOWLEDGMENTS

Martin Finch and associates, Department of Biomedical Graphics, University of Minnesota prepared the illustrations. Janet Sanders prepared the manuscript.

REFERENCES

1. Sutherland D.E.R., Kendall D.: Clinical pancreas and islet transplant registry report. *Transplant. Proc.* 17:307, 1985.
2. Sutherland D.E.R.: Pancreas and islet transplantation registry data. *World J. Surg.* 8:270, 1984.
3. Kelly W.D., Lillehei R.C., Merkel F.K., et al.: Allotransplantation of the pancreas and duodenum along with the kidney in diabetic nephropathy. *Surgery* 61:827, 1967.
4. Brownlee M.C., Cahill G.F.: Diabetic control and vascular complications, vol. 4, in Paoletti R., Gatto A.M. (eds.): Atherosclerotic Reviews. New York, Raven Press, 1979 p. 29.
5. Ungar R.H.: Meticulous control of diabetes: Benefits, risks and precautions. *Diabetes* 31:479, 1982.
6. White N., Skor D.A., Cryer P.E., et al.: Identification or Type I diabetic patients at increased risk for hypoglycemia during intensive therapy. *N. Engl. J. Med.* 308:485, 1983.
7. Gerrish E.W.: Final Newsletter. American College of Surgeons/National Institutes of Health Organ Transplant Registry, June 30, 1977.
8. Sutherland D.E.R.: International human pancreas and islet transplant registry. *Transplant. Proc.* 12(suppl. 2):229, 1980.
9. Sutherland D.E.R., Goetz F.C., Najarian J.S.: 100 pancreas transplants at a single institution. *Ann. Surg.* 200:414, 1984.
10. Lillehei R.C., Ruiz J.O., Acquino C., et al.: Transplantation of the pancreas. *Acta Endocrinol.* 83(suppl. 205):303, 1976.
11. Sutherland D.E.R., Goetz R.C., Najarian J.S.: Recent experience with 89 pancreas transplants between 1978 and 1983. *Diabetologia* 27:149, 1984.
12. Dubernard J.M., Traeger J., Bodi E., et al.: Transplantation for the treatment of insulin-dependent diabetes: Clinical experience with polymer-obstructed pancreatic grafts using Neoprene. *World J. Surg.* 8:262, 1984.
13. Groth C.G., Tyden G., Lundgren G., et al.: Segmental pancreas transplantation with enteric exocrine diversion. *World J. Surg.* 8:257, 1984.
14. Land W., Illner W.D., Abendroth D., et al.: Experience with segmental pancreas transplants in cyclosporine treated diabetic patients using Ethibloc for duct obliteration. *Transplant. Proc.* 16:729, 1984.
15. Calne R.Y., White D.J.G.: The use of cyclosporine in clinical organ grafting. *Ann. Surg.* 196:330, 1982.
16. Baumgartner D., Largiader F.: Simultaneous renal and intraperitoneal segmental pancreatic transplantation. *World J. Surg.* 8:267, 1984.
17. Toledo-Pereyra L.H. Pancreas transplantation. *Surg. Gynecol. Obset.* 157:49, 1983.
18. Sollinger H.W., Cook K., Kamps D., et al.: Clinical and experimental experience with pancreaticocystostomy for exocrine pancreatic drainage in pancreas transplantation. *Transplant. Proc.* 16:749, 1984.
19. McMaster P., Michael J., Adu D., et al.: Experience in human segmental pancreas transplantation. *World J. Surg.* 8:253, 1984.
20. Munda R., First M.R., Webb C.B., et al.: Clinical experience with segmental pancreatic allografts. *Transplant. Proc.* 16:692, 1984.
21. Sutherland D.E.R., Goetz F.C., Najarian J.S.: Pancreas transplantation. *Clin. Endocrinol. Metab.* 11:549, 1982.
22. Sutherland D.E.R., Najarian J.S., Greenberg B.Z., et al.: Hormonal and metabolic effects of an encodrine graft: Vascularized segmental transplantation on the pancreas in insulin-dependent patients. *Ann. Intern. Med.* 95:537, 1981.
23. Pozza G., Traeger J., Dubernard J.M., et al.: Endocrine responses of Type I (insulin-dependent) diabetic patients following successful pancreas transplantation. *Diabetologia* 24:244, 1983.
24. Sutherland D.E.R., Kendall D.: Important issues in clinical pancreas transplantation. *Transplant. Today* 2:56–67, 1985.
25. Standards Committee of the American Society of Transplant Surgeons: Current results and expectations of renal transplantation. *J.A.M.A.* 246:133, 1981.
26. Sutherland D.E.R., Morrow C.E.. Fryd D.S., et al.: Improved patient and primary renal allograft survival in uremic diabetic recipients. *Transplantation* 34:319, 1982.
27. Lillehei R.C., Simmons R.L., Najarian J.S., et al.: Pancreaticoduodenal allotransplantation: Experimental and clinical experience. *Ann. Surg.* 172:405–436, 1970.
28. Calne R.Y.: Paratopic segmental pancreas grafting: A technique with portal venous drainage. *Lancet* 1:595–597, 1984.
29. Gliedman M.L., Gold M., Whittaker J., et al.: Clinical segmental pancreatic transplantation with ureter–pancreatic duct anastomosis for exocrine drainage. *Surgery* 74:171–180, 1973.
30. Dubernard J.M., Traeger J., Neyra P., et al.: A new method of preparation of segmental pancreatic grafts for transplantation: Trials in dogs and in man. *Surgery* 84:633, 1978.
31. Bjorken C., Lundgren G., Ringden O., et al.: A technique for rapid harvesting of cadaveric renal and pancreatic grafts after circulating arrest. *Br. J. Surg.* 63:517–519, 1976.
32. Sutherland D.E.R., Goetz F.C., Najarian J.S.: Living related donor segmental pancreatectomy for transplantation. *Transpl. Proc.* 12(suppl. 2): 33–39, 1980.
33. Chinn P., Sutherland D.E.R., Goetz F.C., et al.: Metabolic effects of hemipancreatectomy in living related graft donors. *Transplant. Proc.* 16:11, 1984.
34. Sutherland D.E.R., Goetz F.C., Najarian J.S.: Pancreas transplants from related donors. *Transplantation* 38:625, 1984.
35. Starzl T.E., Iwatsuki S., Shaw B.W.: pancreaticoduodenal transplantation in humans. *Surg. Gynecol. Obstet.* 159:265, 1984.
36. Sutherland D.E.R., Chinn P.L., Elick B.A., et al.: Maximization of islet mass in pancreas grafts by near total or total whole organ excision without duodenum from cadaver donors. *Transplant. Proc.* 16:111, 1984.
37. Sollinger H., Kalayoglu M., Hoffman R.: Results of segmental and pancreaticosplenic transplantation with pancreatio-cystostomy. *Transplant. Proc.* 17:360–362, 1985.
38. Blanc-Brunat N., Dubernard J.M., Touraine J.L., et al.: pathology of the pancreas after intraductal neoprene injection in dogs and diabetic patients treated by pancreatic transplantation. *Diabetologia* 25:97, 1983.
39. Sutherland D.E.R., Goetz F.C., Najarian J.S.: Intraperitoneal transplantation of immediately vascularized segmental pancreatic grafts without duct ligation: A clinical trial. *Transplantation* 28:485, 1979.
40. Groth C.G., Lundgren G., Arner P., et al.: Rejection of isolated pancreatic allografts in patients with diabetes. *Surg. Gynecol. Obstet.* 143:933–940, 1976.
41. Sutherland D.E.R., Ascher N.L., Najarian J.S.: Pancreas transplantation, in Najarian, J.S., Simmons R.L. (eds.): *Manual of Organ Transplantation.* New York, Springer-Verlag, 1984, p. 237.

42. Sutherland D.E.R., Goetz F.C., Elick B.A., et al.: Experience with 49 segmental pancreas transplants in 45 diabetic patients. *Transplantation* 34:330, 1982.
43. Calne R.Y., White D.J.G.. Rolles K., et al.: Renal and segmental pancreatic grafting with drainage of exocrine secretions and initial continuous intravenous cyclosporin A in a patients with insulin-dependent diabetes and renal failure. *Br. Med. J.* 285:677.
44. Gil-Vernet J.M., Fernandez-Cruz L., Andreu J., et al.: Clinical experience with pancreaticopyelostomy for exocrine pancreatic drainage and portal venous drainage in pancreas transplantation. *Transplant. Proc.* 17:342, 1985.
45. Sutherland D.E.R.: Current status of clinical pancreas and islet transplantation with comments on need for and complications of cyrogenic and other preservation techniques. *Cryobiology* 20:245, 1983.
46. Florack G., Sutherland D.E.R., Chinn P.L., et al.: Clinical experience with transplantation of hypothermically preserved pancreas grafts. *Transplant. Proc.* 16:153, 1984.
47. Najarian J.S., Sutherland D.E.R., Matas A.J., et al.: Human islet transplantation: A preliminary experience. *Transplant. Proc.* 9:233–236, 1977.
48. Sutherland D.E.R., Matas A.J., Najarian J.S.: Pancreatic islet cell transplantation. *Surg. Clin. North Am.* 58:365–382, 1978.
49. Sutherland D.E.R., Matas A.J., Goetz F.C., et al.: Transplantation of dispersed pancreatic islet tissue in humans: Autografts and allografts. *Diabetes* 29(suppl. 1):34, 1980.
50. Sutherland D.E.R., Goetz F.C., Carpenter A.M., et al.: Pancreaticoduodenal grafts: Clinical and pathological observations in uremic versus nonuremic recipients in Touraine J.L., et al. (eds.): *Transplantation and Clinical Immunology*, Amsterdam, Excerpta Medica, 1979, vol. X, pp. 90–195.
51. Sutherland D.E.R., Goetz F.C., Ryansiewicz J.J., et al.: Segmental pancreas tansplantation from living related and cadaver donors: A clinical experience. *Surgery* 90:159, 1981.
52. Sutherland D.E.R., Goetz F.C., Kendall D.M., et al.: Effect of donor source, technique, immunosuppression and presence or absence of end stage diabetic nephropathy on outcome in pancreas transplant recipients. *Transplant. Proc.* 17:325, 1985.
53. Sutherland D.E.R., Chinn P.L., Goetz F.C., et al.: Experience with cyclosporine vs. azathioprine for pancreas transplantation. *Transplant. Proc.* 15:2606, 1983.
54. Rynasiewicz J.J., Sutherland D.E.R., Ferguson R.M., et al.: Cyclosporin A for immunosuppression: Observations in rat heart, pancreas and islet allograft models and in human renal and pancreas transplantation. *Diabetes* 31(suppl. 4):92–108, 1982.
54a. Sibley R.K., Mukai K.: Pathological features in 29 segmental pancreas transplants in 27 diabetic patients. *Lab. Invest.* 48:78A, 1983.
55. Sutherland D.E.R., Sibley R.K., Chinn P.L., et al.: Identical twin pancreas transplants: Reversal and recurrence of pathogenesis in Type I diabetes. *Clin. Res.* 32(2):561A, 1984.
56. Sibley R.K., Sutherland D.E.R., Goetz F.C.: Recurrence of Type I diabetes mellitus in pancreatic allografts and isografts. *Lab. Invest.* 50:54A, 1984.
57. Secchi A., Pontiroli A.E., Traeger J., et al.: A method of detection of graft failure in pancreas transplantation. *Transplantation* 35:344, 1983.
58. Traeger J., Bosi E., Dubernard J.M., et al.: Thirty months experience with cyclosporine in human pancreatic transplantation. *Diabetologia* 27:154–156, 1984.
59. Sutherland D.E.R., Bentley F.R., Mauer S.M., et al.: A report of 26 diabetic renal allograft recipients alive with functioning grafts at 10 or more years after primary transplantation. *Diabetic Nephropathy* 3:39–43, 1984.
60. Barker C.F., Naji A., Perloff L.J., et al.: Invited commentary: An overview of pancreas transplantation—biologic aspects. *Surgery* 92:113, 1982.
61. Faustman D., Hauptfeld V., Lacy P., et al.: Prolongation of murine islet allograft survival by pretreatment of islets with antibody directed to Ia determinants. *Proc. Natl. Acad. Sci. U.S.A.* 78(8):5156, 1981.
62. Clark W.H. (ed.): Proceedings of a workshop on preventing rejection of transplanted pancreas or islets. *Diabetes* 31(suppl. 4):1, 1982.
63. Health Care Financing Administration (HCFA) Office of Special Programs. End-Stage Renal Disease Program Medical Information System, Facility Survey Tables, Department of health and Human Services, USA, HCFA. Jan. 1-Dec. 31, 1981.
64. West K.M.: *Epidemiology of Diabetes and its Vascular Lesions.* New York, Elsevier, 1978.
65. Bart K.J., Macon E.J., Whittier F.C., et al.: Cadaveric kidneys for transplantation: A paradox of shortage in the face of plenty. *Transplantation* 31:374, 1981.
66. Rosenbloom A.L., Silverstein J.H., Lezotte D.C., et al.: Limited joint mobililty in childhood diabetes mellitus indicates increased risk for microvascular disease. *N. Engl. J. Med.* 305:191, 1981.
67. Merimee T.J., Zapf J., Froesch E.R.: Insulin-like growth factors: Studies in diabetes with and without retinopathy. *N. Engl. J. Med.* 309:527, 1983.

37

Endocrine Tumors of the Pancreas

E. Christopher Ellison, M.D.
Peter J. Fabri, M.D.
William R. Gower, Jr., Ph.D.

Hormone-producing tumors of the pancreas are rare, and it can be expected that a single physician would take care of no more than one or perhaps two in his lifetime. However, they are of great interest because each of the clinical syndromes is an experiment in nature, demonstrating the pathophysiologic consequences of excessive GI hormone production. These tumors challenge both diagnosis and treatment. Although the availability of radioimmunoassay has facilitated diagnosis, clinical manifestations are so similar to more common syndromes, such as hypoglycemia, diabetes, gallstones, diarrhea, and peptic ulcer, that identification remains elusive. Treatment is multidisciplinary, involving the principles of endocrinology, gastroenterology, surgery, and oncology. Therapy is directed at correction of the aberrant physiology, then resection of the tumor, and finally control of metastatic disease with chemotherapy.

CLASSIFICATION

Endocrine tumors of the pancreas are classified, named, and defined according to: (1) embryologic characteristics (APUD concept); (2) derivation of the tumor from β or non-β islet cells; (3) whether or not the tumor produces a hormone; (4) the major hormone produced; (5) the clinical syndrome associated with the excessive hormone production; (6) eponyms; and (7) association with multiple endocrine neoplastic syndromes (MEN 1 and MEN 2) (Table 37–1). Figure 37–1 shows the clinical syndromes related to pancreatic APUD tumors.

The APUD Concept

It has been proposed that the endocrine cells of the gut originate from the neural crest and share common biochemical and ultrastructural features related to polypeptide and amine synthesis.[1] These are termed APUD cells. The acronym APUD is derived from the initial letters of the three most important properties of these cells: (1) high content of amine, (2) capacity for amine precursor uptake, and (3) the presence of amino acid decarboxylase. Description of the other characteristics of these cells is beyond the scope of this text. These cells have been identified within the CNS and in the pancreas, intestine, thyroid (parafollicular cells), adrenal medulla, and the urogenital system. APUD cells are found in any organ with the capacity to produce peptide hormones or transmitters.

Tumors arising from the APUD cells are termed apudomas.[2] Pancreatic endocrine tumors are composed of APUD cells and hence may be considered apudomas. Histologically, they may appear as adenomas, carcinomas, or hyperplastic lesions. The neoplastic cells are similar to undifferentiated embryologic precursors and therefore have a multipotential capacity for the production of peptide. This explains, in part, the production of multiple hormones by a single pancreatic endocrine tumor. These APUD cells are distributed throughout the endocrine glands, and a generalized derangement of the APUD system may result in neoplastic change and hyperfunction of multiple endocrine organs, as is observed in the MEN syndromes. Recent acceptable experimental evidence has questioned the neural crest origin of gut and pancreatic APUD cells.[3] In spite of this controversy, the application of the APUD concept explains the diverse and bizarre clinical syndromes that may be associated with endocrine tumors of the pancreas.

Functional-Nonfunctional

Functional endocrine tumors are best named according to the major hormone produced by the tumor. They may be further defined by cell type and associated clinical syndrome (see Table 37–1). Some neoplasms have the gross and histologic appearance of an endocrine tumor, but do not seem to produce a specific hormone. Designation as a nonfunctional islet cell tumor requires the demonstration of normal serum levels of multiple hormones, including insulin, gastrin, vasoactive intestinal peptide (VIP), glucagon, somatostatin, pancreatic polypeptide,[4] neuron-specific enolase,[5] neurotensin, and beta human chorionic gonadotropin (β-HCG). In addition, immunocytochemical staining of the tumor should show no hormone-producing cells. It is important to ascertain whether a hormone is produced by the tumor, since the peptide could serve as a marker to follow response to therapy and disease progression.

TABLE 37–1.—CLASSIFICATION OF PANCREATIC ENDOCRINE TUMORS (APUDOMAS)

TUMOR NAME	CELL TYPE	MAJOR HORMONE(S)	SYNDROMES	EPONYM	ASSOCIATED WITH MULTIPLE ENDOCRINE NEOPLASIA (MEN 1)
Functional tumors					
Insulinoma	β islet cell	Insulin	Hypoglycemic		Yes, MEN 1
Gastrinoma	Non-β islet cell ? D-cell	Gastrin	Ulcerogenic	Zollinger-Ellison syndrome	Yes, MEN 1 & 2
Vipoma	Non-β islet cell	Vasoactive intestinal polypeptide Pancreatic polypeptide	Watery diarrhea, hypokalemia, achlorhydria	Verner-Morrison syndrome	Yes, MEN 1
Glucagonoma	Non-β islet cell α-cell	Glucagon	Hyperglycemic Cutaneous	—	Yes (rare) MEN 1 & 2
Somatostatinoma	Non-β islet cell D-cell	Somatostatin	Hyperglycemic Steatorrhea	—	Yes (rare) MEN 1 & 2
Pancreatic-Polypeptide	Non-β islet cell	Pancreatic polypeptide	No recognized clinical syndrome	—	Yes, MEN 1
Nonfunctional tumors					
—	Islet cell tumor	None	None	None	No

PATHOLOGY

Endocrine tumors of the pancreas have variable gross characteristics and a similar microscopic appearance.

Insulinomas are most frequently small benign adenomas and hence differ from the other endocrine tumors, which are usually malignant. Eighty to ninety percent are single lesions. In the experience from the Mayo Clinic, 70% are smaller than 1.5 cm, hence, localization at operation is difficult.[6] Benign adenomas are evenly distributed throughout the pancreas: head, 30%; body, 35%; tail, 35%. The tumors may be present on the surface of the gland or located within the pancreatic substance. Most of the lesions are covered by a thin rim of normal pancreatic tissue. Characteristically they are more firm than normal pancreas, and on cut section have a typical reddish brown color. Multiple lesions occur in about 10% of cases. This is more common in patients with multiple endocrine neoplasia. Hyperplasia of the islets or nesidioblastosis (neoformation of islet cells from the pancreatic ducts) is present in about 1% of cases. Approximately 10% of insulinomas are malignant and have metastasized at the time of diagnosis. Lesions outside the pancreas are rare. The condition is rare in children. In children less than 1 year of age, hyperplasia and nesidioblastosis are more common than insulinoma. Hypoglycemia and hyperinsulinemia after that age is usually caused by an islet cell adenoma.[7] The nonbeta islet cell tumors differ from insulinomas in that there are frequently multiple primary tumors, and the majority are malignant.

Forty percent of gastrin-producing tumors are associated with multiple primary lesions occurring in the pancreas, duo-

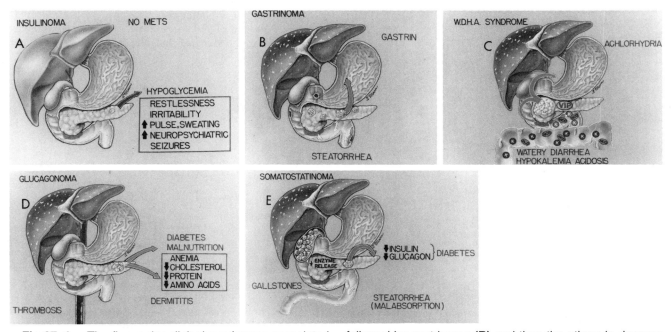

Fig 37–1.—The five major clinical syndromes associated with pancreatic apudomas. Insulinoma **(A)** is most common, followed by gastrinoma **(B)** and then the others in decreasing order of frequency **(C–E).**

denum, pylorus, antrum, or peripancreatic lymph nodes. Both sporadic gastrinomas and those associated with MEN syndromes can be multiple. These tumors are either readily apparent, large lesions or small, less than 1.5 cm in diameter. Occult lesions are coming to be more frequently recognized. Isolated duodenal tumors are found in 10%–15% of cases, and single lesions in the pancreas or peripancreatic lymph nodes in another 10%. In an additional 10% of cases, no primary lesion can be found at laparotomy.

Gastrinomas may be found anywhere in the pancreas or duodenum. Occult and potentially curable lesions are most frequently found within the pancreas, duodenum, or lymph nodes in an anatomical triangle defined by the junction of the cystic and common bile ducts superiorly, the junction of the second and third portions of duodenum inferiorly, and the junction of the neck and the body of the pancreas medially.[8] The tumors have a firm consistency and when sectioned have a reddish brown appearance similar to insulinoma. In unusual cases, the tumor may be cystic. Metastases to lymph nodes or liver are present in nearly one half the patients at the time of diagnosis. Non-β islet cell tumors associated with VIP, glucagon, or somatostatin production are most commonly large lesions that tend to be located in the head of the pancreas. They may be multifocal and similarly may occur as part of a MEN syndrome. Metastases are usually present.

Beta and non-β islet cell tumors have a similar histologic appearance that is typical of nearly all endocrine-related tumors (Fig 37–2). There are three major histologic patterns, including: (1) solid tumors with nodular solid nests and peripheral invading cords; (2) gyriform tumors with a trabecular or ribbon-like structure; and (3) glandular tumors with an acinar or rosette growth pattern.[9] Some tumors may have a mix of these major histologic patterns. All of these lesions have varying degrees of amyloid deposition. Importantly, none of the patterns is characteristic of malignant growth. The histologic diagnosis of malignancy is difficult, but is suggested by vascular or perineural invasion. The most reliable index of malignancy is the presence of metastatic disease.

Routine histologic examination will not predict the behavior or endocrine manifestation of these neoplasms. Immunofluorescence[10] and the peroxidase-antiperoxidase procedure permit the specific demonstration of various pancreatic hormones in tissue section (Fig 37–3). Application of these techniques has shown that (1) the histologic appearance is not predictive of which hormone a tumor will make, (2) a positive stain for a specific hormone correlates well with the abnormal production of that hormone in the patient, and (3) the distribution of hormone cells within a tumor is not uniform.[11–13]

Electron microscopy for investigational purposes has been useful for the demonstration of types of intracellular granules in these various endocrine tumors (Figs 37–4,A and B). When combined with immunocytochemical techniques, EM is a powerful research tool for the study of endocrine tumors.

GENERAL DIAGNOSTIC PRINCIPLES

The evaluation of patients with pancreatic endocrine tumors may be divided into three parts: (1) establishing the abnormal physiology or syndrome (i.e., hypoglycemia, excessive acid secretion), (2) detecting the abnormal serum levels of hormone by radioimmunoassay, and (3) localizing the tumor in preparation for resection. Although some of these steps may vary from tumor to tumor, radioimmunoassay and techniques of tumor localization are common to all of these tumors and will be discussed in this section.

Radioimmunoassay (RIA)

Radioimmunoassay (RIA) has made possible the measurement of minute amounts of circulating peptides, and hence has revolutionized the field of endocrinology. Initially, the technique was described by Berson and Yalow in 1958[112] to measure insulin levels in the blood. For this work Rosalyn Yalow received the Nobel prize in 1977. RIA was subsequently developed for numerous peptide hormones, providing a powerful clinical and research tool.[113] Detection of peptides by RIA is the basis of the diagnosis of apudomas and

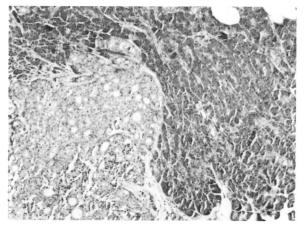

Fig 37–2.—Islet cell carcinoma arising in body of pancreas. Tumor cells resemble normal islet cells and are arranged in solid nests and festoons. (Courtesy of S.E. Tuttle, M.D., Department of Pathology, The Ohio State University College of Medicine.)

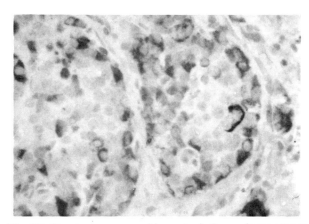

Fig 37–3.—Immunoperoxidase technique demonstrates positive staining of somatostatin in cells composing the islet cell tumor shown in Figure 37–10. Serial sections of the tumor also showed positive immunostaining for calcitonin and glucagon in scattered cells. (Courtesy of S.E. Tuttle, M.D., Department of Pathology, The Ohio State University College of Medicine.)

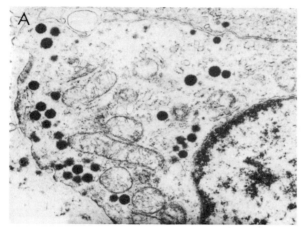

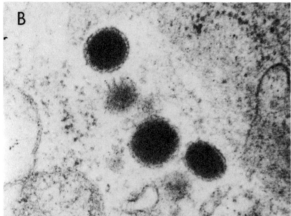

Fig 37–4.—Electron microscopic appearance of secretory granules of the endocrine type from tumor secreting large amounts of vasoactive intestinal peptide (**A,** low magnification). Note dense core granule separated from a single membrane by clear zone (**B,** high magnification). (Courtesy of S.E. Tuttle, M.D., Department of Pathology, The Ohio State University College of Medicine.)

provides a method of following disease progression or detecting cure in these patients.

RIA of peptide hormones is described by the following equation for a "hormone" X:

"hormone"
\+
"hormone" [^{125}I]

\+ antibody

hormone [^{125}I]-antibody
\+
hormone-antibody

The labeled "hormone" [^{125}I] is incubated with unlabeled "hormone" (either a known standard or the serum being tested) and antibody to that hormone. In this system, there is competition between "hormone" and "hormone" [^{125}I] for the specific binding sites on the antibody, reducing the amount of "hormone" [^{125}I] bound to the antibody. After adequate incubation (both equilibrium and dynamic techniques can be used), the bound ("hormone" [^{125}I]-antibody) and the free ("hormone"-^{125}I) fractions are separated by a suitable method (charcoal, exchange resin, second antibody precipitation). The radioactivity in the bound fraction is inversely proportional to the concentration of the hormone in the standard or sample. The level of radioactivity in the bound fraction of the sample is compared to a standard curve established by using different known concentrations of unlabeled "hormone," and the concentration of the unknown is determined by graphic extrapolation or mathematical curve fitting.

RIA for a specific hormone requires the production of antibodies specific for the hormone, availability of a pure form of the peptide for radiolabeling, preparation of a radiolabeled form of the peptide, and an effective method of separating antibody-bound peptide from free peptide. The RIA should be proved to be specific and sensitive, and results should be reproducible. Validation of any technique, whether used as a research or a clinical tool, includes demonstration of the specificity of the antibody used, reproducibility with the within-assay coefficient of variation less than 10% and between-assay coefficient of variation less than 15%. RIAs have been developed for many of the pancreatic and gut hormones, and complete assay kits are available commercially. Prior to basing conclusions on the commercially available kits, validity of the technique must be established. An excellent source of both assay components and kits is Linscott's *Directory of Immunological and Biological Reagents.**

Methods of Tumor Localization

The essential radiologic imaging techniques for tumor localization include CT scan of the abdomen and oral angiography. These are complemented by transhepatic portal venous sampling and intraoperative real-time ultrasonography. Nuclear magnetic resonance may improve detection of the tumor.

CT Scan[14–17]

The accuracy of pancreatic computed tomography in the detection of endocrine tumors varies from 40% to 80%. In general, CT will identify the majority of malignant tumors. Smaller tumors, those less than 2.5 cm in diameter, are not readily detected by standard CT protocols. Rapid-sequence CT scanning (scan every 3 seconds) with bolus contrast material (contrast-enhanced scan) improves the diagnostic accuracy. Tumors as small as 1.0 cm have been detected. Negative CT scan suggests a potentially unresectable small lesion. Angiography should be performed in such cases.

Other noninvasive techniques of imaging the pancreas include ultrasonography and nuclear magnetic resonance (NMR). Ultrasound provides no advantage to CT scan in the prognostic evaluation of the patient with a suspected pancreatic endocrine tumor. NMR is still a research tool, but does distinguish islet cell tumors from normal retroperitoneal structures and may become a valuable pancreatic imaging modality.

Angiography[18–20]

The accuracy of angiography in the detection of pancreatic endocrine tumors varies from 40% to 70%. Sensitivity improves if the angiogram is performed with a bolus of secretin to increase tumor blood flow and enhance the "tumor blush"[19]

*Published by Linscott's Directory, Mill Valley, California.

and with gaseous distention of the stomach.[20] The main reason for performing angiography is to attempt to detect small tumors and as a prerequisite prior to portal venous sampling.

Transhepatic Portal Venous Sampling[21–28]
(Fig 37–5)

Angiography, ultrasound, and CT are perfectly applicable for the large tumor, but by far the majority of these tumors are small and may be multiple at the time of initial presentation. Ingemansson first demonstrated the feasibility of percutaneous transhepatic sampling of blood from the portal venous system for identification of hormone-producing tumors of the pancreas.[21] Serum, sequentially sampled at various sites in the portal system, is assayed for determination of hormone levels. A rise in hormone concentration (usually 100–200 pg/ml over levels in the inferior vena cava) is observed in the serum sampled at the site of the tumor. This technique has been successfully employed by several groups for localization of insulinomas,[21, 23, 27] gastrinomas,[24] and glucagonomas.[27] Application of this technique requires an experienced angiographer and the availability of radioimmunoassays for the hor-

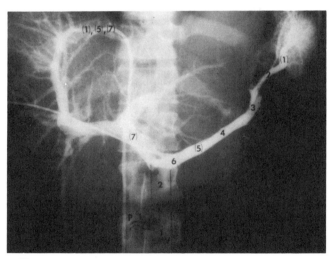

Fig 37–5.—Transhepatic portal venous sampling in a patient with gastrinoma. CT scan and angiogram were normal. Catheters are in the portal vein and hepatic vein for sampling. The numbers indicate points where blood was sampled; those in parentheses were sampled simultaneously. Gastrin results as follows:

| | Gastrin (pg/ml) | | | |
	HEPATIC VEIN	SMV	PANCREATIC (P)	SPLENIC
1	400	400	380	410
2		420		425
3				410
4	425			410
5				410
6				425
7	410			560

There was a rise in the region of the head of the pancreas. The patient had a gastrinoma measuring 1 × 2 cm in the head of the pancreas. (Courtesy of Michael Van Aman, M.D., Department of Radiology, The Ohio State University College of Medicine.)

mones in question. Glaser et al.[25] noted that an appreciation of venous anatomy is critical in the interpretation of the result, since high levels of hormones can be found in sites proximal to the tumor because of venous collaterals. In general, tumors in the head of the pancreas drain into the posterior-superior pancreaticoduodenal vein and high into the portal system. Tumors of the neck drain into the more distal portal vein near the junction of the confluence of the splenic veins and the superior mesenteric. Tumors of the body drain into the proximal splenic, and tumors of the tail drain into the midportion of the splenic vein. Vinik and co-workers[26–28] recommended obtaining celiac artery or peripheral samples simultaneously with portal samples. They also noted that repeated sampling at the same location may yield varied results, which can be attributed either to variability within the radioimmunoassay, a labile hormone secretion, laminar flow within the blood vessels, or errors in estimating catheter location.

Complications of the technique have not been common; however, splenic vein and portal vein thrombosis have been reported. The technique seems to be safe and useful for localization of islet cell tumors and differentiation of single and multiple tumors. In addition, the finding of elevated levels throughout the entire drainage bed of the pancreas would indicate the presence of diffuse microadenomatosis or hyperplasia. In addition, metastatic disease may be detected by this technique.

The practical limitations of this technique obviate wide application. Most of the reports are enthusiastic, but some investigators have been critical. In our experience, the technique has not been helpful and has not replaced thorough operative examination of the pancreas.

Intraoperative Ultrasound[29–32]

Localization of small pancreatic lesions may be difficult by palpation. Several groups have used intraoperative real-time ultrasound to assist the localization of these endocrine tumors of the pancreas. These tumors are hypoechogenic relative to normal pancreas and are usually clearly demarcated. At the present time, the cost of the equipment for intraoperative scanning is excessive, and hence the technique is not cost-effective.

Sequence of Tumor Localization (Fig 37–6)

Using a combination of CT scan, angiography, and portal venous sampling, nearly 80% of pancreatic endocrine tumors can be localized preoperatively. It may not be cost-effective to perform all of these tests in every case. An algorithm for tumor localization is shown in Figure 37–1. In general, if there is any doubt in the interpretation of the test, the next study should be performed. Contrarily, if a study clearly indicates a tumor, there is little benefit to proceeding with additional tests. Finally, if the tumor cannot be localized and there is no question about the diagnosis, the patient should have exploratory surgery.

INSULINOMA

Insulinoma was the first recognized[33] and is the most common apudoma of the pancreas. They produce and secrete in-

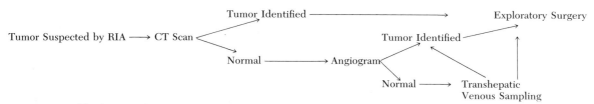

Fig 37–6.—Sequence of radiologic tests for localization of pancreatic apudomas.

sulin autonomously and often at inappropriately low blood glucose levels, which results in spontaneous hypoglycemia and a characteristic clinical syndrome. Symptoms secondary to the hypoglycemia-induced surge of catecholamines include tremor, restlessness, irritability, weakness, hunger, diaphoresis, tachycardia, and sometimes nausea and vomiting. Episodic disturbances in consciousness and aberrant behavior related to hypoglycemia may occur. Progressive and prolonged hypoglycemic attacks cause neuroglycopenia, resulting in symptoms often thought to be neuropsychiatric. These may range from subtle personality changes to confusion, obtundation, and coma. It is not surprising that a neurologic or psychiatric diagnosis is made initially in approximately 20% of cases.[34, 35] Convulsions may intervene, and the illness may be indistinguishable from some forms of epilepsy, particularly temporal lobe seizure. Temporary paralysis is associated with prolonged hypoglycemia in 5% of patients,[36] and another 7% incur irreversible nervous system damage. Death may occur during severe episodes. It is commonly noted by the patient or those close to him that relief of symptoms can be achieved by consumption of carbohydrate-rich foods.

Diagnosis

Differential diagnosis of hypoglycemia in the adult includes reactive or functional hypoglycemia associated with gastrectomy or gastroenterostomy, surreptitious ingestion of insulin, or ingestion of sulfonylureas, chronic pancreatitis, chronic adrenal insufficiency, hypopituitarism, ingestion of denatured alcohol, and, rarely, hepatic insufficiency when more than 80% of the functional hepatocytes have been destroyed (Table 37–2).[37] Patients with reactive hypoglycemia usually have symptoms three to five hours after meals and do not experience fasting hypoglycemia, thereby distinguishing this disorder from insulinoma. Reactive hypoglycemia, in addition, is a nonprogressive disease and usually does not result in loss of consciousness or aberrant behavior.[38]

To differentiate insulinoma from other causes of hypoglycemia, a variety of tests should be performed. Diagnosis of insulinoma depends on the documentation of fasting hypoglycemia with inappropriately elevated insulin levels. It is important to demonstrate Whipple's triad, which includes fast-induced symptoms of hypoglycemia with a blood glucose level of less than 50 mg/100 ml and relief of symptoms following the administration of glucose.[39] A prolonged fast demonstrating Whipple's triad is the most reliable method for diagnosing insulinoma. Blood glucose determinations should be performed every six hours during the fast; simultaneous insulin measurements should also be made. The patient with insulinoma usually shows an insulin level greater than 25 μU/ml by radioimmunoassay. Occasionally, absolute insulin concentra-

tions may be in the normal range of 5–20 μU/ml, but such values are inappropriate in the presence of hypoglycemia. The accuracy of the insulin and glucose measurements can be increased considerably by determining the immunoreactive insulin:glucose ratio. Values greater than 0.3 are found after an overnight fast in 95% of patients with insulinomas and after 72 hours in all patients with tumors.[6, 40] To exclude surreptitious administration of insulin, measurement of C-peptide is necessary. The C-peptide level is usually elevated in the presence of insulinoma, in contrast to the either normal or low levels found in patients giving themselves insulin.[41] Sulfonylurea-induced hyperinsulinism may be suspected when proinsulin and insulin concentrations are proportionately elevated and the ratio of proinsulin to insulin is normal. In addition, plasma sulfonylurea levels may be measured. The proinsulin:insulin ratio is usually elevated when insulinoma is present.[42] After prolonged fasting, further testing is usually not required. Provocative stimulation of insulin release by tolbutamide, glucagon, L-leucine, and calcium is usually not necessary. All of these tests have significant incidence of false negative responses.

The initial imaging procedure of localization of insulinomas is the CT scan. In one study, CT detected 21 of 27 tumors proved at operation (sensitivity, 78%) and correctly excluded the diagnosis in 14 patients.[17] Ultrasound is not helpful. Selective arteriography of the celiac, superior mesenteric, and hepatic arteries is complementary to CT and should be performed to define the position and number of smaller islet cell tumors if CT is negative. Angiography should be used to confirm the presence of hepatic metastases. Successful localization of these tumors by pancreaticoarteriography has ranged between 40% and 90%. The technique of percutaneous transhepatic portal sampling to localize insulinoma and other pancreatic endocrine tumors has been used by several authorities and was discussed in a preceding section.

Treatment (see Fig 37–6)

The treatment of insulinoma is surgical, and complete removal is required for cure. Medical treatment is generally necessary preoperatively in cases of malignant insulinoma.[40] In most cases, hypoglycemia can be avoided with frequent feedings of slowly absorbed forms of carbohydrates. For refractory cases, several pharmacologic agents have been employed, but should be used cautiously, for they may complicate anesthesia of the patient undergoing operation. Diazoxide, which directly inhibits the release of insulin by the β-cell and has an extrapancreatic hypoglycemic effect theoretically related to the release of catecholamines, may be helpful. The usual dose of diazoxide is between 600 and 1,000 mg/day, which may induce hirsutism with long-term treatment,

TABLE 37–2.—CLASSIFICATION OF SPONTANEOUS HYPOGLYCEMIA

I. Organic hypoglycemia*—recognizable anatomical lesion
   A. Pancreatic islet cell disease with hyperinsulinism
     1. Adenoma, single or multiple
     2. Microadenomatosis, with or without macroscopic islet adenomas
     3. Carcinoma, with metastases
     4. Adenoma(s) or carcinoma, associated with adenomas of other endocrine glands, multiple endocrine adenomatosis
     5. Hyperplasia (very rare in adults) in infancy and childhood
       a. Hyperplasia
       b. Nesidioblastosis
       c. Adenoma
   B. Nonpancreatic tumors associated with hypoglycemia
   C. Anterior pituitary hypofunction
   D. Adrenocortical hypofunction
   E. Acquired extensive liver disease
   F. Severe congestive heart failure
   G. Severe renal insufficiency in noninsulin-dependent diabetic patient
II. Hypoglycemia due to identified specific hepatic enzyme defects (infancy and childhood)
   A. Glycogen storage diseases* (deficiency of glucose-6-phosphatase or amylo-1, 6-glucosidase, or phosphorylase)
   B. Fructose-1, 6-diphosphatase deficiency*
   C. Hereditary fructose intolerance (deficiency of fructose-1-phosphate aldolase)
   D. Galactosemia (deficiency of galactose-1-phosphate uridyl transferase)
   E. Aglycogenesis* (deficiency of glycogen synthase)
   F. Familial fructose and galactose intolerance (specific enzyme defect undetermined)
III. Functional hypoglycemia-no recognizable, or no persistent, anatomic lesion
   A. Reactive functional hypoglycemia
   B. Reactive hypoglycemia secondary to mild diabetes
   C. Alimentary hyperinsulinism
   D. Alcohol and poor nutrition*
   E. Deficiency of glucagon*
   F. Transient hypoglycemia in the newborn of low birth weight*
   G. Transient postnatal hypoglycemia in an infant of a diabetic mother*
   H. "Idiopathic hypoglycemia" of infancy and childhood*
     1. Ketogenic hypoglycemia (childhood)
     2. Leucine-sensitive type
     3. Leucine-insensitive type
     4. Others
   I. Erythroblastosis fetalis, transient*
   J. Infantile gigantism with visceromegaly, microcephaly, macroglossia, and omphalocele* (hyperplasia of pancreatic islet cells has been reported in some patients classified under G, H, I, and J)
   K. "Insulin autoimmune syndrome" (no previous insulin administration) and hyperinsulinemia
IV. Hypoglycemia due to exogenous causes
   A. Iatrogenic ⎤ Insulin or sulfonylurea compounds*
   B. Factitious ⎦
   C. Other drugs that may cause hypoglycemia

*Fasting hypolgycemia. From (Fajans S.S., Floyd J.C. Jr., Vij S.K.: Differential diagnosis of hypoglycemia, in Kryston L.J., Shaw R.A., Schwager E. (eds.): *Endocrinology and Diabetes.* New York, Grune & Stratton, 1975. p. 459. By permission.)

and salt and water retention with consequent edema. The simultaneous administration of the thiazide diuretics is helpful in reducing edema and also has a synergistic effect, inhibiting insulin secretion. Phenytoin (Dilantin) given in doses of 300–600 mg/day is effective in reducing insulin secretion in about one third of the patients. D$_l$-propranolol, in doses of 30–240 mg/day is reported successfully to abolish the symptoms of hypoglycemia and normalize blood glucose levels.[43] The mechanism of the drug's effect seems to be suppression of insulin release; however, other mechanisms may be involved, such as increased peripheral insulin resistance.

Preoperative preparation requires adequate hydration, normalization of serum electrolytes, and avoidance of hypoglycemia. An IV infusion of 5% or 10% dextrose with 0.45 normal saline is given the night before operation.

Intraoperatively, glucose levels should be monitored. A midline incision is employed. A general exploration is performed to identify metastatic disease. Preoperative tests guide the exploration of the pancreas. In general, the entire pancreas should be exposed. A generous mobilization of the duodenum is essential for exposure of the head and uncinate process. The body and tail of the gland are exposed through the gastrocolic omentum. The peritoneum along the inferior edge of the body and tail of the gland is incised. Gentle blunt dissection then permits palpation of the distal pancreas between the thumb anteriorly and the index and long fingers posteriorly.

The majority of small adenomas in the body and tail can be enucleated. In such cases, the surrounding pancreatic tissue should be closed. Lesions larger than 3 cm and those in close proximity to the pancreatic duct should not be enucleated, and distal pancreatectomy is advisable. The spleen may be spared, except in cases of obvious malignancy. Lesions in the head of the pancreas should be enucleated. Pancreaticoduodenectomy is reserved for tumors that cannot be locally excised, and hence is rarely needed.

Before the use of angiography and portal venous sampling, no tumor was found at exploration in nearly one quarter of patients. If no tumor is demonstrated intraoperatively, then a blind distal pancreatic resection (to the left of the superior mesenteric vessels) is indicated. If a small adenoma is found in the resected specimen, the operation is terminated. There is some uncertainty as to the most prudent course if no abnormalities are found in the resected pancreas. Some prefer to terminate the procedure, and if symptoms or hypoglycemia occur postoperatively, reevaluate the patient and plan a second exploration. Others perform a 95% pancreatectomy, arguing that the risk of this extent of resection is less than the 18% mortality reported for reoperation in this group of patients. A 95% pancreatectomy is rarely necessary, and a more conservative resection is best.

Intraoperative diagnosis of occult insulinoma may be facilitated by imaging techniques and serum analysis. Real-time ultrasonography is being used to identify small tumors intraoperatively. The equipment is expensive and the cost:benefit ratio is likely to be disproportionate. This technique needs to be investigated further. Monitoring of plasma levels of glucose and insulin during surgery may aid diagnosis.[44, 45] An increase in the serum glucose level and a decrease in the serum insulin level after pancreatic resection confirm an adequate excision. Contrarily, palpation of the pancreas where the tumor is located may lead to increases in insulin and decreases in glucose levels. Detection of slight changes in the blood glucose levels during operation requires a controlled infusion to keep glucose levels near 80 ± 10 mg/dl. In addition, frequent, rapid determinations of blood glucose levels are considered to be important. Rapid radioimmunoassay for insulin has also been applied by two groups of investigators to localize small insulinomas by intraoperative pancreatic vein catheterization.[46, 47] Finally, the artificial pancreas may be used to aid intraoperative localization.[48]

In the presence of malignant insulinoma, local excision of large metastatic lymph nodes or easily accessible tumors in the liver is helpful in reducing hypoglycemia episodes. However, long-term survival is probably not altered. Malignant insulinoma may be treated with chemotherapy using streptozotocin and chlorozotocin.

GASTRINOMA

In 1955, Zollinger and Ellison reported two patients with an unusual triad of symptoms; i.e., primary jejunal ulceration, exaggerated gastric acid hypersecretion, and diarrhea, for which they hypothesized a hormonal basis.[49] It is now unequivocally established that the Zollinger-Ellison syndrome is caused by a pancreatic or duodenal tumor that secretes excessive amounts of gastrin. The Zollinger-Ellison syndrome accounts for less than 0.1% of all peptic ulcer disease and for 2% of recurrent peptic ulcers following standard ulcer operations.[50]

Clinical Manifestations

Gastrinomas have been reported in children and in the elderly, but most patients are between the third and fifth decades. There is no definite sex predilection, nor has a geographical or radial predilection been demonstrated.

The most common presenting symptoms, occurring in 70%–95% of patients, is abdominal pain related to ulcer disease. Approximately 18% of patients have diarrhea as an initial symptom, but three of four of these patients will either simultaneously or subsequently experience ulcer-like symptoms. Regardless of the initial presentation, diarrhea will become manifest in 30% of the patients before their first gastric operation. Although periods of quiescence may occur between exacerbations, most patients have a progressive and relentless course.

Associated endocrinopathies occur in 10%–40% of the patients and may be the first clue to the diagnosis. Association of nonpancreatic endocrine tumors with the Zollinger-Ellison syndrome is called the multiple endocrine neoplasia syndrome type 1 (MEN 1). Parathyroid adenoma is the most commonly associated abnormality, followed by pituitary and adrenal tumors. The syndrome has an autosomal dominant inheritance with a high but variable degree of expression. Clinical manifestations may be synchronous or sequential. The MEN type 2 is characterized by medullary carcinoma of the thyroid, parathyroid adenoma, and pheochromocytoma. There are several cases of pheochromocytoma occurring with gastrinoma.[51] To date, there is only one reported case of Zollinger-Ellison syndrome with medullary carcinoma of the thyroid. The proper evaluation of a patient with Zollinger-Ellison syndrome includes exclusion of coexisting apudomas by complete endocrine screen.

Because of increasing awareness and improved diagnostic techniques, patients with an ulcerogenic tumor are detected much earlier and, as a result, have a less florid form of ulcer diathesis. Several studies indicate that patients diagnosed after 1970 are younger, tend to have a shorter duration of symptoms, often have not had ulcer operations, and frequently have symptoms suggestive of uncomplicated ulcer disease.[52] In addition, more recently diagnosed patients tend to have a lower incidence of virulent ulcer disease and of malignant gastrinoma.

Pathophysiology and Biologic Behavior

Symptoms and complications of the Zollinger-Ellison syndrome are primarily related to the gastrin-induced gastric hypersecretion. Virulent peptic ulcer develops and frequently involves unusual sites. Bleeding, obstruction, and perforation are the inevitable consequences if the hypersecretion is not corrected. Diarrhea is caused by multiple factors, including delivery of excessive amounts of gastric acid to the duodenum, damage to the small-bowel mucosa by acid-rich gastric juice, and shortened intestinal transit time.

Steatorrhea has been reported in many patients with gastrinoma. In addition to small-bowel mucosal damage, inactivation of intestinal lipase by the abnormally low pH of the intestinal lumen occurs, and bile salts precipitate in an acid medium. Gastrointestinal loss of plasma proteins occurs in many patients. The severe diarrhea of malabsorption partially accounts for the poor nutritional status of patients with Zollinger-Ellison syndrome.

Biologically, gastrin-producing tumors are slow-growing, but have a high frequency of multiple primary sites and malignant behavior.[53] More than 60% of patients have malignant tumors, and more than 80% of these have metastases at the time of diagnosis. Thirty-five percent of patients have benign tumors, and 6% have islet cell hyperplasia. Thirteen to fifteen percent of patients have duodenal wall tumors, but only one half have isolated lesions, the others having evidence of multicentricity of the pancreas or metastatic disease.[51, 54] Combining these data, it would seem that the surgeon will have a one-in-four chance of finding an isolated resectable lesion.

Despite the slow growth potential of these neoplasms, the mortality from gastrinoma is high. In the past, complications of gastric hypersecretion accounted for roughly 40% of the deaths, postoperative complications for 25%, and neoplastic progression for 20%.[53] The primary cause of morbidity and death was formerly related to the underlying peptic ulcer diathesis; hence, initial therapeutic efforts must be directed at its correction. The main cause of death in long-term survivors is progression of tumor growth, and, therefore, treatment must also be directed at reduction of the tumor mass.[51]

Diagnosis

Identification of ulcerogenic tumor requires keen suspicion to initiate early medical and surgical treatment. Special attention should be directed to patients who have severe ulcer diathesis refractory to medical management, patients in whom ulcers recur after well-performed standard surgical procedures, elderly patients with persistent ulcer symptoms, children or adolescents with ulcer disease, early postpartum patients with massive GI hemorrhage or perforation, patients who have unexplained protracted diarrhea, patients with a family history of ulcer disease or endocrine disorders, and patients with symptoms of both hyperparathyroidism and GI ulceration.

Before 1970, the diagnosis of the Zollinger-Ellison syndrome was routinely established by radiographic studies, gastric analysis, and gastrin bioassay. The development of the gastrin radioimmunoassay and provocative testing for this hormone has made possible the early and more certain detection of ulcerogenic tumors.

Barium contrast studies of the upper GI tract are almost always abnormal. However, in the majority of patients, the radiographic picture is not distinctively different from that of ordinary peptic ulcer disease. In patients with more florid forms of the disease, upper GI radiographs may be diagnostic[61] (Fig 37–7). Classically, the stomach is characterized by giant, rugal folds and large amounts of retained gastric secretions. Approximately three fourths of the patients will have an ulcer of the duodenal bulb or the immediate postbulbar area. The duodenum may be characterized by lumenal dilatation, justifying the term "megaduodenum." Although found in only a small fraction of patients, distal duodenal and proximal jejunal ulcers are virtually pathognomonic of the Zollinger-Ellison syndrome. The ileum and colon are usually normal. In patients who have had previous gastric operations, the upper GI films may be normal, but stomal ulcerations and prominent gastric and duodenal folds are more often apparent.

Historically, gastric analysis was often the first clue to the

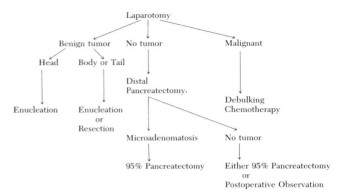

Fig 37–7.—Algorithm of the surgical treatment of insulinoma.

presence of an ulcerogenic tumor. However, it is being replaced as a screening test by the serum gastrin radioimmunoassay. Gastric analysis still has an extremely important role in diagnosis, particularly with regard to the differentiation of hypergastrinemic states. During a 12-hour overnight gastric collection, the patient with an ulcerogenic tumor characteristically has an average output of 100 ml/hr with a fixed acid production of 10 mEq/hr. Approximately 74% of patients with gastrinoma meet these criteria. Two-hour basal acid collections are as accurate as 12-hour studies and are considerably less distressing to the patient. Any patient producing more than 15 mEq/H^+ per hour should be suspected of having an ulcerogenic tumor.

Gastric analysis is best performed by augmentation with pentagastrin administered subcutaneously in a dose of 6 μg/kg. The two measurements that give the best indication of the Zollinger-Ellison syndrome are the rate of basal acid secretion and the ratio of basal to maximum stimulated acid secretion. A basal gastric output of greater than 15 mEq/hr and a ratio of basal acid output to maximum acid output greater than 0.6 strongly favor the diagnosis of gastrinoma. Unfortunately, approximately 40% of patients with the Zollinger-Ellison syndrome will not meet these criteria, and another 10% with ordinary duodenal ulcer disease will have results similar to patients with ulcerogenic tumors.[53, 62] In the postoperative stomach, measurement of acid secretion is quite variable, mainly as a result of technical problems in acid collection and contamination by reflux of alkaline contents from the upper small intestine. However, a basal acid output of greater than 5 mEq/hr after vagotomy and/or gastric resection should be considered suggestive of gastrinoma.

The mainstay of the diagnosis of the Zollinger-Ellison syndrome is the gastrin radioimmunoassay established by McGuigan and Trudeau in 1966 and others.[62–65] Patients with the Zollinger-Ellison syndrome may have serum gastrin levels as high as 1,000 pg/ml. It is generally accepted that a serum gastrin level greater than 500 pg/ml in the presence of ulcer disease and gastric hypersecretion favors the diagnosis of gastrinoma.

In our experience, normal and duodenal ulcer subjects have fasting gastrin concentrations between 20 and 120 pg/ml. Postoperative gastrin levels in patients after vagotomy may range from 250 to 500 pg/ml. Lower fasting values are common after gastric resection or antrectomy, unless the patient has a retained antrum. Although there is no large series that establishes values in patients with recurrent postoperative ulceration, the general experience has been that such patients have serum levels between those of patients who have had vagotomy and antrectomy and those who have not undergone operation.

As clinical experience with gastrin radioimmunoassay has increased, an ever-mounting number of physiologic variations and diseases have been found to be associated with hypergastrinemia. Moderately elevated but reversible levels may be associated with pyloric obstruction or ingestion of a protein meal. However, persistently elevated levels in excess of 250 pg/ml are usually associated with pernicious anemia or atrophic gastritis. Hypergastrinemia may also be associated with retained antrum, carcinoma of the stomach, the short-bowel syndrome, and renal failure. Hypersecretion of gastrin may also result from antral G-cell hyperplasia, an overactivity that is termed "nontumorous hypergastrinemia-hyperchlorhydria".[66]

Serum gastrin levels may be less specific than previously thought. Fasting gastrin determinations in patients with the Zollinger-Ellison syndrome sometimes overlap with those in patients with ordinary duodenal ulcer disease. In borderline cases, as in other syndromes of endocrine hyperfunction, stimulation and suppression tests that distinguish accentuated physiologic secretion from tumor elaboration of hormone have proved useful. Three types of stimulation tests are used, including a standard meal, calcium infusion, and secretin bolus (Fig 37–8).

After a standard test meal, normal persons and most persons with duodenal ulcer disease demonstrate an increase in peripheral serum gastrin (Fig 37–9). The patient with ulcerogenic tumor and an intact stomach, however, will not have a significant rise in gastrin levels. On the other hand, postoperative patients who have had a gastric resection with Billroth II anastomosis or total gastrectomy will have a rise in serum gastrin.[57] Patients with antral G-cell hyperplasia have a large response to a meal. Hence, the magnitude of postprandial response should help to distinguish patients with other disorders from those with gastrinemia.

In patients with the Zollinger-Ellison syndrome, infusion of calcium gluceptate, 12–15 mg/kg over a three-hour period,

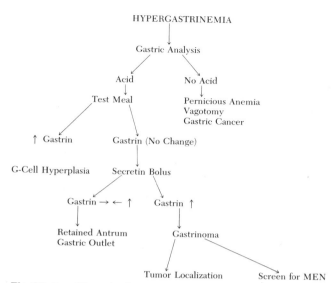

Fig 37–9.—Steps in the evaluation of hypergastrinemia.

will result in a twofold to threefold or greater increase over baseline serum gastrin. However, false positive results occur in 10%–15% of the patients. The frequency of false positive results can be reduced to 2% if a change in serum gastrin of 395 pg/ml is used as the minimal response required for the diagnosis of gastrinoma.[67] Negative responses occur in some cases, however, and should not be considered diagnostically conclusive. Infusion of magnesium sulfate or secretin should be performed in questionable cases and in patients with coexisting hyperparathyroidism or cardiac dysfunction.

Secretin testing is the most reliable and sensitive of the three provocative tests. Secretin, 2 units/kg, is given as a bolus. This test is considered diagnostic for ulcerogenic tumor when serum gastrin increases by at least 110 pg/ml over baseline values. In our experience, a rise of 200 pg/ml above baseline is diagnostic of gastrinoma, with no overlap between these patients and those with nontumorous hypergastrinemia (Fig 37–10). Falsely elevated gastrins have not been reported, and false negative values are estimated to occur in only 5% of the patients. Normal persons, those with duodenal ulcer, with G-cell hyperplasia, and with retained antrum have no response or minimal responses to provocative testing with either calcium or secretin. If one were to select a single provocative test to screen for gastrinoma, a bolus injection of secretin would be favored because it is less time-consuming, is rarely associated with complications, and is the most reliable. The combination of a secretin bolus and a calcium bolus has been suggested as a method to distinguish borderline cases.[68]

After the diagnosis is confirmed by RIA and provocative tests, procedures to localize the tumor may be employed, but frequently are not helpful. These are discussed in the preceding sections.

The diagnosis of Zollinger-Ellison syndrome must be established early because the natural history of this syndrome entails frequent life-threatening complications. The routine performance of serum gastrin determinations in peptic ulcer patients will undoubtedly lead to the more frequent diagnosis of less fulminant forms of the Zollinger-Ellison syndrome.

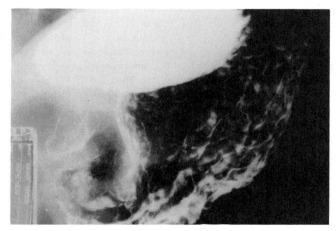

Fig 37–8.—Upper GI series in patient with gastrinoma. Note the multiple gastric ulcers, rugal hypertrophy, and dilution of barium by retained gastric fluid.

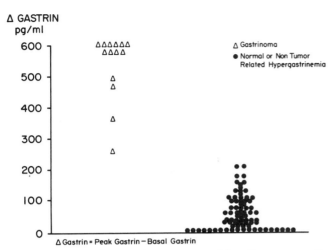

Fig 37-10.—Change in serum gastrin after a secretin bolus. A rise of 200 pg/ml or greater over baseline values is diagnostic of gastrinoma and excludes G-cell hyperplasia.

Treatment

Before the introduction of the H_2-receptor antagonists, which cause a sharp reduction in basal acid output, medical treatment was not successful in patients with gastrinoma. Recent studies have indicated that a large proportion of patients who have gastrinoma have either complete or substantial relief of symptoms with cimetidine in doses of 1,200–2,400 mg/day. Some patients may require large doses, up to 10 gm/day, or the addition of an anticholinergic to maintain pain control, weight gain, and normal formed bowel movements, and to promote ulcer healing.[69] Cimetidine does not alter the serum gastrin levels or tumor progression. Patients with normal ulceration or esophagitis appear to respond well to treatment with cimetidine. Patients with MEN and gross tumor with or without metastases seem to be refractory to cimetidine therapy.[70]

The results of cimetidine therapy initially appeared encouraging, but more trials determined its long-term effectiveness to be limited by side effects, as well as the occurrence of tachyphylaxis.[71] Nearly 50% of patients develop breast tenderness or impotence, which is related to high doses and promptly resolves with cessation of therapy. The overall failure rate in nearly 200 patients treated with cimetidine is about 30%, with over one half of these requiring total gastrectomy. Ranitidine, a newly marketed H_2-receptor antagonist, is more prominent than cimetidine and offers some potential. Failure is usually due to inadequate dose. Control of symptoms is a poor reflection of acid control, and periodic acid determinations should be done.[72] Variable responsiveness indicates the need to individualize the dose of cimetidine or ranitidine. Basal acid secretion should be measured for the one hour prior to the next dose. If acid secretion is less than 10 mEq/hr, the dose should be increased, or anticholingerics, such as isopropamide, should be prescribed. Reassessment of acid inhibition is needed every six months because of changing dose requirements.[69] Esophagogastroduodenoscopy is indicated to prove ulcer healing during treatment. It is reasonable to treat some patients with H_2-receptor antagonists without surgery,

but not routinely. The H_2-receptor antagonists should be used to prepare patients for total gastrectomy and should be offered as an alternative to those who refuse operation or in whom surgical intervention is contraindicated. However, operative treatment remains the most reliable method of controlling the ulcer diathesis and offers the only potential for cure by excision of the gastrinoma. Therefore, all patients should have a exploration, even if medical management is planned.

Surgical therapy should be individualized.[51, 73, 74] Exploration should be recommended to all patients. Laparotomy permits assessment of the presence or absence of tumor and determination of metastatic disease, which allows the physician to give the patient an accurate prognosis. If no gross tumor is found, five-year survival is nearly 100% and ten-year survival is 80%, with deaths not related to tumor. If metastases are present in the liver, five-year survival is about 40%, and ten-year survival rare but possible. Lymph node metastases do not seem to alter survival. If tumor is identified in the pancreas with no spread, 60% of patients live five years, and 40% ten years.[51]

Operative treatment is based on the findings at operation (Fig 37–11). If there is no gross tumor, the minimal operation should be truncal vagotomy and pyloroplasty in the patient who complies with cimetidine therapy and refuses total gastrectomy. Opening the duodenum will permit bi-digital palpation of the duodenal submucosa and possible detection of small gastrinomas which could be resected for cure. Vagotomy will decrease the amount of the H_2-receptor antagonist required postoperatively, as shown by Zollinger and Ellison and more recently by Richardson et al.[75] Postoperatively, gastrin measurements will remain high in this group of patients and will continue to rise over time, indicating the need for periodic radiologic assessment (CT scan). Total gastrectomy is still acceptable treatment in some patients in whom no tumor is found.

When a tumor is found in the pancreas, duodenum, or peripancreatic tissues, it should be excised. Occult tumors are usually found in the "gastrinoma triangle," and careful exploration with biopsy of lymph nodes in this area is necessary (Fig 37–12). If all gross tumor is resected, treatment still must be directed at control of the gastric hypersecretion because the majority of these patients (85%) will continue to have elevated basal and stimulated gastrin levels. In this setting, some prefer a vagotomy and pyloroplasty or vagotomy and antrectomy, with the understanding that the patient may need postoperative cimetidine or ranitidine if hypergastrinemia persists. These lesser gastric operations may be better in patients who have lost a considerable amount of weight and who have coexisting medical problems. In others, total gastrectomy is the most reliable method for controlling gastric acid production.

Several reports indicate that gastrinoma may regress following total gastrectomy. This is infrequent and should not deter the surgeon from attempts at excision of localized tumor.

The extent of pancreatic resection is somewhat controversial. For lesions to the left of the mesenteric vessels, distal pancreatectomy and splenectomy are clearly indicated. In the series of Zollinger and associates,[51] hemipancreatectomy improved survival. Tumors in the head of the pancreas may

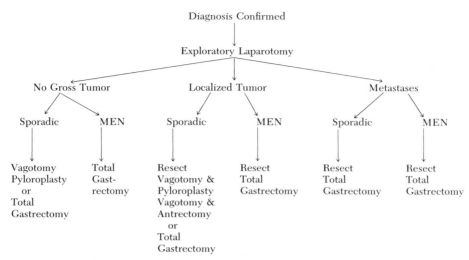

Diagnosis Confirmed

Exploratory Laparotomy

No Gross Tumor | Localized Tumor | Metastases

Sporadic — MEN | Sporadic — MEN | Sporadic — MEN

| Vagotomy Pyloroplasty or Total Gastrectomy | Total Gast-rectomy | Resect Vagotomy & Pyloroplasty Vagotomy & Antrectomy or Total Gastrectomy | Resect Total Gastrectomy | Resect Total Gastrectomy | Resect Total Gastrectomy |

Fig 37–11.—Surgical decision making in gastrinoma.

sometimes be enucleated, but in the majority of cases are unresectable unless a pancreaticoduodenectomy is performed. This operation has been successful in only 23 of 73 patients reported; and one third of the long-term survivors eventually needed gastrectomy. The evidence that patients live many years with residual tumor in the head of the pancreas and total gastrectomy must be balanced against the risk of pancreaticoduodenectomy and the potential for serious medical problems when this operation is combined with total gastrectomy. At present, there are no data to support pancreaticoduodenectomy or total pancreatectomy for gastrinoma.

Metastases should be resected if possible. There are reports of several long-term survivors after removal of isolated liver metastases or large lymph nodes.[51, 57–60] The gastrin levels in these patients remain high, but reduction of the amount of

tumor tends to prolong survival. Total gastrectomy should be performed in patients with metastases because of the potential for excessive gastrin production to overcome acid reduction achieved with lesser gastric resection and vagotomy and cimetidine.

There is some debate about whether those with sporadic gastrinoma and those with MEN should be treated differently.[74] This comes largely from data showing the multicentric nature of gastrinoma in the familial cases, theoretically making them unresectable. There are no clearcut policies in these cases. In Zollinger's experience with 13 MEN patients, the primary tumor was resected in ten, along with metastases in three. The primary tumor was not excised in two. The overall survival at five years was 85% and the ten-year survival 61%, with over half the patients living at least 12 years. Gastrinoma occurring as part of a MEN complex may be biologically less aggressive than sporadic tumor, but it does seem that resection of gross tumor in these cases also improves survival. Attempts to remove the ulcerogenic tumor should be made in MEN patients as well as in those with sporadic gastrinoma. As these patients tend to live for many years and nearly all have persistent hypergastrinemia, even after tumor resection, total gastrectomy seems advisable.

Treatment of gastrinoma must be individualized. In some patients, medical management may be best; in others, radical tumor extirpation; and in others, total gastrectomy. Figure 37–7 offers some guidelines for surgical decision making in the treatment of gastrinoma.

Postoperative Care

After operation, gastrin levels need to be checked periodically. Over five years, these can be expected to rise but not necessarily correlate with the amount of tumor. Complete resection with persistently normal gastrins is possible in 17% of the cases in the literature (see Table 37–2). If gastrin levels continue to rise, radiographic studies to attempt to determine the location and extent of tumor are indicated. The role of second-look surgery in gastrinoma has not yet been defined.

Acid studies should be performed several times per year in patients having less than total gastrectomy who have persis-

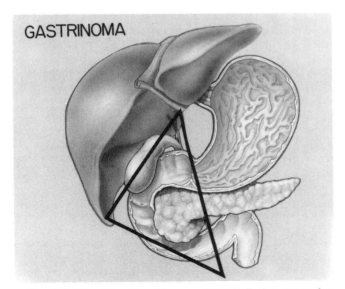

GASTRINOMA

Fig 37–12.—The "gastrinoma triangle," the most frequent location of occult, potentially curable tumors. (Adapted from Stabile B.E., Morrow D.T., Passaro E.: The gastrinoma triangle—operative implications. *Am. J. Surg.* 147:25–31, 1984.)

tent or recurrent hypergastrinemia. The purpose is to check the efficacy of the H$_2$-receptor antagonists. As has been pointed out, symptoms have proved to be poor indexes of cimetidine and probably ranitidine failure.

Chemotherapy is of benefit in those with metastases. Streptozotocin and chlorozotocin have been shown to decrease tumor size and prolong survival.[76]

Following total gastrectomy, monthly B$_{12}$ injections must be continued throughout the patient's life. Also, the patient should be monitored for iron deficiency anemia and dumping, and upper GI studies should be performed to check for stricture of the esophagojejunal anastomosis which may occur late.

All patients and their families should be followed and screened for hyperfunction of other endocrine systems. Serum calcium, parathormone, and prolactin should be checked in all patients and family members. Pancreatic polypeptide may be elevated in some patients and be a useful tumor marker.

G-CELL HYPERPLASIA (NONTUMOROUS HYPERGASTRINEMIA)

Hypergastrinemia arising from hyperplasia of the gastrin-producing cells of the antrum must be distinguished from gastrinoma, for the treatment is clearly different. Nontumorous hypergastrinemia is characterized physiologically by gastric hypersecretion, an exaggerated gastrin response to meals, and no response to secretin stimulation. Pathologically it is characterized by hyperfunctioning hyperplastic G-cells of the antrum. Using cytochemical techniques, Polak and co-workers[114] showed that in nontumorous hypergastrinemia there were over 30 times the G-cell populations seen in normal persons and those with gastrinoma. The incidence of this entity is unknown, but with refinements of diagnostic procedures, including provocative testing, its recognition is increasing. It should be considered in all patients with the possible diagnosis of gastrinoma of both sporadic and MEN types. Friesen and Tomita[115] established that improvement of ulcer symptoms and correction of hypergastrinemia follow antrectomy and vagotomy. G-cell hyperplasia should be treated by antrectomy and vagotomy and not by prolonged H$_2$-receptor antagonist therapy, lesser gastric procedures, or total gastrectomy.

VIPOMA WDHA SYNDROME

Pancreatic tumors associated with watery diarrhea, hypokalemia, and achlorhydria (WDHA) or hypochlorhydria produce a variety of biologically active substances that may cause the WDHA syndrome. The first association between diarrhea and an islet cell tumor was made by Priest and Alexander in 1957.[77] In 1958 Verner and Morrison[78] described two cases. Marks et al. in 1967 coined the acronym WDHA.[79] In 1968 Zollinger and colleagues ascribed a secretin-like bioactivity to tumor extract.[80] The VIP has been measured in the serum of patients with this syndrome and in tumor extract. In addition in 1978 Cooperman and co-workers[82] demonstrated that VIP decreased with tumor resection. Zollinger has had two patients with this disorder, both of whom have elevated levels of VIP, and one of whom produces excessive pancreatic polypeptide. Jaffe and associates in 1977[83] showed that some of

these tumors produce excessive prostaglandins and demonstrated the therapeutic benefit of indomethacin in controlling the diarrhea. Thus, there are various candidates for the active agent in the WDHA syndrome, including VIP, prostaglandins, secretin, and pancreatic polypeptide.[84] By biologic activity and experimental evidence, the two major candidates are VIP and prostaglandins.[84–86]

The clinical features of this disorder are a severe but intermittent diarrhea, often of a watery nature. Patients will have asymptomatic periods. Diarrhea is not relieved by nasogastric suction, as is the diarrhea associated with the ulcerogenic syndrome. Gastric analysis usually indicates hypochlorhydria, although the original description included evidence of achlorhydria. Patients will usually respond with acid production to pentagastrin (6 µg/kg subcutaneously). Often, patients will describe flushing episodes. At the times when their symptoms are most severe, serum measurements of calcium are usually elevated. As the diarrhea subsides, calcium levels return to normal. The etiology of hypercalcemia in this disorder is not well understood, but its presence does seem to correlate with the biologic activity of the tumor.

Treatment of tumors associated with the WDHA syndrome is surgical. A preoperative investigation should be made to localize the tumor. This is facilitated by the standard battery of tests for endocrine tumors of the pancreas, which includes CAT scan, pancreatic angiography, and transhepatic portal venous sampling. Preoperative preparation includes correction of fluid and electrolyte losses, which may take two to three weeks. Hydrocortisone (100 mg every six hours) has been shown to decrease VIP production and lessen the severity of the diarrhea, facilitating preoperative correction of electrolyte abnormalities. Some patients may benefit from preoperative TPN, but in our experience, these patients are usually not as cachectic and malnourished as those with glucagonoma or somatostatinoma.

Exploration should be carried out in all patients, and the findings at operation should guide the surgeon. If no tumor is found, a distal pancreatectomy and search for microadenoma should be carried out. A localized tumor should be resected, which may require pancreaticoduodenectomy. Total pancreatectomy is not recommended in these patients. If tumor is found in the liver and if metastases and lymph nodes are present, there may be some benefit to resecting and debulking the tumor. The reason is to reduce the amount of functional tissue, that is, the amount of tumor producing the VIP, and hence reduce the potential for incapacitating diarrhea. Recurrent symptoms after what is thought to be a complete excision warrant a complete reinvestigation, with a possible second-look operation for further debulking.

In the series recorded by Verner and Morrison in 1974, 20 of the patients had malignant tumors associated with the WDHA syndrome; two of these were helped by operation and one by radiation therapy. Also in this series of 54 patients, 23 had benign tumors, and 16 of these were cured by operation. In 11 other patients, nearly 20% of the total series, no gross tumor could be identified, but diffuse hyperplasia was found in blind pancreatectomy. Surgical cure was achieved in eight of these. The five-year survival of patients, even those with metastatic disease, can be as high as 50%–60%.

Patients with unresectable, recurrent, or metastatic tumor

will have episodic diarrhea with potentially life-threatening hypokalemia. In these patients, long-term steroid therapy has never been shown to be helpful in reducing the diarrhea or hypokalemia. Indomethacin, 25 mg three times daily, may be helpful. More recently, somatomedin (a synthetic somatostatin) has been shown to reduce VIP levels and diarrhea in selected cases. Although still experimental, the clinical use of somatostatin to inhibit hormone release may lessen the severity of the diarrhea in these patients.

GLUCAGONOMA

Pancreatic tumors producing glucagon arise from the alpha cells of the pancreas. The hallmark of this disorder is a severe dermatitis and mild diabetes mellitus. In addition, these patients demonstrate malnutrition with anemia, hypocholesterolemia, hypoproteinemia, and low serum amino acid levels. They also have a tendency to form deep venous thromboses. Historically, the first glucagonoma was probably described by Becker et al.[88] in 1942, when he noted the association between an islet cell tumor and an unusual skin rash. In 1960 Gosner and Korting[89] demonstrated that the tumor extract causes increased glucose. McGavran in 1966 and co-workers[90] described the syndrome of glucagonoma. The largest review series is that of Prinz et al. in 1981.[91]

Glucagonoma may be classified as one of three types: that with the cutaneous syndrome; that without the cutaneous syndrome; and the third type, which occurs as part of the MEN complex.[92] The diabetes characteristic of this disorder is very mild, with elevated basal insulin levels and, rarely, ketoacidosis. The diabetes may either precede or follow the onset of the skin rash. The dermatitis usually affects the lower abdomen, perineum, perioral area, or feet. It appears as a reddened patch with a healing center. It exhibits unusual cyclic migrations, with spreading margins and healing catheters, a cycle that takes about 14 days. The differential diagnosis of this dermatitis includes psoriasis, phemphigus, eczema, and zinc deficiency. Histologically, biopsies of other involved areas of skin commonly show necrosis of the upper half of the epidermis only.

The malnutrition of the glucagonoma syndrome is characterized by anemia thought to be secondary to increased iron turnover. Patients commonly have abnormal amino acid profiles, showing the low levels of the majority of amino acids. The etiology of the hypoaminoacidemia is not clear, but it is speculated that it is due to malabsorption. Weight loss and anorexia are characteristic of this tumor also. Venous thrombosis occurs in nearly 30% of the cases. It is not typical thrombophlebitis migrans associated with adenocarcinoma of the pancreas. Patients usually have a normal coagulation profile.

Patients who do not have the necrolytic migratory erythema usually have severe diabetes, with lower basal insulin levels. In addition to not having a rash, these patients usually do not have anemia or venous thrombosis. The prognosis is worse than for those who have the dermatitis.

Glucagon determinations usually show values in the range of 500–6,000 pg/ml. Normal levels are less than 120 pg/ml. In addition, these patients commonly have elevated basal insulin levels.

Medical therapy consists of treatment of the dermatitis and the diabetes, followed by laparotomy and an attempt to resect the tumor. The primary goal of the treatment of the dermatitis is to prevent secondary infection with a combination of antibacterial and antifungal creams. Steroids have been reported to be of some value, as has methotrexate and iodoquinol. Interestingly, zinc administration has proved to be of benefit to some of these patients. Total parenteral nutrition has also been helpful.[93]

Preoperative assessment should include CAT scan and pancreatic angiography; transhepatic portal venous sampling may be of benefit. Laparotomy should be performed in all patients suspected of having glucagonoma. Complete resection will be possible in only 10%–15%. Metastases are present in 80%. Chemotherapy consists of streptozotocin and chlorozotocin. There have been some reports of successful fluorouracil therapy in combination with dimethyltriazenoimidazole carboxamide (DTIC).

SOMATOSTATINOMA

The clinical features are variable. Some patients have symptoms related to the tumor growth, such as jaundice, vomiting, anemia, and weight loss. In others, there seems to be the characteristic syndrome of gallstones, diabetes, and steatorrhea.[94, 95] It is not clear whether somatostatin is the mediator of this syndrome or merely a marker. Pancreatic tumors causing somatostatinoma arise from the D cells of the pancreas. The syndrome (gallstones, diabetes, and steatorrhea) was described by Ganda et al.[96] in 1977 and Kregs et al.[97] in 1979. They postulated that excessive somatostatin causes these symptoms. Somatostatin is known to inhibit the function of most of the digestive organs: it decreases acid production by the stomach with decreased gastric emptying; decreases absorption of sugar, fat, and amino acids in the small intestine with abnormal motility; decreases contractility of the gallbladder; and decreases bicarbonate and enzyme production from the exocrine pancreas. Somatostatin also has been shown to decrease the production of a variety of hormones from various endocrine systems. Either the administration or excessive production of somatostatin has been associated with diminished growth hormone production by the pituitary gland and deficient insulin and glucagon release. In addition, there have been reports of low serum gastrin levels, low cholecystokinin levels, deficient secretin production, and low renin activity in subjects given exogenous somatostatin and patients with excessive production of this hormone. The hyperglycemia in the somatostatin syndrome seems to be secondary to reduced peripheral glucose utilization owing to a relative insulin deficiency.[98, 99]

Somatostatinoma presents a difficult diagnostic problem, as the early findings are nonspecific. Initial symptoms are secondary to tumor within the pancreas and include pain, weight loss, and diabetes. Symptoms related to excessive somatostatin production seems to be intermittent, making detection difficult.[100] In addition, radioimmunoassay for somatostatin is not widely available, and extreme elevations up to a thousandfold of normal are needed to produce the symptoms. Currently, 12 cases of somatostatinoma have been reported in patients ranging in age from 46 and 70, with an equal male:

female distribution.[96-102] Cholelithiasis occurred in eight of the 12 cases, and diabetes was present in nine as was weight loss. Hypochlorhydria and anemia were present in half the patients. The primary tumor was located in the pancreas in the majority of the patients, and in an ectopic location in one. Duodenal somatostatin-producing tumors have been reported twice. Liver metastases were present in the majority. Tumors produced multiple hormones, including calcitonin in two of the cases, and ACTH in one.

Treatment of somatostatinoma includes control of the diabetes preoperatively and then an exploratory laparotomy. As the majority of these tumors are malignant, resection for cure is rarely possible. Five-year survival is rare. If metastases are present, postoperative chemotherapy may be of benefit. Patients who have not had complete resection of tumor usually require the administration of insulin preoperatively.

CHEMOTHERAPY

The therapy for pancreatic endocrine tumor is initially surgical, with removal of as much tumor as possible. In the presence of unresectable tumor or metastases, chemotherapy may be useful to control symptoms related to local tumor growth and invasion. Successful chemotherapy of functioning tumors may also be associated with decreases in hormone production and hence control of symptoms. The course of islet cell carcinoma is characteristically indolent, and survival from the time of the diagnosis of an unresectable malignant disease to death from metastases frequently exceeds five years. The natural course of these tumors makes determination of response to chemotherapy difficult.

The most frequently used treatment is either streptozotocin (STZ) alone or in combination with fluorouracil (5-FU). Objective responses, defined as decreasing tumor size and decreased hormone levels, have been reported in insulinoma,[103-105] gastrinoma,[76, 106] WDHA syndrome,[107] glucagonoma,[108] and tumor-producing pancreatic polypeptides.[109] STZ alone is associated with a complete remission in about 10% of cases and a partial remission in nearly one third. Combination therapy (STZ + 5-FU) doubles the remission rate. The investigational drug chlorozotocin (CTZ) may improve response rates considerably. It should be released for general use in the near future.

The major side effects of STZ and CTZ are diabetes and renal failure. Hepatic artery infusion has been reported to be complicated by thrombosis of the hepatic artery.[110] Administration of these drugs through the hepatic artery and portal vein should be considered investigational.

Trials to determine the efficacy of DTIC and adriamycin in the treatment of these tumors have begun.[111]

SUMMARY

The principles of diagnosis and the management of these tumors are similar, regardless of the syndrome produced. The presence of an endocrine tumor of the pancreas should be suspected in patients with common symptoms which are refractory to standard treatment and in whom ordinary diseases have been excluded. The physician must have keen suspicion. The diagnosis is confirmed by radioimmunoassay of the hormone in question. Tumor localization should be accomplished preoperatively with CAT scan, angiogram, and portal venous sampling.

Treatment is surgical in most cases and must be directed primarily at control of the tumor. Initially, the effect of the excessive hormone production should be controlled medically by either blocking the end-organ effect of the hormone or by inhibiting hormone release. During this period, supportive care is required to permit tumor localization and to ready the patient for laparotomy. At operation, tumor should be resected if the risk is reasonable. If gastrinoma is present, either a vagotomy with pyloroplasty or total gastrectomy should be performed. In other tumors, attempts to control the excessive function of the target organ are impractical. Postoperatively, continued medical control of the aberrant physiology may be necessary, and chemotherapy should be considered if unresectable tumor and metastases are present.

REFERENCES

1. Wellbourne R.B., Polak J.M., Bloom S.R., et al.: Apudomas of the pancreas, in Bloom S.R. (ed.): *Gut Hormones.* Edinburgh and N.Y., Churchill Livingstone, 1978, pp. 561–569.
2. Friesen S.R.: The APUD syndrome. *Prog. Clin. Cancer* 8:75–87, 1982.
3. Andrew A., Kramer B., Rawdon B.B.: Gut and pancreatic amine precursor uptake and decarboxylation cells are not natural crest derivatives. *Gastroenterology* 84:429–431, 1983.
4. Prinz R.A., Bermes E.W., Kimmel J.R., Marangos P.J.: Serum markers for pancreatic islet cell and intestinal carcinoid tumors: A comparison of neuron specific enolase, beta-human chorionic gonadotropin and pancreatic polypeptide. *Surgery* 94:1019–1023, 1983.
5. Prinz R.A., Marangos P.J.: Serum neron-specific enolase: A serum marker for nonfunctioning pancreatic islet cell carcinoma. *Am. J. Surg.* 145:77–81, 1983.
6. Van Heerden J.A., Edis A.: Insulinoma: Diagnosis and management. *Surg. Rounds* 42–52, November 1980.
7. Zuppinger K.: Disorders of the endocrine pancreas. *Prog. Pediatr. Surg.* 16:51–61, 1983.
8. Stabile B.E., Morrow D.J., Passaro E.: The gastrinoma triangle: operative implications. *Am. J. Surg.* 147:25–31, 1984.
9. Heitz P.V., Kasper M., Polak J.M., et al.: Pancreatic endocrine tumors. *Hum. Pathol.* 13:263–271, 1982.
10. Coons A.H., Leduc S.H., Conolly J.M.: Studies on antibody production: I. A method for the histochemical demonstration of specific antibody and its application to a study of hyperimmune rabbit. *J. Exp. Med.* 102:49–60, 1955.
11. Sternberger L.A.: *Immunocytochemistry,* ed. 2. New York, John Wiley & Sons, 1979.
12. Milkai K., Greider M.H., Grotting T., et al.: Retrospective study of 77 pancreatic endocrine tumors using immunoperoxidase method. *Am. J. Surg. Pathol.* 6:387–399, 1982.
13. Alumels J., Sundler F., Falkner S., et al.: Neurohormonal peptides in endocrine tumors of the pancreas, stomach, and upper small intestine: I. An immunohistochemical study of 27 cases. *Ultrastruct. Pathol.* 5:55–72, 1983.
14. Levitt R.G., Stanley R.J., Sagel S.S., et al.: Computed tomography of the pancreas: 3-second scanning verus 18-second scanning. *J. Comput. Assist. Tomogr.* 26:259–267, 1982.
15. Hosoki T.: Dynamic CT of pancreatic tumors. *Am. J. Radiol.* 140:959–965, 1983.
16. Stark D.D., Moss A.A., Goldberg H.I., et al.: Computed tomography and nuclear magnetic resonance imaging of pancreatic islet cell tumors. *Surgery* 94:1024–1027, 1983.
17. Stark D.D., Moss A.A., Goldberg H.I., et al.: CT of pancreatic islet cell tumors. *Radiology* 150:491–494, 1984.
18. Roche A., Raisonnier A., Gillon-Savoret M.C.: Pancreatic venous sampling and arteriography in localizing insulinoma and gastrinomas: Procedure and results in 55 cases. *Radiology* 145:621–627, 1982.

19. Aldrite J.S., Hon S.Y., Henao F.; Arteriography with simultaneous gastric distention to detect insulin-secreting tumors of the pancreas. *South. Med. J.* 76:1524–1529, 1983.

20. Debas H.T., Soon-Shiang P., McKenzie A.D., et al.: Use of secretin in the roentgenologic and biochemical diagnosis of duodenal gastrinoma. *Am. J. Surg.* 145:408–411, 1983.

21. Ingemansson S., Lunderquist A., Lunderquist I., et al.: Portal and pancreatic vein catheterization with radioimmunologic determination of insulin. *Surg. Gynecol. Obstet.* 141:705–711, 1975.

22. Ingemansson S., Holsh J., Larsson L.I., et al.: Localization of glucagonomas by catheterization of the pancreatic veins and with glucagon assay. *Surg. Gynecol. Obstet.* 145:509–516, 1977.

23. Millan V.G., Vrosa C.L., Molitch M.E., et al.: Localization of occult insulinoma by superselective pancreatic venous sampling for insulin assay through percutaneous tromohepatic catheterization. *Diabetes* 28:249–251, 1979.

24. Burcharth F., Stage J.G., Stadil F.: Localization of gastrinomas by tromohepatic portal catheterization and gastrin assay. *Gastroenterology* 77:44–450, 1979.

25. Glaser B., Valtysson G., Vinile A.C., et al.: Gastrointestinal pancreatic hormone concentrations in the portal venous system in patients with islet cell tumors. *Clin. Res.* 28:556A, 1980.

26. Vinick A.I., Glaser B.: Pancreatic endocrine tumors, in Dent T.L., Echhauser F.E., et al. (eds.): *Pancreatic Disease.* New York, Grune & Stratton, 1981, pp. 427–460.

27. Oho A.J., Vinik A.I., Thompson N.W., et al.: Localization of the source of hyperinsulinism: Percutaneous transhepatic portal and pancreatic vein catheterization with hormone assay. *Am. J. Radiol.* 139:237–245, 1982.

28. Vinik A.I., Glaser B.: Pancreatic endocrine tumors, in Dent T.L., Echhauser F.E., et al. (eds.): *Pancreatic Disease: Diagnosis and Therapy.* New York, Grune & Stratton, 1981, pp. 427–460.

29. Lane R.J., Coupland G.A.: Operative ultrasonic features of insulinomas. *Am. J. Surg.* 144:585–587, 1982.

30. Angelini L., Maceratini R., Bezzi M., et al.: Intraoperative high resolution ultrasonography in the localization of occult endocrine pancreatic tumors. *Ital. J. Surg. Sci.* 13:209–215, 1983.

31. Sigel B., Duarte B., Coelho J.C., et al.: Localization of insulinomas of the pancreas at operation by real-time ultrasound scanning. *Surg. Gynecol. Obstet.* 156:145–147, 1983.

32. Charboneau J.W., Jones E.M., VonHeeden J.A., et al.: Intraoperative real-time ultrasonographic localization of pancreatic insulinoma: Initial experience. *J. Ultrasound. Med.* 2:251–254, 1983.

33. Whipple A.O., Frantz V.K.: Adenoma of islet cells with hyperinsulinism. *Ann. Surg.* 101:1299–1335, 1935.

34. Harrington M.G., McGeorge A.P., Ballantyne J.P., et al.: A prospective survey for insulinomas in a neurology department. *Lancet* 1:1094–1095, 1983.

35. Powers R.D., Robb J.F.: Hyperglycemia due to insulinoma. An unusual cause of altered mental states. *Minn. Med.* 66:13–15, 1983.

36. Jayasinghe K.S., Nimalasuriya A., Dharmadasal C.: A case of insulinoma with peripheral neuropathy. *Postgrad. Med.* 59:689–90, 1983.

37. Fagans S.S., Floyd J.C.: Fasting hypoglycemia in adults. *N. Engl. J. Med.* 294:766–772, 1976.

38. Collin C.F., Bradley E.L.: Pseudoinsulinoma. *Arch. Surg.* 118:1087–1090, 1983.

39. Service F.J., Dale A.J., Elveback L.R., et al.: Clinical and diagnostic features of 60 consecutive cases. *Mayo Clin. Proc.* 51:417, 1976.

40. Fajans S.S., Floyd J.C.: Diagnosis and medical management of insulinoma. *Am. Rev. Med.* 30:313, 1979.

41. Randell M.: The expanding use of C. peptide radioimmunoassay. *Acta Diabetol. Lat.* 20:105–113, 1983.

42. Turner R.C., Heding L.G.: Plasma proinsulin, C-peptide, and insulin in diagnostic suppression tests for insulinomas. *Diabetologia* 13:571–577, 1977.

43. Blum I., Resechi Y., Doron M., et al.: Evidence for a therapeutic effect of d$_l$-propranolol in benign and malignant insulinoma: Report of 3 cases. *J. Endocrinol. Invest.* 6:41–45, 1983.

44. Tutt G.O., Edis A.J., Service F.J., et al.: Plasma glucose monitoring during operation for insulinoma: A critical reappraisal. *Surgery* 88:351–356, 1980.

45. Buysschaert M., Lambotte G., Reynaert M., et al.: Use of extracorporeal glucose monitor for the diagnosis and surgical treatment of an insulinoma. *Br. J. Surg.* 67:841–844, 1980.

46. Teichmann R.K., Spelsberg F., Herberer G.: Intraoperative biochemical localization of insulinoma by quick radioimmunoasssay. *Am. J. Surg.* 143:113–115, 1982.

47. Zick R., Hammer A., Otten G., et al.: Rapid immunoassay for insulin and its application in localized occult insulinoma by intraoperative pancreatic vein sampling. *Eur. J. Nucl. Med.* 7:85–87, 1982.

48. Duncan W.E., Duncan T.G., DeLauerentis D.A., et al.: Artificial pancreas as an aid during insulinoma resection. *Am. J. Surg.* 142:528–531, 1981.

49. Zollinger R.M., Ellison E.H.: Primary peptic ulceration of the jejunum associated with islet cell tumors. *Ann. Surg.* 142:709–728, 1955.

50. Primrose J.N., Jaffe S.N., Ratcliffe J.G., et al.: The prevalence of gastrinoma in recurrent peptic ulceration. *South. Med. J.* 28:328–331, 1983.

51. Zollinger R.M., Ellison E.C., Fabri P.J., et al.: Primary peptic ulceration of the jejunum associated with islet cell tumors: Twenty-five year appraisal. *Ann. Surg.* 192:422–430, 1980.

52. Regan P.T., Malagelada J.R.: A reappraisal of clinical, roentgenographic and endoscopic features of the Zollinger-Ellison syndrome. *Mayo Clin. Proc.* 53:19–23, 1978.

53. Wilson S.W.: Ulcerogenic tumors, in Carey L.C. (ed.): *The Pancreas.* St. Louis, C.V. Mosby, 1973, pp. .

54. Hofmann J.W., Fox P.S., Nilson S.D.: Duodenal wall tumors and the Zollinger-Ellison syndrome. *Arch. Surg.* 107:334–339, 1973.

55. Fox D.S., Hofmann J.W., Wilson S.D., et al.: Surgical management of the Zollinger-Ellison syndrome. *Surg. Clin. North Am.* 54:345– , 1974.

56. Brennan M.F., Jensen R.T., Wesley R.A.: The role of surgery in patients with Zollinger-Ellison syndrome managed medically. *Ann. Surg.* 196:239–245, 1982.

57. Thompson J.C., Lewis B.G., Weiner L., et al.: The role of surgery in the Zollinger-Ellison syndrome. *Ann. Surg.* 197:594–607, 1983.

58. Townsend C.M. Jr., Lewis B.G., Gowsley W.R., et al.: Gastrinoma. *Curr Probl. Cancer.* 7:1–33, 1982.

59. Deveney C.W., Deveney K.E., Stark D., et al.: Resection of gastrinomas. *Ann. Surg.* 198:546–553, 1983.

60. Bonfils S., Landor., Mignon M.: Results of surgical management in 92 consecutive patients with Zollinger-Ellison syndrome. *Ann. Surg.* 194:692–697, 1981.

61. Christoforidas A.J., Nelson S.N.: Radiologic manifestations of ulcerogenic tumor of the pancreas. *J.A.M.A.* 198:97–102, 1966.

62. McGuigan J.E., Trudeau W.L.: Immunochemical measurement of elevated levels of gastrin in the serum of patients with pancreatic tumors of the Zollinger-Ellison variety. *N. Engl. J. Med.* 298:1308–1315, 1968.

63. Malagelada J.R., Davis C.G., O'Fallon W.M.: Laboratory diagnosis of gastrinoma. *Mayo Clin. Proc.* 57:211–218, 1982.

64. Malagelada J.R., Glanzman S.L., Go V.L.W.: Laboratory diagnosis of gastrinoma: A prospective study of gastrin challenge. *Mayo Clin. Proc.* 57:219–226, 1982.

65. Modlin I.M., Brennan M.F.: The diagnosis and management of gastrinoma. *Surg. Gynecol. Obstet.* 158:92–104, 1984.

66. Friesen S.R., Tomita T.: Pseudo-Zollinger-Ellison syndrome. *Ann. Surg.* 194:481–493, 1981.

67. Deveney C.W., Deveney K.S., Way L.W.: The Zollinger-Ellison syndrome 23 years later. *Ann. Surg.* 188:384–394, 1978.

68. Ramanus M.E., Neal J.A., Dilley W.G., et al.: Comparison of four provocative tests for the diagnosis of gastrinoma. *Ann. Surg.* 197:608–617, 1983.

69. Jensen R.T.: Zollinger-Ellison syndrome. Current concepts and management. *Ann. Intern. Med.* 98:59–75, 1983.

70. Stabile B.E.: Failure of historical H$_2$-receptor antagonist therapy in Zollinger-Ellison syndrome. *Am. J. Surg.* 145:17–23, 1983.

71. Jensen R.T., Colleen M.J., Pandel S.J.: Cimetidine-induced impotence and breast changes in patients with gastric hypersecretory states. *N. Engl. J. Med.* 308:883–887, 1983.

72. Raufman J.-P., Collins S.M., Pandol S.J.: Reliability of symptoms in assessing control of gastric acid secretion in patients with Zollinger-Ellison syndrome. *Gastroenterology* 84:108–113, 1983.

73. Malagelada J.R., Edis A.J., Adson M., et al.: Medical and surgical options in management of patients with gastrinoma. *Gastroenterology* 84:1532–1542, 1983.

74. Passaro E., Stabile B.: Of gastrinomas and their management. *Gastroenterology* 84:1621–1673, 1983.

75. Richardson C., Feldman M., McClelland R.N., et al.: Effect of vagotomy in Zollinger-Ellison syndrome. *Gastroenterology* 77:682–686, 1979.

76. Zollinger R.M., Martin E.W., Carey L.C., et al.: Observations on postoperative tumor growth behavior of certain islet cell tumors. *Surgery* 184:525–530, 1976.

77. Priest W.M., Alexander M.K.: Islet cell tumor of the pancreas with peptic ulceration, diarrhea, and hypokalemia. *Lancet* 2:1145–1147, 1957.

78. Verner J.V., Morrison A.B.: Islet cell tumor and a syndrome of refractory diarrhea and hypokalemia. *Am. J. Med.* 25:374–380, 1958.

79. Marks I.N., Banks S., Louw J.: Islet cell tumor of the pancreas with reversible watery diarrhea and achlorhydria. *Gastroenterology* 52:695, 1967.

80. Zollinger R.M., Tompkins R.K., Amerson J.R.: Identification of the diarrheogenic hormone associated with nonbeta islet cell tumors of the pancreas. *Ann. Surg.* 168:502–521, 1968.

81. Said S.I., Falcona G.R.: Elevated plasma and tissue levels of vasoactive intestinal peptide in the watery diarrhea syndrome due to pancreatic, bronchogenic, and other tumors. *N. Engl. J. Med.* 293:155–160, 1975.

82. Cooperman A.M., Desantis D., Winkelman E., et al.: Watery diarrhea syndrome: Two unusual cases and further evidence that VIP is a hormonal mediator. *Ann. Surg.* 187:325–328, 1978.

83. Jaffe B.M., Kopen D.F., et al.: Indomethacin-responsive pancreatic cholera. *N. Engl. J. Med.* 297:817–821, 1977.

84. Jaffe B.M.: To be or not to VIP. *Gastroenterology* 76:419–420, 1979.

85. Modlin I.M., Bloom S.R., Mitchell S.J.: Experimental evidence for vasoactive intestinal peptide as the cause of the watery diarrhea syndrome. *Gastroenterology* 75:1051–1054, 1978.

86. Kane M.C., O'Dorisio T.M., Kregs G.T.: Production of secretory diarrhea by intravenous infusion of vasoactive intestinal peptide. *N. Engl. J. Med.* 309:1482–1485, 1983.

87. Verner J.V., Morrison A.B.: Endocrine pancreatic islet disease with diarrhea. *Arch. Intern. Med.* 133:492–500, 1974.

88. Becker W.E., Kahn D., Rothma S.: Cutaneous manifestations of internal malignant tumors. *Arch. Dermatol.* 45:1069, 1942.

89. Gossner W., Korting G.W.: Metastasierendes inzellen karzinom vom A zelltyp bei einen fall von pemphigus foliaceous mit diabetes renalis. *Dtsch. Med. Wochenschr.* 85:434, 1960.

90. McGavran M.H., Unger R.H., Recant L., et al.: A glucagon-secreting alpha cell carcinoma of the pancreas. *N. Engl. J. Med.* 274:1408, 1966.

91. Prinz R.A., Dorsch T.R., Lawrence A.M.: Clinical aspects of glucagon-producing islet cell tumors. *Am. J. Gastroenterol.* 76:125–131, 1981.

92. Mallinson C., Bloom S.R.: The hyperglycemic cutaneous syndrome: Pancreatic glucagonoma, in Friesen S.R. (ed.): *Surgical Endocrinology: Clinical Syndromes.* Philadelphia, J.B. Lippincott, 1978, pp. 171–201.

93. Amon R.B., Swenson K.H., Hanifin J.M.: The glucagonoma syndrome and zinc (letter). *N. Engl. J. Med.* 295:962, 1976.

94. Stackpoole P.W., Kasselberg A.G., Berklowitz M., et al.: Somatostatinoma syndrome: Does a clinical entity exist? *Acta Endocrinol.* (Copenhagen) 102:80–87, 1983.

95. Pipeleers D., Couturier E., Gepts W., et al.: Five cases of somatostatinoma: Clinical heterogeneity and diagnostic usefulness of basal and tolbutamide-induced hypersomatostatinemia. *J. Clin. Endocrinol. Metab.* 56:1236–1242, 1983.

96. Ganda O.P., Weis G.C., Soeldner A.: Somatostatinoma: A somatostatin-containing tumor of the endocrine pancreas. *N. Engl. J. Med.* 296:963–967, 1977.

97. Kregs G.J., Orci L., Conlon M., et al.: Somatostatinoma syndrome. *N. Engl. J. Med.* 301:285–292, 1979.

98. Lowry S.F., Brennan M.F.: Glucose turnover and gluconeogenesis in a patient with somatostatinoma. *Surgery* 89:309–312, 1981.

99. Axelrod L., Bush M., Hirsch H.J., et al.: Malignant somatostatinoma: Clinical features and metabolic studies. *J. Clin. Endocrinol. Metab.* 52:886–896, 1981.

100. Sommers G., Pipeleers-Marichal M., Gepta W., et al.: A case of duodenal somatostatinoma: Diagnostic usefulness of calcium-pentagastrin test. *Gastroenterology* 85:1192–1198, 1983.

101. Kelly T.R.: Pancreatic somatostatinoma. *Am. J. Surg.* 146:671–673, 1983.

102. Sakazaki S., Umeyama K., Nakagawa H., et al.: Pancreatic somatostatinoma. *Am. J. Surg.* 146:674–679, 1983.

103. Murray-Lyon I.M., Eddlestone S.L.W.F., William R., et al.: Treatment of multiple hormone producing malignant islet cell tumor with streptozotocin. *Lancet* 2:895–898, 1968.

104. Broder L.E., Carter S.K.: Pancreatic islet cell carcinoma: Results of therapy with streptozotocin in 52 patients. *Ann. Intern. Med.* 79:108–118, 1973.

105. Herbai G., Lundin A.: Treatment of malignant metastatic pancreatic insulinoma with streptozotocin. *Acta Med. Scand.* 220:447–452, 1976.

106. Ruffner B.W.: CHemotherapy for malignant Zollinger-Ellison tumors. *Arch. Intern. Med.* 135:1032–000, 1976.

107. Gagel R.F., Costanza M.E., Pehellis R.A., et al.: Streptozotocin-treated Verner-Morrison syndromes: Plasma vasoactive intestinal peptide and tumor responses. *Arch. Intern. Med.* 136:1429–1435, 1976.

108. Danforth D.N., Triche T., Doppman J.C.: Elevated plasma proglucagon-like component with glucagon-secreting tumor: Effect of streptozotocin. *N. Engl. J. Med.* 297:242–245, 1976.

109. Friesen S.R., Stephens R.C., Heard S.: Effective streptozotocin therapy for metastatic pancreatic polypeptide apudoma. *Arch. Surg.* 116:1090–1092, 1981.

110. Holt S., Raysmith A., Reid J., et al.: Hazards of hepatic artery infusion of streptozotocin. *Scot. Med. J.* 24:163–165, 1979.

111. Awrich A.E., Peetz M., Fletcher W.S.: Dimethyltriazendimidazole carboxamide therapy of islet cell carcinoma of the pancreas. *J. Surg. Oncol.* 17:321–326, 1981.

112. Berson S.A., Yalow R.S.: Isotopic tissues in the study of diabetes, in Tobias C.A., Lawrence J.H. (eds.): *Advances in Biological and Medical Physics.* New York, Academic Press, 1958, pp. 350–430.

113. McGuigan J.E., Wolfe M.M.: Gastrin radioimmunoassay. *Clin. Chem.* 28:368–373, 1982.

114. Polak J.M., Stagg B., Pearse A.G.E.: Two types of Zollinger-Ellison syndrome: Immunofluorescent, cytochemical, and ultrastructural studies of the antral and pancreatic gastrin cells in different clinical states. *Gut* 13:511–512, 1972.

115. Friesen S.R., Tomita T.: Pseudo Zollinger-Ellison syndrome: Hypergastrinemia, hyperchlorhydria without tumor. *Ann. Surg.* 194:481–493, 1981.

PART VII

Diseases of the Intestinal Tract

38

Intestinal Pseudo-Obstruction and Paralytic Ileus

JAMES CHRISTENSEN, M.D.

INTRODUCTION

Definitions

"Paralytic ileus" is a term of very long standing, while "intestinal pseudo-obstruction" is of more recent vintage.[1] The former term is usually used to refer to an acute physiologic state that is assumed to be temporary or at least potentially reversible, while the latter implies a diagnosis that has a degree of permanence. Ileus is usually considered to be the consequence of the activation of a normal inhibitory mechanism, like an inhibitory reflex, while pseudo-obstruction usually refers to some abnormal process that affects the function of GI nerve and/or muscle. There can be little doubt, however, that the two terms have been used interchangeably in the past and continue to be. Both ileus and pseudo-obstruction are characterized by many of the features of GI obstruction, when a concrete mechanical obstruction to flow is not, in fact, present.

This is an area where precise physiologic and pathologic definitions are not yet possible. Ileus and pseudo-obstruction, whether acute or chronic, can be used to describe syndromes, clinical states, that may have several causes. Thus, "paralytic ileus" and "intestinal pseudo-obstruction" resemble many other terms (e.g., "congestive heart failure" and "malabsorption syndrome") that have a certain everyday utility without in themselves being precisely defined in respect to specific pathophysiologic processes.

The intent of this chapter is to review the features of these syndromes, to set forth a current classification of their recognized causes, and to describe the current means to establish diagnoses and apply treatment. These matters have been treated in several reviews in recent years.[1-13]

This subject does not have a long history. Though there were casual reports of pseudo-obstruction about 50 years ago, publications on the topic have been numerous only in about the past decade. Ileus, as well, was not a subject for much study before the early part of the century. The science of GI motility is evolving rapidly and may be expected to further explain these clinical syndromes in the next few years.

A Classification of the Syndromes

It is now clear that the syndromes of pseudo-obstruction and ileus can come about through a variety of mechanisms that lead to a common defect. The common defect is one of ineffective propulsion of the GI contents by the movements of the muscular walls of the gut. Such ineffective motion represents abnormal contractions of the smooth muscle that makes up the muscular walls of the GI viscera. These abnormalities can arise from disturbances within the muscle itself, disturbances in the autonomic nerves that supply this muscle, or disturbances in the biochemical and hormonal milieu of the muscle. Some of these disturbances are genetic in origin and others are iatrogenic, but many remain idiopathic. Thus, a classification is both complex and tentative.

A classification that has proved to be of some utility follows.

I. Primary or idiopathic pseudo-obstruction
  A. Familial syndromes
    1. Familial visceral myopathies
    2. Familial visceral neuropathies
  B. Nonfamilial (or sporadic) syndromes
    1. Visceral myopathies
    2. Visceral neuropathies
II. Secondary pseudo-obstruction (related to recognized diseases)
  A. Diseases of gastrointestinal muscle
    1. The "collagen diseases"
      a. Scleroderma
      b. Dermatomyositis/Polymyositis
      c. Systemic lupus erythematosus
    2. Amyloidosis
    3. Generalized disease of muscle
      a. Myotonic dystrophy
      b. Progressive muscular dystrophy
    4. Ceroidosis ("brown bowel syndrome")
  B. Diseases of gastrointestinal nerves
    1. Parkinson's disease
    2. Hirschsprung's disease
    3. Chagas' disease
    4. Primary autonomic dysfunction
  C. Endocrine diseases involving the gastrointestinal tract
    1. Myxedema
    2. Diabetes mellitus
    3. Hypoparathyroidism
    4. Pheochromocytoma
  D. Drug-induced syndromes
    1. Psychotropic drugs
    2. Anti-parkinsonian drugs
    3. Cathartics
  E. Miscellaneous causes
    1. Jejunoileal bypass
    2. Jejunal diverticulosis
    3. Inflammatory bowel diseases

III. Paralytic ileus
  1. Related to intra-abdominal disease
  2. Related to extra-abdominal disease

FAMILIAL FORMS OF IDIOPATHIC PSEUDO-OBSTRUCTION

Familial Visceral Myopathy

HISTORICAL REVIEW.—There have been several reports of cases of pseudo-obstruction syndromes that cluster in families. The early reports were incomplete so that precise definitions of the syndromes—the organs involved, the patterns of inheritance, and the pathology—were not made. Later reports have been more comprehensive and have depicted syndromes that better approach a precise definition.

The first such report was that of Weiss[14] in 1938, a paper which was not widely noted at that time and only came to general attention 40 years later, when interest in the subject increased. Weiss described six cases in a German family. All of them had megaduodenum. Some had esophageal dilatation, gastric dilatation, and megacolon as well. The symptoms were somewhat variable, but included episodic abdominal distress, abdominal distention, nausea, and vomiting. Symptoms rarely occurred before middle age.

Law and Ten Eyck[15] described nine members in two generations of a family of Italian descent. These cases had megaduodenum and an enlarged urinary bladder. Abdominal and urinary tract symptoms did not develop until adulthood. Duodenal motility studies were abnormal in two of the patients. Microscopic examination of resected tissue was possible only in one case: both the dilated duodenum and the uninvolved jejunum in that case showed normal smooth muscle and normal-appearing ganglia by light microscopy in conventionally stained specimens.

Newton[16] described two black American brothers with megaduodenum, one of whom also had megacystis. Microscopic examination of resected specimens showed normal-appearing smooth muscle and ganglion cells.

Schuffler and Pope[17] described a 15-year-old girl with intestinal atony who had six relatives with lesser evidence of a motility disorder; in four of them there was esophageal motor dysfunction as revealed by manometry, and two others had urinary bladder dysfunction. The resected intestine in the index case showed degeneration of the smooth muscle but normal-appearing nerve tissue.

Lewis et al.[18] studied relatives of a young patient with megaduodenum and found abnormal esophageal motor function in one sibling. The authors did not have the opportunity to examine tissues histologically.

Maldonado et al.[19] had two patients with intestinal pseudo-obstruction with positive family histories, but more detailed studies were not reported.

Faulk et al.[20] reported a large kindred of Scottish descent in whom at least 18 members in five generations had evidence of pseudo-obstruction. The most prominent manifestations were megaduodenum, megacolon, and megacystis. Esophageal motor dysfunction was detected in several cases, and duodenal motor dysfunction was demonstrated manometrically. Resected tissues from several cases showed marked attenuation of the smooth muscle of the outer longitudinal layer

with replacement of the muscle by collagen. The nerves of the myenteric plexus appeared to be normal.

Shaw et al.[12] described a family in which children were involved with pseudo-obstruction that affected the esophagus, duodenum, and colon. Histologic examination of resected intestine showed degeneration and fibrosis of the longitudinal muscle layer.

Jacobs et al.[21] described members of a family with gastric and intestinal pseudo-obstruction in whom there was degeneration and fibrosis, especially of the muscles of the longitudinal muscle layer of the intestine.

Anuras et al.[22] described a family in which there was gastric atony, dilation of the entire intestine, and multiple jejunal diverticulosis, associated with external ophthalmoplegia. In the intestine, the longitudinal muscle layer was especially affected by degeneration and fibrosis; the nerve plexuses appeared to be normal. Transmission was autosomal and recessive.

The clinical features, pathology and apparent mode of inheritance of the syndromes in these families is summarized in Table 38–1 and in Figure 38–1.

CLINICAL FEATURES—SOME GENERALIZATIONS.— From the reports cited above, it is now possible to make some generalized statements about the clinical features of familial visceral myopathy.

First, the organs involved and the pathology found tend to be similar in most cases within each family. Thus, in some families megaduodenum and megacolon occur commonly (Fig 38–2), while in others there is generalized involvement of the whole of the GI tract. Similarly, the pathology (Fig 38–3) tends to be similar in patients within a single kindred. It appears, however, that the apparently genetic abnormality is expressed somewhat differently among individual affected members of a single family, so that not all such cases in one family are identical in the location of the disease or in the degree of symptoms. This variability in expression is more apparent in the severity than it is in the extent of the lesion.

Second, the disorder appears to be a primary disorder of the muscle rather than a muscular lesion secondary to neuropathy, because in none of these families have pathologic features of the myenteric or submucosal plexuses been reported. It should be noted, however, that the inspection of the plexuses is a relatively crude approach in routinely stained cross sections of the intestine, and it might miss a subtle or incomplete neuropathologic process because of sampling error.

Third, familial visceral myopathy is not a single nosological entity, since there are important differences among the several families reported in the extent of the lesions, in the age of onset of symptoms, and in the apparent pattern of transmission.

Fourth, the fundamental pathologic process appears to be one that proceeds very slowly, so slowly in some cases that it appears to be static.

SYMPTOMS.—The symptoms vary considerably, depending both on the extent of the involvement and on the severity or degree of muscular degeneration that has occurred.

When the esophagus is affected, the organ may be rather dilated, but esophageal retention and dysphagia are not

TABLE 38–1.—A SUMMARY OF FAMILIAL SYNDROMES OF PRIMARY VISCERAL MYOPATHY

AUTHOR(S)	YEAR	CONFIRMED/NO. FAM. INVEST.	MODE OF INHERITANCE	GI LESIONS	UROLOGIC LESIONS	MICROSCOPIC LESIONS
Byrnes et al.[4]	1977	13/21	Autosomal dominant	Esophageal aperistalsis megaduodenum, segmental dilatation of small bowel, dilatation & redundancy in colon	Neurogenic bladder	Microscopic lesions, patchy areas of mild villous abnormality with increased numbers of lymphocytes in the lamina propria
Schuffler et al.[23]	1978	2/4	Probably autosomal recessive	Esophageal aperistalsis, dilated esophagus, stomach, & small bowel, extensive colonic diverticulitis	Not studied	Degeneration of the intestinal myenteric plexus with intranuclear inclusion bodies present (composed of filamentous material)
Schuffler and Pope[10]	1977	5/16	Autosomal dominant	Esophageal aperistalsis, megaduodenum, dilated proximal jejunum, redundant colon	Megacystis	Degeneration and fibrosis of both intestinal muscle layers
Lewis et al.[18]	1978	5/12	Autosomal dominant	Esophageal aperistalsis, megaduodenum, dilated proximal jejunum	Not studied	Mild patchy atrophic changes and fibrosis of jejunum
Faulk et al.[20]	1978	18/93	Autosomal dominant	Esophageal aperistalsis megaduodenum, redundant colon	Megacystis	Degeneration and fibrosis of intestinal muscle; longitudinal layer is more involved
Shaw et al.[12]	1979	9/39	Autosomal dominant	Esophageal aperistalsis, megaduodenum, redundant colon	Not studied	Degeneration and fibrosis of intestinal muscle; longitudinal layer is more involved
Jacobs et al.[21]	1979	2/5	Autosomal recessive	Gastric atony, tubular featureless small bowel	Not studied	Degeneration and fibrosis mainly of longitudinal muscle layer
Weiss[14]	1938	6/11	Autosomal dominant (sex-linked dominant cannot be ruled out)	Megaduodenum, megacolon	Not studied	Not studied
Law and Ten Eyck[15]	1962	8/36	Autosomal dominant	Megaduodenum	Megacystis	Smooth muscle normal?
Newton[16]	1968	2/10	Probably autosomal dominant	Megaduodenum	Megaureter, megacystis	Smooth muscle normal?
Anuras et al.[22]	1983	3/3 carriers/63	Autosomal recessive	Gastric atony, dilatation of entire small bowel with multiple diverticula	No clinical manifestation	Degeneration and fibrosis mainly of longitudinal muscle layer

prominent symptoms because the esphagogastric sphincter is atonic. Thus, the esophageal abnormality more closely resembles that of scleroderma than it does that of achalasia. One might expect reflux esophagitis to be present, but that has not been a conspicuous feature of reported cases.

When the stomach is involved, the symptoms resemble those of gastric outlet obstruction. Early satiety, postcibal abdominal distention, dyspepsia, nausea, and vomiting all may occur. There may be bezoar formation and gastritis.

With small-intestinal involvement, whether localized or generalized, early satiety, distention, dyspepsia, and vomiting may also be accompanied by episodic or continuous diarrhea. The diarrhea is a manifestation of bacterial overgrowth in the small intestine that comes about from the inability of the small intestine to clear itself of bacteria of either oral or colonic origin.

When the colon is involved alone, there is likely to be severe constipation, but bacterial overgrowth in the small intestine may tend to avert the constipation when small-intestinal disease is also present.

Megacystis is commonly asymptomatic, or so slightly symptomatic as not to bring the patient to the physician.

Malnutrition may be evident as a vitamin-deficiency syndrome and extensive weight loss. Steatorrhea may be promi-

nent in cases with extensive small-intestinal disease. Dysfunction of other kinds of muscle, striated muscle, cardiac muscle, and vascular smooth muscle, have not been reported except for the external ophthalmoplegia in the recessive syndrome described by Anuras et al.[22]

Familial Visceral Neuropathy

REPORTED CASES.—Visceral neuropathic syndromes that seem to be familial have been rarely reported. When the syndrome is a manifestation of a generalized autonomic dysfunction, it should be considered to be a secondary form of pseudo-obstruction (see below). In other cases, however, the syndrome has not appeared to be part of a generally recognized syndrome, and the intestinal pseudo-obstruction has appeared to be the major manifestation. An early report was of four siblings with intestinal pseudo-obstruction with steatorrhea.[24] They also suffered from mental retardation and had cerebral calcifications. The intestinal myenteric plexus in one patient was found to show a degeneration of nerve cell bodies on silver-impregnation staining. In another report, three sisters had deficient motility of the gastric antrum dilatation, and multiple jejunal and ileal diverticula.[25] They also suffered from deafness and a progressive peripheral sensory neuropathy. No histologic study was made of the smooth

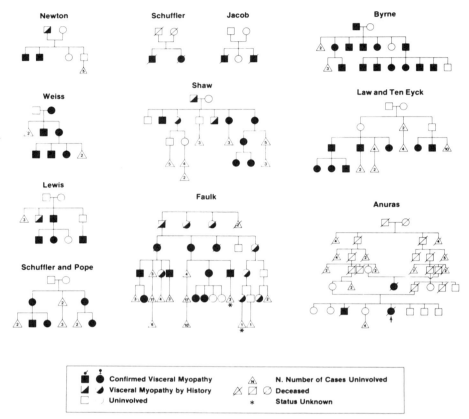

Fig 38–1.—The family trees of 11 families reported with familial visceral myopathy. These families are designated by the name of the first author of the report (see reference list).

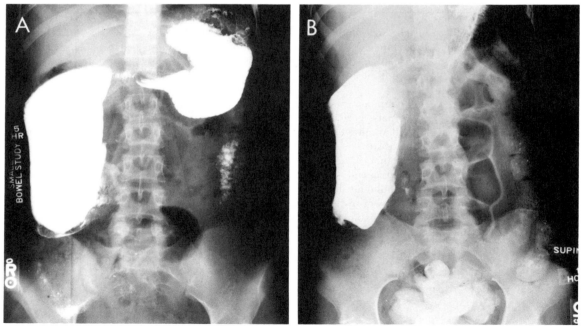

Fig 38–2.—Megaduodenum in a grandmother **(A)** and granddaughter **(B)** to indicate the identity of the segmental duodenal disease. The mother in this family (Faulk) had an identical lesion. Only the granddaughter was symptomatic.

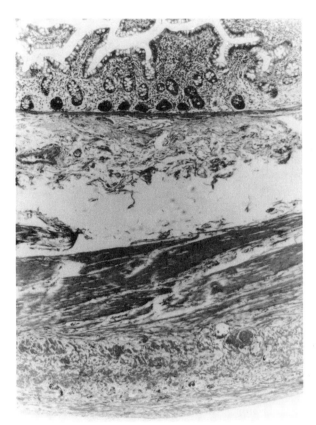

Fig 38–3.—The pathology of the muscle in familial visceral myopathy. The circular muscle layer is intact, but the longitudinal muscle layer is degenerated. The submucosa shows edema. (Photograph courtesy of F.A. Mitros, M.D.)

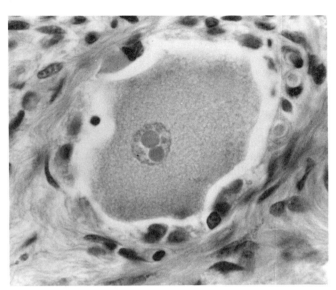

Fig 38–4.—Intranuclear inclusion bodies in neurons of the myenteric plexus in a case of visceral neuropathy. (Photograph courtesy of M.D. Schuffler, M.D.)

muscle or of the myenteric plexus in the affected organs.

The most complete description of an idiopathic or familial neuropathy that seemed to involve primarily the nerves of the myenteric plexus is the report by Schuffler et al.[23, 26] of two adult siblings who had had intestinal pseudo-obstruction manifested as abdominal pain and distention and vomiting for many years. They also had ataxia, constricted poorly-reactive pupils, dysarthria, absent deep tendon reflexes, and impaired peripheral sensation on physical examination. Autonomic dysfunction was present, as manifested by orthostatic hypotension, defective sweating, and abnormal pupillary reflexes. Esophageal manometry showed abnormal motility and positive responses to methacholine. At autopsy, degeneration of the nerves of the myenteric plexus was observed in the esophagus, small intestine, and colon. Round eosinophilic intranuclear inclusion bodies were found in many neurons of the myenteric plexus as well as in nerves and glial cells of the brain, spinal cord, dorsal root ganglia, and celiac plexus ganglia (Fig 38–4).

DISCUSSION.—It is impossible to discuss in general terms a situation that has been reported so rarely and that seems to be so heterogeneous. It is noteworthy that, in all three reports, the neurologic disorder was generalized, extending beyond the autonomic innervation of the gut alone. From the descriptions given, it appears that in all three instances, the disease involved a considerable extent of the gut, but that

small-intestinal involvement was most evident.

These three instances are so different that they must be considered to be separate entities. They do not fit any of the recognized syndromes of generalized peripheral neuropathy, and so they are best currently viewed as three separate isolated instances of previously unrecognized diseases.

It should be noted that, in all three cases, the familial nature of the disease was supported only by concurrence in siblings. Thus, one cannot firmly conclude that these are hereditary disorders. Siblings share a common environment, and so these syndromes could as well be environmental as hereditary in origin. When a syndrome spans several generations, a hereditary disorder is more strongly implied. Thus, these cases must be considered only tentatively to be examples of a hereditary disorder. Familial visceral neuropathy as a cause of pseudo-obstruction must be considered to be rare.

NONFAMILIAL OR SPORADIC IDIOPATHIC PSEUDO-OBSTRUCTION

HISTORICAL REVIEW.—The occurrence of nonfamilial cases of idiopathic pseudo-obstruction has been recognized for a long time. Some of these develop signs of an underlying disease like scleroderma with time, but some do not. With suitably careful investigation of families, such cases are not found to have affected relatives. One is forced to the conclusion that many truly sporadic idiopathic cases occur, perhaps representing the action of undefined environmental influences like infectious agents or toxins. These cases have received much less attention than have the familial cases, but they appear to be at least as frequent. Little more can be said on this subject than was said by Faulk et al. in 1978.[5]

CLINICAL FEATURES—SOME GENERALIZATIONS.—Several generalizations can be made about the sporadic forms of idiopathic pseudo-obstruction, even though they certainly represent a heterogeneous group of disorders.

First, it is much less likely that the disordered motor function will be found to be confined to one or a few organs. Extensive disease is almost the rule, and the small intestine is the most commonly involved organ (Fig 38–5).

Second, in contrast to the familial forms of pseudo-obstruction, the nonfamilial forms commonly show evidence of progression of the disease, though the progression may be rather slow. We have seen cases, for example, in which only the colon was thought to be involved at first, and in which partial or total colectomy relieved symptoms for a period before the small intestinal disorder became evident.

Third, the pathologic abnormalities found are highly variable and hence unpredictable. Muscle degeneration has been described in the longitudinal layer alone, in the circular layer alone, and in both layers together. Some cases have been described that have neuropathic findings on histology. In one case, the disorder appeared to be a paraneoplastic syndrome related to a small-cell carcinoma of the lung.[27]

One interesting and rare form of pseudo-obstruction that affects only the stomach has been called *tachygastria*. This disorder is not yet well-defined, but it seems to represent the consequences of a tachyarrhythmia of the gastric antrum. The normal 20-second rhythm of the antrum, paced by the antral pacesetter potentials or slow waves, is reported to be disrupted with both abnormal patterns of migration and rapid frequencies; the consequent disruption of orderly antral peristalsis leads to gastric retention and vomiting. The cause is unknown. It is possible that similar dysrhythmias can occur in other parts of the gut where pacesetter potentials establish an orderly pattern of contraction, the small intestine and colon, but this has not been established.

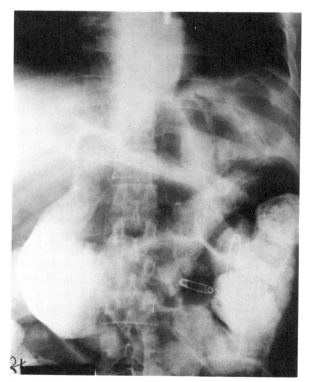

Fig 38–5.—Generalized small-intestinal dilatation in a case of sporadic (or nonfamilial) intestinal pseudo-obstruction with generalized visceral disease.

CLINICAL FEATURES—SYMPTOMS.—These patients have symptoms that, as described above, reflect the major organs of involvement. For reasons that are not entirely clear, the symptoms in these cases frequently show spontaneous exacerbations and remissions, with attacks that may closely mimic acute intestinal obstruction. It is not surprising that these patients are frequently operated upon early in the course of the illness. Subsequent attacks are thereafter blamed on obstruction due to adhesions, though repeated lysis of adhesions does not cause the attacks to abate. Fortunately, the attacks are usually self-limited and regress after a period of nonoperative management, such as is commonly done for partial intestinal obstruction, only to recur again and again. A history of such a course is almost the rule in patients with nonfamilial pseudo-obstruction.

As in the case of the familial forms of pseudo-obstruction, a wide variety of symptoms is described. Symptoms may include those of esophagitis, gastric retention, and partial bowel obstruction; weight loss, malnutrition syndromes and episodic diarrhea and constipation are common; the exact constellation of manifestations depends on the organs that are involved.

SECONDARY PSEUDO-OBSTRUCTION

Drug-induced Pseudo-obstruction

Many drugs have been thought to cause pseudo-obstruction. The commonest of these, atropine, may be responsible for a false diagnosis of gastric retention when its ingestion has been unsuspected. Such parasympatholytics as atropine, taken in the usual dosage, seem rarely to affect intestinal or colonic motor function enough to cause symptoms.

Most of the drugs that have been related to pseudo-obstruction are neurotropic drugs, and many of them are psychotropic agents. Given the widespread use of psychotropic drugs, and given the fact that pseudo-obstruction, particularly colonic atony, seems to be especially common among patients who are long-term residents of institutions for the mentally ill, it is difficult to accept unqualifiedly that any of these agents is directly responsible. Both chlorpromazine and other phenothiazines,[28] including trifluoperazine and thioridazine, have been cited as offenders. The antidepressant agents imipramine, amitriptyline, and nortriptyline have also been reported to produce the picture of pseudo-obstruction. All of these associations arise from case reports. Remission upon withdrawal of the agents has been the usual criterion for establishing the relationship; rechallenge has not been done in general. Pathologic examinations of resected tissues have not been reported, nor have physiologic studies been done beyond routine radiographic assessment.

Anti-parkinsonian drugs like benztropine and trihexyphenidyl are known to cause occasional constipation, an effect often attributed to their parasympatholytic actions. The syndrome of pseudo-obstruction has been described in patients with Parkinson's disease, even in untreated patients, and so it is difficult to know whether the syndrome is caused by the drugs used or whether it is part of the neurologic syndrome itself.

Antagonists of ganglionic transmission were once used commonly in the treatment of hypertension, and their use was often associated with severe colonic atony and intestinal and gastric dilatation. Recent reports have also suggested that the antihypertensive agent, clonidine, may induce a severe colonic motor dysfunction that is reversed when the agent is withdrawn.

A variety of new agents used in cancer chemotherapy can produce the syndrome. Adriamycin and vincristine are common offenders. Methotrexate, accidentally taken in very large doses, has been reported to cause it. Since these agents also cause a peripheral neuropathy, it is presumed that they induce GI motor dysfunction by altering the actions of the nerves that supply the gut. Direct evidence for that is lacking.

The abuse of laxatives, especially those containing the anthraquinones, is widely accepted as a cause of chronic colonic dilatation, and, sometimes, such symptoms as chronic abdominal distention, abdominal pain, and vomiting. Dozens of over-the-counter laxative formulations containing these substances are available in the United States, usually being advertised as "natural" or "vegetable" laxatives. The laxative substance is metabolized by the colonic microflora to produce a brown pigment that is taken up by mucosal macrophages to produce the picture of melanosis coli. The motor dysfunction is thought to represent the toxic effect of a metabolite upon the action of the intramural nerves of the colon, but the evidence for that is sparse.

The "Collagen" Diseases

It has long been recognized that patients with the collagen diseases may develop localized or generalized GI motor dysfunction.

The commonest of these diseases is *scleroderma*, or diffuse systemic sclerosis, a term that encompasses, in fact, a rather wide spectrum of clinical syndromes that share a number of features. An acronym in common use that describes the various clinical features found in scleroderma is the "CREST" syndrome, signifying subcutaneous calcinosis (C), Raynaud's phenomenon (R), esophageal motor dysfunction (E), sclerodactyly (S), and telangiectasia of the face and fingertips (T). These five features are found in various combinations in such patients, and the presence of widespread GI motor dysfunction may be associated with any combination of them. One form of scleroderma, localized scleroderma, or morphea, seems never to be associated with the syndrome of GI pseudo-obstruction.

Not all patients with scleroderma develop GI motor dysfunction, but about half do. The incidence undoubtedly varies with the enthusiasm with which it is sought. We have seen one case in which the diagnosis became clear only when a vagotomy and pyloroplasty (done for ulcer disease) induced nearly complete gastric retention because the effect of the operation was added to that of the scleroderma. Undoubtedly, many patients with scleroderma have a subclinical degree of motor malfunction in one or more segments of the gut. In scleroderma, it is the esophagus that is most commonly and most severely affected. Gastric retention is less frequent, and small-intestinal and colonic motor disorders are rather uncommon.

The pathology of the GI lesion in scleroderma is well-known. There is patchy fibrosis of smooth muscle in both layers in affected organs, accompanied by fibrinous vascular narrowing. Schuffler and Beegle[8] pointed out the histologic features that distinguish scleroderma from idiopathic visceral myopathy (Table 38–2). This table shows that visceral myopathy is characterized by both vacuolar degeneration and fibrosis of the smooth muscle, while only fibrosis is found in scleroderma. Subserosal and submucosal fibrosis are not important diagnostic findings, both occurring in some normal tissues. In scleroderma, there appears to be some selectivity for involvement of the circular over the longitudinal muscle layer, while both muscle layers may be involved in visceral myopathy.

Patients with *dermatomyositis* frequently have oropharyngeal dysphagia because of striated muscle dysfunction. Visceral smooth muscle is much less commonly affected, certainly less often than it is in scleroderma. Still, there are several reports of instances in which there was radiographic evidence of esophageal dilatation, megaduodenum, delayed intestinal transit, and colonic dilatation. Patients with dermatomyositis are frequently very ill, and radiographic study of the GI tract may seem to be an unnecessary step, so that it is possible that subclinical cases of GI motor malfunction in dermatomyositis are missed. Also, dermatomyositis, like scleroderma, is a heterogeneous disorder, and some forms may be more likely to develop pseudo-obstruction than others. Pathologic examination has revealed degeneration and fibrosis of both muscle coats and fibrinous narrowing of blood vessels.

There is one report of fatal *polymyositis* accompanied by intestinal pseudo-obstruction. The stomach and small intestine were both affected, with degeneration and fibrosis of both somatic muscle and GI smooth muscle. That patient had some features of scleroderma, so that the nosological picture is clouded. Certainly, most patients with polymyositis have little evidence of visceral muscle involvement.

In *lupus erythematosus*, the pseudo-obstruction syndrome may occur, though the incidence is certainly low. In those cases reported, abnormal motor functions occurred in the stomach and intestine, and fibrosis of the smooth muscle was found, along with an arteritis.

Diseases of Muscle

In *myotonic dystrophy*, abnormal motility of the smooth-muscled segment of the esophagus is very common, though it does not commonly produce major symptoms. Much less

TABLE 38–2.—A COMPARISON OF HISTOLOGIC FINDINGS IN THE SMALL INTESTINE IN PROGRESSIVE SYSTEMIC SCLEROSIS (PSS), VISCERAL MYOPATHY (VM), AND NORMAL (N) CONTROL PATIENTS*

| | DIAGNOSIS, % | | |
HISTOLOGIC ABNORMALITY	N	VM	PSS
Submucosal fibrosis	11	0	5
Fibrosis of circular muscle	0	50	75
Vacuolization of circular muscle	0	67	0
Fibrosis of longitudinal muscle	0	100	8
Vacuolization of longitudinal muscle	0	83	0
Subserosal fibrosis	23	77	17

*Compiled from data in reference 7. Numbers refer to the proportion of tissue specimens from each group found to contain the abnormality.

commonly, radiographic evidence of dilatation of the stomach, intestine, and colon has been found, and it has been suggested that the visceral myopathy may sometimes antedate the other, more familiar manifestations of the disease. The only histological study reported indicates that fat-containing vacuoles separated the muscle bundles in the gut wall. Muscle cells were observed to have degenerated. The nerves of the gut wall were intact.

In *progressive muscular dystrophy*, the whole of the GI tract may be involved in the generalized muscle disease. Pathologic findings include degeneration of the muscle in both layers and separation of muscle fibers and bundles by edema. Very little fibrosis occurs. Infiltration of the myenteric plexus by fat is also described.

Ceroidosis, or the "brown bowel syndrome," is a rare disorder characterized by the deposition of a brown lipofuscin pigment, called ceroid, in the musculature of the bowel (Fig 38–6). It has been observed in two diseases characterized by fat malabsorption, celiac disease and chronic pancreatitis, and one theory relates the pigment deposition to vitamin E deficiency. We have seen one case in a patient who suffered the ravages of chronic alcohol abuse, and at least one case has occurred in scleroderma. Ceroidosis has been found in several cases of intestinal pseudo-obstruction, but the cause-and-effect relationship is not clear. One proposal is that the pigment alters visceral muscle function. Alternatively, the malnutrition associated with the related diseases could lead to the

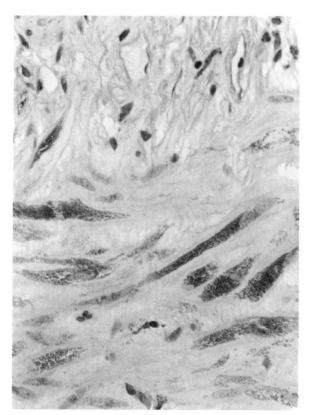

Fig 38–6.—The appearance of ceroid pigment in the muscle of the small intestine in a case of ceroidosis. (Photograph courtesy of F.A. Mitros, M.D.)

ceroid deposits. Also, the muscle dysfunction and the pigment could be, in common, secondary to the state of malnutrition.

Endocrine Diseases

In *myxedema*, intestinal pseudo-obstruction, called myxedema ileus, has long been recognized as a trap for the unwary surgeon.[29] It is much rarer now than in former times, because of improved diagnostic and therapeutic means, but it remains an important consideration in patients who seem to have chronic ileus. The ileus may long precede the other symptoms and signs of the disease, or it may dominate the clinical picture. The stomach, intestine, and colon may all be involved, but the colon is usually the most strikingly affected. Accordingly, constipation is the usual complaint, but abdominal distention may also be pronounced, in part from the dilated gut and in part from the accumulation of peritoneal fluid. Vomiting is not commonly associated with the syndrome. Histologic examination of the resected bowel has revealed edema of the whole of the bowel wall from the accumulation of mucopolysaccharide, with an infiltration of the mucosa with lymphocytes and plasma cells. The muscle itself and the myenteric plexus are normal in appearance. The pseudo-obstruction resolves fully when the myxedema is corrected. The reason for the diffuse abnormal motor function is not clear. While stiffening of the wall of the gut by the edema could alone account for defective motility, it has been proposed as well that intramural nerve function is deranged, that a relative intestinal ischemia (due to reduced cardiac output) could be responsible, and that defective motility may reflect altered calcium metabolism.

In *diabetes mellitus*, symptoms suggestive of disturbed GI motor function are common. Constipation is the most frequent GI complaint and it may be severe. Nausea, vomiting, abdominal distention, abdominal distress, and diarrhea all occur. These complaints are more common in those patients who have diabetes of long-standing with well-developed vascular and neurologic complications of the disease. In such patients, radiographic studies frequently reveal dilatation of the viscera, delayed transit, and abnormal flow patterns. All organs may be affected, and abnormalities may be present even in the absence of symptoms. Abnormalities of movement in the smooth-muscled part of the esophagus are frequent, but this rarely causes symptoms. The gastric atony, however, is frequently symptomatic; besides complicating the management of the diabetes, the delayed gastric emptying may lead to bezoar formation and gastritis. When stasis occurs in the intestine, bacterial overgrowth occurs leading to diarrhea, often with considerable steatorrhea. These abnormalities in motor function characteristically fluctuate in severity, being particularly severe in diabetic ketoacidosis, which can produce a picture very suggestive of acute intestinal obstruction. The mechanism of the motor abnormality is not known, but it is usually attributed to an autonomic neuropathy; the few histopathologic studies that are reported are conflicting. Some authors have detected degeneration of nerves and a lymphocytic infiltration in the intramural plexuses, while others find no such damage. Demyelination of fibers in the vagus and altered morphology of the sympathetic ganglia have also been found. In experimental diabetes in rats, dysfunction of nerves in the myenteric plexus of the intestine has been demonstrated.

Single instances have been reported of pseudo-obstruction in association with *hypoparathyroidism* and with *pheochromocytoma*. These must certainly be rare occurrences, however, and one is not presently justified as listing these firmly among recognized causes.

Primary Disorders of Nerves

Chagas' disease, an infection with *Trypanosoma cruzi,* is a disorder not to be encountered in North America except in immigrants from those regions of Latin America, where the disease is endemic, mainly in Brazil. The organism is contracted in youth from the bite of its intermediate host, a beetle, and produces an acute self-limiting illness, followed months or years later by the development of lesions that represent autonomic denervation. The GI manifestations of the disease may involve any part of the gut, but the esophagus and colon seem to be more commonly affected than the stomach and intestine. The affected organs become greatly dilated, and the flow of the GI content is correspondingly retarded. The esophageal lesion resembles that of achalasia. Histopathologic examination of resected tissues reveals variably diminished numbers of ganglion cells in the intramural plexuses and, to a variable degree, smooth muscle hypertrophy. The mechanism by which the chronically harbored organism brings about this destruction of the intrinsic nerves of the gut is not clear.

In *Hirschsprung's disease,* the obstruction is organic, but functional in the sense that it represents dysfunction of a segment of the colon. This congenital disorder represents the consequences of a developmental defect in the innervation of the distal colon. The incidence of the disease is high, about 0.2 per 1,000 live births. It occurs predominantly in males. Although most cases are florid, being evident within the first few days or weeks of life, it is now evident that lesser degrees of defective innervation occur, so that occasional patients may live to the second or third decade of life before the diagnosis is made. The denervated segment of the distal colon is tonically contracted to produce a functional obstruction to the passage of feces, and the internal anal sphincter fails to relax in reflex response to rectal distention. The affected segment is highly variable in length—it may constitute only the last few centimeters of the colon, or it may extend well up into the abdominal colon. The obstructing segment always extends to the anus. The obstruction leads to dilation of the colon above the obstruction. Histopathologic examination reveals an absence or deficit of ganglion cells in the myenteric and submucosal plexuses in the constricted segment. There are also bizarre hypertrophic nerve bundles in the affected region. Other parts of the gut do not seem to be affected. The diagnosis is made by seeking ganglion cells in the submucosal plexus from rectal biopsy, and by assessing the reflex relaxation of the internal anal sphincter in response to rectal distention.

Achalasia, an idiopathic disease of the esophagus, resembles Hirschsprung's disease in the sense that it, too, is a real obstruction, but a functional one because of neurogenic dysfunction of smooth muscle. It may begin at any age and affects both sexes equally, so that it appears to be an acquired rather than a congenital lesion. Most patients are in mid-life when the diagnosis is made. The disease may assume several forms. In the classic form, the whole of the esophagus is dilated while the esophagogastric sphincter is contracted at rest, so that ingested food and fluid are retained for long periods in the esophageal body. Physiologic studies indicate that the esophagogastric sphincter fails to relax on swallowing and that the smooth muscle segment of the esophageal body fails to contract. Other cases manifest slightly different features, but these cases are assumed to be variants of achalasia. Thus, some patients may show rather little esophageal dilatation with spontaneous nonpropulsive contractions of the esophageal body, a variant often called "vigorous achalasia." Still other cases may show very strong spontaneous and nonpropulsive contractions of the esophageal body, so that they are at first falsely diagnosed as cases of esophageal spasm. If such patients are observed over a period of time, they are occasionally seen to evolve to the state of classic achalasia. This neuropathic disorder seems to be confined to the esophagus, for other segments of the gut seem to function normally, despite some recent reports of delayed gastric emptying in some patients. The histopathologic lesion has not been well described, for tissue is rarely obtained. Diminished numbers of ganglion cells and lymphocytic infiltration of the myenteric plexus have been described.

Generalized autonomic dysfunctions include several very rare and ill-defined syndromes, some of which are familial. Many of these are diseases of infancy and childhood and the cardiovascular abnormalities dominate the clinical picture. Megacolon and, to a lesser extent, more generalized atony of the GI musculature have been described in some such patients.

Miscellaneous Causes of Pseudo-obstruction

In *amyloidosis,* both in the primary disease and in that form that is secondary to such chronic diseases as multiple myeloma, pseudo-obstruction has been reported to occur rarely.[30] The esophagus, stomach, intestine, and colon may all be involved. The pathogenesis of the generalized motor abnormality is a matter of speculation. Stiffening of the bowel wall from amyloid deposition, neuropathy from amyloid deposits in nerves, vascular insufficiency from vascular infiltration with amyloid, and separation of muscle bundles by amyloid deposits all could contribute (Fig 38–7).

The *jejunoileal bypass* operation, done for the control of morbid obesity, is known now to lead commonly to a variety of undesirable consequences. Among them are megacolon and generalized intestinal dilatation.[31] These abnormalities have often led to reoperation in search of organic obstruction. Cultures taken from the lumen of the bypassed bowel have revealed the overgrowth of anaerobic bacteria, and the dilatation has been observed to regress with treatment of the bacterial overgrowth. The limited histopathology that is reported indicates only blunting of the mucosal villi and inflammatory cell infiltration of the mucosa; abnormalities of muscle and intramural nerves have not been described. It seems, therefore, that the motor abnormalities are a consequence of bacterial overgrowth, probably related to the blind loop that is formed by the operation.

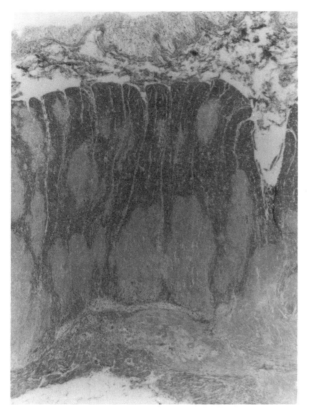

Fig 38–7.—The appearance of amyloid in the small intestine in a case of amyloidosis. Amyloid is seen as pale areas in both muscle layers. (Photograph courtesy of F.A. Mitros, M.D.)

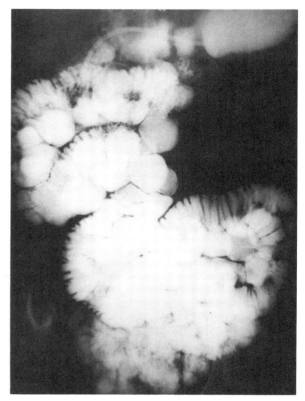

Fig 38–8.—Multiple jejunal diverticulosis associated with the pseudo-obstruction syndrome.

Jejunal diverticulosis[32] is well-known to predispose to the development of a blind-loop syndrome related to the overgrowth of colonic microflora in the intestine. Many patients with multiple jejunal diverticula develop symptoms and signs suggestive of intestinal obstruction (Fig 38–8). The interrelationships among the three features—the diverticula, the bacterial overgrowth, and the pseudo-obstruction syndrome—are conjectural. The diverticula could be primary, with secondary bacterial overgrowth within the pockets as a result of stasis and, as a result of that, depressed motor function due to toxic products elaborated by the bacteria. Alternatively, a motor abnormality, intestinal dyskinesia, could be primary, the diverticula being produced by pulsion and leading to the bacterial overgrowth from stasis. It is proposed that nerve dysfunction underlies the formation of the diverticula.

Several *inflammatory diseases* of the bowel may cause a clinical picture suggestive of obstruction. This has occurred in celiac sprue, in eosinophilic gastroenteritis, in Crohn's disease, and in radiation enteritis. The toxic megacolon that sometimes develops in ulcerative colitis may also be considered to be a form of pseudo-obstruction. It is usually not difficult to detect the underlying disease in such cases, so that there is rarely a misdiagnosis, but there may be. The mechanism of the ileus in such situations is unknown.

THE DIAGNOSTIC APPROACH TO PSEUDO-OBSTRUCTION

When a patient presents symptoms and signs of obstruction to flow at any level of the GI tract, the first consideration is the question as to whether the obstructed flow is the result of a lesion that can be removed or bypassed at operation. The answer to this question requires accuracy in nonoperative diagnosis, and the circumstances of the illness obviously limit severely the objective methods that can be employed, particularly radiographic methods.

In any case in which obstruction to flow along the gut is suspected, the distinction that must be made is between mechanical obstruction and functional obstruction. Mechanical obstruction refers to the presence of mass lesions, like tumors, adhesions, or compressions produced by torsion, that obstruct the flow produced by normally operating neuromuscular apparatus of the gut wall. Functional obstruction (ileus or pseudo-obstruction) refers to the impairment of flow because of abnormal movements of the gut wall. Operative intervention may be appropriate in both cases, but the nature of the operation is dictated by the nature of the lesion. The distinction can be made on the basis of the features that can be identified at all stages of the clinical approach to the patient.

The History

Mechanical obstruction is clinically characterized by the sudden onset of symptoms and rapid progression to the point of complete obstruction. Functional obstructions, in contrast, usually develop slowly, progress slowly, may occur in distinct episodes widely separated in time, and only reach the point of complete cessation of flow after the passage of months or years. This distinction, though a very useful one, is not infallible. Slowly growing tumors may mimic functional obstruction, but it is rare that a functional obstruction presents the picture of acute complete obstruction that characterizes torsion of the gut, for example.

Mechanical obstructions often appear as discrete events in time, while functional obstructions, being chronic, are usually characterized by remissions and exacerbations. Again, this distinction in not infallible, for incomplete obstruction due to adhesions may produce episodic symptoms over months or years.

In patients in whom functional obstruction is suspected, the history should include a complete assessment of all the usual components of the history, with a special search for features that might support the diagnosis of functional obstruction. Thus, the family history, the history of drug use, and the history of concomitant illnesses all may quickly point to a specific pathophysiologic process. The failure to make this simple sort of enquiry still leads to inappropriate operations.

The Physical Examination

In mechanical obstruction, the acute onset and rapid progression to complete obstruction presents a classic and familiar set of signs on physical examination. In functional obstruction, these signs are usually less characteristic. That is, the abdominal tenderness, distention, and altered bowel sounds are often significantly more moderate in functional obstruction than they are in mechanical obstruction. Again, this is not a sharp distinction, for incomplete obstruction due to adhesions or slowly growing tumors may produce a rather mild set of signs.

The physical examination in cases of suspected functional obstruction often proves valuable in identifying secondary pseudo-obstruction. Thus, for example, the classic peripheral signs of scleroderma and myxedema should be looked for. It is not unusual for such systemic illnesses first to become manifest as an episode of functional obstruction, so that it is such an episode that leads to the correct diagnosis.

Radiographic Observations

Radiographs of the abdomen are routinely taken in cases of suspected mechanical obstruction. Although they are always helpful to support the clinical impression, they are not often fully diagnostic except in the case of volvulus or torsion, where well-known configurations of gas-filled loops may occur. The distribution of gas and fluid levels is useful to help to decide the general location of a mechanical obstruction or the extent of involvement of a functional obstruction.

Contrast radiography is usually done with considerable caution when both mechanical obstruction and functional obstruction are suspected. This caution is related to the fear of producing barium impaction and to the belief that the impaired flow will rarely allow the contrast medium to define the obstruction. Unless complete mechanical obstruction is very strongly suspected from the clinical picture or is defined by plain radiographs, contrast radiography should be done.

The likelihood of barium impaction can be circumvented by the use of water-soluble contrast mediums. The ability of conventional radiography to outline the lesion in mechanical obstruction is much greater with modern techniques using air-contrast with small volumes of contrast medium. The air-contrast technique and the small-bowel enema (or enteroclysis technique) have proved very useful in our hands in defining both incomplete mechanical obstructions and functional obstructions.

Laboratory Evaluations

Laboratory evaluation should always be guided by clinical impressions derived from the history and physical examination. The consequences of the obstruction or pseudo-obstruction should be evaluated in the usual ways. Diagnostic laboratory tests are less easily dealt with when a functional obstruction is suspected.

In the case of familial or sporadic idiopathic pseudo-obstruction, there are no specific laboratory examinations that will establish the diagnosis. In the case of paralytic ileus and secondary pseudo-obstruction, there are, but their use, too, should be guided by the history and physical examination. Still, because some systemic diseases or conditions may be so subtle as to reveal themselves mainly as an ileus or a secondary pseudo-obstruction, some routine tests to investigate the causes of secondary pseudo-obstruction ought to be done in all cases of suspected functional obstruction. Jejunal manometry may soon come to have a place in such investigations.[33]

THE TREATMENT OF PSEUDO-OBSTRUCTION

The treatment of functional obstruction can take the form of three approaches: (1) correction of the underlying cause, (2) operative removal or bypass of the offending segment of the gut, or (3) the maintenance of nutrition by parenteral means with no attempt to alter GI flow.

Treatment of the Underlying Cause

In paralytic ileus and secondary pseudo-obstruction, the underlying cause can usually be treated with resolution of the obstruction. In cases where it cannot, physicians often resort to the use of drugs that are thought to alter the movements of the gut.

The drugs that have been used are cholinergic agonists, cholinergic antagonists, and new agents whose mechanism of action is unknown. In cases where intestinal bacterial overgrowth is present, antibiotics are used as well.

CHOLINERGIC AGONISTS.—The long-acting cholinergic agonist, bethanechol, is often used in an attempt to stimulate motor activity when it appears to be depressed in any part of the gut. Its use is logical inasmuch as the excitatory nerves to much of the gut are cholinergic and much of the GI musculature contains excitatory muscarinic receptors. Its use is illogical inasmuch as not all parts of the gut are excited equally well by cholinergic agonists; also, when disordered motility rather than hypoactivity is the problem, cholinergic agonists cannot restore normal patterns; finally, in conditions where the muscle is degenerated or fibrotic or in which muscle function is impaired by infiltrative processes (as in amyloidosis and myxedema) such drugs cannot have any effect. Of course, cholinergic agonists have no place in the management of mechanical obstruction.

In fact, cholinomimetic agents have proved to be of very little benefit in practice. They are most often tried in diabetic enteropathy when delayed gastric emptying is the major problem. Even in this situation, it is not at all clear that such treatment is helpful.

CHOLINERGIC ANTAGONISTS.—Cholinergic antagonists are sometimes tried in the treatment of the situation where localized spasm seems to be producing a functional obstruction; this occurs only in achalasia and pylorospasm (an ill-defined clinical entity). They do not work.

NEW AGENTS WHOSE MECHANISM OF ACTION IS NOT CLEAR.—Two rather new agents are currently being promoted as effective agents to normalize gastrointestinal motor function: metoclopramide and domperidone. The former has a long history of use as an antiemetic, while the latter is of more recent introduction. Some of their actions may be simply as cholinergic agonists, but another mechanism (not well-defined) relating to dopamine is postulated as well. The evidence that they can, in fact, help to relieve the symptoms of pseudo-obstruction is poor. They have been used mainly in diabetic gastropathy, where some report considerable benefit but others find little. In a condition like diabetic gastropathy, which is characterized by spontaneous exacerbations and remissions, long-term, double-blind trials are required to eliminate the placebo effect and to avoid the confusion that arises from the inconstancy of the abnormal motor function. Such clinical trials have not been made with these agents. The use of these agents, as in the case of cholinomimetic drugs, is illogical in diseases characterized by muscle degeneration, fibrosis, or infiltration.

ANTIBIOTICS.—In patients with bacterial overgrowth in the small intestine, such as occurs in diabetic enteropathy, jejunal diverticulosis, and the iatrogenic blind-loop syndrome of the jejunoileal bypass operation, antibiotic therapy certainly relieves the diarrhea and steatorrhea, but the effect is transient. It is not clear that abnormal motility is affected. The concept that toxic products of bacterial metabolism alter motility is interesting but unproved.

There is one clear indication for antibiotic therapy in the treatment of pseudo-obstruction syndromes. Antibiotic therapy directed toward the colonic flora should always be a part of the preoperative treatment when it is anticipated that the gut will be opened. Severe, even fatal, sepsis can be expected if the contents of a chronically atonic stomach or intestine are allowed to contaminate the peritoneum, because the contents of such organs may contain an abundant colonic flora, even when diarrhea is not a prominent part of the clinical syndrome.

Operative Removal or Bypass of the Diseased Segment

Patients with pseudo-obstruction are often operated on early in the course of the illness because an incomplete mechanical obstruction is suspected. Subsequent episodes are then attributed to adhesions (which, of course, will be present

to some degree), and a long series of operations to break up adhesions may then ensue. This prospect alone is ample reason for the surgeon to be cautious in operating to find a mechanical obstruction when it has not been objectively demonstrated, or when the clinical picture is not wholly convincing that a mechanical obstruction exists.

When pseudo-obstruction is suspected and the cause is established to be one that cannot be affected by nonsurgical means, the place of operative treatment becomes problematical. The surgical attack must be highly individualized according to the exact nature of the problem—the location and extent of the lesion, the likelihood of progression, and the degree of disability it produces must all be considered.[34-37] It is not possible to deal in this chapter with all situations, given the complexity of the problem, but some generalizations can be made.

LOCALIZATION OR EXTENT OF THE LESION.—When the disease is sharply localized, operation can be beneficial. In idiopathic pseudo-obstruction due either to familial or to sporadic visceral myopathy, the dysfunctional segment may affect mainly one segment of the gut. This is particularly true in the case of megaduodenum (as occurs in some of the familial visceral myopathies) and in isolated colonic dysfunction. In the case of megaduodenum, duodenojejunostomy has successfully relieved symptoms in some cases. In the case of isolated colonic atony, subtotal colectomy has also been practiced successfully.

Operations to resect or bypass dysfunctional segments should be undertaken only when the motor function of the whole of the gut has been assessed as completely as possible. In most cases of pseudo-obstruction, the disease affects far more of the gut than is suspected by routine radiographic studies that show localized dilatation. When operation is done in such cases, the symptomatic relief achieved may only be partial and transient.

THE PROGRESSIVE NATURE OF THE DISEASE.—The idiopathic visceral myopathies and neuropathies do not, in general, appear to be rapidly progressive. It should be noted, however, that clinical experience with these is very limited, both in the number of cases and in the time over which they have been observed. Only when the pathologic process appears to be reasonably stable should operations to resect or bypass be done.

THE DEGREE OF DISABILITY.—It is remarkable that patients who have the pseudo-obstruction syndromes are not more severely disabled by their illness. Patients often learn to adjust their eating habits or to accept limited degrees of chronic constipation, diarrhea, abdominal pain, and distention quite well. The diarrhea, steatorrhea, and malnutrition that characterize the intestinal lesions can often be effectively relieved, though temporarily, by antibiotic therapy. When, however, this tactic proves to be unsuccessful, operative bypass of localized disease can be of real benefit. Similarly, in patients who have isolated colonic dysfunction, the management of the constipation by dietary adjustments and laxative agents can be successful for long periods. Subtotal colectomy in cases of isolated colonic dysfunction should be reserved until everyone concerned is assured that nonsurgical management has failed.

Some Generalizations about Operation in Pseudo-obstruction

From the preceding sections, it might be concluded that the surgeon has rather little to offer the patient with functional obstruction of the gut. This is, of course, not true, for the surgical treatment of certain entities such as achalasia and Hirschsprung's disease is clearly highly successful. With respect to the idiopathic visceral myopathies, the principles outlined above have proved to be a useful guide to us, at least. As for the two commonest forms of secondary pseudo-obstruction, the following guidelines are suggested, based on personal observation.

1. *Patients with diabetic gastroenteropathy are not often benefited by operation:* Subtotal gastrectomy might be thought to be of use in those diabetic patients in whom gastroparesis appears to be the major motor problem. Experience has indicated that subtotal gastrectomy is not very helpful. Similarly, the megacolon of diabetic enteropathy might be thought to be an indication for subtotal colectomy, but it has not proved to be beneficial. The lack of success of such operations arises from the fact that the lesion is generalized and progressive.

2. *Patients with scleroderma of the gut are rarely helped by operations:* This is the case, as in diabetic enteropathy, because the lesion is generalized and progressive. The only exception is in the surgical treatment of reflux esophagitis due to involvement of the esophagus in scleroderma. Some surgeons attempt to treat the reflux by one or another form of fundoplication. This can be disastrous, for the esophageal body, in such a situation, may not be able to generate sufficient force after a swallow to breach the mechanical obstruction presented by the fundoplication. Nevertheless, a "loose" fundoplication may be created to provide a barrier to reduce reflux without obstructing the antegrade flow that is brought about by hydrostatic forces. Both extensive experience and luck are required to achieve this. An attempt to accomplish this should only be made in those cases in which the esophagitis is complicated by ulcer or stricture formation and in which prolonged and enthusiastic nonoperative management has failed. Such cases are very rare.

PARALYTIC ILEUS

Introduction

As pointed out in the Introduction, the term "paralytic ileus" is usually used to refer to an acute and potentially reversible physiologic state that leads to complete or partial GI motor deficit. It is, of course, much commoner than pseudo-obstruction, but it is much less well understood as regards pathogenesis except for what can be inferred from the circumstances of its occurrence.

Description

Paralytic ileus is characterized by several features that distinguish it from pseudo-obstruction. *First,* ileus usually occurs in a previously-well patient, one who has not been subject to antecedent unexplained episodes suggesting partial ileus. *Second,* ileus is usually sudden in onset, progressing rapidly to a picture of complete cessation of gut motor function, as opposed to the episode of pseudo-obstruction, which has, often, an imperceptible beginning and a slow progression. *Third,* ileus usually occurs in a setting in which ileus, from previous experience, is known to occur, in relation to recognized causes of ileus (see below). *Fourth,* ileus involves all of the gut except the esophagus; esophageal atony has not been described in paralytic ileus, although it is not likely that esophageal motility is often examined, even superficially, in a syndrome that so clearly centers in the intra-abdominal viscera. Thus, paralytic ileus is characterized by the sudden appearance of abdominal distress and distention, cessation of the passage of stool or flatus, nausea, vomiting, and a silent abdomen. The syndrome can be distinguished from that of organic (mechanical) obstruction by the difference in the degree of abdominal pain, pain usually being much more severe and often more focal in mechanical obstruction than it is in paralytic ileus. This criterion is, of course, not fully reliable, for slowly developing mechanical obstruction, as in a slowly growing carcinoma of the colon, can be virtually painless.

The Circumstances of Paralytic Ileus

INTRA-ABDOMINAL DISEASE.—The commonest circumstance in which paralytic ileus occurs is abdominal operation. Ileus is routine after any operation in which the abdomen is opened, and it usually lasts only a few days. It may occasionally be prolonged, a circumstance that suggests mechanical obstruction. But ileus also can occur with blunt abdominal trauma, with intra-abdominal sepsis, with spontaneous perforation, as in perforated ulcer, and with bile peritonitis.

EXTRA-ABDOMINAL DISEASE.—Ileus is well-known to occur in association with a variety of extra-abdominal disorders. Lobar pneumonia and myocardial infarction both can cause ileus. Any kind of fracture may also do so, though ileus is more likely to accompany severe or widespread trauma than it is a simple isolated fracture. Severe generalized sepsis may be complicated by ileus. These nonabdominal causes of ileus have all been recognized for decades by clinicians, but they are not often discussed formally, knowledge of them seeming to pass from generation to generation as clinical wisdom rather than as a subject for scholarly study.

Ileus can also be an acute occurrence in patients with electrolyte imbalance such as hypophosphatemia and, in particular, hypokalemia, as can be produced by the enthusiastic use of the modern potent diuretics.

The Pathogenesis of Paralytic Ileus

The pathogenesis of paralytic ileus can only be inferred from what is known of the physiology of GI motility and from the circumstances in which ileus is seen.

Ileus is commonly believed to be usually, if not always, neurogenic; it is generally considered to be attributable to the action of the adrenergic innervation of the gut. There is much to favor this view—ileus begins and ends suddenly, it occurs often in response to severely painful situations, and it does not seem to involve the esophagus (in which the influence of the adrenergic nerves is slight). But there is also some difficulty with this view—ileus is not always accompanied by a generalized sympathetic discharge, and it usually seems to be confined to the GI tract (seeming often to spare, for example, the urinary bladder); the treatment of prolonged postoperative ileus with adrenergic antagonists does not seem to be beneficial (at least, it has not come into widespread clinical use), and ileus does not always arise in apparent consequence of a severely painful disorder.

Ileus probably does come about mainly by neurogenic mechanisms. Neurogenic (including adrenergic) inhibition may be one such mechanism, brought about by reflexes excited in response to severe pain at any location. Similar reflex responses seem to be excitable by peritoneal irritation which may involve stimulation of pain receptors. It appears that some of these reflexes are centrally mediated, while purely local reflexes may operate in some instances. The ileus related to electrolyte imbalances may also be neurogenic, representing some undefined neural dysfunction, but it also could be due to dysfunction of smooth muscle.

The Diagnosis and Treatment of Paralytic Ileus

The most important factor in the treatment of paralytic ileus is to make the diagnosis; to identify the cause and to treat the cause can only follow the clinical recognition of the syndrome. To treat the cause is to treat the ileus. It is common that paralytic ileus is recognized and distinguished from mechanical obstruction solely on the basis of the identification of the cause, like an unsuspected pneumonia or myocardial infarction.

Often, the precipitating cause of ileus is obvious from the routine steps in diagnosis, but it may not be. We have seen one case in which the cause, painless infarction of the gallbladder, was not evident for many weeks, being manifest only as a slight hyperbilirubinemia that was falsely attributed to total parenteral alimentation.

The aggression with which the paralytic ileus itself is treated depends on its cause and its anticipated duration, and on the degree of distress produced by the ileus. Evacuation of the stomach should always be done to obviate the risks of vomiting and aspiration. When the ileus is expected to be prolonged, a small intestinal drainage tube is to be preferred to simple gastric drainage.

Drugs that are thought to affect GI nerve and muscle seem to have found no widespread use in the treatment of paralytic ileus. Adrenergic antagonists and cholinergic agonists have certainly been tried, especially in prolonged postoperative ileus, but they are not predictably beneficial. One can have no confidence in anecdotal accounts of the successful use of such agents, because prolonged postoperative paralytic ileus is an unstable situation tending to improve spontaneously, and because the situation is heterogeneous as to cause and severity. The question of the value of such treatments would be a difficult one to answer.

CONCLUDING REMARKS

This chapter has attempted to survey the wide variety of disorders that can mimic the clinical picture of mechanical obstruction along the GI tract, to outline the approach that can be made to their distinctions from one another and from mechanical obstruction, and to state some general principles as to their management.

The rise in interest in functional obstruction in the gut in recent years, together with the popularization of the term "pseudo-obstruction," has been both beneficial and detrimental. On the one hand, physicians are more aware of the existence of the various forms of pseudo-obstruction, and so they are less likely to recommend or perform abdominal operations on insufficient grounds. On the other hand, the term has come to be thought of as a diagnosis rather than a syndrome; this has tended to retard careful scholarly investigation of such cases. Also, in some patients who in fact have partial mechanical obstruction with subtle symptoms, operation may be delayed.

The idiopathic forms of pseudo-obstruction seem to be commoner than was once supposed, and the recent study of such cases suggests that there are several pathologic processes in existence whose nature is not yet clear. Those physicians who encounter such cases have an obligation to study them as fully as possible if we are to be able to improve what we can offer to them, to their families, and to future generations.

REFERENCES

1. Dudley H.A.F., Sinclair I.S.R., McLaren I.F., et al.: Intestinal pseudo-obstruction. *J. R. Coll. Surg. Edinb.* 3:206, 1958.
2. Anuras S., Christensen J.: Primary (or idiopathic) chronic intestinal pseudo-obstruction. *Prog. Gastroenterol.* 4:269, 1983.
3. Anuras S., Crane S.A., Faulk D.L., et al.: Intestinal pseudoobstruction. *Gastroenterology* 74:1318, 1978.
4. Byrne W.J., Cipel L., Euler A.R., et al.: Chronic idiopathic intestinal pseudo-obstruction syndrome in children—clinical characteristics and prognosis. *J. Pediatr.* 90:585, 1977.
5. Faulk D.L., Anuras S., Christensen J.: Chronic intestinal pseudoobstruction. *Gastroenterology* 74:922, 1978.
6. Faulk D.L., Anuras S., Freeman J.B.: Idiopathic chronic intestinal pseudo-obstruction. *J.A.M.A.* 240:2075, 1978.
7. Lane R.H.S., Todd I.P.: Idiopathic megacolon: A review of 42 cases, *Br. J. Surg.* 64:305, 1977.
8. Schuffler M.D., Beegle R.G.: Progressive systemic sclerosis of the gastrointestinal tract and hereditary hollow visceral myopathy: Two distinguishable disorders of intestinal smooth muscle. *Gastroenterology* 77:664, 1979.
9. Schuffler M.D., Lowe M.C., Bill A.H.: Studies of idiopathic intestinal pseudo-obstruction: 1. Hereditary hollow visceral myopathy: Clinical and pathological studies. *Gastroenterology* 73:327, 1977.
10. Schuffler M.D., Pope C.E. II: Studies of idiopathic intestinal pseudo-obstruction: II. Hereditary hollow visceral myopathy: family studies. *Gastroenterology* 73:339, 1977.
11. Schuffler M.D., Rohrman C.A., Chaffee R.A., et al.: Chronic intestinal pseudo-obstruction. *Medicine* 60:173, 1981.
12. Shaw A., Shaffer H., Teja K., et al.: A perspective for pediatric surgeons: Chronic idiopathic intestinal pseudo-obstruction. *J. Pediatr. Surg.* 14:719, 1979.
13. Smith B.: The neuropathology of intestinal pseudo-obstruction, in Chey W.H. (ed.): *Functional Disorders of the Gastrointestinal Tract.* New York, Raven Press, 1983, pp. 231–236.
14. Weiss W.: Zur Atiologie des Megaduodenums. *Dtsch. Z. Chir.* 251:317, 1938.
15. Law D.H., Ten Eyck R.A.: Familial megaduodenum and megacystis. *Am. J. Med.* 33:911, 1962.
16. Newton W.T.: Radical enterectomy for hereditary megaduodenum. *Arch. Surg.* 96:549, 1968.
17. Schuffler M.D., Pope C.E.: Esophageal motor dysfunction in idiopathic pseudo-obstruction. *Gastroenterology* 70:677, 1976.
18. Lewis T.D., Daniel E.E., Sarna S.K., et al.: Idiopathic intestinal pseudo-obstruction: Report of a case, with intraluminal studies of mechanical and electrical activity and response to drugs. *Gastroenterology* 74:107, 1978.
19. Maldonado J.E., Gregg J.A., Green P.A., et al.: Chronic idiopathic intestinal pseudo-obstruction. *Am. J. Med.* 49:203, 1970.

20. Faulk D.L., Anuras S., Gardner G.D., et al.: A familial visceral myopathy. *Ann. Intern. Med.* 89:600, 1978.
21. Jacobs E., Ardichvili D., Perissino A., et al.: A case of familial visceral myopathy with atrophy and fibrosis of the longitudinal muscle layer of the entire small bowel. *Gastroenterology* 77:745, 1979.
22. Anuras S., Mitros F.A., Nowak T.V., et al.: A familial visceral myopathy with external ophthalmoplegia and autosomal recessive transmission. *Gastroenterology* 84:346, 1983.
23. Schuffler M.D., Bird T.D., Sumi S.M., et al.: A familial neuronal disease presenting as intestinal pseudo-obstruction. *Gastroenterology* 75:889, 1978.
24. Cockel R., Hill E.E., Purliton D.I., et al.: Familial steatorrhea with calcifications of the basal ganglia and mental retardation. *Q. J. Med.* 42:771, 1973.
25. Hirschowitz B.I., Groll A., Ceballos R.: Hereditary nerve deafness in three sisters with absent gastric motility, small bowel diverticulitis and ulceration and progressive sensory neuropathy. *Birth Defects* (Original Article Series) 8:27–41, 1972.
26. Schuffler M.D., Jonak Z.: Chronic idiopathic intestinal pseudoobstruction caused by a degenerative disorder of the myenteric plexus: The use of Smith's method to define the neuropathology. *Gastroenterology* 82:476, 1982.
27. Schuffler M.D., Baird H.W., Fleming C.R., et al.: Intestinal pseudoobstruction as the presenting manifestation of small-cell carcinoma of the lung: A paraneoplastic neuropathy of the gastrointestinal tract. *Ann. Intern. Med.* 98:129, 1983.
28. Sriram K., Schumer W., Ehrenpreis S., et al.: Phenothiazine effects on gastrointestinal tract function. *Am. J. Surg.* 137:87, 1979.
29. Abbasi A.A., Douglass R.C., Bissell G.W., et al.: Myxedema ileus: A form of intestinal pseudo-obstruction. *J.A.M.A.* 234:181, 1975.
30. Wald A., Kichler J., Mendelow H.: Amyloidosis and chronic intestinal pseudo-obstruction. *Dig. Dis. Sci.* 26:5:462, 1981.
31. Barry R.E., Chow A.W., Billesdon J.: Role of intestinal microflora in colonic pseudo-obstruction complicating jejunoileal bypass. *Gut* 18:356, 1977.
32. Krishnamurthy S., Kelly M.M., Rohrmann C.A., et al.: Jejunal diverticulosis: A heterogeneous disorder caused by a variety of abnormalities of smooth muscle or myenteric plexus. *Gastroenterology* 85:538, 1983.
33. Summers R.W., Anuras S., Green J.: Jejunal manometry patterns in health, partial intestinal obstruction and pseudo-obstruction. *Gastroenterology* 85:1290, 1983.
34. Anuras S., Shirazi S., Faulk D.L., et al.: Surgical treatment in familial visceral myopathy. *Ann. Surg.* 189:306, 1979.
35. Klatt G.R.: Role of subtotal colectomy in the treatment of incapacitating constipation. *Am. J. Surg.* 145:623, 1983.
36. McCready R.A., Beart R.W.: The surgical treatment of incapacitating constipation with idiopathic megacolon. *Mayo Clin. Proc.* 54:779, 1979.
37. Watkins W.L.: Operative treatment of acquired megacolon in adults. *Arch. Surg.* 93:620, 1966.

39

Crohn's Disease

VICTOR W. FAZIO, M.B.

REGIONAL enteritis (Crohn's disease) is a chronic inflammatory condition of the intestinal tract of unknown etiology. The disease tends to occur in young people presenting with the common triad of abdominal pain, diarrhea, and weight loss. All parts of the intestinal tract may be involved, but most commonly the disease affects the terminal ileum, with or without colonic involvement, or the colon and rectum alone. Pathologically, the disease is transmural and is associated with inflammation of all layers of the bowel, penetrating fissures, increased inflammatory cells in the mucosa and submucosa, thickening of the bowel wall, and granuloma formation, both in the bowel wall and in the adjacent lymph nodes. Characteristically, the ulcerative process in the colon is patchy, with normal or near-normal segments between areas of ulceration. The rectum is usually spared.

In the small intestine, the disease affects the ileal segment more or less evenly, with gradual changes to a normal mucosa in a proximal direction. However, a patchy distribution of the disease may also be seen in the small intestine, ranging from scattered, minute, shallow, pale, aphthous ulcers, to short or long segments of frank ulceration and stricture (skip lesions).

Manifestations of the disease relate to narrowing of the bowel lumen, to local, intra-abdominal, and perineal septic complications due to penetrating ulceration of the bowel wall, and to a variety of extraintestinal systemic conditions. These are related to either the activity of the disease (especially the colitis pattern) or to pathophysiology of the small bowel.

HISTORICAL BACKGROUND

While Morgagni in 1761 described instances of inflammation of the ileum and associated large lymph nodes, Combe and Saunders in 1813 described the first probable case of Crohn's disease of the ileum. They said: "The lower part of the ileum as far as the colon, was contracted for the space of three feet to the size of a turkey quill." In 1828 Abercrombie described a number of cases (postmortem) of ileal as opposed to colonic disease. Specifically, thickening and induration of all coats of the ileum were associated with luminal stricturing; tuberculosis was excluded, making the diagnosis of ileocecal tuberculosis unlikely. In 1853 Bristow described a patient with thickening of the ileum and lower jejunum with a stricture and ileoileal fistula; the colon was also ulcerated. Tuberculosis was excluded. In 1888 Hale and White described 29 cases of ulcerative colitis in their case report. There were

eight probable cases of Crohn's disease, one of which had Crohn's disease of the duodenum.

In the 20th century, Braun (1909) described several cases of inflammatory masses involving the ileum. In 1913 Kennedy Dalziel reported nine patients on whom he had operated, "who had chronic, interstitial enteritis, and not tuberculosis." In 1923 Moschowitz and Wilensky described four cases of nonspecific granuloma of the intestine; one of these four had both colon and small intestine involvement. In 1932 Crohn delivered a presentation entitled "Terminal Ileitis" in New Orleans. This forbidding title was changed to "Regional Ileitis" at the suggestion of Bargen, and was published by Crohn, Ginzberg, and Oppenheimer. In 1952 Wells described segmental colitis, paving the way for the description by Brooke in 1959 and Lockhart-Mummery and Morson (1960) of Crohn's disease in the colon.

INCIDENCE AND ETIOLOGY

The problems in case reports relate to a number of areas. First, the gathering of reliable data depends on accurate case identification. In societies where functional GI complaints are common, it is clear that accurate case identification requires the appropriate use of objective diagnostic aids such as roentgenographic, endoscopic, and biopsy material. Furthermore, the era of particular studies may make information unreliable. Prior to the mid-1960s, it was not widely recognized that Crohn's disease could occur in the colon. To this day, diagnostic difficulties arise even with the more sophisticated of methods. In a substantial number of instances, even with histologic examination of a resected segment of bowel, there can be difficulty in distinguishing ulcerative colitis from Crohn's disease. Incidence range of Crohn's disease is 0.8–5.0/100,000 population as reported from different countries. In the United States the incidence increased from 1.8 to 3.7/100,000 (1963 to 1973).

There appear to be changes in the incidence of Crohn's disease. In Sweden 1955–59, the incidence was 1.5/100,000 population. Heller's 1979 report of the Stockholm experience noted a gradual rise from 2.2 in 1960–64 to 4.5/100,000 in 1972–74. He used the date of definitive diagnosis in measuring disease incidence. He also noted a reduction in the interval between onset of symptoms and time of definitive diagnosis. Heller concluded that there had been a steady increase in disease incidence from 1 to 4.5 cases per 100,000 population from 1955 to 1969, but that after that, the incidence had been stationary.

Factors noted as possibly playing a role in the etiology include the following.

AGE AND SEX.—Although there have been variations described from various authors, the sex ratio is about equal. Crohn's disease has its greatest incidence in early adult life, although later peaks have been described in elderly patients.

URBAN AND RURAL DIFFERENCES.—Kyle in 1971 and Mendeloff in 1966 described a relatively low incidence of Crohn's disease in rural populations. Others, however (Heller in 1979), have observed no differences.

SOCIOECONOMIC FACTORS.—In Baltimore, Maryland, Crohn's disease was slightly more common among persons of high educational levels. There was no such distinction in an Aberdeen Study.

ETHNIC VARIATIONS.—The patients are more commonly Western than Oriental. Among the Western populations, it is much more common in Northern Europeans, Anglo-Saxons, or those from northern portions of Eastern Europe. The disease is more common among Caucasians than amongst non-Caucasian groups. The disease is more common among Jews living in Europe and North America, than among non-Jews, but not as common among Israelis. These differences remain unexplained. It has been suggested that Jews are susceptible to inflammatory bowel disease because of environmental rather than genetic factors.

DIET.—There is suggestive evidence of an association between high intake of sugar and low-fiber diet and the higher incidence of Crohn's disease.

BACTERIAL AND VIRAL INFECTIONS.—Animal transmission studies suggest that a transmissible agent may be present in Crohn's tissues, but the studies have failed to show the specificity of this proposed agent or its etiologic significance. Early reports of Bargen's *Streptococcus bovis* as an etiologic agent have not been borne out. Recently, there has been interest in the variability of *E. coli* subtypes producing intestinal disease in man; however, no specific organism has consistently been isolated in patients or produced disease in experimental animals. There is a possibility that transient enteric infection might induce a change which continues in some self-perpetuating manner. Another variant of enteric bacteria is that of the cell wall defective agent. Orr reported that the direct injection of the terminal ileum of rabbits with a stable L-form of *Streptococcus faecalis* was able to induce focal granulomatous lesions. In a study by Berent and Mitchell, high titers of serum antibody against *Pseudomonas aeruginosa* was found in high titers in patients with Crohn's disease. In 1978 Burnham described the growth of an acid-fast organism of the *Mycobacterium kansasii* after long-term culture of lymph node materials in one of 27 patients with Crohn's disease.

With respect to viruses, several investigators have now reported the presence of cytopathic agents from tissues involved with inflammatory bowel disease. There remains considerable controversy concerning the specificity of these findings and whether these cytopathic agents are indeed viruses. It has not proved possible to classify the proposed viral agents into a single group, and there is no convincing demonstration of viral particles under electromicroscopic examination of disease tissue.

GENETICS.—At The Cleveland Clinic Foundation, Farmer, Michener, and Mortimer reviewed 316 patients with ulcerative colitis, and found that 29% had family histories positive for inflammatory bowel disease. Of 522 patients with Crohn's disease, 185 (35%) had family histories positive for inflammatory bowel disease. In the Crohn's disease group, 15% had immediate family members affected and 7.5% had siblings affected.

IMMUNOLOGIC MECHANISMS

Initial studies were based on a hypothesis that an exaggeration of normal immune mechanisms directed against either normal gut-associated antigens (bacterial flora) or against gut mucosa resulted in chronic inflammation and tissue damage. Observations on circulating antibodies and peripheral blood lymphocytes in both ulcerative colitis and Crohn's disease showed abnormal immune responses directed against the gut, suggestive of autoimmune conditions.

In both disorders, humoral activity is activated, active disease being accompanied by normal or slightly elevated levels of IgA, IgM, and IgE. In contrast to lymphocytes from normal subjects, intestinal mononuclear cells in inflammatory bowel disease patients show decreased spontaneous antibody synthesis. However, peripheral blood monocytes in inflammatory bowel disease show enhanced in vitro antibody synthesis, especially of IgA. Clearly, there is an abnormality of regulation of immunoglobulin synthesis by intestinal mononuclear cells in inflammatory bowel disease, but its pathophysiologic significance is unclear.

There is a striking increase in IgG plasma cells in the mucosa of both ulcerative colitis and Crohn's disease patients, extending somewhat deeper into the mucosa in the latter case. Some of the IgG produced has antibody specificity for colonic bacteria, suggesting the formation of local antigen/antibody complexes with tissue destruction, as the result of activation of complement and neutrophils. This may account for some of the sequelae of inflammatory bowel disease, but requires preliminary loss of integrity of the mucosa.

Thus there is no good evidence that immunologic abnormalities are the primary cause of inflammatory bowel disease, but they may contribute to the inflammatory process.

PATHOPHYSIOLOGY

The manifestations of disease relate to the location, extent, and severity of the diseased segment or segments of the GI tract involved. Intestinal obstruction and the septic sequelae of penetrating ulceration are direct results of the pathologic process. Further manifestations depends on the adequacy of functional reserve of the small bowel, nutritional deficiencies and deficiencies of absorption, and the presence of extraintestinal manifestations.

Assuming adequate digestion, absorption of carbohydrates, protein, and fat occurs rapidly from the proximal small bowel; therefore, a considerable amount of intestine may be diseased, bypassed, or resected before nutritional absorption is compromised. A process of adaptation may occur over a period of a year or two following intestinal resection, so the residual, unaffected gut can increase its absorptive function.

Nutritional deficiencies occur when there is inadequate intake of calories or when there are abnormalities of digestion and absorption. Ileal Crohn's disease and ileal resection for Crohn's disease are frequently associated with bile acid malabsorption and excessive fecal bile acid excretion. In one study of patients with nonoperative Crohn's disease, 44% had bile acid malabsorption. A major factor affecting bile acid metabolism is that of bacterial overgrowth in the small bowel. This results from the potential of many species of bacteria, especially anaerobes, to deconjugate bile acids. Unconjugated bile acids are absorbed rapidly from the intestine by diffusion, leading to micellar bile acid deficiency and fat malabsorption. Ileal resections smaller than 100 cm produce marked bile acid diarrhea, since hepatic synthesis is able to maintain the bile acid pool. Larger resections of small bowel result in depletion of the pool, and then fat maldigestion and malabsorption dominate the clinical picture. Extensive ileal disease or the combination of ileal resection and residual disease may produce such profound bile acid malabsorption that hepatic synthesis cannot maintain a normal bile acid pool. Under these circumstances, hepatic bile acid secretion is diminished, which can lead to further profound disturbances of fat digestion, and absorption.

When intestinal strictures or adhesions are producing partial, closed loops, or when enteric fistulas between small and large bowel occur, bacterial overgrowth may be a major factor in producing fat, protein, carbohydrate, and vitamin malabsorption. The incidence of lactose malabsorption in Crohn's disease is similar to that in a controlled population. This suggests the coexistence of Crohn's disease and hereditary lactase deficiencies. With respect to protein absorption, the presence of mucosal disease and bacterial overgrowth could interfere with peptide amino acid absorption. Severe protein malnutrition can occur from small-bowel bacterial overgrowth.

Folic acid malabsorption can occur in approximately one quarter of patients with Crohn's disease, especially those with jejunal involvement, but also in patients with disease apparently confined to the colon. This malabsorption appears to be a true transport defect rather than a failure to hydrolyze polyglutamyl folate. It is not clear whether a given case of folate malabsorption invariably indicates an abnormal jejunum. Vitamin B_{12} malabsorption may occur in up to 60% of unoperated Crohn's patients, even with quite localized ileal disease or when the ileum is radiologically normal. There is poor correlation between vitamin B_{12} absorption and disease activity. Even after ileal resection, the magnitude of vitamin B_{12} absorption is only roughly correlated with a surgical assessment of the length of bowel removed. Vitamin D absorption relates to deficiencies in fat digestion and absorption. Vitamin D deficiency frequently occurs in patients with Crohn's disease. Those with small-intestine involvement have the lowest levels of cholecalciferol. Deficiency of vitamin D is probably a consequence of both reduced diet intake and of malabsorption. Hypocalcemia may be secondary to vitamin D deficiency. Iron deficiency is a frequent accompaniment of Crohn's dis-

ease, as is zinc deficiency and, occasionally, magnesium deficiency. Deficiencies in chromium, copper, and nicotinic acid, as well as vitamins A, B, C, and K, have also been described. Plasma protein depletion can occur from protein-losing enteropathy. Losses from the gut can occur as a result of increased mucosal cell loss and turnover of inflamed tissues. The colon has a very limited capacity for reabsorption of amino acid, so loss of protein into the ileum may lead to hypoalbuminemia and deficiencies of plasma and tissue amino acids. Other metabolic effects of small-bowel Crohn's disease include retardation of growth and development and delay in sexual maturation. Growth retardation occurs in about 20% of patients who have onset of the disease in childhood. In such patients, deficient caloric intake and low serum albumin are invariably found. It is now accepted that diminished caloric intake rather than malabsorption or even use of corticosteroids is the major factor in growth retardation. Steroid therapy in lower dosage, especially alternate-day therapy, may control disease and promote growth acceleration. There is controversy with respect to the role of surgical resection of diseased bowel in promoting growth. The increase in ability to add to caloric intake is probably the effective agent with respect to surgery. Increase in gallstones and oxalate renal calculi has also been observed in patients with Crohn's disease.

Extraintestinal Manifestations

Practically every system may be affected by the local and systemic effects of Crohn's disease or its therapy, in addition to which numerous associations of other maladies have been described (Table 39–1). Rankin et al. in 1979[1] reported extraintestinal manifestations in reviewing 569 patients in the National Cooperative Crohn's Disease Study. The prevalence of these manifestations was estimated for the three major clinical patterns of the disease—ileitis, ileocolitis, and colitis. For these three patterns, there was a prevalence for arthritis/arthralgia of 17.9, 18.9, and 26.7%, respectively; for iritis/uveitis of 2.8, 3.4, and 6.7%; for erythema nodosum/pyoderma gangrenosum, 2.8, 5.1, and 8.3%, respectively. It is unusual for such conditions to be the sole or even the major indication for surgery of Crohn's disease. In the study by Greenstein et al.,[2] which included 498 patients with Crohn's disease and 202 patients with ulcerative colitis, they observed two main groups of complications—"colitis related" and "related to the pathophysiology of the small bowel." The colitis-related group comprised joint, skin, mouth, and eye disease. There was a close association with active inflammation, and the manifestations often responded to medical or surgical treatment of the bowel disease. These complications occurred more frequently in colitis (42%) than in disease confined to the small bowel (23%). The second group of complications included: malabsorption, gallstones, kidney stones, and acalculous obstructive uropathy. There was a relationship to the severity of the disease in the small bowel and a tendency to persist even in the absence of active inflammation. Malabsorption was mostly confined to patients with small-bowel disease (10% incidence), while gallstones and renal stones were also both more frequent in Crohn's disease (11% and 9%, respectively), the latter usually in association with small-bowel resection or ileostomy.

TABLE 39–1.—EXTRAINTESTINAL ASSOCIATIONS AND COMPLICATIONS OF CROHN'S DISEASE

Skin	Aphthous ulcers of the mouth Cutaneous vasculitis Erythema multiforme Erythema nodosum Lichen planus Pellagra Psoriasis Pyoderma gangrenosum Stevens-Johnson syndrome	Liver	Amyloidosis Biliary cirrhosis Fatty infiltration Hepatic abscess Hepatitis—chronic—active Pericholangitis Portal hepatic fibrosis Postnecrotic cirrhosis Sclerosing cholangitis
Eyes	Conjunctivitis Episcleritis Iridocyclitis Iritis Orbital pseudotumor Retrobulbar Secondary glaucoma Uveitis	Vascular	Arterial thrombosis Necrotizing vasculitis Takayasu's arteritis Thrombophlebitis
Bones and Joints	Clubbing Intestinal arthritis Osteoarthropathy Osteomalacia Osteomyelitis Osteonecrosis Osteopenia Osteoporosis Polychondritis Rheumatoid arthritis Synovitis Tenosynovitis	Renal Neoplasms Others	Glomerulonephritis Hydroureter, hydronephrosis Pyelonephritis Stones (phosphate, oxalate, urate) Urinary fistulas Carcinoma (large and small bowel) Carcinoma in fistulous tracts Leukemia Lymphoma (small and large bowel) Drug complications Pancreatitis, thyroiditis, cardiomyopathy

DIAGNOSIS

The diagnosis of Crohn's disease may be delayed for considerable periods, even years, in certain patients. Unlike ulcerative colitis, where affected patients will usually present with bleeding and characteristic inflammatory changes on proctoscopic examination, Crohn's disease in most cases has no such specific findings or symptoms. Abdominal pain, diarrhea, and weight loss can be associated with irritable bowel syndrome, yet these three symptoms are the cardinal ones occurring in Crohn's disease. The persistence of this triad of symptoms, in contrast to their intermittent nature in irritable bowel syndrome, should raise the clinician's level of suspicion. A specific manifestation of the illness becomes evident usually within three to six months. Depending on the anatomical pattern of disease, i.e., small bowel alone (ileitis), small bowel and colon (ileocolitis), and colon and/or rectum (colitis), one or more specific symptoms or signs will dominate the clinical picture. For example, patients with ileitis usually present with intestinal obstructive symptoms, such as abdominal pain, nausea, and distention. Patients with ileocolitis will present in a similar way, but are also likely to develop fever and evidence of a phlegmon or mass due to intestinal perforative complications. Patients with Crohn's colitis may manifest symptoms and signs related to perianal fistula/abscess, colonic bleeding, toxic reaction due to megacolon, and extraintestinal manifestations of disease. Children may present with fever of unknown origin with little or no diarrhea. Growth retardation may be the sole presentation in children or adolescents.

Abdominal Pain

In Crohn's disease abdominal pain is usually cramping, located in the lower abdomen, and in the case of ileitis or ileocolitis, is often associated with nausea and abdominal distention. Vomiting is relatively uncommon. Response to anti-inflammatory agents is usually dramatic initially, but most patients develop exacerbations of the disease. The pain is often worse after meals, and the patient will refrain from "normal" eating, even though hungry, because of the predictable outcome of an even moderate-sized meal. A more constant pain, especially in the right lower quadrant, implies a perforative process, and a mass may be found on examination. Uncommonly, the patient may develop low back or hip pain due to retroperitoneal sepsis secondary to a perforated viscus. A psoas abscess (Fig 39–1) can be diagnosed in a patient with Crohn's disease who has such pain accompanied by fever, lower quadrant mass, and a fixed flexion deformity of the hip. Obstructive uropathy may also be present from ureteric compression.

With colonic Crohn's disease, pain may also be colicky and is basically indistinguishable from the pain of ulcerative colitis. Rectal involvement may also be associated with tenesmus. Anal pain occurs from perianal abscess and fistula. Anal ulcer is discussed in a later section.

Rarely, patients with Crohn's disease may present with an "acute abdomen" that is difficult to distinguish from an acute appendicitis. More commonly, this presentation is that of acute ileitis (see below). Biliary colic and renal colic are other

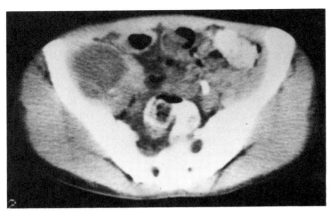

Fig 39–1.—CT scan shows a large psoas abscess in the right lower quadrant secondary to retroperitoneal perforation of ileocecal Crohn's disease.

types of pain a patient may experience. Peptic ulcer disease occurs in 6%–10% of patients with Crohn's disease.

Diarrhea

Initially, diarrhea is usually transient, with accompanying bouts of abdominal discomfort or pain. Diarrhea becomes more severe and persistent. Stools are small, frequently occur at nighttime, and are loose to watery, although usually not bloody. If severe, diarrhea may be accompanied by incontinence.

Buchmann and Alexander-Williams[3] studied continence in 39 Crohn's disease patients, 20 of whom had urgency. Interestingly, this symptom occurred only in patients with small-bowel involvement. None of seven patients with colonic Crohn's disease had urgency. Degrees of proctitis, anal sphincter basal pressure and squeeze pressure, and response to rectal filling, were equally abnormal in those with and without urgency. Urgency correlated strongly with frequency and the liquid consistency of stool. The conclusions of the study were that rapid rectal filling, not proctitis, produced urgency.

Weight Loss

Reluctance to eat (because of accompanying pain or anorexia) results in weight loss. Other mechanisms for weight loss were discussed in the section on pathophysiology (bacterial overgrowth, bowel obstruction, etc.).

Retardation of Growth

Lack of weight gain, delay in onset of puberty, and cessation of bone development were found to occur in 18%–30% of children with inflammatory bowel disease, and are more common in patients affected with Crohn's disease than ulcerative colitis. Growth retardation may precede by several years the onset of symptoms, specifically for inflammatory bowel disease. While steroid therapy has been indicted in the past as a major contributor to growth retardation, there is a general consensus now that retardation is due to inadequate caloric intake. In some patients, normal growth resumes when the disease is controlled medically. If this is not possible, surgery generally is indicated. Bowel resection does not always provide the hoped-for growth spurt, perhaps because of the delay in surgery; resection after the age of 16 years may be too late.

Other Symptoms

Bleeding is an uncommon symptom in Crohn's disease. Anemia, however, may occur for a variety of reasons, including occult bleeding, iron deficiency, and folic acid deficiency. Hemolytic anemia, Heinz body anemia from sulfasalazine, thrombocytopenia purpura, anaphylactoid purpura, and hyposplenism have been described in association with Crohn's disease. Massive hemorrhage is rare in Crohn's disease and is discussed below.

EXAMINATION OF THE PATIENT

The patient may show evidence of anemia, weight loss, dehydration, electrolyte imbalance, vitamin deficiency, and any number of extraintestinal manifestations of disease. Usually, however, the signs elicited relate to the GI tract.

Abdominal tenderness, especially in the right lower quadrant, indicates an inflamed, sometimes palpable loop of intestine. Abdominal distention may be present with small-bowel obstruction or colonic dilatation. Free perforation is rare; in such cases, signs of generalized peritonitis may be present. An enterocutaneous fistula may be present, frequently presenting through an old appendix scar. Flexion deformity of the hip may indicate the presence of a psoas abscess. Borborygmus and visible peristalsis indicate an obstruction process.

Examination of the perineum may show stigmas of Crohn's disease. Hypertrophied, tender anal tags (external hemorrhoids) are commonly seen. Perianal abscesses and fistulas occur frequently. In the National Cooperative Crohn's Disease Study, perianal complications were found in 25.5% of patients with small-bowel involvement, 41.4% of those with both small- and large-bowel involvement, and 46.7% of those with colon involvement alone. Perianal lesions may be the sole manifestations of Crohn's disease in 5% of patients. Fistulas are often multiple and can be associated with extensive tracking into the groin, scrotum, labia, vagina, urethra, prostate, or seminal vesicles (Fig 39–2). Tissue destruction by sepsis may produce sphincter impairment and incontinence. Anorectal stricture may result with transient resolution of the sepsis. Fissures are characteristically large, indolent, laterally sited, and relatively painless. Acute, painful anal fissures may be seen in the characteristic posterior and anterior positions. These may be more a feature of chronic diarrhea than of an active Crohn's process in the anal canal. An anal canal ulcer may be a variant lesion that affects an entire quadrant or more of the anal canal extending into the rectum. This is an exquisitely painful lesion that frequently requires fecal diversion for symptomatic relief. While the figures cited from the National Cooperative Crohn's Disease Study group are typical of many reports, the incidence of perianal disease has been reported as high as 32% and 92% for Crohn's disease of the small bowel and colon, respectively.

Oral ulceration is indistinguishable from aphthous ulcers and has been described as a common finding in Crohn's disease. Oral lesions may precede GI symptoms by as much as one year in 30% of patients.

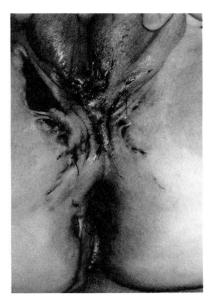

Fig 39–2.—Extensive perianal fistulae are seen tracking into the groins and base of scrotum.

Endoscopic Examination

With all endoscopic maneuvers of the lower intestinal tract for patients with Crohn's disease, there is the possibility that local pain and tenderness will thwart an adequate examination. This may dictate a need for examination using anesthesia, but with most patients this is unnecessary. Much information can be gained from such an examination. Time spent in allaying the patient's fears is well invested.

Anoscopy

This is the only adequate method of assessing the lower rectum and anal canal for anoperineal, anovaginal, or rectovaginal fistula.

Proctoscopy

The rectum affected with Crohn's disease may show a spectrum ranging from minute (2–3 mm) aphthous ulcers to severe disease. The disease is usually patchy or discontinuous (as opposed to ulcerative colitis). Granularity and friability are less commonly seen than in ulcerative colitis, but this by no means excludes the diagnosis of Crohn's disease. Large ulcers of a serpiginous nature are sometimes seen usually running in the longitudinal plane of the bowel. These are well-circumscribed and deep. Several parallel ulcers (bear claw effect) may be seen. Cobblestone appearance is more commonly seen in the colon but is occasionally seen in the rectum. Strictures or symmetric narrowing of the rectum may be present. Pseudopolyps may occur but are less common than in ulcerative colitis. Edema and thickened, rugose, mucosal folds with loss of the sharp valves are commonly seen in Crohn's disease. However, it is the patchy nature of the mucosal abnormality, with intervening areas of apparent or relative normalcy, that is the most useful endoscopic aid to the diagnosis.

The role of colonoscopy is somewhat controversial with respect to its specific indications. Most patients can be managed without it, especially if a good-quality barium enema is available.

Esophagogastroduodenoscopy is used for both visual assessment and the obtaining of material for histologic examination. Patients with Crohn's disease and who complain of dysphagia may have Crohn's disease of the esophagus. This can be difficult to distinguish from reflux esophagitis. In Crohn's disease of the esophagus the lesions are typically shallow, flat, irregular ulcers or erosions surrounded by a red margin in an otherwise healthy esophageal mucosa.

With gastroduodenal Crohn's disease, thickening of antral mucosal folds, erythema, friability, and cobblestone appearance of the mucosa may be seen. Usually, ulcers are multiple, small, and pale, but may coalesce to form a large, irregular ulcer. Biopsies are best taken as deeply as possible from the ulcer edge. Duodenal intubation may be difficult because of stricture. Crohn's disease may affect the duodenum alone with changes similar in appearance to those in the stomach. Endoscopic and even histologic examination may prove inadequate to the task of excluding conventional peptic ulcer disease. Radiographic contrast studies of the upper GI tract may show characteristic extensive stricturing or fistulas that assist in making the diagnosis.

Biopsy

In addition to biopsy material from the upper intestinal tract, the practice of rectal biopsy is advised when performing the initial diagnostic proctoscopic examination or if a change in appearance of the mucosa is noted on subsequent examinations. There is controversy about the value of such biopsies if the rectum appears normal. Korelitz and Sommers[4] found rectal inflammation in 58%, 28%, and 21% of patients with Crohn's disease confined to the colon, patients with ileitis, and patients with ileocolitis, respectively; in all cases, the rectum was endoscopically normal. Granulomas were present in 4.2% of patients and microgranulomas in 8.0%. The significance of these findings and prognosis in terms of future rectal disease has yet to be determined. A personal view is that restoration of intestinal continuity or definitive anal surgery should not necessarily be withheld from patients when the rectal mucosa appears normal and there is histologic evidence of disease.

RADIOLOGIC STUDIES

Barium Enema

Lesions may be distributed throughout the entire colon and rectum or may involve specific segments, leaving intervening, normal-appearing mucosa, or may affect an isolated segment, such as the sigmoid or transverse colon (Figs 39–3 and 39–4). Reflux of barium into the small intestine may demonstrate ileal involvement or anastomotic stricture.

Typically, the mucosal changes are less uniform than in ulcerative colitis. A nodular appearance termed cobblestoning is due to the combination of deep, longitudinal ulceration and narrow, transverse, slit ulceration. The presence of extracolonic barium in an abscess cavity or extending into another viscus serves to differentiate from ulcerative colitis, where such perforation/fistulas do not occur. Using high-quality air-

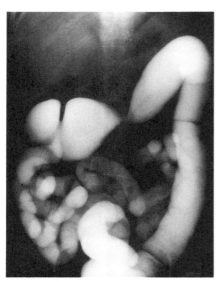

Fig 39–3.—Barium enema with a tight, benign, stricture of the midtransverse colon.

contrast techniques, fine mucosal detail can be observed and even aphthoid ulcers diagnosed. Spiculation of the bowel wall (rose thorn appearance) may be seen especially in Crohn's disease of the left colon. Longitudinal submucosal and subserosal fistulous tracts (Marshak's sign), while not pathognomonic of Crohn's disease, are certainly suggestive. Contraction of the colonic lumen may be symmetric or isolated (stricture). Typically, there is less contraction of the colon and less evident descent of the splenic flexure than in ulcerative colitis, and pseudopolyps are less likely.

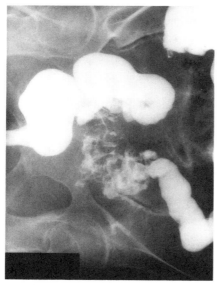

Fig 39–4.—Barium enema shows a diffuse, irregular, stricture of the sigmoid colon with mucosal irregularity and retroperitoneal perforation. Laparotomy revealed the presence of both Crohn's colitis and diverticular disease isolated to the sigmoid segment.

Barium Meal and Small-Bowel Series

The appearance of gastroduodenal Crohn's disease was described in an earlier section. The small intestine may demonstrate all of the mucosal abnormalities as listed for the colon (Fig 39–5). Additionally, a variety of fistulas, such as enteroenteric, enterocolic, enteroduodenal, enterocutaneous, enterovesical may be seen. Typically, the terminal ileum is affected with luminal narrowing and mucosal irregularity due to ulceration, and degrees of proximal small-bowel dilatation are seen. Skip lesions of the proximal ileum and jejunum occur in up to 25% of cases. Diffuse jejunoileitis may occur in about 5% of patients, as may Crohn's disease of the small bowel with sparing of the terminal ileum. A reliable sign is the filling defect in the right lower quadrant and right midabdomen, producing compression of the small bowel proximal to ileal disease upward and to the patient's left side. This is caused by the gross mesenteric adenopathy and fat wrapping of the ileum.

Other Investigations

Ultrasound and CT scan have been used in the diagnosis of Crohn's disease as well as for the localization of abscesses sec-

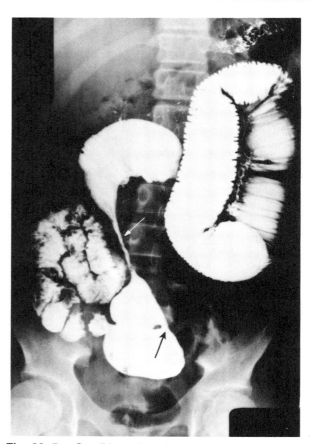

Fig 39–5.—Small-bowel series showing several distal strictures with intervening dilated loops in the terminal ileum. (From Fazio V.W.: Regional enteritis (Crohn's disease): Indications for surgery and operative strategy. *Surg. Clin. North Am.* 63:27–48, 1983. Used by permission.)

ondary to the disease. The thick-walled ileum with narrowed lumen can be identified. Using ultrasound imaging in the diagnosis of Crohn's disease, sensitivity and specificity rates of 76% and 88% have been achieved.

Scintiscanning with indium-111-labeled autologous leukocytes has been reported to be as accurate as a barium enema in localizing the site of inflammatory involvement in the colon, both in ulcerative colitis and Crohn's disease—a potential use is to distinguish active from quiescent disease.

ACTIVITY OF THE DISEASE

The site of the disease is probably the most important clinical determinant of the course of Crohn's disease. Attempts at quantifying activity of Crohn's disease have been made to see whether guidelines could be established with respect to alterations of therapeutic modalities at any particular point in the course of the disease and to provide a basis for comparison of treatments within and between groups of patients. Symptoms, signs, and laboratory abnormalities were assigned and agreed on as a somewhat arbitrary and unobjective score for computer analysis. Not all that is significant is measurable, and not all that is measurable is significant. Experience with the National Cooperative Crohn's Disease Study and the development of a Crohn's Disease Activity Index has shown the difficulties of such assessment. Use of colonoscopy in Crohn's disease is more helpful in the initial evaluation of the patient and in the differential diagnosis than as a sequential measure of activity. Anemia and hypoalbuminema generally correlate with the nutritional status, and the signs of intoxication help in assessing the severity of the disease. Fever and associated complications are useful indices, but the most helpful aid lies in the assessment of the patient's symptoms. The patient with an otherwise quiescent state of Crohn's disease may have a fibrotic stricture of the ileum and obstructive symptoms.

MEDICAL TREATMENT

General Measures

In the past, a high-protein, low-residue diet was prescribed. Currently, the patient is advised to take a regular diet with as few restrictions as possible. Patients with significant (20% or greater below ideal body weight) malnutrition or whose symptoms are difficult to control medically may require TPN. While the value of TPN as primary therapy is at best limited, its adjunctive use in preparing patients for surgery is of undoubted value.

Deficiencies of iron, vitamin B_{12}, folic acid, various minerals, and trace elements can be remedied. The widespread use of multiple vitamins has unproved value. Patients are advised to have regular review for early detection of complications (or recurrence after surgery) as well as for emotional support. Selective use of antidiarrhea and analgesic medication may be required.

Medication

The method of action for most drugs used in Crohn's disease is unknown. Sulfasalazine (salicyl-azo-sulfapyridine) is degraded by enteric bacteria into 5-aminosalicylic acid and sulfapyridine. The drug inhibits prostaglandin formation, may have an antibacterial action on enteric flora, inhibits metabolic processes in granulocytes, and inhibits cytopathic effect of lymphocytes on other cells. Controlled trials have demonstrated that the drug is effective in active ileocolitis and Crohn's colitis. There is an uncertainty as to the length of time the drug should be used, as further benefit is doubtful after initial improvement is seen. Perhaps courses of three to four months' duration are best.

Steroids are used systemically and topically in the treatment of Crohn's disease. Beneficial effect occurs when steroids are used systemically for active ileal Crohn's disease, ileocolitis, and probably for severe active colitis. In the National Cooperative Crohn's Disease Study, Crohn's colitis was not benefited by steroids. There seems to be little difference between the effect of ACTH and corticosteroids. The latter is preferred in treating reactivation or acute flare of the disease if the patient was previously taking corticosteroids. There has been no preventive effect in the incidence of relapse or recurrence rates as the result of using prophylactic, low-dose steroids.

The main role of steroids is to settle a relapse of inflammation over the course of days or weeks.

Combination of corticosteroid and sulfasalazine has failed to increase rates of remission in active disease as compared with corticosteroid alone, and relapse rates are similarly unaffected.

The role of azathioprine is debatable. Critics of the National Cooperative Crohn's Disease Study (which failed to identify a beneficial effect of azathioprine) point out that the duration and dose of the drug may have been inadequate. Patients with Crohn's disease have a significantly lower K-cell activity when treated with azathioprine or prednisone compared to untreated patients. Additionally, there is a nonspecific, anti-inflammatory effect and possible antibacterial action against enteric anaerobes. Because of its steroid-sparing effect, many clinicians use the drug when their patients' maintenance steroid requirements become excessive. A common view among surgeons is to confine use of the drug to situations in which surgery is particularly hazardous and undesirable.

Disodium cromoglycate was advanced as an agent for use in Crohn's disease, in that histamine liberation in the gut and release of slow-reacting substance from mast cells may be prevented and, therefore, inflammations prevented. No conclusive benefit has yet been realized in trials so far.

The role of metronidazole has received considerable recent attention. One prospective study found it to be as effective as sulfasalazine in effecting clinical improvement in Crohn's disease and superior to sulfasalazine in producing a fall in the level of plasma orosomucoid, an acute-phase reactant indicative of inflammatory activity. Patients with colitis fared better than those with ileitis. Beneficial effects have been noted with metronidazole given to patients with perianal septic disease and those with postoperative perianal sinuses.

No drug is curative in the treatment of Crohn's disease, and the hazards of steroid use as well as other immunosuppressives are documented. By intelligent manipulation of these medications, however, with bipartisan involvement of the internist and the surgeon (and with the knowledge that the placebo effect of medication in Crohn's disease is considerable), the patient may be carried through relapses with minimal side effects of the drug or at least have timely surgery.

Surgical treatment

Crohn's disease is curable neither by medical nor surgical treatment. It behooves the surgeon to regard the disease from several perspectives. On the one hand, aggressive surgical management will rid the patient of the disease, prevent serious complications, restore health, and free the patient from the need for steroid medication. On the negative side are the risks associated with an operation, the metabolic and nutritional effects of intestinal loss, and the occasional need for an ileostomy. With relapse (recurrence) of the disease comes the possibility of future operations and development of a short-bowel syndrome. The aim of the surgeon should be to deal with the current problem as simply as possible and to maintain a strategic view of the pathologic process, since it may affect the rest of the patient's life.

In general terms, surgery is performed for complications of the disease (Table 39–2) and less commonly for failure of medical management. This is not to say that one must wait for a complication to develop to advise surgery. Malnutrition, growth retardation, chronic disability or bleeding, the need for long-term, large-dose steroid therapy or its side effects, are all relative indications for surgery. Other indications for surgery are listed in Table 39–3. The operation addresses the complication(s) that provided the indication for surgery. For example, a patient may be advised to have surgery for intestinal obstructive symptoms due to ileal Crohn's disease, yet may also be proved endoscopically to have asymptomatic duodenal Crohn's disease. It would be inappropriate to direct any operative procedure to the duodenum at the time of laparotomy for ileal resection.

Since Crohn's disease of the small bowel is more widely distributed than clinically appreciated, the concept of curative excision is fallacious, except in the limited sense of defining resections that encompass all visible evidence of disease. The concept of persistence of Crohn's disease, flare of which may be termed recurrence, can be supported by the histochemical evidence of diminished brush border and cytoplasmic en-

TABLE 39–2.—INTESTINAL COMPLICATIONS OF CROHN'S DISEASE

Obstruction	Colonic	Fulminant disease	With and
	Gastroduodenal		without
	Rectal stricture		colonic
	Small bowel		dilatation
Sepsis	Free perforation		
	Ileocecal abscess		
	Paracolic	Hemorrhage	
	Perianal/pelvic		
	Psoas abscess		
Fistulas	Choledochoenteric		
	Colocutaneous		
	Enterocolic		
	Enterocutaneous	Carcinoma	In fistulous tracts
	Enteroduodenal		Large bowel
	Enteroenteric		Small bowel
	Enteroperineal		
	Enteroureteric		
	Enterouterine		
	Enterovaginal		
	Enterovesical		
	Gastrocolic		
	Perineal	Lymphoma	Colon
	Rectovaginal		Small bowel

zymes, reflecting damage to intestinal microvilli in otherwise normal-appearing bowel; by colonoscopic evidence of early disease—aphthoid ulcers; by the altered bidirectional fluxes through histologically normal intestinal mucosa and the decreased bile salt pool in nonoperative patients with Crohn's disease of the intestine. The rule, therefore, is not to perform resection only because a particular segment exhibits features of Crohn's disease. Bowel conservation must be kept in mind. Stricture should be dealt with (see below for techniques of resection, bypass, and strictureplasty), even if the strictures occur in excluded or bypassed segments.

Even among clinicians experienced in the management of Crohn's disease views differ about some aspects of surgery—not only as to choice of operation, but whether resectional surgery is needed at all. Internal fistulas, skip lesions, diffuse jejunoileitis, perianal disease, and even enterovesical fistulas may or may not be indications for surgery, depending on the patient and the bias of the clinician supervising the care. Also controversial is the timing of surgery, especially when an ileostomy is contemplated. It is sometimes hoped that with more time and more medical treatment, ileostomy can be

TABLE 39–3.—PRIMARY INDICATION FOR INITIAL OPERATION AT CLEVELAND CLINIC HOSPITAL, No. (%)*

	ILEOCOLIC		PATTERN SMALL INTESTINE		COLON		ANORECTAL
Indication for operation							
Perianal disease	22	(15)	6	(7)	17	(23)	8
Internal fistulas and abscess	56	(38)	24	(29)	19	(25)	
Toxic megacolon	5	(3)	0		14	(19)	
Intestinal obstruction	54	(37)	45	(54)	9	(12)	
Other (including severe disease; poor response to therapy; growth retardation)	9	(6)	8	(9)	16	(21)	4
Total in group	252		176		166		21
Patients with operation	183		90		85		12
Operations at Cleveland Clinic	146		83		75		12
Operations before Cleveland Clinic	75		36		19		0
Elsewhere	37		7		10		
Both	38		29		9		

*Adapted from Farmer R.G., et al.[5]

avoided. The specter of recurrence may give both the gastroenterologist and the patient pause before agreeing to an operation. A more tenuous argument is that resectional surgery itself may increase the chance of further recurrence. As a result medical treatment may be prolonged until serious complications, occasionally life-threatening, manifest themselves.

Indications for Operation

These are rarely absolute in Crohn's disease with the exception of undrained, intra-abdominal abscesses, free perforation of the intestine, impending perforation (most cases of toxic megacolon), and uncontrolled intestinal hemorrhage (see Table 39–3). The anatomical pattern of the disease has clinical significance with respect to the frequency distribution of various indications for surgery, the clinical course, operative rate, and recurrence rates.[5]

In general, intestinal obstruction and internal fistulas associated with sepsis are the main indications for surgery of ileitis and ileocolitis. Perianal disease assumes a significant role as an indication for operation in all three major patterns of disease. For Crohn's colitis, the major reasons for surgery include toxicity (including toxic dilatation), poor response to medical therapy, debility, bleeding, and extraintestinal manifestations of disease. Sepsis and obstruction are also indications, but are not as commonly encountered with ileitis and ileocolitis. At ten years from diagnosis, we have found an operative rate of 90% for patients with ileocolitis. Two thirds of patients with the small-bowel pattern and with the colitis pattern have undergone operative treatment in the same period.

COMPLICATIONS FOR WHICH OPERATION IS COMMONLY DONE

Bowel Obstruction

Usually, the patient will give a history of several episodes of subacute obstruction alleviated by decreasing oral intake or increasing corticosteroid medication. The surgeon may often be asked to advise whether the surgery is indicated. The considerations include: duration of the disease; the association of their complications; whether or not an adequate trial of medical therapy has been used; the frequency of the obstructive bouts, and the ease with which recovery occurs; extent of the disease; and radiologic appearance. The leaning is to surgery if the disease has been present for several years (with chronic disease, mural fibrosis occurs with diminished capacity for recovery of the bowel). Surgery is advised if the patient has associated problems, such as a right lower quadrant mass; evidence of sepsis or internal fistulas; or if the obstructive episodes have been increasing in frequency, with prolonged recovery, or if these episodes occur despite the patient's receiving optimal medical treatment. If the disease is localized rather than diffuse, this is a relative indication for surgery.

For an acute, obstructive episode, IV fluids and nasogastric suction usually are successful in avoiding emergency surgery. After relief of the acute episode, a much safer resection can be done at an elective time or even at hospital admission. The problem of obstructing skip lesions is discussed later.

Sepsis

Intra-abdominal abscesses develop in 12%–28% of patients with Crohn's disease.[6] The principle for drainage of abscesses applies to Crohn's disease, as does the need to do emergency surgery for bowel perforation, an uncommon though occasional problem with small-bowel Crohn's disease. A more common presentation is the phlegmon of terminal ileum, with or without cecal involvement, which reflects a gradually developing septic process due to transmural penetration of fissures. Adjacent viscera, parietes or omentum attempt to seal off this perforation, which is accompanied by a varying degree of abscess formation. While at this stage, during which a mass may be felt in the right lower quadrant, there is still a capacity for resolution, since internal drainage of the septic process back into the bowel may occur. One relies on this when managing such conditions conservatively with IV fluids and antibiotics and bactericidals for aerobic and anaerobic gram-negative organisms. However, because of loculation of pus, extension into other tissue planes (such as behind the psoas fascia) or, occasionally, intraperitoneal perforation of the abscess, surgery becomes necessary. For this ileocecal phlegmon, the operation involves bowel resection and drainage, although exclusion-bypass procedures can be considered in the desperately ill individual who tolerates anesthesia poorly. Unless tender, a right lower quadrant mass does not constitute an indication for surgery. The entity does constitute a relative indication, however, as it is a harbinger of things to come.

Free perforation occurs in 1%–2% of patients with Crohn's disease and necessitates excision of the involved segment, including the obstructing area.[7] Surgical judgment will then dictate whether anastomosis is safe or whether an end stoma is made. The latter approach is my preference. Steinberg et al. (1973)[8] reckoned that perforation occurred during an acute flare of the disease and was associated with obstruction due to a chronic, stenosing lesion. Since most of these perforations occur in the ileum rather than jejunum (a 10:1 ratio reported by Nasar et al. 1969[7]), a temporary stoma may be made without undue concern about short-bowel syndrome.

Fistula

Most fistulas are associated with sepsis to a variable extent, but for purposes of discussion, are here looked at separately. The mechanism of formation is similar to that of an abscess, namely, the transmural penetration of the bowel by a fissure with escape of enteric content, formation of an abscess which penetrates into an adjacent viscus or through a wound.

Enterocutaneous Fistula

These may be single or multiple and usually arise from the affected segment of bowel. Spontaneous fistulas are uncommon and arise from external drainage of an abscess, usually secondary to perforative ileocecal Crohn's disease. More usual is the occurrence of fistulas through an abdominal incision site, the source being an area of recurrent disease at an ileocolic anastomosis. Frequently, there are associated problems such as enteroenteric or enterovesical fistulas. A further variety is the fistula that occurs early in the postoperative period.

The indications for surgery depend on the extent to which the fistula is causing a problem for the patient; the presence of undrained sepsis; other complications relating to the Crohn's disease, such as obstruction; the presence of residual Crohn's disease; and the degree of difficulty expected in obtaining a reasonable result for the patient. In the patient who has to wear a pouch for collecting fistula output, where unresolved sepsis persists or distal obstruction exists, surgery is indicated. One could add that the obstruction is frequently at or within a few centimeters distal to the site of the fistula, making radiographic identification of distal obstruction quite difficult. If the patient is content to wear a pad and change it as necessary, presumably with little other problems symptomatic of the disease, this is a reasonable course to follow, provided one understands that almost *never* does the fistula close when associated with the disease. Total parenteral nutrition may allow for significant subsidence of fistula output in such cases, and even temporary healing, but is followed by fistula recurrence shortly after cessation of TPN. This is quite the reverse of what one might expect with postoperative fistulas after the diseased segment has been removed, in which case, provided there is no distal obstruction or undrained sepsis, complete healing with TPN can be anticipated.

One encounters the rare, albeit memorable patient who develops multiple enterocutaneous fistulas has a history of multiple abdominal operations for Crohn's disease, and whose proximal fistula is in proximity to the duodenojejunal junction. One is inclined to place such patients on a long-term, home hyperalimentation program, reserving surgery for the establishment of a pouchable stoma. With the passage of time (at least four months), further consideration can be given to restoring bowel length, after investigations show such bowel to be usable. Enterocutaneous fistulas may also occur following appendectomy for acute regional ileitis. These may arise from either the appendiceal stump or from the terminal ileum. The author has treated four patients whose fistula occurred after laparotomy alone. The referring surgeons had noted previously undiagnosed Crohn's disease of the ileum but had performed no procedure. Presumably, handling of the involved segment itself may be enough to provide drainage for occult, sealed, mini-perforations. The treatment of these fistulas is resection of the underlying Crohn's disease.

Enteroenteric Fistula

Fistulas from one small-bowel loop to another are commonly encountered. These may be recognized or suspected preoperatively on contrast studies of the intestinal tract. Of themselves, they do not constitute an absolute indication for surgery but, if associated with other indications, such as failure to thrive, obstruction, or sepsis, surgery is indicated. At operation both loops of ileum may be involved with the disease but, commonly, one may be free of disease, and if located at a distance from the diseased segment, a localized resection and anastomosis is done in addition to dealing with the primary pathologic process.

Ileocoloduodenal Fistula

This is a relatively uncommon entity, but assumes importance because of the degree of difficulty associated with the operative procedure (Fig 39–6). Wilk et al. (1977)[9] reviewed

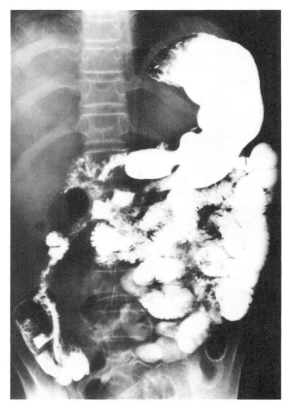

Fig 39–6.—Ileoduodenal fistula is present secondary to Crohn's disease recurrent in the terminal ileum and at an ileotransverse anastomosis.

our experience with nine such cases. In the main, the entity occurred as the result of recurrent disease at an ileocolic anastomosis which overlay the second part of the duodenum with secondary fistulization. These patients were particularly debilitated; several needed TPN prior to surgery. Apart from the technical difficulties of dissecting the diseased ileocolic anastomosis from the duodenum and head of the pancreas, there are also difficulties in dealing with the fibrotic, inflamed duodenal defect. We have favored a localized, limited resection of the anterior duodenal wall around the fistula and anastomosing a loop of proximal jejunum to this segment, a side-to-side duodenojejunostomy.

Attempts at closing the duodenal defect primarily or use of a serosal patch are likely to lead to a postoperative duodenal fistula. No fistulas were encountered using the duodenojejunostomy. Ileosigmoid fistula (Fig 39–7) and ileo-right colic fistulas also occur. The latter offers no exceptional difficulties in terms of operative treatment in that the adjacent colon may be removed in continuity with the ileal Crohn's disease. However, ileosigmoid fistulas are frequently associated with severe nutritional depletion and sepsis in the right iliac fossa and require additional attention.

Other fistulas (enterocutaneous, enterovesical) are sometimes in evidence with the ileosigmoid fistula. In contrast to diverticulitis, the small intestine, is the source of the fistula, and, invariably, the sigmoid colon is free of Crohn's disease. Usually, these patients will require preoperative nutritional restitution, unless fulminant sepsis dictates earlier interven-

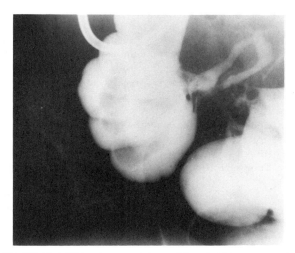

Fig 39–7.—This close-up view of the right lower quadrant following barium enema shows reflux of dye into a strictured terminal ileum with a fistula tract extending to the antimesenteric aspect of the sigmoid colon.

tion. At surgery, one commonly encounters a phlegmon in the ileocecal area plastered onto the antimesenteric aspect of the sigmoid colon.

An inflammatory nest, or abscess, is often found in the pelvis involving the right leaf of the sigmoid mesentery. If the antimesenteric surface of the sigmoid colon is involved, the colon segment is removed, even if the fistula cannot be demonstrated at operation. So often one is able to demonstrate this later in the laboratory, when it was far from clear at operation, that the conservative approach is sigmoid resection in addition to ileocecal resection. Only a short segment is removed until a soft, noninflamed colon wall is identified for subsequent anastomosis; one will then complete the ileoascending colon anastomosis or make an ileostomy and oversew the ascending colon. In this latter instance, the final anastomosis is made three months later. We have reviewed our experience with 27 cases[10] and found no mortality and no instances of postoperative fistulas following the above procedures. Thirteen of 27 patients had temporary fecal diversion. In the case of fibrous nonseptic fistula, the sigmoid defect may be handled by simple suture closure.

Does ileosigmoid fistula always constitute an indication for surgery? Cure of such internal fistulas has been reported with medical management including azathioprine. The difficulty in establishing healing of the fistula is reflected in our experience, where preoperative contrast roentgenograms were effective in demonstrating a fistula in fewer than 20% of the cases; yet in all cases, a fistula could be demonstrated in the specimen. Certainly, patients may be rendered asymptomatic or significantly improved by medical treatment and, indeed, by *no* treatment on occasion. One may speculate that the fistula could act as a spontaneous internal bypass operation. Currently the author is following three such patients who are essentially asymptomatic.

Enterovesical Fistula

Because of the likelihood of progressive ascending urinary tract infection with permanent renal impairment, this entity constitutes an absolute indication for surgery in the individual who can tolerate a general anesthetic agent. The principles of surgery are resection of the diseased bowel; curettage and debridement of the associated inflammatory nest; no attempt at partial bladder resection; and constant catheter drainage of the bladder for seven to ten days. One may be fortunate in being able to find healthy serosal tissue adjacent to the bladder defect or omentum to oppose over the defect. If not, and provided the defect is minimal (as is usually the case), then bladder drainage and intraperitoneal drainage is adequate.

Enterogenital Fistula

Fistulas from the ileum to the apex of the vagina occur and are frequently associated with other internal fistulas. The principles of surgery include resection of the diseased segment, drainage of vaginal apex, and interposition of healthy tissue, such as omentum between the bowel anastomosis and the vaginal cuff. Surgery is indicated in most cases because of the disabling drainage per vagina. Occasionally, a fistula is seen between the ileum and the right fallopian tube, sometimes with tubo-ovarian abscess. Again, surgery is usually necessary, involving bowel resection of the involved segment and salpingo-oophorectomy. Rarely, a fistula is seen from ileum to the lumen of the uterus. The author has treated one such case where an ileo-uterine-cutaneous fistula was present, presenting as cyclic bleeding onto the anterior abdominal wall. This was treated by bowel resection, curettage of the fistula opening in the uterus, and interposition of a vascularized pedicle of omentum with a salutary result.

Peri-ileostomy Fistula

Greenstein et al. (1983)[11] reported 15 cases in 214 patients who underwent an ileostomy for Crohn's disease. The fistulas were frequently multiple. Local (using the same site) revision is appropriate for most superficial fistulas, but deep fistulas require ileostomy resection and neoileostomy with relocation.

Perineal Fistula

These occasionally constitute an indication for surgery when associated with small-bowel Crohn's disease. We have observed that these fistulas, particularly the perianal type, will be the initial manifestation of the disease in about 7% of cases. While conservative procedures are usually favored, one is impressed with the frequency with which one sees nicely healed scars at old anal fistulotomy sites, when seeing the patients with ileal Crohn's or ileocolitis. This has given one pause and encouragement to consider definitive fistulotomy procedures in patients where the rectum is overtly normal and whose fistulas are particularly troublesome. In the case of rectovaginal fistula in association with proximal Crohn's disease, we have performed ileocecal resection, ileostomy, and over-sewing of the ascending colon, and definitive rectovaginal fistulectomy with sphincter repair in four patients. All patients had later restoration of the intestinal tract without recurrence of the fistula or incontinence. Another patient, in whom diversion was not done, had a recurrent rectovaginal fistula; this was treated successfully a second time using a temporary ileostomy. Many patients elect to tolerate degrees of discomfort associated with small rectovaginal fistulas, especially when the proximal disease is well-controlled by medications.

Obstructive Uropathy

We reviewed the Cleveland Clinic experience with 2,368 patients with Crohn's disease.[12] Of the 958 patients undergoing intravenous pyelography (IVP), 45 patients (4.7%) had a hydroureter or hydronephrosis. Gastrointestinal symptoms usually overshadowed genitourinary complaints. In our series, 44% had an abdominal mass or fistula. Psoas spasm may be associated with the retroperitoneal inflammation. The obstruction to the ureter is produced by compression of an ileocecal phlegmon or abscess. Retroperitoneal and periureteric scarring may add to this obstruction. Block et al. (1973)[13] reckoned this was a common occurrence and recommended adding ureterolysis to bowel resection. They described the occurrence of persistent, symptomatic hydronephrosis after intestinal resection alone requiring later ureterolysis. While this may occur, it is uncommon in our experience; and since ureterolysis is not without hazard, we adopt a highly selective attitude with respect to ureterolysis, reserving it for those situations where a dense, fibrous retroperitoneal encasement of the ureters is seen. Only three patients of ours underwent ureterolysis, although a variety of procedures, including temporary diversion or abscess drainage, was used. Resolution of the obstructive uropathy was seen in 87% of our patients (Table 39–4).

This experience, notwithstanding the sound principles of surgery advocated by Block et al. (1973),[13] may allow the surgeon some latitude in operative strategy, so that internal bypass or diversion does not of necessity have to be excluded from surgical choices in a particular difficult case.

Acute or massive hemorrhage is a rare complication (about 1%) of Crohn's disease and may occur in all three major patterns of the disease: ileitis, ileocolitis, and colitis. Since associated peptic ulcer disease is so commonly seen with Crohn's disease, there may be considerable difficulty in identifying the bleeding source. High rates of rebleeding following surgery have been reported, a finding with which we concur. The identification of the bleeding point is often difficult, especially in the small intestine, although in certain cases intraoperative angiography through an indwelling, superior mesenteric artery catheter has been helpful in allowing limited, specific resection of the bleeding segment.[14] In certain situations, where continued bleeding occurs, the problem is compounded by a bleeding tendency related, in part, to multiple transfusions. In these situations, the use of fresh whole blood may be very helpful. In a literature review, Homan et al. (1976)[15] found that surgical treatment controlled hemorrhage in 14 of 17 patients, sounding a more optimistic note with respect to such therapy, as opposed to the views of Sparberg and Kirsner (1966).[16] It seems reasonable to advocate resectional surgery, if the patient's hemodynamic state cannot be sustained by transfusion, or if another indication for resection exists. This is probably the correct approach as well for the patient who is stable but who has received 4 to 6 units of blood and is still bleeding, and for the patient with recurrent massive hemorrhage. These latter two options are controversial. In our own experience of 14 patients presenting with massive hemorrhage between 1970 and 1974, 6 were treated with blood transfusion and no surgery; 7 patients with transfusion and then elective resection; and 1 patient with emergency resection after 12 units of blood transfusion failed to stabilize her condition. There was no mortality in the group.

Carcinoma

This is a rare complication of Crohn's disease of the small intestine, and it would be uncommon for any clinician to have encountered more than two or three cases. Hoffman et al. (1977)[17] reviewed their own experience (two cases) and collected 49 cases from the literature. These 51 patients were contrasted with a group of patients with small-bowel adenocarcinoma not associated with Crohn's disease. The Crohn's group were younger at the time of diagnosis (46 vs. 64 years); more cancers occurred in the ileum than in the proximal small intestine (76% vs. 27%); diagnosis was less successful; the cure rate was worse (6.7% vs. 20%–30%); cancer occurred 60–300 times more frequently in patients with Crohn's ileitis than in patients of the same age without Crohn's disease. The bypassed, small intestine has been considered cancer prone in the past, and in about a third of these cases a bypass operation had been done. Since in two thirds the bypass procedure had *not* been done, and since this is such a rare entity, the selective use of bypass procedures, in particular the diffi-

TABLE 39–4.—RESULTS OF SURGERY FOR OBSTRUCTIVE UROPATHY*

PROCEDURE	NO. OF PROCEDURES WITH PREOPERATIVE IVP	POSTOPERATIVE IVP UNAVAILABLE	RESOLUTION POSTOPERATIVE IVP	UNCHANGED IVP	WORSE
Bypass, decompression, or both	12	2	8	2	
Intestinal resection	23	9	13§		1
Intestinal resection and ureterolysis	3		2		1
Other surgery†	5	1	2§	2	
Medical therapy	6	3	2	1	
Total	49‡	15	27	5	2

*(Copyright permission: Siminovitch, J.M.P., Fazio, V.W.: Ureteral obstruction secondary to Crohn's disease: a need for ureterolysis? *Am. J. Surg.* 139:96, 1980).
†Five patients had drainage of an abscess, with two patients also receiving nephrostomy tubes.
‡Three patients had seven procedures.
§One patient with bilateral hydronephrosis had resolution in one ureter with intestinal resection; the other ureter with abscess drainage.

cult situations, should not be dismissed unconditionally on the score of its being a cancer preparation. Because of the difficulty in following up such patients, elective resection of the bypassed segment is indicated.

Colonic cancer occurs more commonly in Crohn's disease than in the non-Crohn's disease population, but the risk does not approach that of ulcerative colitis.[18]

Extraintestinal Manifestations of Crohn's Disease

This was discussed in an earlier section of this chapter.

Toxic Megacolon Due to Crohn's Disease

Following resuscitation of the patient and institution of medical therapy, certain situations call for an immediate operation. These include pneumoperitoneum, gram-negative endotoxemia, massive hemorrhage, and evidence of general peritonitis. Additionally, severe, localized tenderness or deterioration in the patient's condition and massive colonic dilatation are relative indications for surgery. In less extreme situations, the patient is observed at frequent intervals over the next 24–48 hours. Deterioration in clinical laboratory parameters of toxicity or further colonic dilatation are indications for prompt surgical intervention at our institution. Failure to improve within 72 hours in the context of toxic dilatation is an indication for surgery. Goligher et al.[19] showed improved survivorship when operating for ulcerative colitis by operating early in the course of the acute attack (within seven days of intensive treatment).

The operative procedures advised for toxic megacolon include total proctocolectomy and ileostomy, subtotal colectomy with ileostomy and rectal mucous fistula, and diverting loop ileostomy with decompressive skin-level (blow-hole) colostomy.

Total proctocolectomy as a one-stage procedure is an attractive proposition, but is technically demanding and is generally reserved for patients who are good operative risks, without evidence of free perforation. Block et al.[20] showed a superiority for subtotal colectomy over total proctocolectomy when operating for toxic megacolon, with mortality of 6.1% and 14.3%, respectively. The differentiation of Crohn's disease from ulcerative colitis can be extremely difficult in toxic dilatation even with full histologic examination of the specimen. With the current interest in intestinal restoration and pelvic reservoir for ulcerative colitis, the case for rectal preservation in toxic dilatation is compelling. Fry and Atkinson[21] found that intra-abdominal abscesses and enterocutaneous fistula occurred more commonly following proctocolectomy than for subtotal colectomy.

Subtotal colectomy and ileostomy is the most widely used procedure for toxic dilatation. It is the procedure of choice when free perforation of the colon has occurred, for patients with a mobile and not grossly distended colon, and when there is no evidence of sealed perforation of the colon. Similarly, when colonic hemorrhage is associated, abdominal colectomy is advised. At a later date, abdominoperineal proctectomy or ileorectal anastomosis can be performed. When sealed perforations exist or where the colon is particularly fragile, and mobilization of a high splenic flexure is difficult, iatrogenic fecal spill may occur with disastrous results. Precautions should be taken to minimize the effects of fecal spill.

Maximal exposure is obtained, and the distended, transverse colon and splenic flexure is decompressed by placing a large-bore needle through a taenia and applying aspiration. The rest of the abdomen is quarantined with packs while mobilizing the splenic flexure. Rather than make a primary mucous fistula, the surgeon is well advised to exteriorize the lower sigmoid stump and wrap it in gauze to prevent retraction. A mucous fistula can be safely made seven to ten days later.

The third alternative is a procedure advocated by Turnbull et al.[22]; namely, loop ileostomy and blow-hole colostomy (Fig 39–8). Turnbull argued that the fragile colon, especially one associated with a high splenic flexure, was prone to iatrogenic perforation during the course of its mobilization. The finding of thickened, inflamed omentum (Fig 39–9) attached to the antimesenteric aspect of the descending or sigmoid colon was a sign that walled off perforations were present and could be disrupted even with gentle handling. Although ileostomy alone had fallen into disrepute because of its attendant high mortality (the colon could still perforate despite diversion), ileostomy and blow-hole colostomy have proved to be valuable adjuncts in the above-cited circumstance.

The opponents to the blow-hole procedure note certain disadvantages. It is a staging procedure much like a preliminary colostomy for an obstructive sigmoid colon cancer, and further surgery is almost always required. However, the same can be said for subtotal colectomy, where rectal resection is usually needed in the future. Second, if colonic bleeding was a feature preoperatively, there was a 25% chance of further significant hemorrhage postoperatively. In most situations transfusion is sufficient management, but even if colectomy is required to control bleeding, as has occurred in three patients, the patient's toxicity and colonic dilatation are usually resolved, and the colectomy is not excessively difficult. A further argument is that a grossly infected organ is left behind

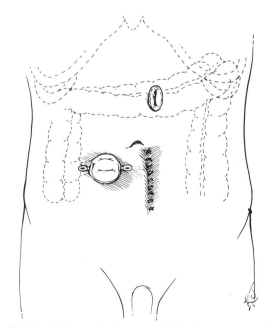

Fig 39–8.—Schematic diagram of the decompressed and diverted colon (the Turnbull blow-hole colostomy and loop ileostomy).

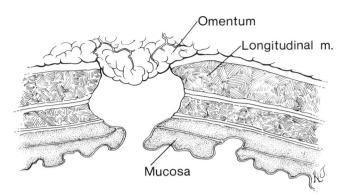

Fig 39–9.—Schematic representation of perforation of the colon associated with toxic megacolon where omentum has walled off the perforation. Mobilization of this segment with detachment of the omentum can lead to fecal spill.

and could lead to persistent sepsis and toxicity. In our experience, this has not been the case, with the possible exception of one patient. That patient had developed multiple perforations of the ileum and jejunum due to necrotizing enteritis.

There are, however, distinct advantages of the procedure. It is simple, rapid, and associated with detoxification within 24 hours. It is an attractive alternative for the surgeon who only occasionally sees or operates on patients with toxic dilatation. The mortality rate is lower. The procedure is contraindicated in the presence of free perforation of the colon or severe hemorrhage.

We have reviewed our experience with toxic megacolon due to ulcerative colitis and Crohn's colitis at the Cleveland Clinic.[23] Seven of 115 patients with diagnoses of toxic dilatation were discharged from the hospital having had successful medical management. Fifty of the remaining patients had Crohn's colitis. The operations performed fell into two major groups. Abdominal colectomy with ileostomy was performed in 26 patients and decompression diversion procedures were performed in 83 patients. Nine patients in a series of 115 died, yielding a mortality of 7.8%. Three patients (11.5%) died after subtotal colectomy compared with three patients (3.6%) after decompression diversion procedures. Two other patients died following elective colectomy, for an overall mortality of 6% in the decompression diversion group. Another patient died following surgery for small-bowel obstruction. He had been discharged from the hospital after an uneventful recovery from subtotal colectomy for toxic megacolon.

Free perforation of the colon occurred preoperatively in 17 patients (14.8%), with five deaths, for a mortality of 29.4%.

Perianal Disease

Many surgeons have cautioned against any radical operations for perianal Crohn's disease, since the results of treatment are more disabling than the original problem. Others, including McKay and McMahon[24] and Lockhart-Mummery,[25] have advocated active, if not aggressive, surgical intervention. In specific situations, fistulotomy operations may be performed. In general, perianal lesions are not treated unless they are producing significant symptoms, notably, pain. Abscesses are treated by simple incision and drainage, although,

if recurrent, they may be treated by long-term use of small mushroom catheter or even loosely applied setons. Should this fail to be effective, and a course of metronidazole produce minimal response, a case for fistulotomy can be made, if the rectum appears normal and the fistula does not transgress significant parts of the internal and external sphincter mechanism. For high or multiple fistulas, conservative drainage procedures are used. In selected cases, where an internal opening is easily seen and where there is concern regarding the amount of sphincter muscle that would be divided in the conduct of a fistulotomy, an advancement rectal mucosal flap with a covering stoma is advised, provided the rectum appears normal. The ileostomy can be closed approximately two to three months later. These operations are reserved for patients who have sufficient disability from their perineal Crohn's disease that fecal diversion has already been contemplated. Sphincter plication has been done by us and others, under similar circumstances, when anal incontinence following fistulotomy caused the patient to present to the institution. If extensive perianal disease or rectovaginal fistulas are associated with rectal Crohn's disease, radical surgery is not advised. Sphincter repairs will become disrupted, and perianal wounds will fail to heal. Surgical maneuvers here are confined to simple unroofing of abscesses or insertion of setons. If these measures and conventional therapy such as metronidazole fail to keep the patient reasonably comfortable, fecal diversion is usually necessary. Subsequently, or even at the same time, proctocolectomy may be required.

Anal fissures are not treated, unless associated with pain. In this situation, Crohn's disease of the rectum is usually absent. Dilatation using anesthesia or, in selected cases, conservative sphincterotomy may be used.

CLINICAL SUBPATTERNS OF CROHN'S DISEASE OF THE SMALL BOWEL

Acute Ileitis

This entity is probably unrelated to Crohn's disease but can be difficult to differentiate from chronic ileitis (Crohn's disease). Typically, the patient presents with signs of acute appendicitis, usually with pain of less than seven days' duration, located in the right iliac fossa. At operation the ileum is inflamed, edematous, and beefy-red in color. The lumen is not constricted. An intense serositis is present, associated with mesenteric lymph node enlargement. The appendix looks normal. An association with *Yersinia enterocolitica* is common. In a literature review and a report of 34 patients of their own with acute ileitis, Gump et al.[26] made a strong case for the entity's being separate from Crohn's disease. They found it was self-limiting. They collected 369 cases from 17 series; 60% had a preoperative diagnosis of appendicitis, and only 35 patients (9%) subsequently developed chronic Crohn's disease. Abnormalities are rarely found in contrast x-ray studies in patients with acute ileitis. If there is ileal narrowing, the patient is likely to progress to chronic ileitis. Given the laparotomy appearance of acute ileitis and a normal cecum, appendectomy seems to be safe. Enterocutaneous fistulas occurred only once in the 24 patients undergoing appendectomy in the Gump series, and once in the 68 patients in the series of Kewenter et al. (1974).[27]

However, if there is evidence of an underlying chronic ileitis with fibrosis, there is a likelihood of a fistula if appendectomy is performed. Ordinary appendicitis may complicate Crohn's ileitis, but is rare. In that circumstance, resection of the diseased bowel segment seems to be safer than appendectomy alone. Yang et al. (1979)[28] advised appendectomy for patients with Crohn's disease confined to the appendix. In my experience, granulomatous appendicitis occurring in isolation is rare, and I would caution the surgeon to look for evidence of adjacent intestinal Crohn's disease before performing appendectomy alone. It seems that resection may be the safer course to follow.

Diffuse Jejunoileitis

Nutritional iron and folic acid deficiencies commonly accompany this variety of diffuse Crohn's disease (Fig 39–10). Frequently, the colon is involved as well. Cooke and Swan (1974)[29] found 18 cases of this condition in 330 patients with Crohn's disease. Six patients, all men, died two to 18 years after the onset of the disease. Extensive surgical resection was not beneficial, but excision limited to short obstructing segments seemed to be of value. Patients with this condition usually present with intestinal obstruction and require multiple hospitalizations. Most have had a number of courses of TPN prior to having surgery. One would agree with the advice of Cooke and Swan with respect to conservative surgery confined to short obstructing segments. It is in this group of patients where the operation of strictureplasty, as proposed by Lee[30] and Alexander-Williams,[31] may have particular benefit.

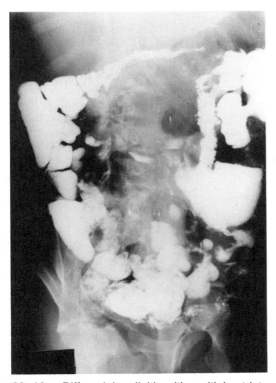

Fig 39–10.—Diffuse jejunoileitis with multiple strictures in a 30-year-old man. The patient's obstructive symptoms resolved with multiple strictureplasties without resection.

Home hyperalimentation programs have been of major benefit to patients with this condition.

Skip Lesions

These occur in about 25% of patients with Crohn's disease (Fig 39–11). The incidence of such lesions requiring surgical treatment is not so clear. If the lesion is in proximity (10 cm) to the main lesion in the terminal ileum, the intervening normal segment is sacrificed, and a single anastomosis is made. Diffuse or multiple skip lesions are individually assessed at laparotomy as to the extent to which they are causing a problem. Dilatation of the bowel above this stricture indicates surgical treatment. At the other end of the spectrum, little more than slight fat wrapping of the mesentery or thickening of the mesenteric margin may be in evidence. In general terms, the surgeon will treat the symptomatic skip lesion by resection or bypass, using side-to-side autosuture techniques. If the skip lesions are few and short, several resections and end-to-end anastomosis may be done. When skips are numerous, bypass procedures are preferred.

In recent years, Lee[30] and Alexander-Williams[31] have advocated the selective use of strictureplasty (Fig 39–12) on either long or short segments, claiming no significant incidence of fistula or enteric leak. Alexander-Williams has used the maneuver of strictureplasty (Heineke-Mikulicz type) on 32 occasions for simple, short strictures and in a smaller number of patients with stenoses of greater than 10 cm, using a Finney pyloroplasty technique. I have used the former method in four patients and can attest to its value in the short term. Certainly, it is a simple technique and seems especially suited for patients with numerous strictures. While the segment is certainly diseased, much of the disease appears confined to the mesenteric margin as opposed to the antimesenteric margin. The procedure may be combined with resection of distal phlegmonous or perforated segments.

Gastroduodenal Crohn's Disease

Gastroenterostomy alone has been a valuable method of treating refractory symptoms due to gastroduodenal Crohn's disease. Previous reports have shown that symptomatic relief has been good and anastomotic ulceration infrequent.[32] Ear-

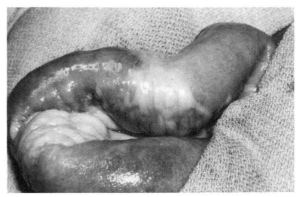

Fig 39–11.—Skip lesions in the terminal ileum with classic fat wrapping. (From Fazio V.W.: Regional enteritis (Crohn's disease): Indications for surgery and operative strategy. *Surg. Clin. North Am.* 63:27–48, 1983. Used by permission.)

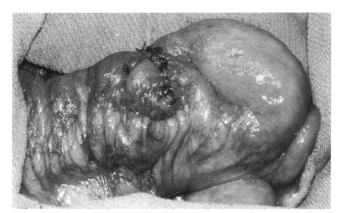

Fig 39–12.—Shows a completed strictureplasty on a narrowed jejunal segment due to Crohn's disease.

lier studies from the Cleveland Clinic supported this view with five-year follow-up, but in a recent review of the same patients with 14-year follow-up, this early enthusiasm was not borne out.[33] Anastomotic ulceration was common when gastroenterostomy alone was performed. The addition of vagotomy prevented recurrent peptic ulceration, but some patients did develop anastomotic stricture, probably due to Crohn's disease. We therefore now recommend that vagotomy be used routinely when performing gastroenterostomy. Despite the need for revisionary surgery in these patients, quality of life, as measured by the Karnofsky performance scale, remains remarkably good. Recently, Alexander-Williams[31] has advocated the use of a Roux-en-Y loop or strictureplasty for obstructing duodenal Crohn's disease.

PRINCIPLES OF OPERATIVE MANAGEMENT

Preoperative Preparation

Dehydration, electrolyte imbalance, coagulopathy, and anemia, are corrected preoperatively. Ideally, malnutrition would also be corrected, but this is often not possible. Corticosteroid coverage is provided to the patient who has been using these drugs in the preceding six months. The patient is given a minimum-residue diet for three to four days prior to surgery, using a modified elemental diet such as Ensure Plus, and in the elective cases this preparation can be given to the patient on an outpatient basis. Unless obstructive or acute severe disease is present, 10% mannitol solution, 500 ml, is given orally over four hours on the afternoon before surgery. Neomycin and erythromycin base, 1 gm each, are given orally at 1 P.M., 2 P.M., and 10 P.M. on the day before surgery. Systemic antibiotics to cover enteric pathogens are given IV immediately before surgery and for 24 hours thereafter. If operative contamination occurs, the antibiotics are continued for a further five days. The antibiotic products most commonly used at our institution are cefotaxime and metronidazole. In elective cases, patients have a preoperative urogram. An ileostomy may be required as part of the definitive or staged surgical treatment of Crohn's disease.

Extent of Resection in Small Bowel Crohn's Disease

Using the foregoing guidelines, one will resect bowel about 10 cm proximal to the line of clinical involvement (Fig 39–13). For ileal disease extending to or within 10 cm of the ileocecal valve, the cecum is resected in continuity. There is controversy concerning the extent of resection. Many surgeons, perhaps most, favor a relatively conservative clearance, as outlined. Bergman and Krause (1977)[34] reckon that extensive resection should be done. In an uncontrolled trial, they found a recurrence of 29% after radical operations as compared with 84% after nonradical procedures with 7½–9½ years of follow-up. A recent study from Johns Hopkins University does not support this.[35] Pennington et al. (1980)[35] in a retrospective study of 103 operative specimens looked at the presence or absence of inflammatory changes at the lines of resection (and anastomoses) and found no statistical differences in recurrence and reoperation rates. Others have found lessened rates of recurrence where the margins are disease-free. Colcock (1960)[36] advocated wide resection of the small-bowel mesentery where there were enlarged lymph nodes on the basis that leaving them behind may predispose to recurrence. The proviso was that this be done only if lymphadenectomy could be done without sacrificing more intestine than was clinically indicated. Most surgeons would agree with this approach, although there is no evidence that leaving enlarged lymph nodes behind favors a higher likelihood of recurrence. Suppurative lymphadenopathy, both before and after bowel resection has been observed, so that removal of very large nodes is desirable vis-à-vis Colcock's disclaimer.

TYPE OF OPERATIONS FOR CROHN'S DISEASE OF THE SMALL BOWEL

Bypass or Resection

Current attitudes strongly favor intestinal resection, since improvement with anesthesia techniques and pre- and post-operative management have dispelled the claim of high morbidity and mortality with resection. Notwithstanding the clear superiority of resection over bypass in recent retrospective studies,[37] the lack of randomization, the use of bypass surgery for the more severe cases, and the fewer numbers of bypass procedures in the past two decades do not permit valid conclusions to be drawn. Homan and Dineen (1978)[38] point out that in their series, the indications for surgery were similar in their three groups: resection, bypass in continuity, and exclusion bypass. Selectivity by the surgeon was minimized with respect to both types of bypass vs. resection in that the operations, with few exceptions, were done in sequence. Expressed as 15-year follow-up of 115 patients, they found recurrence rates of 65%, 82%, and 94% for resection, bypass with exclusion, and simple bypass, respectively.

Most surgeons perform bowel resection for Crohn's disease. A bypass operation is still considered a reasonable procedure in specific situations. For certain types of ileocecal Crohn's disease with associated abscess or phlegmon densely adherent to the retroperitoneum, exclusion bypass with extraperitoneal

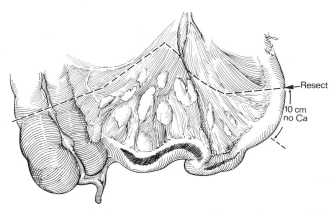

—Resect

10 cm
no Ca

Fig 39–13.—Extent of resection in Crohn's disease of the small intestine, provided there is no underlying malignancy. A 10-cm margin of bowel above obvious disease is chosen for the proximal line of resection; distally, the cecum is removed. Enlarged mesenteric lymph nodes are removed provided this does not produce a risk of a wider resection because of undermining of blood supply.

abscess drainage is reasonable. In such situations, the proximal end of the bypassed bowel is brought to the abdominal wall as a mucous fistula, as the bypassed segment with over-sewn proximal end may perforate or form a huge, infected mucocele. Most forms of ileocecal Crohn's disease, even with such septic complications, can still be handled well by resection.

In continuity (simple) bypass procedures can be done for gastroduodenal Crohn's disease; for the rarely seen Crohn's patient with a fibrotic rather than inflammatory stenosis of the ileum, especially when the patient's condition is poor; and for patients with multiple obstructing skip lesions.

Ileostomy

This may be done in certain cases either alone or as a complement to intestinal resection. Indications for ileostomy alone are similar to those for exclusion bypass; namely, ileocecal perforative Crohn's disease, although even for this, it is an uncommon operation. A loop ileostomy may be used in such circumstances and has further application in salvaging patients with anastomotic breakdown following resection of their Crohn's disease. A loop ileostomy may also be used above an ileocolic anastomosis where the surgeon is concerned that the proximity of the anastomosis to a draining abscess cavity may cause the anastomosis to break down. In such circumstances, however, one would prefer to resect the diseased segment, construct an end ileostomy, close over the proximal colon, and implant that end into the wound in proximity to the ileostomy. This allows for an easy, subsequent, ileocolic anastomosis. This approach was reflected in our surgical experience, as reported by Farmer et al. (1976)[39] in the periods 1966–69 and 1972–73 (Table 39–5). Ileostomy alone was not used for ileitis or ileocolitis but in conjunction with resection in 9 cases (7%) and 77 cases (34.2%) of patients operated on for ileitis and ileocolitis, respectively.

TABLE 39–5.—NUMBER AND TYPES OF OPERATIONS PERFORMED*

OPERATION	PATTERN			
	Ileocolic	Small intestinal	Colonic	Anorectal
Ileostomy only	0	0	2	
Ileostomy and resection	77	9	96	18
Resection only	132	106	9	
Bypass	13	13	2	
Ileorectal anastomosis	3	2	18	
Total	225	130	127	

*(Copyright permission: Farmer R.G., Hawk W.A., Turnbull R.B. Jr.: Indications for surgery in Crohn's disease: Analysis of 500 cases. *Gastroenterology* 71:245–260, 1976.)

CROHN'S DISEASES OF THE COLON WITH AND WITHOUT RECTAL INVOLVEMENT— REVIEW OF PROCEDURES

Total Proctocolectomy and Ileostomy

This operation may be done as a one-stage procedure several months after initial abdominal colectomy and ileostomy with rectal preservation. For all practical purposes, other varieties of staging such as initial diverting loop ileostomy followed by later proctocolectomy are rarely used. Perhaps there is a role for this latter operation in the patient who has severe rectal and suppurative perineal Crohn's disease, who is not willing to have a permanent ileostomy at a particular time. Should the patient insist on having the ileostomy closed, it is possible to do so. Reactivation of the disease usually follows. Invariably, patients appreciate the value of the ileostomy, find it not quite as horrible as they had thought, and have developed lessened perianal sepsis, allowing for a safer proctocolectomy. In such circumstances, my preference would be for abdominal colectomy and ileostomy with later proctectomy, but on several occasions, we have used the approach described above.

The one-stage operation is not usually done for patients with fulminant disease, toxic megacolon, or with severe malnutrition or perianal sepsis. Some surgeons advocate total proctocolectomy even for fulminant disease with or without megacolon. It has been pointed out that construction of a rectal mucous fistula or simple oversew is not without hazard and that the experienced surgeon can remove the rectum safely and expeditiously. This may be true in certain instances, but I would caution against it as a general rule. A more pressing argument for primary proctocolectomy may be made when severe colonic hemorrhage is a feature of the disease. Even in this circumstance, unless proctoscopic evidence of significant rectal hemorrhage is present, I have usually chosen abdominal colectomy over proctocolectomy.

Technique

Unless there is evidence for or suspicion of cancer in the colon or rectum, conservative colorectal resection is practiced. Excessive raw retroperitoneal spaces are avoided. The mesentery of the right, transverse and left colon are divided close (about 1–2 cm) to the colon edge. The author's preference is to preserve the entire omentum. While less operative time is taken to sacrifice the omentum than to preserve it, the preserved omentum is useful in a variety of ways. The pedicle of omentum may be used to occupy the pelvis after proctectomy and, by its absorptive and buffer effect, minimize collection of exudate, hematoma, and obstruction due to adherent loops of small intestine. Furthermore, future laparotomy for recurrence is possible and reentry of the abdomen is facilitated if a veil of omentum is interposed between the abdominal incision and the underlying loops of small intestine.

Delivery of the splenic flexure is facilitated by approaching the area from both the transverse colon and the descending colon. In the latter instance, an incision is made along the white line of Toldt and carried upward to the lower pole of the left kidney. At that point, the incision in the retroperitoneum is carried parallel to the lateral colon edge, about 1 in. away. The assistant surgeon facilitates delivery of the flexure by gentle traction on both the transverse colon and the descending colon, producing an effect like peeling the colon out of its mesentery. This minimizes the risk of splenic injury.

The technique of proctectomy also causes disagreement. The goals that surgeons would agree are desirable include: (1) primary healing of the perineal wound or at least no undue delay in healing; (2) avoidance of pelvic sepsis (and therefore, avoidance of inadvertent entry into the rectum); (3) avoidance of injury to ureters, bladder, prostate, or vagina; (4) preservation of sex function; and (5) avoidance of pelvic hemorrhage.

Primary closure of the perineal wound is an attractive proposition avoiding the several weeks to months (or longer) of persistent discharge, when the perineum is left open. If this can be achieved with a minimal risk of pelvic sepsis, the approach is favored by our group. This presupposes that extensive perianal sepsis is not present preoperatively; that pelvic hemostasis has been effective; that saline irrigation and sump suction of the presacral space is carried out for three to five days after surgery; that parenteral antibiotics have been given preoperatively and in the immediate postoperative period; that rectal content did not contaminate the presacral space during the course of proctectomy. Otherwise, the alternative technique of closure of the pelvic peritoneum and packing of the pelvis through the open perineal wound is performed.

In a previous report,[40] the mechanism of injury to the nerves governing sexual function in the male were outlined. This has a bearing on the techniques of proctectomy. The conservative resection involves close dissection of the pararectal tissues including close dissection along the mesenteric aspect of the rectum. This certainly is commendable with respect to taking all possible precautions in avoiding nerve interruption. However, this is a tedious and bloody procedure, much more difficult than a modified conservative approach. The author finds that by dissecting in the bloodless plane between the investing layer of fascia of the rectum and Waldeyer's fascia to the lower border of the third sacral vertebra, this posterior dissection can be done without risk to the nervi erigentes and the sacral sympathetic nerves. At that point, completion of rectal mobilization is carried out by dissecting immediately against the rectal wall. This facilitates the proctectomy considerably, and blood loss is minimal. It is em-

phasized that this is not a proctectomy as for cancer, since the lateral rectal dissection is kept in close proximity to the rectal wall, especially at the level of the lateral ligaments. Anteriorly, the dissection is carried out on the rectal side of the fascia of Denonvilliers, exposing the vertical fibers of the rectal muscle wall but not the seminal vesicles. The perineal proctectomy is completed by the endoanal technique.[41] An intersphincteric dissection is made preserving anal skin, external sphincter, and levator muscles. Primary closure of the perineal wound is accomplished by suturing together the right and left halves of the levator and external sphincter complex. The skin is closed with 30 Dexon sutures. While this has been our preferred method, others believe that excision of external sphincters is desirable.

Variations of total proctocolectomy other than intersphincteric dissection of the rectum have been proposed in an attempt to avoid the disabling problem of a persistent draining perineal sinus. Extended anterior resection of the rectum to the level of the levators has been proposed. The rectum is transected and closed by sutures or staples at the levator level. This leaves a small anorectal segment that is purported to be trouble free, in relative terms, and avoids a perineal wound altogether. A variation of this in the form of mucosal proctectomy, with or without closure of the stump, has been advocated by Hulten.[42] Certainly, these alternatives avoid major perineal wounds, but drainage from the anus may occur, and even with removal of anorectal mucosa, perianal fistulas may persist.

Technique of Ileostomy Construction

Primary mucocutaneous maturation of the stoma is followed based on the principles outlined by Brooke and Turnbull. Earlier reference was made to the importance of preoperative marking of the stoma site. Over this site a disk of skin approximately 3.5 cm in diameter is excised. Countertraction is provided on the wound edge at the fascial and subcutaneous level opposite the stoma. The subcutaneous fat and fascia of the anterior rectus sheath is incised vertically rather than cored out. The muscle is separated and the posterior sheath incised so that a two-finger-width aperture is constructed. Too wide an opening predisposes to formation of parastomal hernia and possible prolapse; too narrow an opening produces obstructive symptoms. The oversewn end of ileum is brought through the aperture so that 5–6 cm of ileum projects beyond skin level without tension. Following eversion and primary maturation, a 2.5–3-cm stoma is produced. Ensurance of an adequate blood supply is obtained by observing arterial bleeding from the cut edge of the small-bowel mesentery. The small bowel mesentery from the cephalad end of the internal ileostomy aperture is approximated to the anterior abdominal wall, an inch to the right of the incision up to the level of the falciform ligament. In this way, internal volvulus is prevented. The end of the ileum is not transected and matured until the main abdominal wound is closed.

Loop ileostomy is used in the surgery of colitis in several circumstances. This may be the definitive stoma constructed primarily at the time of proctocolectomy for obesity (loop-end ileostomy) or by conversion of a loop ileostomy to a loop-end ileostomy. This latter instance obtains if the initial operation was an ileostomy alone or if combined with a blow-hole colostomy for toxic megacolon, or if a planned temporary ileostomy (as may be used above an ileorectal anastomosis) is converted to a permanent one because of downstream disease or complications. Loop ileostomy is used as in the instance cited above, covering an ileorectal anastomosis, but is also used whenever the surgeon is concerned about the integrity of the distal anastomosis, as in associated sepsis. Additionally, in the situation where anastomotic breakdown occurs postoperatively, loop ileostomy is valuable in preventing further intra-abdominal contamination.

The loop ileostomy is constructed by drawing the loop of ileum through the abdominal wall aperture using a linen tape as a tractor (Fig 39–14). A plastic rod is placed through the mesentery and allowed to rest on the parastomal skin without tension. The loop is oriented so that the proximal functional end lies caudad and the nonfunctional end cephalad. A ⅘ incision of the antimesenteric aspect of the bowel is made on the recessive limb about 15 mm from the skin surface. This allows the proximal end to escape from its fellow. Primary maturation is performed, and the plastic rod is removed at seven days.

Subtotal (Abdominal) Colectomy

This operation is common in certain circumstances. For fulminant colitis or toxic megacolon, where the addition of proctectomy may be hazardous by virtue of added operating time in a severely ill patient and of breaching additional extraperitoneal spaces (with risk of contamination and later pelvic sepsis), abdominal colectomy is chosen over total proctocolectomy. Severe perianal sepsis, malnutrition, concurrent major medical illness, and relative rectal sparing of Crohn's disease are other common reasons for avoiding rectal resection at this time.

Where abdominal colectomy is proposed, a line of transection of the distal colon is chosen that will allow the rectosigmoid stump to reach the anterior abdominal wall. For situations other than fulminant colitis or toxic megacolon, stapled closure of the distal segment using the TA55 device is used. This end is then brought to the subcutaneous level and quarantined from the peritoneal cavity by placing 20 chromic gut sutures circumferentially between the peritoneum and the mesentery and serosa of the stump, about 1 in. below the stapled end. This allows for easy identification of the rectal stump if future proctectomy or ileorectal anastomosis is planned. It obviates the problem of collection of mucus or exudate from a sigmoid mucous fistula. Any perforation of the

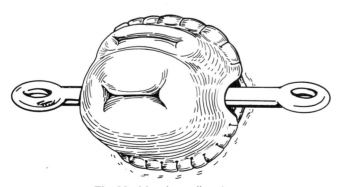

Fig 39–14.—Loop ileostomy.

stump will be extraperitoneal, preventing peritonitis. The experienced surgeon may deem it safe to proceed with proctectomy at the time of abdominal colectomy, even in severe malnutrition, fulminant colitis, toxic megacolon, or major perianal sepsis. In general, in these cases the author follows the more conservative practice of abdominal colectomy alone. When abdominal colectomy is required for toxic megacolon, the bowel wall is so fragile that any suture material used for either closure of the end or construction of a primary mucous fistula results in tearing out of the sutures, with recession of the fistula into the abdomen. In that instance I prefer to exteriorize a sigmoid segment, wrap it with a gauze roll to prevent its recession, and after the serositis has diminished sufficiently (about seven to ten days), amputate the stump with delayed construction of a mucous fistula.

In certain cases, abdominal colectomy and ileostomy becomes the definitive operation for Crohn's proctocolitis. We reported on the fate of the rectum after such a procedure in 101 patients.[43] Four patients died postoperatively; 6 patients had the rectum in situ at death in later years; 46 patients underwent completion proctectomy for continuing symptoms due to Crohn's disease (one of whom had rectal cancer); 12 patients underwent ileorectal anastomosis, of whom 6 had later rectal resection. Thirty-three patients still have the rectum in situ. It is for this asymptomatic group of patients where guidelines on follow-up have not been forthcoming in the literature. We have observed dysplasia in Crohn's colitis. The significance of dysplasia has been studied less well in Crohn's disease than in ulcerative colitis, but merits attention because of reported cases of cancer.[44] The finding of severe dysplasia in an excluded rectal segment (or in circuit for that matter) constitutes an indication for proctectomy. This represents the author's opinion and is not based on a known high association of dysplasia and cancer in Crohn's disease. To carry this argument further, the patient at risk would be advised to have endoscopic evaluation and biopsy of the rectum at regular intervals, say, every one to two years. Our policy has been to do such endoscopy using the pediatric flexible gastroscope. Should rectal stricture prevent adequate surveillance, a relative indication for surgery is present.

Ileorectal Anastomosis

The operation is considered when the rectum is spared of disease; distensibility of the rectum is present on air insufflation; sphincter tone is adequate; there is a lack of perianal sepsis or fistula; and extensive ileal disease is absent. None of these criteria is absolute, and experience and philosophy can lead the surgeon to favor the operation in an individual case, when one or more of the above criteria are lacking. Alexander-Wiliams and Buchmann[45] reported that patients undergoing ileorectal anastomosis where the ileum was affected with Crohn's disease fared no worse than those whose ileum was free of disease; a functioning anastomosis was present in 67% and 61%, respectively, of those two groups. Also, they reported that in the mean follow-up period of six years, there was no difference in functional results, whether or not perianal disease was present at the time of ileorectal anastomosis. The authors have provided a caveat that the perianal disease is asymptomatic before advising the operation.

With respect to staged vs. primary anastomosis, again,

there is some disagreement. Most surgeons avoid primary anastomosis (where the rectum is otherwise suitable) in toxic colitis with or without megacolon, where there is associated intra-abdominal sepsis or significant malnutrition. Alexander-Williams advises against the operation altogether if the rectal mucosa looks abnormal, since the hope that it will improve with diversion is usually a forlorn one. I agree with this in general, but in severely toxic colitis or megacolon, the inflammation in the rectum may be more apparent than real, and subsequent anastomosis, after initial abdominal colectomy, may be possible. My feeling is that primary anastomosis without proctecting loop ileostomy is usually safe, unless the patient is in a toxic state or malnourished. Rather than staging the operation by a covering ileostomy above the ileorectal anastomosis in suboptimal circumstances, I prefer to do the abdominal colectomy and ileostomy, with subsequent anastomosis of the ileum to the rectal stump. The rectal tissue is less fragile in such a situation than in the initial operation.

This operation has also the merit of being able to deal with rectovaginal fistula or perianal fistula in a definitive way, with or without sphincter repair/plication prior to anastomosis. This presupposes that there is no endoscopic or histologic evidence of rectal Crohn's disease.

If the colonic disease extends distally to the splenic flexure or descending colon, the surgeon will preserve as much distal bowel as possible, and construct, for example, an ileosigmoid anastomosis. Both for ulcerative colitis and Crohn's disease, the principles of construction of the ileorectal anastomosis involve the union of both ends of bowel that are free of disease, where the blood supply is excellent. The anastomosis is free of tension and widely patent. This may involve making an antimesenteric slit on the small bowel side to equalize the circumference of the bowel ends. The level of the rectal transection is that of the sacral promontory in the case of ulcerative colitis, so that monitoring of the rectum with the rigid proctoscope is facilitated. Both hand and end-to-end stapled anastomoses have been done in our unit with satisfactory results. In a personal series, of 21 consecutive stapled anastomoses, there was one radiologic leak and no clinical leaks. In a review of the Cleveland Clinic experience, approximately 50% of patients had long-term satisfactory results.[46]

Segmental Resection of the Colon

While segmental resection of the ileum in continuity with involved colon is the accepted treatment of choice for ileocolitis with distal sparing of variable amounts of the colon and rectum, the management of segmental colitis is less clear. In general, a high rate of recurrence has been seen. In the case of Crohn's disease confined to the transverse or sigmoid colon (a rare pattern of disease), it is tempting to perform segmental colonic resection and colocolic or colorectal anastomosis. Indeed, this has been done where the preoperative diagnosis of diverticulitis was made. My impression is that a high rate of recurrence (on the proximal side) follows such procedures and that probably resection of all colon proximal to the diseased segment, as well as the involved segment, should be done. Glotzer and Silen have advocated ileocolic resection and segmental resection of the sigmoid colon when the disease affects the ileum with a skip lesion in the sigmoid.

Colostomy

This is not a common operation for Crohn's disease. For Crohn's disease confined to the rectum, rectal excision with iliac colostomy has been advocated[47] without any significant increase in recurrence of Crohn's disease in the stoma compared to similar cases where proctocolectomy and ileostomy was done. However, attitudes in North America generally favor this latter operation because of perceptions that recurrences in colostomies not only are commoner than in ileostomy, but also are usually associated with major parastomal sepsis or fistulaes. A case can be made for colostomy construction in the patient who has undergone extensive small-bowel resection, now has significant dehydration, and needs fecal diversion because of the rectal or perianal Crohn's disease. Here the risks are outweighed by the advantage of having more intestinal absorptive surface than if proctocolectomy was performed. Skin-level, blow-hole colostomy has already been discussed.

Postoperative Management

Following operation, IV fluids and nasogastric tube suction are continued until signs of bowel activity are present and the patient is able to tolerate oral liquids. Total parenteral nutrition is continued after a day or two, if TPN was used preoperatively or if a prolonged ileus precludes oral feeding. Prophylactic systemic antibiotics are discontinued after 24 hours, unless operative contamination has occurred or sepsis was found at surgery. In that event, antibiotics are continued for five days and the patient is then reassessed.

Patients who are taking corticosteroids preoperatively continued on to take them postoperatively. In general terms, IV hydrocortisone, 100 mg every 12 hours, is given for two to three days, and is then reduced to 50 mg every 12 hours until the patient can absorb prednisone by mouth. The dose is reduced until the patient's usual (preoperative) maintenance level is reached, generally within seven to ten days. Over the next three months, the dose is tapered and then stopped.

Sump drains are used in patients having rectal resection. Saline irrigation, 3 L/24 hours, is provided for one to three days until the return from the suction drains is clear. The sump drains are then placed to suction for only 24 hours and then removed. Penrose drains or latex rubber sheets are used in patients with established intra-abdominal abscesses. These drains are sutured lightly into position with 4–0 plain catgut. The drains are removed after seven to ten days.

No special care of the abdominal wound is required over that of incisions for other conditions. Delayed primary closure techniques are sometimes useful: in patients with established abdominal sepsis; where there has been major abdominal or wound enteric contamination; for obese patients; where multiple laparotomies have been done using the same incision; or for the immunosuppressed or malnourished patients.

The perineal wound is almost always closed primarily following proctocolectomy. Postoperative pain in that region is usual and normally becomes more noticeable after three to four days. Erythema, local tenderness, or pain that seems out of proportion to the findings signals further investigation. The simplest, best technique is to produce cutaneous anesthesia and then pass a 17-gauge needle attached to an aspirating syringe through the perineal wound into the presacral space. If pus or malodorous, altered blood is found, a mushroom catheter may be inserted into the space, after heavier infiltration of the sphincters with lidocaine (Xylocaine). Material is sent for culture and sensitivity studies.

Postoperative ileostomy management is discussed only briefly. All pouches placed on stomas in the postoperative period should be transparent so that the quality of the effluent as well as the appearance of the ileostomy can be evaluated. Numerous appliances are available, but the two-piece (Sure-Fit, System II) or Hollister pouch with Stomahesive skin barrier are particularly useful. Ileostomy output can be quite deceptive in the early postoperative period. More than 1 L/day of succus entericus and mucus may be passed despite the presence of a major ileus. If a loop ileostomy has been used, the plastic supporting rod is removed at seven days. The stoma therapist begins instruction in the care of the ileostomy about the fifth to seventh postoperative day. Homegoing equipment is provided, along with appropriate printed handout materials and a phone number so that patients can reach an enterostomal therapist at any time. A postoperative stoma check is provided for four weeks after discharge. Remeasurement of the diameter of the stoma and possible equipment alterations are done during this time.

Outpatient Visits

Aside from assessment of a stoma, the abdominal and/or perineal wound, the patient is checked for evidence of anemia, malnutrition, electrolyte imbalance, or dehydration. Usually the diet has been light until the first postoperative visit. At this point, further latitude is given to the patient in terms of fiber and protein intake. Highly refined carbohydrate is probably best avoided. Vitamin B_{12}, folic acid, or iron supplements may be needed depending on presumed or known defects.

Diarrhea is usual after most bowel resections. The patient may volunteer that this is manageable by diet or by eating smaller meals more frequently. Otherwise, until intestinal adaptation occurs, the patient may need antidiarrhea medication. The first-line drugs include Metamucil, Lomotil, and Loperamide. If these (singly or in combination) are ineffective, one will use liquid codeine phosphate, up to 60 mg every six hours, or tincture laudanum, 10–15 drops, every six hours.

Later follow-up is provided at six months and then annually. There is no hard evidence to support a particular regimen of follow-up over, say, having the patient return only if further symptoms occur. With a chronic disease, however, and one that is prone to recurrence as well as to exhibiting later complications, such as gallbladder or renal calculus formation, malnutrition, electrolyte problems, anemia, analgesic abuse, and depression, I believe that routine annual follow-up is indicated.

Routine endoscopy and contrast roentgenography are not indicated, unless the patient shows signs or symptoms of disease. The exception might be in patients who have had abdominal colectomy with a rectum left in situ and no further operation is planned. There is no information in the literature to my knowledge on this matter, but my practice is to perform endoscopy and rectal biopsy annually (a pediatric endoscope is often required due to rectal stricturing) to exclude dysplasia.

RESULT

Morbidity

Patients undergoing major abdominal surgery for Crohn's disease are susceptible to numerous complications. The most serious factors relate to ileostomy function, sexual and bladder function, perineal wound healing, and anastomotic complications.

Ileostomy Complications

Most reports relate to the surgery of ulcerative colitis or to series combining ulcerative colitis and Crohn's disease. While recurrence in the ileostomy is the commonest complication affecting the stoma in Crohn's disease (see below under Recurrence), the non-Crohn's related complications are still considerable and estimated to require revisionary surgery in 10%–15% of cases. Complications include ileostomy recession, ileostomy fistula, stricture, prolapse, parastomal hernia, ischemic necrosis, paraileostomy abscess/ulcer, internal hernia and volvulus, and ileostomy diarrhea. Additionally, skin reaction (dermatitis) may occur with a receded, flush or poorly sited stoma or as a sensitivity reaction to skin barriers, adhesive agents, tape, or pouch material. In general, modern stoma therapy techniques and equipment will resolve many of these dermatitis problems, even for some stomas that are receded. For others (including ischemic or strictured stomas), formal revision is required. Ileostomy relocation is required for prolapse, hernia, deep or multiple fistulas, and for a poorly sited stoma.

Sexual and Bladder Dysfunction

These complications are largely preventable by employing conservative resection techniques when removing the rectum. Following proctectomy for inflammatory bowel disease, rates of male sexual dysfunction as high as 25% have been reported. However, rates of permanent impotence in patients under 50 years of age, are considerably less, ranging to 5%. In a personal series of 108 patients undergoing proctocolectomy for ulcerative colitis (approximately half being men), none developed impotence.

Bladder dysfunction occurs in up to 16% of patients following proctocolectomy. After urography, cystometrogram evaluation, and a failed trial of voiding, cholinergic stimulation and or self-catheterization for four to six weeks are usually effective in allowing return of function. Rarely, transurethral resection of the prostate is required if prostatic enlargement contributes to the problem.

Perineal Wound Healing

Delayed healing or persistent perineal sinus is a common complication following proctocolectomy. Incidences of 7%–70% have been cited. Factors that seem to enhance these rates include proctectomy in females, pelvic sepsis, the practice of packing the perineal wound from below as opposed to primary closure, Crohn's disease (vs. ulcerative colitis), multiple perianal fistulas or sepsis, and lack of good pelvic hemostasis.

The problem ranges from a small, narrow, virtually asymptomatic sinus to a complex, indurated, deep granulation tissue-lined cavity that may penetrate the posterior wall of the vagina or even extend to and communicate with the anterior abdominal incision. The surgeon will exclude the presence of a foreign body and in selected cases obtain a sinogram to define the limits of the cavity, as well as exclude an enteroperineal fistula. For the larger cavities, radical debridement and split-thickness skin grafting has been our preferred method of management. Others have employed vascularized pedicles of gracilis or gluteus maximus muscle to fill in the cavity.

Anastomotic Complications

Anastomotic dehiscence may occur following any type of anastomosis or enterotomy closure in Crohn's disease, but overall, is relatively uncommon. Leakage is perhaps more common when intra-abdominal sepsis is found at surgery or after ileorectal anastomosis. The judicious use of a temporary ileostomy proximal to an anastomosis will prevent the catastrophic sequelae of a nonintact anastomosis. In the unprotected state, a defective enterocolic anastomosis requires urgent recognition and treatment. In the early postoperative course, laparotomy with separation of the anastomosis exteriorizing the proximal end as an ileostomy and the distal end as a mucous fistula is advised. If the degree of obliterative peritoneal reaction precludes easy mobilization of the anastomosis, then a loop enterostomy proximal to the dehiscence and drainage, is appropriate. This is the procedure of choice for a disrupted ileorectal anastomosis. Enterocutaneous fistulas appearing after ten days may be managed with *TPN*, and if of low output (less than 200 ml/day), healing can be anticipated without surgery.

Other complications, such as intra-abdominal abscesses, bowel obstruction, venous thrombosis, and wound complications, are not uncommon but are beyond the scope of this chapter.

Mortality

Postoperative mortality is due to intra-abdominal sepsis and bacteremia, although venous thrombosis may be a cause. Crude mortality rates of 7%–18.3% were reported in a review by Higgens and Allan.[48] They cited a total mortality and Crohn's disease-related mortality of 14.9% and 7%, respectively, in their own series. In our own series[49] operative mortality among 361 patients was 2%. Overall disease-related mortality was 5.8%. Goligher[50] noted a mortality rate of 4.1% for primary operations and 8.3% for subsequent operations. Mortality is adversely affected by advancing age of the patient, the severity of the disease, the emergency nature of surgery, and the preoperative state of the patient. Mortality has declined in the past decade.

Recurrence

The definitions of recurrent disease are different in different reports (Fig 39–15). The commonly used definitions include: (1) recurrent symptoms such as diarrhea, weight loss, and pain; (2) recurrent symptoms with radiologic and/or sur-

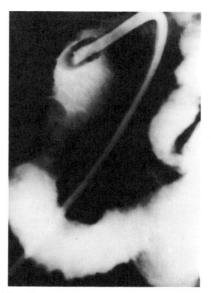

Fig 39–15.—Contrast roentgenogram by ileostomy injection demonstrates recurrent, prestomal disease manifested by spiculation and mucosal ulceration.

gical evidence of recurrent disease; and (3) further resection for Crohn's disease.[51]

As expected, the more stringent the criteria of recurrence, the lower are rates of recurrence reported. Furthermore, the methodology of reporting influences the results, as values for crude recurrence rates are lower than those for cumulative recurrence rates.

Other factors reported to influence recurrence rates include:
1. The age of the patient at onset of symptoms
2. Previous operations for Crohn's disease
3. The site of the disease
4. Bypass operations
5. Leaving behind large lymph nodes
6. Leaving residual diseased bowel

1. The younger the patient, the more likely it is that recurrence will occur sooner.[52, 53] A short pre-resection history of Crohn's disease favors recurrence,[50] although in the report of Higgens and Allan (1980)[48] this was only true in the short term.

2. Surgical procedures directed at Crohn's disease have been indicated as possibly favoring recurrence.[54] This was disputed in an actuarial study by Higgens and Allan (1980),[48] as it had been by Colcock and Vansant[36, 55] and Atwell et al.[56] Using actuarial methods to obtain cumulative recurrence rates, Greenstein et al. (1975)[57] and Lennard-Jones and Stalder (1967)[51] showed an increase in reoperations and recurrences after sequential procedures—although in these series numbers were small.

3. The more favorable outlook after surgery for pure Crohn's colitis or ileitis compared with that for ileocolitis has been noted by Farmer et al.,[39] Hellers,[58] and Mekhijan et al.[59] Gump et al.[60] found a statistically significantly greater risk of recurrence if patients had perianal disease. Fifty-two percent of 29 patients with recurrent disease and 17% of 35

patients without recurrent disease had had previous perianal suppurations. They also found a positive association between length of bowel involved and likelihood of recurrence, a finding supported by (Atwell et al.[56] and Schofield[61]).

4–6. The controversies related to resection vs. bypass leaving behind enlarged lymph nodes at time of resection and the presence of residual disease at the line of anastomosis have already been considered.

There is general agreement that recurrence rates are related to the length of follow-up. This may explain the apparent anomaly of such a wide range of reported recurrence rates after primary resection and anastomosis for ileocolitis, from 40% (de Dombal et al.[52]) to 100% (Korelitz et al.[62]). Hellers [58] found that the cumulative recurrence rates after the first curative operation were 30% at 5 years, 50% at 10 years, and 60% at 15 years. After the second resection, they were 45% at 5 years and 65% at 10 years. Reviewing our experience of patients undergoing their initial definitive operation at the Cleveland Clinic,[43] we found an overall incidence of recurrence, defined as the need for a further resection, as 35% after a mean follow-up of 11.4 years. We also found that recurrence rates varied at different sites. At 14 years after the initial operation, the cumulative risk of recurrence for patients with ileocolic disease was 50% ($\pm$ 9.6%), whereas for terminal ileal disease alone it was only 38% ($\pm$ 6%) and for large bowel disease alone only 32% ($\pm$ 7%).

The importance of using actuarial studies instead of crude recurrence rates was emphasized by Greenstein et al.[57] Crude data implied that reoperation rate diminished with each succeeding operation from 58%, after the first operation to 47% after the fourth. However, actuarial analysis showed that at the three-year follow-up point, the cumulative chance of reoperation increased from 37% after the first resection to 60% after the fourth.

This view of inexorable tendency for recurrences with more surgical procedures is challenged in the report of Higgens and Allan.[48] In their study using actuarial analysis, reoperation rates were similar after the first, second, and third resections.

Philosophy of Management

In general, the indications for operation for recurrent Crohn's disease follow the same guidelines as those for the initial operation. The clinician is perhaps somewhat cautious in advising another operation, especially if much small intestine has been removed previously or if there have been multiple resections. Nevertheless, operations will be indicated if there are persistent symptoms or intra-abdominal sepsis. My impression is that the medical treatment of recurrent Crohn's disease is not as satisfactory as the same treatment for primary Crohn's disease.

Increasing attention is being given to attempts to measure the follow-up quality of life in studies of patients with Crohn's disease. Such studies partly dispel the gloom traditionally associated with recurrent disease. Farmer and Michener[63] felt that the patient's assessment of his or her quality of life related to the activity of the disease rather than to whether an operation became necessary. The current state of health was assessed in a report of the Cleveland Clinic experience of 522 patients whose disease onset occurred under age 21 years

with a mean follow-up of 7.7 years. They rated health as good in 23%, fair in 67%, and poor in only 6%. Nonoperative patients with ileitis fared better as a group than did those with colitis; this evened out in the two groups after operation. Bergman and Krause,[64] using similar categories, assessed 87% as in perfect health, some 9% as having restriction of work or leisure capacity, and only 4% as being severely incapacitated.

The patient who has had an operation for Crohn's disease remains at risk of developing problems other than recurrence. These include diarrhea, vitamin B_{12} deficiency, malnutrition, gallstones, renal calculi, and bile salt deficiency. The withdrawal of steroid therapy after a successful operation may unmask extraintestinal manifestations especially arthritis. The clinician should follow the patient at regular intervals, not only to assess general health and possible recurrence, but also to attain a relationship with the patient that is conducive to trust and credibility. Regular meetings also allow the clinician to give the patient reassurance and support that are so necessary in the long-term management of this chronic disease.

REFERENCES

1. Rankin G.B., Watts H.D., Melnyk G.S., et al.: Extraintestinal manifestation and perianal complications. *Gastroenterology* 77:914–920, 1979.
2. Greenstein A.J., Janowitz H.D., Sachar D.B.: The extraintestinal complications of Crohn's disease and ulcerative colitis: a study of 700 patients. *Medicine* 55:401–412, 1976.
3. Buchmann P., Alexander-Williams J.: Classification of perianal Crohn's disease. *Clin. Gastroenterol.* 9:323–330, 1980.
4. Korelitz B.I., Sommers S.C.: Rectal biopsy in patients with Crohn's disease. Normal mucosa on sigmoidoscopic examination. *J.A.M.A.* 237(35):2742–44, June 20, 1977.
5. Farmer R.G., Hawk W.A., Turnbull R.B. Jr.: Clinical pattern in Crohn's disease: a statistical study of 615 cases. *Gastroenterol.* 68:627–635, 1975.
6. Steinberg D.M., Cooke W.T., Alexander-Williams J.: Abscess and fistulae in Crohn's disease. *Gut* 14:865–869, 1973.
7. Nasar K., Morowitz D.A., Anderson J.G.: Free perforation in regional enteritis. *Gut* 10:206–208, 1969.
8. Steinberg D.M., Cooke W.T., Alexander-Williams J.: Free perforation in Crohn's disease. *Gut* 14:187–190, 1973.
9. Wilk P.J., Fazio V.W., Turnbull R.B. Jr.: Ileoduodenal fistula complicating Crohn's disease. *Dis. Colon Rectum* 20:387–392, 1977.
10. Fazio V.W., Wilk P.J., Turnbull R.B. Jr.: The dilemma of Crohn's disease. Ileosigmoid fistula complicating Crohn's disease. *Dis. Colon Rectum* 20:387–392, 1977.
11. Greenstein A.J., Dicker A., Meyers S., Aufses A.J. Jr.: Peri-ileostomy fistulae in Crohn's disease. *Ann. Surg.* 197:179–182, 1983.
12. Siminovitch J.M., Fazio V.W.: Ureteral obstruction secondary to Crohn's disease: a need for ureterolysis? *Am. J. Surg.* 139:95–98, 1980.
13. Block G.E., Enker W.E., Kirsner J.B.: Significance in treatment of occult obstructive uropathy complicating Crohn's disease. *Ann. Surg.* 178:322–330, 1973.
14. Fazio V.W., Zelas P., Weakley F.L.: Intraoperative angiography and the localization of bleeding from the small intestine. *Surg. Gynecol. Obstet.* 151:637–640, 1980.
15. Homan W.P., Tang C.S., Thorbjarnarson B.: Acute massive hemorrhage from intestinal Crohn's disease: Report of seven cases and review of the literature. *Arch. Surg.* 111:901–905, 1976.
16. Sparberg M., Kirsner J.: Recurrent hemorrhage in regional enteritis. Report of three cases. *Am. J. Dig. Dis.* 2:652–657, 1966.
17. Hoffman J.P., Taft D.A., Wheelis R.G.: Adenocarcinoma in regional enteritis of the small intestine. *Arch. Surg.* 112:606–611, 1977.

18. Weedon D.D., Shorter R.G., Ilstrup D.M., et al.: Crohn's disease and cancer. *N. Engl. J. Med.* 289:1099–1103, 1973.
19. Goligher J.C., Hoffman D.C., de Dombal F.T.: Surgical treatment of seven attacks of ulcerative colitis with special reference to the advantage of early operation. *Br. Med. J.* 4:703–706, 1970.
20. Block G.E., Moossa A.R., Simonowitz D., et al.: Emergency colectomy for inflammatory bowel disease. *Surg.* 82:531–537, 1977.
21. Fry P.D., Atkinson K.G.: Current surgical approach to toxic megacolon. *Surg. Gynecol. Obstet.* 143:26–30, 1976.
22. Turnbull R.B. Jr., Hawk W.A., Weakley F.L.: Surgical treatment of toxic megacolon—ileostomy and colostomy to prepare patients for colectomy. *Am. J. Surg.* 122:325–331, 1971.
23. Fazio V.W.: Toxic megacolon in ulcerative colitis and Crohn's colitis. *Clin. Gastroenterol.* 9:389–407, 1980.
24. McKay J.L., McMahon W.: Crohn's disease of the anal region. *Northwest Med.* 71:111–112, 1972.
25. Lockhart-Mummery H.E.: Crohn's disease; anal lesions. *Dis. Colon Rectum* 18:200–203, 1975.
26. Gump F.W., LePore M., Barker H.G.: A revised concept of acute regional enteritis. *Ann. Surg.* 166:942–946, 1967.
27. Kewenter J., Hulten L., Kock N.G.: The relationship and epidemiology of acute terminal ileitis in Crohn's disease. *Gut* 15:801–804, 1974.
28. Yang S.S., Gibson P., McCaughey R.S., et al.: Primary Crohn's disease of the appendix: Report of 14 cases and a review of the literature. *Ann. Surg.* 189:334–339, 1979.
29. Cooke W.T., Swan C.H.: Diffuse jejunoileitis of Crohn's disease. *Quart. J. Med.* 43:583–601, 1974.
30. Lee E.: Personal communication. March 1984.
31. Alexander-Williams J.: Overview of surgical management and directions of future research in Allan R.N., Keighley M.R.B., Alexander-Williams J., et al. (eds.): *Inflammatory Bowel Disease.* New York, Churchill Livingstone, 1983, pp. 496–504.
32. Nugent F.W., Richmond M., Park S.K.: Crohn's disease of the duodenum. *Gut* 18:115–120, 1977.
33. Ross T., Fazio V.W., Farmer R.G.: Long-term results of surgical treatment for Crohn's disease of the duodenum. *Ann. Surg.* 197:399–406, 1983.
34. Bergman L., Krause U.: Crohn's disease: A long-term study of the clinical course. *Scand. J. Gastroenterol.* 12:937–944, 1977.
35. Pennington L., Hamilton S.R., Bayless T.M., et al.: Surgical management of Crohn's disease: Influence of disease at margin of resection. *Ann. Surg.* 192:311–318, 1980.
36. Colcock B.P., Vansant J.H.: Surgical treatment of regional enteritis. *N. Engl. J. Med.* 262:435–439, 1960.
37. Alexander-Williams J., Fielding J.F., Cooke W.T.: A comparison of results of excision and bypass for ileal Crohn's disease. *Gut* 13:973–974, 1972.
38. Homan W.P., Dineen P.: Comparison of the results of resection bypass and bypass with exclusion for ileocecal Crohn's disease. *Ann. Surg.* 187:530–535, 1978.
39. Farmer R.G., Hawk W.A., Turnbull R.B. Jr.: Indications for surgery in Crohn's disease: Analysis of 500 cases. *Gastroenterology.* 71:245–250, 1976.
40. Fazio V.W., Turnbull R.B. Jr.: Ulcerative colitis in Crohn's disease of the colon. A review of surgical options. *Med. Clin. North Am.* 64:1135–1159, 1980.
41. Turnbull R.B. Jr., Fazio V.W.: Endoanal proctectomy and two-directional myotomy—ileostomy, in Nyhus L.M. (ed.): *Surgery Annual.* New York, Appleton-Century-Crofts, 1975, pp. 315–329.
42. Hulten L.: Personal communication. June 1982.
43. Lock M.R., Fazio V.W., Farmer R.G., et al: Proximal recurrence and the fate of the rectum following excisional surgery for Crohn's disease of the large bowel. *Ann. Surg.* 194:98–104, 1981.
44. Lavery I.C., Jagelman D.G.: Cancer in the excluded rectum following surgery for inflammatory bowel disease. *Dis. Colon Rectum* 25:522–524, 1982.
45. Alexander-Williams J., Buchmann P.: Criteria for assessment for suitability and results of ileorectal anastomosis. *Clin. Gastroenterol.* 9:409–417, 1980.
46. Lefton H.B., Farmer R.G., Fazio V.W.: Ileorectal anastomosis for Crohn's disease of the colon. *Gastroenterology* 69:612–617, 1975.
47. Ritchie J.K., Lockhart-Mummery H.E.: Nonrestorative surgery in the treatment of Crohn's disease of the large bowel. *Gut* 14:263–269, 1973.
48. Higgens C.S., Allan R.N.: Crohn's disease of the distal ileum. *Gut* 21:933–940, 1980.
49. Lock M.R., Fazio V.W., Farmer R.G., et al.: Recurrence and reoperation for Crohn's disease. *N. Engl. J. Med.* 304:1586–1588, 1981.
50. Goligher J.C.: Crohn's disease (granulomatous enteritis), in Goligher J.C. (ed.): *Surgery of the Anus, Rectum and Colon,* ed. 4. London, Bailliere Tindall, 1980.
51. Lennard-Jones J.E., Stalder G.A.: Prognosis after resection of chronic regional ileitis. *Gut* 8:332–336, 1967.
52. de Dombal F.T., Burton I.L., Goligher J.C.: Recurrence of Crohn's disease after primary excisional surgery. *Gut* 12:519–527, 1971.
53. Stahlgreen L.H., Ferguson L.K.: The results of surgical treatment of chronic regional enteritis. *J.A.M.A.* 175:986–989, 1961.
54. Bockus H.L.: Regional enteritis. *Gastroenterology* 21:226–310, 1964.
55. Colcock B.P.: Operative technique in surgery for Crohn's disease and its relationship to recurrence. *Surg. Clin. North Am.* 53:375–380, 1973.
56. Atwell J.D., Duthie H.L., Goligher J.C.: The outcome of Crohn's disease. *Br. J. Surg.* 52:966–972, 1965.
57. Greenstein A.J., Sachar D.B., Pasternack B.S., et al.: Reoperation and recurrence in Crohn's colitis and ileocolitis: Crude and cumulative rates. *N. Engl. J. Med.* 293:685–690, 1975.
58. Hellers G.: Crohn's disease in Stockholm County 1955–1974: A study of epidemiology: Results of surgical treatment and longterm prognosis. *Acta Chir. Scand. Suppl.* 490, 1979.
59. Mekhijan H.S., Sweitz D.M., Watts H.D., et al.: National Cooperative Crohn's Disease Study. Factors determining recurrence of Crohn's disease after surgery. *Gastroenterology* 77:907–913, 1979.
60. Gump F.E., Sakellariadis P., Wolff M., et al.: Clinical pathological investigation of regional enteritis as a guide to prognosis. *Ann. Surg.* 176:233–242, 1972.
61. Schofield P.F.: The natural history and treatment of Crohn's disease. *Ann. R. Col. Surg. Engl.* 36:258–279, 1965.
62. Korelitz B., Gribetz D., Kopel F.: Granulomatous colitis in children: Study of 25 cases in comparison with ulcerative colitis. *Pediatrics* 42:446–457, 1968.
63. Farmer R.G., Michener W.M.: Prognosis of Crohn's disease with onset in childhood or adolescence. *Dig. Dis. Sci.* 24:752–757, 1979.
64. Bergman L., Krause U.: Crohn's disease: A long-term study of clinical course in 186 patients. *Scand. J. Gastroenterol.* 12:937–944, 1977.

40

Tumors of the Small Bowel

DONALD C. MCILRATH, M.D.

INTRODUCTION

Because neoplasms of the small intestine occur infrequently, relative to other GI tumors, the average physician encounters only a few cases during his professional career. Therefore, he must depend on information accumulated from many institutions, particularly those with large series of cases, for guidance in diagnosing and managing these patients. It has taken the contributions of many surgeons over time to establish the background knowledge needed to understand the clinical patterns associated with small-bowel tumors and to deal appropriately with them. The magnitude of the challenge of understanding the natural history of these relatively rare neoplasms is appreciated by the realization that there are at least 35 histologic types of benign and malignant tumors and many different clinical manifestations. The purpose of this chapter is to emphasize the clinical and pathologic features of these tumors, appropriate surgical management, and the prognostic implications.

HISTORY

The first reported case of a small-bowel tumor was a duodenal carcinoma described by Hamburger in 1746.[1] The first review of the subject was by Leichtenstern in 1876.[2] He reported 780 carcinomas of the intestinal tract of which 16 were primary in the ileum. In 1920, Johnson[3] reported the statistics of 41,838 autopsies at the Vienna General Hospital, in which 3,585 cases of carcinoma were revealed, 343 of these were intestinal, of which 10 were in the small bowel. Judd[4] reported in 1919 that in a number of clinics, 3% of intestinal carcinomas were found in the small bowel.

Comprehensive reviews, especially the early ones, were made on autopsy data, and consequently are of limited value in providing clinical perspective. The report of Rankin and Mayo[5] in 1930, which involved the clinical management of 55 patients with carcinoma of the small intestine, stimulated modern interest in this subject.

A thorough compilation of all published cases of benign tumors of the small intestine in the world literature was made by River et al.[6] in 1956. They found 1,399 such tumors had been discovered either at operation or at autopsy. In another review of the world literature, Rochlin and Longmire[7] accumulated cases of malignant tumors of the small bowel.

The comparative frequency of benign and malignant tumors

is different in autopsy series than in operative series. Darling and Welch[8] found that malignant neoplasms constituted only 26% of small-bowel tumors discovered at autopsy compared with 75% among patients who had symptomatic tumors found at operation. This difference in incidence is explained by the fact that many benign tumors remain asymptomatic and undetected, a point emphasized further by the observation that many of them are found incidentally in surgical series. Another explanation for the different incidences is that the great majority of malignant tumors become symptomatic and are detected during life. Unfortunately, recognition too often is delayed until the malignancy has reached an advanced stage. One third of 370 Mayo Clinic patients[9] with malignant neoplasms developed signs or symptoms of partial bowel obstruction one year before diagnosis was established.

CLINICAL RECOGNITION: SYMPTOMS

Symptoms associated with primary neoplasms of the small intestine often are insidious in onset and nonspecific, including dyspepsia, anorexia, malaise, and mild discomfort in the midepigastric area. Commonly there is a history which stimulates to a degree duodenal ulcer, biliary tract disease, or other GI disease. The sometimes vague, nonspecific nature of the symptoms may not impress either the patient or the physician until serious complications develop. The long interval from onset of symptoms to diagnosis noted in all reported series can be reduced by maintaining a high index of suspicion about the possibility of small-bowel tumor as a cause of a variety of unimpressive symptoms. In some cases, symptoms and signs are truly absent until a significant complication develops and/or the chance of cure by complete excision of the malignancy has passed.

The two most common complications of both benign and malignant tumors are bleeding and obstruction.

Obstruction, either partial or complete, results from the presence of an intraluminal mass, volvulus, compression of the bowel, or intussusception (Fig 40–1). The main features of acute intestinal obstruction are a sudden attack of severe, cramping abdominal pain, varying degrees of distention, and eventually nausea and vomiting. The first episode is usually short, a matter of hours, and often is followed by complete recovery. Weeks or even months may pass before another bout of acute intestinal obstruction occurs. With advancement of the disease, the tendency is for greater severity and shorter

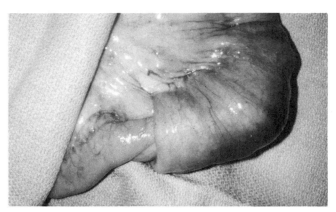

Fig 40–1.—Intussusception of the ileum secondary to fibrous histiocytoma, a rare type of malignant tumor of the small bowel.

intervals between episodes. Late in the course, symptoms become continual.

One should appreciate that the patient who relates a history of colicky abdominal pain or discomfort following intake of food and associated with abdominal bloating, distention, and sometimes vomiting, has bowel obstruction until proved otherwise, and the possibility of small-bowel neoplasm should be included in the differential diagnosis. Problems related to suspecting this diagnosis are that all these classic symptoms may not be present, the patient may be a poor historian, or the physician may not pursue the correct line of questioning to elicit the symptoms. Sometimes the tip-off to diagnosis of obstruction is the history of weight loss owing to the patient's fear of eating because he knows the act will initiate abdominal pain. Constipation is more frequently complained of than diarrhea. Diarrhea often alternates with constipation and simulates a clinical pattern sometimes noted with carcinoma of the large intestine.

Bleeding from small-bowel tumors often is occult or is manifested by intermittent melena. Therefore, the patient with microcytic-hypochromic, iron-deficiency anemia may harbor a neoplasm in the small intestine. If investigation for more common causes such as carcinoma of the colon or peptic ulcer disease is negative, a barium x-ray examination of the small intestine should be performed. Tests of stool for occult blood, which are being used more frequently today, may aid in earlier recognition asymptomatic small-bowel tumors. Massive or life-threatening hemorrhage may occur, particularly from leiomyomas and hemangiomas, and necessitate emergency laparotomy. When the patient's condition permits, angiography may be helpful in diagnosing and localizing the bleeding tumor. The astute physician will consider benign or malignant small-bowel neoplasm in the differential diagnosis of GI bleeding, even when it is of great magnitude.

Some types of benign tumors are more prone to bleed, and at least one third of all tumors diagnosed clinically have bleeding. Leiomyomas and hemangiomas are particularly prone to develop this complication. As leiomyomas enlarge, they outgrow their blood supplies and develop necrosis of the tips. Approximately 25% of malignant tumors present with

bleeding. Adenocarcinomas and lymphosarcomas are the two neoplasms in this category that tend to bleed.

PHYSICAL EXAMINATION

Results of physical examination of the abdomen depend on the stage of the disease at which it is made and the complications caused by the intestinal tumor. Because partial or complete obstruction of the intestine is common, physical signs noted most often are abdominal distention, hyperactive bowel sounds, visible peristalsis, and signs of peritoneal irritation. Palpation of an intra-abdominal mass usually is an ominous finding, because it often indicates malignancy and/or a late stage of disease and suggests that the neoplasm is not amenable to curative resection. An exception is malignant lymphoma, which often presents as a palpable mass and yet is resectable because the lesion, even though quite large, is still localized to a segment of small intestine. Most palpable masses are movable unless the tumor has invaded surrounding structures and become fixed. The most favorable type of palpable mass is intussusception associated with benign small-bowel tumors. Signs of intestinal perforation, including abdominal distention, peritoneal irritation, hypoactive bowel sounds, or silent abdomen, usually are associated with malignant lymphomas or adenocarcinomas of the small intestine.

DIAGNOSTIC STUDIES: ROENTGENOLOGIC EXAMINATIONS

When clinical findings suggest the possibility of small-bowel tumor, the diagnosis may be confirmed by roentgenologic examination, but differential diagnosis of the specific pathologic type of neoplasm is not always possible on the basis of radiologic features alone. Review of roentgenographic examinations in which at least a lesion was suspected indicates that a diagnosis of small-bowel tumor can be made in 60%–90% of cases. In the past, such an examination has been performed prior to discovery of a tumor at operation, in only about 50% of symptomatic patients.

If significant obstruction has occurred, a roentgenogram of the abdomen without the use of contrast material may show evidence of it. The characteristic gaseous distention, "ladder effect," and presence of multiple fluid levels may be sufficient for diagnosis and a warning that other roentgenologic procedures are inadvisable.

Contrast material such as barium in suspension or a water-soluble iodinated compound can be employed in a number of ways. It can be given by mouth, introduced into the duodenum through a tube, or injected into a long tube that has been allowed to progress as far down the intestine as possible. In some cases, tumors in the terminal ileum can be visualized on barium enema when the contrast material refluxes into this segment of bowel.

Good[10] described the characteristic roentgenologic patterns seen with intestinal neoplasms. They include: (1) complete obstruction which is not specific for tumor but suggests the possibility; (2) intussusception of the small bowel which is identified by a narrow channel of barium with a "concentric ring" effect (although intussusception can be produced by lesions other than tumors, this finding in an adult commonly is secondary to either a benign or a malignant tumor; and (3) local filling defects in the opacified intestinal lumen which are either intraluminal (mucosal or ulcerating) or intramural.

Villous tumors are neoplasms that arise from columnar epithelium and account for approximately 1% of duodenal neoplasms (9 of 750 duodenal tumors at the Mayo Clinic).[10] On barium x-ray examination, their characteristic appearance consists of multiple radiolucent, rounded areas interspersed in a fine lacework of radiopaque material. This results from the barium entering clefts between the fine, frond-like projections of the tumors. This appearance has been called the "soap bubble." In contrast, smooth-walled defects in the proximal duodenum seen on roentgenograms suggest adenoma, leiomyoma, lipoma, neurogenic tumor, aberrant pancreatic tissue, prolapsed pyloric mucosa, and antegrade intussusception of pedunculated antral polyp.

Adenomatous polyp, leiomyoma, fibroma, and ganglioneuroma are seen most commonly as an intraluminal filling defect. The mucosal or ulcerating pattern indicates adenocarcinoma or malignant lymphoma whereas the intramural defect suggests benign or malignant leiomyomas, lipoma, hemangioma, and carcinoid.

It should be remembered that failure to demonstrate a tumor by roentgenologic examination of the small bowel does not exclude the diagnosis, because false negative results occur in 15%–30% of examinations.[10] Therefore, one must remain concerned about the patient with unexplained blood-loss anemia or symptoms of intestinal obstruction, even though initial roentgenographic studies are normal.

Objective evidence of partial or intermittent intestinal obstruction sometimes can be obtained by performing flat and upright x-rays of the abdomen the next time the patient has the onset of abdominal pain or discomfort. A few dilated loops of small intestine may be demonstrated by this technique even in patients who have had one or more negative barium studies.

OTHER DIAGNOSTIC STUDIES

Other studies such as hypotonic duodenography, enteroscopy with flexible fibroscope, ultrasonography, CT scanning of the abdomen, or angiography may be necessary to establish a diagnosis. Endoscopy has assumed an increasingly useful role for lesions in the duodenum, proximal jejunum, and even in the distal ileum. Angiography is of value in diagnosing and localizing tumors of vascular origin, such as hemangiomas, and some actively bleeding tumors. The rate of bleeding usually is lower than can be seen on angiography.

CT scanning of the abdomen is of particular value in demonstrating extraluminal tumors such as leiomyomas, leiomyosarcomas, and some lymphomas. This examination also can show large metastases in the small-bowel mesentery which may be associated with a carcinoid tumor so small that it cannot be seen on barium x-ray examination. Some tumors with definitive vascular patterns can be outlined when contrast material is injected. An example is one of the tumors of smooth muscle origin.

Despite all the diagnostic studies available today, there are

still some patients in whom exploratory laparotomy will be necessary to establish the diagnosis of neoplasm in the small intestine.

BENIGN TUMORS

Many benign tumors of the small bowel are asymptomatic and found only incidentally at laparotomy or autopsy. In the River et al.[6] review of 1,399 benign tumors, they noted that such tumors are found 15 times more frequently at autopsy than at surgery. When symptomatic, they produce the same array of symptoms and signs found with malignant neoplasms. In fact, there is little difference between the clinical manifestations of the two groups of tumors.

The six most common types of benign neoplasms are shown in Table 40–1. In many series, adenomatous polyp occurs most frequently. The more rare types of benign tumors include neurofibroma, Brunner's gland adenoma, adenomyoma, adenofibroma, lipoleiomyoma, cystadenoma, ganglioneuroma, myxoma, and nodular fibroma. A photograph of the latter type is shown in Figure 40–2.

Adenomatous polyps are the second most common benign neoplasm of the small bowel in surgical cases and they typically occur singly and are pedunculated. Good[10] reported a rather even distribution of these polyps with 21% in the duodenum, 36% in the jejunum, and 43% in the ileum. Because they often are pedunculated, they have a tendency to produce intussusception. In addition to this complication, bleeding is the other major problem. Clinical symptoms or signs occurred in fewer than 50% of patients in the Mayo Clinic series.[9]

LEIOMYOMAS

Leiomyomas arise from the muscular coat of the small intestine, and with growth they become predominantly subserosal, submucosal, or intraluminal. The major clinical concern with these tumors is bleeding, which River et al.[6] found in 67% of cases. Because central necrosis may erode an artery of significant size, this tumor is a frequent cause of the rare presentation of massive hemorrhage. The intraluminal type is another cause of intussusception.

LIPOMAS

Only 13% of lipomas of the GI tract occur in the small bowel, particularly the ileum. Their growth patterns are sim-

TABLE 40–1.—INCIDENCE OF BENIGN TUMORS OF THE SMALL BOWEL

TYPE OF NEOPLASM	NO. OF CASES (%)
Leiomyoma	120 (33.5)
Lipoma	67 (18.7)
Adenomatous polyp	67 (18.7)
Hemangioma	57 (15.9)
Lymphangioma	16 (4.5)
Fibroma	11 (3.1)
Other	20 (5.6)
Total	358 (100)

Moertel et al.[11]

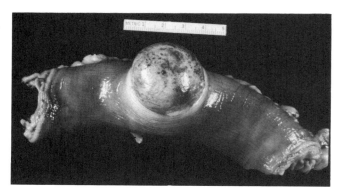

Fig 40–2.—Nodular fibroma of the jejunum, a rare benign tumor of the small intestine.

ilar to leiomyomas in that they may be located subserosally, submucosally, or become pedunculated within the lumen of the intestine.

BRUNNER'S GLAND ADENOMAS

Brunner's gland adenomas occur in the first and second parts of the duodenum and account for fewer than 10% of benign tumors in the duodenum. They are usually less than 1–2 cm in diameter. Occasionally, they become very large and produce symptoms of obstruction. The most common complication is bleeding. In 157 cases in the world literature (32 seen at the Mayo Clinic), malignancy was not noted.[12] Since these lesions are benign, the small adenomas can be removed by endoscopic means; if too large, they can be removed transduodenally, with care taken to avoid injury to the papilla or Vater.

GASTROINTESTINAL POLYPOSIS SYNDROMES

Of the various GI polyposis syndromes, there are four with which multiple polyps in the small bowel have been noted. They are familial polyposis coli, Gardner's Peutz-Jeghers, and Cronkhite-Canada.

The most common of these syndromes is familial polyposis coli, estimated to occur once in 8,300 births. There have been a few cases of this syndrome in which adenomatous polyps were noted in the small intestine.[13]

With Gardner's syndrome, adenomatous polyps also are located primarily in the colon, but they may occur occasionally in the stomach and small intestine. This syndrome, transmitted as an autosomal dominant trait, is reported to occur in 14,025 births.[13] Approximately 150 cases of Gardner's syndrome or closely related variants have been reported in the literature.[13] Features other than polyps are: (1) a variety of cutaneous and subcutaneous tumors, including epidermoid cysts and fibromas, (2) bone lesions, especially osteomas of the mandible and skull and exostoses and cortical thickening of the long bones, and (3) desmoid tumors in the abdominal wall and mesentery of the small bowel. The latter can cause serious problems of ureteral obstruction and intestinal obstruction, either of which can be extremely difficult to correct surgically. Schnur et al.[14] stated that the propensity to develop these fibrous masses is so great that such a complication

should be the first consideration when an incisional mass is present. The same authors reported that patients with Gardner's syndrome may develop duodenal polyps or adenocarcinomas or both. They recommend that roentgenograms of the upper portion of the GI tract be made a routine part of the follow-up examination of these patients. They further recommend that these patients should be advised to consult a physician on the development of any symptoms referable to the upper part of the GI tract.

Although the adenomatous polyps in both familial polyposis coli and Gardner's syndrome are of clinical significance, primarily because of the high incidence of colonic carcinoma developing over time, it should be remembered that occasionally, with these rare syndromes, polyps may be present in the small intestine.

Of more clinical interest in discussion of small-bowel tumors is the Peutz-Jeghers syndrome in which the tumors are hamartomas rather than adenomatous polyps, and they occur throughout the GI tract, but are most common in the jejunum and ileum (Fig 40–3). This polyposis syndrome is inherited as a single dominant pleiotropic gene with a high degree of penetrance. The other features are mucocutaneous pigmentation (melanin spots) on the face, lips, buccal mucosa, palms, soles, and perianal area. An association of carcinomas of the GI tract is uncommon and is estimated to occur in only 2%–3% of cases. Treatment should be conservative and directed only at complications caused by the hamartomas in the small bowel, the most common of which are bleeding from infarction of the intraluminal hamartomas or obstruction of the intestine by intussusception. Preventive surgery does not seem warranted and often is not feasible. There is a recent report[15] of endoscopic removal of polyps in a patient with this syndrome who required operation for removal of a large polyp. An endoscope was passed both directions through an enterotomy, and four smaller polyps were removed satisfactorily using electrosurgical technique.

There are fewer than 50 documented cases of Cronkhite-Canada syndrome,[13] in which polyps are generalized, especially in the stomach and colon, but sometimes in the small bowel. This syndrome, which does not seem to be inherited and has an average onset of 60 years, also included cutaneous

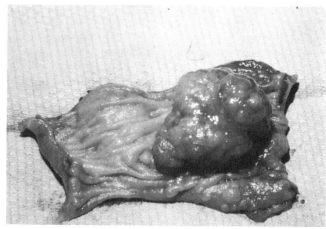

Fig 40–3.—Hamartoma of the jejunum from a patient with Peutz-Jeghers syndrome.

hyperpigmentation, alopecia, and onychodystrophy.

Patients with neurofibromatosis may have neurofibromas in the small intestines, particularly the jejunum.

ADULT COELIAC DISEASE AND MALIGNANT SMALL-BOWEL TUMOR

It is now recognized that patients with coeliac disease are at greater risk than the general population to develop malignant neoplasms of the small intestine, especially lymphomas. The association of small-bowel lymphoma with established coeliac disease was reviewed recently by Swinson and co-workers.[16] Of 259 histologically confirmed malignancies in 235 patients with histologically proven coeliac disease, 133 were malignant lymphomas. Patients with coeliac disease also are at increased risk of developing adenocarcinoma of the small intestine. As reported by Swinson et al.,[16] the mucosal damage in coeliac disease may make the small intestine more permeable to environmental carcinogens.

MALIGNANT TUMORS

Malignant tumors are found most commonly in the fifth to seventh decades of life and occur in approximately equal distribution between males and females. The clinical presentation of malignant tumors of the small bowel include weight loss, abdominal pain, obstruction, GI bleeding, and perforation. There is no symptom complex that is specific. Wilson and co-workers[17] reported the most frequent symptoms in 808 patients were weight loss (39%), obstruction (30%), bleeding (23%), and abdominal pain (20%).

Duration of symptoms varies from a few days to several years before diagnosis. The delay in diagnosis is less with duodenal than with more distal small-bowel tumors. This probably reflects the fact that tumors in the duodenum may have more specific associated problems, such as jaundice, and the tumors in this location are easier to visualize by x-ray examination or endoscopy.

In a collected series[7] of 2,144 malignant small bowel tumors, the distribution of the major histologic types was adenocarcinoma (50%), carcinoid (39%), and sarcoma (11%). The relative types of tumors in a collected series compiled by the author is shown in Table 40-2.

Less common malignant tumors include hemangiopericy-toma, fibrosarcoma, plasmacytoma, angiosarcoma, liposarcoma, hemangioendothelioma, and lymphangioendothelioma.

Malignant small bowel tumors have been reported in association with Crohn's disease, villous adenoma, adult coeliac disease, and Gardner's syndrome. The distribution of the four major types of malignant tumors in the small intestine is shown in Table 40-3.

Adenocarcinomas

Primary adenocarcinoma of the small bowel, first reported by Hamburger in 1746,[1] accounts for 0.3% of all malignant neoplasms of the GI tract and is the most common of the malignant tumors of the small bowel that produce symptoms or signs. Arising from the mucosa of the intestine, they tend to enlarge as a polypoid endoluminal mass or as an anular constricting lesion.

Some adenocarcinomas appear to arise from villous adenomas in the small intestine. In a series[27] of 20 patients with villous adenomas of the duodenum collected from the literature by Miller and Herrman, 5 contained invasive carcinoma, 2 focal cancer, and 1 in situ carcinoma.

As of 1976, 35 patients with adenocarcinoma associated with regional enteritis had been reported.[28]

Lymphomas

Malignant lymphoid tumors may involve the GI tract either as primary growths or as manifestations of generalized lymphomatous disease. The nomenclature of these tumors varies because of differences in interpretation of cell types, cell maturity, and practical difficulties of distinguishing early neoplastic changes from hyperplastic changes. Naqvi et al.[29] reported 162 cases of lymphoma of the gastrointestinal tract and classified them as follows: stage I: a tumor confined to a single focus in the GI tract without nodal involvement; stage II: a tumor confined to a single focus in the GI tract with node involvement, but without perforation or peritonitis; stage III: a tumor confined to a single focus in the GI tract but invading adjacent structures, such as the pancreas, without free perforation or peritonitis; and stage IV: a tumor in the GI tract with distant metastasis. Of the 162 cases they reported, 27% were in the small intestine, and the overall five-year survival in this subgroup was 33%. Within each stage, results were better with Hodgkin's disease and giant follicular lymphoma

TABLE 40-2.—Pathologic Types of Malignant Tumors of Small Intestine

SERIES	ADENOCARCINOMA	CARCINOID	LYMPHOMA	LEIOMYOSARCOMA
Aranha et al.[18]	9	23	8	2
Awrich et al.[19]	26	28	18	9
Braasch and Denbo[20]	60	16	8	7
Brookes et al.[21]	55	32	43	13
Darling and Welch[8]	33	15	29	9
Ebert and Zuidema[22]	20	5	—	4
Goel et al.[23]	21	15	9	10
Pagtalunan et al.[9]	92	46	39	33
Miles et al.[24]	16	31	15	10
Norberg and Emas[25]	11	8	—	9
Silberman et al.[26]	19	8	1	4
Wilson et al.[17]	48	37	25	11
Total (%)	410 (41)	264 (26)	195 (20)	121 (13)

TABLE 40–3.—DISTRIBUTION OF MALIGNANT
TUMORS OF SMALL INTESTINE*

TUMOR	DUODENUM	JEJUNUM	ILEUM	TOTAL
Adenocarcinoma	157	140	69	366
Carcinoid	24	17	174	215
Lymphoma	2	74	80	156
Leiomyosarcoma	16	48	35	99

*Collected series of cases.[8, 9, 18–26]

than with lymphosarcoma or reticulum cell sarcoma. They recommend removal of the tumor and as much of the secondary spread as possible, and consideration of postoperative radiation therapy and/or chemotherapy. These measures are usually applied when nodes are positive or resection is incomplete.

The four main types of lymphomas by histology are lymphocytic or lymphoblastic, reticulum cell sarcoma or lymphosarcoma, follicular, and Hodgkin's disease. All types may produce chronic intestinal obstruction or may present with malabsorption, intussusception, or perforation.

Leiomyosarcoma

Leiomyosarcomas are the fourth most common malignancies of the small bowel, and they occur most commonly in the jejunum (see Table 40–3). These neoplasms, usually round or ovoid, arise from the muscular layers of the intestinal wall and, therefore, usually are subserosal or exoenteric. Starr and Dockerty[30] studied 41 leiomyosarcomas of the small intestine and found that the majority were of low histologic degree of malignancy (Broder's grades 1 or 2). This fact suggests a favorable prognosis might be anticipated with treatment, but it also accounts for the long interval before the patient becomes aware of this slow-growing tumor.

There is a high incidence of bleeding from leiomyosarcomas because these tumors have a tendency to outgrow their blood supplies and develop central necrosis and mucosal ulceration. Of all small-bowel tumors, leiomyosarcomas are most likely to cause intussusception of the small intestine. Therefore, acute intestinal obstruction with a palpable intra-abdominal mass is the second most common type of clinical presentation.

Although these neoplasms are slow-growing, they do metastasize via the bloodstream in the advanced stages and produce peritoneal implants. The lack of lymphatic metastases eliminates the need for extensive removal of the mesentery when segmental small-bowel resection is performed.

In the duodenum, leiomyosarcoma occurs one tenth less commonly than adenocarcinoma in this location. Even when located in the second part of the duodenum, jaundice is infrequently a presenting sign. If the leiomyosarcoma is in the first or second part of the duodenum, pancreaticoduodenectomy is usually the procedure of choice. If the tumor is small and is in the third or fourth portions of the duodenum, a distal duodenal resection with preservation of the pancreas may be done. Even though the neoplasm is often large at the time of operation, distant metastasis may not have occurred. For this reason, aggressive surgical treatment is indicated in the management of patients with leiomyosarcomas.

Carcinoids

Carcinoid tumors arise from the argentaffin cells situated in the crypts of Lieberkühn. In the older literature there are reports of "benign" carcinoids, but today it is appreciated that these tumors are malignant. Because they have the tendency to grow slowly and remain small in size, many are asymptomatic. The most common clinical presentation is chronic progressive construction of the bowel usually due to kinking of the intestinal wall caused by mesenteric fibrosis and retraction of tumor infiltration.

Carcinoids commonly are smaller than 2 cm in diameter, submucosal in location, and multiple in one third of patients. They tend to spread via the lymphatics to the liver, but more distant metastases are uncommon.

The frequency of occurrence of carcinoids increases from duodenum to ileum, particularly the distal ileum. More than 90% of 152 carcinoids in the Mayo Clinic series[31] were located in the latter site. Of 158 patients with GI carcinoids diagnosed and treated at the Mayo Clinic between 1972 and 1982,[32] 43% were in the ileum, 6% in the jejunum, and 2% in the duodenum; 59% of these patients were asymptomatic. In the collected series shown in Table 40–3, the major site of occurrence was the ileum (81%).

Carcinoid tumors secrete a variety of biochemical substances including serotonins, kinins, histamine, and ACTH. This capability underlies the fascinating malignant carcinoid syndrome that was first documented by Cassidy[33] in 1934. This syndrome, which occurs in about 10% of patients with carcinoid tumors, represents the final clinical stage of the tumor, the most "benign" malignant neoplasm of the small intestine. It usually occurs only in patients with hepatic metastases, but can occur with tumors in the retroperitoneum, ovary, testicle, or lungs from which venous drainage bypasses the hepatic portal system.

Cutaneous flushing is the clinical hallmark, and classically this is an episode of erythema involving the face, neck, and upper chest and having the appearance of a blush. Flushing often is precipitated by ingestion of food or alcohol or by pressure on the abdomen. This may be accompanied by a fall in the systolic and diastolic blood pressure and an increase in heart rate. Patients may have respiratory distress similar to asthma or digestive disturbances such as diarrhea, the most common symptom. Far too often patients with carcinoids are regarded as having psychosomatic problems during the years they suffer from intermittent symptoms of small-bowel obstruction and the nature of the disease is recognized only when flushing heralds incurability.

Thorson and co-workers[34] established the precise correlation between carcinoid tumor and the clinical manifestations of the malignant carcinoid syndrome. Serotonin, the principal active product of ileal carcinoid is the mediatro of the syndrome. The principal excretory product of serotonin metabolism is 5-hydroxyindoleacetic acid (5-HIAA), and increased concentration of this in the urine establishes the diagnosis of carcinoid syndrome.

Metastatic Tumor: Solitary

Single metastatic lesions to the small bowel are encountered less frequently than primary malignancy, but the clinical presentations are similar; that is, obstruction or bleeding. Malignant melanoma, hypernephroma, and Kaposi's sarcoma are the three most common neoplasms that produce isolated or single metastases in the small intestine. Malignant melanoma is found more commonly in the duodenum than in the jejunum or ileum (Fig 40–4). If a patient's life expectancy is reasonably good, operation to relieve hemorrhage or obstruction may achieve significant palliation.

SURGICAL TREATMENT

Surgical treatment of malignant tumors of the small intestine is resection. For lesions in the jejunum and proximal ileum, en bloc resection of a segment of small bowel, with adequate margins of clearance on each end and adjacent wedge of mesentery to include regional lymph nodes, is the procedure of choice. The latter is less important in cases with leiomyosarcoma because the lymph nodes usually are not involved. Excessive mesenteric resection should be avoided in all cases to reduce extensive loss of small intestine. Tumors in the terminal part of the ileum are managed by right hemicolectomy and ileotransverse colostomy. For malignant lesions in the duodenum, radial pancreaticoduodenectomy (Whipple procedure) is the procedure of choice. For neoplasms in the third and fourth parts of the duodenum, distal duodenal resection with preservation of the pancreas is an attractive alternative.

When curative resection is not deemed possible because of widespread metastases, less radical resection of malignant tumors in the jejunum or ileum may offer significant palliation by relieving obstruction and eliminating a site of bleeding or the possibility of subsequent perforation.

Intussusception secondary to malignant tumor should be resected, but if this complication is associated with a benign tumor, it is possible sometimes to reduce the intussusception

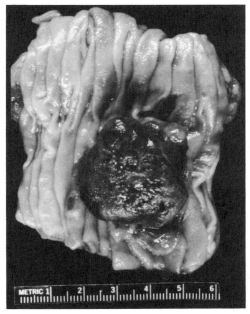

Fig 40–4.—Metastatic malignant melanoma of the jejunum.

and then locally remove the tumor through an enterotomy.

Benign tumors in the small bowel frequently can be removed by local resection, but when they involve a large area of the intestinal wall, limited resection of a segment of bowel and enteroenterostomy (end-to-end) is preferable.

The dramatic symptoms associated with the malignant carcinoid syndrome may be abolished by surgical treatment which includes hepatic resection of the metastases and hepatic artery ligation with or without infusion of a chemotherapeutic agent. Of five patients who underwent hepatic resection at the Mayo Clinic,[35] all but one had metastases confined to a single lobe of the liver. The procedures included wedge resection, subsegmental resection of the left lobe, and formal left lobectomy. All patients experienced cessation of facial flushing and diarrhea. In four patients the 5-HIAA level returned to normal and remained so. Two patients died during the follow-up period (mean 32 months), one of metastatic carcinoid tumor after 31 months and the other of myocardial infarction after 46 months. The other three patients were alive 12, 39, and 45 months after operation.

Seven patients with carcinoid tumors metastatic to the liver, six with primaries in the ileum, underwent hepatic artery ligation and cholecystectomy, a concept of management that has become of interest in recent years. All patients had relief of symptoms and improvement in quality of life, but the duration of response to ligation was only five to seven months.

The best response rates with chemotherapy[35] have been only about 26% for a single agent (fluorouracil) and 33% for combination treatment (fluorouracil and streptozotocin), with median duration of response of three and seven months, respectively.

Currently, Martin and co-workers[35] are using a combination of hepatic devascularization and infusion chemotherapy. After ligation of the hepatic artery, a catheter is inserted distal to the ligature and positioned proximal to the hepatic artery bifurcation. Initially, the liver is perfused with heparinized saline; after the liver function returns to normal, chemotherapy is begun. They are using a single course of doxorubicin by hepatic artery infusion plus systemic dacarbazine. This is followed by alternating courses of systemic fluorouracil plus streptozotocin and systemic doxorubicin plus dacarbazine. It will be interesting to review the results of this new approach to management of patients with malignant carcinoid when they become available.

Although infrequent in occurrence, metastases of small-bowel carcinoid into the adjacent mesentery can be so extensive that they will produce ischemia of a long segment of the small intestine. Patients with this rare complication present with signs and symptoms of intestinal ischemia and a large, firm, palpable mass secondary to the extensive mesenteric involvement. This problem has been diagnosed accurately as metastatic carcinoid by radiologists performing angiography on patients thought to have ischemic bowel disease.

ENDOSCOPIC POLYPECTOMY

Recently, fiberoptic endoscopic polypectomy has been reported by Sweeney and Anderson.[15] Polyps in the duodenum, jejunum, and distal ileum have been removed and retrieved by this technique. Patients included have had single duodenal polyps and polyps associated with Gardner's syndrome and Peutz-Jeghers syndrome. The safety and efficacy of endoscopic polyp removal should be satisfactory. With the availability of the two-channel enteroscope, polypectomy in the small intestine undoubtedly will become more common in the future.

PROGNOSIS

Prognosis with benign tumors is excellent. Exceptions to this general statement are vascular tumors (hemangiomas), which may be difficult to locate in the small intestine, and complications that can develop with Gardner's syndrome.

Prognosis with malignant neoplasms is another matter. Because there is considerable variation in the behavior or natural history of malignant small-bowel tumors, overall five-year survival figures for all patients are not particularly useful. Such data emphasize the magnitude of the problem and the advanced stage of disease when operation is performed.

Overall five-year survival rates for all patients with malignant tumors is approximately 30%–35%. The five-year survival rates for patients with malignant duodenal tumors ranges from 0% to 30%,[29, 36] whereas they range from 29% to 33% for ileal lesions.[20,36]

Information about survival after surgery for each type of malignancy is of greater clinical value than knowledge of survival for all patients with the various types of tumors. The report of Awrich et al.[19] emphasizes this point and illustrates the fact that long-term results following curative resection of malignant tumors, particulary carcinoids, are quite rewarding (Table 40–4).

Reduced survival rates in most series are attributed to delay in diagnosis and the presence of metastases at the time of diagnosis. Ebert and Zuidema[22] reported that 69% of their patients had metastasis at the time of operation.

ADENOCARCINOMAS

Adenocarcinoma, which constitutes about 40% of all primary malignancies of the small bowel, carries the worst prognosis. In Morgan and Busuttil's series,[37] the median survival from time of diagnosis was only 10.5 months, and 55% of the patients were dead within 24 months. There were no five-year survivors. Goel and co-workers[23] noted a median survival of 25.5 months. Sixty-five percent (42 of 62 patients) in Ouriel and Adams' series[36] were considered amenable to curative resection, and the overall five-year survival was 30% by actuarial methods. When nodes were negative, 70% of patients were alive at five years, whereas only 13% of patients with

TABLE 40–4.—MALIGNANT TUMORS OF SMALL BOWEL: FIVE-YEAR SURVIVAL AFTER SURGERY (%)*

TUMOR TYPE	OVERALL	AFTER CURATIVE RESECTION
Adenocarcinoma	26	50
Carcinoid	47	100
Lymphoma	33	33
Leiomyosarcoma	37	50

*Awrich et al.[19]

positive nodes lived as long. These results compare favorably with the 19%–31% survival following resection reported by others.[7, 8, 23, 25]

CARCINOIDS

In a recent survey (1972–82) at the Mayo Clinic,[32] the overall five-year survival for patients with ileal carcinoid was 62%. Unfortunately, 18 patients (13%) with ileal carcinoid had hepatic metastases and 50% of them were dead within five years. These statistics are similar to those reported by others and they emphasize that the chance of survival after surgery depends on the stage of disease at time of operation. When the carcinoid is localized to the primary site, the five-year survival approaches 100%.

Leiomyosarcomas

In the largest single published group,[9] 15% of 31 patients (48%) survived five years after diagnosis. This more favorable result may relate to the fact that the majority of these tumors are of low histologic degree of malignancy (Broder's grades 1 or 2), and distant metastases occurred less commonly at time of operation.

Lymphomas

Naqvi and co-workers[29] reported a 33% overall five-year survival of 43 patients who had lymphomas of the small intestine. Within each stage, results were better with Hodgkin's disease and giant follicular lymphoma than with lymphosarcoma or reticulum cell sarcoma. One of the best five-year survival rates (48%) was reported by Fu and Perzin.[38] These authors advocate radical surgical resection as the primary treatment, with addition of radiotherapy if the regional lymph nodes or surgical margins are involved.

Survival statistics also depend on the stage of disease. As one might expect, the best results occur when the tumors are contained locally and the worst results when the lesions have invaded surrounding structures or there is evidence of disease elsewhere.

HELPFUL DIAGNOSTIC TIPS

1. Perforation of the small bowel suggests leiomyosarcoma, lymphoma, or adenocarcinoma.

2. Bleeding as a presenting sign often is associated with hemangioma, leiomyosarcoma, and adenocarcinoma.

3. Intussusception may indicate leiomyoma or adenomatous polyp.

4. A palpable intra-abdominal mass suggests leiomyosarcoma, lymphoma, or intussusception may be the cause.

5. Obstruction in the ileum is most often due to carcinoid, whereas obstruction in the jejunum or proximal ileum usually is secondary to adenocarcinoma, leiomyosarcoma, or lymphoma.

6. Upper GI series are almost uniformly unsuccessful in detecting hemangiomas or nonobstructing carcinoids.

7. Pigmentation in derioral or buccal distribution suggests Peutz-Jeghers syndrome.

8. Angiomas of the mouth or skin indicate the possibility of angiomas in the small bowel (Rendu-Osler-Weber syndrome).

9. Neurofibromas in small bowel occur with von Reckling-hausen's disease, or neurofibromatosis.

10. Flushing of skin of the head and neck, diarrhea, and asthma should alert one to the malignant carcinoid syndrome.

SUMMARY

Although tumors of the small intestine occur infrequently, they invariably present difficult problems in diagnosis and treatment. Many of them, particularly the malignant ones, produce serious complications, and the associated mortality is greater than with malignant neoplasms in other sites in the GI tract.

The critical factor in reducing morbidity and mortality associated with small bowel tumors is early recognition of the lesions. Unfortunately, diagnosis often is delayed or missed in many cases for the following reasons: (1) Symptoms are frequently absent until significant complications have developed. When symptoms are present, they may be so vague and nonspecific that a tumor is not suspected. (2) Physical examination may not provide any valuable clues to diagnosis other than signs of bowel obstruction or chronic anemia. (3) Roentgenologic examination of the small intestine may fail to demonstrate an existing tumor. (4) The numerous types of neoplasms found in the small bowel produce various clinical manifestations, many of which are not recognized as clues to diagnosis.

The only adequate treatment of tumors of the small intestine is complete surgical excision. When a definitive type of procedure is possible, segmental resection of the bowel including as much of the adjacent mesentery as reasonable, is the treatment of choice for lesions located in the jejunum and proximal ileum. Malignancies located in the distal part of the ileum require a right hemicolectomy to ensure adequate removal of the venous and lymphatic drainage field. Malignant neoplasms of the duodenum are treated best by radical pancreaticoduodenectomy (Whipple procedure).

Unfortunately, 30%–50% of malignant tumors of the small bowel are not excisable with the hope of cure at the time of surgical intervention, because they have already metastasized widely to mesenteric lymph nodes or beyond. In these cases, palliative resection should be performed, if possible, to eliminate a site of bleeding or to relieve obstruction.

Surgical removal of benign tumors is indicated under most circumstances because complications occur frequently and the benign character of the lesion cannot be determined with certainty. Although local excision suffices in most instances, segmental resection sometimes is required because of the size of the tumor.

The future challenge in the management of patients with tumors of the small intestine is earlier recognition of their presence. It is hoped that physicians will have a higher index of suspicion and a greater awareness to pursue the diagnosis even when initial studies are normal. Only in this way will it be possible for surgical treatment to provide more satisfactory results.

REFERENCES

1. Hamburger G.: *De Ruptura Intestine Duodeni.* Jena Ritterianis, 1746.

2. Leichtenstern O.: *Handbuch des speciellen Pathologie and Therapie.* Leipzig, F.C.W. Vogel, 1876, p. 523.

3. Johnson R.: Carcinoma of the jejunum and ileum. *Br. J. Surg.* 9:422, 1921.

4. Judd E.S.: Carcinoma of the small intestine. *Lancet.* 39:159, 1919.

5. Rankin F.W., Mayo C. II.: Carcinoma of the small bowel. *Surg. Gynecol. Obstet.* 50:939, 1930.

6. River L., Silverstein J., Tope J.W.: Benign neoplasms of the small intestine: A critical comprehensive review with reports of 20 new cases. *Int. Abstr. Surg.* 102:1, 1956.

7. Rochlin D.B., Longmire W.P. Jr.: Primary tumors of the small intestine. *Surgery* 50:586, 1961.

8. Darling R.C., Welch C.E.: Tumors of the small intestine. *N. Engl. J. Med.* 260:397, 1959.

9. Pagtalunan P.J.G., Mayo C.W., Dockerty M.B.: Primary malignant tumors of small intestine. *Am. J. Surg.* 108:13, 1964.

10. Good C.A.: Tumors of the small intestine: Caldwell Lecture, 1962. *A.J.R.* 89:685, 1963.

11. Moertel C.G., Sauer W.G., Dockerty M.B., et al.: Life history of carcinoid tumor of small intestine. *Cancer.* 14:901, 1961.

12. Orkin B.A., McIlrath D.C. Unpublished data.

13. Schwabe A.D., Lewin K.J.: Gastrointestinal polyposis syndromes, in *Viewpoints on Digestive Disease.* vol. 12, No. 1, January 1980.

14. Schnur P.L., David E., Brown P.W., et al.: Adenocarcinoma of the duodenum and the Gardner's syndrome. *J.A.M.A.* 223:1229, 1973.

15. Sweeney B.F., Anderson D.S.: Endoscopic removal of duodenal polyp in a patient with Gardner's syndrome. *Dig. Dis. Sci.* 27:557, 1982.

16. Swinson C.M., Slavin G., Coles E.C., et al.: Coeliac disease and malignancy. *Lancet* 1:111, 1983.

17. Wilson J.M., Melvin D.B., Gray G.F., et al.: Primary malignancies of small bowel: A report of 96 cases and review of the literature. *Ann. Surg.* 180:175, 1974.

18. Aranha G.V., Reyes C.V., Lindert D.J., et al.: Primary tumors of small intestine. *Am. Surg.* 45:495, 1979.

19. Awrich A.E., Irish C.E., Vetto R.M., et al.: A twenty-five year experience with primary malignant tumors of the small intestine. *Surg. Gynecol. Obstet.* 151:9, 1980.

20. Braasch J.W., Denbo H.E.: Tumors of the small intestine, *Surg. Clin. North Am.* 44:791, 1964.

21. Brookes V.S., Waterhouse J.A.H., Powel D.J.: Malignant lesions of the small intestine. *Br. J. Surg.* 55:405, 1968.

22. Ebert P.A., Zuidema G.D.: Primary tumors of the small intestine. *Arch. Surg.* 91:452, 1965.

23. Goel I.P., Didolkar M.S., Elias E.G.: Primary malignant tumors of the small intestine. *Surg. Gynecol. Obstet.* 143:717, 1976.

24. Miles R.M., Crawford D., Duras S.: The small bowel tumor problem. *Ann. Surg.* 189:732, 1979.

25. Norberg K., Emas S.; Primary tumors of the small intestine. *Am. J. Surg.* 142:569, 1981.

26. Silberman H., Crichlow R.W., Caplan H.S.: Neoplasms of the small bowel. *Ann. Surg.* 180:157, 1974.

27. Miller E.R., Herrman W.W.: Argentaffin tumors of small bowel: Roentgen sign of malignant change. *Radiology* 39:214, 1942.

28. Tyers G.F.O. Steiger E., Dudrick S.J.: Adenocarcinoma of the small intestine complicating regional enteritis: Case report and review of the literature. *Ann. Surg.* 169:510, 1969.

29. Naqvi M.S., Burrows M.D., Kark A.E.: Lymphoma of the gastrointestinal tract. *Ann. Surg.* 170:221, 1969.

30. Starr G.F., Dockerty M.B.: Leiomyomas and leiomyosarcoma of the small intestine. *Cancer* 8:101, 1955.

31. Moertel C.G., Dockerty M.B., Judd E.S.: Carcinoid tumors of the vermiform appendix. *Cancer* 21:270, 1968.

32. Thompson G.B., van Heerden J.A., Martin J.K. Jr., et al.: Unpublished data.

33. Cassidy M.A.: Abdominal carcinomatosis associated with vasomotor disturbances. *Proc. R. Soc. Med.* 27:220, 1934.

34. Thorson A., Bjork G., Bjorkmann G., et al.: Malignant carcinoid of the small intestine with metastases to liver, valvular disease of the right side of the heart (pulmonary stenosis and tricuspid re-

gurgitation without septal defects), peripheral vasomotor symptoms, bronchoconstriction, and an unusual type of cyanosis. *Am. Heart J.* 44:795, 1954.

35. Martin J.K. Jr., Moertel C.G., Adson M.A., et al.: Surgical treatment of functioning metastatic carcinoid tumors. *Arch. Surg.* 118:537, 1983.

36. Ouriel K., Adams J.T.: Adenocarcinoma of the small intestine. *Am. J. Surg.* 147:66, 1984.

37. Morgan D.F., Busuttil R.W.: Primary adenocarcinoma of the small intestine. *Am. J. Surg.* 134:331, 1977.

38. Fu Y., Perzin K.H.: Lymphosarcoma of the small intestine, a clinicopathologic study. *Cancer* 29:645, 1972.

41

Acute Appendicitis

Robert E. Condon, M.D.

The appendix is a vestigial, dispensable organ. Its major importance in human medicine is the propensity of this bit of intestine to cause major mischief through the clinical syndrome we recognize as acute appendicitis. Acute appendicitis is a relatively common cause of abdominal pain at all ages, and is the most frequent cause of an "acute abdomen" in teenagers. Because it is relatively so common, and because all of its manifestations can prove so diagnostically confusing, acute appendicitis has become the classic disease on which teaching of the differential diagnosis of an "acute abdomen" is based.

The incidence of acute appendicitis has been decreasing steadily during the past half century.[1, 2] The yearly incidence of appendicitis is now about 10 per 100,000 population, and the overall future risk of developing appendicitis has fallen to approximately 7%. The comparable figures at the turn of the century were 15 in 100,000, with a future risk of about 15% during lifetime. Although appendectomy in past years accounted for up to 5% of all surgical operations, at present much fewer than 1% of all general surgery operations are for appendicitis.[3–5] Data for recent years in one of the teaching hospitals of the Medical College of Wisconsin are presented in Figure 41–1.

Appendicitis is relatively rare in infancy, becomes increasingly common during childhood, and reaches its maximal incidence in the late teens and early twenties (Fig 41–2). The incidence then declines throughout adulthood, although appendicitis continues to occur at old age. Among teenagers and young adults there is a slight excess of males affected, but after age 25 this differential incidence also progressively declines: from the fourth decade onward, the sex ratio is equal.

Mortality has decreased to less than 1 in 100,000 persons annually. The mortality risk of acute but not gangrenous appendicitis is less than 0.1%; in gangrenous appendicitis, this risk rises to about 0.6%. The mortality of perforated appendicitis is approximately 5% today, much less than the risk of over 50% a half century ago. Although mortality of appendicitis has declined progressively, morbidity of appendicitis continues to be high. Overall, complications occur in 10% of all patients with appendicitis; wound infection accounts for one third of all morbidity. The presence of gangrene increases the morbidity risk fivefold, and the presence of perforation increases it more than tenfold; wound infection rates of 20%–40% are reported with perforated appendicitis.

Over the past two decades, there has been a changing clinical pattern in appendicitis. Patients at the extremes of age tend to come to the hospital at later stages of appendicitis with a concomitant increase in the incidence of perforation and its associated morbidity (Fig 41–3). While the current overall mortality risk of appendicitis is less than 1%, the proportion of fatal cases is six times as great in perforated appendicitis as in those operated on at an earlier stage.[6, 7] Death in those with a perforated appendix is usually due directly to appendicitis, while death in patients with an unperforated appendix is most commonly related to the effects of a concomitant disease. The role that delay in diagnosis and treatment plays in mortality and serious morbidity needs to be emphasized. In cases in which the diagnosis is uncertain, observation until typical or definite symptoms appear is often ill-advised. Exploration to discover the cause of more minimal but unexplained symptoms, especially in poor-risk patients at the extremes of life, is safer than waiting.[7, 8]

HISTORICAL ASPECTS

The history of appendicitis is a curiosity. Although man presumably has carried an appendix and been subject to appendicitis for millenia, appendicitis as a diagnosed entity was not recorded in the medical literature until about 500 years ago. Meade,[9] in his review of the surgical history of appendicitis, credits the French physician Jean Fernel with the first description of a case of perforated appendicitis. The first appendectomy, according to Richardson,[10] was performed by Claudius Amyand, Master of the Company of Barber Surgeons, in 1736. Amyand operated on a boy with a fecal fistula of the scrotum: on opening the scrotum, he found an appendix perforated by a pin; he removed both, repaired the hernia, drained the fistula, and the boy recovered. Over the years, despite isolated reports of similar instances, if any diagnosis was applied in cases of appendicitis it was typhlitis, or inflammation of the cecum, and it resulted in the death of the patient. The position prior to the 19th century is epitomized by the remark of John Hunter that "it was impossible to diagnose appendicitis during life."

In 1824, Louyer-Villermay[11] reported two cases of appendicitis, and Melier in 1827[12] reported four additional cases of acute appendicitis and first correctly described the origin of "purulent iliac tumor," in reality a periappendiceal abscess,

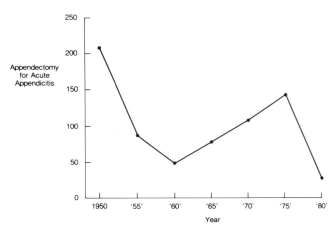

Fig 41–1.—The incidence of acute appendicitis and of appendectomy in Milwaukee County General Hospital shows a generally downward trend over the past 30 years.

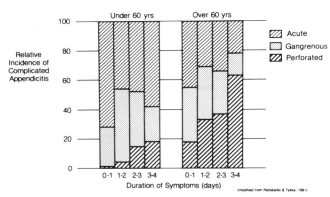

Fig 41–3.—At all ages, the risk of developing perforated appendicitis increases with the duration of symptoms. However, the relative risk of developing perforation regardless of the duration of symptoms is much higher in patients who are over 60 years of age.

as beginning with inflammation in the appendix. But Dupuytren, the leading surgeon of the day in Paris, vigorously opposed the new notion of acute appendicitis and, by weight of his authority, succeeded in preventing acceptance of appendicitis as a disease entity by his generation of physicians.

Throughout the 19th century, largely as the result of increased use of autopsy examinations, there began to be increasing awareness of the various stages of appendicitis, correlated with a more accurate perception of the early clinical signs and symptoms of appendicitis. But surgeons were still reluctant to treat appendicitis until an abscess had formed and could be drained. Reginald Fitz,[13] in 1886, defined clinical appendicitis and strongly suggested that early appendectomy was essential to cure; thereafter, surgeons began to operate with less reluctance although controversy continued into the 20th century. Nicholas Senn,[14] Professor in the Milwaukee Institute of Anatomy and Surgery, was the first surgeon to correctly diagnose acute appendicitis prior to rupture, to perform an urgent appendectomy and have the patient recover, and to report his experience.

By the end of the 19th century, acute appendicitis routinely was being diagnosed prior to rupture, and appendectomy was being performed at earlier and earlier stages in the disease. In 1902, just before his scheduled coronation, Edward, the

Prince of Wales, developed appendicitis. He had an appendectomy, recovered rapidly, and was crowned six weeks later. The future king's rapid recovery greatly helped acceptance of early appendectomy as the proper treatment of acute appendicitis.

There continued to be differences of opinion among surgeons regarding management of patients with generalized peritonitis following rupture of the appendix. The two schools of thought can be epitomized by the names of two prominent Chicago surgeons, John B. Murphy and A. J. Ochsner. Murphy[15] taught that the appendix always should be removed whether generalized peritonitis was present or not. Ochsner,[16] on the other hand, counseled delay of operation, bedrest, opiates to paralyze the bowel, and clyses to maintain fluid balance. Only when the inflammatory process had localized was operation performed and the abscess drained. Debate about management of a perforated appendix continues to some degree today.

ANATOMICAL FEATURES

The appendix arises from the inferior tip of the cecum. Suppression of development of this apical segment of the cecum during fetal growth causes appendicular hypoplasia or agenesis.[17, 18] Doubling of the appendix may occur as a part of intestinal duplication,[19] or by persistence of an outgrowth from the cecal wall which characterizes the 32-mm embryo but which normally disappears subsequently.[20]

At birth, the cecum and appendix have an infantile contour in which the appendix is shaped like an inverted pyramid, broad at its junction with the cecum but narrow at its tip; differential growth produces the typical tubular appendix by about age 2 years. During infancy and early childhood, more rapid growth of the right and anterior portions of the cecum results in rotation of the appendix posteriorly and medially to its adult intraperitoneal but retrocecal position.

The appendix averages 10 cm in length in adults, although it is not uncommon to find an appendix that is shorter or one more than 20 cm in length. The narrow lumen of the appendix is lined by colonic epithelium. At birth, there are a few

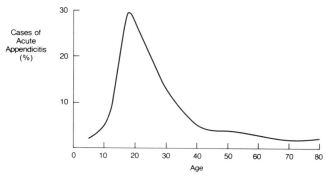

Fig 41–2.—Appendicitis is most common among teenagers and young adults. Nearly one third of patients with appendicitis are between ages 17 and 20.

lymphoid follicles present in the submucosa: these gradually increase to a peak of approximately 200 submucosal lymphoid follicles between the ages of 12 and 20. After age 30, there is a relatively abrupt reduction in the number of follicles to fewer than 100, and thereafter a progressive decrease to a trace or total absence of lymphoid tissue in the appendix after age 60.

The appendix has muscular walls; the inner circular layer is a continuation of the same muscle in the cecum; the outer longitudinal muscle coat is formed by coalescence of the three taeniae coli at the junction of the cecum and appendix. Thus, the taeniae, particularly the anterior taeniae, may be used to find an elusive appendix: the anterior taeniae is followed until the junction of appendix with the cecum is apparent.

The mesentery of the appendix passes behind the terminal ileum to join the mesentery of the small intestine. The main artery to the appendix, a branch of the ileocolic artery, runs in the free inferior border of the mesoappendix. In many patients, an additional accessory branch from the posterior cecal artery supplies the base of the appendix at its junction with the cecum. Unless specifically sought and ligated, this accessory appendiceal artery can be a source of troublesome bleeding during appendectomy.

The relation of the base of appendix to the cecum is constant, but the tip of the appendix may be found in a variety of locations. Most commonly, the appendix lies behind the cecum but still within the peritoneal cavity. This retrocecal, intraperitoneal position characterizes two thirds of patients, and is due to the fact that several inches of cecum usually remain in an intraperitoneal position, the reflection of peritoneum from the right colon to the parietes occurring opposite the ileocecal junction. The second most common position of the tip of the appendix, found in about one fourth of patients, is at the brim of the pelvis. An appendix in the pelvis may be associated with an increased likelihood of development of acute appendicitis.

In about 5% of patients, the tip of the appendix lies extraperitoneally, either behind the cecum and ascending colon, or passing behind the distal ileum along the right margin of the ascending colon. Appendicitis in such a retroperitoneal appendix gives rise to very atypical symptoms and signs, and the diagnosis in such cases rarely is made before rupture or another complication has occurred.

Malrotation or maldescent of the cecum is associated with an abnormal position of the appendix as well as of the cecum; in such cases, the appendix may be found anywhere between the right iliac fossa and the left infrasplenic area. In cases of situs inversus, the appendix will be found in a mirror image of the various positions described for the normal appendix. As is true of a retroperitoneal appendix, abnormal intraperitoneal positions of the cecum and appendix introduce diagnostic difficulties should appendicitis supervene.

MICROBIOLOGY

The bacteria which grow in the lumen of the appendix are those of the fecal flora, a mixture of aerobic and anaerobic organisms. The anaerobic appendiceal flora was first described by Veillon and Zuber.[21] But, for reasons which are not immediately apparent, these early observations were lost,

and for many years the bacteria in the appendix were thought to be primarily coliforms and aerobic streptococci. The true polymicrobic nature of the appendiceal flora was emphasized again by Altemeier[22] in 1938. Once more, this accurate description of the mixed aerobic and anaerobic nature of the appendiceal flora was largely ignored. It has been only recently, when methods for recovery of anaerobes became readily available in most hospitals, that the polymicrobic nature of appendicitis has become widely appreciated and accepted.

The flora recovered from infectious complications of acute appendicitis are representative of the flora found in the appendix lumen (Table 41–1). More than 90% of wound infection cultures are polymicrobic. The most common result is to grow five different species of bacteria. *Bacteroides* is the most frequent pathogen, followed by *E. coli*, other gram-negative aerobes, and anaerobic and aerobic streptococci. Clostridia, although regularly present in the appendix, account for only about 10%–15% of bacterial isolates in appendicitis.

PATHOPHYSIOLOGY

The cause of acute appendicitis is infection, the bacteria involved being those of the fecal flora normally occupying the appendix lumen. Over the years, a number of hypotheses have been proposed concerning the pathophysiologic mechanisms leading to appendicitis, but most have either been disproved or are highly implausible. The possibility that appendicitis is related to a change in the fiber content of the modern Western diet is a popular topic today, but was suggested as long ago as 1920 by Short,[23] who provides a balanced discussion of the topic. In a recent epidemiologic study of acute appendicitis, the decreasing incidence of the disease could not be correlated with an increase in mean dietary fiber intake.[24] In some cases, there seems to be a familial factor in the genesis of appendicitis.[25]

Among the various hypotheses about initiation of infection in appendicitis, the one which has the most clinical and experimental evidence in its support is that appendicitis is the result of obstruction. The obstruction theory was championed by van Zwallenberg[26] and extensively investigated in the experimental laboratory by Dennis and associates.[27, 28] Obstruction seems to be essential in the development of gangrene and perforation, and can be demonstrated in a proportion, but not all, cases at earlier stages of appendicitis. Dennis[28] noted that the pressure required to perfuse the lumen of the appendix in any stage of appendicitis was increased compared to a normal appendix, even when complete obstruction was not yet present.

TABLE 41–1.—BACTERIAL FLORA OF THE APPENDIX (RELATIVE PREVALENCE, %)*

AEROBES		ANAEROBES	
Escherichia coli	80	*Bacteroides fragilis* group	89
Klebsiella-Enterobacter	57	Other *Bacteroides*	25
Str. faecalis group	26	Streptococci	64
Other gram-positive cocci	8	Clostridia	13
Other aerobes	43	Other anaerobes	41
No growth	1	No growth	4

*Data from the Surgical Microbiology Research Laboratory, Medical College of Wisconsin.

The major objection to the obstructive theory of the etiology of appendicitis is the demonstration[8, 29] that sometimes the lumen of the appendix is open and can be perfused in early stages of acute appendicitis. At least in some cases it appears that obstruction follows rather than precedes the onset of the disease. There is no doubt, however, in cases that progress from gangrene to perforation, that obstruction is present prior to the onset of the complicated stages of gangrenous or perforated appendicitis. The initiating factor in those cases of appendicitis which begin without apparent complete obstruction is unknown.

Further insight into the association of obstruction and the genesis of appendicitis may be gained from patients with cystic fibrosis, nearly all of whom have hyperplastic appendiceal mucosa; in about one fourth of these patients, the appendix is firm and dilated but inflammation is absent; appendicitis occurs in only 1%–2%. Therefore, mucosal swelling as the sole cause of obstruction seems to be an insufficient process to bring about acute appendicitis.[30]

It seems quite clear that appendicitis is not a specific bacterial disease in the sense that it is due to a single identifiable microorganism. But there are instances reported in which bacteria alone, without significant obstruction, seem to have been responsible for the initial stages of inflammation which evolve into appendicitis; such cases have been reported involving pneumococci.[31] Whether these organisms reach the appendix by being swallowed or via the bloodstream during a pneumonia is not entirely clear. Trauma is not a cause of acute appendicitis, but a blow may burst an inflamed appendix.[32]

Lymphatic hyperplasia which leads to obstruction is most frequent in children. Lymphoid follicles in the submucosa of the appendix respond to a variety of infections, especially viral and bacterial infections of the GI tract, so that appendicitis may follow; the association of measles and appendicitis is well recognized. Obstruction due to a fecalith is frequent in adults but does occur in children.[33] A foreign body or parasite or a stricture or tumor of the appendix or the adjacent cecum are other causes of appendicitis.

Once obstruction occurs, continued secretion leads to accumulation of mucus in the lumen. Fecal bacteria convert the accumulating mucus into pus. Continued secretion combined with the relative inelasticity of the appendiceal serosa leads to a rise in lumen pressure, eventually causing obstruction of lymphatic drainage. Edema begins, and diapedesis of bacteria through the intact mucosa ensues. As lumen pressure rises further, mucosal ulcers begin to appear. Acute *catarrhal appendicitis* is present.

Continued secretion causes a further rise in intraluminal pressure, bringing about venous obstruction and beginning ischemia in the wall of the appendix. Bacterial invasion spreads through the wall, until inflammation involves the serosa. This is the stage of acute *suppurative appendicitis.* There is some bacterial contamination of periappendiceal tissues, but the process is still largely confined to the appendix.

If not treated by appendectomy, continuation of the secretion pressure cycle eventually leads to venous thrombosis and compromise of the arterial blood supply. These vascular events occur first along the midportion of the antimesenteric border of the appendix, since this is the area with the poorest blood supply. With the appearance of tissue infarctions, the stage of *gangrenous appendicitis* has developed. Morbidity increases, since the infarcted tissues of the appendix functionally act as a perforation, permitting escape of bacteria from the lumen to contaminate the adjacent peritoneal cavity.

Necrosis coupled with high intraluminal pressure finally leads to perforation through a gangrenous infarct, spilling the pus which has accumulated in the appendix lumen. *Perforated appendicitis* is now present; both morbidity and mortality increase. The length of time from onset of symptoms to perforation may be influenced by the point in the appendix at which obstruction occurs. When obstruction is near the tip, the perforation is earlier than when the obstruction is near the base.[34] In most cases, the obstruction that initiated appendicitis blocks retrograde spillage of feces from the cecum.

If the progression of the appendicitis has not been too rapid, inflammatory adhesions form between loops of bowel, peritoneum, and omentum to wall off the infective process around the appendix from the general peritoneal cavity. The perforation is contained as a localized peritonitis, and a periappendiceal abscess eventually forms. But, in a small percentage of patients, particularly those who are very young or very old, peritoneal defense mechanisms are ineffective, and the disease is more rapidly progressive so that generalized peritonitis ensues when the appendix perforates.

CLINICAL SYNDROMES

Typical Appendicitis

Typical appendicitis involves the "classic" symptom sequence of dull, aching pain perceived initially in the central abdomen, accompanied by anorexia and some nausea, later increasing in intensity, then shifting and becoming sharply localized in the right lower quadrant. This classic presentation characterizes only about two thirds of all patients with appendicitis, and may occur with other intra-abdominal disorders.[35] In another fourth of cases, pain is confined to the right lower quadrant from the beginning. Anorexia is almost always present in appendicitis in teenagers and adults, although it is a less frequent complaint in children. Nausea, at least of some degree, is reported by nine of ten patients with appendicitis. Vomiting occurs in only about one fourth of patients, mostly children, and usually is not persistent or prolonged. It is important to recognize that vomiting in appendicitis appears only after the onset of pain; if vomiting precedes pain, appendicitis is less likely.

The physical signs to be sought in suspected cases of appendicitis are local tenderness, rebound tenderness, muscle guarding, and muscle rigidity. Systematic gentle palpation of the abdomen will detect the presence of tenderness, usually maximal overlying the inflamed appendix, and, of course, most often localized in the right lower quadrant at or near McBurney's point.[36] Rebound tenderness can be elicited by the usual maneuver of sudden release of abdominal palpation pressure, but more reliable information concerning the presence of rebound tenderness is obtained by gentle percussion of the abdomen in the area of tenderness. A marked increase in pain induced by light percussion is evidence of peritoneal irritation.

If symptoms have been present for more than a few hours, careful inspection may disclose some limitation of muscular movement in the lower half of the abdomen during respiration, a reflection of muscle guarding. The degree of guarding, or voluntary resistance to abdominal palpation, increases as local inflammation increases. Eventually, voluntary muscle guarding is replaced by reflex involuntary muscle rigidity, indicating the presence of regional inflammation of the peritoneal serosa. True rigidity is not diminished during expiration, a finding that allows it to be differentiated by palpation from voluntary guarding: the palpating hand is placed on the abdominal wall, exerting slight pressure, and variations in tone of the underlying muscles are noted through several respiratory cycles. Voluntary contractions of the abdominal musculature relax slightly during expiration (guarding); if this fails to occur, the muscle is being maintained reflexly in contraction (rigidity).

Other physical signs occasionally may be elicited, including cutaneous hyperesthesia, Rovsing's sign, or a psoas or obturator sign. Cutaneous hyperesthesia, a perceptible difference in sensation elicited by light stroking of the skin in the right and left lower quadrants of the abdomen, will be reported by an occasional patient but is beyond the discriminatory capacity of most patients with appendicitis. Rovsing's sign, pain noted in the right lower quadrant when palpation pressure is exerted in the left lower quadrant, is a manifestation of referred rebound tenderness. The psoas sign, elicited by active flexion of the right hip against resistance or by passive extension of the hip, may be positive if an inflamed appendix is in contact with the psoas muscle. The obturator sign, hypogastric or thigh adductor region pain elicited by passive internal rotation of the flexed thigh, may be positive if an inflamed appendix is lying in the pelvis against the obturator internus muscle. Both the psoas and obturator signs rarely are present early in appendicitis and, by the time they can be easily elicited, other clinical signs of appendicitis usually are quite clear. As appendicitis progresses, any movement which must be undertaken is done slowly. The right hip is often maintained in a slightly flexed position.

Once the appendix ruptures, physical signs change. Tenderness, which was well localized at McBurney's point now spreads to encompass the entire right lower abdomen. Rebound tenderness and muscular rigidity become more marked. A boggy, tender mass, representing omentum and loops of bowel adherent in a periappendiceal phlegmon, may become palpable.

Appendicitis may cause a rise in temperature to 38°C (100.4°F), but higher fever is unusual, unless gangrene or perforation has occurred. Early high fever is more suggestive of a urinary tract infection. The temperature may be normal, even with very advanced appendicitis. The pulse usually remains normal or only slightly elevated until rupture and peritonitis occur.

Rectal examination is essential in every patient suspected of having appendicitis, primarily to exclude disease of pelvic organs. Since some degree of discomfort is usual during a rectal examination, a baseline for discomfort should be established initially by palpating the sacrum and coccyx. Without changing the degree of pressure being exerted on the perineum and the anal canal, the tip of the examining finger then gently palpates first the right and then the left sides of the rectum and pelvis, noting if the patient reports any increase in discomfort. Some patients may appreciate an increase in tenderness high on the right side, but this finding will be absent in most patients with typical appendicitis.

Laboratory examinations are unnecessary to make a diagnosis of appendicitis, but may be obtained to provide secondarily supporting information. The diagnosis of appendicitis should never be excluded simply because laboratory work is normal. In cases of suspected appendicitis, clinical findings should take precedence whenever there is disagreement between clinical observations and the results of laboratory examinations. Most patients with typical appendicitis have a modest elevation of up to 15,000/cu mm in the total leukocyte count. In interpreting the WBC count, it is well to recall that up to one third of patients, particularly older adults and blacks, will have a normal total leukocyte count in the presence of acute appendicitis.[37] Further, even when the total leukocyte count is elevated, the degree of elevation does not correlate with the degree of abnormality in the appendix.[38] In most patients, even if the total leukocyte count is normal, there will be a left shift in the differential white count. Fewer than 4% of patients with appendicitis will have both a normal differential and a normal total leukocyte count. Therefore, the differential count is more helpful than the total leukocyte count in supporting a diagnosis of acute appendicitis. The hematocrit is normal in appendicitis. If an older patient presents with clinical appendicitis and has a significant anemia, carcinoma of the cecum should be suspected.

Minimal albuminuria, and the presence of a few white and red blood cells in the urine, is not unusual in a patient with appendicitis. It is not necessary for the inflamed appendix to be in contact with the ureter or bladder for the urinalysis to be abnormal. The presence of some WBCs in a voided urine specimen is so common in women that this finding is of no diagnostic value. Identification of significant numbers of microorganisms in the urinary sediment confirms the presence of a urinary tract infection but does not exclude a diagnosis of appendicitis. But, if more than 30 RBCs or more than 20 WBCs per high-power field are seen, the diagnosis is less likely to be appendicitis and more likely to be a primary urinary tract abnormality.[39]

X-ray examination of the abdomen is unnecessary in typical appendicitis. If obtained, x-rays may show an air-fluid level of the cecum early in appendicitis (cecal ileus), but there are no pathognomonic early findings with the exception of demonstration of an appendiceal fecalith. In the later stages of appendicitis, particularly after gangrene or perforation has supervened, a number of positive x-ray signs of appendicitis may be seen. These include gas in the lumen of the appendix, a mass extrinsic to the cecum, scoliosis, absence of the right psoas shadow, absence of small-bowel gas in the right lower quadrant (though abundant elsewhere in the abdomen), edema of the abdominal wall, or interruption of the preperitoneal fat line in the flank.

A barium enema, although contraindicated in the early

stages of suspected appendicitis because of the risk of spilling barium should the appendix perforate, is useful in the diagnosis of patients with atypical or desultory symptoms, and may be carried out safely after an initial period of 6–12 hours of observation.

Atypical Appendicitis

Atypical appendicitis refers to the absence of the classic shifting pain sequence or to failure of pain to localize in the right lower quadrant, and is present in at least one fourth of all patients with appendicitis. Atypical pain is more frequent in older patients, in whom the severity of pain is always less intense. The clinical signs and symptoms may be atypical because the appendix is in an unusual position (pelvic, retroperitoneal, malrotated), or because the progression of appendicitis has been sufficiently rapid, or, conversely, sufficiently desultory that perforation is already present when the patient is first seen (much more frequent in aged patients).

Keep in mind that all physical signs are fallible in appendicitis. An acutely inflamed appendix located entirely within the true pelvis may never produce symptoms or signs referable to the anterior abdomen, except for mild distention reflecting some paralytic ileus. Instead, there may be only suprapubic discomfort, rectal tenesmus, and bladder irritability. Rectal examination is essential in every patient suspected of having appendicitis, primarily to exclude an ovarian cyst, tubal abscess, and similar pelvic lesions. In those few patients in whom the appendix is located in an abnormal position, central pain in the abdomen may shift initially to a more sharply localized focus corresponding to the geographical location of the appendix. If the appendix is retrocolic or retroperitoneal in location, pain may be located only in the loin or flank. It is usual for the diagnosis of appendicitis in such cases to be delayed, often not being made until rupture and periappendiceal abscess have ensued. Patients who are receiving long-term antibiotic therapy, such as teenagers being treated for acne, also often will report less intense and later localization of pain. As is true of typical appendicitis, only modest fever and leukocytosis are present in cases of atypical appendicitis prior to gangrene and perforation.

Appendicitis may first appear as a mechanical small-bowel obstruction, a mode of presentation particularly prevalent in elderly patients. The disease process initially has progressed to gangrene but with minimal signs of peritoneal irritation on physical examination. The late abdominal inflammatory response, including development of adhesions, is responsible for the occurrence of mechanical small-bowel obstruction.

Laboratory examinations in cases of atypical appendicitis are similar to those in typical appendicitis. The temperature and white count are only modestly elevated prior to the onset of complications. The differential white count is always more helpful than the total white count.

The possible role of laparoscopy in reducing both missed early appendicitis and exploration with finding a normal appendix is currently undergoing evaluation. Laparoscopy may prove to be particularly helpful in young women with right lower quadrant symptoms, the group in whom the diagnostic error rate is highest. Routine laparoscopy in this patient group has reduced the number of negative explorations[40] and

also has been effective in young patients.[41] At present, it appears that laparoscopy is a worthwhile diagnostic maneuver in patients in whom the diagnosis is in doubt. If a normal appendix can be visualized, appendicitis obviously is excluded. Some pelvic pathology may be identified as the cause of symptoms and appropriate therapy can be undertaken. If the appendix is not visualized, and no alternative explanation for the symptoms is forthcoming as the result of laparoscopic examination, exploration to rule out appendicitis is still necessary.

X-ray examination of patients with atypical complaints, in particular a barium enema, done after a period of 6–12 hour's observation without progression or resolution of symptoms, is safe and may eliminate appendicitis as a possible cause of the symptoms.[42] An abnormal location of the cecum and appendix may be demonstrated and will clarify the diagnosis.[43] It must be remembered that compete filling of the cecum and the appendix, and subsequent emptying of the barium from the appendix, is required if the barium enema is to be interpreted as eliminating acute appendicitis as the cause of the symptoms.[44–46] Because of difficulty in being sure the appendix is filled entirely to its tip, the false negative rate of an apparently normal barium enema in appendicitis is 10%. A barium swallow as an alternative to barium enema also has been reported.[47]

The great difficulties in diagnosing atypical appendicitis have stimulated attempts to devise computer algorithms or other similar scoring systems to improve diagnostic accuracy.[48–51] While these schemes have modestly improved the accuracy of diagnosis in young women, they do not appear to have had any major impact in other clinical settings of atypical appendicitis. The best that can be done in this clinical situation is to maintain a high index of suspicion, and to explore patients with suspected appendicitis if the diagnosis cannot be excluded. The rationale is that the morbidity and mortality of a negative exploration or of appendectomy conducted prior to gangrene or rupture is low. But, once gangrene or perforation have ensued, mortality and morbidity markedly increase. To remove the appendix reliably whenever it is inflamed and before it leads to complications, exploration of a certain number of patients who prove not to have appendicitis is necessary. Overall, negative exploration rates of up to 30% are considered acceptable.[35, 52]

Appendix Mass

On occasion, especially in patients who seek care relatively late in the course of appendicitis, a periappendiceal mass may be palpated in the right lower quadrant. The mass may be due to an abscess or to adherent omentum and coils of bowel about the inflamed appendix. If the patient is showing little or no local or systemic reaction (muscle spasm, fever, leukocytosis) in the presence of a palpable periappendiceal mass, and symptoms have been present for more than three days and seem to be stable or subsiding, treatment by bedrest, bowel rest (nasogastric suction), IV antibiotics and IV fluids may permit resolution of the acute process.[53–55] Such patients, if nonoperative treatment initially is elected, must be observed very closely. Drainage of the abscess, usually with appendectomy, should be undertaken if symptoms progress or fail to resolve. Nonoperative treatment of an appendix mass should not be considered in children, pregnant women, or elderly patients.

Appendicitis in the Very Young

In infancy, the broadly open base of the appendix and its conical shape make obstruction of the lumen unlikely. Appendicitis is, therefore, uncommon in infants. If perforated appendicitis does occur in very young infants, it often is associated with Hirschsprung's disease.[56] An accurate diagnosis of appendicitis is very difficult to establish in infants and young children. Nonspecific abdominal pain is common in infants and young children; physicians, therefore, often do not consider early enough the possibility that appendicitis may be the cause of the symptoms. Very young patients, for obvious reasons, are unable to give a history of their illness or to describe their complaints.

The symptoms to be sought in infants and very young children are vomiting, fever, irritability, flexing of the thighs, and diarrhea. The most consistent finding on physical examination is distention of the abdomen. "Beware of diarrhea in the child whose illness begins with abdominal pain." Leukocyte counts are not reliable in this age group. The presence of a fecalith found on x-ray of a child with acute abdominal symptoms is sufficient evidence to consider the diagnosis of appendicitis established. Among children who have a negative laparotomy for suspected appendicitis, routine cultures are positive in 40%, evidence that mild acute primary peritonitis might explain some symptoms.[57]

The incidence of perforation is very high in this age group, approaching 100% in infants less than 1 year of age and remaining above 50% up to the age of 5 years. The higher mortality of this age group often has been attributed to absence of a fully developed omentum with consequent generalized peritonitis following perforation. While the omentum is a factor, the most important element is a delay in establishing the diagnosis, permitting rupture to occur. Up to 40% of children with gangrenous or perforated appendicitis have been seen early in their illness by a physician who failed to appreciate the nature of the disease process. Stone et al.[58] identified four factors indicating the probable presence of gangrenous or perforated appendicitis in children: duration of symptoms longer than 36 hours, fever of 102°F or more, presence of diffuse abdominal tenderness, and leukocystosis of 13,000/cu mm or more. When all four of these features were present, the incidence of complicated appendicitis rose from 2% to more than 50%.

Despite identification of the group at risk, there continues to be controversy among pediatric surgeons about when an appendectomy should be conducted. All agree that fluid resuscitation, control of hyperthermia, and initiation of antibiotics are needed. Those favoring early operation then perform appendectomy with an overall complication rate of about 7% and no mortality.[59] Those favoring initial non-operative management, with appendectomy being performed if the clinical situation deteriorates or as an interval operation after 4–6 weeks, report complication rates of the order of 8%.[60] Nonoperative management seems to succeed best in those children who present relatively late, often more than 4–5 days into their illness, who often have a palpable appendiceal mass, and who do not show progression of clinical signs or symptoms during the initial period of observation.

Nonoperative management should not be applied to children seen relatively early in the course of appendicitis who do not yet have signs of perforation; these patients should have a prompt operation to avoid the consequences of perforation. But, if they appear later for treatment, when perforation has already occurred, there is less to be gained by immediate appendectomy unless the situation is clinically progressing and deteriorating.

Appendicitis in Young Women

Young women, 20–35 years of age, have the highest rate of error in diagnosing appendicitis. While the overall incidence of negative laparotomy in all adults with suspected appendicitis is of the order of 15%–20%, the incidence in young women is more than twice as high. Diagnostic difficulty is generated by the fact that pain and discomfort associated with ovulation (Mittelschmerz), and primary diseases involving the ovary, fallopian tubes, or the uterus, as well as infections and other disorders of the urinary system, may produce symptoms which closely mimic those of acute appendicitis.

In many young women, the clinical signs and symptoms will be those of typical appendicitis and diagnosis is not really in doubt; such patients should be prepared for appendectomy. But, when faced with the problem of possible appendicitis in a young woman in whom the symptoms are not classic, careful observation may be in order if pain is atypical, there is no muscular spasm in the right lower quadrant on physical examination, and fever and leukocytosis are absent. If the symptoms seem sufficiently acute that operative exploration seems warranted even though there is doubt about the diagnosis, laparoscopy to clarify the diagnosis should be entertained. Laparoscopic examination, if it visualizes a normal appendix or establishes the presence of alternative pelvic pathology as the cause of the symptoms, may avoid a negative exploration.

If symptoms and signs do not progress over several hours of observation, a careful barium enema which visualizes the appendix may be helpful in ruling out appendicitis as the cause of the symptoms. When following a program of observation and additional diagnostic studies, it must be remembered that a negative exploration in a healthy young woman is to be preferred, in most circumstances, to permitting evolution of acute appendicitis to the stage of perforation with its consequent increase in morbidity.

Appendicitis in the Elderly

Although the overall incidence of appendicitis is decreasing, the incidence in patients over age 65 seems to be rising, probably a reflection of improved longevity among the aged. As is true of infants, acute appendicitis among older patients has a mortality risk much greater than that of young adults. This increased mortality risk is due both to delay by the patient in seeking medical care and to delay by physicians in removing the appendix. Classic appendicitis occurs in the elderly but is much less common than an atypical sequence of symptoms and signs. Pain, anorexia, and nausea are present in most elderly patients but are less pronounced than in younger adults. Pain usually is felt in the lower abdomen or diffusely in the right lower quadrant, often is very mild, and may cause little initial concern. Pain may never become well localized.

Physical examination in the early course of appendicitis in the elderly is remarkable for the paucity of findings in the presence of a relatively advanced disease. Initial examination may reveal nothing abnormal, although some tenderness in the right lower quadrant eventually can be elicited in most patients. Distention of the abdomen, as is also true of infants, is a prominent early symptom in elderly patients, usually occurring before perforation. Symptoms and signs suggesting the presence of a partial mechanical small-bowel obstruction are not uncommon. Fever may be entirely absent in an aged patient with appendicitis; subnormal temperatures also are more frequently encountered in this age group, especially with perforated appendicitis which has led to generalized peritonitis or an appendiceal abscess.

Occasionally, an older patient will enter the hospital with a painless right lower quadrant mass, denying any previous history suggestive of appendicitis. Conversely, some elderly patients initially present generalized peritonitis of an obscure etiology; they, too, deny previous acute symptoms.

More than a third of elderly patients (see Fig 41–3) have a ruptured appendix at the time of operation. Relatively impaired blood supply is said to be responsible, at least in part, for earlier perforation in older patients. Although poor vascular supply undoubtedly plays a role, delay in accomplishing appendectomy really accounts for the high rate of perforation. Part of this delay is the responsibility of the patient, who does not perceive the gravity of the situation because of the relatively minimal symptoms, and a part of the delay occurs because physicians do not advise early exploration in doubtful cases, citing the presence of concomitant diseases that increase operative risk. It must be remembered that if an elderly patient probably has acute appendicitis, an urgent operation should be advised. More elderly patients die from misdiagnosis and delay in appendectomy than die from an error in diagnosis and removal of a normal appendix.

Whenever a patient develops appendicitis in the sixth decade of life or later, a concomitant carcinoma of the right colon may be present and should be specifically sought during exploration. The association in the elderly of carcinoma involving the cecum or right colon and of acute appendicitis seems to be higher than chance association of these two diseases warrants.

Appendicitis During Pregnancy

Appendicitis is the most common extrauterine condition requiring an abdominal exploration during pregnancy. The fact of pregnancy does not change the risk of developing appendicitis, so that appendicitis occurs about once in every 2000 pregnancies.

The symptoms of appendicitis depend on the location of the appendix. For the first half of a pregnancy, the appendix is not significantly displaced from its usual location in the right lower quadrant, and the symptoms of appendicitis do not differ much from those of a nonpregnant woman. As the preg-

nancy progresses through the last trimester, the cecum and appendix are displaced superiorly and rotated laterally. The pain of appendicitis then may be vague and localized in the right flank.[61] Therefore, the localization of pain in appendicitis during the later stages of pregnancy is higher and more lateral than in a nonpregnant woman.

Appendectomy should be performed on suspicion of the presence of appendicitis, just as if the pregnancy were not present. If performed before the appendix ruptures, appendectomy often does not disturb the pregnancy, particularly during the first or second trimester. Appendicitis during the final trimester tends to be more serious, since the displaced omentum often is unable to reach the area of the inflamed appendix to help contain infection. In addition, induced contractions of the nearby uterus serve to impair localization. Premature labor occurs in about half of women who develop appendicitis during the third trimester. The prognosis for the infant in uncomplicated appendicitis is directly related to birth weight. Should rupture of the appendix occur, it is often followed by diffuse peritonitis. In this situation, fetal loss is much higher due not only to prematurity but also to the effects of sepsis on the fetus. Cesarean section should be advised if generalized peritonitis is present, since fetal death secondary to sepsis and premature labor occurs with a high incidence in this clinical setting.

Chronic or Subacute Recurrent Appendicitis

There are a few patients in whom appendicitis is a clinically subacute or chronic syndrome, with attacks subsiding spontaneously, sometimes more than once. Characteristically, these patients are free of symptoms between attacks, and physical examination is then normal. However, if the patient is examined while symptoms are present, there usually is some tenderness in the right lower quadrant, although the findings rarely will allow an unequivocal diagnosis of acute appendicitis. If abdominal x-rays demonstrate the presence of a fecalith, if a barium enema shows nonfilling of the appendix, or if observation of repeated attacks provides evidence that the patient is truly suffering from recurrent subacute appendicitis, elective appendectomy may be undertaken.

To sustain a diagnosis of chronic appendicitis as justification for elective appendectomy in a patient with persistent, recurrent right lower abdominal complaints, the resected appendix must show evidence of preceding attacks of appendicitis: fibrosis in the muscular wall of the appendix, partial to complete obstruction of the lumen resulting from mucosal scarring, and infiltration of the muscular wall of the appendix by chronic inflammatory cells.[62] A few subserosal or intramuscular polymorphonuclear leukocytes within an excised appendix are not sufficient to establish a diagnosis of chronic appendicitis. This latter degree of "inflammatory response" can be elicited by the manipulations required for excision of a normal appendix. It also is not sufficient to establish this diagnosis to identify histologically only mucosal edema or intramucosal collections of acute inflammatory cells.

DIFFERENTIAL DIAGNOSIS

Because appendicitis may mimic so many other diseases, and so many other diseases may mimic appendicitis, any disease or disorder which may produce an acute abdomen may enter into the differential diagnosis in a case of suspected acute appendicitis. While a long list of alternative diagnostic possibilities has to be kept in mind, the essential differential diagnostic maneuver in suspected acute appendicitis is to eliminate those diseases that do not need operative therapy, such as acute pancreatitis, basilar pneumonia, myocardial infarction, and similar entities which may be made worse if abdominal exploration is undertaken. It must also be remembered, such entities apart, that most of the diagnostic possibilities which enter into the differential diagnosis of appendicitis require operative therapy or, if not, usually are not made worse by an exploratory operation. So, while a judicious period of observation may be indicated to improve the surety of diagnosis, the time and effort so expended should be limited to reduce the risk of perforation of the appendix.

In young children, diseases which most frequently produce signs and symptoms masquerading as appendicitis are acute gastroenteritis, mesenteric lymphadenitis, pyelitis, Meckel's diverticulitis, intussusception, enteric duplication, Henöch-Schonlein purpura and primary peritonitis. Basilar pneumonia, even on the left side, may produce abdominal symptoms suggestive of appendicitis in this age group. Acute gastroenteritis is usually associated with cramping abdominal pain and watery diarrhea. Gastroenteritis may be viral in origin, but may also involve infection by *Shigella* or similar enteric pathogens. In mesenteric adenitis, an upper respiratory infection is often present or has recently subsided. Measles and other viral infections may also cause a reaction in the submucosal lymphoid tissue of the appendix leading to symptoms which may or may not progress to a true appendicitis. Intussusception usually occurs below age 2; appendicitis is uncommon in that age group. The intussuscepted mass may be palpable in the right lower quadrant. Gentle barium enema will demonstrate the intussusception and usually succeeds in its reduction. Children with cystic fibrosis may have an engorged appendiceal mucosa and develop low-grade right lower quadrant symptoms; usually this syndrome does not evolve to acute appendicitis. Infectious hepatitis is particularly important to differentiate in children. In the preicteric phase, abdominal pain, nausea, or vomiting may be associated with tenderness under the right costal margin similar to that of a subhepatic appendicitis. Bile may be recognizable in the urine at this stage and may help to make a correct diagnosis.

Repeated examinations over a period of a few hours are the most valuable diagnostic test. If appendicitis is present, signs will develop, persist, and increase, and the pulse rate will usually eventually rise. In other noninfectious conditions, the picture will tend to fluctuate from time to time and the point of maximum tenderness will vary in position on repeated examination. In acute lymphocytic leukemia in children, inflammation progressing to necrosis and perforation of the cecum, appendix, or adjacent ileum may occur. This entity, for which the ancient term "typhlitis" has been resurrected, is more properly called the leukemic-ileocecal syndrome. It is important because it exactly mimics an acute appendicitis. Controversy exists concerning surgical intervention; without an operation, most children die; the prognosis is still grim,

although better when aggressive surgical therapy is undertaken.[63–66]

In a young woman, a ruptured graafian follicle may produce acute symptoms in midmenstrual cycle. Other entities to be considered include salpingitis (pelvic inflammatory disease), torsion of an ovarian cyst, ruptured ectopic pregnancy, and endometriosis. In most patients with a ruptured ectopic pregnancy, there is a palpable tubal mass on pelvic examination, and culdocentesis yields nonclotting blood. Endometriosis can be differentiated by the repetitive recurrence of pain with each menses. Salpingitis may present the greatest diagnostic difficulty, but usually the pain is bilateral and low in the abdomen; the older concept[67] that salpingitis and appendicitis were more common in the latter half of the menstrual cycle has recently been challenged by an extensive study[68] showing no significant difference between the various phases of the menstrual cycle and the onset of appendicitis or of salpingitis. Women taking hormones for contraception sometimes report right lower quadrant abdominal discomfort at the end of the second week of each cycle; pain is diffuse, but leukocytosis and fever are absent, helping to differentiate this entity.

In a young man, the list of alternative diagnoses is smaller: acute regional enteritis, right renal or ureteral calculus, testicular torsion, and acute epididymitis. Renal or ureteral calculi characteristically cause severe pain, much more severe than that of acute appendicitis, but pain does not usually persist or progress, since it is related to movement of the calculus; there will be associated microscopic hematuria. Testicular torsion and acute epididymitis are diagnosed by examination of the external genitalia. Regional enteritis can be a confusing entity. Cramps and diarrhea are frequent, and anorexia usually is infrequent, clues that the process is regional enteritis rather than appendicitis.

In adults, diseases that must be considered in the differential diagnosis are diverticulitis, perforated duodenal or gastric ulcer, acute cholecystitis, recurrent pancreatitis, intestinal obstruction, perforating cecal carcinoma, perforated ileal or cecal diverticulum, mesenteric vascular occlusion, rupturing aortic or iliac aneurysm, and idiopathic infarction of an epiploic appendage or the omentum. Deep venous thrombosis involving the iliac venous system may produce symptoms mimicking a pelvic appendicitis. Inflammatory pseudotumors are a rare group of nonneoplastic reactive lesions which may be confused with a malignant tumor. These tumors share certain features with fibrocystocytoma and plasma cell granuloma. Simple appendectomy is sufficient treatment.[69]

Gastrointestinal infection with *Yersinia enterocolitica* causes a gastroenteritis-like syndrome that may mimic appendicitis. The usual finding is of hyperemia of the terminal ileum, appendix and cecum, associated with mesenteric lymphadenitis. On occasion, the inflammatory response may look like terminal ileitis. Confirmation of the nature of the infection can be obtained by measurement of serum antibody titers. A mesenteric lymph node should also be obtained for culture, although the organism is not always recovered even when the rise in antibody titer indicates the probability that *Yersinia* was the infecting organism.[70] Infections with the related organism *Y. pseudotuberculosis* produce caseating granulomas in involved tissues and lymph nodes.

CLINICAL MANAGEMENT

Preoperative Preparation

All patients need intensive preoperative preparation over a period of two to four hours. Fluid replacement should be carried out as rapidly as possible with the objective of establishing good urinary output. Nasogastric suction is helpful in all patients with appendicitis but particularly so in infants and the elderly, who tend to develop more profound paralytic ileus, and in patients with generalized peritonitis. High fever leading to febrile convulsions may be a problem in children and should be treated with antipyretics. If the fever does not subside, a cooling mattress may be required. Anesthesia should not be induced in patients whose temperature is over 39°C.

Patients who have generalized or spreading peritonitis when first examined should undergo general abdominal exploration promptly once resuscitation has been accomplished. A midline incision is preferred in such cases. The objectives of therapy are those of management of generalized peritonitis: control of the source of peritonitis (appendectomy), removal of pockets of infected fluid or pus and debridement of gross fibrinous exudate without inducing bleeding, followed by thorough lavage and aspiration of the lavage fluid. Drainage of localized collections of pus which have created potential dead spaces is indicated but prophylactic placement of multiple drains is not warranted. Such drains are rapidly walled off, and so do not succeed in draining the peritoneal cavity,[71] and are detrimental rather than helpful, since they perpetuate inflammation and provide a route for reinfection.

Patients who appear for treatment more than three days into the course of their appendicitis, who do not have fever above 39° C (102° F), whose clinical condition seems stable, and in whom the disease appears to be resolving are candidates for initial nonoperative management. Similarly, patients in whom the diagnosis is unclear, who are not apparently having progressive disease, and in whom the symptoms are atypical, also are candidates for initial treatment by observation. Fine clinical judgment is required in this situation so that a decision to operate can be made prior to the occurrence of perforation but also so that operation will not be undertaken in those patients who do not have appendicitis.

Antibiotic Therapy

A half century ago, prior to the introduction of antimicrobial drugs into clinical practice, the mortality of acute appendicitis was of 8%–15%, while the incidence of perforation was approximately 30%. Today, the overall mortality risk of acute appendicitis is less than 1%, while the incidence of perforation continues to be high, about 20% overall. Not all of the improvement in mortality can be attributed simply to the availability of antimicrobial drugs, since other aspects of improved management of anesthesia and surgical care also play a role. But, mortality has declined in spite of the continuing high incidence of perforation; antibiotic therapy has been an important factor in this happy result.

The bacteria associated with appendicitis were recorded in Table 41–1. The organisms are a polymicrobic aerobic-anaer-

obic mixture derived from the fecal flora. It has long been recognized that the risk of developing an infection becomes progressively greater as the stage of appendicitis worsens (Table 41–2). The risk of a wound infection after removal of a normal appendix, or an appendix affected only by early catarrhal appendicitis, is of the order of 5%. When gangrene supervenes, the risk increases three- or four-fold, and when the appendix is perforated, the risk of wound infection rises to one of every two or three patients.[73]

The increased risk of wound infection and other septic complications of appendicitis is widely understood in association with the complicated forms of appendicitis—gangrenous and perforated appendicitis—and there is little argument about administration of antibiotics in these patients. But, despite the fact that the wound infection risk for the removal of a normal appendix, and certainly for the removal of an early acutely inflamed appendix, is distinctly above the wound infection risk of a strictly clean operation, there is reluctance among many surgeons to recognize the need for antibiotic prophylaxis in this clinical setting.

A number of clinical trials have been conducted to measure the effects of antibiotics in appendicitis. These data are summarized in Table 41–3. When pooled, the conclusion from these data that antibiotics reduce the incidence of infectious complications at all stages of appendicitis is established.

Many antimicrobial and antiseptic substances have been used as wound and cavity irrigants during appendectomy. These data are summarized in Table 41–4. Antibiotics are more efficacious than antiseptics; their effect is probably due to a high antibiotic concentration in the wound tissues following irrigation. Postoperative peritoneal lavage with diluted ampicillin solution has been shown in cases of perforated appendicitis to have no effect on the incidence of intra-abdominal abscess or of wound infection.[73]

Since appendicitis-related infections are polymicrobic infections in which aerobe-anaerobe synergy plays a pathogenic role, antibiotic therapy which affects only aerobes or only anaerobes permits a residual incidence of infections due to the untreated microorganisms. Therefore, in choosing an antibiotic for prophylaxis or therapy in appendicitis, a drug with activity against both aerobes and anaerobes is preferred. We currently prescribe cefoxitin for patients with suspected ap-

TABLE 41–2.—APPENDIX PATHOLOGY AND
WOUND INFECTION RISK

SENIOR AUTHOR, YEAR	NO. OF PATIENTS	STATE OF APPENDIX (INFECTION RATE, %)			
		Normal	Acute	Gangrenous	Perforated
Bird 1971	84	27	30	27	50
Gilmore 1973	84	14	6	15	70
Bates 1974	100	10	28	—	42*
Gilmore	151	11	8	19	60
Everson 1977	63	10	0	—	84*
Leigh 1978	491	15	14	—	69*
Pashby 1978	72	28	29	82	89
Gottrup 1980	206	3	4	24	45
Nystrom 1980	143	6	3	11	38
Renvall 1980	238	3	4	12	36
Foster 1981	22	14	16	—	70*
Gaffney 1984	100	—	2	—	0*

*Includes gangrenous plus perforated cases.

TABLE 41–3.—Clinical Trials of Parenteral Antibiotics in Appendicitis

SENIOR AUTHOR, YEAR	ANTIBIOTIC(S) STUDIED	INFECTION RATE (%) Placebo	INFECTION RATE (%) Treated
Pulaski 1956	Tetracycline	6	1
Magarey 1971	Amp or tetra	34	23
Evans 1973	Cephaloridine	23	16
Leigh 1976†	Lincomycin	17	6*
Willis 1976	Metronidazole	24	10
Everson 1977	Cephaloridine	29	11*
Foster 1978	Cephaloridine	12	1*
Fine 1978	Genta-clinda	10	5
Pashby 1978	Metronidazole	34	2*
Donovan 1979	Clindamycin	33	17*
	Cefazolin		35
Greenall 1979†	Metronidazole	24	2*
Rodgers 1979	Metronidazole	15	5
Bates 1980	Metronidazole	25	20
Gottrup 1980	Metronidazole	12	1*
Pinto 1980	Metronidazole	8	5
Tanner 1980	Metronidazole	22	2*
Morris 1980	Cefazolin	30	20
	Metronidazole		21
	Cefazolin-metron		3*
Busuttil 1981	Cefamandole	13	2*
	Cefamondole-carben		0*
Foster 1981	Metronidazole	24	12*
Gottrup 1981	Metronidazole	45	3*
Kortelainen 1982	Metronidazole	11	1*
Brennan 1982	Metronidazole	19	11
Winslow 1983	Cefoxitin	10	0*
Keiser 1983	Metronidazole	10	7
Gledhill 1983†	Cefamandole	12	24
Yamauchi 1983	Pen-gentamicin	11	13
	Pen-genta-clinda		8
	Ceforanide-clinda		9
McLean 1983	Metronidazole	12	4*
Sherlock 1984†	Genta-clinda	25	0*

*Significant difference between groups (p<0.05).
†Topical povidone-iodine used in all patients in this study; amp = ampicillin; carben = carbenicillin; clinda = clindamycin; genta = gentamicin; metron = metronidazole; tetra = tetracycline.

TABLE 41–4.—Clinical Trials of Topical Antimicrobials in Appendicitis

SENIOR AUTHOR, YEAR	ANTIMICROBIAL(S) STUDIED	PLACEBO Infected Total	PLACEBO %	TREATED Infected Total	TREATED %
Noon 1967	Kana-bacitracin	22/41	52	11/50	22*
Rickett 1969	Ampicillin	8/39	21	1/36	3*
Crosfil 1969	Chlorhexidine	12/91	13	11/90	12
Mountain 1970	Ampicillin	18/24	24	7/76	9
Bird 1971	Noxythiolin	25/84	30	22/64	34
Longland 1971	Tetracycline	12/50	24	1/50	2*
	Neo-baci-poly	9/50	18	9/50	18
Andersen 1972	Ampicillin	42/245	17	10/245	6
Benson 1973	Tetracycline	7/30	23	3/41	7
Gilmore 1974	Povidone-iodine	24/151	16	12/149	8
	Neo-baci-poly			14/150	9
Bates 1974	Ampicillin	16/100	16	3/100	3*
	Neo-baci-poly			14/150	9
Stewart 1978	Tetracycline	21/72	29	5/59	9*
	Noxythiolin			19/59	32
Tanphiphat 1978	Ampicillin	12/124	10	4/122	3
	Savlon			12/128	10
Viljanto 1980	Povidone-iodine	7/82	9	1/38	3
Lau 1981	Hydrogen peroxide	26/108	24	21/109	19
Foster 1981	Povidone-iodine	27/115	24	29/119	24
Sherlock	Povidone-iodine	9/36	25	6/39	15

*Significant difference between groups (p < 0.05). Kana = kanamycin; neo = neomycin; baci = bacitracin; poly = polymixin.

pendicitis, administering 2 gm IV in adults (proportionately smaller doses in children) as soon as a decision to conduct appendectomy has been reached, and repeating this dose every three to four hours, to a total of four doses. In patients with acute but otherwise uncomplicated appendicitis, administration of antibiotics is stopped within 24 hours postoperatively. For patients with gangrenous or perforated appendicitis, antibiotic administration is continued until clinical evidence suggests that any infection is under control. This usually entails about a week of antibiotic therapy, somewhat longer in children. Whether topically applied antimicrobials should be used in conjunction with or in place of systemic antibiotic therapy in cases of appendicitis remains an open issue; convincing data from controlled trials regarding this issue is lacking, and no recommendation can be made at this time.

Examination Using Anesthesia

For most patients, the abdominal examination is repeated after induction of general anesthesia. If examination using anesthesia does not show a definite appendiceal mass, appendectomy is performed. If an appendiceal mass is detected by examination with anesthesia, the objective of the operation becomes drainage of the abscess (with appendectomy, if it can be accomplished without difficulty). On occasion, examination using anesthesia shows acute cholecystitis or other disease to be the real cause of the patient's symptoms, and the operation then can be properly directed toward management of that disorder.

Presumed Uncomplicated Acute Appendicitis

The so-called McBurney incision is the time-honored and most widely used incision for appendectomy. It has the advantage of being a gridiron type of muscle-splitting incision, but that is its only advantage. Exposure through this incision is less adequate than through a transverse incision, and it cannot easily be extended if the diagnosis is incorrect. The only reason this incision is so widely used is that it is traditionally taught, from one surgeon to another, and those who employ it have not apparently thought about alternatives. For those who desire to use this incision, a description will be found in reference 36.

Transverse incision.—Exposure of the appendix through a transverse incision is better, particularly in obese patients and in those with a retroperitoneal appendix. The incision is made at a level 1–3 cm below the umbilicus and is centered on the midclavicular-midinguinal line. This incision lies in the direction of the skin wrinkle lines and yields a cosmetically superior scar, even if, of necessity, it is not sutured primarily. The incision must be long enough for the surgeon to be able to insert his hand into the abdominal cavity. The aponeuroses and muscles of the abdominal wall are split or incised in the direction of their fibers, which at this level also will be close to the direction of the skin wound (Fig 41–4).

The rectus sheath should not be opened routinely, but there should not be any hesitation about opening 1 or 2 cm of the anterior and posterior rectus sheath at its lateral border if be necessary to obtain appropriate exposure.

MOBILIZATION OF THE APPENDIX.—After the peritoneum is opened transversely, the location of the appendix is identified by following the anterior cecal taenia, and the inflamed appendix is coaxed into the wound, cupped in the palm of the hand. If the appendix is retrocecal (common) or retroperitoneal (uncommon), or if local inflammation or edema is intense, exposure is improved by dividing the lateral peritoneal reflection of the cecum. If mobilization is done properly, the cecum is rotated anteriorly and lies within the abdominal wound. The appendix will be at the level of the

anterior abdominal wall, and it will be unnecessary for vigorous retraction to be maintained throughout the operation.

EXCISION.—The mesoappendix is transected beginning at its free border, taking small bits of tissue between pairs of hemostats placed approximately 1 cm from and parallel to the appendix. A suture should be placed through the mesoappendix and into the wall of the cecum close to the base of the appendix to secure the intramural accessory branch to the posterior cecal artery.

On occasion, the appendix cannot be delivered into the wound because it is fixed in a retroperitoneal position. In these cases, retrograde removal of the appendix is accomplished, beginning by transecting the appendix at its base and followed by progressive division of the mesoappendix between clamps until the entire appendix has been mobilized and excised.[74]

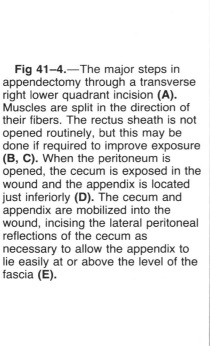

Fig 41–4.—The major steps in appendectomy through a transverse right lower quadrant incision **(A)**. Muscles are split in the direction of their fibers. The rectus sheath is not opened routinely, but this may be done if required to improve exposure **(B, C)**. When the peritoneum is opened, the cecum is exposed in the wound and the appendix is located just inferiorly **(D)**. The cecum and appendix are mobilized into the wound, incising the lateral peritoneal reflections of the cecum as necessary to allow the appendix to lie easily at or above the level of the fascia **(E)**.

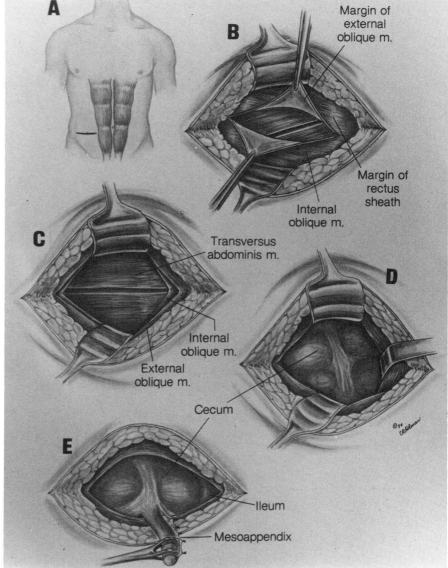

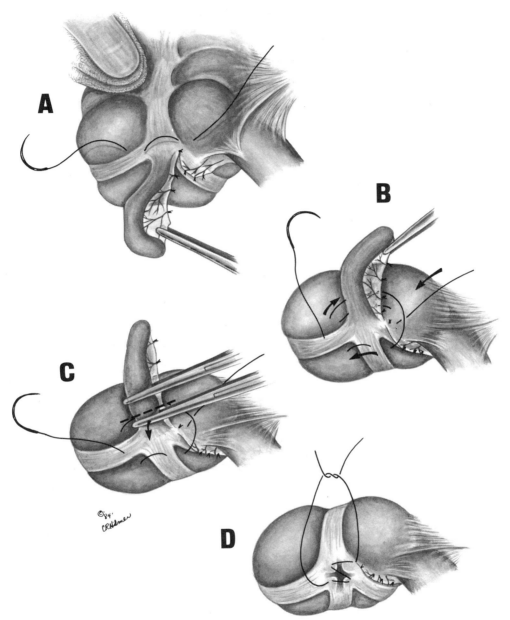

Fig 41–5.—A "Z" stitch is utilized to close the base of the cecum after excision of the appendix and inversion of the unligated appendiceal stump. Two bites of the suture are taken through the anterior wall of the cecum approximately one centimeter away from the appendix **(A).** The suture is then brought around the appendix medially and two additional bites are taken in the same direction in the posterior wall of the cecum **(B).** The appendix is then transected between clamps **(C).** The unligated stump of the appendix is inverted by pushing the tip of the hemostat holding the stump into the cecum and tightening the stitch **(D).** (From Adams J.T.: Z-Stitch suture for inversion of the appendiceal stump. *Surg. Gynecol. Obstet.* 127:1321, 1968.)

CLOSING THE STUMP.—Inversion of the unligated stump using a "Z" stitch, rather than the more conventional purse-string suture, is preferred (Fig 41–5). This maneuver accomplishes inversion of the appendiceal stump without spillage of cecal content. An appendix to be inverted should not be ligated, since ligation plus inversion does not reduce the risk of infectious complications, but creates conditions conducive to development of an intramural abscess or mucocele. In addition, the ligated plus inverted appendiceal stump may later appear as a cecal tumor and be a vexing source of diagnostic difficulties. If the appendix is edematous, turgid or otherwise unsuitable for inversion, it should be doubly ligated at its base, the distal ligature being placed as a suture ligature. It is unnecessary to paint the appendix with alcohol or iodophor or to suture the mesoappendix or omentum over the base of the cecum.

UNEXPECTED ABNORMALITIES IN THE APPENDIX.—On occasion, the operative findings are not those of appendicitis but of another entity in the appendix. The presence of a yellow-gray bulbous mass suggests a carcinoid tumor or mucocele. In the absence of metastases, simple appendectomy with a 2-cm border is sufficient therapy for most of these lesions; if a carcinoid is greater than 2 cm in diameter, right hemicolectomy should be done. Carcinoma of the appendix or cecum, or an appendiceal metastasis from a primary lesion elsewhere, can be associated with symptoms mimicking appendicitis. Patients with a large appendiceal mass or abscess also are particularly suspect of harboring a hidden right colon cancer; right hemicolectomy is usually required.

FINDING A NORMAL APPENDIX.—If an appropriate threshold for the decision to operate is maintained, a finite number of patients will be found to have a normal appendix at the time of exploration. This situation is due to the difficulty of firmly establishing the diagnosis in some patients, and in others is due to the presence of another intra-abdominal conditions producing symptoms mimicking appendicitis. In this clinical situation, the term "unnecessary appendectomy" is sometimes used but is inaccurate. Removal of a normal appendix in appropriate clinical circumstances never constitutes an unnecessary appendectomy. Active surgical intervention on the basis of minimal clinically suspicious symptoms and signs reduces both the morbidity and mortality associated with appendicitis.

When a normal appendix is found, an orderly investigation for the cause of the symptoms must be carried out. The first maneuver is to obtain a specimen of any peritoneal fluid or exudate for Gram stain to determine whether bacteria are present; this specimen also should be cultured for aerobes and anaerobes. Next, the cecum and adjacent ileum should be inspected looking for a tumor, perforated diverticulum, or regional enteritis. The small intestine is next examined in retrograde fashion, seeking a Meckel's diverticulum. The pelvic organs are palpated and inspected, seeking disease in that area. The intra-abdominal colon should be palpated next, after which the gallbladder and duodenum in the right upper quadrant should be visualized.

If enlarged lymph nodes are present in the mesentery, perhaps accompanied by some serositis, a representative node should be excised and sent for culture. Enteric pathogens will be recovered in a proportion of these cases of apparent mesenteric adenitis. Exploration of the abdomen should not cease until the cause of the acute abdominal symptoms has been identified or the surgeon is certain that no remedial lesion is present within the abdominal cavity. If no obvious cause of the appendicitis is identified intraoperatively, postoperative measurement of serum antibody titers for *Yersinia* may be in order.

WOUND CLOSURE.—The right iliac fossa and the wound margins are irrigated copiously; irrigation should be repeated after the muscles and aponeuroses have been sutured. The lavage solution should be suctioned away as completely as possible. Closure of the peritoneum is not necessary. Each musculofascial layer is closed with nonabsorbable sutures. If pus has been encountered intraoperatively, the skin and subcutaneous tissues should be packed open for 24–48 hours after which secondary wound closure is permitted.[58, 75] Otherwise, the skin wound should be closed primarily. The subcutaneous fat need not be sutured; a locking mattress suture can be used, if needed, to obliterate dead space in the subcutaneous portion of the wound.

Drainage of either the deep or of the subcutaneous portions of the wound, or of the abdominal cavity is not only unnecessary, but increases the risk of infection and other wound complications.[71, 76, 77] The patient may be discharged from the hospital when afebrile and a normal diet has been resumed, usually about two or three days postoperatively.

Appendiceal Mass Noted During Examination With Anesthesia

In these patients, there is gangrenous or locally perforated appendicitis with a developing phlegmon. Usually the duration of symptoms is too short for a fully developed periappendiceal abscess to have formed. Appendectomy is still the objective of this operation. The transverse incision, however, should be made directly over the most prominent portion of the mass. The muscles and aponeuroses are split in the direction of their fibers. The peritoneum at the lateral margin of the wound is bluntly mobilized medially and the mass entered from its lateral aspect. Fluid and pus, if present, are aspirated away after a specimen has been obtained for culture and sensitivity tests. The tissues are bluntly dissected sufficiently to expose the appendix. Care should be taken not to disturb adherent coils of intestine or omentum on the medial side of the mass while accomplishing the appendectomy. More often than not, the base of the appendix will be turgid, and double ligation of the stump, rather than inversion, will be selected.

The question of whether or not to drain in these cases remains a subject of debate. In most patients with a gangrenous but unperforated appendix, and without a defined collection of appendiceal pus, closure without subfascial drainage is indicated. If a periappendiceal abscess is present such that the turgid tissues have created a potential dead space, the cavity should be drained with a suction drain brought out through a separate stab incision. The suction drain need remain in place only for one–three days. The right iliac fossae and the wound should be irrigated prior to layer closure of the muscles with interrupted nonabsorbable sutures. The skin and subcutaneous wound should not be sutured. Parenteral antibiotic therapy is continued postoperatively as clinically indicated. A rectal examination should be done daily to detect any developing postoperative pelvic abscess. Discharge from the hospital is delayed until the patient has been afebrile for two days, has not been receiving antibiotics for the preceding three days, and has no evidence of an intraperitoneal or pelvic abscess.

Management of An Appendix Mass Noted on Admission to Hospital

Patients who are first seen when symptoms are subsiding and in whom a well localized periappendiceal mass can be detected on physical examination should be managed initially without an operation. Considerable clinical judgment needs to be exercised in selecting patients for this form of management. It should be kept in mind that children, pregnant women, and many elderly patients will have a high failure rate when treated in this expectant fashion.

The patient should be put to bed, treated with IV fluids, nasogastric suction and IV antibiotics. In two thirds of adults in whom expectant treatment is carried out, symptoms continue to subside, the periappendiceal mass resolves, and a subsequent interval appendectomy can be accomplished after four to six weeks. In one third of patients, however, symptoms do not subside, but persist or worsen. In these patients, prompt drainage of the periappendiceal abscess must be carried out.

The incision for drainage is made just medial to the iliac crest at the level of the most prominent aspect of the periappendiceal mass. The muscles are split and the lateral edge of the peritoneum is exposed. The mass surrounding the appendix is approached from its lateral retroperitoneal aspect. If pus is present under pressure, the abscess may rupture spontaneously. If not, a finger should be slowly introduced into the abscess and its loculations broken down by blunt dissection. Care must be taken not to break down adhesions walling off the medial aspect of the appendix mass from the peritoneal cavity. If the appendix is readily accessible, appendectomy can be performed. The incidence of recurrent appendicitis within two years after nonoperative treatment, or drainage of an appendiceal abscess without appendectomy, is 25%. This fact urges interval appendectomy which should be conducted six to eight weeks later.[78, 79]

A suction drain should be inserted into the abscess cavity and extracted through a stab wound in the flank. The abscess cavity is irrigated, the muscular layers are approximated with absorbable sutures, and the subcutaneous tissues and skin incision are packed open. The sump tube should be left undisturbed until it is draining less than 2 oz. each day. The tube should then be twisted but not advanced. If drainage does not resume, a sinogram should be obtained. Only when the abscess cavity has collapsed around the drain, should the drain be progressively advanced and removed.

Parenteral antibiotic therapy is continued as clinically indicated. A daily rectal examination is made to detect any developing pelvic abscess. The patient will often be more comfortable if the head of the bed is elevated 15°–30°, but this maneuver does not necessarily promote localization of a subsequent abscess in the pelvis.

If, after a week or so, the patient is afebrile and shows no signs of developing complications, continued treatment in the hospital is not necessary simply because the drain remains in place. When the patient is consuming an adequate oral diet, has not been receiving antibiotics for 72 hours, and has not had a temperature exceeding 37.5°C (99.5°F) for 48 hours, hospital discharge and management of the resolving abscess as an outpatient are in order.

Incidental Appendectomy

Incidental appendectomy is performed under two circumstances: first, during an operation done for suspected acute appendicitis but the appendix is found to be normal and, second, as an addition to another elective abdominal operation, typically hysterectomy or cholecystectomy. Opinion regarding appendectomy in the first instance is reasonably well-settled: the appendix should be removed. The reason is that the incision suggests an operation for appendicitis, but the patient's memory in the future may not be entirely clear about either the nature of the disease which lead to the operation or whether the appendix was removed, thus setting the stage for future diagnostic and therapeutic confusion should the appendix remain in place. It is better to remove the appendix in these circumstances and to inform the patient clearly that the appendix has been excised.

Opinion regarding removal of the appendix as an incidental addition to other routine intra-abdominal operations is not unanimous.[80] Some studies[81, 82] indicate that incidental appendectomy slightly increases the risk of wound infection. Other studies indicate little impact on morbidity and that incidental appendectomy is safe.[83, 84] The risk of future appendicitis (Fig 41–6), although small, is probably greater than any risk associated with incidental appendectomy in younger patients.[85] After age 50, however, the future risk of developing appendicitis is balanced by the morbidity and mortality risks of incidental appendectomy, and the rationale in older adults for routine incidental appendectomy, therefore, is less clear.

Several conditions must be present if elective incidental appendectomy is to be conducted with minimal risk. There must be adequate exposure, without undue additional dissection, through the incision made for the primary operation. The patient must have tolerated the main operative procedure well, and there should be no existing complications resulting from the main procedure. Incidental removal of the appendix in patients who have Crohn's disease is generally safe if the patient has had acute bowel symptoms for less than one week; if symptoms have been present for longer than this, incidental appendectomy is followed by a high incidence of fistula.[86, 87]

Incidental appendectomy has been objected to on the basis that the appendix may have an immune function and serve as a source of immunologically competent lymphocytes. There is no evidence that appendectomy results in any deficit in any

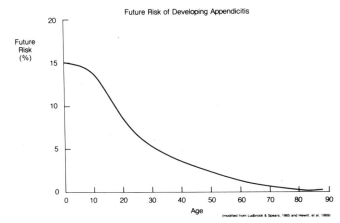

Fig 41–6.—The future risk of developing appendicitis is approximately 15% at birth and declines steadily throughout life. After middle age, the risk of developing appendicitis at any time in the future is quite small. (From Hewitt D., Milner J., LeRiche W.H.: Incidental appendectomy: a statistical appraisal. *Can. Med. Assoc. J.* 100:1075, 1969; and Ludbrook J., Spears G.F.S.: The risk of developing appendicitis. *Br. J. Surg.* 52:856, 1965.)

lymphocyte-mediated function in man. Objections also have been raised to incidental appendectomy on the basis that appendectomy may predispose to subsequent development of cancer. Extensive population studies have now discredited this objection.[88]

One of the curious observations in reported series of incidental appendectomy is that 15%–25% of incidentally excised appendices show evidence of concurrent or antecedent abnormality. In many cases, the diagnosis established is mucosal inflammation, an entity whose clinical significance is not established and which probably does not serve as a harbinger of future appendicitis.[89] However, in about 10% of incidentally excised appendices, abnormalities which might lead to the future development of appendicitis have been identified, adding weight to the rationale of conducting routine incidental appendectomy in patients below age 40.

COMPLICATIONS OF APPENDECTOMY

Most complications of appendicitis, both immediate and delayed, are due to perforation. This is the reason why it is important to diagnose appendicitis and conduct appendectomy prior to perforation. It also is the justification for exploration whenever appendicitis is suspected and cannot be ruled out, and for finding a proportion of normal appendices at such explorations.

Wound infection is the most common complication following appendectomy. The organisms involved are those of the polymicrobic fecal flora found in the appendix lumen; aerobic coliforms and streptococci tend to predominate among the bacteria recovered from an infected subcutaneous wound; anaerobes become more frequent if the muscular or subfascial planes are involved. Classic signs of infection often are not present. A painful wound associated with modest edema and slight erythema is usually detected by the end of the first postoperative week. When such signs are present, the skin sutures should be removed and the wound opened. A thin, serous discharge of small volume is a more common result than a rush of pus.

Intra-abdominal abscesses, including pelvic and subphrenic abscesses, occur in up to 20% of patients who have suffered perforation of the appendix. These abscesses are due to preoperative contamination of the peritoneal cavity by organisms leaking from the appendix. Less often, contamination by intraoperative spillage during appendectomy results in an abscess. Occasionally, an abscess forms around a retained fecalith or other foreign body. The organisms involved in intra-abdominal abscesses also are derived from the polymicrobic fecal flora; in this instance anaerobic organisms, such as *Bacteroides* species and anaerobic streptococci, predominate over aerobic organisms.

The presence of an abscess is manifest by the usual signs: recurrent fever, eventually becoming spiking in pattern, associated with malaise and anorexia, usually beginning toward the end of the first postoperative week and becoming more obvious by the end of the second postoperative week. A pelvic abscess may, in addition, cause diarrhea and often can be palpated on vaginal or rectal examination. Subphrenic abscess, in addition to the usual signs, frequently produces an

effusion in the overlying hemithorax and immobility of the involved diaphragm.

Computed tomography is a great help in diagnosing an intra-abdominal abscess. If the abscess if suitably accessible, percutaneous drainage may be effected; if not, operative surgical drainage is required. A pelvic abscess, on occasion, may be drained through the rectum or vagina. In patients suspected of having an abscess in whom diagnostic efforts are unavailing, abdominal exploration after the second postoperative week may be appropriate.

Fecal fistula is not a common complication following appendectomy; should it occur, the underlying presence of Crohn's disease should be suspected. Fecal fistulas also may be due to a retained foreign body or to a purse-string suture tied too tightly around the base of the appendix, leading to necrosis and perforation of the cecum. Necrosis from a periappendiceal abscess, retention of the tip of the appendix, or an undetected neoplasm also may lead to a postoperative fecal fistula. Fecal fistulas close spontaneously in most cases. All that is required is to ensure that the track remains open until all drainage ceases. Fecal fistulas which do not close spontaneously are those in which the tip of the appendix or foreign body has been retained, bowel beyond the fistula is partially or completely obstructed, or mucous membrane of the gut becomes continuous with the skin. In such cases, closure of the fistula requires an operation.

Pylephlebitis is a serious illness associated with gangrenous or perforated appendicitis and characterized by high fever, chills, and jaundice. It is due to septicemia of the portal venous system, and leads to development of liver abscess. Pylephlebitis may appear either preoperatively or postoperatively. The infecting organism usually is *E. coli*. Fortunately, now that antibiotics are utilized before and after appendectomy, this complication has become relatively rare.

Hepatic abscess as a complication of appendicitis usually is a consequence of pylephlebitis. In a rare case, a subacute appendicitis may settle, the consequent hepatic abscess causing symptoms only several weeks later. The symptoms of hepatic abscess are those of any bacterial abscess: spiking fever and intermittent chills, usually accompanied by relatively profound anorexia; sometimes liver tenderness to palpation is also present. A CT examination of the liver is the most useful diagnostic test. Blood cultures are positive during episodes of chills and rigors; the alkaline phosphatase is usually elevated, and leukocytosis is also always present.[90]

Intestinal obstruction, initially paralytic but occasionally progressing to true mechanical obstruction, may occur with slowly resolving peritonitis in complicated appendicitis. Mechanical obstruction is seen most frequently in elderly patients, and its development usually requires operative relief.[91]

Perforated appendicitis occurring in teenaged girls may have an adverse subsequent effect on fertility. Although the incidence of such problems is small,[92] recognition that tubal infertility may result from appendicitis rather than from ascending genital tract infection provides a further imperative for early appendectomy in suspected appendicitis.[93]

Appendectomy may subsequently increase the incidence of right inguinal hernia, particularly if the hernia repair is performed through a McBurney or other low-abdominal incision.[94]

REFERENCES

1. Castleton K.B., Puestow C.B., Sauer D.: Is appendicitis decreasing in frequency? *Arch. Surg.* 78:794, 1959.
2. Jessop J.H.: Falling incidence of appendicitis. *Br. J. Surg.* 68:445, 1981.
3. Lewis F.R., Holcroft J.W., Boey J., et al.: Appendicitis: A critical review of diagnosis and treatment in 1,000 cases. *Arch. Surg.* 110:677, 1975.
4. Noer T.: Decreasing incidence of acute appendicitis. *Acta Chir. Scand.* 141:431, 1975.
5. Raguveer-Saran M.K., Keddie N.C.: The falling incidence of appendicitis. *Br. J. Surg.* 67:681, 1980.
6. Peltokallio P., Tykka H.: Evolution of the age distribution and mortality of acute appendicitis. *Arch. Surg.* 116:153, 1981.
7. Silberman V.A.: Appendectomy in a large metropolitan hospital: Retrospective analysis of 1,013 cases. *Am. J. Surg.* 142:615, 1981.
8. Howie J.G.R.: Death from appendicitis and appendicectomy. *Lancet* 2:1334, 1966.
9. Meade R.H.: The evolution of surgery for appendicitis. Surgery 55:741, 1964.
10. Richardson R.G.: *The Surgeon's Tale.* New York, Charles Scribners Sons, 1958.
11. Louyer-Villermay J.B.: Observations pour servir a l'histoire de inflammations de l'appendice du caecum. *Arch. Gen. Med. Paris.* 5:246, 1824.
12. Melier F.: Mémoire sur des tumeurs phlegmoneuses occupant la fosse de l'appendice cecal. *J. Gen. Med. Chir. Pharm.* 100:317, 1827.
13. Fitz R.H.: Perforating inflammation of the vermiform appendix, with special reference to its early diagnosis and treatment. *Trans. Assoc. Am. Physicians* 1:107, 1886.
14. Senn N.: A plea in favor of early laparotomy for catarrhal and ulcerative appendicitis, with report of two cases. *J.A.M.A.* 12:630, 1889.
15. Murphy J.B.: 2,000 Operations for appendicitis—deductions from his personal experience. *Am. J. Med. Sci.* 128:187, 1904.
16. Ochsner A.: The conservative treatment of appendiceal peritonitis. *J. La. State. Med. Soc.* 87:32, 1934.
17. Collins D.C.: Agenesis of the vermiform appendix. *Am. J. Surg.* 82:689, 1951.
18. Host W.H., Rush B., Lazaro E.J.: Congenital absence of the vermiform appendix. *Am. Surg.* 38:355, 1972.
19. Saleeby R.G., Zollinger R.M., Ellison E.E.: Acute appendicitis in an adult with two separate vermiform appendices. *Surgery* 36:306, 1954.
20. Kelly A.J., Hurdon E.: *The Vermiform Appendix and Its Diseases.* Philadelphia, W.B. Saunders Co., 1905.
21. Veillon A., Zuber A.: Sur quelques microbes strictement anaerobies et leur role en patholgie. *Arch. Med. Exp.* 10:517–545, 1898.
22. Altemeier W.A.: The bacterial flora of acute perforated appendicitis with peritonitis: A bacteriologic study based upon one hundred cases. *Ann. Surg.* 107:517, 1938.
23. Short A.R.: *The Causation of Appendicitis.* Bristol, John Wright, 1946.
24. Arnbjornsson E., Asp N.-G., Westin S.I.: Decreasing incidence of acute appendicitis with special reference to the consumption of dietary fiber. *Acta Chir. Scand.* 148:461, 1982.
25. Arnbjornsson E.: Acute appendicitis: A familial disease? *Curr. Surg.* 39:18, 1982.
26. van Zwalenburg C.: The relation of mechanical distention to the etiology of appendicitis. *Ann. Surg.* 41:437, 1905.
27. Wangensteen O.H., Dennis C.: Experimental proof of obstructive origin of appendicitis in man. *Ann. Surg.* 110:629, 1939.
28. Dennis C.: Physiologic behavior of the human appendix and the problem of appendicitis: Reaction of the appendix to drugs. *Arch. Surg.* 43:1021, 1941.
29. Arnbjornsson E., Bengmark S.: Obstruction of the appendix lumen in relation to pathogenesis of acute appendicitis. *Acta. Chir. Scand.* 149:789, 1983.
30. McCarthy V.P., Mischler E.H., Hubbard V.S., et al.: Appendi-

ceal abscess in cystic fibrosis; A diagnostic challenge. *Gastroenterology* 86:564, 1984.
31. Dimond D.M., Proctor H.J.: Concomitant pneumococcal appendicitis, peritonitis and meningitis. *Arch. Surg.* 111:888–889, 1976.
32. Fowler R.H.: Rare incidence of acute appendicitis resulting from external trauma. *Ann. Surg.* 107:529–539, 1938.
33. Schisgall R.M.: Appendiceal colic in childhood: The role of inspissated casts of stool within the appendix. *Ann. Surg.* 192:687, 1980.
34. Deck K.B., Pettitt B.J., Harrison M.R.: The length-time correlate in appendicitis. *J.A.M.A.* 244:806, 1980.
35. Buchman T.G., Zuidema G.D.: Reasons for delay of the diagnosis of acute appendicitis. *Surg. Gynecol. Obstet.* 158:260, 1984.
36. McBurney C.: The incision made in the abdominal wall in case of appendicitis with a description of a new method of operating. *Ann. Surg.* 20:38, 1894.
37. Hyman P., Westring D.W.: Leukocytosis in acute appendicitis: Observed racial difference. *J.A.M.A.* 229:1630, 1974.
38. Bolton J.P., Craven E.R., Croft R.J., et al.: An assessment of the value of the white cell count in the management of suspected acute appendicitis *Br. J. Surg.* 62:906, 1975.
39. Kretchmar L.H., McDonald D.F.: The urine sediment in acute appendicitis. *Arch. Surg.* 87:209, 1963.
40. Deutsch A.A., Zelikovsky A., Reiss R.: Laparoscopy in the prevention of unnecessary appendicectomies: A prospective study. *Br. J. Surg.* 69:336–337, 1982.
41. Leape L.L., Ramenofsky M.L.: Laparoscopy for Questionable Appendicitis: Can it reduce the negative appendectomy rate?. *Ann. Surg.* 191:410, 1980.
42. Rajagopalan A.E., Mason J.H., Kennedy M., et al.: The value of the barium enema in the diagnosis of acute appendicitis. *Arch. Surg.* 12:531, 1977.
43. Smith D.E., Jacquet J.M., Virgilio R.W.: Left upper quadrant appendicitis. *Arch. Surg.* 109:443, 1974.
44. Jona J., Belin R., Selke A.: Barium enema as a diagnostic aid in children with abdominal pain. *Surg. Gynecol. Obstet.* 144:351, 1977.
45. Hatch E.I. Jr., Naffis D., Chandler N.W.: Pitfalls in the use of barium enema in early appendicitis in children. *Curr. Surg.* 39:356, 1982.
46. Smith D.E., Kirchmer N.A., Stewart D.R.: Use of the barium enema in the diagnosis of acute appendicitis and its complications. *Am. J. Surg.* 138:829, 1979.
47. Schisgall R.M.: Use of the barium swallow in the diagnosis of acute appendicitis. *Am. J. Surg.* 146:663, 1983.
48. DeDombal F.T., Leaper D.J., Horrocks J.C., et al.: Human and computer-aided diagnosis of abdominal pain: Further report with emphasis on performance of clinicians. *Br. Med. J.* 1:376, 1974.
49. Van Way C.W., Murphy J.R., Dunn E.L., et al.: A feasibility study of computer aided diagnosis in appendicitis. *Surg. Gynecol. Obstet.* 155:685, 1982.
50. Teicher I., Landa B., Cohen M., et al.: Scoring system to aid in diagnosis of appendicitis. *Ann. Surg.* 198:753, 1983.
51. Edwards F.H., Davies R.S.: Use of a Bayesian algorithm in the computer-assisted diagnosis of appendicitis. *Surg. Gynecol. Obstet.* 158:219, 1984.
52. Jess P., Bjerregaard B., Brynitz S., et al.: Acute appendicitis: Prospective trial concerning diagnostic accuracy and complications. *Am. J. Surg.* 141:232, 1981.
53. Foran B., Berne T.V., Rosoff L.: Management of the appendiceal mass. *Arch. Surg.* 113:1144, 1978.
54. Jordan J.S., Kovalcik P.J., Schwab C.W.: Appendicitis with a palpable mass. *Ann. Surg.* 193:227, 1981.
55. Skubo-Kristensen E., Hvid I.: The appendiceal mass: Results of conservative management. *Ann. Surg.* 196:584, 1982.
56. Martin L.W., Perrin E.V.: Neonatal perforation of the appendix in association with Hirschsprung's disease. *Ann. Surg.* 166:799, 1967.
57. Bell M.J., Bower R.J., Ternberg J.L.: Appendectomy in childhood: Analysis of 105 negative explorations. *Am. J. Surg.* 144:335, 1982.

58. Stone H.H., Sanders S.L., Martin J.D. Jr.: Perforated appendicitis in children. *Surgery* 69:673, 1971.

59. Schwartz M.Z., Tapper D., Solenberger R.I.: Management of perforated appendicitis in children. *Ann. Surg.* 197:407, 1983.

60. Powers R.J., Andrassy R.J., Breenan L.P., et al.: Alternate approach to the management of acute perforating appendicitis in children. *Surg. Gynecol. Obstet.* 152:473, 1981.

61. Baer A.L., Reis R.A., Erens R.A.: Appendicitis in pregnancy with changes in position and axis of the normal appendix in pregnancy. *J.A.M.A.* 98:1359, 1932.

62. Grossman E.B. Jr.: Chronic appendicitis. *Surg. Gynecol. Obstet.* 146:596–598, 1978.

63. Sherman N.J., Woolley M.M.: The ileocecal syndrome in acute childhood leukemia. *Arch. Surg.* 107:39, 1973.

64. Ver Steeg K., LaSalle A., Ratner I.: Appendicitis in acute leukemia. *Arch. Surg.* 114:632, 1979.

65. Shaked A., Shinar E., Freund H.: Neutropenic typhlitis: A plea for conservatism. *Dis. Colon Rectum* 26:351, 1983.

66. Schaller R.T., Schaller J.F.: The acute abdomen in the immunologically compromised child. *J. Pediatr. Surg.* 18:937, 1983.

67. Arnbjornsson E.: Varying frequency of acute appendicitis in different phases of the menstrual cycle. *Surg. Gynecol. Obstet.* 155:709, 1982.

68. Robinson J.A., Burch B.H.: An assessment of the value of the menstrual history in differentiating acute appendicitis from pelvic inflammatory disease. *Surg. Gynecol. Obstet.* 159:149, 1984.

69. Narasimharao K.L., Malik A.K., Mitra S.K., et al.: Inflammatory pseudotumor of the appendix. *Am. J. Gastroenterol.* 79:32, 1984.

70. Saebo A.: The Yersinia enterocolitica infection in acute abdominal surgery. *Ann. Surg.* 198:760, 1983.

71. Yates J.L.: An experimental study of the local effects of peritoneal drainage. *Surg. Gynecol. Obstet.* 1:473, 1905.

72. Gottrup E., Hunt T.K.: Antimicrobial prophylaxis in appendectomy patients. *World J. Surg.* 6:306, 1982.

73. Uden P., Eskilsson P., Brunes L., et al.: A clinical evaluation of postoperative peritoneal lavage in the treatment of perforated appendicitis. *Br. J. Surg.* 70:348, 1983.

74. Ker H.: Retrograde appendicectomy. *Lancet* 2:889, 1964.

75. Grosfeld J.L., Solit R.W.: Prevention of wound infection in perforated appendicitis. *Ann. Surg.* 168:891, 1968.

76. Haller J.A. Jr., Shaker I.J., Donahoo J.S., et al.: Peritoneal drainage versus non-drainage for generalized peritonitis from ruptured appendicitis in children. *Ann. Surg.* 177:595, 1973.

77. Stone H.H., Hooper C.A., Millikan W.J. Jr.: Abdominal drainage following appendectomy and cholecystectomy. *Ann. Surg.* 187:606, 1978.

78. Befeler D.: Recurrent appendicitis: Incidence and prophylaxis. *Arch. Surg.* 89:666–668, 1984.

79. Arnbjornsson E.: Management of appendiceal abscess. *Curr. Surg.* 41:4, 1984.

80. Hays R.J.: Incidental appendectomies: Current teaching. *J.A.M.A.* 238:31, 1977.

81. Cruse P.J.E.: Incidence of wound infection on surgical services. *Surg. Clin. North Am.* 55:1269, 1975.

82. Pollock A.V., Evans M.: Wound sepsis after cholecystectomy. Effect of incidental appendicectomy. *Br. Med. J.* 1:20, 1977.

83. Cromartie A.D. Jr., Kovalcik P.J.: Incidental appendectomy at the time of surgery for ectopic pregnancy. *Am. J. Surg.* 139:244, 1980.

84. Strom P.R., Turkleson M.L., Stone H.H.: Safety of incidental appendectomy. *Am. J. Surg.* 145:819, 1983.

85. Mulvihill S., Goldthorn J., Woolley M.M.: Incidental appendectomy in infants and children. *Arch. Surg.* 118:714, 1983.

86. Fonkalsrud E.W., Ament M.E., Fleisher D.: Management of the appendix in young patients with Crohn's disease. *Arch. Surg.* 117:11, 1982.

87. Simonowitz D.A., Rusch V.W., Stevenson J.K.: Natural history of incidental appendectomy in patients with Crohn's disease who required subsequent bowel resection. *Am. J. Surg.* 143:171, 1982.

88. Moertel C.G., Nobrega F.T., Elveback L.R., et al.: A prospective study of appendectomy and predisposition to cancer. *Surg. Gynecol. Obstet.* 138:549, 1974.

89. Pieper R., Kager L., Nasman P.: Clinical significance of mucosal inflammation of the vermiform appendix. *Ann. Surg.* 197:368, 1983.

90. Cooperman M.: Complications of appendectomy. *Surg. Clin. North Am.* 63:1233–1247, 1983.

91. Harris S., Rudolf L.E.: Mechanical small bowel obstruction due to acute appendicitis: Review of 10 cases. *Ann. Surg.* 164:157–161, 1966.

92. Puri P., Guiney E.F., O'Donnell B., et al.: Effects of perforated appendicitis in girls on subsequent fertility. *Br. Med. J.* 288:25, 1984.

93. Reiss H.E.: Effect of perforated appendicitis in girls on subsequent fertility. *Br. Med. J.* 288:570, 1984.

94. Arnbjornsson E.: Development of right inguinal hernia after appendectomy. *Am. J. Surg.* 143:174, 1982.

42

Chronic Ulcerative Colitis

KEITH A. KELLY, M.D.
ROGER R. DOZOIS, M.D.

DEFINITION AND OVERVIEW

Chronic ulcerative colitis is a cryptogenic, inflammatory, ulcerating disease of the mucosa of the large intestine for which no specific medical therapy exists. Patients with severe and progressive forms of the disease often come to operation, at which excision of the large intestine and permanent end-ileostomy have usually been performed. After operation, the patients must wear an external bag day and night to collect the output from the GI tract. Newer operative approaches are being used today, however, that allow proctocolectomy without the need of the bag. The newer approaches include colectomy, mucosal rectectomy and ileal pouch-anal anastomosis, continent ileostomy, and the ileostomy occluding device. This chapter will contrast the standard operative approach to the newer approaches and to other operations for ulcerative colitis.

HISTORICAL BACKGROUND

Patients with ulcerative colitis were seldom operated on prior to the 20th century. With the 1913 report of Brown,[1] who did ileostomy alone for this condition, bypassing the diseased large intestine, interest in the surgical approach was kindled. The ileostomy Brown made was a straight, end-on ileostomy, the terminal portion of which projected above the skin surface. Intestinal content was discharged onto the serosal surface of the ileum and onto the abdominal skin. The exposed serosa of the terminal ileum and the skin became acutely and chronically inflamed, leading to serositis and ileostomy dysfunction. Ileostomy care was primitive. The bypassed but still diseased large intestine, moreover, continued to cause symptoms and result in disability. The need for resection of the diseased bowel and for improvements in ileostomy construction and care was increasingly recognized.

Resection came to be accepted in the 1920s, '30s, and early '40s, but improvements in ileostomy construction and care were not brought about until the work of Dragstedt's team[2] and Brooke[3] in the late 1940s and '50s. These advances made the end results of the operation more acceptable.[4] Kock's concept of a continent ileal pouch proximal to an end ileostomy in the 1960s[5] further stimulated interest in the search for alternatives to the incontinent Brooke ileostomy or to an ileostomy of any type. These efforts have led to the endorectal ileal pouch-anal anastomosis.[6-8] With this novel procedure,

the entire disease can be removed, while the usual transanal route of fecal discharge and anal continence are nearly completely preserved.

INCIDENCE

Ulcerative colitis is an uncommon disease, estimated to occur in about 5 of 100,000 individuals at risk per year.[9] The disease is as common in men as in women and can strike persons of any age, although the peak age of onset is in the second decade of life. The disease is more common among whites than among blacks or orientals, and may be more common among certain ethnic groups, such as Jews. A familial tendency has been noted, but the disease is not inherited in an autosomal dominant pattern. Persons who live in temperate climates are at greater risk than those who live in tropical climates.

ETIOLOGY

No etiology has been established for ulcerative colitis. Infectious causal agents, especially bacteria and viruses, have long been sought, but none has yet been clearly identified. An autoimmune origin has been proposed, the immune response perhaps being triggered by the consumption of bovine milk instead of human mother's milk in susceptible infants, but again no clear-cut causal relationship has been established. A psychogenic origin of ulcerative colitis has also been proposed. There is no doubt that some patients with ulcerative colitis have personality disorders. Whether these are the cause of the colitis or the result of it is unknown. Clearly, having 20 to 30 bowel movements per day, feeling ill, and being confined to close quarters because of the need for toilet facilities stresses the psyche. Moreover, many if not most patients will resolve their personality disorders when their disease has been removed, suggesting that the personality disorder is the result of the disease rather than its source.

PATHOLOGY

The early and characteristic lesion of ulcerative colitis is an acute inflammatory infiltrate surrounding the crypts of the mucosal glands of the large intestine. The infiltrate is accompanied by edema, hyperemia, and abscess formation, the crypt abscess (Fig 42–1). Hemorrhagic necrosis and ulceration

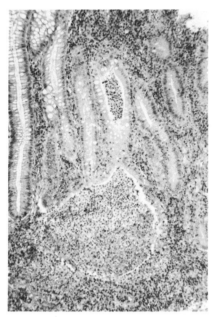

Fig 42–1.—Photomicrograph of colonic mucosa in ulcerative colitis showing crypt abscess.

of the mucosa develop, but extension of the inflammatory process into or even through the tunica muscularis usually does not develop. When the ulcerations are large and confluent, the remaining islands of less involved mucosa may mimic polyps; hence, the term pseudopolyps (Fig 42–2).

The disease most often begins in the rectum and sigmoid colon, where it is usually most severe. The disease may extend proximally into the descending colon, the transverse colon, the ascending colon, the cecum, and the appendix, although these areas may be spared. The involvement is usually continuous from the rectum proximally, rather than patchy or segmental.

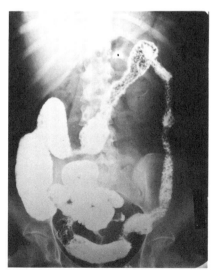

Fig 42–2.—Radiograph of large intestine using BaSO$_4$ showing ulcerative colitis. Ulceration and pseudopolyps are especially prominent on the left side of the colon.

Progression of the disease leads to loss of blood, protein, fluid, and electrolytes via the stools. Weight loss, inanition, and malnutrition ensue. Severe progression of the inflammatory progress may result in marked dilatation, subsequent necrosis, and even perforation of the bowel wall. The enlargement of the colon is accompanied by signs and symptoms of peritonitis and systemic toxicity, a picture called "toxic megacolon."

Long-standing inflammation can lead to stricture of the colon or to malignant transformation of the mucosa. Among patients with onset of the colitis in childhood and with universal involvement of large intestine, the risk of adenocarcinoma developing in the diseased mucosa is about 2% of the population at risk per year after the first ten years of the disease. Such cancers are often multiple, high grade, infiltrating, and metastatic.

PREVENTION OF DISEASE

No specific preventive measures are known because no specific etiology has been identified. Because of the increasing risk of cancer ten years after the development of universal disease in children or young adults,[10] many surgeons have recommended prophylactic proctocolectomy in such individuals. An alternative recently suggested is endoscopic surveillance and multiple biopsies, advising operation only for those patients with cancer or dysplasia of the sampled mucosa. The effectiveness of the latter approach remains unproved.

SYMPTOMS AND SIGNS OF DISEASE

Patients with ulcerative colitis develop diarrhea. Stools are frequent, watery, and usually bloody. The passage of 20 or 30 stools per day is not uncommon. Blood loss via the stools may be acute enough to require transfusion to maintain the circulating blood volume. When the loss is less acute but continuing, chronic anemia and hypoproteinemia may result. Urgency, abdominal cramps, and tenesmus accompany the call to stool. Urgency is such that incontinence is not uncommon. The cramps and tenesmus are disabling. Patients are often so restricted by their diarrhea that they fear leaving their houses.

When strictures appear, increased cramping and abdominal distention indicate partial intestinal obstruction. The development of adenocarcinoma of the large-intestinal mucosa is often insidious, being masked by the symptoms and signs of the colitis. With continued growth, however, such cancers will produce bleeding, obstruction, and perforation on their own, as they do in patients without ulcerative colitis.

Patients with toxic megacolon appear acutely ill with fever, tachycardia, a thready pulse, and a decreased blood pressure. Respirations are shallow and rapid. Abdominal pain is diffuse. The abdomen is tense, tender, and tympanitic. Bowel sounds are absent.

Extraintestinal manifestations may complicate the disease (Table 42–1). Erythema nodosum, erythema multiforme, and pyoderma gangrenosum may involve the skin, while iritis and uveitis appear in the eye. Arthritis may be migratory and involve the peripheral joints or may be central, involving the spine with ankylosing spondylitis. The characteristic liver le-

TABLE 42–1.—COMPLICATIONS OF
ULCERATIVE COLITIS

Intestinal
    Stricture, obstruction
    Perforation
    Hemorrhage
    Adenocarcinoma
Extraintestinal
    Skin
        Erythema nodosum
        Erythema multiforme
        Pyoderma gangrenosum
    Eyes
        Uveitis, iritis
    Joints
        Migrating polyarthritis
        Ankylosing spondylitis
    Liver
        Sclerosing cholangitis
        Cirrhosis
        Cancer of the bile ducts
    Blood
        Thrombocytosis
        Thrombosis and
           embolism

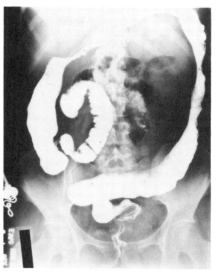

Fig 42–3.—Radiograph of large intestine using $BaSO_4$ showing ulcerative colitis. Diffuse mucosal ulceration and shortening of the entire large intestine are present.

sion is hepatic triaditis, an acute and chronic inflammation of the portal triad that can progress to cirrhosis. Sclerosing cholangitis and cancers of the bile ducts are more common among patients with ulcerative colitis than controls. Thrombocytosis may develop and result in thrombosis and occlusion of the venous and arterial vessels. With chronic debility, amyloidosis may develop.

DIAGNOSIS

The onset of the characteristic symptoms and signs arouses suspicion of the disease. The diagnosis can usually be confirmed by endoscopy, biopsy and radiologic examination of the colon with $BaSO_4$. On endoscopy, the mucosa is granular, friable, bleeds easily when touched or rubbed, and may be ulcerated. The normal vascular pattern is effaced. Biopsy shows acute inflammation of the mucosa with the characteristic crypt abscess. The ulcerative and diffuse nature of the mucosal disease can be confirmed by the radiologist, who usually finds the most severe involvement in the rectum and sigmoid colon, with continuous but lesser involvement as the right side of the colon is visualized (Fig 42–3). Pseudopolyps, strictures, and cancers may be noted by either the endoscopist or the radiologist.

The accumulation of air in any or all segments of the colon suggests toxic megacolon (Fig 42–4), as does gas in the wall of the bowel or in the adjacent vessels. Free air in the abdominal cavity may be found when perforation has occurred, although most often the perforation is sealed.

Infectious causes of colitis must be ruled out by microscopic examination and culture of the stool and by serologic tests (Table 42–2). Crohn's disease of the large intestine can usually, but not always, be excluded by history, physical examination, endoscopy, and radiology (Table 42–3). Anal symptoms and signs, with fissures, abscesses, and fistulas, are more common with Crohn's than ulcerative colitis, as discussed in chapter 39. Crohn's disease is usually segmental or discontinuous and transmural, while ulcerative colitis is diffuse, contin-

uous, and mucosal. Crohn's disease more commonly has an ileal and right colonic distribution than does ulcerative colitis, and more often results in intra-abdominal fistulas and abscesses. Crohn's disease causes a granulomatous inflammatory response, while ulcerative colitis is characterized by crypt abscesses. Nonetheless, while careful study will usually establish whether the patient has Crohn's disease or ulcerative colitis, not every patient can be clearly categorized. Some patients have features of both diseases, and only the subsequent clinical course will eventually establish the true nature of the disease.

MEDICAL TREATMENT

Medical treatment is nonspecific and supportive. Most patients usually receive either sulfasalazine or prednisone or

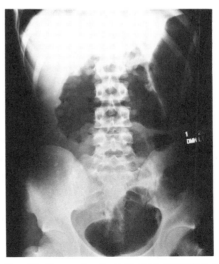

Fig 42–4.—Radiograph of abdomen showing marked dilatation of the large intestine in patient with "toxic megacolon" secondary to ulcerative colitis.

TABLE 42–2.—SPECIFIC CAUSES OF
INFLAMMATORY BOWEL DISEASE

Campylobacter fetus subspecies jejuni
Eosinophilic gastroenteritis
Shigellosis
Salmonellosis
Amebiasis
Gonorrhea
Schistosomiasis
Syphilis
Tuberculosis
Lymphogranuloma venereum
Histoplasmosis
Balantidium coli
Cytomegalic inclusion disease
Antibiotic colitis
Radiation colitis
Ischemic colitis
Vasculitis
Scleroderma
Amyloidosis
Systemic lupus erythematosis
Hemolytic uremic syndrome
Chemical proctitis
Gold-induced enterocolitis
Yersinia enterocolitis
Behçet's syndrome
Chronic lymphocytic leukemia
Lymphoma-lymphosarcoma

both. More recently, mercaptopurine and 5-aminosalicylic acid have been tried, but their value and role remain to be elucidated. Patients are frequently placed on bland diets, with restrictions on intake of dairy products and fiber. Anemia is treated with iron and blood transfusions. Diarrhea may require loperamide HCl. Medical treatment is continued until the disease subsides and the patient enters a remission or until it is clear that operation is indicated.

INDICATIONS FOR OPERATION

Complications of the colitis and intractability to medical therapy are the main reasons for operation.

Complications of Colitis

Both intestinal and extraintestinal complications of ulcerative colitis may lead to operation (see Table 42–1). Chronic intestinal complications that require surgical intervention include stricture with intestinal obstruction and cancer of the large intestine. Cancer is more likely to appear in patients whose disease had its onset in childhood, involves the entire large intestine, and has been present for greater than ten years.[10] About 2% of such patients develop cancer each year after the first decade of the disease. Acute intestinal complications, such as bleeding, perforation, toxic megacolon, and acute obstruction, also may lead to operation.

Extraintestinal complications may also require surgery. Pyoderma gangrenosum, erythema nodosum, aphthous stomatitis, iritis, thrombocytosis, and peripheral arthritis usually clear promptly after excision of the diseased large intestine. Inflammation of the liver (hepatic triaditis), cirrhosis, sclerosing cholangitis, ankylosing spondylitis, chronic nephropathies, and amyloidosis usually do not improve after operation.

Intractability to Medical Therapy

While complications of the disease may lead to operation, more commonly patients are operated on because of intractability to medical therapy. In spite of persistent and adequate medical therapy, many patients with colitis continue to have disabling enteric symptoms. Malaise, weight loss, anemia, and hypoproteinemia appear. Work and play become difficult. Children experience growth failure. These continuing symptoms and signs require operative intervention.

Medical therapy itself may result in complications. Sulfasalazine sometimes causes diarrhea and peripheral neuropathy. Prolonged steroid therapy can cause osteoporosis, diabetes mellitus, psychosis, obesity, hirsutism, Cushinoid features, acne, and hypertension. Development of the complications of medical therapy may necessitate its discontinuance and lead to operation.

Most patients have had their disease about eight years by

TABLE 42–3.—CLINICAL DISTINCTION BETWEEN ULCERATIVE AND CROHN'S COLITIS

OBSERVATIONS	ULCERATIVE COLITIS	CROHN'S COLITIS
Symptoms and Signs		
Diarrhea	80%–90%	70%–90%
Rectal bleeding	Prominent	Less common
Abdominal pain (cramps)	Mild	Moderate to severe
Palpable mass	No (unless large cancer)	At times
Anal complaints	Infrequent (<20%)	Frequent (>50%)
Radiologic findings		
Ileal disease	Rare (backwash ileitis)	Common
Nodularity, fuzziness	Yes	No
Distribution	Rectum extending upward and continuously	Skip areas
Ulcer	Collar-button	Linear, cobblestone, fissures
Toxic dilatation	Yes	Yes
Proctoscopic findings		
Anal fissure, fistula, abscess	Rare	Common
Rectal sparing	Rare (5%)	Common (50%)
Granular	Yes	No
Ulceration	Superficial erosion	Linear, deep

the time they come to operation. The mean age at which operation is performed in adults at Mayo is 32 years for both men and women.

SURGICAL TREATMENT

Overall Rationale

The rationale is that by excising the diseased mucosa of the large intestine, the patients can be cured of their disease and their health improved. Patients and physicians, however have been reluctant to act on this rationale, and operations for ulcerative colitis have often been delayed or even postponed indefinitely in the past despite strong indications for surgical therapy. Reluctance has arisen because of the fear of ileostomy and its physical, social, and psychological consequences.

The conventional ileostomy leaves the patient with complete fecal incontinence. An appliance must be worn day and night to collect the output from the stoma. The appliances are unsightly, uncomfortable, and odoriferous. Noises may issue from the stoma during times of fecal discharge, causing embarrassment to the patient. There is also the ever-present danger of leakage of stool or gas at the site of attachment of the appliance to the skin. The peristomal skin may become irritated.[4] In addition, the appliances are expensive. Some patients estimate the cost of maintaining the appliance and servicing the ileostomy to be in the neighborhood of $300–$400 per year. Thus, alternatives to an incontinent Brooke ileostomy are needed.

Today, alternative operations are available that allow the disease to be removed and yet preserve fecal continence and avoid ileostomy. The newer operative approaches to ulcerative colitis include the ileoanal anastomosis, the continent ileostomy (Kock pouch), and the continent ostomy device. These procedures are used in patients requiring elective operation for their disease.

CHOICE OF OPERATION

In elective operations for chronic ulcerative colitis, we usually employ colectomy, mucosal rectectomy and ileal pouch-anal anastomosis for nonobese patients who are less than 55 years of age and who have a competent anal sphincter. Obese and older patients usually require proctocolectomy and Brooke ileostomy. An alternative for these patients may be a prestomal ileal pouch with a continent ostomy valve. Ileorectostomy, another continence-preserving operation, is reserved for those few patients with mild rectal disease who do not wish complete excision of their disease for fear of an ileostomy. Proctocolectomy and Brooke ileostomy are done for those patients not wishing the more extensive continence-preserving operations. The continent ileal pouch of Kock is used mainly for those patients who already have a Brooke ileostomy after proctocolectomy.

PREPARATION FOR OPERATION

The nutritional status of the patient is stabilized before operation. This sometimes, but not often, requires parenteral supplementation. Anemia is treated by blood transfusion. For patients currently on or recently receiving steroid therapy, additional steroids—usually 100 mg of hydrocortisone IV every eight hours—are given to ensure adequate supply during the operative stress. The bowels are cleansed with laxatives and enemas for two days prior to operation. Alternatively, 4 L of an electrolyte solution (GoLYTLEY) can be given by mouth the night before operation. Diet is restricted to clear liquids the day before operation.

The growth of enteric bacteria is suppressed by giving neomycin, 0.5 gm every 4 hours, and tetracycline, erythromycin or metronidazole, 250 mg every 4 hours, for two days prior to operation. Cefazolin, 0.5 gm, is given IV just prior to the operation and is continued every 8 hours for two more doses.

OPERATIVE TREATMENT

Elective Operations

PROCTOCOLECTOMY AND BROOKE ILEOSTOMY.—Proctocolectomy with Brooke ileostomy is the standard procedure for patients with ulcerative colitis who require operation. The ileostomy is made from the terminal ileum and is positioned in the right lower quadrant of the abdomen. The patient's fecal effluent discharges through the stoma and is collected by an appliance which the patient wears continuously, day and night. These ileostomies, when properly constructed and managed, have proved remarkably safe and trouble-free.

Rationale.—The rationale is that excision of the entire large intestine will cure the patient of ulcerative colitis, while the establishment of a Brooke ileostomy will result in a satisfactory lifestyle.

Type of patient.—The operation can be done in patients of any age who require excision of the large intestine. Because of the advent of continence-preserving operations, however, we at Mayo use the operation today mainly in older patients or in obese patients who are not candidates for the continence-preserving procedures.

Special preoperative preparation.—At a preoperative interview, the exact description of the procedure and an understanding of the new anatomy produced by the operation is thoroughly discussed with the patient. The patient must understand that the ileostomy provides a permanent abdominal stoma, and that an appliance must be worn continuously to collect the fecal effluent. A visit with a person who already has made a successful adjustment to an ileostomy is also most helpful. The old patient can frequently dispel the new patient's fears and misconceptions about the operation.

In addition, before operation, an appropriate site should be selected for the ileostomy by actually positioning an appliance on the patient's abdomen. The site is usually just lateral to and inferior to the umbilicus, midway between the midline and the right anterior iliac spine. This position allows the patient to bend and move the body in all directions without dislodging the appliance. The site should also be selected to avoid abdominal skin folds, creases, and scars that might hinder effective sealing of the appliance to the skin. The assistance of a competent stomal therapist is invaluable.

Technique.—The patient is placed in a modified lithotomy position to allow the surgeon access to both the abdomen and the perineum. A catheter is inserted into the urinary bladder for continuous drainage, and the skin is prepared with a dilute solution of povidone-iodine (Betadine) or another suitable antiseptic.

Through a vertical midline abdominal incision, a thorough inspection of the abdominal content is made to confirm the presence or absence of disease. The diseased large intestine is then excised, making every effort to preserve as much of the small intestine as possible. Usually, all but a few centimeters of terminal ileum can be saved. The surgeon should also carefully preserve the mesentery of the small intestine and of the right colon for later use in closing the peritoneal space lateral to the terminal ileum.

The terminal ileum is next prepared for construction of the stoma by dividing its secondary and tertiary vascular arcades, while preserving its marginal artery and vein. This "trimming down" of the mesentery allows the bowel to be more easily turned inside out during later construction of the stoma.

The surgeon then moves to the cutaneous surface of the right lower abdomen to begin the construction of the stoma. The abdominal skin at the exact center of the site selected for the ileostomy is grasped with a Kocher clamp and elevated into the operative field. Using a knife passed in the plane parallel to the surface of the abdomen, a circular defect of approximately 2 cm in diameter is created in the skin. A 1-cm circle of the anterior rectus sheath is then excised, and the dissection continued posteriorly through the rectus muscle and into the abdominal cavity. The surgeon should assure himself that the defect created in the abdominal wall will easily admit the index and middle finger simultaneously, a defect with a diameter of about 4 cm. Smaller defects may narrow and obstruct the terminal ileum, while larger defects may predispose to parastomal hernia.

A noncrushing clamp is then passed from the exterior through the defect, and into the abdominal cavity. The distal cut end of the ileum is grasped in the blades of the clamp, and the ileum brought through the anterior abdominal wall to the skin surface. The ileum should project above the skin surface for a distance of about 5 cm. The ileum is then anchored to the abdominal wall from the peritoneal side using three interrupted 4–0 Dacron sutures. These sutures approximate the seromuscular layer of the ileum to the endoabdominal fascia at the site of exit of the ileum from the abdomen. This prevents prolapse or retraction of the stoma in the postoperative period.

Next, the space lateral to the terminal ileum is closed by approximating the ileal mesentery to the retroperitoneum and to the right lateral parietal peritoneum, using a continuous 3–0 absorbable suture. This maneuver prevents later internal herniation and obstruction of the small intestine at this site.

The stoma is then constructed by turning the terminal ileum inside out, so that its mucosal surface is exposed, and its serosal surface is covered by the eversion, thus preventing ileostomy dysfunction. Because 5 cm of terminal ileum has been pulled through to the exterior from the abdomen, when the terminal ileum is turned inside out, a stoma 2.5 cm in length results. A stoma of this length projects well into an ileostomy bag; leakage and slippage of the bag are minimized; yet it is not long enough to be excessively bulky or physically unattractive. The distal cut edge of the everted ileum is sewn

to the dermis at the site of the stoma using eight interrupted absorbable sutures. Some of these sutures also include the seromuscular layer of the inner wall of ileum at the skin level. The stoma should be bright red at the completion of its construction. This assures the surgeon that the blood supply to the stoma is satisfactory.

The abdomen is then irrigated with an isotonic saline solution to remove blood, necrotic tissue, enteric content, and other debris that may remain after the resection of the intestine and the construction of the ileostomy. The abdominal incision is closed, using absorbable sutures. We place a subcuticular catheter in the wound for suction and irrigation of the wound with antibiotics in the postoperative period.[11] This technique has reduced our incidence of wound infections to approximately 1% of operated patients. After the wound is closed, an ileostomy appliance is applied immediately to cover the stoma. The appliance protects the skin from irritation by ileal content discharged in the postoperative period.

The rectum and anus are excised in the intersphincteric plane.[12] The perineal wound is closed primarily, leaving a double-lumen suction-irrigation catheter in the presacral space. Suction-irrigation of the wound in the postoperative period with 154 mM NaCl, 50 ml/hr, removes blood, serum, necrotic debris, and intestinal content, and minimizes the possibility of wound infection.[13]

Postoperative care.—Postoperatively, the patient is kept on nothing by mouth and given nourishment by IV fluid and electrolyte solutions. The stomach is aspirated via a nasogastric tube. The urinary catheter is left in place, and the patient is ambulated beginning the day after operation.

The ileostomy often begins discharging content on about the third or fourth postoperative day, at which time the nasogastric tube can be removed. The urinary and perineal catheters are usually removed on about the fifth day, and at this time the patient is ready to begin taking oral feedings. We begin with a pure liquid diet, gradually increasing the solid content, so that by the seventh day the patients are usually taking a general diet. At this point, the patient is ready to learn self-care of the ileostomy, assisted by the stomal therapist.

Ileostomy output should be carefully monitored in the early postoperative period to ensure that the patient does not have excessive losses. The output from a healthy ileostomy is about 600 ml/day. If volumes greater than 1 L/day are passed, the patient may need IV supplementation of the oral intake to ensure that water and electrolyte depletion do not result.

The patient is usually ready for hospital discharge on approximately the tenth day after operation. After discharge, we encourage the patients to eat all types of food, but caution them to thoroughly masticate indigestible fiber. Undispersed fiber may obstruct an ileostomy. Food such as mushrooms, raw vegetables, and nuts are of particular concern. The patients generally require no long-term medications. In particular, vitamin B_{12} is usually not needed, provided not more than a few centimeters of terminal ileum have been resected.

The patients must care properly for their stoma to protect the skin from the ileostomy content. The skin becomes irritated, and a peristomal dermatitis will develop if the content gets on it. This problem can be prevented by adequate stomal care.

Patients generally return to an active physical life after operation and resume their previous work. They can pursue sports such as tennis, swimming, golf. There is no contraindication to an active sexual life, including pregnancy for women. Most patients adjust satisfactorily to the presence of the stoma and enjoy an active social life. There may be noises and occasionally odors from the stoma, which are embarrassing, but the patients and friends learn to deal with these without undue dismay. Still, approximately 20% of patients may experience mild to moderate (15%) or severe restrictions (10%) on their activities (Table 42–4).[4]

Complications.—Complications from the operation are infrequent. Infection, abscess, and bleeding may occur in the early postoperative period, but they are usually prevented by careful attention to preoperative preparation and operative detail. Stomal obstruction, diarrhea, retraction of the stoma, prolapse of the stoma, perforation, hemorrhage, and peristomal hernia may appear in the later postoperative period, but they are also rare (5% of patients or fewer) when the techniques described above are employed.[14] Should they occur, revision of the stoma is often required.

Patients with Brooke ileostomies, however, are susceptible to two long-term metabolic complications: urinary stones and gallstones. In regard to urinary stones, these patients are in a state of chronic water and sodium depletion because of the loss of ileal content through their stoma. The colon in health ordinarily absorbs water and electrolytes. The loss of this absorptive capacity leads to loss of more water, sodium, chloride, potassium, and bicarbonate through the stoma than in health. Mild chronic dehydration and slight acidosis develop.[15] The ensuing low output of acidic urine may lead to precipitation of uric acid stones in the urinary tract. To prevent this, the patients should be encouraged to drink adequate amounts of fluids. The taking of an alkali may also be indicated.

With regard to gallstones, the loss of bile salts through the stoma, especially in patients who have had more extensive resections of portions of their terminal ileum, may deplete the bile salt pool and hence make them susceptible to the formation of gallstones. No adequate form of prophylaxis has proved efficacious to date, but the oral ingestion of bile salts might be considered. Should gallstones appear, cholecystectomy may be indicated.

Urinary and sexual dysfunction may be long-term sequelae when nerves to these organs are damaged by the operative dissection. These complications are minimized when the excision of the rectum and anus is done in the intersphincteric plane close to the anorectal lumen.[12]

Outcome.—Patients are restored to good health. While the Brooke stoma is incontinent and requires the patients to wear an appliance day and night to collect the outflow from the enteric tract, these ileostomies are compatible with a satisfactory life-style over the long term.

COLECTOMY, MUCOSAL RECTECTOMY, ILEAL POUCH-ANAL ANASTOMOSIS.—A current, attractive, operation for ulcerative colitis is colectomy, mucosal rectectomy, and ileal pouch-anal anastomosis.

Rationale.—The rationale behind the operation is that it entirely removes the disease via the colectomy and mucosal rectectomy, yet it preserves anal sphincteric function, transanal fecal flow, and anal continence. No permanent ileostomy is required. The ileal pouch provides sufficient reservoir to prevent excessive stooling. Because the mucosal rectectomy is done from the luminal side of the rectum, injury of the perirectal nerves to the bladder and genitalia is minimized. Thus, there is little likelihood of urinary or sexual dysfunction after the operation. In addition, because the anus and rectum are not excised, no perineal wound is present after the procedure, a wound which is sometimes difficult to heal.

Type of patient.—This operation can be done on children and on young or middle-aged adults. Patients older than 55 years are less likely to be candidates, because their anal sphincters may be less competent than those of younger patients. Patients should have good anal sphincteric function and continence prior to operation. The operation is more likely to be successful if there is no perianal disease, such as abscesses or anal fistulas, and if there has been no previous anal surgery. Candidates should not be obese. Obese patients often have a thick, short intestinal mesentery which prevents the terminal ileum from being easily brought down to the dentate line for the ileoanal anastomosis. Patients with severe illness and inanition, however, and those who take corticosteroids should not be barred from consideration.

Operative technique.—The patient is anesthetized and placed in a modified lithotomy position to provide access to both the abdomen and the perineum. A vertical, midline ab-

TABLE 42–4.—INFLUENCE OF ABDOMINAL ILEOSTOMY ON DAILY ACTIVITY

| ACTIVITY | DEGREE OF IMPACT (% OF 685 PATIENTS) | | | |
| | Restricted | | No Restriction | Improved |
	Moderate-Severe	Mild		
Social	7	14	51	28
Sports	17	26	42	15
Work at home	4	8	68	20
Recreation	8	21	48	23
Family relationships	3	5	68	24
Sexual	14	15	56	15
Travel	8	18	48	26
Mean ± SEM, all categories	9 ± 2	15 ± 3	54 ± 4	22 ± 2

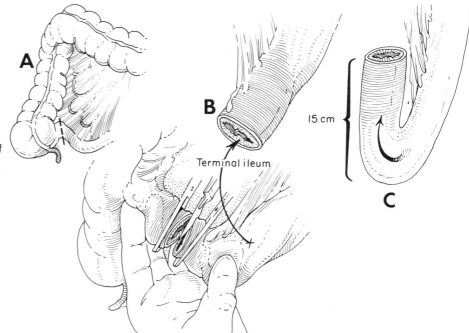

Fig 42–5.—Construction of ileal pouch. **A** and **B,** division of terminal ileum, removal of cecum and colon. **C,** fashioning ileum into a "J" shape with 15-cm limbs.

dominal incision is made, the abdominal content inspected, and the presence of ulcerative colitis verified. The large intestine is mobilized from the cecum to the levator ani and its blood supply divided. The rectum is transected using a stapling apparatus at a point about 7 cm proximal to the levator ani, and the cecum, colon, and proximal rectum removed.

The operator then constructs an ileal pouch from the terminal 30 cm of ileum (Figs 42–5 and 42–6). The terminal ileum is fashioned into the shape of a "J," and the anterior and posterior layers of the "J" anastomosed together, using two layers of continuous absorbable suture or stainless steel staples.

The mucosal rectectomy can be performed in one of two ways. In the first method, the operator positions himself at the perineum. The anus is effaced by placing Gelpi self-retaining retractors at right angles to the dentate line. The operator then everts the distal rectum onto the perineum and strips the diseased distal rectal mucosa from the underlying tunica muscularis using the cautery (Figs 42–7 and 42–8). A dilute (1:100,000) solution of epinephrine is injected into the submucosa immediately above the dentate line to facilitate separation of mucosa from muscularis and to reduce bleeding. The dissection begins at the dentate line and extends to a point 5 cm orad to the dentate line. The bowel is transected at this point and the specimen removed. The everted rectal tunica muscularis is then repositioned in its usual anatomical location.

In the second method, the mucosa of the anal canal and lower rectum are stripped endorectally from the underlying muscular layer without everting the distal rectum onto the perineum (Fig 42–9). Using either scissors or electrocautery probe, the dissection is started at the dentate line and continued to a level just proximal to the levator ani muscle. The full-thickness of the rectal wall is then transected at this level and the specimen removed.

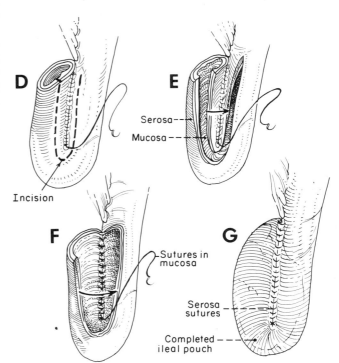

Fig 42–6.—Construction of ileal pouch (continued). **D,** suturing of ileal limbs with 2-0 absorbable suture. **D** and **E,** division of antimesenteric border of ileum. **F,** suturing of posterior mucosal layer of pouch. **G,** completed closure of anterior layer of pouch with two rows of 2-0 absorbable suture.

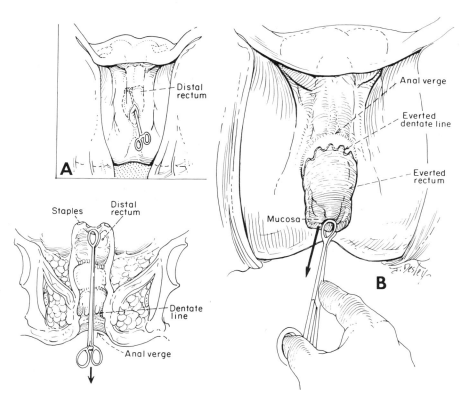

Fig 42–7.—Technique of mucosal rectectomy. **A,** transanal grasp of midrectum with sponge forceps. **B,** eversion of rectum and dentate line onto perineum.

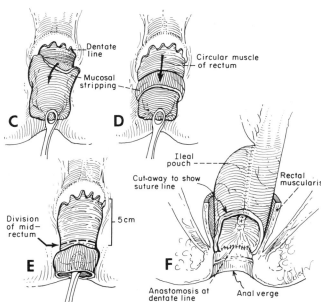

Fig 42–8.—Technique of mucosal rectectomy *(continued)* and ileal pouch-anal anastomosis. **C** and **D,** stripping of rectal mucosa from underlying circular muscle. **E,** site of division of rectal wall at *dotted line.* **F,** ileal-pouch anal anastomosis to dentate line.

The previously constructed "J" pouch is then brought down endorectally and anastomosed to the dentate line with continuous 2-0 absorbable suture (see Figs 43–8 and 43–9). A suction drain is placed through the left flank and into the presacral space alongside the pouch to drain the presacral and peripouch space in the postoperative period. The drain should be placed well away from the ileal-anal anastomosis so as not to hinder healing of the anastomosis. A proximal diverting loop ileostomy is established in the right lower quadrant.

The patient is allowed two months to recover from the initial procedure, at which time digital examination of the anorectum, proctoscopy, roentgenographic studies of the ileoanal anastomosis, and sometimes anorectal manometry are performed to ascertain the degree of healing and recovery of anorectal function. With a well-healed anastomosis, no sign of intrapelvic sepsis or fistulas, and a competent anal sphincter being present, the diverting ileostomy can be taken down and ileal continuity reestablished at a second operation.

Postoperative care.—After closure of the ileostomy, the patients are given loperamide hydrochloride and a psyllium preparation until thickening of the enteric content is obtained and satisfactory stooling frequency is present. These medications can usually be gradually decreased over a three- to four-month period.

Side effects.—The patients are usually completely continent during the day, but they do pass larger quantities of stool after operation than do individuals in health. The fecal output of the patients averages about 650 ml/day, a quantity passed as four to six bowel movements during the day and perhaps one at night.[16–19] The discrimination of gas from feces is generally satisfactory, but is not quite as good as in health. In addition, at night during sleep, there may be some minor fecal leakage because of the decrease in the reservoir function of the distal bowel after the colectomy, the more fluid nature

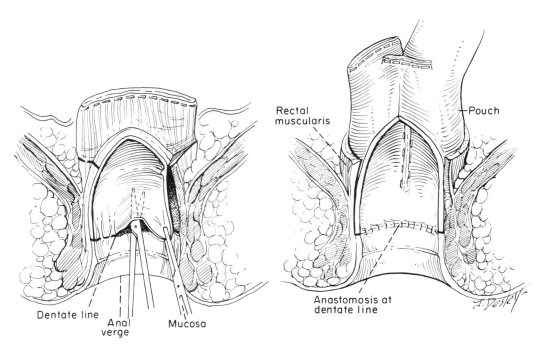

Fig 42–9.—Left, technique of mucosal rectectomy using the transanal, endorectal technique. **Right,** anastomosis of ileal pouch made with staples to dentate line.

and larger volume of the enteric content, and the propulsive force of the distal ileal contractions.[18]

Complications.—The main complications of the operation are perianastomotic sepsis (11% of patients at risk) and intestinal obstruction (9% of patients).[19] Perianastomotic sepsis can be minimized by using the bowel preparation outlined above and by constructing the diverting ileostomy. Obtaining excellent hemostasis prior to abdominal closure and the use of the presacral drains to remove serum and blood in the area of operation will minimize abscess formation.

Intestinal obstruction is combatted again by careful hemostasis prior to closure, intra-abdominal irrigation to remove necrotic material, debris, and blood, and careful construction of a loop ileostomy in the right lower quadrant. The proximal ileum is positioned intra-abdominally to the left of the stoma, and the distal ileum is placed to the right of the stoma and laterally. This positioning of the bowel helps to prevent herniation and volvulus of the proximal bowel into the space lateral to the ileostomy. The likelihood of herniation and volvulus is further diminished by splinting the proximal ileum via a 16 F catheter inserted through the stoma and advanced into the proximal bowel for a distance of 50 cm.

Outcome.—The procedure does achieve its objective of maintaining fecal control without the need for permanent ileostomy and with transanal passage of fecal content.[7, 8] Our patients have all been able to evacuate their neorectum spontaneously. None has required catheterization of the pouch, as has sometimes been necessary when an "S"-shaped ileal pouch has been used.[6] The resting and squeeze pressures of the anal sphincters are preserved by the operation. The rectal-anal inhibitory reflex is abolished, but this has pro-

duced no apparent clinical disability.[16] The "J"-shaped ileal pouch provides a satisfactory reservoir for stool and may even improve capacity over that noted preoperatively by the patients. Moreover, the greater the neorectal capacity, the fewer the propulsive contractions with filling of the distal bowel and the better the clinical result. Patients with a compliant neorectum and a capacity of 400 ml or greater have few propulsive contractions in the neorectum, and the contractions that they do have are of small amplitude. These patients have fewer bowel movements per day, require less "anti-diarrhea" medication, and have less incontinence than patients with smaller, less compliant, more contractile pouches.

Urinary and sexual function are also preserved well by the procedure.[17] None of the 38 male patients we studied had postoperative impotence or failure to have orgasm, although nine had retrograde ejaculation.[8, 19] Seven of our female patients have become pregnant, and six of these have delivered healthy infants to date, five per vaginam and one via cesarean section. Digestion and absorption of nutrients has been good. No supplemental dietary or vitamin therapy has been needed. Endoscopic biopsies of the distal ileum have shown only mild, chronic inflammation of the mucosa, which has assumed a "colonic" morphology.

The main disadvantages of the procedure are frequent bowel movements, occasional leakage of stool at night, and a perianal irritation associated with such leakage. These problems are most common among patients with postoperative weakness of the anal sphincters, poor neorectal compliance, and small pouch capacity. Inability to evacuate the pouch completely may also aggravate these symptoms and be complicated further by pouchitis. In this condition, patients develop a bacterial overgrowth in the ileal pouch and perhaps in the bowel proximal to the pouch. Unusual organisms may appear, such as *Clostridium difficile* or *Campylobacter*, which in turn may result in diarrhea, fever, weakness, and malaise. This problem can usually be treated satisfactorily with an antibacterial agent, such as metronidazole, 250 mg four times per day, for ten days.

THE CONTINENT ILEOSTOMY (KOCK POUCH).—The continent ileostomy or Kock pouch consists of three parts: a reservoir or pouch made of distal ileum, a valve made of terminal ileum interposed between the pouch and the exterior, and an efferent ileal limb leading from the valve to the stoma. For patients who require an ileostomy, the Kock pouch provides fecal continence and eliminates the need for an ileostomy appliance.[5] Because of this, the stoma can be fashioned flush with the skin and placed nearer the groin to make it less conspicuous.

Rationale.—The rationale behind the procedure is that the pouch collects and holds fecal content until it is emptied by passing a catheter through the stoma and valve into the pouch. The content then drains through the catheter directly into the toilet bowl, after which the catheter is removed. The catheter is rinsed after its use and placed in a purse to be carried in the patient's pocket during the day. A small dressing is placed over the stoma after drainage to prevent mucus secreted by the surface epithelium of the ileum from soiling the clothes. In between intubations, no gas or stool leaks, and so no ileal appliance need be worn. The patient has complete control over his/her fecal discharge.

Type of patient.—This operation is suitable for young or middle-aged adults who already have an incontinent Brooke ileostomy or who require proctocolectomy but wish to avoid the increased frequency of stooling with ileoanal anastomosis. Patients must have sufficient understanding, intelligence, and physical capabilities to deal with catheterization and care of the pouch. Thus, children or patients over 70 years of age are often not candidates. Also, construction of a Kock pouch is difficult in obese patients.

Technique.—The operation is done in one stage and is performed with the patient in the modified lithotomy position. The proctocolectomy is accomplished, after which the pouch is fashioned from the terminal 45 cm of ileum. The anterior and posterior walls of the pouch are constructed with two layers of continuous 2-0 absorbable suture. The terminal ileum is intussuscepted into the newly formed pouch for a distance of 5 cm to form the valve. The intussuscepted ileum is anchored in place with four cartridges of stainless steel staples (Fig 42–10). Additional sutures of 4-0 Dacron are placed at the exit of the efferent limb from the pouch to further anchor the valve in place (Fig 42–11). We have not used fascia lata or plastic mesh to enhance fixation of the valve, but we are currently using polyglycolic acid mesh. The efferent ileal limb leading to the stoma is made as short as possible, and the stoma placed just above the hairline in the right lower quadrant. The pouch is sewn to the anterior abdominal wall just beneath the stoma, again with interrupted 4-0 Dacron sutures (Fig 42–12). The ileostomy is made flush with the skin. The space lateral to the pouch is closed by approximat-

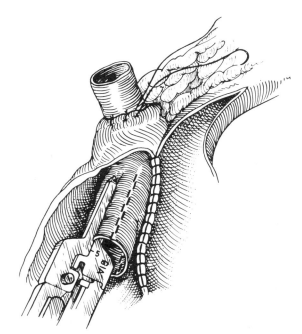

Fig 42–10.—Construction of valve of Kock pouch using staples.

ing the ileal mesentery to the parietal peritoneum of the right lower quadrant of the abdomen. This obviates volvulus of the pouch and peripouch herniation of the more proximal small intestine.

Postoperative care.—The pouch is intubated postoperatively for a period of one month to ensure that the pouch and valve remain in the appropriate position while the fibrous tissue of healing fixes the structures in place. The tube is then removed, and the patient begins intermittent intubation of the pouch. At first, the intubations are done every two hours during the day, while the catheter is left in place continuously

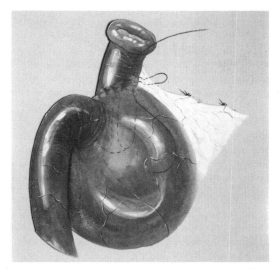

Fig 42–11.—Valve of Kock pouch is anchored in pouch with 4-0 Dacron sutures at site of exit of efferent ileal limb.

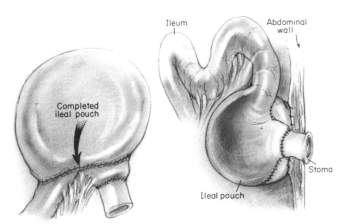

Fig 42–12.—Completed ileal pouch is sewn to the anterior abdominal wall. The ileal stoma is made flush with the skin.

overnight. The interval between intubations is increased gradually, so that after the second month, the patient is intubating the pouch four times a day but not at night. The patients require no medication and can eat a general diet provided that they masticate thoroughly. Poorly masticated, indigestible materials, such as mushrooms, kernels of corn, string beans, and cabbage, may plug the catheter during intubations and interfere with emptying.

Outcome.—The procedure does achieve its objective of providing complete control over fecal discharge. The patients, however, do have an ileostomy, and they must intubate the ileal pouch to empty it. In addition, two complications of the Kock pouch have appeared: malfunction of the valve and diarrhea.

Malfunction of the valve occurs because the intussuscepted terminal ileum used to make the valve sometimes reduces partially, resulting in a tortuous tract leading from the pouch to the exterior. The patient then has two problems: difficulty intubating the pouch and leakage of content from the pouch. Reoperation is usually required, at which time the valve must be replaced within the pouch and reanchored with stainless steel staples and sutures. Reoperation is necessary today in about 15%–20% of patients and is usually successful.[20] However, reoperation does not guarantee that the valve will function perfectly henceforth. A second reoperation may be required in an additional 15%–20%.

Diarrhea, which occurs in about 7% of patients, likely results from bacterial overgrowth in the pouch. The diarrhea, when symptomatic, can usually be managed satisfactorily with antibiotics. Other possible causes of diarrhea, such as partial small-bowel obstruction and lactase deficiency, may be responsible and require correction.

ILEOSTOMY-OCCLUDING DEVICE.—The artificial, ileostomy-occluding device provides control over fecal discharge in ileostomy patients and eliminates the ileostomy bag.

Rationale and plan of use.—The rationale of the ileostomy-occluding device is to provide a mechanical blockage to the outflow from an ileal pouch or an end-ileostomy and so provide control over fecal discharge from the intestinal tract.[21]

Moreover, the possibility of valvular malfunction requiring reoperation, as is the case with the Kock pouch, is avoided.

The device consists of a 28 F catheter that has a soft, inflatable balloon affixed to its internal end (Fig 42–13). The catheter is inserted into the pouch, the balloon inflated, and the inflated balloon pulled up against the anterior abdominal wall just beneath the stoma. A disk slipped over the external end of the catheter and pushed down to the skin keeps the balloon snug up against the anterior abdominal wall and occludes fecal outflow from the pouch. The catheter is folded over and fixed to the disk to prevent leakage of fecal content.

Type of patient.—The ileostomy occluding device can be used in patients of almost any age or body habitus. For example, it can be employed in elderly patients and in obese patients not ordinarily good candidates for ileoanal anastomosis or the continent ileostomy of Kock.

Technique.—An ileal pouch is constructed from the terminal 35 cm of ileum, as with a Kock pouch. However, the biologic valve of the Kock type is not made. Instead, the efferent limb from the ileal pouch is simply brought through the anterior abdominal wall and the stoma constructed. The device is then passed through the stoma and positioned in the pouch (Fig 42–14). The device is connected to straight drainage for the first postoperative month to allow the pouch to heal before it is distended. Intermittent occlusions using the device are begun thereafter, and continence is achieved immediately.

Outcome.—The main advantages of the procedure are its simplicity and its lack of complications. The device can be removed and reinserted at will. Reoperation to change the device is not necessary. The main disadvantage of the procedure is the need to wear the device and the discomfort thereof. The appliance itself, while not large, does provide some bulk on the anterior abdominal wall. In addition, the presence of the appliance stimulates the production of mucus from the terminal ileum, so that absorbent pads must be worn between the appliance and the skin.

ILEORECTOSTOMY.—Ileorectostomy has been used infrequently at Mayo. The operation does not excise the diseased rectal mucosa, which continues to ulcerate, bleed, and cause pain and diarrhea. In addition, the risk of carcinoma is not entirely eliminated.

Type of patient.—Nonetheless, some patients have such minimal involvement of the rectum that an ileorectostomy is a reasonable choice, especially if these patients are young and

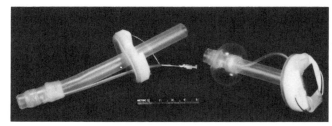

Fig 42–13.—Ileostomy occluding device. **Left,** occluding balloon deflated. **Right,** occluding balloon inflated.

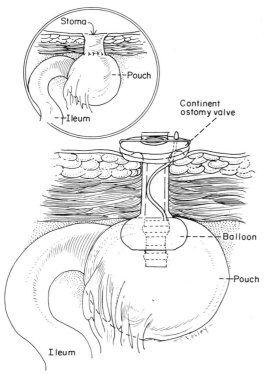

Fig 42–14.—Diagram of ileostomy occluding device in place in patient with prestomal ileal pouch. *Inset:* Ileal pouch prior to insertion of the device.

eager to avoid any type of ileostomy and its disabilities or any risk of sexual or urinary dysfunction occasioned by a proctectomy.[22]

Technique.—The operation is done with the patient in the supine position through a midline abdominal incision. After excision of the cecum and colon, the ileum is anastomosed end-to-end or side-to-end to the rectum using continuous 3-0 absorbable sutures on the mucosa and interrupted 4-0 Dacron sutures on the seromuscular layer.

Outcome.—Our experience at Mayo has shown that fewer than one half of patients undergoing this operation will have a satisfactory result over a five-year to 15-year follow-up.[23] Those with a good result experience fewer than eight bowel movements/day, are continent, require no systemic steroids, and maintain a satisfactory style of life. They require yearly

proctoscopic examinations to ascertain the presence or absence of continuing inflammation in their rectal mucosa and also of dysplasia or frank malignancy. The other one half of the patients have more disabling symptoms that require treatment, threaten life, and eventually mandate excision of the remaining rectal mucosa. The overall risk of carcinoma in the remaining rectum is about 5%.

Other Elective Operations

ILEOSTOMY WITHOUT RESECTION.—Ileostomy without resection was initiated early by Brown[1] and was continued later by others.[24] The rationale was that diversion of the stool from the diseased colon would allow the ulcerative colitis to heal, after which the ileum could be reanastomosed to the colon and the continuity of the fecal stream restored. However, in only a few patients with fecal diversion has the disease become quiescent enough to allow restoration of intestinal continuity. Most patients subjected to diversion only have required subsequent excision of the diseased intestine.

SEGMENTAL RESECTION OF THE COLON.—Occasionally, patients will present with ulcerative colitis which seems to be confined to one area of the large intestine. In these patients, resection of the involved area with either an end colostomy, an ileocolostomy or a colocolostomy, depending on the portion resected, might seem a reasonable approach. Most patients who undergo such limited resections, however, will experience a flare-up of their colitis in the remaining colon or rectum, which requires further medical or surgical therapy. Segmental resections, therefore, are seldom indicated.

Pros and Cons of the Elective Operations

The pros and cons of the various operations for ulcerative colitis are outlined in Table 42–5. On the balance, most patients at Mayo today elect the ileal pouch-anal anastomosis. The major advantages of this operation include total excision of the disease, avoidance of a permanent ileostomy, maintenance of transanal fecal flow, and reasonable continence.

Emergency Operations

COLECTOMY, RECTAL CLOSURE, BROOKE ILEOSTOMY.—Operations for colonic bleeding, perforation, or toxic megacolon from ulcerative colitis almost always require excision of the abdominal colon, closure of the proximal rectum, and construction of a terminal Brooke ileostomy. The

TABLE 42–5.—OUTCOME OF OPERATIONS FOR ULCERATIVE COLITIS

PROCEDURE	FECAL CONTINENCE PRESERVED	STOMA PRESENT	INTUBATIONS REQUIRED	DISADVANTAGES
Ileal pouch-anal anastomosis	Yes	No	No	Frequent stooling, occasional fecal leakage
Kock pouch	Yes	Yes	Yes	Valve malfunction, diarrhea
Ileostomy occluding device	Yes	Yes	No	Device discomfort, mucus discharge
Ileorectostomy	Yes	No	No	Rectal mucosa remains to cause symptoms and cancer
Brooke ileostomy	No	Yes	No	Ileostomy bag required

operation excises the areas of perforation and major bleeding and the areas most severely involved with toxic megacolon. The advantage of leaving the rectum in place is that the patient can subsequently undergo mucosal rectectomy and ileoanal anastomosis should he or she so desire. The operation is also shorter and simpler than a proctocolectomy and/or the continence-preserving operations, an advantage in these patients, who are usually desperately ill.

PROCTOCOLECTOMY, BROOKE ILEOSTOMY.—An exception to preserving the rectum during an emergency operation is the case in which the operation is done for massive bleeding from the rectum. Proctocolectomy and Brooke ileostomy or ileal pouch-anal anastomosis are then required.

"BLOW HOLE" COLOSTOMY.—Some surgeons have recommended creation of an ileostomy and one or more colostomies in the distended portions of the toxic megacolon to allow feces and gas to escape. The resulting decompression is thought to allow defervescence of the disease and to permit later medical or surgical treatment on an elective basis. The effectiveness of this approach has yet to be established. In the series of Turnbull's group, nearly half of the patients did not detoxify.[25] Moreover, some patients whose colon is not removed after a bout of toxic megacolon will develop a second episode of toxic megacolon.[26]

PROGNOSIS

Once the ulcerative colitis has been resected, the life expectancy of the patients is restored to that of other healthy individuals of the same sex and age, provided that patient has no complications of the disease or the operation. The presence of complications such as sclerosing cholangitis or cancer of the large intestine can affect the long-term outlook.

FUTURE TRENDS

The future trends are toward complete excision of the disease at a point early enough in its course to avoid the development of serious complications such as cancer of the large intestine, cirrhosis of the liver, or perforation of the colon. Moreover, newer, better techniques for maintaining transanal fecal discharge and anal continence will likely emerge.

Acknowledgment

Thanks are expressed to O.H. Beahrs, who contributed greatly to the development of much of the work described in this chapter.

REFERENCES

1. Brown J.Y.: The value of complete physiological rest of the large bowel in the treatment of certain ulcerative and obstructive devices of this organ, with descriptions of operative technique and report of cases. *Surg. Gynecol. Obstet.* 16:610–613, 1913.
2. Dragstedt L.R., Dack G.M., Kirsner J.B.: Chronic ulcerative colitis: A summary of evidence implicating bacterium necrophorium as the etiologic agent. *Ann. Surg.* 114:653–662, 1941.
3. Brooke B.N.: The management of an ileostomy: Including its complications. *Lancet* 2:102–104, 1952.
4. Roy P.H., Sauer W.G., Beahrs O.H., et al.: Experience with ileostomies: Evaluation of long-term rehabilitation in 497 patients. *Am. J. Surg.* 119:77–85, 1970.
5. Kock N.G.: A new look at ileostomy. *Surg. Annu.* 8:241–256, 1976.
6. Parks A.G., Nicholls R.J., Belliveau P.: Proctocolectomy with ileal reservoir and anal anastomosis. *Br. J. Surg.* 67:533–538, 1980.
7. Utsunomiya J., Iwama T., Imajo M., et al.: Total colectomy, mucosal proctectomy, and ileoanal anastomosis. *Dis. Colon Rectum* 23:459–466, 1980.
8. Taylor B.M., Cranley B., Kelly K.A., et al.: A clinico-physiological comparison of ileal pouch-anal and straight ileoanal anastomosis. *Ann. Surg.* 198:462–468, 1983.
9. Mendeloff A.I.: The epidemiology of idiopathic inflammatory bowel disease, in Kirsner J.B., Shorter R.G. (eds.): *Inflammatory Bowel Disease.* Philadelphia, Lea & Febiger, 1980, pp. 3–19.
10. Devroede G.J., Taylor W.F., Sauer W.G., et al.: Cancer risk and life expectancy of children with ulcerative colitis. *N. Engl. J. Med.* 285:17–21, 1971.
11. McIlrath D.C., van Heerden J.A., Edis A.J., et al.: Closure of abdominal incisions with subcutaneous catheters. *Surgery* 80:411–416, 1976.
12. Lyttle J.A., Parks A.G.: Intersphincteric excision of the rectum. *Br. J. Surg.* 64:413–416, 1977.
13. Schwab P.M., Kelly K.A.: primary closure of the perineal wound after proctectomy: A new technique. *Mayo Clin. Proc.* 49:176–179, 1974.
14. Pemberton J.H., Phillips S.F., Dozois R.R., et al.: Conventional ileostomy—current clinical results, in: Dozois R.R. (ed.): *Alternatives to Conventional Ileostomy.* Chicago, Year Book Medical Publishers, 1985, pp. 40–50.
15. Kennedy H.J., Al-Dujaili E.A.S., Edwards C.R.W., et al.: Water and electrolyte balance in subjects with a permanent ileostomy. *Gut* 24:702–705, 1983.
16. Heppell J., Kelly K.A., Phillips S.F., et al.: Physiolgic aspects of continence after colectomy, mucosal proctectomy, and endorectal ileo-anal anastomosis. *Ann. Surg.* 195:435–443, 1982.
17. Neal D.E., Williams N.S., Johnston D.: Rectal, bladder and sexual function after mucosal proctectomy with and without a pelvic reservoir for colitis and polyposis. *Br. J. Surg.* 69:599–604, 1982.
18. Taylor B.M., Beart R.W. Jr., Dozois R.R., et al.: Straight ileoanal anastomosis versus ileal pouch-anal anastomosis after colectomy and mucosal proctectomy. *Arch. Surg.* 118:696–701, 1983.
19. Metcalf A., Beart R.W. Jr., Dozois R.R., et al.: Clinical outcome of ileal "J" pouch-anal anastomosis for ulcerative colitis and polyposis coli. Submitted for publication.
20. Dozois R.R., Kelly K.A., Ilstrup D., et al.: Factors affecting revision rate after continent ileostomy. *Arch. Surg.* 116:610–613, 1981.
21. Pemberton J.H., van Heerden J.A., Beart R.W. Jr., et al.: A continent ileostomy device. *Ann. Surg.* 197:618–626, 1983.
22. Oakley J., Fazio V., Jagelman D., et al.: Complications and quality of life after ileorectal anastomosis for ulcerative colitis. *Am. J. Surg.* In press.
23. Farnell M.B., van Heerden J.A., Beart R.W. Jr., et al.: Rectal preservation in nonspecific inflammatory disease of the colon. *Ann. Surg.* 192:249–253, 1980.
24. Truelove J.C., Ellis H., Webster C.U.: Place of a double-barreled ileostomy in ulcerative colitis and Crohn's disease of the colon: A preliminary report. *Br. Med. J.* 1:150–153, 1965.
25. Turnbull P.B. Jr., Hawk W.A., Weakley F.L.: Surgical treatment of toxic megacolon: Ileostomy and colostomy to prepare patients for colectomy. *Am. J. Surg.* 122:325–331, 1971.
26. Grant C.S., Dozois R.R.: Toxic megacolon: Ultimate fate of patients after successful medical management. *Am. J. Surg.* 147:106–110, 1984.

43

Diverticulosis and Diverticulitis of the Large Intestine

THOMAS A. CASTILLE, M.D.
ISIDORE COHN, JR., M.D.

DIVERTICULOSIS COLI is perhaps the most common condition affecting the colon in modern times. As much as a third of Western man has acquired the condition by the sixth decade and two thirds by the eighth decade. Though often asymptomatic, simple diverticulosis may have a variety of sequelae. Among these are inflammation ranging from mild and localized infection to abscess, perforation, and fistula formation, hemorrhage, and obstruction.

The diverticulum itself is a herniation of the colonic mucosa through a defect in the muscular coat, most commonly at the site of penetration of nutrient vessels, and occurs as a consequence of increased intraluminal pressure. Therefore, these are pulsion type diverticula. Although descriptions of these colonic outpouchings antedate the industrial age, they were not recognized until the late 19th century. Decreased dietary fiber has been implicated as the primary inciting agent, with its corresponding diminution of stool bulk and the increased intraluminal pressure required to ensure stool transit. Chronologically, this theory dovetails nicely with the use of roller-milling of flour, which greatly decreased the bran content of white bread in the 1870s, and an approximate latent period of 30 years required for diverticula to develop.[1] In less developed nations even today, diverticular disease is decidedly uncommon and relatively insignificant as a clinical entity in both autopsy and radiologic series.[2]

The incidence of diverticulosis increases with age within a given population. When individuals below the age of 40 present with symptoms, this usually indicates a greater likelihood of medical failure and the need for surgical resection. Otherwise, the great majority of patients with symptomatic diverticular disease can be managed nonoperatively.

PATHOGENESIS

It is generally conceded that the formation of colonic diverticula commences with a dietary intake lacking in adequate fiber to provide bulk to the stool. The propulsion of the fecal stream thereby requires greater effort, and muscular hypertrophy results. Eventually, muscular dyskinesia occurs. Contraction of muscle in an effort to propel the fecal stream against a more distal spastic region results in segmental high

pressure bladders within which pulsion-type pseudodiverticula form. These consist of outpouchings of mucosa through anatomical weak points, the most common being sites of penetration of nutrient arteries between the mesenteric taenia and the two antimesenteric taeniae (Fig 43–1). Diverticula are almost invariably found in the sigmoid colon. They are found in decreasing frequency as one progresses proximally in the colon, being next most common in the descending colon, then in the transverse, and then in the right colon. The taenia coalesce into a continuous longitudinal muscular coat in the rectum, and there is no mesentery as such; hence, diverticula are rare though not unknown in that anatomical site.

Solitary congenital cecal diverticula are true diverticula in that they contain all layers of the bowel wall. These occur in younger individuals and have no relation to increased age or diet, though they may exist concomitant with acquired diverticula. Presumably this lesion arises as an outgrowth of the cecum in the first six weeks of gestation and persists into adulthood or until the time of symptomatic presentation.

ASSOCIATED CONDITIONS

Owing to similarity of presentation or common etiologic factors, diverticular disease of the colon is associated with several other pathologic conditions. The initial association of colonic diverticula with cholelithiasis and hiatal hernia is attributed to Charles Saint.[3] All three have in common an increased prevalence in industrial nations and a presumptive relation to dietary habits. Parks noted an incidence of cholelithiasis of 13.8% among patients with diverticular disease and an incidence of hiatal hernia of 7.3%.[4] Capron et al.[5] in a prospective case-control study found the prevalence of gallstones was higher in patients with diverticular disease of the colon (45%) than in control subjects matched for age, sex, weight and number of pregnancies (22%).

The differentiation of inflammatory bowel disease from diverticular disease is an occasional problem. Though patients with inflammatory bowel disease often present at a younger age, there is a subset of patients who do not present until their latter years, in whom concomitant diverticular disease may easily confuse the picture clinically and even histologi-

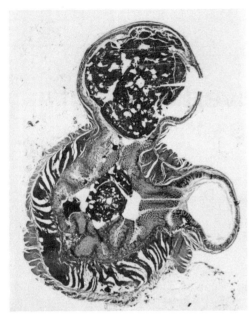

Fig 43–1.—Photomicrograph of whole section of bowel with diverticular disease. Continuity of mucosal layer is demonstrated, as is lack of muscular covering of diverticula. (Courtesy of Ronald Welsh, M.D., Department of Pathology, Louisiana State University, New Orleans.)

cally. Similarly, the differentiation of diverticular disease from colonic malignancy poses a special set of problems, both on preoperative assessment and intraoperative decision making. Parks[4] noted coincident carcinoma of the large bowel in 3.1% of patients presenting with diverticular disease.

Diverticula of the jejunum and ileum also may accompany diverticulosis coli and may be the actual symptomatic source leading to operative intervention for bleeding or inflammatory disease. These diverticula are more common in the proximal small bowel and decrease in frequency as one progresses distally. They tend to be widemouthed, are often located within the mesentery, are less apparent than colonic diverticula, but are found in 3%–7% of patients with diverticulosis coli.[6]

Since the majority of these patients are elderly, specific attention must be given to the inevitable diseases acquired through the years. Cardiovascular reserve must be assessed preoperatively, for it may influence the choice of operative procedure. Renal function must be assessed, acute changes differentiated from the patient's baseline state, and output must be maintained at optimal levels. Hepatic function should be screened chemically prior to any operative therapy. Elderly patients can be operated on safely, but attention to the details of their management is necessary. Even patients undergoing urgent surgery can benefit from a little extra time for medical repair.

CLINICAL SPECTRUM

Diverticulosis is present in about 5% of the populace of the United States, and increases with age until the eighth decade, when two thirds of the populace has diverticula demonstrable on barium enema or colonoscopy. The clinician faced with a

patient with incidentally discovered diverticula should be aware of the natural history of the process, the likelihood of complications and the best means of management. Only about 20% of patients with diverticular disease require surgical intervention. Ouriel and Schwartz[7] found that 55% of patients younger than 40 who were initially managed medically required further hospitalization, and 45% of these required subsequent operation. Thus, the young patient with asymptomatic diverticula may require close follow-up, and the young symptomatic patient might be best served by elective resection at an earlier stage.

The symptomatology associated with diverticular disease covers a wide spectrum, and the "asymptomatic" patient may not really be so. Chronic constipation is almost invariable, sometimes with laxative dependence as an added factor. If carefully questioned, most patients will give a history of intermittent, crampy lower abdominal pain though it may be quite mild, and even of subjective fever in conjunction with the pain. The presence of crampy left lower quadrant abdominal pain with tenderness is strongly suggestive of diverticulitis, as is barium enema evidence of spasm and the so-called concertina deformity of the sigmoid colon. Not infrequently at operation there is no gross correlation with the extent of the symptoms or the radiologic picture, and even histologic examination of the specimen may reveal diverticula without evidence of acute inflammation. Therefore, it may be better to speak of symptomatic diverticular disease rather than diverticulitis in this circumstance.

The asymptomatic and the minimally symptomatic patient are managed in the same manner as the patient who presents with more severe symptomatology and responds to initial medical management. All should be given dietary counseling, with added dietary fiber. For that matter, most patients approaching their fifth decade should also be given added fiber in view of the near ubiquity of this process with increasing age. Simply described, the diet should include eating bran-containing cereals, whole-meal bread, and plenty of fruits and vegetables. Dry bran can be added to the diet as a topping on cereals and salads, a thickener in cooking, and to baked products such as muffins and pancakes. Painter[1] emphasized that bran should be added to the diet and increased until the individual is having soft and bulky stools without straining. The proper dose is the one that obtains the desired effect.

INFLAMMATORY SYMPTOMS

The spectrum of symptoms due to inflammation of diverticula is fairly broad. The pathogenesis of inflammation involves obstruction of the narrow neck of the diverticulum, usually by fecal material, and the consequent overgrowth of bacteria within the obstructed sac. Drainage can occur spontaneously through the neck of the sac or back into the bowel lumen through the wall adjacent to the inflamed diverticulum, or an abscess may be formed in the mesentery, against the abdominal wall or against a contiguous organ or structure. The fate of an abscess at any of these sites depends on local and systemic factors, but any may rupture into the free peritoneum, causing diffuse peritonitis, or erode into structures in contiguity, causing fistulas or complex abscesses. Each of these will be examined individually.

DIVERTICULITIS

Presentation

Diverticulitis or "symptomatic diverticular disease" is the most common inflammatory condition to complicate diverticulosis. Symptoms most commonly reflect sigmoid disease. The typical history is of a middle-aged or elderly patient with hours to days of cramping left lower quadrant pain. This may be exacerbated by bowel movement and accompanied by subjective fever. There may be a history of laxative dependence or chronic constipation. The patient may relate prior similar episodes and may attribute onset of symptoms to the consumption of specific foods.

Physical findings include fever, usually low grade, and lower quadrant tenderness with or without rebound. Sometimes a sausage-shaped mass will be palpable in the left lower quadrant and may persist for several days after other symptoms resolve. Rectal examination may reveal some pelvic tenderness but no mass or fluctuance. Should a pelvic mass, fluctuance, or diffuse tenderness with rebound be present, the patient has perforated a diverticulum or a diverticular abscess has formed, and surgical therapy will be necessary on an urgent basis once medical repair is complete.

Initial serum chemistry analysis should be obtained and used as a basis for correction of defects of hydration or electrolyte status. Leukocytosis is common but usually not marked in this mild form of the disease. Proctoscopy may be attempted, but it is difficult to identify the diverticular openings with the rigid scope and often extremely uncomfortable for the patient as well. Flexible sigmoidoscopy more successfully demonstrates the openings, but this also may be tolerated poorly. Barium enema will demonstrate the presence of diverticula and may reveal a region of bowel in spasm. Radiologic and endoscopic procedures are deferred until after resolution of acute symptoms unless the diagnosis is seriously in doubt or the patient is responding atypically or not responding to management.

Management

The majority of patients presenting as described above can be managed by nonoperative measures. These should include bowel rest, with or without nasogastric suction, IV hydration and IV antibiotics, at least initially until the patient responds and symptoms begin to resolve. Choice of antibiotic could occupy a lengthy discussion, but we usually use cefoxitin in a dosage of 1 gm every six hours, and most patients respond to this. Failure of symptoms to resolve within 24–36 hours may indicate that a more complicated process is present, and operative exploration should be considered.

With resolution of symptoms, diet can be resumed and advanced as tolerated. At this point, an added-fiber diet should be explained to the patient. Bulk-type laxatives also may be prescribed. Surgical intervention is not indicated unless there are repeated episodes of similar complaints, medical management fails, or unless the patient is in the young age group, where there is a greater tendency to progress to complicated disease.

Surgical therapy should be elective and done during a quiescent stage of the disease if possible. Preoperative management should include assessment of the extent of diverticular disease within the colon. Barium enema and colonoscopy are complementary in this respect. They will alert the surgeon to areas of active inflammation and enable him to estimate the margins of resection as well as help in eliminating the possibility of concomitant neoplasm. Intravenous pyelography (IVP) is strongly recommended, as the ureters are often involved in contiguous inflammation and fibrosis, and knowledge of their course and of bilateral renal function is of some importance.

Prior to elective resection, mechanical bowel preparation is desirable if it can be accomplished without activating an acute episode. When possible, consideration should be given to the traditional three days of low-residue diet, cleansing enemas, and, with some patients, cathartics or the one-day preparation with saline or osmotic solutions. Perioperative parenteral antibiotics and preoperative intraluminal antibiotics should also be used in accordance with the various described regimens.[8, 9] The patient should be advised preoperatively of the possible necessity for a stoma, though in these circumstances one is rarely indicated.

A lower midline incision serves well in most patients. Intraoperative assessment sometimes contradicts preoperative impressions, as the patient may have little gross evidence of acute or chronic inflammation, but more often a localized segment of sigmoid will be seen bearing the stigmas of inflammatory episodes. Resection with primary anastomosis should be possible with disease at this stage. The extent of resection should provide for anastomosis in bowel which is free of disease, but this does not imply that the patient with diffuse diverticula but evidence of inflammation only in the sigmoid should undergo subtotal colectomy. Conservation of bowel not involved in inflammatory disease should be the rule. Often anastomosis can be accomplished safely above the peritoneal reflection in the very distal sigmoid.

Postoperatively the patient is maintained on nothing by mouth until flatus is passed, at which time diet is begun and advanced as tolerated. Prior to discharge, the added-fiber diet is explained again.

DIVERTICULAR ABSCESS

Presentation

The patient with diverticular abscess may be clinically indistinguishable from the patient with acute diverticulitis and may only be recognized as such when there is a failure of response to medical therapy. The cramping and pain may be more frequent or more constant, and often there is alteration of bowel habits consistent with paralytic ileus or extrinsic obstruction of colon or small bowel. Difficulty with or pain at micturition may be present if the abscess is adjacent to the bladder. The symptoms may be gradual, prolonged, and associated with weight loss.

On physical examination, the patient appears distressed and commonly has fever and tachycardia. Abdominal distention is often present due to local obstruction or paralytic ileus and a lower quadrant mass may be evident. Rectal examination may elicit pelvic tenderness or fluctuance and pelvic examination in the female may also elicit tenderness on manipulation of the uterus or an adnexal mass.

Serum electrolytes reflect the extent of dehydration, and leukocytosis with a left shift is the rule. Proctoscopy, colonoscopy, and barium enema should be used with great caution, if at all, as the distortion and acute inflammation make all three procedures technically difficult and unduly hazardous. Furthermore, they are usually unnecessary, as it is evident that the patient has an acute process requiring surgical intervention. CT scan and/or ultrasonography might be useful in categorizing the extent and anatomical relations of the abscess. If the patient's renal status permits, IVP should be obtained, though CT scan with contrast can provide the same information with more detail about anatomical relations.

Management

Preparation of the patient for operation includes hydration and restoration of optimal renal function, correction of any electrolyte or clotting abnormalities, and careful consideration of the patient's physiologic reserve to determine his ability to tolerate an extensive procedure. Mechanical and antibiotic bowel preparation are not feasible in most cases, but parenteral antibiotics should be given. Metronidazole or clindamycin plus an aminoglycoside are preferable to any single drug. The possibility of a stoma should be mentioned.

The operative approach is dependent to some extent on the physiologic reserve of the patient. The severely septic patient in multiple organ failure might be treated best by drainage of the abscess and proximal colostomy, recognizing that the fecal contents in the bowel distal to the stoma are a source of continuing contamination and accepting that to avoid an intraoperative mortality. However, in the patient who is able to tolerate a more extensive procedure, resection is the wiser course. Eng and others[10] in a collected series showed a much higher mortality and morbidity for those with stoma and drainage alone as opposed to those who had primary resection of the diseased segment (Table 43–1). Even in view of the greater attendant hazard to contiguous structures, such as the ureters and bladder, resection should be pursued. In actuality, an abscess is not amenable to resection as such unless it is located within the leaves of the mesentery. Instead, the abscess wall is debrided of necrotic tissue and appropriate drainage used at the site. At times the surgeon will be unable to differentiate diverticular abscess from perforated malignancy with abscess. Preoperative fine-needle aspiration has been recommended in the evaluation of rectosigmoidal stenosis;[11] however, we would treat the disease as a malignancy, including the appropriate nodal drainage area in the resection.

Once resection is accomplished, the question of how best to manage the bowel arises. Primary anastomosis in the presence of infection is hazardous but, if successful, reduces hospital stay. Schrock et al.[12] cited these single variables as factors associated with increased colonic anastomotic leakage: age greater than 80, steroid therapy, intraoperative hypotension, prolonged operative period, transfusions of more than two units of blood, emergency operations, extraperitoneal anastomoses, and infection—that is, peritonitis, abscess, or fistula. The experienced surgeon may elect to perform primary anastomosis in patients who are stable intraoperatively, with minimal contamination from their abscess and healthy bowel available for anastomosis. In malnourished or steroid-dependent patients or in those who are unstable at operation, end colostomy and mucous fistula or Hartmann's closure may be the more prudent decision. In the Schrock review, the mortality for anastomotic leak was 33%. A compromise to this is primary anastomosis protected by a proximal colostomy with a second-stage colostomy closure. This might even be the preferable approach in the patient in whom the distal margin of resection is well below the peritoneal reflection, and a Hartmann procedure would render subsequent attempts at reanastomosis technically very difficult. The site of the previous abscess cavity should be drained adequately but attention should be given drain placement. Suction drains in proximity to an anastomosis can induce leakage. If possible, the omentum or similar tissue should be interposed to protect the suture or staple line.

Postoperatively, antibiotics should be continued for five to seven days or longer if the patient's clinical status dictates. Nasogastric suction should be used to ensure bowel rest until the passage of flatus or stool signals the return of bowel func-

TABLE 43–1.—MORTALITY BY SURGICAL APPROACH FOR PERFORATED DIVERTICULAR DISEASE

AUTHOR	COLOSTOMY/ DRAINAGE		COLOSTOMY/ RESECTION		RESECTION/ ANASTOMOSIS		RECOMMENDATION
	Cases	Mortality No. (%)	Cases	Mortality No. (%)	Cases	Mortality No. (%)	
Eng[10] (collected series)*	86	28(31)	44	4(9.1)	50	5(10)	Colostomy/Resection
Madden	20	7(35)	—	—	37	3(8)	Resection/Anastomosis
Madden[14] (collected series)*	313	143(46)	—	—	115†	11(9)	Resection/Anastomosis
Rodkey, Welch[28]							
1964–73	16	5(31)	1	1(100)	—	—	Colostomy/Resection
1974–83	16	8(50)	35	3(8)	?Anastomosis in any?		Colostomy/Resection
Welch, Welch (collected series)*	—	—	152	10(6.5)	88	6(6.8)	Colostomy/Resection

*Collected series overlap one another.
†Colostomy/Resection and Resection/Anastomosis groups not separated.

tion. Diet can then be instituted and advanced as tolerated. Readmission and restoration of bowel continuity should be deferred until the inflammatory process is well resolved, a time interval on the order of two to six months. Prior to operative reconstruction, the patient should have proctoscopy and barium enema to identify any residual active disease and to eliminate the possibility of obstruction distal to the proposed anastomotic site. There is an inescapable morbidity and even mortality to reconstruction, 2.9% in one series,[13] but the staged procedure remains the safer course in many situations.

PERFORATION

Presentation

Perforation into the free peritoneal cavity is relatively uncommon. It is usually preceded by formation of an abscess which subsequently perforates, but may commence with free perforation of a diverticulum. Presenting complaints are similar to those for abscess—gradual onset of progressive malaise, with cramping lower quadrant pain and alteration of bowel habit. When free perforation takes place, there is diffuse abdominal pain, general deterioration of the patient's status, and perhaps altered sensorium.

Physical findings usually include fever, tachycardia, often tachypnea, and not uncommonly respiratory distress with or without hypotension. Typically, the abdomen is distended, diffusely tender, with absent bowel sounds and demonstrable rebound. Elderly patients may have a raging peritonitis but a remarkable lack of signs and symptoms. This is especially true in steroid-dependent and in diabetic and uremic patients.

Serum electrolytes, hematocrit, and clotting studies should be obtained and gross abnormalities corrected prior to operation. Endoscopy and radiologic studies are rarely necessary in the patient who presents with a surgical abdomen, prior history of diverticular disease or progressive deterioration despite attempts to correct hydration or electrolyte problems. These patients should be readied rapidly for their procedure and operated on without delay. Occasionally, the surgeon will be faced with a patient who, in retrospect, probably experienced a free perforation several hours to several days prior to recognition and who is stable and apparently responding to medical therapy, implying that the perforation has sealed spontaneously. Additional time can be spent on these patients, and CT scan can be useful in identifying isolated collections.

Management

Most of these patients would be well served by central venous pressure monitoring, and in some Swan-Ganz monitoring would be necessary. Antibiotic choice is broad-spectrum coverage for anaerobes, especially *Bacteroides*, and aerobes. Therefore, clindamycin and an aminoglycoside are probably the most appropriate, though metronidazole is an adequate substitute for clindamycin, and the dosage of aminoglycoside may have to be curtailed due to antecedent renal dysfunction.

At operation, the same arguments referable to the advantages of immediate resection and reestablishment of continuity pertain, except that here, the caveat against primary anastomosis should be even stronger. Many very experienced surgeons[14] have spoken in favor of primary anastomosis in this instance, but it is doubtful whether the average surgeon could duplicate results or select patients with the same degree of judgment. Any abscesses or loculations encountered should be disrupted sufficiently to allow peritoneal bathing of the walls, and those which are adjacent to the abdominal wall should be drained with a Penrose or a sump drain as seems appropriate. Irrigation of the peritoneal cavity to evacuate gross debris and dilute frank pus should be accomplished. Hovnanian and Saddawi[15] concluded that their experimental studies "prove the unequivocal harmlessness of irrigation. We have demonstrated that the spread of organisms by the act of irrigation does not add to the mortality rate of the host." The report of Dunn et al.[16] that dilution of the peritoneal contents by saline may be deleterious may not be as contradictory as it seems, since their report deals with instillation of additional fluid into the peritoneal cavity in an experimental setting, in contrast to its value as an irrigant in other studies. Postoperative antibiotic administration should continue for seven to ten days, to militate against the development of recurrent abscesses and against the growth of resistant strains of bacteria. Failure to improve clinically should direct the surgeon's attention to reevaluation of antibiotic coverage, the possibility of undrained or reaccumulated pus and the likelihood of breakthrough sepsis by an organism with little sensitivity to the specific regimen, the most common such microorganism being *Streptococcus faecalis*.

Provided primary anastomosis is deferred or protected with a proximal colostomy, intestinal continuity should be reestablished only after a suitable period of recovery and after reassessment of the bowel distal to the proposed anastomotic site to avoid distal obstruction.

FISTULA

Presentation

Fistula occurs in diverticular disease when an abscess drains into some contiguous hollow viscus. The process rarely presents acutely and usually originates in sigmoid diverticular inflammation as opposed to cecal or transverse colon disease. In men the most common fistula is to the bladder. In women the intervention of the uterus and vagina make colovaginal fistula more common, though colovesical fistula[17, 18] may occur even without prior hysterectomy. The incidence of fistula in patients with symptomatic diverticular disease is reported as 3%–5%. Diverticular abscesses have also eroded into the ischiorectal spaces and presented as perirectal abscess and fistula-in-ano.

Though fistula may be the first presentation of diverticular disease, the rule is a long prior history of cramping, lower quadrant pain with pelvic discomfort and associated suprapubic pain as the process progresses. Exacerbation of symptoms at voiding is common. Pneumaturia is virtually pathognomonic but is not necessarily an early feature, even in established colovesical fistula. Eventually, all patients with colovesical fistula will experience pneumaturia. A common presenting history is of persistent or recurrent urinary tract infections despite what should be appropriate therapy. Any male presenting with this history should be suspected of having colovesical fistula, as should a reasonable percentage of females, especially if they are within the sentinel age group and have had no prior history of genitourinary infection as young adults. In females, persistent, foul-smelling vaginal discharge may trouble the patient for some time before the presence of feces in the vagina is appreciated.

Physical findings may include fever from urinary tract infection, but often the patient is afebrile, with minimal signs of septic complaints. The abdomen is soft and nontender, unless there is concomitant acute diverticulitis. Rectal examination may be entirely unremarkable. Vaginal examination usually discloses a posteroapical source of the feces, emphasized with staining.

Abnormal laboratory findings include an altered WBC count and urinalysis consistent with infection, i.e. bacteruria, with white cells, fecaluria at times, and, in about 20% of cases, hematuria. Sigmoidoscopy and barium enema are rarely useful in localizing the fistula opening. Cystoscopy and the cystogram usually will identify the urinary aspect of the fistulous tract. Intravenous pyelogram is useful in describing the course of the ureters, identifying any preoperative ureteral obstruction, and verifying bilateral renal function. Though the fistulous tract may not be apparent on sigmoidoscopy, the procedure is important in assessing the distal GI tract for obstruction and in identifying the occasional carcinoma.

Management

Preoperatively the patient should be placed on a low-residue diet and mechanical bowel preparation. This may be the traditional three-day approach or one of the briefer preparations utilizing an osmotic enteral load. Intraluminal antibiotics should be used in the perioperative period as should perioperative parenteral antibiotics. Broad coverage and efficacy against both anaerobic and aerobic organisms should be used. In the occasional patient where radiologic or endoscopic findings suggest the possibility of extreme difficulty with the ureteric course, stents placed at cystoscopy can guide the surgeon safely away from ureteric injury.

Resection for fistula is often more difficult than resection for malignancy due to the attendant chronic fibrosis as well as whatever acute inflammatory changes are present. The guiding principle should be resection of the diseased bowel, the fistulous tract and a core of normal tissue around the tract's drainage site. This means a margin of bladder should be included around the fistulous tract in the treatment of colovesical fistula and that hysterectomy should be a basic part of the treatment of colovaginal fistula. In the patient who is very ill or has serious cardiac, renal, or neurologic disease which might preclude the safe performance of primary resection, simple proximal colostomy should allow resolution of symptoms. Primary resection is the preferable course. The hope that the bowel can be restored to continuity without recurrence of the fistula after simple colostomy alone is unrealistic and is mentioned only to be condemned.

If resection of only a small portion of bladder wall is required to excise a colovesical fistula, two-layer closure with absorbable suture is acceptable management, provided Foley catheter drainage is maintained for a period of seven to ten days to decompress the closure. Larger bladder defects can be closed in essentially the same manner, but a suprapubic catheter should be placed as well, so that if prolonged urinary drainage is required, Foley catheter-induced epididymitis and prostatitis can be avoided. Fistulas to the bladder originating from the tranverse and right colon are usually to the region high on the dome of the bladder and consequently easier to resect and to repair. Fistulas from the sigmoid to the bladder may be deep in the pelvis and more difficult to manage. Urologic consultation is useful in the preoperative and intraoperative periods in many cases. The majority of these patients can undergo a safe primary reanastomosis without proximal decompression, provided the anastomosis is in normal bowel, is performed carefully, and soft tissue, such as omentum, can be interposed between the anastomotic suture line and the closure of the bladder or the posterior vagina.

The most common major postoperative complication of this approach is colocutaneous fistula, but this complication is even more common when anastomosis is performed in the face of abscess or peritonitis.

The postoperative care should follow sound principles of surgical care as discussed earlier.

DIVERTICULAR HEMORRHAGE

Presentation

Of the complications of diverticular disease of the colon, the most frustrating to deal with is hemorrhage. Even well-conceived efforts at accurate identification of the source of bleeding are not always rewarding, and the surgeon is led into more extensive resection than he may wish or than the patient may tolerate easily. Localio and Stahl[19] credit Koch with the first description of hemorrhage complicating diverticulosis coli in 1903, but it was much later that diverticular bleeding was well appreciated as a clinical entity. The acute onset of painless rectal bleeding is the hallmark of this process. It is not commonly associated with inflammatory symptoms, and while usually self-limited, it may be exsanguinating. The process is more dangerous within the age group it affects than the absolute volume of blood loss might indicate, since most patients will have preexisting coronary artery and cerebrovascular disease markedly reducing physiologic reserve. Although the sigmoid colon is the most common site for colonic diverticula, bleeding is thought to occur more commonly from the right colon.

Typically, the patient presents with painless rectal bleeding, most characteristically maroon in color, though it may be bright red if it is brisk or from relatively close to the rectum, or black and tarry if it has remained intraluminally for enough time to allow bacterial action on the hemoglobin. Bleeding may be persistent and slow or rapid and exsanguinating. Diverticulosis is also responsible for occult rectal bleeding, which must be differentiated from that due to carcinoma, but carcinoma is rarely responsible for massive hemorrhage as described above.

Physical findings may be remarkably few. If the patient is hypovolemic as well as anemic, there may be tachycardia and hypotension. The abdomen is soft and nontender. Rectal examination discloses grossly bloody stool or clots within the rectum without mass or tenderness. Bowel sounds may be hyperactive due to the cathartic effect of intraluminal blood.

Serum electrolytes are perused in search of electrolyte imbalances which may require correction. The BUN is some-times elevated, particularly if the ileocecal valve is incompetent and there is gross reflux of blood into the small intestine with increased nitrogen reabsorption. The initial hematocrit may be within normal limits if the bleeding is acute and extracellular space redistribution has not occurred, or if the blood loss was relatively minor and self-limited. In the past, barium enema to demonstrate diverticulosis, sigmoidoscopy to document bleeding from above the limits of the scope, and some maneuver—e.g., nasogastric lavage—to eliminate an upper GI source of hemorrhage led to the diagnosis of diverticular hemorrhage by exclusion. Diagnostic maneuvers now are contingent on the rate of hemorrhage. Massive rectal bleeding precludes colonoscopic inspection but lesser degrees of hemorrhage are best assessed by colonoscopy.[20] At the same time esophagogastroduodenoscopy can be performed to eliminate an upper GI source of hemorrhage presenting per rectum. Upper GI endoscopy should be used as well when hemorrhage is too great to allow adequate colonoscopy. More than one patient has been subjected to operation for lower GI bleeding when the true culprit was a duodenal ulcer.

In acute hemorrhage when adequate endoscopic visualization is not possible, radiologic measures come to the fore. When the rate of hemorrhage exceeds 0.5. ml/minute, angiography may demonstrate extravasation at the bleeding site, either directing the surgeon to a site for segmental resection or providing access for therapeutic intervention. The superior mesenteric arterial tree should be injected first, in view of the preponderance of bleeding from the right side of the colon, and if that fails to reveal a site of hemorrhage, the inferior mesenteric system should be injected next. If neither site shows evidence of extravasation, then some[21] advocate reinjection in view of the vasodilatory effects of the contrast medium. However, the renal effects of the contrast load should be considered prior to this and the decision based on the individual patient's renal function and hydration status. Another approach in this circumstance is the injection of an isotope, followed by large-field gamma camera scanning of the entire abdomen. This method may not be quite so precise as angiography, localizing the site generally to the right or left colon, but it is more sensitive, detecting bleeding at rates of as little as 0.1 ml/minute. In spite of all these techniques, there will continue to be a subset of patients whose source of bleeding cannot be identified preoperatively.

Management

In the patient in whom bleeding stops spontaneously and minimal transfusion is required, no further therapy is indicated, provided the physician is comfortable with the diagnosis of diverticular bleeding. The patient should begin eating the added-fiber diet and may be followed up in the manner most suitable to the patient and his physician. The patient with recurrent lower GI bleeds should undergo elective resection of the portion of the colon bearing the bleeding point provided that has been identified. Failing that, the patient should undergo subtotal colectomy with ileoproctostomy presuming his physical state is such that he will tolerate it and his anticipated lifespan and quality of life suggest that he may live long enough to require an emergency procedure if it is not done electively.

The patient with more extensive bleeding identified at angiography can be controlled at least transiently by selective catheter administration of intra-arterial vasopressin at an initial rate of 0.2 units/minute (Table 43–2). Repeated contrast injection to document vasoconstriction and cessation of hemorrhage follows at an interval of about 30 minutes. If necessary, the dose may be increased to a maximum of 0.3 units/minute infused over an eight- to 12-hour period, or if hemorrhage is controlled, the dose can be reduced to 0.1 units/minute, and continued for the same eight- to 12-hour interval. Electrocardiographic monitoring is wise during this therapy, as the coronary arteries may present signs of ischemia from continued vasopressin administration. Bleeding may recur hours to days after this therapy, but it allows time for stabilization of the patient and some patients will avoid surgery entirely. An alternative approach to vasopressin infusion is angiographic embolization with any of a variety of substances including Gelfoam, Teflon spheres, and tiny metal coils. As with any procedure, there is risk to these. Chronic ischemia in the embolized or thrombosed segment can result in stricture[22]; we can relate an anecdote wherein acute ischemia following embolization resulted in perforation of the colon, necessitating emergency laparotomy.

The patient with bleeding localized at angiography who does not respond to angiographic therapy should be prepared for operation with replenishment of blood, repair of any clotting deficits, and, at operation, segmental resection of the involved bowel should be performed. Primary anastomosis can be accomplished safely, as blood acts as a cathartic and the fecal load generally is diminished markedly. Perioperative parenteral antibiotics are indicated. Determining the point at which conservative measures have failed is not always straightforward, but if the patient persists in bleeding and requires transfusion beyond 6 units of blood, further delay is more likely to result in deterioration of the patient and render operation that much more hazardous.

The most difficult patient with which one has to deal is the one in whom all diagnostic maneuvers have been unsuccessful in localizing a source of hemorrhage but who persists in bleeding. Depending on the skill of the radiologists and the whim of fortune, this subgroup can be quite large. Hagihara and co-workers[23] reviewed 14 colonic bleeders, 11 of whom underwent angiography, and in five of the 11 localization of

TABLE 43–2.—VASOPRESSIN INFUSION FOR
ARTERIOGRAPHICALLY IDENTIFIED BLEEDING SOURCE

The solution

To 5% dextrose, 1,000 ml, add 200 units of vasopressin and infuse at appropriate rate to deliver 1 ml/min; or: To 5% dextrose, 250 ml, add 200 units of vasopressin and infuse at rate to deliver 0.25 ml/min (15 gtts./min).

Administration

After selective catheterization of the bleeding vessels, infuse vasopressin at 0.2 units/min. Repeated contrast injection at 30 minutes should confirm cessation of hemorrhage. If hemorrhage controlled, reduce vasopressin infusion to 0.1 units/min and continue for 8–12 hr. If hemorrhage not controlled, increase vasopressin infusion to 0.3 units/min and continue for 8–12 hours, provided patient responds to this dose.

Caveats

Cardiac monitoring imperative as vasopressin may constrict these vessels also. Splanchnic ischemia can result in bowel necrosis.

---

the bleeding site was not accomplished by radiologic measures in spite of persistent hemorrhage. Faced with this situation at laparotomy, the surgeon may try to localize the bleeding segment of bowel by segmental isolation with non-crushing clamps or ties, by multiple colostomies and intra-operative endoscopy or by transillumination of the bowel wall using an endoscope, but emergency subtotal colectomy as advocated by Drapanas et al.[24] in 1973 is the most conservative course in spite of its apparent radical nature. The time saved by proceeding with resection rather than futile maneuvers redounds to the patient's benefit. Ileocolostomy is a safer anastomosis than colo-colostomy, especially in patients with distal aortic atherosclerotic disease, and the surgeon can usually rest assured he has resected the hemorrhagic lesion. This is especially true if the ileocecal valve is competent and the small bowel is devoid of intraluminal blood. When blood has refluxed into the small bowel, there is always the possibility that it originated from a jejunoileal diverticulum or vascular ectasia or some other proximal source. Postoperatively, the patient must be observed closely. Perioperative myocardial infarction is not uncommon, and impaired renal function due to hypovolemia and hypotension, and exacerbated by angiographic contrast studies may complicate fluid management. Patients recovering from subtotal colectomy and ileoproctostomy generally experience multiple liquid stools for a period of two to six months before they stabilize at two to three semisolid stools per day.

OBSTRUCTION DUE TO DIVERTICULAR DISEASE

Presentation

Complete obstruction of the colon due to diverticular disease is uncommon, particularly in comparison with the more common malignant obstruction. The differential evaluation of obstructive diverticular disease is a problem, primarily in terms of identifying a concomitant malignancy or demonstrating the benign histologic nature of the disease process. The mechanism of stricture formation is fibrotic resolution of prior inflammatory diverticular disease. Intramural abscesses drain spontaneously back into the lumen or resolve without drainage, but result in relatively thickened bowel. With progressive fibrosis, there is progressive stenosis. Clinically, the change in bowel habits, alteration in stool caliber, and sensation of incomplete evacuation are no different from the presentation of a sigmoid or rectal malignancy. Prior history of diverticular disease should be of no comfort to the patient or physician, as a diagnosis of a malignant process must be presumed until proved otherwise. Sigmoidoscopy and barium enema may define the lesion without clearly establishing a benign or malignant nature. Biopsy is only possible at the most accessible point. Technical difficulty such as pelvic adhesions at 12–15 cm from the anal verge may frustrate the procedure. Adequate bowel preparation may be impossible due to the obstructive process. Therefore, the patient may come to laparotomy with an obstructed colon and no clear diagnosis.

Even at operation, it may not be possible to differentiate a thickened sigmoid due to chronic inflammation from a sigmoid neoplasm. When in doubt, the lesion should be treated as though it were neoplastic. After resection of the obstructing lesion, colostomy with Hartmann's closure or mucous fistula is the safest course. Primary left colon anastomosis at operation for obstruction is fraught with hazard in even the best of hands.

GIANT DIVERTICULA OF THE COLON

Presentation

A rare complication of diverticular disease is the giant diverticulum. Slightly more than 50 cases have been reported in the literature.[25, 26] They are most commonly antimesenteric in origin and limited almost exclusively to the sigmoid colon. They probably arise within a preexisting diverticulum with a ball-valve mechanism acting to inflate gradually the diverticulum into a balloon-like cyst.

Patient complaints are centered around left lower quadrant abdominal pain and cramping. A mass may be palpable but more commonly is not. Physical examination in fact may be quite unremarkable. Plain film of the abdomen is usually diagnostic, revealing a large air-containing cyst in the lower abdomen. Intravenous pyelogram or CT scan will demonstrate that the cyst is not retroperitoneal.

Management consists of elective resection of that portion of the sigmoid containing the cyst. Otherwise, the patient may present with an acute complication. Volvulus, perforation and small-bowel obstruction due to adhesions all have been described.

SOLITARY CECAL DIVERTICULUM

A different clinical problem is posed by the solitary cecal diverticulum. This is a true diverticulum containing all layers of the bowel wall and has a congenital origin. Therefore, it is not age-related or related to diet.

Presenting complaints are similar to those of appendicitis with which the process is most often confused preoperatively. A ten-year review[27] of the experience at the hospitals affiliated with the Louisiana State University Medical Center of New Orleans disclosed 19 patients presenting with cecal diverticulitis. There were 10 men, 9 women, and the age range was 23 to 73 years, with an average of 39 years. All these patients complained of right lower quadrant pain of varying duration. Ten patients had nausea, six reported vomiting. Anorexia and melena also were reported. Fever was common at presentation. All patients had right lower quadrant tenderness, with rebound in six patients, palpable mass in two, and rectal tenderness in five patients. Laboratory and radiologic studies were nonspecific.

The correct diagnosis was made preoperatively in only two patients, each of whom had undergone prior appendectomy. A correct intraoperative diagnosis was made in 11 patients (58%), neoplasm or inflammatory mass mimicking neoplasm being the intraoperative diagnosis in the remainder.

Local resection of the diverticulum with concurrent appendectomy is usually advocated. Hemicolectomy is reserved for cases which are recurrent, those without a clear differentiation from neoplasm or where there may be compromise of the ileocecal valve. Sixteen of the patients in our series were managed with right hemicolectomy and had a shorter hospital stay and less morbidity than the three patients who had local resection, although the numbers are too small for any statistical analysis. Nonetheless, hemicolectomy can be performed safely and quickly, and we advocate it as the procedure of choice for cecal diverticulitis.

SUMMARY

Diverticulosis coli is a common clinical entity with a broad range of related complications, though most patients have minimal difficulty. The etiologic background is related to an inadequate dietary intake of fiber and a series of colonic abnormalities developed in response to the subsequent constipation. Prophylaxis and therapy for the mild case are the same: increased dietary fiber and modest exercise.

Complications of diverticulosis coli include diverse inflammatory problems ranging from mild local inflammation to abscess, perforation, and fistulization to adjacent structures. Recurrent mild cases and virtually all the more serious cases will require surgical extirpation of the involved bowel. Most often this means segmental sigmoidectomy. Hemorrhage, usually self-limited, may be exsanguinating. In these patients, localization of the bleeding site is the clinical goal and subsequent therapy is directed at local control or, failing that, surgical extirpation. Stricture is a rare complication of recurrent inflammatory episodes of diverticulitis and must be differentiated from inflammatory bowel disease and malignancy prior to resection.

The management of diverticular disease and its complications is marked by a morbidity and mortality that are distressingly high. The elderly patients suffering from this condition require the utmost in care and consideration and a very keen sensitivity to physiologic reserve if they are to weather their storm safely.

REFERENCES

1. Painter N.S.: Diverticular disease of the colon: The first of the Western diseases shown to be due to a deficiency of dietary fibre. *South Afr. Med. J.* 61:1016, 1982.
2. Ajao O.G.: Differences between surgical colorectal conditions seen in the temperate and tropical regions. *Dis. Colon Rectum.* 25:795, 1982.
3. Muller C.J.B.: Hiatus hernia, diverticula and gall stones: Saint's Triad. *South Afr. Med. J.* 22:376, 1948.
4. Parks T.G.: Reappraisal of clinical features of diverticular disease of the colon. *Br. Med. J.* 4:642, 1969.
5. Capron J.-P., Piperaud R., Dupas J.-L., et al.: Evidence for an association between cholelithiasis and diverticular disease of the colon: A case-controlled study. *Dig. Dis. Sci.* 26:523, 1981.
6. Altemeier W.A., Bryant L.E., Wulsin J.H.: The surgical significance of jejunal diverticulosis. *Arch. Surg.* 86:732, 1963.
7. Ouriel K., Schwartz S.I.: Diverticular disease in the young patient. *Surg. Gynecol. Obstet.* 156:1, 1983.
8. Cohn I. Jr.: *Intestinal Antisepsis.* Springfield, Ill., Charles C Thomas Publishers, 1968.
9. Clarke J.S., Condon R.E., Bartlett J.G., et al.: Preoperative oral antibiotics reduce septic complications of colon operations: Results of prospective, randomized, double-blind clinical study. *Ann. Surg.* 186:251, 1977.
10. Eng K., Ranson J.H.C., Localio S.A.: Resection of the perforated segment: A significant advance in treatment of diverticulitis with free perforation or abscess. *Am. J. Surg.* 133:67, 1977.
11. Axelsson C.K., Francis D.: Preoperative fine-needle aspiration biopsy: An aid to differential diagnosis between diverticular disease and colonic cancer? A preliminary report. *Dis. Colon Rectum* 21:319, 1978.
12. Schrock T.R., Deveney C.W., Dunphy J.E.: Factors contributing to leakage of colonic anastomoses. *Ann. Surg.* 177:513, 1973.
13. Bell G.A.: Closure of colostomy following sigmoid resection for perforated diverticulitis. *Surg. Gynecol. Obstet.* 150:85, 1980.
14. Madden J.L., Tan Y.T.: Primary resection and anastomosis in the treatment of perforated lesions of the colon with abscess or diffusing peritonitis, *Surg. Gynecol. Obstet.* 113:646, 1961.
15. Hovnanian A.P., Saddawi N.: An experimental study of the consequences of intraperitoneal irrigation. *Surg. Gynecol. Obstet.* 134:575, 1972.
16. Dunn D.L., Barke R.A., Ahrenholz D.H., et al.: The adjuvant effect of peritoneal fluid in experimental peritonitis. Mechanism and clinical implications. *Ann. Surg.* 199:37, 1984.
17. Boles R.S., Jordan S.M.: The clinical significance of diverticulosis. *Gastroenterology* 35:579, 1958.
18. Hafner C.D., Ponka J.L., Brush B.E.: Genitourinary manifestations of diverticulitis of the colon: A study of 500 cases. *J.A.M.A.* 179:76, 1962.
19. Localio S.A., Stahl W.M.: Diverticular disease of the alimentary tract: The colon. *Curr. Probl. Surg.* 4:1–78, 1967.
20. Tedesco F.J., Waye J.D., Raskin J.B., et al.: Colonoscopic evaluation of rectal bleeding: A study of 304 patients, *Ann. Intern. Med.* 89:907, 1978.
21. Eisenberg H., Laufer I., Skillman J.J.: Arteriographic diagnosis and management of suspected colonic diverticular hemorrhage, *Gastroenterology.* 64:1091, 1973.
22. Shenoy S.S., Satchidanand S., Wesp E.H.: Colonic ischemic necrosis following therapeutic embolization. *Gastrointest. Radiol.* 6:235, 1981.
23. Hagihara P.F., Sachatello C.R., Mattingly S.S., et al.: Massive rectal bleeding of colonic origin: Localization of the bleeding site. *Surgery* 92:589, 1982.
24. Drapanas T., Pennington D.G., Kappelman M., et al.: Emergency subtotal colectomy: Preferred approach to management of massively bleeding diverticular diaese. *Ann. Surg.* 177;519, 1973.
25. Gallagher J.J., Welch J.P.: Giant diverticula of the sigmoid colon: A review of differential diagnosis and operative management. *Arch. Surg.* 114:1079, 1979.
26. Heimann T., Aufses A.H. Jr.: Giant sigmoid diverticula. *Dis. Colon Rectum* 24:468, 1981.
27. Wyble E.J., Lee W.C.: Cecal diverticulitis: Changing trends in management. Submitted for publication.
28. Rodkey G.V., Welch C.E.: Changing patterns in the surgical treatment of diverticular disease. Presented at the 104th Annual Meeting of the American Surgical Association, Toronto, Canada, April 25–27, 1984.

44

Malignant Disorders of the Anorectum

KIRBY I. BLAND, M.D.
EDWARD M. COPELAND III, M.D.

CANCER OF THE ANUS

The anal canal is composed of columnar epithelium of colorectal type in the upper third and squamous epithelium in its lower third. The middle zone is called the anal transitional zone (ATZ). The anal canal extends between the superior and inferior border of the internal anal sphincter. Thus, the ATZ is interposed between uninterrupted columnar epithelium above and intact squamous epithelium below.

Epithelial malignancies of the anal canal are quite rare and account for 1%–2% of all large bowel carcinoma.[1-5] The various histologic patterns that are recognized in this anatomical site account for the multitude of terms that have been applied to lesions of this area (e.g., squamous, basosquamous, transitional, cloacogenic, basaloid, mucoepidermoid). While histologically distinct and separable on the basis of histochemical and microsectioning analyses,[6] these lesions have similar clinical presentations and management. The aforementioned lesions are therefore *variants of epidermoid carcinoma* and can be divided into two groups on the basis of their microscopic appearance: *keratinizing* (squamous) and *nonkeratinizing* (basal, cloacogenic, basaloid, Bowen's, Paget's).

Keratinizing (Squamous) Carcinoma of the Anus

The anatomical anal canal is defined as the terminal 2–2.5 cm of the large intestine and extends from the dentate line to the anus. The relative incidence of epidermoid carcinoma of the anorectum has been reported by Morson and Volkstadt.[7] Of 3,672 patients with cancers of the anorectum, 3,535 (96.3%) were adenocarcinoma, and 122 (3.3%) were epidermoid carcinoma. The remaining 15 (0.4%) were melanoma. Of malignant tumors of the perianal skin, anal canal, and distal 2 cm of the rectum, approximately two thirds were adenocarcinoma and one third epidermoid carcinoma.[8]

Demographic data suggest that in essentially all series there is a preponderance of women. Clinical symptoms appear typically in the late fifth or sixth decades of life.[9] Predisposing factors to the development of epidermoid carcinoma of the anus include: chronic inflammation (fistulas, fissure, lymphogranuloma venereum, condyloma acuminatum), irradiation, and poor hygiene.[4, 9, 10]

The *clinical presentation* usually consists of more than one symptom, such as rectal bleeding, mucous discharge, pain, mass, tenesmus, and change in bowel habits. Rectal bleeding continues to be the single most common symptom. In a series

reported by Singh and coauthors,[11] duration of symptoms extended from two weeks to two years (mean, five months). The majority of patients had associated benign conditions (e.g., hemorrhoids, fissures, fistulas). Rarely, a patient may present with a chronic inflammatory process (Crohn's disease) or venereal disease (syphilis, condyloma, etc.). Approximately one third of epidermoid carcinomas are mistakenly diagnosed as benign lesions until disproved by biopsy.

Diagnosis is first established by realizing the possibility of anal carcinoma in a patient presenting with any anal symptom or associated disease. Many patients have been treated for benign, chronic inflammatory disease (hemorrhoids, fissure) for a considerable duration prior to diagnosis by digital rectal examination, anoscopy, and/or proctosigmoidoscopy. Early lesions have flat, raised, or warty surfaces. As the neoplasm enlarges, the surface may ulcerate and develop indurated margins fixed to adjacent tissues. A polypoid lesion on gross visual inspection may be mistaken for an adenocarcinoma of the anorectum. Biopsy and histologic sectioning is confirmatory.

Morson[12] found the amount of keratin formation (Fig 44–1) useful to classify tumors as undifferentiated or differentiated and suggested that the usual histologic staging was of lesser value. When correlated with prognosis, this classification has greater merit than the application of Broder's classification or of mitoses, fibrosis, inflammatory response, and necrosis. Cancers of the anal margin tend to be more keratinizing than anal canal lesions.

Prognosis with epidermoid carcinoma directly relates to size of the primary, a situation different from adenocarcinoma of the colorectum. Kuehn et al.[13] reported no survivors when the primary tumor exceeded 6 cm in diameter. Dillard and associates[14] noted 75% five-year survival in 12 patients with tumor size $\leq$ 8 cm^2; while 47% survival was observed in 38 patients with tumor size > 8 cm^2.

The importance of a staging system for epidermoid carcinoma of the anal region has been confirmed by Paradis et al.,[15] who suggest that prognosis of perianal and anal canal lesions are similar. Richards et al.[16] observed that Broder's grades were a good prognostic indicator; however, the Morson grading system is preferred by most pathologists.

TREATMENT.—*Surgical therapy* depends on the location and extent of invasion of the primary lesion, and clinical evidence of inguinal lymph node involvement. Tumors of the

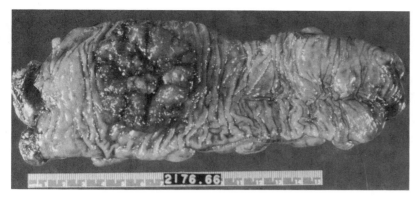

Fig 44–1.—Keratinizing (squamous) carcinoma of anus. (Courtesy D.A. Franzini, M.D., Department of Pathology, University of Florida.)

perianal skin are managed identical to those for epidermoid carcinoma in other sites of the body.[15] Beahrs and Wilson[1] evaluated 27 patients with superficial lesions of the perianal skin; all survived for five years when treated by local excision. These patients are at risk for the development of inguinal nodal metastases (bilateral) and close follow-up. Superficial groin dissection is indicated if inguinal nodes become clinically positive.

Three groups of lymphatics surround and drain the lower part of the large intestine.[16] These zones include: (1) the *inferior* group, which drains the perianal skin and anal canal; (2) the *central* group, which drains the terminal bowel several centimeters immediately superior to the dentate line and accompanies the inferior and middle hemorrhoidal vessels to terminate in the internal pudendal and hypogastric nodes, and (3) the *superior* group, which drains the rectum with efferent flow to lymphatics coursing along the superior hemorrhoidal and inferior mesenteric vessels. Various interconnections exist among these groups of lymphatics. Hematogenous routes of metastases are infrequent.[13, 17] The lymphatic system represents the primary mechanism of dissemination. Patients with primary tumors of the anorectum studied by Kuehn's group[13] had a 41% incidence of lymphatic metastases to perirectal, mesenteric, or inguinal nodes. Klotz et al.[17] observed metastases to at least one or more of the three nodal groups in approximately one third of his patients, the perirectal group being most frequent (75%).

Abdominal-perineal resection (APR) of the rectum and anal canal remains the standard therapy for invasive lesions of the anal margin and for all infiltrating lesions of the anal canal or the anorectum.[9] The variations in treatment results reported by various institutions depend on the design of the operation. Differentiation of an *anal verge* from an *anal canal* epidermoid carcinoma is crucial to appropriate management. Wolfe and Bussey[18] note that wide local excision only is appropriate management of an anal verge lesion, since metastases to lymph nodes of the superior and central groups are rare. This recommendation differs from that of other series.[14, 19] The difference is best explained by the variations of staging and anatomical location of the primary lesion. For example, Dillard et al.[14] reported the five-year survival for 46 patients with epidermoid carcinoma of the anal verge or canal following curative APR to be only 58%. Certainly for anal canal lesions APR is appropriate and Goligher[20] advocates APR with wide margin of perianal skin, muscle and fat. Additionally, in fe-

males, if the posterior vaginal wall is involved, it should be resected *en bloc.*

Epidermoid anal carcinomas are usually radiosensitive. In years past, radiation therapy was considered ineffective because of limitations of orthovoltage and its detrimental effects on anal function. Damage to the perianal skin and anal sphincter often necessitated colostomy after curative doses of radiation therapy. More recently, Papillon et al.[21] have utilized interstitial irradiation alone or in combination with external beam radiation therapy in selected patients with anal malignancies and have achieved a cure rate equal to that of surgical resection. Size of tumors significantly influences the prognosis and probability of preservation of anal function utilizing this technique. At three years, for 39 patients with tumor size ≤ 4 cm, 79% had no recurrence, and 93% had normal anal function. For tumors > 4 cm, a 64% control rate was achieved, and 65% of patients had preservation of anal sphincter function.

The preliminary application of multimodal approaches was reported by Nigro et al.[22] Preoperative external-beam irradiation and a short course of fluorouracil (5-FU) and mitomycin C were followed by APR. No residual tumor was identified in two of three APR specimens, and a third patient who refused operation had no recurrence after prolonged follow-up. Thereafter, Buroker et al.[23], Newman and Quan,[24] Wanebo et al.,[25] Sischy et al.[26] and Cummings et al.[27] utilized variations of this protocol to achieve control rates and survival similar to radical surgical procedures alone. The initial results of these pilot studies are encouraging, but extended follow-up is required before this formal therapy, particularly without APR, can be recommended.

TREATMENT OF REGIONAL LYMPHATIC METASTASES.— There are advocates of *prophylactic pelvic lymphadenectomy* in conjunction with APR in good-risk patients.[4] However, Quan et al.[28] observed little improvement in the overall survival when this surgical procedure was added to standard APR.

In virtually all surgical series reported, dissemination to inguinal nodes bears an ominous prognosis. Patients with clinically palpable nodes at the time of initial presentation of the neoplasm are rarely cured. In a review by Sugarbaker et al.,[29] only 16% of patients with synchronous inguinal nodal metastases survived five years. The futility of the *prophylactic (elective) lymph node dissection* (LND) has been confirmed in many series. Kuehn et al.[13] did synchronous prophylactic LND on 11 patients at the time of APR or within one month of the procedure. Microscopic disease was present in six patients, all of whom were dead of metastatic disease within six months. Likewise, Klotz et al.[17] recorded no survivors in patients treated with APR and synchronous prophylactic LND when microscopic foci of metastatic disease was found in the lymph nodes.

The interval presentation of palpable inguinal nodes after local control of the primary disease necessitates *therapeutic regional LND*. Radiation therapy infrequently controls gross nodal disease. Patients should be instructed to examine their inguinal areas on a weekly basis. Physician follow-up is recommended every two months for the first two years postoperatively, quarterly for years three and four, and annually thereafter. Appropriate selection of medically suitable patients is essential, as morbidity and mortality are real and identifiable with regional LND.[30] Therapeutic LND for inguinal adenopathy provided satisfactory control and cure for 60% of the patients in the series by Stearns and Quan.[8] Superficial and deep pelvic dissections have been advocated by several authors and appear to offer the greatest probability for local and regional control. The combination of both a superficial and deep dissection, however, almost ensures that symptomatic lymphedema will occur in the ipsilateral leg. For patients with large metastatic deposits fixed to skin, radiation therapy should be considered in conjunction with LND better to ensure local control. If the defect in the skin cannot be closed or skin flap viability is questionable, the sartorius muscle should be transposed over the femoral vessels and the skin defect grafted.

Unresectable epidermoid carcinomas of the anus represent difficult management problems. Large, painful, necrotic, odoriforous lesions are rarely excised and locally controlled with surgery alone. External irradiation in moderate doses (2,000–4,000 rad) may initiate regression with reduction of pain and discharge. Cryosurgery may also be effective for cytoreduction of large exophytic lesions.

Curative resections of intrapelvic recurrences are rarely successful. These patients have pain secondary to spinal and nerve root compression from extensive pelvic disease. These lesions are best managed by fractionated doses of irradiation. Newer techniques of brachytherapy with exact localization of radiotherapy implants is warranted in select cases. Ineffective control of intrapelvic metastases with irradiation or chemotherapy may necessitate neurosurgical intervention with sacral intrathecal alcohol block or cordotomy.

Colostomy rarely provides relief of pain and seldom obviates the malodorous discharge and bleeding which accompany such lesions. Inoperable anal epidermoid cancers usually do not obstruct and are thus best managed by radiotherapy, often in combination with chemotherapy.

Nonkeratinizing Epidermoid Carcinoma of the Anus

According to the histologic criteria previously established by Grinvalsky and Helwig,[31] Klotz et al.,[17] Pang and Morson,[32] and Kheir et al.,[33] the terms *transitional cell, mucoid adenocarcinoma, basal,* and *basaloid* are all appropriately classified as *cloacogenic carcinoma*. The remnants of the cloa-

cal membrane in adults is found proximal to the pectinate line and consists of a narrow zone of transitional epithelium penetrated by the anal glands. The anal transitional zone (ATZ) is characterized by an epithelium that bears a resemblance to that of the anal glands and has few goblet cells.[6] The ATZ incorporates features of both urothelium and squamous epithelium and is not considered specialized. Cloacogenic carcinoma is a specific morphological entity and can be readily distinguished from urothelial and squamous carcinoma, as well as the keratinizing variant of epidermoid carcinoma. The transitional type is composed of cells similar to the intermediate zone cells of ATZ, an observation which confirms the concept that the transitional form of cloacogenic carcinoma is derived from the ATZ. Pleomorphic variants and basaloid carcinoma appear to represent differentiated forms of the cloacogenic neoplasm.[34]

Histologically, transitional variants display a papillary structure with stratification of uniform, columnar cells that simulate urothelial carcinoma. Basaloid forms are characterized by clusters of smaller, ovoid cells with scant cytoplasm and hypochromatic nuclei. Pleomorphic tumors display greater nuclear and cellular atypism with an increased mitotic rate. The large polygonal cell is typical of pleomorphic tumors with highly irregular nuclear profiles.

In a collective review of 373 cloacogenic carcinomas by Klotz and co-workers,[17] these carcinomas accounted for 2.7% of the anal neoplasms with a female:male ratio of 2:1. Kheir et al.[33] recorded a similar female:male ratio (2.3:1) and incidence (2.4%). Serota et al.[35] and Nielson and Koch[36] classified cloacogenic tumors as to predominance of basaloid *squamous elements* (squamous pearls, cell keratinization, and basaloid features) or predominance of *glandular elements* (adenoid cystic, mucoepidermoid patterns). In the series by Serota and coinvestigators, the basaloid squamous type was most common.

Histologic characteristics of the tumor correlated with biological behavior. The *basaloid squamous* type of cloacogenic neoplasm was more common in women and had a more favorable course in both sexes (mean survival = 5.0 years). *Glandular variants* of this neoplasm, with a mucoepidermoid or adenocystic pattern, occurred predominantly in males and tended to have a more aggressive clinical course. The glandular type manifested early metastases to inguinal and mesenteric lymph nodes, liver, and lung and had a mean survival of 2.5 years. Five-year survival was observed in 82% of patients with the basaloid squamous histologic pattern when treated by APR or pelvic exenteration. Over one half of these prolonged survivors also received postoperative radiotherapy. These authors conclude that the histologic pattern of anal cloacogenic carcinoma provides a useful prognostic indicator for the subsequent clinical course. The importance of histologic differentiation and its effect on end results is worthy of future studies.

CLINICAL PRESENTATION AND DIAGNOSIS.—The presentation of cloacogenic carcinoma is the same as that for the keratinizing variant of epidermoid carcinoma, and diagnosis is established in a similar fashion. The entire anorectum should be inspected closely for proximal extension of the neoplasm. The circumference of the anorectal wall should be palpated for transmural penetration and involvement of pararectal nodes. Both inguinal areas should be examined for metastatic involvement. Associated benign disease (hemorrhoids, fissures, fistulas, Crohn's, radiation proctitis, syphilis) was noted in all the malignant epithelial tumors of the anal canal reported by Singh et al.[11] These patients may be followed up for various durations with presumed benign diseases, thus, suspicion of possible malignancy is important for diagnosis. In females, thorough pelvic examination of the adnexa and uterus is mandatory to document the superior and lateral limit of extension and to determine evidence of rectovaginal fixation or fistulas.

TREATMENT.—A uniform staging system for this malignancy has not been universally adopted since the Dukes classification is not applicable to cloacogenic neoplasms.[15] Treatment is aimed at extirpation of the primary neoplasm *en bloc* with the anorectal segment and management of potential lymph node metastases to the perirectal, iliac, and inguinal sites. It the past, therapy was similar to that used for the keratinizing epidermoid carcinoma. For invasive, locally advanced tumors, APR *en bloc* with a 4–5-cm wide margin of perianal skin represented standard therapy. In women with vaginal invasion and tumor fixation, *en bloc* resection of perianal skin with APR and posterior vaginectomy were necessary to decrease the high incidence of local recurrence. Singh et al.[11] documented that the lowest recurrence rates occurred when APR accompanied posterior exenteration with wide pelvic and perineal excision of advanced primary neoplasm (invasion of contiguous soft tissue, i.e., ischiorectal fossa, vagina, bladder, urethra). Once the neoplasm infiltrated muscle or soft tissue, the local recurrence rate was 60% and distant metastases were found in 30% of patients. Patterns of recurrence appear to be slightly different for each sex and histologic type.

More recently, Svenson and Montague[37] stressed the importance of *pelvic* and *perineal irradiation* combined with surgical ablation and documented improved local control and survival in patients with cloacogenic carcinoma. Both preoperative and postoperative irradiation were delivered with 22–25 meV photons through parallel-opposed fields that covered the pelvis with beam fall-off over the perineum. Preoperative radiation doses of 4,000 rad or postoperative radiation in 5,000 rad tumor-dose at 1,000 rad/week were administered. All patients treated with irradiation alone or combined with surgery have remained well.

Small cloacogenic carcinomas do not require combination with radiation therapy prior to surgical extirpation. Large lesions should be treated with preoperative radiation therapy prior to APR. The specimens from several patients treated by this method have revealed no remaining cloacogenic carcinoma in the specimen. This observation has stimulated several centers now to treat small lesions with radiation alone. When lesions have totally regressed, no surgical therapy has been used and lesions have not recurred. Too few patients have been followed up for too short a time for radiation therapy alone to be recommended as primary therapy. However, the follow-up of this subset of patients will be interesting, since, clearly, saving the anal sphincter is desirable when an equal chance of cure exists.

TREATMENT FOR NODAL METASTASES.—Management of *inguinal* lymphatic metastases represent an integral part of the treatment of cloacogenic carcinoma. Serota et al.[35] found lymph node metastases less common in *basaloid* squamous disease than in the cloacogenic glandular variant. For both sexes with basaloid squamous disease, *lymph node metastases* occurred in six (25%) of 24 patients. In distinction, the *glandular* type had lymph node metastases in ten (91%) of 11 cases. Sink et al.[38] noted inguinal nodal metastases in 50% of patients at some time during the course of their disease. Distant metastases in both series were noted most commonly in the liver and lungs.

In medically stable patients and in the absence of remote metastases, *therapeutic inguinal* lymph node dissection *(LND)* is indicated for clinically palpable disease. Preferably, this procedure is done four to six weeks following treatment of the primary neoplasm. *Prophylactic inguinal LND* for cloacogenic carcinoma is not recommended, since no report confirms any advantage in disease-free or overall survival with this approach in the presence of microscopically involved nodes.[8, 12, 16, 28, 35, 39] Further, a considerable number of patients may be subjected to operation without therapeutic benefit and exposure to the potential complications of postoperative morbidity related to regional LND. Likewise, the efficacy of prophylactic inguinal nodal radiation therapy has not been established.

Premalignant Dermatoses of the Anus

BOWEN'S DISEASE.—This precancerous dermatosis was described in 1912 by Bowen. The condition may mimic a wide variety of chronic minor skin irritations. Histologically, this lesion represents a slowly progressive *intraepidermal squamous cell carcinoma* with low-grade invasive and metastatic potential. The perianal lesion may be so small that it is found only with incidental, histologic examination of perianal tissues removed for other purposes (fissures, hemorrhoids, etc.). On occasion, the presentation will be as a large, irregular, erythematous or pigmented zone of fissured, scaly, plaquelike skin that extends over large areas.

Bowen's disease may be confused with benign perineal lesions that include psoriasis, eczema, keratoses, anal skin tags, external hemorrhoids, nevi, and condylomata.[40] Biologically, this entity represents a slowly maturing *in situ* squamous carcinoma and has a tendency to invade and metastasize in <5% of reported cases.[41, 42] Strauss and Fazio[43] emphasized a systematic approach to the diagnosis and treatment of perianal Bowen's disease. Biopsies are performed to locate affected areas, so that involved skin may be identified prior to definitive therapy. Goligher[20] noted that preservation of sensitive anal skin and lower rectal mucosa is important to continence of the anal sphincteric mechanism. Therapy is directed at total macroscopic and microscopic resection with frozen-section analysis to determine adequacy of marginal excision of the skin. Closure with split-thickness skin graft is often necessary for areas of widely excised skin.

Bowen's disease has been associated with other *visceral cancers*. In the series reported by Strauss and Fazio,[43] a diagnosis was confirmed incidentally in one half the patients following histologic examination of anorectal tumor removed for other purposes. Fifty-eight percent of patients previously had a systemic or cutaneous cancer removed or developed visceral malignancies at metachronous intervals. Thus, when

Bowen's disease is discovered, a careful search for other primary cancers is warranted. *Multicentric pigmented Bowen's disease* as a variant of the clinically benign squamous cell carcinoma *in situ* was recently described by Bhawan.[44] This multicentric type differs from the usual Bowen's disease by occurring in younger individuals, at multiple sites, and in the penile or vulvar areas. Further, the lesions are pigmented and may undergo spontaneous regression.[45] Ultrastructural evaluation by Friedrich[46] suggested a viral etiology. However, no useful, reliable histologic criteria have been found to differentiate this variant from Bowen's disease. Treatment with local excision and, if needed, the application of split-thickness skin grafts is curative.

EXTRAMAMMARY PAGET'S DISEASE.—Extramammary Paget's has a disputed histogenesis; some consider origin from localized epidermal cellular dedifferentiation that subsequently spread downward to involve gland ducts or apocrine glands themselves. An anorectal carcinoma is always an associated finding and has an ominous prognosis. The Pagetoid cells may represent an extra-anatomical extension of a rectal primary. The perianal skin may be erythematous and pruritic. Goligher[20] documented the well-recognized association of this entity with long-standing anal fistula tracts. Both squamous carcinoma and colloid adenocarcinoma of the anorectum take origin from the fistulas.

The prominent clinical features of extramammary Paget's disease of the perianal region is the absence of symptoms within the anal canal—thus, the term *extramucosal adenocarcinoma*. These lesions, when mature, spread in an annular, centrifugal fashion with extensive infiltration of perianal tissues. Metastases are often demonstrated via regional (perirectal, pelvic, and inguinal) nodes. Extensive Pagetoid involvement of the skin may lead to eruption with an exophytic, scaly eczema of the perianal region similar to Paget's disease of the nipple-areola complex.

As the skin presentation is remote from the origin of the primary tumor, this lesion may be confused with Bowen's disease, cloacogenic carcinoma, or malignant melanoma. Visual inspection and full-thickness biopsy of the infiltrative lesion is diagnostic. The mucin-positive pagetoid cells associated with a pale, vacuolated cytoplasm are pathognomonic and easily distinguished histologically from the surrounding squamous epithelium. This lesion may also be confused with other inflammatory conditions, such as pruritus ani and Crohn's disease.

TREATMENT.—Treatment of extramammary Paget's is identical to that of epidermoid cancer of the anal canal. For medically suitable patients, APR with wide removal of perianal tissues is necessary. Lymphatic dissemination represents the primary route of metastases. Approximately 50% of patients will have evidence of *inguinal lymphatic involvement*,[47] and in suitable candidates a therapeutic inguinal lymph node dissection is indicated. Hematogenous metastases are uncommon. Evidence of inguinal adenopathy necessitates therapeutic inguinal LND for control of metastatic disease and to obviate skin and vascular infiltration and necrosis. The submucosal presentation of these lesions, with infrequent anorectal obstruction, rarely prompts the decision for diverting colostomy. Advanced cases, considered inoperable on the basis of extensive regional and distant spread, may be managed by irradiation.

Malignant Melanoma of the Anorectum

INCIDENCE.—Melanoma of the anorectum represents an extremely virulent neoplasm that takes origin from the melanocytes of the anal canal mucosa. The incidence of melanoma was 0.4% in 3,672 patients with cancers of the anorectum and anal canal reviewed by Morson and Volkstadt.[7] Quan et al.[48] described an identical incidence for 4,500 malignant tumors of the anorectum. Remigio et al.[49] noted that melanoma of all sites in the body constituted 1.1%–2% of all cancers in the United States, while anorectal melanoma accounted for 1.6% of all melanomas, 1% of all anal cancer, and 0.25% of all anorectal malignancies.

DEMOGRAPHIC DATA.—Distribution of melanoma of the anorectum appears equal in the two sexes,[48, 49] and age at diagnosis may range from 27 to 85 years old (mean age = 55 years). Past reviews[48–50] note predominance of white patients, although recent reports document anal melanoma in blacks,[51, 52] arising from the mucocutaneous junction.

CLINICAL PRESENTATION.—The symptoms of squamous carcinoma and benign diseases of the anorectum are similar to those of anorectal melanoma. Typically, the patient has the sensation of an abnormal mass that is presumed to be benign disease, such as fissures or hemorrhoids. Stearns and colleagues[9] observed bleeding in 47% of 59 patients, a "mass" in 17%, and pain with defecation in 10%. Symptoms occur with increasing size of the anorectal neoplasm. On occasion, the disease initially manifests itself as inguinal metastasis, and the cryptic primary in the anal canal may be unsuspected. Neurologic complications (sciatica, disorders of micturition) are indicative of direct invasion of pelvic structures.[49, 53]

DIAGNOSIS.—The primary lesions may vary greatly in appearance from small, benign-appearing exophytic masses to ulcerated, bleeding, pigmented lesions with near or complete obstruction of the anus. In the Quan[48] series, the largest tumor diameter was 6 cm, and the size range of nonulcerative melanomas varied between 3 and 5 cm. An exophytic or elevated, pigmented lesion in the perirectum or anal canal tissues should be considered melanoma until histologically proved otherwise. On occasion, amelanotic lesions will mimic benign growths such as hemorrhoids, skin tags, papillomas, condylomata, and dermatitis. Differentiation from benign lesions or from cloacogenic and keratinizing epidermoid carcinoma requires biopsy. Excisional biopsy of small lesions is appropriate; however, the majority are ≥3 cm at presentation and may require incisional biopsy prior to initiating definitive therapy.

BIOLOGIC BEHAVIOR AND METASTASES.—Many investigators[7, 48, 49, 52, 53] document the cephalad dissemination of melanoma via submucosal perirectal lymphatics once the lamina propria of the anal canal has been penetrated. Additionally, melanoma cells may enlarge in the submucosal plexus and fill the columns of Morgagni to cross the pectinate line and involve the mucosa and submucosa of the terminal rectum (Fig 44–2).

The introduction of tumor thickness (mm) as an accurate staging guide and prognostic indicator by Breslow[54] provided an objective method to evaluate melanoma. Using the Breslow classification for deepest vertical growth phase of the neoplasm, Stearns et al.[9] and Wanebo et al.[50] have applied this technique as a guide to therapy. Stearns et al. reported no five-year survivors for tumors ≥1.7 mm in thickness. Wanbeo and associates adopted a radical resection with APR, wide perianal excision, and pelvic node dissection for melanomas ≤3 mm and reported a few apparent cures. A prophylactic LND was not included in this radical, ablative effort.

The data by Wanebo et al.[50] suggest that survivorship directly correlates with tumor thickness, and this observation was confirmed by Stearns et al.[9] The prognosis associated with anorectal melanomas thicker than 2 mm is dismal. No patients with lesions >2.0 mm survived longer than five years, and 85% lived two years or less. Three evaluable patients with melanoma <1.7 mm were free of disease at follow-up (13–26.5 years).

Melanoma of the anorectum can also produce hematogenous metastases via portal and inferior vena caval systems. Quan and associates[28] document metastases of anal melanoma in order of diminishing frequency to be: liver, spine, lungs, groins, long bones, brain, and subcutaneous tissue.

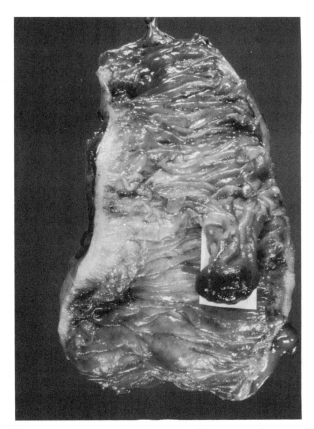

Fig 44–2.—Malignant melanoma of the anorectum; ×40. (Courtesy D.A. Franzini, M.D., Department of Pathology, University of Florida.)

THERAPY.—Surgery continues to represent the major therapeutic modality. Quinn and Selah,[51] in a review of the medical literature, found 107 cases with long-term follow-up, of whom 74 (69%) were managed by radical surgical procedures. Despite these aggressive surgical approaches, only five patients (6.7%) lived five years or longer. These authors observed that melanoma of the anus disseminated by obturator, inguinal, iliac, and aortic nodes. However, systemic involvement of visceral organs and the CNS may be apparent in the absence of regional (pelvic) nodal disease. Quinn and Selah[51] concluded that treatment of this aggressive neoplasm had little effect on prognosis.

For thicker lesions, at minimum, wide excision should be attempted. For locally advanced lesions in medically suitable patients not easily controlled by local measures, APR provides the most effective palliation. It is rare to achieve prolonged disease-free intervals or cure following either local excision or APR for this virulent neoplasm. Regardless, in appropriately selected patients with tumor thickness ≤2 mm, APR with dissection of the pelvic and obturator nodes appears to be the most reasonable choice of therapy and to offer the highest probability of cure. For the majority of patients, however, few therapeutic options exist, as APR is *not* decisively advantageous over excision alone to control local and regional disease, particularly when thickness of the primary exceeds 2 mm. In a series of patients reported by Cooper et al.,[55] the determinant survival for patients treated by APR, local excision, or incomplete excision was evaluated. No statistical differences in survival were apparent for patients treated by APR vs. local excision only. However, those having incomplete excision did significantly worse than the APR or local excision groups ($P = 0.001$). Tumor size did not appear to affect choice between local excision and APR in this series, although patients were not microstaged by Breslow classification. Rarely is local irradiation effective for palliating large, invasive lesions. Chemotherapy and immunotherapy may be considered in the treatment of distant or regional metastases; however, addition of these therapeutic agents rarely influences survival.

Prophylactic inguinal or *pelvic LND* is not advised, yet the interval appearance of inguinal nodal metastases after curative APR is best managed by superficial and/or deep inguinal nodal dissection to prevent subsequent ulceration, hemorrhage, etc. The appearance of inguinal metastases usually indicates mesenteric nodal spread and advanced metastatic disease. We advocate therapeutic inguinal node dissection, although we realize this procedure is only palliative. Pelvic lymphadenectomy, in conjunction with APR, may be necessary to encompass the grossly positive iliac-obturator lymph nodes; lymphedema will occur in about two thirds of patients and may be severe 30% of the time.[56]

Melanoma of the anorectum and anal canal metastatic from extrarectal sites may initiate obstructive symptoms necessitating emergency diverting colostomy, APR, or small-bowel resections in select patients. Das Gupta and Brasfield[57] summarized the experience of melanoma metastatic to the GI tract. Of 100 autopsies, 58 cases had metastases to small bowel, 22 to colon, 5 to rectum, and 1 to anus. In every patient, the true pelvis (iliac, hypogastric, obturator sites) had extensive metastatic involvement. These metastases from extra-anatomical sites may prompt the medical decision for small- or large-bowel resections to palliate advanced disease. Melanoma of the anus remains the most aggressive malignancy of the GI tract. Better methods of treatment must be sought to improve survival.

REFERENCES

1. Beahrs O.H., Wilson S.M.: Carcinoma of the anus. *Ann. Surg.* 184:422, 1976.
2. Corman M.L., Haggitt R.C.: Carcinoma of the anal canal. *Surg. Gynecol. Obstet.* 145:674, 1977.
3. Golden G.T., Horsley J.S. III: Surgical management of epidermoid carcinoma of the anus. *Am. J. Surg.* 131:275, 1976.
4. Welch J.P., Malt R.A.: Appraisal of the treatment of carcinoma of the anus and anal canal. *Surg. Gynecol. Obstet.* 145:837, 1977.
5. Sawyers J.L.: Current management of carcinoma of the anus and perianus. *Am. Surg.* 43:424, 1977.
6. Fenger C., Filipe M.I.: Mucin histochemistry of the anal canal epithelium: Studies of normal anal mucosa and mucosa adjacent to carcinoma. *Histochem. J.* 13:921, 1981.
7. Morson B.C., Volkstadt H.: Malignant melanoma of the anal canal. *J. Clin. Pathol.* 16:126, 1963.
8. Stearns M.W. Jr., Quan S.H.O.: Epidermoid carcinoma of the anorectum. *Surg. Gynecol. Obstet.* 131:953, 1970.
9. Stearns M.W. Jr., Urmacher C., Sternberg S.S., et al.: Cancer of the anal canal. *Curr. Probl. Cancer* 4(12):1, 1980.
10. Sturm J.T., Christenson C.E., Uecker J.H., et al.: squamous-cell carcinoma of the anus arising in a giant condyloma acuminatum: Report of a case. *Dis. Colon Rectum* 18:147, 1975.
11. Singh R., Nime F., Mittelman A.: Malignant epithelial tumors of the anal canal. *Cancer* 48:411, 1981.
12. Morson B.C.: The pathology and results of treatment of squamous cell carcinoma of the anal canal and anal margin. *Proc. R. Soc. Med.* 53:416, 1960.
13. Kuehn P.G., Eisenberg H., Reed J.F.: Epidermoid carcinoma of the perianal skin and anal canal. *Cancer* 22:932, 1968.
14. Dillard B.M., Spratt J.S. Jr., Ackerman L.V., et al.: Epidermoid cancer of anal margin and canal. *Arch. Surg.* 86:772, 1963.
15. Paradis P., Douglass H.O. Jr., Holyoke E.D.: The clinical implications of a staging system for carcinoma of the anus. *Surg. Gynecol. Obstet.* 141:411, 1975.
16. Richards J.C., Beahrs O.H., Woolner L.B.: Squamous cell carcinoma of the anus, anal canal, and rectum in 109 patients. *Surg. Gynecol. Obstet.* 114:475, 1962.
17. Klotz R.G. Jr., Pamukcoglu T., Souilliard D.H.: Transitional cloacogenic carcinoma of the anal canal. *Cancer* 20:1727, 1967.
18. Wolfe H.R.I., Bussey H.J.R.: Squamous-cell carcinoma of the anus. *Br. J. Surg.* 5:295, 1968.
19. Hardy K.J., Hughes E.S.R., Cuthbertson A.M.: Squamous cell carcinoma of the anal canal and anal margin. *Aust. N.Z. J. Surg.* 38:301, 1969.
20. Goligher J.C.: Carcinoma of the anal canal and anus, in *Surgery of the Anus, Rectum and Colon.* London, Bailliére Tindall, 1980, pp. 667–677.
21. Papillon J., Mayer M., Montbarbon J.F., et al.: A new approach to the management of epidermoid carcinoma of the anal canal. *Cancer* 51:1830, 1983.
22. Nigro N.D., Vaitkevicius V.K., Buroker T., et al.: Combined therapy for cancer of the anal canal. *Dis. Colon Rectum* 24:73, 1981.
23. Buroker T.R., Nigro N.D., Bradley G., et al.: Combined therapy for cancer of the anal canal: A follow-up report. *Dis. Colon Rectum* 20:677, 1977.
24. Newman H.K., Quan S.H.O.: Multi-modality therapy for epidermoid carcinoma of the anus. *Cancer* 37:12, 1976.
25. Wanebo H.J., Futrell W., Constable W.: Multimodality approach to surgical management of locally advanced epidermoid carcinoma of the anorectum. *Cancer* 47:2817, 1981.
26. Sischy B., Remington J.H., Hinson E.J., et al.: Definitive treat-ment of anal-canal carcinoma by means of radiation therapy and chemotherapy. *Dis. Colon Rectum* 25:685, 1982.
27. Cummings B.J., Harwood A.R., Keane T.J., et al.: Combined treatment of squamous cell carcinoma of the anal canal: Radical radiation therapy with 5-Fluorouracil and Mitomycin-C, a preliminary report. *Dis. Colon Rectum* 23:389, 1980.
28. Quan S.H.O., Magill G.B., Leaming R.H., Hajdu S.I.: Multidisciplinary preoperative approach to the management of epidermoid carcinoma of the anus and anorectum. *Dis. Colon Rectum* 21:89, 1978.
29. Sugarbaker P.H., Gunderson L.L., MacDonald J.S.: Cancer of the anal region, in DeVita V.T. Jr., Hellman S., Rosenberg S.A. (eds.): *Cancer: Principles and Practice of Oncology.* Philadelphia, J.B. Lippincott Co., 1982, pp. 724–731.
30. Bland K.I., Klamer T.W., Polk H.C. Jr., et al.: Isolated regional lymph node dissection: Morbidity, mortality and economic considerations. *Ann. Surg.* 193:372, 1981.
31. Grinvalsky H.T., Helwig E.B.: Carcinoma of the anorectal junction: I. Histological considerations. *Cancer* 9:480, 1956.
32. Pang L.S.C., Morson B.C.: Basaloid carcinoma of the anal canal. *J. Clin. Pathol.* 20:128, 1967.
33. Kheir S., Hickey R.C., Martin R.G., et al.: Cloacogenic carcinoma of the anal canal. *Arch. Surg.* 104:407, 1972.
34. Gillespie J.J., MacKay B.: Histogenesis of cloacogenic carcinoma: Fine structure of anal transitional epithelium and cloacogenic carcinoma. *Hum. Pathol.* 9:579, 1978.
35. Serota A.I., Weil M., Williams R.A., et al.: Anal cloacogenic carcinoma: Classification and clinical behavior. *Arch. Surg.* 116:456, 1981.
36. Nielson O.E., Koch F.: Carcinomas of the anorectal region of extramucosal origin with special reference to the anal ducts. *Acta Chir. Scand.* 139:299, 1973.
37. Svenson E.W., Montague E.D.: Results of treatment in transitional cloacogenic carcinoma. *Cancer* 46:828, 1980.
38. Sink J.D., Kramer S.A., Copeland D.D., et al.: Cloacogenic carcinoma. *Ann. Surg.* 188:53, 1978.
39. Stearns M.W. Jr.: Epidermoid carcinoma of the anal region: Inguinal metastases. *Am. J. Surg.* 90:727, 1955.
40. Visaya R. Jr., Papadakis L., Calem W.S.: Bowen's disease in anoperineal region. *N.Y. State J. Med.* 68:306, 1968.
41. Grodsky L.: Bowen's disease of the anal region (squamous cell carcinoma in situ). *Am. J. Surg.* 88:710, 1954.
42. Herold W.C., Cooper Z.K.: Bowen's disease, an intra-epidermal carcinoma: Report of cases from the Barnard Free Skin and Cancer Hospital. *Surg. Clin. North Am.* 24:1033, 1944.
43. Strauss R.J., Fazio V.W.: Bowen's disease of the anal and perianal area: A report and analysis of twelve cases. *Am. J. Surg.* 137:231, 1979.
44. Bhawan J.: Multicentric pigmented Bowen's disease: A clinically benign squamous cell carcinoma in situ. *Gynecol. Oncol.* 10:201, 1980.
45. Berger B.W., Hori Y.: Multicentric Bowen's disease of the genitalia. *Arch. Dermatol.* 114:1698, 1978.
46. Friedrich E.G. Jr.: Reversible vulvar atypia: A case report. *Obstet. Gynecol.* 39:173, 1972.
47. Spjut H.J.: Pathology of neoplasms, in Spratt J.S. (ed.): *Neoplasms of the Colon, Rectum, and Anus: Mucosal and Epithelial,* Philadelphia, W.B. Saunders Co., 1984, pp. 159–204.
48. Quan S.H.O., White J.E., Deddish M.R.: Malignant melanoma of the anorectum. *Dis. Colon Rectum* 2:275, 1959.
49. Remigio P.A., Der B.K., Forsberg R.T.: Anorectal melanoma: Report of two cases. *Dis. Colon Rectum* 19:350, 1976.
50. Wanebo H.J., Woodruff J.M., Farr G.H., et al.: Anorectal melanoma. *Cancer* 47:1891, 1981.
51. Quinn D., Selah C.: Malignant melanoma of the anus in a negro: Report of a case and review of the literature. *Dis. Colon Rectum* 20:627, 1977.
52. Hambrick E., Abcarian H., Smith D., et al.: Malignant melanoma of the rectum in a negro man: Report of a case and review of the literature. *Dis. Colon Rectum* 17:360, 1974.
53. Mikal S.: Malignant melanoma of the anus and rectum. *Am. J. Surg.* 103:191, 1962.

54. Breslow A.: Tumor thickness, level of invasion and node dissection in Stage I cutaneous melanoma. *Ann. Surg.* 182:572, 1975.

55. Cooper P.H., Mills S.E., Allen M.S. Jr.: Malignant melanoma of the anus: Report of 12 patients and analysis of 255 additional cases. *Dis. Colon Rectum* 25:693, 1982.

56. Papachristou D., Fortner J.G.: Comparison of lymphedema following incontinuity and discontinuity groin dissection. *Ann. Surg.* 185:13, 1977.

57. Das Gupta T.K., Brasfield R.D.: Metastatic melanoma of the gastrointestinal tract. *Arch. Surg.* 88:969, 1964.

45

Malignant Diseases of the Colon and Rectum

Kirby I. Bland, M.D.
Edward M. Copeland III, M.D.

ADENOCARCINOMA OF THE COLON AND RECTUM

Epidemiology, Carcinogenic Theory, and Genetics

Epidemiology.—Carcinoma of the colon and rectum continues to be a major source of morbidity and mortality in the United States. In 1984, an estimated 130,000 new cases will have been diagnosed, and an estimated 59,400 cancer deaths (13.2%) related to carcinoma of this anatomical site. A static, age-adjusted mortality has existed for colorectal carcinoma in men since 1950, while a slight trend toward decreased mortality has occurred in the female. Current trends in survival project an overall five-year survival of 50% and 42% for white and black subjects, respectively. This represents a 10% enhancement in five-year survival relative to comparable stages reported in 1960–63 for both groups. Presently, colorectal carcinoma constitutes 11.6% of the estimated cancer death-rates for males and is second only to lung cancer in site-specific mortality. In the female, colorectal carcinoma is responsible for 14.8% of cancer-related mortality and follows breast and lung, respectively, in frequency.[1]

The incidence and mortality of colorectal carcinoma has great variation in distribution throughout the world. Of 48 industrialized nations reporting colorectal-related mortality, the United States ranked 15th. This age-adjusted death rate for 1978–79 noted deaths at 26.5/100,000 males and 20.2/100,000 females. These high death rates are characteristic of well-developed countries in the West, the United Kingdom, and Scandinavia. Lower death rates were observed in Eastern Europe, the Orient, and Third World countries. These epidemiologic data identify marked variations in the international distribution of this entity with dependence on geographic, ethnic and socioeconomic status. Even within industrialized and nonindustrialized nations, marked discrepancies occur in the frequency of cancers of the large intestine and rectum. In the United States, death from cancer of the colorectum show marked concentration in the Northeast for both sexes, whereas in the South and Southwest, incidence of colorectal cancer is significantly below the United States average.[2]

A detailed analysis of large-bowel cancer mortality by counties in the United States from 1950–69 was undertaken by Blot et al.[3] in an effort to explain the above regional differences. High cancer rates were primarily related to counties

with a large population, higher educational levels, higher income, and a greater proportion of the population reported to be of German, Irish, or Czech descent. A further analysis to separate "urbanness" or "ruralness" did not provide explanation of the mortality differences observed. Regional variation between the Northeast and Southeast persisted after adjustment for socioeconomic differences. Higher rates of rectal cancer had a somewhat similar distribution.

Although substantial differences in the mortality rates for this disease exist in the United States, the variability is not readily accounted for by demographic factors. Per capita consumption of specific foodstuffs is distributed uniformly throughout the United States, but mortality differences may also reflect nondietary factors. In the United States and Canada, colonic cancer incidence rates are substantially higher than corresponding rates of rectal cancer and represent a shift from the distal rectal mucosal site to a predominance in the colon.[4, 5] While incidence data are limited for South America, annual rates for both colonic and rectal neoplasms are essentially identical in Colombia. Demographic variations exist which confirm that highly populated and industrialized areas sustain the greatest incidence rates and are significantly different from economically deprived and less densely populated areas. The mechanisms of colon carcinogenesis are poorly understood and are, perhaps interrelated with dietary (beef consumption), genetic, environmental or other undetermined factors.[6]

Genetics and the hereditary predisposition to the development of colorectal carcinoma.—Genetic factors have been implicated in site-specific colon cancer (with or without polyposis) and in syndromes associated with tumors and disorders of other organs and organ systems. The great number of colon cancer-related syndromes are probably monogenic, polyposis syndromes. These disorders include all of the *familial adenomatous polyposis syndromes* and, perhaps, syndromes associated with nonneoplastic polyps (*Peutz-Jeghers* and *juvenile polyposis*). As a group, the polyposis syndromes account for approximately 1%–5% of the colon cancer disorders.[7, 8] The inherited nonpolyposis colon cancers occur with greater frequency and may comprise upward of 20%–25% of all colon cancers.[8] These nonpolyposis syndromes (*herditary colonic cancer, hereditary gastrocolonic cancer, hereditary adenocarcinomatosis,* and *Muir's [Torre's] syndrome*) are autosomally dominant inheritance with onset in the early to mid-forties and an increase frequency of multiple primary carcinomas. *Inherited* colonic carcinomas occur more frequently in the right colon while the *noninherited* types are most frequent in the descending and rectosigmoid colon areas.[8–10] Albano et al.[11] and Lynch and Lynch[12] observed a significantly improved ($P < 0.05$) overall five-year survival for the hereditary nonpolyposis cancer population (52.8%) as compared to the American College of Surgeon's audits of the general colon cancer population (35.3%). Knowledge of cancer genetics provides the surgeon with a useful mechanism for recognizing patients who may profit from highly targeted cancer surveillance/management programs.

Table 45–1 enumerates both familial and nonfamilial populations who are considered at increased risk for the subsequent development of carcinoma of the colorectum. As noted previously, adenomatous polyps represent preneoplastic neoplasms with projections of malignancy correlating with grade of dysplasia and size of the adenoma. Specifically, the malignant transformation potential of villous adenomas of all sizes is much greater (40%) than that for tubular adenomas (5%). Further, this risk is escalated in patients with multiple adenomas.[12] Copeland et al.[13] observed 23% of patients with a single colonic carcinoma to have associated polyps. These polyps were multiple in 42% of the cases (Table 45–2). When focal carcinoma was discovered in a tubular polyp, a separate invasive carcinoma of the colon occurred in 20% of cases and other benign polyps were present in 48% of the colons. Benign polyps were associated with carcinoma within a villous adenoma in 25% of the subjects. Of 110 patients with colon cancer and an associated single polyp, 7.3% had a synchronous colonic malignancy, and 2:7% developed a metachronous colon cancer. In patients with colonic cancer and associated multiple polyps, secondary synchronous colon cancers were observed in 14.6%, while 12.4% developed metachronous invasive lesions. Such a high association between colonic polyps and colon cancer is another indication of the existence of the "neoplasm-prone colon." Copeland's study is important because patients who had familial syndromes or inflammatory bowel disease were not included in the case reviews.

CANCER FAMILY SYNDROME (CFS).—The first description of CFS is attributed to a 1913 report by Warthin. In this initial description, modest familial clusters of carcinoma of the uterus and gastrointestinal tract were described. Subsequently, the autosomal dominant inheritance of the site-specific *colorectal carcinoma* and *cancer family syndrome* was described in patients with colorectal carcinoma and female genital tumors. As the number of CFS reports enlarged and details of the clinical and pathologic evaluation of involved families were investigated more thoroughly, the following criteria for the syndrome were established: (1) a high frequency of adenocarcinoma of the colon, endometrium, and ovary. Carcinoma of the breast and stomach and lymphomas are additional components of the neoplastic spectrum; (2) a significant excess of proximal colonic involvement; (3) early age of cancer onset (mean = 45 years); (4) an excess of multiple primary neoplasms in affected subjects; (5) the infrequent occurrence of sebaceous adenomas, epitheliomas, and other carcinomas (Torre's syndrome); and (6) prolonged survival in cancer-prone patients.[14]

Clearly, an important mechanism operative for the development of colon cancer is the genetic predisposition for risk. Estimation of the risk for development of colonic carcinoma in the first-degree relatives of patients with CFS exceeds that of the general population.[15]

Although popular theses suggest that the development of colorectal neoplasms is influenced largely by environmental factors, the identity of such factors and their modes of action in carcinogenesis has not been forthcoming. Yet, inheritance is believed to play a less significant role in the overall genesis of the neoplasm than is environmental or otherwise undescribed biochemical processes. The association with neoplasms of other organs suggests that inherited factors may have a greater role in genesis than believed previously. For women, the probability of developing a *new primary* colorectal carcinoma is increased if the patient has had a previous colorectal carcinoma or polyps and cancer of the female genital tract, breast, or bladder. This relative increase in risk is also operative in male patients with a prior history of colorectal carcinoma, polyps, or bladder cancer. In persons with previous colorectal carcinoma the probability for developing a second (metachronous) lesion approaches three times that of the general population.[15, 16]

Management perspectives of the CFS are directed toward

TABLE 45–1.—FAMILIAL AND NONFAMILIAL POPULATIONS WITH INCREASED PREDISPOSITION (RISK) FOR CARCINOMA OF THE COLON AND RECTUM

Neoplastic polyposis
  Adenomas
    Tubular (adenomatous)—multiple > 2 cm
    Tubulovillous (mixed)—multiple
    Villous
  Familial adenomatous polyposis syndromes
    Familial polyposis coli
    Gardner's syndrome
    Oldfield syndrome
    Turcot's syndrome
    Muir's (Torre's) syndrome
  Nonfamilial polyposis syndromes
    Cronkhite-Canada syndrome
Cancer family syndromes
Familial site-specific colon cancer
Inflammatory bowel disease
Prior history of female genital/breast cancer
Prior history of colon/bladder cancer (both sexes)
Demographically increased risk of resident population
Immune deficiency states

TABLE 45–2.—NUMBER OF POLYPS CONCURRENT WITH CARCINOMA OF THE COLON

NO. OF POLYPS	SINGLE CANCER, No. (%) (n = 169)	CANCER IN VILLOUS ADENOMA, No. (%) (n = 20)	FOCAL CANCER IN ADENOMATOUS POLYP, No. (%) (n = 35)
1	98 (57.9)	15 (75)	18 (51.4)
2–5	63 (37.2)	5 (25)	16 (45.7)
>5	8 (4.9)	0	1 (2.9)

Courtesy of Copeland E.M., Jones R.S., Miller L.D.: Multiple colon neoplasms. *Arch. Surg.* 98:141, 1969. Copyright 1969, American Medical Association.

three distinct clinical settings: (1) appropriate screening of asymptomatic high-risk family members, (2) clinical management of diagnosed malignancies in family members, and (3) specific follow-up of cancer-affected family members.[12, 14] At present, no specific clinical feature, mechanism, immunologic, or biochemical precursor will identify a given patient harboring the genotype for the CFS. A detailed family history evaluation and geneology search will provide the clinician a mechanism to appropriately categorize high-risk family members. While the prognosis for the CFS patient is improved over that for sporadic forms of familial colonic cancer, appropriate cancer therapy directed at cure is mandatory. When a malignancy is diagnosed in kindred of the CFS, a complete evaluation is essential to rule out other synchronous tumors, e.g., other colonic, genitourinary and endometrial sites. Additionally, as these patients have a higher incidence of metachronous colonic lesions, the scope of the initial surgery should be extended to include a total abdominal colectomy with ileorectal anastomosis as the preferred procedure rather than standard radical hemicolectomy.[17] This approach appears to be preferable to total abdominal colectomy with proctectomy, as rectal carcinoma has *not* been observed with the CFS. However, the risk of endometrial and ovarian carcinomas are real, thus, total abdominal hysterectomy with bilateral salpingo-oophorectomy is advised at the time of colonic resection in medically suitable patients. Extended operations are not advisable when metastatic disease is encountered at exploration.

MECHANISMS OF CARCINOGENESIS.—While the preceding section supports the positive relationships of genetic influence in colonic carcinogenesis, environmental and dietary factors appear to be the major etiologic mechanism for carcinoma of this organ. The international variations are graphically depicted by Haenszel and Kurihara,[18] who observed much higher colonic cancer rates within the same generation of Japanese who immigrated to the United States. Also, offspring of immigrants from low-risk countries of Europe assume similar risk rates as U.S. whites. The Western diet, with its high fat and beef content, is implicated as a major etiologic factor. Mortality rates for colon and rectal carcinoma continue to escalate primarily due to increased incidence in previously low-risk countries. England and Scotland, considered high-risk population areas, are observing diminution in colon cancer mortality rates. Thus, alterations of environmental and/or dietary factors are being translated into a changing risk for this neoplasm.[19]

International studies suggest that large-bowel cancer risk has been primarily linked to dietary variation secondary to *economic development*. The evidence for this is as follows:

1. *Low fiber—refined carbohydrate diet.* Burkitt,[20] in his extensive studies of African subpopulations, developed the theory that highly refined carbohydrate dietary components associated with low-fiber intake are related to colonic carcinogenesis. Such diets reduce the bulk and volume of stool and decrease transit time in the gut. Burkitt postulates that the low-fiber diet allowed greater duration of contact and higher concentrations of carcinogens in foodstuffs to initiate carcinogenesis. While this theory is novel, additional variables including nondietary, environmental, and genetic must be included.

2. *Bile acids* and *promoters.* Biliary and cholesterol metabolites of bacterial digestion could be operative as "promoters" of carcinogenesis. Fecal bacteria containing 3-oxocholanoyl Δ 4-dehydrogenase and 7-hydroxycholanoyl dehydroxylase are capable of converting primary bile acids to a potential carcinogenic substance.[21] This latter compound may collaborate with both unsaturated and saturated bile acids to initiate mucosal malignant transformation.[22] Bile acid and neutral sterol fecal concentrations are altered by the ingestion of unsaturated fatty acids.[23]

3. *Concentrations of acid and neutral fecal sterol.* Individuals on high- and low-meat diets have great variations in the concentrations of fecal acid and neutral sterols. Patients with colonic carcinoma were observed to have much higher fecal bile-acid concentrations (82%) than control subjects (17%).[23] Presence of higher concentrations of sterols in stools was more common in patients with colon cancer than controls, as were higher concentrations of sterol conversion products (lithocholic and deoxycholic acid and cholesterol metabolites). It appears also that the activity of a 7-α-dehydroxylase, which initiates the conversion of cholic and chenodeoxycholic acid to deoxycholic and lithocholic acids, is greatest in patients with colonic cancer.[21, 22, 24] Acid sterol concentrations increase as a result of consumption of diet with a high concentration of unsaturated fat, typical of the diet of Britain and the United States. Fecal acid metabolites are lower in populations with a reduced risk of colon carcinoma, as is the ingestion of unsaturated fat.[25]

4. *Microbiotic floral alterations.* Additional epidemiologic data suggest that colorectal carcinoma is associated with variations of the intestinal flora and that these microorgansims are responsible for the synthesis of initiators and promoters of carcinogenesis. The substrate elements are probably derived from foodstuffs or from intestinal secretions such as bile acids. The composition of the diet may initiate alterations of the intestinal microflora and provide the substrates for the production of carcinogens.[25]

Perhaps all of the above etiologic mechanisms of cancer are correct and are synergistic with other, undefined mechanisms. Definitive proof that any given dietary factor is causally related to variations of the incidence of colon cancer has not been established.

Pathology

GROSS APPEARANCE.—Adenocarcinoma of the colon is the most frequent histologic type, accounting for over 95% of all cancers of this organ. Five variants of the gross appearance of adenocarcinoma of the colorectum are described:

1. *Ulcerative carcinoma.* This is the most frequent and is often associated with colonic obstruction. These lesions present with a raised, irregular, inverted edge and an ulcerated base. This variant is elongated in a transverse axis but rarely extends more than two quadrants of the bowel circumference (Fig 45–1). As the neoplasm infiltrates the bowel wall, deformity and progressive narrowing is evident. These lesions are most common in the left colon.

2. *Polypoid carcinoma.* This neoplasm is the second most frequent and presents as a cauliflower-like, fungating mass which projects into the bowel lumen. The protruding surface may be coarsely or finely nodular with segmented areas of

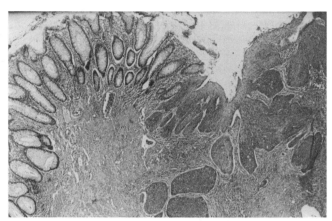

Fig 45–1.—Gross pathologic specimen of proximal and distal rectum with large (5.5-cm) ulcerative carcinoma. Patient presented with symptoms of partial obstruction and passage of bright blood per rectum. (Courtesy D.A. Franzini, M.D., Department of Pathology, University of Florida.)

ulceration (Fig 45–2). These lesions are typically well differentiated and have a prolonged doubling time. Their most common location is in the right colon, where obstruction may occur.

3. *Annular or scirrhous (stenosing) carcinoma.* This variant is less common than the aforementioned types and occurs most commonly in the sigmoid and rectum. It may extend into the long axis of the bowel and initiate a stenotic or circumferential growth, with the characteristic appearance of an anular ("applecore") configuration on barium enema (Fig

45–3). These lesions commonly present with partial or complete obstruction of the left colon.

4. *Infiltrating (linitis plastica) carcinoma.* These lesions are characteristically diffuse and transmurally infiltrate the intestinal wall for a variable length (5–8 cm). An intact mucosa may be visualized since this aggressive malignancy extends submucosally much like linitis plastica of the stomach.

5. *Colloid carcinoma.* This lesion is characterized by an abundance of mucus-laden cells, which initiate a bulky growth with a gelatinous appearance. Ulceration and infiltration may coexist with the colloid neoplasm.

HISTOLOGY.—The spectrum ranges from well-differentiated to highly anaplastic variants. The initial Dukes' histologic grading classification (1940) arbitrarily distinguished five microscopic features from the lowest (grade I) to the highest (grade VI) with regard to anaplasticity, glandular formation, and infiltration. An additional classification for colloid (mucoid) tumors has been added to correspond to that of Grinnell (1939), and thus several histologic grades are utilized today.

Adenocarcinoma of the large bowel may present with multiple variants; however, histologically this neoplasm resembles colonic epithelium with multilayering of columnar and cuboidal cells and attempted glandular differentiation (Fig 45–4). The ratio of epithelium to stroma varies with the gross pathologic appearance. An abundant stroma is apparent in

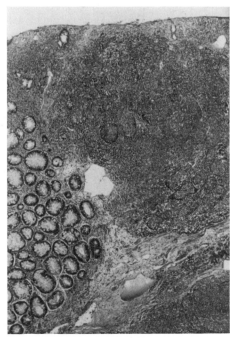

Fig 45–2.—Gross section of left colon wall with typical appearance of a polypoid carcinoma. This cauliflower-like, fungating lesion projects into the bowel lumen on a well-defined pedicle.

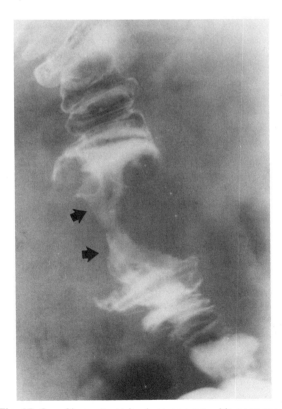

Fig 45–3.—Air-contrast barium enema with spot magnification view of anular (applecore) carcinoma in left transverse colon. Early obstructive symptoms were present in the patient secondary to this intermediate-grade obstruction. (Courtesy F. Clore, M.D., VA Medical Center, University of Florida.)

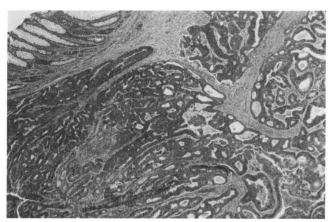

Fig 45–4.—Low-power (×40) view of typical microscopic appearance of adenocarcinoma of the colon. Transmural involvement of the colonic wall with nodal metastases (Dukes C) was apparent. Microscopic extension of well-differentiated neoplastic glands infiltrate the submucosa. (Courtesy D.A. Franzini, M.D., Department of Pathology, University of Florida.)

stenosing (annular) lesions but is scant in polypoid tumors.

Adenocarcinomas are classified as mucinous if over 60% of the surface area is occupied by mucus. *Signet-ring carcinoma,* a less frequent histologic variant, produces intracellular mucin with the resultant microscopic appearance of a signet ring and is associated with poor survival. *Epidermoid carcinoma* of the rectum takes origin from epithelium of the anoderm and occurs primarily at the anorectal junction. Less frequent histologic cell types can take origin from the epithelium of the transitional zone between squamous and columnar mucosa. These histologically distinct variants are classified according to the epithelium of origin, e.g., *transitional cell* or *cloacogenic.* Other rare lesions of the anorectum include basal cell carcinoma, basosquamous carcinoma of the perianal apocrine glands, and malignant melanoma.

ROUTES OF METASTASES.—Adenocarcinoma may disseminate via local, lymphatic, or hematogenous routes (Fig 45–5). Dukes formulated the concept that cancer of the rectum advanced locally by penetration of the bowel wall and noted that lymphatic metastases rarely occurred prior to penetration of the muscularis propria into perirectal tissues. Dukes also observed that the progression of lymphatic metastases was orderly and predictable for each echelon of lymph nodes in the epicolic, colic, para-aortic, and distant sites. The lymphatic drainage characteristically parallels the blood supply of the colon and rectum. Thus, the blood supply to the large bowel, i.e., the superior mesenteric artery, the inferior mesenteric artery, and the hypogastric (internal iliac) arteries, have corresponding lymphatic nodal drainage. The superior mesenteric artery gives rise to the right colic, ileocolic, and middle colic vessels. The corresponding left colon, sigmoid, and upper rectum are supplied via the left colic, sigmoidal and superior hemorrhoidal artery, all of which take origin from the inferior mesenteric artery. The hypogastric arteries supply the middle and distal rectum at the level of the lateral ligaments and the levator ani muscles via the middle and in-

terior hemorrhoidal vessels. The marginal artery of Drummond provides an anastomotic channel through which all vessels supplying the abdominal colon may communicate. It lies just beneath the colon wall in the mesentery.

Approximately one third of patients with carcinomas of the colon have clinical evidence of hematogenous metastases at the time of initial presentation. The most common site of visceral disease is the liver, accounted for by invasion of the tributaries of the portal vein. Hematogenous routes also account for the presentation of bony metastases to the vertebral bodies, often via Batson's plexus. Distant metastases may also occur to the lung, brain, and adrenal glands.

Intraperitoneal implantation may occur following exfoliation of tumor cells from a primary lesion that penetrates the serosa of the colon. Exfoliation of tumor cells within the bowel lumen represents the most important cause of anastomotic suture-line recurrences following colon resection. *Suture line recurrence* is most common in left colon lesions probably because of the more vigorous operative manipulation required prior to resection and anastomosis when compared to right colon cancer.[26] For this reason, tape ligatures should be placed around the colon proximal and distal to the cancer before manipulation is undertaken. Any exfoliated cells will then be removed with the specimen; none should be in the area of bowel prepared for anastomosis.

CLINICAL PRESENTATION.—When diagnosed, the majority of patients with adenocarcinoma of the colorectum are symptomatic. The presentation of carcinoma of this organ is dependent on: (1) the anatomical site of the tumor; (2) the gross morphological features of the neoplasm; and (3) the consistency of feces. A frequent complaint is change in bowel habits which is related to the growth characteristics and/or obstructive symptoms of large, bulky lesions. Patients may present with an irritable bowel syndrome and with gaseous complaints alternating with diarrhea or constipation. Complaints of colicky abdominal pain are common.

Table 45–3 documents the signs and symptoms of colorectal cancer relative to site of origin of the neoplasm. Typically, patients with carcinoma of the cecum or ascending colon present with an occult anemia, and approximately one third of anemic patients exhibit symptoms such as fatigability, weakness, lethargy, shortness of breath, or cardiac symptoms. An additional one fourth to one half of patients have documented weight loss. Diarrhea was observed in one quarter of rectosigmoid lesions, while it was present in only 16% of individuals with cecal cancer.[27]

The observation of grossly bloody stools occurred in 77% of rectal lesions and almost one half of the sigmoid lesions. This finding is the sine qua non of rectal carcinoma until proved to the contrary. In a series of patients reviewed by Copeland et al.,[27] 27% of patients with rectal cancer had had some form of treatment for hemorrhoids prior to the primary rectal neoplasm was recognized.

PHYSICAL EXAMINATION.—Physical findings may occupy a great spectrum, from absent to extensive, and are dependent on the stage, site, and nutritional status of the patient at presentation. The insidious presentation of anemia is common in the presence of right colon lesions and is detected by skin pallor and absence of color from mucous membranes. The ap-

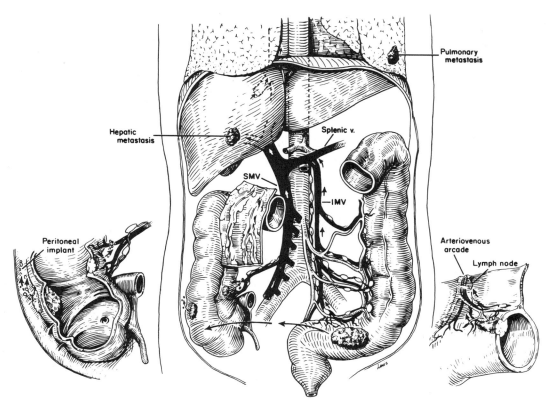

Fig 45–5.—Pathophysiologic mechanism of metastasis of colorectal neoplasms. Neoplastic cells of colonic mucosal origin transmurally invade the bowel wall to enter the lymphatic afferent or venous arcades. Subsequent tumor implantation in regional or distant sites is a function of the biologic parameters of the tissue of origin. Neoplastic cells may implant in regional lymphatics, liver, or distant sites (lung, bone, brain, etc.). Serosal and peritoneal metastases follow exfoliation of extramural neoplastic proliferation and deposition with neovascularization in remote sites. (From Bland K.I., in Fry D.E. (ed.): *Reoperation in Abdominal Surgery,* New York, Marcel Dekker. In press.)

pearance of jaundice, ascites, palpable hepatic metastases, and abdominal masses are ominous signs of advanced local, regional, and systemic disease. Metastases to the cul-de-sac may be palpated as a nodule(s) or firm mass (Bloomer's shelf) on rectal examination and follows direct extension or intraperitoneal implantation of the tumor. On occasion a rectovaginal

fistula may be the presenting complaint with vaginal discharge of feculent contents. Careful pelvic examination is advisable to evaluate involvement of the uterus, vagina, or adnexal structures. Also, extension of rectal cancer to the lateral pelvic side walls can often best be evaluated by vaginal examination.

TABLE 45–3.—SIGNS AND SYMPTOMS (%) OF COLONIC OR RECTAL CARCINOMA RELATIVE TO SITE OF ORIGIN*

SIGN	RECTUM	RECTOSIGMOID	SIGMOID	DESCENDING COLON	SPLENIC FLEXURE	TRANSVERSE COLON	HEPATIC FLEXURE	ASCENDING COLON	CECUM
Patients in series, no.	432	79	253	74	39	59	32	58	55
Asymptomatic	5.3	2.5	4.4	0	2.6	5.1	9.4	0	1.8
Abdominal pain	24.4	45.6	60.5	77.0	77.0	74.5	78.0	76.0	54.5
Anemia	22.2	22.8	21.3	27.0	33.3	35.6	31.2	77.8	74.6
Weight Loss	36.0	30.4	28.8	28.4	38.5	40.5	40.5	40.0	47.4
Change in bowel habits	45.5	49.5	48.0	55.5	38.5	34.0	34.4	19.0	18.0
Diarrhea	16.3	25.4	12.7	4.0	11.0	6.8	9.4	13.8	16.4
Blood in stool	77.2	73.5	48.5	33.8	36.0	29.0	22.0	25.5	23.6
Hemorrhoids	27.4	10.1	5.5	8.1	2.5	3.4	3.1	1.7	0
Abdominal mass	4.2	15.2	24.2	32.5	18.0	37.4	44.0	62.0	58.0
Rectal mass	65.6	28.0	7.9	0	0	0	0	0	0
Obstruction	2.3	10.1	17.0	28.4	41.0	29.0	12.5	13.8	16.4
Appendicitis	0.5	1.3	0.8	1.4	5.1	0	6.2	3.5	5.5

*From unpublished observations, Copeland E.M., Miller L.B., Jones R.S., in Sleisenger M.H., Fordtran J.S. (eds.): Gastrointestinal Disease: Pathophysiology, Diagnosis and management. Philadelphia, W.B. Saunders, 1978, p. 1787.

Diagnosis of Colorectal Carcinoma

The identification of groups at high risk for colorectal carcinoma necessitates appropriate screening measures. Success with the Hemoccult test (Smith-Kline Diagnostics) is attributed to its sensitivity. However, nearly as many adenomas are undetected by the fecal occult blood testing as are identified by it, and approximately 20% of colon cancers are not detected when individuals completing the Hemoccult test undergo proctoscopy or fiberoptic sigmoidoscopy. While the most reports favor continuing the fecal Hemoccult test, Winawer et al.[28] noted that only 50% of neoplasms of the colon were detected by Hemoccult testing. The false positive rate of this screening tool is fortunately quite low, 0.5%. It should not replace digital and endoscopic evaluations, but can be used as a first stage of screening: when positive, further workup is required.

Physical examination should be the initial part of the evaluation process for patients with colorectal cancer, and should include pelvic examination in women. Patients should have a complete blood hemogram and serum chemistries. The laboratory tests currently applied to detect hepatic metastases include measurement of serum alkaline phosphatase, 5'-nucleotidase, SGGT, lactic dehydrogenase (LDH), SGOT, SGPT, bilirubin, and leucine aminopeptidase. Carcinoembryonic antigen (CEA) has value as an early biologic marker of colorectal malignancy of all stages, and increasing serum values may parallel tumor burden. LDH was found by Ranson et al.[29] to be the most sensitive laboratory test for the presence of hepatic metastases. LDH was elevated in 81% of patients with occult metastases and in 80% with palpable metastatic disease. The role of CEA as a diagnostic and monitoring parameter of recurrent disease will be dicussed subsequently. Additionally, all patients should have routine chest radiograph (PA and lateral views) to evaluate the pulmonary interstitium for metastatic and/or concurrent disease. Evaluation of equivocal metastatic pulmonary disease on routine chest x-ray may be resolved with whole lung tomography or computed tomography (CT). CT is also of value to assess hepatic or locoregional extension of disease recognized with serum enzyme, CEA, or other chemical abnormalities.

The digital rectal examination and sigmoidoscopy are prerequisites for evaluating any symptomatic patient. Digital examination can be confusing in the presence of fissures, fistulas, hypertrophic papillae, and hemorrhoids. Approximately 60% of patients have large-bowel neoplasms within reach of the conventional 25-cm sigmoidoscope. While the trend to more proximal colonic neoplasms continues, the addition of the 60-cm flexible fiberoptic sigmoidoscopy to the diagnostic armamentarium allows visual examination of the entire rectum and sigmoid colon. Channels within this instrument allow biopsy and polypectomy when indicated. An electrocautery unit is also available to secure hemostasis. Large polypoid or ulcerative lesions that present in the rectum are best biopsied via the conventional sigmoidoscope. Smaller polypoid or sessile lesions can be extricated using cautery snare. The complications of conventional or fiberoptic sigmoidoscopic biopsy include bowel perforation, active hemorrhage, and infrequent explosion of flammable methane/nitrogen bowel gases.

Routine plain abdominal films in a flat and upright projec-

tion have special merit for evaluation of intestinal obstruction. Usually, these roentgenograms permit differentiation of small-bowel vs. colonic intestinal obstruction. Diagnosing anatomical obstruction, however, may require a barium enema. In patients presenting with partial or nearly complete colonic obstruction, care must be exercised in the filling of the dilated proximal colon with barium, for a complete obstruction can be precipitated. Except patients with obstructing lesions, barium enema should be performed to detect synchronous mucosal primary neoplasms. When obstruction is suspected, Gastrografin (Squibb) should be instilled initially into the colon. The quality of the films is not of the quality produced with barium, but the chance of precipitating a complete obstruction is much less.

Roentgenographic detection of a colonic primary is suggested by repeated demonstration of an intraluminal radiolucent mass on fluoroscopic examination of the barium column. Typical radiographic stigmas of colorectal carcinoma include the appearance of an anular (applecore) lesion (Fig 45–6), distortion of the muscosal pattern, incomplete filling of the lumen, rigidity, and segmental defects with or without the presence of obstruction. The confirmation of these findings is best made by multiple projections of the barium-filled colon at different angles.

While diagnostic accuracy of barium enema examination is excellent, exceptions occur at the extreme ends of the large bowel, e.g., the cecum, ileocecal valve, and anorectum. A low-lying rectal lesion may be obscured by the rectal balloon that is inflated to secure the contrast dye. This reinforces the necessity of careful digital and sigmoidoscopic examination of the distal colon and rectum. Determination of normalcy of the

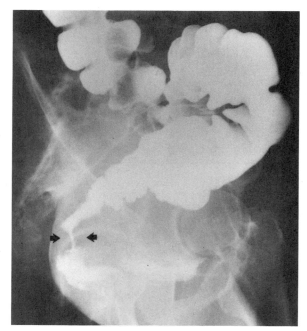

Fig 45–6.—Typical barium enema oblique projection for extensive carcinoma of the proximal and mid-rectum. *Arrows* denote the circumferential anular stenotic lesion with high-grade obstruction. Dilated proximal colon is identifiable. (Courtesy F. Clore, M.D., VA Medical Center, University of Florida.)

ileocecal valve and cecum may be difficult, as filling is often incomplete in this portion of the organ. Further, previous surgical procedures (appendectomy, adnexal procedures, etc.) may produce radiographic distortions of the cecum or terminal ileum and make adequate roentgenographic interpretation impossible.

The air-contrast barium study with a dual column increases the sensitivity above that of the single-column roentgenogram. Colonoscopy is indicated to provide confirmation of the x-ray findings and to evaluate possible synchronous lesions, especially when the barium column cannot be advanced proximal to a partially obstructed primary lesion. Colonoscopy should be avoided in the presence of near-complete obstructive lesions of the left colon, as the risk of perforation and peritoneal contamination exceeds the potential value of the procedure.

Luminal lavage cytology does not appear to increase the yield above that of conventional sigmoidoscopic or endoscopic biopsy. Additionally, lavage and brush cytology are often difficult to interpret because of the large number of exfoliated nonviable cells. Lavage cytology appears to have value to evaluate multiple polypoid lesions of the colon in the absence of local neoplastic lesions or in the course of surveillance of inflammatory bowel disease.[28]

The fiberoptic colonoscope provides direct visual inspection of the entire colon. This instrument should be considered a noncompetitive complement to air-contrast barium enema examinations. Colonoscopy is useful to detect mucosal and submucosal lesions not identified radiographically, and histologic documentation of the disease process may be obtained. The value of this instrument in follow-up of high-risk individuals with polyposis, colonic strictures, and inflammatory bowel disease represents a major advancement.[30]

Due to the proximity of the genitourinary tract to the colon and rectum, an IVP is advisable to define the anatomical variations of the ureters in the pelvis and their relationship to the descending colon, sigmoid, and rectum. Patients with hematuria, frequency, or other micturition dysfunction should have cystography and possibly cystoscopy to identify bladder invasion by the colon neoplasm. Segmental involvement of the wall of the bladder should be identified preoperatively to plan en bloc resections with the colon and cystoureteral reconstructions. Invasion of the trigone of the bladder may require concomitant cystectomy and total urinary diversion.

Liver metastases result in progressive hepatomegaly. Extensive hepatic involvement produces chronic pain from distention of the liver capsule and eventual compromise of hepatic function producing hepatic failure, ascites, and coma. Synchronous hepatic metastases are found in 10%–30% of patients at the time of laparotomy for resection of their primary neoplasm. Computed tomography has many of the same limitations as technetium liver scans with an overall concordance of x-ray findings with the surgical results in 85% and 81%, respectively. The false positive rate for hepatic metastases approaches 5% for CT and 6% for liver scan[31] when both procedures are done and evaluated by experts.

Staging

Currently, no universally accepted system exists for staging of colorectal carcinoma. The majority of current staging methods represent modifications of the 1932 Dukes classification, which was initially based on the clinical classification of Lockhart-Mummery. Despite its modification, the Dukes classification represents a practical, anatomical, clinical staging system. This system divides adenocarcinoma of the colon and the rectum into three stages: (A) limitation of the neoplasm to the colonic or rectal mucosa; (B) extension of the neoplasm direct continuity into extrarectal tissues with absence of lymph gland metastases; and (C) metastases to regional lymphatics. In the report by Dukes and Bussey,[32] the five-year survival rates differed significantly among the aforementioned staging groups. Survival rate in stage A was 81.2%, stage B, 64.0%, and stage C, 27.4%. Despite the rigidity and simplicity of the original Dukes classification, it remains a very practical staging classification system. However, the multifactorial relationships of prognostic variables on end result classification and prognosis have obvious limitations. Thus, a system based purely on transmural penetration and regional lymphatic involvement has undergone revision with reclassification by the TNM system.

The TNM system which attempts to bring together a great number of variables that have impact on survival has been supported by the UICC and the American Joint Committee for Cancer Staging and End-Result Reporting (Table 45–4). Still, the Astler-Coller (1954) modification of the Kirklin et al. (1949) classification is the most commonly employed staging of colorectal lesions. Significant variations of the Astler-Coller with the original Dukes classification were that C_1 and C_2 subdivisions were made to separate tumors with lesser or greater penetration of the bowel wall. Subsequently, Dukes[7] C_1 and C_2 subdivisions were made to distinguish tumors with greater and lesser lymphatic involvement (Fig 45–7). While there may be important reasons for adoption of a uniform system such as the TNM system, especially in a research setting, the general acceptance of the Dukes system is so widespread and simplistic that its abandonment for the TNM system may be ill-advised. Another system, the DNMG (depth, nodes, metastases, grade) system, has been proposed (1980) in an effort to address additional prognostic variables which affect the prognosis for cancer of this organ.

THERAPY OF CARCINOMA OF THE COLON AND RECTUM.—Adequate preoperative staging should be completed by radiography, CT, and/or photoscanning. The majority of patients will have established histologic diagnosis prior to the planned therapy; however, surgical intervention may be necessary on the basis of history and clinical and radiographic findings (e.g., obstruction, perforation).

For elective procedures, dehydration, hypoproteinemia, and anemia should be corrected preoperatively. Appropriate medical evaluation of compromised organ systems (cardiovascular, pulmonary, renal, hepatic) will avoid unnecessary morbidity and mortality. Mechanical reduction of the endogenous bacterial flora with cathartics and saline enemas is a prerequisite to reduction of wound morbidity and potential mortality. Classically, enemas and cathartics (castor oil, magnesium citrate, bisacodyl) have been given for two-three days preoperatively. A 24-hour preparation of the bowel using hypertonic cathartics (e.g., mannitol) is gaining popularity. Oral nonabsorbable antibiotics utilizing neomycin and erythromycin base or kanamycin over a period of 24–36 hours preoperatively appears to be of benefit to further diminish wound

TABLE 45–4.—STAGING SYSTEMS FOR CARCINOMA OF THE COLORECTUM

AJCC 1982*	UICC† 1978 (3rd ed)	DUKES (1932, 1935)‡	ASTLER-COLLER§
Stage 0	Stage 0		Stage 0
Carcinoma in situ			
Tis N_0 M_0	Tis, N_0, M_0		0
Stage I	Stage I	A	Stage I
IA Tumor confined to mucosa or submucosa	1A		
T_1, N_0, M_0			
IB Tumor involves muscularis propria but not beyond	T_1, N_0, M_0 1B	A	A
T_2, N_0, M_0	T_2, N_0, M_0	A	B1
Stage II	Stage II		Stage II
Involvement of all layers of bowel wall with or without invasion of immediately adjacent structures T_3, N_0, M_0	T_3, T_4, N_0, M_0 (T_{3a} with fistula) (T_{3b} without fistula)		B2
Stage III	Stage III	C (1932)	Stage III
Any degree of bowel wall with regional node metastasis	Any T, N_1, M_0	C_1 (1935) C_2 (1935)	C_1 C_2
Any T, N_1–N_3, M_0			
Extends beyond contiguous tissue or immediately adjacent organs with no regional lymph node metastasis			
T_4, N_0, M_0			
Stage IV	Stage IV	Type 4	Stage IV
Any invasion of bowel wall or without regional lymph node metastasis but with evidence of distant metastasis	Any T, any N, M_1	(so-called D)	D
Any T, any N, M_1			

*American Joint Committee on Cancer, in Beahrs O.H., Myers M.H.: *Manual for Staging of Cancer*, ed. 2. Philadelphia, J.B., Lippincott Co., 1983.
†UICC-Union International Contre le Cancer.
‡Dukes: A = limited to bowel wall; B = spread to extramural tissue; C = involvement of regional nodes (C_1: near primary lesion; C_2: proximal node involved at point of ligation); type 4 (so-called D) = distant metastasis.
§Astler-Coller: A = limited to mucosa; B_1 = Same as AJCC stage IB (T_{2b}); B2 = same as AJCC Stage IB (T_{2a}); C_1 = limited to wall with involved nodes; C_2 = through all layers of wall with involved nodes. Spratt J.S.: *Neoplasms of the Colon, Rectum, and Anus.* Philadelphia, W.B. Saunders, 1984.

infection rate by reducing colonic bacterial flora. More recently, perioperative and immediate postoperative systemic antibiotic agents (second/third-generation cephalosporins) have been shown to be of similar value. Preoperative antibiotic therapy is indicated in both *elective* and *emergent* circumstances necessitating colorectal resections.

Emergency operations for perforation or obstruction (complete or partial) necessitate prompt intervention to obviate progressive peritoneal contamination with its ominous consequences. Nichols et al.[33] indicated that the entire spectrum of peritonitis, from overwhelming sepsis to resolution with an abscess, is a dose-related phenomenon and correlates directly with the total number of pathogenic bacteria introduced into the peritoneum. Further, experimental evidence suggests that mixed fecal flora, which is found in peritonitis, acts synergistically to enhance total bacterial virulence. Appropriate resuscitation with replacement of fluid, electrolyte, and blood product deficits represent *a priori* management to reduce the significant mortality from perforation or obstruction.

TECHNIQUE.—Surgical resection of the involved colorectal segment is the most effective form of therapy. Modern concepts to ensure a curative procedure include an *en bloc* removal of: (1) the malignant neoplasm and contiguous colonic segments in the distribution of the major arterial and venous supply, (2) resection in continuity with the primary lymphatic drainage of the colonic segment, (3) mechanical and technical attempts to reduce local implantation and venous embolization. Original support for radical lymphadenectomy and the "no-touch" technique by Turnbull and colleagues[34] demonstrated a five-year survival rate for Dukes C lesions of 58%, compared with 28% for historical controls treated with "conventional" operative principles. This technical maneuver provided control of possible metastases by ligation of the lymphovascular mesenteric supply *prior* to operative manipulation of the involved colonic segment. Subsequently, Stearns[35] has emphasized that results for comparable stages of disease are identical to those of Turnbull et al.[34] in a group of patients in whom the "no-touch" technique was not applied. Rather, extent of the operative procedure done by Stearns was designed and initiated on the basis of origin and distribution of regional blood supply. These concepts have subsequently been confirmed by others.[36] Stearns' data confirm the hypothesis that survival advantage is related primarily to the radical, anatomical resection and lymphadenectomy which encompasses the origins of the arterial blood supply to the involved segments

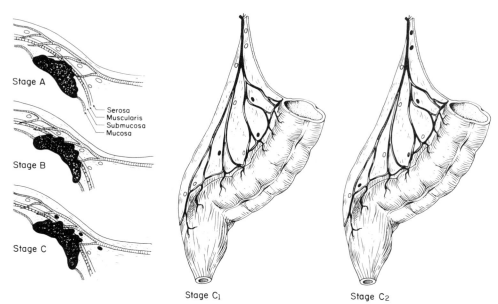

Fig 45–7.—Modified Dukes' classification (1932) for carcinoma of the colorectum with correlation of pathologic stage of disease: *Stage A,* carcinoma limited to wall of rectum, no extension to extrarectal tissue, no nodal metastases. *Stage B,* carcinoma extension by continuity to extrarectal tissues, no nodal metastases. *Stage C,* transmural colonic extension of carcinoma with positive regional lymphatics. Dukes and Bussey (1935) enlarged the A, B, C classification to include extent of lymphatic mestastases: C_1, lymphatic involvement with extension which has not reached glands at the highest point of ligature of blood vessels. C_2, positive lymphatics, glandular spread to highest point of ligature. Five-year survival was 40.9% for C_1 lesions and 13.6% for C_2 lesions. Dukes C_1 and C_2 are to be differentiated from Kirklin et al. and Astler-Coller subdivisions which separate tumors with lesser or greater penetration of the bowel wall. (From Dukes C.E., Bussey H.J.R.: *Br. J. Cancer* 12:309, 1958. Used by permission.)

of the intestine. Further, similar radical efforts for rectal carcinoma has reduced the incidence of local recurrence.

For *adenocarcinomas of the veriform appendix, cecum, ascending colon, hepatic flexure,* and *right transverse colon,* a *right hemicolectomy* is indicated. Proper radical resection of the mesentery as noted above is essential and necessitates ligation of the vasculature as near the origin of the aorta as possible. While the "no-touch" technique has not shown benefit in critical analysis by Stearns,[35] the authors continue to employ isolation and ligation of the lymphaticovascular supply and manipulation of the involved neoplastic process only after this maneuver is accomplished. Ligatures placed proximal and distal to the neoplasm also appear advisable to avoid intraluminal exfoliation of neoplastic cells and potential suture line recurrences. Intestinal continuity is reestablished by end-to-end or end-to-side ileotransverse colostomy. Anastomosis may be constructed by two-layer suture technique or by stapling methods.

Neoplasms of the *midtransverse colon* are best resected with adequate mesentery to ensure resection of the entire transverse colon and the distal ascending colon and proximal descending colon. This resection necessitates the section of the middle colic artery and the terminal branches of the right colic artery. The left colon is supplied solely by the marginal artery of Drummond from the left colic artery. Many surgeons have begun treating lesions of the transverse colon by complete resection of the right, transverse, and descending colon with ileosigmoid anastomosis. The functional result is similar to the more limited resection, and the possibility of

anastomotic breakdown is less. Blood supply to the anastomosed ends of the bowel is unaffected as is the quality of the tissue to be approximated. A classical *left colectomy* is appropriate for tumors of the *left transverse colon,* the *splenic flexure, proximal descending colon,* and *upper sigmoid.*

Anterior resections are reserved for neoplasms of the distal sigmoid and upper rectum (6–11 cm). As resection margins should be a minimal of 5 cm beyond the distal leading edge of the tumor, lesions of the rectum with lesser marginal clearance above the levator sling will require an abdominoperineal resection (APR) and permanent end-sigmoid colostomy. In similarly matched patients with carcinomas of the rectum at 6–7 cm above the dentate line, no survival advantage of APR appears evident over the lower anterior resection (55% vs. 51%, respectively).[37] Thus, in some patients, permanent colostomy can be avoided and low anterior resection done when the cancer is in this area of the rectum. Factors to be considered when selecting APR vs. lower anterior resection include the curative or palliative intent of the procedure, contiguous organ involvement, tumor size and configuration, tumor fixation, and pelvic configuration. The possibility of cure should not be sacrificed in favor of maintaining the anal sphincter.

At the time of the operative procedure and definitive colonic resection, thorough exploration of the abdominal cavity is essential to document metastatic spread. Examination of periaortic lymphatics, peritoneum, small-bowel and large-bowel serosa, and the liver are important to confirm the absence or presence of metastatic disease. The liver should be carefully palpated and inspected to determine the presence of synchronous hepatic metastases that must be resected, if technically feasible, and, when minimal operative morbidity and mortality can be ensured. The large bowel should be carefully palpated to detect the presence of second primary colonic lesions. Consideration should be given for total abdominal colectomy with ileoproctectomy in the individual with synchronous colonic cancers or the presence of confirmed colonic cancer and associated multiple tubular or villous polyps.

The presence of extracolonic tumor in patients with colorectal cancer is often determined by preoperative roentgenographic or biochemical studies. When metastases were not suspected preoperatively, they were found by Silverberg et al.[1] to be localized in 44% of patients, regional in 26%, and metastatic in 25% at the time of surgical exploration. Despite the presence of extracolonic neoplasm, patients should always be considered candidates for *palliative colonic resection* to obviate the inevitable consequences of obstruction, perforation, and hemorrhage.

When colonic resection *cannot* be done with *curative intent*, adequate surgical resection and anastomosis or proximal diversion of the fecal stream is necessary. Temporary proximal decompressing colostomy is advisable for insecure anastomoses. In the presence of extensive *intra-abdominal carcinomatosis*, proximal diverting end colostomy with or without resection is indicated.

Carcinoma of the large bowel is the most common etiology for obstruction of this organ. The presentation of *colonic obstruction* requires prompt surgical intervention to avoid perforation. Following resuscitation of fluid, electrolyte, and blood product deficits and the administration of systemic antibiotics, operation is directed to relieve the obstruction by resection or fecal diversion. Upper intestinal decompression by intubation is accomplished as expeditiously as possible, but it must not delay operation. For lesions obstructing the *right colon*, immediate right hemicolectomy with restoration of intestinal continuity as an ileotransverse colostomy is appropriate in most patients. For distal *transverse* and *left colonic* obstructive lesions, resection of the lesion and construction of an end-colostomy and mucous fistulas with the two cut ends of the bowel is optimal treatment in the stable patient. No attempt to anastomose an unprepared bowel should be done, for obstructing lesions distal to the right transverse colon for medically-unstable patients or when a proper oncologic operation cannot be done, a proximal diverting colostomy is indicated. For emergent obstructive *rectosigmoid* and *rectal* cancers, the presence of extensive local and/or regional extension of pericolonic disease usually requires a diverting proximal colostomy, since resectability is either questionable or impossible. Should resection be possible and the distal segment too short to exteriorize as a mucous fistula, a *Hartmann pouch* is fashioned with closure of the distal segment by suture or staple technique. Mucus and blood that collect in this segment are easily evacuated via the anus. The distal segment should never be closed if the obstructing lesion remains intact, for proximal closure of this segment with a retained obstructing lesion distally produces a closed-loop obstruction destined to rupture. Most patients with rectal obstruction will require postoperative radiotherapy before an attempt is initiated to resect the primary lesion. APR or anterior resection should be done, if possible, however, for irradiation alone rarely achieves satisfactory palliation. Determination of advanced local/regional disease, in the absence of distant metastases, justifies an exenterative procedure.

Colonic perforations necessitate emergent surgical control of the site of peritoneal soilage to obviate the inevitable mortality associated with this condition. *Perforations of the cecum* occur at or just proximal to obstructing lesions of the right colon.[38] Therapy for perforations of the *right colon* includes resection, temporary ileostomy, and mucous fistula. Thorough debridement and irrigation, systemic antibiotics, and extensive drainage are requisite for prudent management. Annular infiltrative lesions of the *left colon* or *rectosigmoid* may perforate locally with adjacent abscess formation. Localized perforation with fecal and bacterial contamination initiates less physiologic derangements than free perforations with continual soilage of the peritoneum. The cecum is the most common site of perforation of a closed-loop obstruction that occurs as a result of a competent ileocecal valve proximally and an obstructing colon cancer distally.

Interval resection of the primary cancer with establishment of colonic continuity is advised in medically unstable patients. Initial management should only be proximal diverting colostomy. In stable patients, locally contained perforations of the *left colon* may be primarily resected with the establishment of proximal colostomy diversion, distal mucosa fistula, and drainage of the abscess. When the perforative lesion is low in the pelvis, a proximal end-sigmoid colostomy and mucous fistula are performed. Interval anterior resection or APR should be done if anatomically possible, since selected subsets of patients achieve long-term survival and/or more satisfactory palliation from this aggressive approach. *Radiotherapy* may provide palliation for patients with advanced regional pelvic disease and/or distant metastases who are *not* considered candidates for staged resections of the rectosigmoid lesion after diversion of the fecal stream, drainage of the perforation, and resolution of the inflammatory process.

EXTENDED RESECTIONS FOR SELECTED CARCINOMAS.—Spratt and Spjut[39] recognized that only 46% of all *resectable* carcinomas metastasize to lymphatics regardless of size of the primary lesion (54% are a nonmetastasizing biologic variant). Polk et al.[40] have emphasized that tumor size, unlike breast carcinoma, is not a determinant of regional metastases for colorectal carcinoma. These seemingly advanced neoplasms often have invaded contiguous organs; however, their favorable biologic characteristics dictate a therapeutic approach that includes mobilization of contiguous organs to achieve adequate *en bloc* resection. In the absence of metastases, this extended technique for patients with extensive local and regional disease allowed Polk[41] to achieve a tumor-free survival rate of 42% (mean = 25 months). Objective improvement in quality of life was obtained for individuals who ultimately died of their colonic carcinoma. Extended resections for colon carcinomas which invade contiguous organs are indicated in 6%–19% (mean = 12%) of cases and can be done expeditiously; morbidity and mortality rates are acceptable.[41–43] Several organs may require partial removal or extirpation, and such procedures should not be undertaken unless reconstruction can be achieved. Lysis of adhesions to adjacent organs, whether neoplastic or inflammatory, is to be discouraged. If tumor spillage occurs, recurrence is inevitable except when principles of *en bloc* resection are followed.

A variant of the extended procedure is *total colectomy*. This procedure is often advocated as a measure to extirpate colonic mucosa which may generate subsequent malignant lesions (e.g., villous, tubular, tubulovillous polyps) and for purposes of resecting synchronous primary neoplasms. Previous data[43] suggest that patients cured of a first colonic tumor and followed up for more than 25 years have a 32% chance of developing a metachronous colonic cancer. Additionally, this study suggested that operative mortality for colonic resection was unrelated to the length (> 7 cm) of the intestinal resection ($P = 0.9$), multiple organ resections ($P = 0.9$), or the maximal cordal dimension of the tumor ($P > 0.9$). Positive and negative correlates for factors which effect operative mortality for carcinoma of the colon and the rectum after extended procedures are summarized in Table 45–5.[43, 44]

Prognostic Factors for Carcinoma of the Colon and Rectum

Copeland and associates[45] evaluated 1,084 patients with carcinoma of the colon and rectum, of which 826 (76.4%) were estimated to be cured by the operative procedure. Palliative resections were done in 186 patients (17.1%), of whom one half died within the first 12 postoperative months and 87% died within 36 months. Anatomical site of the neoplasm served as a guide to survival. Lesions of the rectosigmoid and rectum had a poorer prognosis than more proximal lesions. The five-year survival for all patients was 37.3%. These authors confirmed that the presentation of an obstructing carcinoma, venous invasion, and degree of tumor differentiation were important prognostic determinants for survival when the local margin of resection was ≤ 5 cm. Further, the number of lymph node metastases was related prognostically to survival. In the absence of regional lymphatic involvement, 51.5% had five-year survival, whereas involvement with one to four nodes was associated with an approximate 25% survival. When ≥ 5 lymph node metastases were detected, the

TABLE 45–5.—FACTORS AFFECTING OPERATIVE MORTALITY FOR CARCINOMA OF THE COLON AND RECTUM WHICH INFLUENCE EFFORTS AFTER EXTENDED PROCEDURES

NEGATIVE CORRELATION	P VALUE	POSITIVE CORRELATION	P VALUE
Tumor diameter > 7 cm	$>.900$	Lymph nodes resected, ≤ 10	.009
Length of intestine resected	.900	Resection for palliation	.009
Multiple organ resections	.900	Heart disease requiring digitals	.015
Antimicrobial intestinal preparation	.350	Age > 69 yr	.019
Lymph node metastases	.325	Presence of inflammatory mass	.029
Intestinal obstruction	.153		
Associated colonic disease (diverticular disease)	.076		

Adapted from Bland K.I., Polk H.C. Jr.: The curative and palliative control of colorectal carcinoma, in Nyhus L.M. (ed.): *Surgery Annual*, New York, Appleton-Century-Crofts, vol. 15, p. 127, 1983.

five-year survival declined to 10.0% (Table 45–6). The depth of penetration of the bowel wall, with or without nodal spread as delineated by an Astler-Coller classification was integrally related to prognosis (Table 45–7). Extension of an invasive tumor was most frequent through the muscular wall of the colon (379 cases). Patients in this category had a five-year survival of 43% in the absence of nodal involvement and 15% when nodal metastases were present. Bowel penetration alone was an important prognostic determinant. Tumors penetrating into, but not through, the muscularis had a 65% five-year survival compared to 43% survival when the entire muscular coat was invaded. Because of the method by which patients die, five-year survival figures for colon cancer differ among large series. In Copeland's series, patients dying with and without cancer are included in the survival statistics; thus, the determinant five-year survival for all other categories are less than those in other reports.

DELAY IN DIAGNOSIS.—Several investigators have suggested that patients with acute onset of symptoms necessitating emergency therapy have a poor prognosis. Data to support this contention were presented by Devlin et al.,[46] who confirmed that individuals who present early with symptoms represented a subset of patients with a poor prognosis. Of 61 patients with colicky abdominal pain, 36 (59%) presented with acute obstruction and the ominous prognosis that follows near-circumferential involvement of the bowel lumen. An association between short duration of symptoms and high histologic grade of the tumor was noted. In a study of 200 patients with colon and rectal cancer, Rowe-Jones and Aylett,[47] found a statistically significant increased proportion of Dukes C lesions for a subset of individuals in whom diagnosis was delayed. Only two (0.5%) of the patients presented with intestinal obstruction. This study emphasized that the effect of medically related delay (nonpatient-related) was important in diminishing prognosis. It appears that patients who attach little significance to their symptoms (rectal bleeding or anemia) have biologically more favorable lesions. Conversely, patients who seek help early because of advanced symptomatology often have aggressive tumors. Thus, Rowe-Jones and Aylett suggest a relationship between medically-induced *delay of diagnosis* and *stage of disease*. An important distinction is apparent between delay in diagnosis for patient subsets with poor prognosis who *must* seek medical services early because of symptomatic lesions and for those individuals who have *diagnostic delay* for (physician) medically induced reasons. One must consider delay in diagnosis important, as these patients fail to benefit from the potential advantages of early curative and noncurative colonic resections. It is this subset which necessitates a greater number of *emergency resections* and *fecal diversions*. Also, it is this subset that sustains an increased morbidity and mortality related to the stage of presentation.[47]

COLON AND RECTAL OBSTRUCTION.—Obstructive colorectal carcinoma portends a poor prognosis. In an exhaustive review, Sugarbaker[48] confirmed that approximately 50% of patients are not candidates for potentially curative operations because of distant metastases found at the time of exploratory laparotomy. Operation was uniformly accompanied by high morbidity and mortality (11%–39%). Surgical complications were observed in one third to one half of the patients. Five-

TABLE 45–6.—CORRELATION OF REGIONAL NODAL INVOLVEMENT AND FIVE-YEAR SURVIVAL
OF PATIENTS WITH CARCINOMA OF THE COLON, %

STATUS	NO NODES INVOLVED (n = 584)	ONE NODE INVOLVED (n = 112)	TWO NODES INVOLVED (n = 68)	THREE NODES INVOLVED (n = 40)	FOUR NODES INVOLVED (n = 24)	FIVE OR MORE NODES INVOLVED (n = 110)
Alive with no carcinoma	48.5	26.8	25.0	15.0	29.1	9.1
Alive with carcinoma	3.0	3.5	2.9	2.5	4.2	0.9
Dead with no carcinoma	17.6	6.2	5.9	2.5	4.2	4.5
Dead with carcinoma	31.9	63.5	66.2	80.0	62.5	85.5

Copeland E.M., Miller L.D., Jones R.S.: Prognostic factors in carcinoma of the colon and rectum. *Am. J. Surg.* 116:875, 1968.

year survival following surgery with curative intent rarely exceeded 30%. Ragland et al.[49] observed that obstructive lesions had a reduction in five-year survival (58.8%) even when lymph nodes were negative. When one to five positive nodes were resected in the surgical specimen, five-year survival diminished to 16.7%. No survivors with $\geq$ 6 positive lymph nodes were observed.

PERFORATION.—Glenn and McSherry[50] reported that 99 of 1,815 patients (5.5%) with colorectal carcinoma presented with perforations. For 41% of the patients in this series, the perforation was free with gross peritoneal soilage. Of these patients, a curative operative procedure was done in 66% with a mortality of 19.2%, whereas 33% had palliative procedures with a mortality of 27.3%. Patients with free perforation of the carcinoma with peritoneal soilage had a five-year survival of 7.3%. Conversely, the five-year survival for 58 patients with localized perforations was 41.4%. In an analysis of 70 patients with perforative cancer, Miller and associates[38] noted a similar five-year survival rate (14%) for patients presenting with free perforations. In a review of five surgical series, Sugarbaker[48] reported hospital mortality for 20%–74% (median 43%) in 176 patients with free colonic perforations. In this review of 8,252 patients, 232 (2.8%) had localized perforations. Overall, five-year survival was two- to six-fold greater in subjects who presented with localized perforation compared with free perforations and subsequent peritoneal soilage. The ominous prognosis of a perforative carcinoma following operation with curative intent allows a five-year survival that approximates 30%.

Age at Diagnosis

ELDERLY POPULATION.—The presumption that advancing age portends an ominous prognosis for adenocarcinoma of the large bowel and rectum has not been substantiated. Jensen et al.,[51] in a study of patients $\geq$ 70 years of age, reported an operative mortality of 13%. Overall five-year survival was 37%. Patients > 70 years of age had a 69.2% $\pm$ 7.0 five-year survival compared to patients $\leq$ 70 years of age, whose survival rate was 59.4% $\pm$ 3.6 (P = ns). These data have been substantiated by Block and Enker.[52] In their study, postoperative mortality for patients > 70 years old was 15%, and age-adjusted five-year survival rate was 67.2%. In contradistinction, a 60.9% survival rate was noted for rectal cancer patients $\leq$ 69 years. These authors conclude that elderly patients surviving conventional curative operations for colorectal carcinoma have a relative five-year survival which exceeded that of the general population. Sugarbaker[48] concluded that the operative mortality with aged patients is two to three times that of the younger population; nonetheless, survival rates following curative surgery exceed that of the younger patient group.

YOUNG AGE ($\leq$ 30 YEARS).—A review of ten surgical series by Sugarbaker[48] indicates that patients $\leq$ 30 years of age have a larger proportion of poorly differentiated neoplasms, more mucinous tumors, and present with a more advanced stage of disease. These prognostic determinants account for the poor prognosis in younger patients with colorectal carcinoma. In the large series by Recio and Bussey,[53] 1.2% of

TABLE 45–7.—TUMOR PENETRATION OF COLORECTAL WALL WITH AND WITHOUT NODAL METASTASIS
RELATIVE TO FIVE-YEAR SURVIVAL, %

STATUS AT FIVE YEARS	INVOLVEMENT OF MUCOSA WITHOUT NODES (n = 66)	INVOLVEMENT OF MUCOSA WITH NODES (n = 3)	INVOLVEMENT INTO BUT NOT THROUGH MUSCLE WITHOUT NODES (n = 150)	INVOLVEMENT INTO BUT NOT THROUGH MUSCLE WITH NODES (n = 58)	INVOLVEMENT THROUGH MUSCLE WITHOUT NODES (n = 379)	INVOLVEMENT THROUGH MUSCLE WITH NODES (n = 329)
Alive with carcinoma	3	0	3	5	3	2
Alive with no carcinoma	71	67	61	48	39	13
Alive; no details available	0	0	1	0	1	0
Dead; no details available	0	0	0	0	2	2
Dead with no carcinoma	20	33	16	0	16	3
Dead with carcinoma	6	0	18	47	40	80

Copeland E.M., Miller L.D., Jones R.S.: Prognostic factors in carcinoma of the colon and rectum. *Am. J. Surg.* 116:875, 1968.

4,430 patients with colon and rectal carcinomas presented before the age of 30. Five-year survival was remarkably reduced; only 19.5% survived ≥ five years. In these younger patients, tumor histology revealed a high-grade malignancy in over one half of the specimens. This figure compares to the usual 20% with undifferentiated tumors in most large series. In younger patients, survival is based on the same prognostic indicators as those in older individuals. Those series reported, however, show that younger patients usually present with a more advanced stage of disease. Possibly symptoms in the young are ignored longer by both patient and physician. Physicians should be cautioned to evaluate critically a young patient with symptoms suggestive of a carcinoma in a manner similar to that for older subjects.

CEA AND THE SECOND-LOOK PROCEDURE.—Gold and Freedman[54] identified a glycoprotein antigen common to malignant neoplasms that arose from the epithelium of the human digestive tract. They originally thought this antigen was specific for adenocarcinoma of colorectal origin. Subsequently, it has been determined that carcinoembryonic antigen (CEA) is not specific for colorectal or other GI neoplasms. While CEA has less value as a screening tool for colon cancer than was originally proposed, its value does reside in monitoring the detection of residual or recurrent colon cancer.[55] Also, CEA levels correlate with prognosis and stage of disease.[48]

Martin and associates[56] were early advocates of CEA as an indicator of recurrent colorectal carcinoma and as a tool for selection of individuals for second-look operations. In an analysis of 60 patients reoperated over a seven-year interval using the CEA value as a biochemical marker of tumor recurrence, they found recurrent or residual colon cancer in 93% of reoperated patients. They next entered patients into a prospective study beginning in 1976 (Table 45–8). Thirty-eight patients had a second-look procedure based on a rising CEA value. Resectable, localized disease was observed in 48% and the CEA was misleading (false positive or negative) in only 7% of patients. These authors have since reported an unprecedented resectability rate of 61% in this prospective series of 60 patients conducted from 1976 to the present. The mean observed delay between a rise in CEA value and reoperation in patients studied with *unresectable* tumor was 5.5 months. In those patients with resectable disease at second look, the delay was 3.2 months. A CEA nomogram can be plotted to establish a range of values within 95% confidence limits of normal for any radioimmunoassay level. When CEA values exceed the limits of confidence of this nomogram, additional assays are performed to determine reproducibility. Elevations in the CEA levels at intervals between assays of 1.5–2 months are considered positive. These patients are then subjected to comprehensive staging with gastrointestinal barium contrast studies, colonoscopy, computed tomography of the abdomen, pelvis, and lungs, and hepatic function tests. These radio-

TABLE 45–8.—A COLLECTIVE REVIEW OF SURGICAL SERIES UTILIZING CEA AS GUIDE
TO SECOND-LOOK PROCEDURES

AUTHOR (YR)	NO. SECOND-LOOK PROCEDURES	RESECTABLE LOCALIZED DISEASE, No. (%)	FALSE POS/NEG PROCEDURES, No. (%)	INTERVAL (MO.) CEA ELEVATION AND REOPERATION (MEAN)		CURRENT NED STATUS, No. (%)	RESECTABLE TUMOR SURVIVAL NED (MO.), Range (Mean)
				Resected	Unresected		
Martin et al. (1980)†,‡	60	29 (48)	4 (7)	1.8	5.4	21 (35)	NA*
(1972-75)	22†	6 (27)	3 (14)	3.5	7.0	2 (9)	24–84 (54)
(1976-79)	38‡	23 (61)	1 (3)	1.4	4.5	19 (50)	≤36 (NA)
Nicholson and Aust (1978)†	3	1 (33)	0 (0)	3.0	3.0	1 (33)	24
Mach et al. (1978)†	4	1 (25)	0 (0)	11.0	15.7	1 (25)	2
Staab et al. (1978)‡	28	10 (36)	0 (0)	3.8	4.4	7 (25)	9–15 (NA)
Evans et al. (1978)‡	11	2 (18)	3 (27)	2.0	NA	1 (9)	12
Wanebo et al. (1978)‡	16	7 (44)	2 (13)	3.0	3.0	4 (25)	12–37 (21.5)
Steele et al. (1980)‡	16	4 (25)	1 (6)	2.0	2.5	2 (12)	13–24 (18.5)
Attiyeh and Stearns (1981)‡	37	16 (43)	4 (11)	2.5	6.0	8 (25)	2–61 (15)
Sugarbaker (1982)‡,§	10	5 (50)	0 (0)	1.0	≤3.0	2 (20)	6–48 (27)
Total	185	75 (41)	18 (10)	3.2	5.5	68 (37)	

*NA = Not available.
†NED = No evidence of disease.
‡Retrospective study.
§Personal communication to author, 1982.
Modified from Bland K.I., Polk H.C. Jr.: The curative and palliative control of colorectal carinoma, in, Nyhus L.M. (ed.), *Surgery Annual*, Connecticut, Appleton-Century-Crofts, 1983.

graphic procedures potentially enhance localization of recurrent or residual disease. A second-look procedure is then performed.

The NED (no evidence of disease) status for 50% of patients, in the most recent prospective series by Martin et al.[56] suggests an enhanced survival (≤ 36 months) can be achieved with minimal morbidity and mortality, but must be viewed with cautious optimism. Neither long-term survival nor the quality of survival can be ascertained for the second-look procedure without well-designed, randomized, prospective trials with concurrent controls.

Most obvious in this collective analysis of nine surgical series reported between 1972 and 1982 is the increased incidence of resectable neoplasms when delay is minimized following elevation of the CEA and reoperation. False negative/positive procedures were performed in 0%–27% of the second-look operations (mean = 10%) of this series.[42]

Polk and Spratt[57] defined a subgroup of patients in whom curative reexcision of the perineum, with or without associated resection of viscera, achieved excellent pain control with acceptable morbidity and mortality. Each of these patients had previously undergone a Miles APR. Recurrence without palpable disease was disclosed microscopically in one third of the patients. In this series of patients reoperated *without* the benefit of variations in the plasma CEA values, disease-free survival (range = 3–36 months, median = 12 months) was disappointing and tempered our enthusiasm for aggressive diagnosis and treatment of locally recurrent colorectal carcinoma in the pelvic musculature and perineum. These data suggest that the control of locally recurrent cancer of the pelvis and perineum is unique after an apparently *standard* primary operative excision when CEA determinations are not available. These early efforts should be recognized as palliative rather than curative measures initiated through a well-defined follow-up regimen and an aggressive treatment alternative.

Operative Therapy for Hepatic Metastases

NATURAL HISTORY OF HEPATIC METASTASES.—Secondary liver cancer is considered incurable in most cases. Jaffe et al.[58] documented that metastatic liver cancer was the primary etiologic mechanism that most often related to death in patients with malignant diseases. For 177 patients with colon and rectum cancer, the mean survival of 5.0 months was statistically different ($P < 0.001$) for metastatic gastric, pancreatic, and biliary tract carcinoma. These authors reported that the intrinsic factors that most often influence survival include the primary tumor site, the histologic tumor type, and the degree of tumor differentiation. The extent of hepatic involvement with metastatic disease is also important in determining prognosis, as patients with limited (solitary) disease have improved survival regardless of the therapy employed.[58–62] Wood and associates[62] reported a one-year survival of 60% in patients with solitary, untreated metastases from colorectal carcinoma, whereas only 5.7% survival was evident when both hepatic lobes contained diffuse disease. The mean survival for patients with minimal (solitary) disease was 16.7 months, while only 3.1 months for patients with extensive hepatolobar disease. Pettavel and Morgenthaler[61] cite the value of the serum alkaline phosphatase and hepatomeg-

aly to categorize extent of metastases. In the absence of both criteria, 27 patients were observed to have a mean survival of 16 months, whereas 30 patients with both clinical indices present survived an average of 1.4 months. The majority of patients who are found to have hepatic metastases are observed to harbor these lesions at diagnosis, at resection of their primary tumor, or within 24 months of treatment of the primary neoplasm.[59]

Synchronous hepatic metastases are observed in 10%–30% of patients at the time of initial laparotomy for resection of their primary colonic or rectal neoplasm. The hepatic lesion is resectable in 25% of these patients and is either a solitary nodule or is limited to a single segment or lobe of the liver.[59]

SURGICAL THERAPY.—Survival for as great as two years following demonstration of metastatic hepatic disease is unusual. Essentially all five-year survivors with biopsy-proved metastases from primary colorectal carcinomas have had appropriate *surgical therapy* for their disease. These efforts to improve survival by hepatic resections have been recently reviewed by Bland and Polk.[42] Foster[59] has previously emphasized that patients undergoing resections for hepatic metastases of colorectal origin are highly selected and in many cases would have a more favorable prognosis than the general patient with liver metastases even if left unresected.

Woodington and Waugh[63] observed a 20% five-year survival rate and an acceptable operative mortality (4%) following resection of hepatic metastases from various visceral neoplasms. This experience has been updated by Wilson and Adson[64] for liver metastases of primary colorectal origin. Solitary lesions were resected from the liver in 40 patients, and multiple lesions were resected in 20 individuals. Operative mortality rate was only 1.7%. Of 54 patients eligible for five-year survival analysis, 28% lived five years or greater, and 15% were alive without evidence of recurrent disease ten years or more following operation. No patients survived five years after excision of multiple hepatic lesions. These data suggest that aggressive surgical therapy for solitary hepatic metastases of colorectal origin is justified.

The recent analysis for the survival rates of patients with biopsy-proved *unresected* hepatic metastases, which were the only evidence of residual disease, revealed the extent to which the natural history, rather than resection may determine length of survival. Wagner et al.[65] studied 141 patients having resection of hepatic metastases and confirmed the five-year survival of 25%. Although excision of metastatic disease palliated some patients who died, one-half of the patients in this series had no relief of symptoms and were not benefited by resection. In this report, *stage* of the primary lesion, female *sex*, and *the absence of extrahepatic metastases* were the most significant determinants of a favorable prognosis following resection of hepatic metastases.

Patients with untreated hepatic metastases have limited survival (mean = 6.0 months). In the 1974 Liver Tumor Survey (LTS) by Foster and Berman,[66] 88 patients were available for five-year survival analysis. Of these patients, 16 (18%) were alive five years following hepatic resection. Twenty percent of 45 patients at risk with resected *solitary* metastases, and 16% of 43 patients with excised *multiple* metastases (unilobar and bilobar) from colorectal primaries lived five years. Statistical analysis disclosed no difference between these operative groups with regard to survival. Additional analysis noted that prognosis was not altered by the presence of more than one tumor nodule, unless multiple metastases were evident in both anatomical lobes. This analysis has been further updated by Foster[67, 68] to include the combination of multi-institutional collective reviews, the LTS, and the author's experience. Of 259 patients considered survivors of hepatic resection for colorectal carcinoma, 108 solitary and 54 multiple nodules in 162 patients were at risk of recurrence for five years. Patients operated for solitary lesions had a 30% five-year survival compared to 13% for subjects undergoing resection of multiple hepatic metastases (Table 45–9). A prolonged disease-free interval had a nonbeneficial effect on prognosis after liver resection for liver metastases. Observation of hepatic metastases for disease progression to determine resectability was not warranted. Additionally, survival after simultaneous resection of the colon primary and liver metastases was essentially identical to that for metachronous hepatic resections when the interval following resection of the primary colon neoplasm exceeded two years. These cumulative reviews[66–68] also suggest that survival does not correlate with the status of mesenteric lymph nodes of the primary colonic neoplasm at the time of initial resection or with extent of hepatic parenchyma resected; size and number of the secondary hepatic tumors relate directly to curability by resection.

To determine the size of metastatic lesion as a determinant of prognosis following hepatic resection, Adson and Van-Heerden[69] evaluated 34 patients managed since 1973 by major hepatic resection of large metastases. Two hospital deaths (5.8%) were recorded. The one-, two-, and three-year or greater survival rates were 82%, 58%, and 41%, respectively. These authors conclude from a critical analysis of duration and quality of survival that at least 20%, and perhaps 30%, of the patients in this series were benefited by resection of large hepatic metastases.

In summary, approximately one fifth of patients with primary colorectal carcinoma have metastatic hepatic involvement, and only one fourth of these secondary lesions are solitary or unilobar. Thus, only 5% of patients with intraoperative metastatic hepatic disease will prompt the intraoperative decision for potential resection. Further, over 50% of these patients will have undetectable metastases at operative evaluation. The above data strongly favor the operative decision to initiate hepatic resection when limited unilobar or solitary

metastases are encountered at operation. When the primary colorectal neoplasm is controlled in the absence of extrahepatic involvement, resection of metastases should be attempted if technically feasible. These decisions must be tempered by the technical expertise and experience of the surgeon, the medical status of the patient, and the availability of adequate blood products and anesthesia support. Data do not exist to support anatomical (total) lobectomy as the procedure preferred over simple excision or wedging of the primary lesion. Solitary or unilobar metastases are best managed by resection with an adequate margin of normal tissue which well encompasses the metastatic neoplasm.

Chemotherapy for Advanced Carcinoma of the Large Bowel and Rectum

The future of chemotherapy for advanced colorectal cancer is dependent on synthesis of new chemotherapeutic drugs which have specific activity and response rates. The most extensively investigated chemotherapeutic agent for the treatment of this neoplasm has been fluorouracil (5-FU). Carter[70] reviewed a collective series of over 2,000 patients treated with this agent and calculated response rates to be approximately 21%. Previously reported individual series observed response rates which varied from 8% to 85%.[71] The Central Oncology Group[72] conducted a study of 198 patients with colorectal carcinoma randomized to receive 5-FU via four dosage schedules:

1. *IV loading:* 12 mg/kg/day × 5 days. Eleven half-doses are given on alternate days until a toxic reaction is observed. Maintenance doses of 15 mg/kg/week were continued.

2. *Weekly IV:* 15 mg/kg/week as a bolus injection × 4 days. Increase to 20 mg/kg in absence of intoxication.

3. *Nontoxic IV:* 500 mg/day × 4 days, followed with 500 mg/week.

4. *Oral:* 15 mg/kg/day × 6 days, followed by 15 mg/kg/ week.

An overall objective remission of 18% was demonstrated. Duration of response was significantly longer with IV loading; however, toxic reactions were highest with this schedule. Nonetheless, the survival advantage was not enhanced with this more toxic regimen. The application of other *single-agent chemotherapeutics* (chlorozotocin, MeCCNU, BCNU, CCNU) had response rates in the range of 10%–20%. Thus, the role of single-agent chemotherapy for advanced colorectal carcinoma appears limited.

The utility of *combination chemotherapy* for the treatment of this neoplasm has met with varying response results. Combinations employing 5-FU with MeCCNU, BCNU, vincristine, CTIC, hydroxyurea, adriamycin, mitomycin C, and streptozocin have had mixed results. Presently, no drug schedule or combination of drugs with or without 5-FU have apparent benefits when compared to the 5-FU regimen alone.[73] The GI Tumor Study Group[74] recently reported the results of 621 patients with Dukes stage B_2, C_1 or C_2 colon cancer randomly assigned to one of four chemoimmunotherapy programs. The administration of 5-FU with semustin, immunotherapy with methanol extraction residue of bacillus Calmette-Guérin (BCG), combination therapy with 5-FU, semustin, and BCG, or close follow-up without adjuvant therapy were evaluated. In follow-up (median = 5.5 years), no

TABLE 45–9.—SUMMARY OF SURVIVAL DATA FOLLOWING HEPATIC RESECTIONS FOR METASTATIC COLORECTAL CARCINOMA

SURVIVAL	NO. OF PATIENTS (%)	
Operative survivors		
2-Year survival	259	
5-Year survival	84/192 (44)	
Dead of disease	46/206 (22)	
≥ 5 years	12 (5)	
Postresection		
	SOLITARY NODULE	MULTIPLE NODULE
Patients at risk	108	54
Operative mortality (%)	1 (1)	7 (13)
5-Year survival (%)	33 (30)	7 (13)

Adapted from Foster J.H.: *Am. J. Surg.* 135:389, 1978.

significant differences were observed for either recurrence or survival rates among the four treatment programs. These data did not support the use of chemotherapy or its combination with immunotherapy as an adjuvant treatment program for patients at high-risk for recurrent colon carcinoma.

Bland and Polk[42] reported a review of 15 major series which described the various vascular infusional techniques for treating hepatic metastases. This study was a mix of 904 patients utilizing variable drug schedules, routes, and dosages. Patients treated by infusional therapy survived an average of 10.2 months, while control patients survived 5.4 months. Variance was considerable. These individual studies must be cautiously interpreted as no dramatic responses were demonstrable. The encouraging studies by Taylor[75] utilizing hepatic arterial ligation with hepatic arterial and umbilical vein perfusion with 5-FU are noteworthy. Trials are being initiated to determine the advantages of synchronous arterial and venous infusions of active cytoxic drugs (5-FU, FUDR).

The current application of totally implantable drug infusion devices to deliver regional hepatic chemotherapy via hepatic artery catheterization for treatment of *unresectable* hepatic neoplasms is under evaluation in several centers. Balch et al.[76] completed a phase II prospective evaluation of regional FUDR chemotherapy utilizing a totally implantable drug infusion pump. In comparison of 81 patients with colorectal metastases to the liver treated with this regional delivery system vs. 129 patients who served as historical controls, pump patients demonstrated an 88% response rate as evidenced by a fall in serum CEA levels by $\geq$ one third after two cycles of chemotherapy. Utilizing four evaluation criteria, regional chemotherapy patients had improvement and better survival rates than controls. The one-year survival and median survival were better for the entire group of pump patients vs. controls (82% vs. 36%, 26 months vs. 8 months; $P < 0.0001$). Survival for the regional chemotherapeutic patients was not influenced by extent of tumor involvement or the presence of symptoms of hepatic disease. These authors conclude that regional chemotherapy with this implantable pump prolonged life by 12–18 months greater than matched historical controls. Similar data have been confirmed in two studies.[77, 78] These results suggest significant improvement in survival over previously published reports utilizing externalized arterial catheters and portable pumps.[79] Significant advantage of the totally implantable delivery system is that long-term chemotherapy could be administered on a continual basis with little risk of thrombosis, infection, and catheter migration.

Utilization of the drug delivery system appears to provide palliative control of disease in a significant percentage of patients with hepatic metastases; however, major cause of death resulted from progression of disease at extrahepatic sites (e.g., lung and abdomen). Finally, it is to be emphasized that regional hepatic arterial delivery systems represent palliative therapy and essentially all patients eventually relapse unless new drugs or combinations of drugs are developed. While the results of the aforementioned clinical trials are encouraging, a randomized control series utilizing conventional systemic therapy must be conducted to confirm its efficacy. The ultimate improvement of duration and quality of survival using aggressive regional therapy will only be determined following randomized prospective trials.

Radiotherapy

Currently, 50%–70% of patients with colorectal carcinoma and extension through the bowel wall (Dukes C) suffer from metastases, recurrence, and death when treated by operation alone. Radiation therapy has been employed primarily for patients at highest risk for recurrence. Additionally, this therapeutic modality has marked palliative benefit in patients with local/regional symptoms initiated by recurrent disease.

The greatest stimulus for the scientific evaluation of benefit with *adjuvant preoperative radiotherapy* was initiated by Stearns et al.[80] at Memorial Hospital in 1959. Initial enthusiasm for low-dosage (1,500–2,000 rad) radiation occurred as a result of the preliminary indication of benefit to Dukes C patients over nonirradiated controls. However, in subsequent publications by Quan et al.[81, 82] and Stearns et al.[83] the evaluation of a prospectively randomized study of 700 patients reversed this consensus of therapeutic advantage with preoperative radiation therapy in similar dosages. A report[84] by the Veterans Administration Surgical Adjuvant Group (VASAG) noted therapeutic benefit to preoperatively irradiated patients (2,000–2,500 rad in 10 fractions over 12 days) having APR compared with controls. A reduction in lymph node invasion, in local recurrence and in distant metastases with an improved five-year survival was reported. The subsequent analysis by Higgins[85] described differences in survival times for patients in the two treatment groups managed by colonic resection and APR; however, statistical differences were not evident. A substantial reduction (13.4%) in the proportion of patients with Dukes' C cancers was observed in the adjuvantly treated group. However, this trial failed to confirm any specific benefit to patients at highest risk. A separate study by Rider and associates[86] utilized a randomized trial of 500 rad given as a single dose preoperatively within eight hours of planned surgery. No differences in *overall* survival benefit was noted in irradiated and control groups; however, patients with Dukes' C lesions were observed to have a statistically significant difference ($P < 0.014$) in five-year survival for irradiated vs. control groups (34% vs. 18%).

Trials of preoperative radiotherapy for management of high-risk (B_2 and C) lesions are difficult to design from the standpoint of adequate stratification, randomization, and control. Future trials are necessary to identify subsets at high-risk for recurrence who benefit from this adjuvant preoperative modality.

Cass et al.[87] in a retrospective analysis of 165 patients with recurrent colorectal carcinoma, observed local recurrence in 60%, concomitant local recurrence and remote metastases in 14%, and distant metastases alone in 26%. The rate of local recurrence directly correlated with degree of tumor anaplasia and depth of bowel wall penetration. Local recurrence without clinical evidence of distant metastases represented the most common mechanism of death (29%) within the first five years following diagnosis of recurrence. Further, local recurrences developed in structures contiguous with the operative sites or abdominal incision in 92%. Thus, postoperative radiotherapy trials have been instituted to reduce the risk of recurrence of the resected tumor bed. Selection of patients for *postoperative irradiation* is dependent on the orientation of the tumor to contiguous structures, lymph node involvement, and penetration through the bowel wall. In general, tumors of the abdominal colon are not considered for irradiation unless they are adherent to unresectable structures (pelvic wall, anterior abdominal wall, bladder, etc.). However, portions of the rectum and rectosigmoid that are affixed to pelvic retroperitoneal organs or structures have definitive criteria for irradiation. As catalogued by Gunderson,[88] the criteria for postoperative irradiation are : (1) known inadequate margins of resection; (2) adherent to retroperitoneum, sacrum, or pelvic sidewalls; (3) macroscopic transmural tumor penetration of the bowel wall; and (4) extensive microscopic tumor penetration and/or the presence of positive lymph nodes. Additionally, patients who are considered to have nodal metastases at the highest level of surgical resection (Dukes C_2) may be considered candidates for therapy to residual principal, intermediate, or paraaortic lymphatics. Radiation therapy may be valuable as an adjuvant for resectable rectal carcinomas. Low-dose preoperative irradiation and curative operations followed by postoperative radiotherapy (*Sandwich technique*) is being evaluated.

Radiotherapy has also been used to treat suture line and pelvic recurrences. Low dose hepatic irradiation may be occasionally of benefit for patients with hepatic metastases who have failed chemotherapy, particularly if they have pain related to distention of Glisson's capsule. Radiation is also of benefit in 50%–80% of patients as a palliative measure to treat bony metastases of colorectal origin.[89]

Screening and Follow-up

The ultimate goal of screening is to detect the cancerous or precancerous state before dissemination into regional or remote sites. Therefore, the yield from screening techniques is best directed in a cost-effective manner to high-risk groups. Techniques employed in *screening* are CEA, rigid or flexible fiberoptic proctosigmoidoscopy, barium contrast examinations, and fecal occult blood testing. *CEA is an insensitive indicator of early cancer.* Only 4% of patients with Dukes A cancer and 26% of patients with Dukes B lesions have abnormal values.[15, 90] Proctosigmoidoscopy remains valuable, even though colon cancer appears to be less localized to the rectum and rectosigmoid than in previous years. The more recent introduction of the flexible fiberoptic sigmoidoscope (30 and 60 cm long) provides a convenient method for examination of the entire rectum and sigmoid and left colon.

Knutson and Max[91] identified a group of patients who had positive fecal occult blood tests or gross blood per rectum in the presence of negative rigid proctoscopic and standard barium enema examinations. Colonoscopic examination was done in 139 of these patients. A total of 41 unsuspected lesions were detected in 35 patients (25%); 9 (22%) of these lesions were carcinomas. Nonetheless, the barium contrast enema remains the primary diagnostic modality for confirming colonic lesions. The frequency of false positive examinations with routine barium contrast studies was 17% in 230 consecutive patients who had endoscopic evaluation for the radiographically identifiable polypoid colonic lesions. False positive tests can be minimized, and the need for colonoscopic examinations reduced if appropriate preradiographic colonic preparation is emphasized[92] and air contrast is added to the study.

Hemoccult testing of the stool for occult blood is a gross screening tool. Most series report a large number of both false positive and false negative tests. Thus, the test should not be considered as a diagnostic indicator of early GI malignancies. Some chemical indicators (guaiac and benzidine) used earlier recognized the hemoglobin regardless of the animal source. Thus, lack of dietary restrictions and the absence of quality control of reagents increased the errors in diagnosis.[93]

The most common patterns of metastases, according to data from Whiteley,[93] are local (33%), intra-abdominal (14%), hepatic (33%), and systemic (20%). Systemic metastases commonly involve hepatic and pulmonary sites. Additional common sites include the ovaries (22%–25%),[42, 94] bone, and brain. Patients should be followed up every three months with careful physical examinations, CEA, and rectal or colostomy examinations. Chest x-ray should be done every six months. Two years after treatment, the frequency of follow-up can be decreased to every six months. Sixty percent of recurrences will take place in the first two years after resection and 94% will occur by five years. Yet, this remaining colon should be examined by barium enema and/or colonoscopy annually for the remainder of the patient's life. In a review by Polk and Spratt,[95] symptoms of recurrent colon cancer were nonspecific and contributed little to diagnosis, emphasizing the need for careful follow-up examinations. Symptoms of dull perineal discomfort aggravated by sitting preceded the detection of recurrent rectal cancer in the perineal scar by one to nine months in 84% of patients evaluated. A prospective evaluation by Sugarbaker et al.[96] was done to determine the most sensitive method to detect recurrent disease. Analysis of CEA values, quarterly physical examinations, and monthly biochemical and radiologic tests were utilized in this evaluation sequence. Serial CEA values emerged as the *earliest* indicator of recurrent disease, followed by physical examination results.

Currently, surgeons are moderately successful in the treatment of primary colorectal cancer. An integration of the prognostic significance of the pathologic characteristics of the primary neoplasm, the techniques of the original operation, and the duration of risk for recurrent disease are essential to planning follow-up and subsequent therapy. Re-resections for recurrence after a standard procedure rarely result in cure. However, the majority of patients who are candidates for such procedures are palliated. The future role of CEA and of the second-look procedure and its relationship to potential cure has not been fully determined. Prospective randomized trials are necessary. Effective adjuvant and therapeutic cytotoxic agents specific for colorectal cancer should be developed. The surgical oncologist has possibly reached his maximum ability to cure this disease.

CARCINOIDS OF THE COLON AND RECTUM.—These neoplasms of enterochromaffin and argentaffin cell-origin were originally described in 1899 by Kulchitzky. These apudoma cells are located in the crypts of Lieberkühn and may be diffuse in the GI tract or present in extraintestinal sites (bronchus, ovary).

In most collective series, three-fourths of all abdominal carcinoid apudomas originate from the midgut. In a comparative series, carcinoids were the most frequent tumors of the appendix (77%), and this organ was the most common site for this neoplasm (35%–45%).[97] Carcinoids of colonic origin are most commonly located in the cecum and, like adenocarcinoma, remain occult, until their appearance with obstructive, invasive, or metastatic symptoms indistinguishable from those of carcinoma. The rectum and rectosigmoid represented the third most frequent site (Table 45–10).

The typical carcinoid tumor of colorectal origin is < 2 cm in size. These lesions may be recognized on barium enema or endoscopic studies as *submucosal* nodules with intact mucosa. Their gross configuration can be intraluminal, polypoid, anular, or infiltrative with transmural involvement of the bowel wall. With fixation of the polypoid growth to the underlying muscularis, the serosa becomes tethered and shortened. Occasionally, the lesion is deceptively mobile and unattached.

Histologically, the lesion is composed of small nests and strands (ribbons) of regular, polygonal to cuboidal epithelial cells that occasionally form glandlike patterns (Fig 45–8). Difficult diagnostic dilemmas may arise by the benignity of the microscopic appearance of monotonous sheets of cells with uniform nuclear size and shape. The distinguishing features of the malignant colonic carcinoid are, therefore, not histologic but morphological; i.e., size and the presence of extraintestinal metastases. *Metastatic potential* is clearly related to *size* and the *depth of local invasion*. Of the carcinoids 2 cm or greater in size, metastatic disease was observed in 80%–100%.[98–100] Bates[100] reported that 82% of rectal carcinoids > 2 cm were metastatic at diagnosis compared to 10% of lesions 1–2 cm in size and only 1.7% neoplasms < 1 cm in diameter.

The vasomotor effects of serotonin and bradykinin produce the *carcinoid syndrome* and are rarely observed in carcinoids of hindgut origin. Rather, these lesions present with symptoms identical to carcinomas of colorectal origin with obstruction, hemorrhage, or extraintestinal metastases to regional and distant sites. The liver is the organ most commonly involved with metastases, although lung and bone metastases occur.

Diagnosis of the colorectal carcinoid is established by sig-

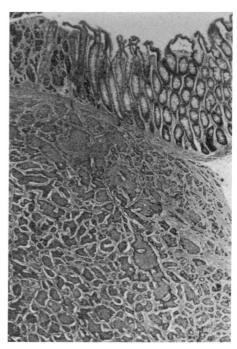

Fig 45–8.—Cross-sectional low-power (×40) view of malignant carcinoid tumor of left colon. Nests of uniform, round cells are present within the mucosa and submucosa of the colonic wall. (Courtesy D.A. Franzini, M.D., Department of Pathology, University of Florida.)

moidoscopic or endoscopic biopsy. Tumors < 2 cm which demonstrate no evidence of microscopic invasion may be treated by local excision and vigilant proctosigmoidoscopic or endoscopic follow-up. More extensive radical procedures are indicated for larger (≥ 2 cm) neoplasms with evidence of fix-

TABLE 45–10.—COLLECTIVE ORGAN DISTRIBUTION OF CARCINOID TUMORS

ORGAN	ABSOLUTE NUMBER			% OF ALL CARCINOIDS			% OF ALL LOCAL TUMORS
	A	B	C	A*	B†	C‡	
Esophagus and stomach	94	42	19	2.53	2.25	1.96	0.3
Small bowel							
Duodenum	135	33	22	3.63	1.77	2.27	33.7
Jejunum		19	19	—	1.02	1.96	
Ileum	1,074§	202	134	28.89	10.82	13.81	
NOS‖	0	99	70	0	5.30	7.22	
Ileocecum	0	14	0	0	0.75	0	
Appendix	1,686	820	340	45.35	43.92	35.05	77.3
Colon (except appendix)	91	122	65	2.45	6.53	6.70	0.3
Rectum & rectosigmoid	592	296	121	15.92	15.85	12.47	1.3
Lungs & bronchi	ND¶	191	137	ND	10.23	14.12	0.6
Biliary tract	10	2	0	0.27	0.11	0	ND
Ovary	34	0	3	0.91	0	0.31	ND
Pancreas	2	0	0	0.05	0	0	ND
Other sites	0	27	40	0	1.45	4.12	ND
Total	3,718	1,867	970	100	100	100	

*A = Wilson et al. series.
†B = End Results Group.
‡C = Third National Cancer Survey.
§Includes both jejunal and ileal carcinoids, and Meckel's diverticulum.
‖NOS = not otherwise specified.
¶ND = no data available.
Bland K.I., Polk H.C.: The apudomas: The concept and associated neoplasms, in Copeland E.M. (ed.): *Surgical Oncology.* John Wiley & Sons, 1983, pp. 385–422.

ation and muscular invasion of the bowel wall. Radical surgical resection which encompasses the involved colorectal segment *en bloc* with the mesentery is indicated. Colonic carcinoids proximal to or near the peritoneal reflection require colonic resections or anterior resections with colocolostomy. Malignant carcinoids with demonstrable invasion below the peritoneal reflection necessitate abdominoperineal resection.

When technically feasible, attempts should be made to resect carcinoid tumor in metastatic sites. Liver metastases amenable to approach by virtue of their anatomical distribution may be resected by traditional hepatic lobectomy. Lesions in the peripheral aspects of either hepatic lobe may be managed by wedge resections, partial lobectomy, and/or enucleation.[97, 101] Partial hepatectomy or lobectomy is impractical and ill-advised with diffuse metastatic involvement of multiple hepatic segments. While no trials have been reported utilizing continuous hepatic arterial infusional chemotherapy for metastatic carcinoids, the application of this technique for unresectable neoplasms may be beneficial.

Responses to single or combination cytotoxic agents given by systemic IV route for carcinoid metastases have met with variable success. Palliation may be established by systemic administration of the single agents 5-FU, cyclophosphamide, or thiotepa. Mengel[102] reported success with the parenteral administration of methotrexate alone and in combination with oral cyclophosphamide. Schein et al.[103] report inconsistent response rates for streptozotocin, which has specific anti-β islet-cell activity. Davis and associates[104] suggest that the combination of streptozotocin and 5-FU offers the best overall response rate (66%) of the available chemotherapeutics. Radiation therapy has been of little value in the therapy of this traditionally radioresistant neoplasm.

METASTATIC (SUBMUCOSAL) TUMORS.—Neoplasms of extraintestinal origin may present as polypoid intraluminal or transmural invasive types in the submucosa of the colorectum. The distribution may be solitary, patchy, or diffuse. These lesions may represent metastases from extracolorectal sites (*melanoma, sarcoma, carcinoma of the breast, ovary, lung,* or *other GI organs*), or may present as invasive submucosal lesions of contiguous organs (*prostate, small bowel, pancreas, stomach, retroperitoneum*).[105] Diagnosis may be achieved following pursuit of the symptoms of colorectal obstruction or bleeding with mucosal invasion or following workup, diagnostic evaluation, and staging of the primary neoplasm. Endoscopic visualization confirms elevation of an intact, overlying mucosa surrounding the mass effect. Diagnosis may be established by submucosal biopsy of the identifiable colorectal lesion.[106] Therapy, when required, is primarily surgical and may necessitate colonic resections of the involved colorectal wall and its mesentery with colocolostomy or sigmoid colostomy. Radical colon or abdominoperineal resections are indicated only if the primary neoplasm is controlled and extraintestinal metastatic disease is not demonstrable at surgical exploration.

REFERENCES

1. Silverberg E.: Cancer statistics, 1984. *CA* 34(1):7, 1984.
2. Mason T.J., McKay F.W., Hoover R., et al.: Atlas of cancer mortality among U.S. nonwhites: 1950–1969. DHEW publication no. (NIH)76–1204, 1976.
3. Blot W.J., Fraumeni J.F. Jr., Stone B.J., et al.: Geographic patterns of large bowel cancer in the United States. *J.N.C.I.* 57:1225, 1976.
4. Schottenfeld D., Haas J.F.: Epidemiology of colorectal cancer, in Lipkin M., Good R.A. (eds.): *Gastrointestinal Tract Cancer.* New York, Plenum Medical Book Co., 1978, pp. 207–240.
5. Rhodes J.B., Holmes F.F., Clark G.M.: Changing distribution of primary cancers in the large bowel. *J.A.M.A.* 238:1641, 1977.
6. Sugarbaker P.H., Macdonald J.S., Gunderson L.L.: Colorectal cancer, in: Devita V.T. Jr., Hellman S., Rosenberg S.A. (eds.): *Cancer: Principles and Practice of Oncology.* Philadelphia, J.B. Lippincott Co., 1983, pp. 643–723.
7. Schimke R.N.: *Genetics and Cancer in Man.* Edinburgh, Churchill Livingstone, 1978.
8. Anderson D.E.: Familial predisposition, in Schottenfeld D., Fraumeni J.F. (eds.): *Cancer Epidemiology and Prevention.* Philadelphia, W.B. Saunders Co., 1982, pp. 483–493.
9. Knudson A.G. Jr., Kelly P.T.: Genetics and cancer: Genetic counseling with the cancer patient's family. *Curr. Probl. Cancer.* 7(12):15, 1983.
10. Lynch H.T., Organ C.H. Jr., Harris R.E., et al.: Familial cancer: Implications for surgical management of high-risk patients. *Surgery* 83:104, 1978.
11. Albano W.A., Recabaren J.A., Lynch H.T., et al.: Natural history of hereditary cancer of the breast and colon. *Cancer* 50:360, 1982.
12. Lynch H.T., Lynch P.M.: Tumor variation in the cancer family syndrome: Ovarian cancer. *Am. J. Surg.* 138:439, 1979.
13. Copeland E.M., Jones R.S., Miller L.D.: Multiple colon neoplasms. *Arch. Surg.* 98:141, 1969.
14. Lynch H.T., Krush A.J., Guirgis H.: Genetic factors in families with combined gastrointestinal and breast cancer. *Am. J. Gastroenterol.* 59:31, 1973.
15. Winawer S.J., Sherlock P.: Malignant neoplasms of the small and large intestine, in Sleisenger M.H., Fordtran J.S. (eds.): *Gastrointestinal Disease: Pathophysiology, Diagnosis and Management.* Philadelphia, W.B. Saunders Co., 1983, pp. 1220–1249.
16. Morson B.C.: Genesis of colorectal cancer. *Clin. Gastroenterol.* 5:505, 1976.
17. Ekelund G.R.: Cancer risk with single and multiple adenomas: Synchronous and metachronous tumors, in Winawer S.J., Schottenfeld D., Sherlock P. (eds.): *Colorectal Cancer: Prevention, Epidemiology and Screening,* Progress in Cancer Research and Therapy. New York, Raven Press, 1980, vol. 13.
18. Haenszel W., Kurihara M.: Studies of Japanese migrants: I. Mortality from cancer and other diseases among Japanese in the United States. *J.N.C.I.* 40:43, 1968.
19. Haenszel W., Correa P.: Cancer of the colon and rectum and adenomatous polyps: A review of epidemiologic findings. *Cancer* 28:14, 1971.
20. Burkitt D.P.: Epidemiology of cancer of the colon and rectum. *Cancer* 28:3, 1971.
21. Hill M.J.: The role of colon anaerobes in the metabolism of bile acids and steroids, and its relation to colon cancer. *Cancer* 36:2387, 1975.
22. Weisburger J.H., Reddy B.S., Spingarn N.E., et al.: Current views on the mechanisms involved in the etiology of colorectal cancer, in Winawer S.J., Schottenfeld D., Sherlock P. (eds.): *Colorectal Cancer: Prevention, Epidemiology and Screening,* Progress in Cancer Research and Therapy. New York, Raven Press, 1980, vol. 13, pp. 19–41.
23. Hill M.J., Drasar B.S., Williams R.E.O., et al.: Faecal bile-acids and clostridia in patients with cancer of the large bowel. *Lancet* 1:535, 1975.
24. Reddy B.S., Weisburger J.H., Wynder E.L.: Effects of high risk and low risk diets for colon carcinogenesis on fecal microflora and steroids in man. *J. Nutr.* 105:878, 1975.
25. Lipkin M., Sherlock P., DeCosse J.J.: Risk factors and preventive measures in the control of cancer of the large intestine. *Curr. Probl. Cancer* 4(10):1–57, 1980.

26. Beal J.M., Cornell G.N.: A study of the problem of recurrence of carcinoma at the anastomotic site following resection of the colon for carcinoma. *Ann. Surg.* 143:1, 1956.

27. Copeland E.M., Miller L.B., Jones R.S.: unpublished observations, in Sleisenger W.H., Fordtran J.S. (eds.): *Gastrointestinal Disease: Pathophysiology, Diagnosis and Management.* Philadelphia, W.B. Saunders, 1978, pp. 1784–1800.

28. Winawer S.J., Andrews M., Flehinger B., et al.: Progress report on controlled trial of fecal occult blood testing for the detection of colorectal neoplasia. *Cancer* 45:2959, 1980.

29. Ranson J.H.C., Adams P.X., Localio S.A.: Preoperative assessment for hepatic metastases in carcinoma of the colon and rectum. *Surg. Gynecol. Obstet.* 137:435, 1973.

30. Hunt R.H., Waye J.D.: Indications for colonoscopy, in *Colonoscopy: Techniques, Clinical Practice and Color Atlas.* London, Chapman & Hall. 1981.

31. Temple D.F., Parthasarathy K.L., Bakshi S.P., et al.: A comparison of isotopic and computerized tomographic scanning in the diagnosis of metastasis to the liver in patients with adenocarcinoma of the colon and rectum. *Surg. Gynecol. Obstet.* 156(2):205–208, 1983.

32. Dukes C.E., Bussey H.J.R.: The spread of rectal cancer and its effect on prognosis. *Br. J. Cancer* 12:309, 1958.

33. Nichols R.L., Smith J.W., Balthazar E.R.: Peritonitis and intraabdominal abscess: An experimental model for the evaluation of human disease. *J. Surg. Res.* 25:129, 1978.

34. Turnbull R.B. Jr., Kyle K., Watson F.R., et al.: Cancer of the colon: The influence of the no-touch isolation technic on survival rates. *Ann. Surg.* 166:420, 1967.

35. Stearns M.W. Jr.: Benign and malignant neoplasms of colon and rectum: Diagnosis and management. *Surg. Clin. North Am.* 58:605, 1978.

36. Enker W.E., Laffer U.T., Block G.E.: Enhanced survival of patients with colon and rectal cancer is based upon wide anatomic resection. *Ann. Surg.* 190:350, 1979.

37. Stearns M.W. Jr.: The choice among anterior resection, the pull-through, and abdomino-perineal resection of the rectum. *Cancer* 34:969, 1974.

38. Miller L.D., Boruchow I.B., Fitts W.T.: An analysis of 284 patients with perforative carcinoma of the colon. *Surg. Gynecol. Obstet.* 123:1212, 1966.

39. Spratt J.S. Jr., Spjut H.J.: Prevalence and prognosis of individual clinical and pathologic variables associated with colorectal carcinoma. *Cancer* 20:1976, 1967.

40. Polk H.C. Jr., Spratt J.S. Jr., Bennett D., et al.: Surgical mortality and survival from colonic carcinoma. *Arch. Surg.* 89:16, 1964.

41. Polk H.C. Jr.: Extended resection for selected adenocarcinomas of the large bowel. *Ann. Surg.* 175:892, 1972.

42. Bland K.I., Polk H.C. Jr.: Therapeutic measures applied for the curative and palliative control of colorectal carcinoma, in Nyhus L. (ed.): *Surgery Annual.* Norwalk, Appleton-Century-Crofts, 1983, vol. 15, pp. 123–161.

43. Polk H.C. Jr., Spratt J.S. Jr., Butcher H.R. Jr.: Frequency of multiple primary malignant neoplasms associated with colorectal carcinoma. *Am. J. Surg.* 109:71, 1965.

44. Baughman B.B., Knutson C.O., Ahmad W., et al.: The surgical treatment of carcinoma of the colon and rectum: An index of quality care and sociologic and geographic distribution. *Ann. Surg.* 183:550, 1976.

45. Copeland E.M., Miller I.D., Jones R.S.: Prognostic factors in carcinoma of the colon and rectum. *Am. J. Surg.* 116:875, 1968.

46. Devlin H.B., Plant J.A., Morris D.: The significance of the symptoms of carcinoma of the rectum. *Surg. Gynecol. Obstet.* 137:399, 1973.

47. Rowe-Jones D.C., Aylett S.O.: Delay in treatment in carcinoma of colon and rectum. *Lancet* 2:973, 1965.

48. Sugarbaker P.H.: Carcinoma of the colon: Prognosis and operative choice. *Curr. Probl. Surg.* 18(12):753–826, 1981.

49. Ragland J.J., Londe A.M., Spratt J.S. Jr.: Correlation of the prognosis of obstructing colorectal carcinoma with clinical and pathologic variables. *Am. J. Surg.* 121:552, 1971.

50. Glenn F., McSherry C.K.: Obstruction and perforation in colorectal cancer. *Ann. Surg.* 173:983, 1971.

51. Jensen H.E., Nielsen J., Balslev I.: Carcinoma of the colon in old age. *Ann. Surg.* 171:107, 1970.

52. Block G.E., Enker W.E.: Survival after operations for rectal carcinoma in patients over 70 years of age. *Ann. Surg.* 174:521, 1971.

53. Recio P., Bussey H.J.R.: The pathology and prognosis of carcinoma of the rectum in the young. *Proc. R. Soc. Med.* 58:789, 1965.

54. Gold P., Freedman S.O.: Demonstration of tumor-specific antigens in human colonic carcinomata by immunological tolerance and absorption techniques. *J. Exp. Med.* 121:439, 1965.

55. Moertel C.G., Schutt A.J., Go V.L.W.: Carcinoembryonic antigen test for recurrent colorectal carcinoma: Inadequacy for early detection. *J.A.M.A.* 239:1065, 1978.

56. Martin E.W. Jr., Cooperman M., Carey L.C., et al.: Sixty second-look procedures indicated primarily by rise in serial carcinoembryonic antigen. *J. Surg. Res.* 28:389, 1980.

57. Polk H.C. Jr., Spratt J.S. Jr.: The results of treatment of perineal recurrence of cancer of the rectum. *Cancer* 43:952, 1979.

58. Jaffe B.M., Donegan W.L., Watson F., et al.: Factors influencing survival in patients with untreated hepatic metastases. *Surg. Gynecol. Obstet.* 127:1, 1968.

59. Foster J.H.: Survival after liver resection for secondary tumors. *Am. J. Surg.* 135:389, 1978.

60. Bengmark S., Hafstron L.: The natural course for liver cancer. *Prog. Clin. Cancer* 7:195, 1978.

61. Pettavel J., Morgenthaler F.: Protracted arterial chemotherapy of liver tumors: An experience of 107 cases over a 12-year period. *Prog. Clin. Cancer* 7:217, 1978.

62. Wood C.B., Gillis C.R., Blumgart L.H.: A retrospective study of the natural history of patients with liver metastases from colorectal cancer. *Clin. Oncol.* 2:285, 1976.

63. Woodington G.F., Waugh J.M.: Results of resection of metastatic tumors of the liver. *Am. J. Surg.* 105:24, 1963.

64. Wilson S.M., Adson M.A.: Surgical treatment of hepatic metastases from colorectal cancers. *Arch. Surg.* 111:330, 1976.

65. Wagner J.S., Adson M.A., Van Heerden J.A., et al.: The natural history of hepatic metastases from colorectal cancer: A comparison with resective treatment. *Ann. Surg.* 199:502, 1984.

66. Foster J.H., Berman M.M.: Resection of metastatic tumors, in Ebert P.A. (ed.): *Solid Liver Tumors,* Major Problems in Cinical Surgery. Philadelphia, W.B. Saunders Co., 1977, vol. 22, pp. 209–234.

67. Foster J.H.: Survival after liver resection for secondary tumors. *Am. J. Surg.* 135:389, 1978.

68. Foster J.H.: Treatment of metastatic cancer to liver, in DeVita V.T. Jr., Hellman S., Rosenberg S.A. (eds.): *Cancer: Principles and Practice of Oncology.* Philadelphia, J.B. Lippincott Co., 1982, pp. 1553–1563.

69. Adson M.A., VanHeerden J.A.: Major hepatic resections for metastatic colorectal cancer. *Ann. Surg.* 191:576, 1980.

70. Carter S.K.: Large-bowel cancer—the current status of treatment (editorial). *J.N.C.I.* 56:3, 1976.

71. Moertel C.G.: Large bowel, in Holland J.F., Frei E. III (eds.): *Cancer Medicine.* Philadelphia, Lea & Febiger, 1973, pp. 1597–1627.

72. Ansfield F., Klotz J., Nealon T., et al.: A Phase III study comparing the clinical utility of four regimens of 5-fluorouracil. *Cancer* 39:34, 1977.

73. Wolmark N., Haller D., Allegra J.: Chemotherapy of colorectal cancer, in Spratt J.S. (ed.): *Neoplasms of the Colon, Rectum and Anus: Mucosal and Epithelial.* Philadelphia, W.B. Saunders Co., 1984, pp. 347–362.

74. Gastrointestinal Tumor Study Group. Adjuvant Therapy of Colon Cancer—Results of a Prospectively Randomized Trial. *N. Engl. J. Med.* 310:737, 1984.

75. Taylor I.: Cytotoxic perfusion for colorectal liver metastases. *Br. J. Surg.* 65:109, 1978.

76. Balch C.M., Urist M.M., Soong S.J., et al.: A prospective Phase II clinical trial of continuous FUDR Regional Chemotherapy for colorectal metastases to the liver using a totally implantable drug infusion pump. *Ann. Surg.* 198:567, 1983.

77. Ensminger W., Niederhuber J., Gyres J., et al.: Effective control of liver metastases from colon cancer with an implanted sys-

tem for hepatic arterial chemotherapy. *Proc. A.S.C.O.* 1:94, 1980.

78. Oberfield R.A., McCaffrey J.A., Polio J., et al.: Prolonged and continuous percutaneous intra-arterial hepatic infusion chemotherapy in advanced metastatic liver adenocarcinoma from colorectal primary. *Cancer* 44:414, 1979.

79. Cady B.: Hepatic arterial patency and complications after catheterization for infusion chemotherapy. *Ann. Surg.* 178:156, 1973.

80. Stearns M.W. Jr., Deddish M.R., Quan S.H.O.: Preoperative roentgen therapy for cancer of the rectum. *Surg. Gynecol. Obstet.* 109:225, 1959.

81. Quan S.H.O., Deddish M.R., Stearns M.W. Jr.: The effect of preoperative roentgen therapy upon the 10- and 5-year results of the surgical treatment of cancer of the rectum. *Surg. Gynecol. Obstet.* 111:507, 1960.

82. Quan S.H.O.: A surgeon looks at radiotherapy in cancer of the colon and rectum. *Cancer* 31:1, 1973.

83. Stearns M.W. Jr., Deddish M.R., Quan S.H.O., et al.: Preoperative roentgen therapy for cancer of the rectum and rectosigmoid. *Surg. Gynecol. Obstet.* 138:584, 1974.

84. Roswit B., Higgins G.A. Jr., Keehn R.J.: Preoperative irradiation for carcinoma of the rectum and rectosigmoid colon: Report of a national Veterans Administration randomized study. *Cancer* 35:1597, 1975.

85. Higgins G.A. Jr.: Adjuvant radiation therapy in colon cancer. *Int. Adv. Surg. Oncol.* 2:1, 1979.

86. Rider W.D., Palmer J.A., Mahoney L.J., et al.: Preoperative irradiation in operable cancer of the rectum: Report of the Toronto trial. *Can. J. Surg.* 20:335, 1977.

87. Cass A.W., Million R.R., Pfaff W.W.: Patterns of recurrence following surgery alone for adenocarcinoma of the colon and rectum. *Cancer* 37:2861, 1976.

88. Gunderson L.L.: Combined irradiation and surgery for rectal and sigmoid carcinoma. *Curr. Probl. Cancer* 1(5):40, 1976.

89. Leaming R.: Radiation therapy in the clinical management of neoplasms of the colon, rectum and anus, in Stearns M.W. Jr. (ed.): *Neoplasms of the Colon, Rectum and Anus.* New York, John Wiley & Sons, 1980, pp. 143–153.

90. Winawer S.J.: Colorectal cancer screening and early diagnosis, in Brodie O.R. (ed.): *Screening and Early Detection of Colorectal Cancer.* Consensus Development Conference Proceedings. Washington, NIH publication no. 80–2075, 1979.

91. Knutson C.O., Max M.H.: Value of colonoscopy in patients with rectal blood loss unexplained by rigid proctosigmoidoscopy and barium contrast enema examinations. *Am. J. Surg.* 139:84, 1980.

92. Knutson C.O., Williams H.C., Max M.H.: Detection of intracolonic lesion by barium contrast enema. The importance of adequate colon preparation to diagnostic accuracy. *J.A.M.A.* 242:2206, 1979.

93. Whiteley H.W. Jr.: Advanced colon and rectum cancer, in Stearns M.W. Jr. (ed.): *Neoplasms of the Colon, Rectum, and Anus.* New York, John Wiley & Sons, 1980, pp. 101–113.

94. MacKeigan J.M., Ferguson J.A.: Prophylactic oophorectomy and colorectal cancer in premenopausal patients. *Dis. Colon Rectum* 22:401, 1979.

95. Polk H.C. Jr., Spratt J.S. Jr.: Recurrent colorectal carcinoma: Detection, treatment and other considerations. *Surgery* 69:9, 1971.

96. Sugarbaker P.H., Zamcheck N., Moore F.D.: Assessment of serial carcinoembryonic antigen (CEA) assays in postoperative detection of recurrent colorectal cancer. *Cancer* 38:2310, 1976.

97. Bland K.I., Polk H.C. Jr.: The apudomas: The concept and associated neoplasms, in Copeland E.M. III (ed.): *Surgical Oncology.* New York, John Wiley & Sons, 1983, pp. 385–422.

98. Moertel C.G., Sauer W.G., Dockerty M.B., et al.: Life history of the carcinoid tumor of the small intestine. *Cancer* 14:901, 1961.

99. Crowder B.L. II, Judd E.S., Dockerty M.B.: Gastrointestinal carcinoids and the carcinoid syndrome: Clinical characteristics and therapy. *Surg. Clin. North Am.* 47(4):915, 1967.

100. Bates H.R. Jr.: Carcinoid tumors of the rectum. *Dis. Colon Rectum* 5:270, 1962.

101. Quan S.H.O., Bader G., Berg J.W.: Carcinoid tumors of the rectum. *Dis. Colon Rectum* 7:197, 1964.

102. Mengel C.E.: Malignant carcinoid: Effect of parenteral methotrexate (NSC-740) therapy alone and in combination with cyclophosphamide (NSC-26271) orally. *Cancer Chemother. Rep.* 51:239, 1967.

103. Schein P., Kahn R., Gorden P., et al.: Streptozotocin for malignant insulinomas and carcinoid tumor: Report of eight cases and review of the literature. *Arch. Intern. Med.* 132:555, 1973.

104. Davis Z., Moertel C.G., McIlrath D.C.: The malignant carcinoid syndrome. *Surg. Gynecol. Obstet.* 137:637, 1973.

105. Fry D.E., Amin M., Harbrecht P.J.: Rectal obstruction secondary to carcinoma of the prostate. *Ann. Surg.* 189:488, 1979.

106. Spjut H.J., Perkins D.E.: Endometriosis of the sigmoid colon and rectum. *A.J.R.* 82:1070, 1959.

46

Benign and Premalignant Lesions of the Large Intestine

Kirby I. Bland, M.D.
Edward M. Copeland III, M.D.

The prevalence, morbidity, and mortality of cancer of the colon and anus make this disease worthy of attention and surveillance. Despite remarkable refinements in surgical techniques, and innovative diagnostic and therapeutic approaches with the advent of colonoscopy, radioimmunoassay methodology, and advancements in radiotherapeutic and chemotherapeutic principles, the age-adjusted death rate for cancer of the colon and anus was static for the American male for three decades.

Recent data from surveys conducted by the Commission on Cancer of the American College of Surgeons suggest that cancer care in the United States has adapted rapidly to these advances in technology and to the findings of the research community.[1] The clinical stage of disease for colorectal carcinoma was observed to change little between 1973 and 1978; however, a significant change toward earlier stage of disease at diagnosis was observed for certain ethnic groups. The increasing application of multimodal diagnostic and therapeutic measures for colorectal neoplasms portends the capability for diagnosis of benign and premalignant neoplasms prior to development of an invasive or metastatic clinical stage. This chapter reviews the contemporary efforts available to diagnose and treat the multiplicity of benign and malignant neoplasms common to the mucosa of the colorectum and anus.

NEOPLASTIC POLYPS

The term "polyp" (Greek *poly* ["many"] and *pous* ["foot"]) denotes a focal (localized) tissue mass which projects into the lumen of the bowel. These neoplasms are an important consideration in the genesis of cancer of the colon, rectum, and anus. Because of their intraluminal position, polyps can initiate a multiplicity of symptoms and may be characteristically associated with specific hereditary and nonfamilial syndromes. To conceptualize thoroughly the carcinogenic potential and the varying presentations of specific polyps, one must appreciate the pathogenesis and the natural history of distinct pathologic classifications for these benign and malignant neoplasms. Table 46–1 characterizes the various types of polyps which take origin from the mucosa of the colon and rectum. Classically, *neoplastic polyps* may be tubular (adenomatous), tubulovillous (mixed), or villous adenomas and may share fea-

tures as a malignant variant with carcinoma *in situ* (intramucosal) or can be invasive, with extension through the muscularis mucosae. In distinction, the *nonneoplastic polyp* is characteristically of hamartomatous (mixed mesodermal) or inflammatory origin (Fig 46–1). An additional classification distinguishes the polyp which represents normal mucosal excrescence (hyperplastic/metaplastic) from those of submucosal etiology (carcinoids, metastatic, and heterotopic origin).

Tubular Adenoma (Adenomatous Polyps)

INCIDENCE.—*Tubular adenomas* are the most common neoplastic polyps of the mucosa of the colon and rectum. These circumscribed proliferations of benign epithelium are observed to increase in frequency with aging and occur approximately eight times more frequently than villous adenomas. The majority (80%) are located in the rectosigmoid with a uniform distribution in the remaining proximal colon. The best estimate of frequency suggests that approximately 5% of adults have colorectal mucosa that harbors at least one tubular adenoma. Remarkable variations of the distribution of this polyp within the various segments of the colon and rectum are apparent, and this distribution varies with genetic, environmental, and ethnic background.

In an extensive review of 1,856 adenomas and papillomas of colonic and rectal mucosa in 1,335 patients, Grinnell and Lane[2] noted multiplicity in 26% of the patients with tubular adenomas. In 311 patients with a separate coexisting carcinoma, 34% had multiple polyps. In 17% of the cases in which carcinomas were not found, polyps were observed to be multiple. Site of origin was sigmoid in 51.0%, rectum 28.4%, cecum or ascending colon 5.6%, transverse colon 7.4%, and splenic flexure or descending colon 6.8%. As with villous adenomas and carcinomas, a major portion of tubular adenomas appear to be within reach of the 25-cm proctoscope. Autopsy studies of patients dying of noncolonic tumors have demonstrated a more even distribution of tubular adenomas throughout the colon when compared to other colonic neoplasms.

HISTOLOGY.—Typically, the tubular adenoma is a firm, pedunculated (68%) growth of densely-packed colonic glands that may resemble normal colonic epithelium (Fig 46–2,A),

TABLE 46–1.—CLASSIFICATION FOR
POLYPS OF COLORECTAL ORIGIN

Neoplastic polyps
  Adenoma
    Tubular (adenomatous)
    Tubulovillous (papillary, mixed)
    Villous
  Familial Adenomatous polyposis syndromes
    Multiple familial polyposis
    Gardner's syndrome
    Oldfield syndrome
    Turcot's syndrome
    Muir's (Torre's) syndrome
  Nonfamilial polyposis syndromes
    Cronkhite-Canada syndrome
Nonneoplastic polyps
  Hamartomatous (mixed mesodermal) polyposes
    Juvenile (mucus retention) polyp
    Juvenile polyposis syndrome
    Peutz-Jeghers syndrome
    Neurofibromas (von Recklinghausen's disease)
    Lipomas
    Leiomyomas
    Hemangiomas
  Inflammatory polyps (pseudopolyps)
    Inflammatory polyp
    Benign lymphoid polyp
    Colitis cystica profunda/superficialis
Additional (unclassified) polypoid lesions
  Hyperplastic (metaplastic)
  Pneumatosis cystoides intestinalis
  Carcinoids
  Metastatic (submucosal) tumors
  Heterotopic (endometriosis)

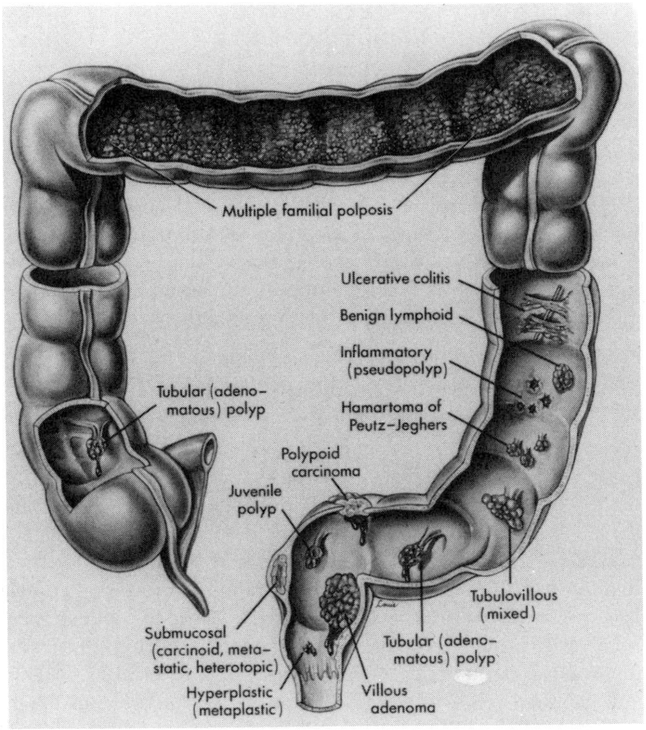

Fig 46–1.—Morphological variations of polyps and polypoid lesions of mucosal and submucosal origin in the colon and rectum.

while variants show loss of goblet cell mucin, branching of glands, and variable amounts of nuclear atypia (Fig 46–2,B). The average size of adenomatous polyps is 1.2 cm (range, 0.2–7.0 cm).[2] The pedunculated tubular adenoma has a stalk bridged with normal large-bowel mucosa and includes an uninterrupted projection of the muscularis mucosae (Fig 46–3). Blood vessels, lymphatics, and connective tissues provide nutrient supply and support to the head of the polyp, occupy the submucosal position, and are in direct continuity with the submucosa of the contiguous bowel. This morphological feature is of great importance in considering the polyp-carcinoma hypothesis. The adenomatous epithelium is superficial to the muscularis mucosa in all tubular adenomas, and invasion of the muscularis mucosae represents the pathologic criterion of an invasive malignancy. According to Lipkin,[3] tubular and villous adenomas occur as a result of failure of the maturation process during cellular proliferation and differentiation. In phase I, colonic epithelial cells incompletely repress the synthesis of DNA, and resultant proliferative components of the cellular compartments expand onto the mucosal surface. The normal mucosal surface is smooth, and the cell production rate equates with the rate of cell extrusion (Fig 46–4). In phase II, undifferentiated cells of the epithelium initiate growth on the mucosal surface with resultant retention of this undifferentiated cell population, now recognized as a polypoid growth. Lipkin noted the phase II lesion in pure tubular adenomas, while the phase I proliferative lesion was present in the morphologically normal-appearing mucosa of subjects who subsequently developed adenomas. Phase I lesions were also present in the apparently normal mucosa of affected family members with familial polyposis who had not yet developed polyps. This clinicopathologic observation suggests that mutational, proliferative, and differentiational events of colonic mucosal cells initiate growth of mucosal polyps.

The average size of a colorectal polyp is < 1 cm, and the majority are purely *tubular* representing 77% of the polyps in the series reported by Muto et al.[4] (Table 46–2). In lesions > 2 cm, the *tubulovillous* adenoma was noted approximately 50% of the time, the remainder being purely *villous*. The tubulovillous or papillary adenoma represents a mixture of the histologic features of the tubular and villous types. This intermediate pattern of growth has branching villous processes with a substantial proportion of tubular epithelium (Fig 46–5). The villous component has a higher degree of dysplasia and atypia and, thus, may be more frequently associated with carcinoma. These polyps may have foci of cells that have irregular nuclei, loss of polarity, and cribriform glands within densely-packed cell populations. Loss of normal histologic features leads to the interpretation of a malignant foci. The polyp contains carcinoma *in situ* when only the epithelial component is involved without evidence of extension through the muscularis mucosae to the lymphovascular supply. Day and Morson[5] noted carcinoma *in situ* in 10% of tubular polyps, mild atypia in 60%, and moderate atypia in 30%. An increasing probability of atypia and carcinomatous transformation parallels an increasing size of the polyp[4, 5] (Table 46–3).

CLINICAL PRESENTATION.—The majority of patients with tubular or mixed tubulovillous adenomas are asymptomatic or have nonspecific symptoms relative to the GI tract. The most common symptom is bleeding per rectum or occult

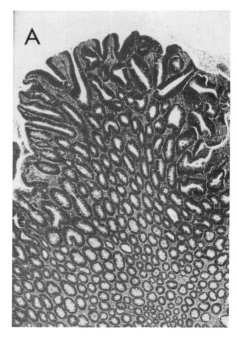

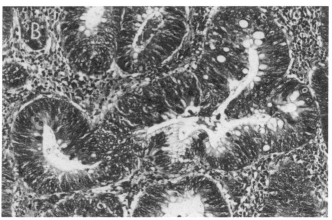

Fig 46–2.—Tubular (adenomatous) adenoma. **A,** closely-packed glands with crowded nuclei and variable amounts of mucin; ×40. **B,** moderate atypia (dysplasia) in tubular adenoma revealing marked cellular stratification with enlarged vesicular nuclei; ×100. (Courtesy D.A. Franzlni, Department of Pathology, University of Florida.)

hemorrhage with hematochezia. The frequency, duration, and amount of blood loss is difficult to correlate with size of the polyp. Stool guaiac testing of an asymptomatic population will lead to false positive evaluation in approximately one half the patients, while false negative results will be obtained in an undetermined proportion of people with proved adenomatous polyps later confirmed by barium enema, sigmoidoscopy, or colonoscopy.[6, 7] Port wine or mahogany-colored, blood-tinged stool suggests origin from the cecum or right colon, whereas bright red blood per rectum indicates origin from the left colon, rectum, or anus. Rarely, large adenomatous or mixed tubulovillous polyps may initiate colicky, hypogastric, abdominal pain as a result of intermittent intussusception. The large stalked polyp which arises proximal to the dentate line may infrequently present with prolapse through the anus and be thought initially to be a prolapsed hemorrhoid. As the majority of these lesions are asymptomatic, their presence is confirmed via adjunctive diagnostic procedures; e.g., sigmoidoscopy, colonoscopy, or barium enema (Fig 46–6).

Villous Adenoma

INCIDENCE.—The villous adenoma is most commonly solitary. In the series by Grinnell and Lane,[2] only 8 (3.7%) of 216 patients had multiple villous adenomas. Of these 216 patients, 10% were associated with synchronous cancers of the colon or rectum and an additional 30% had concomitant tubular adenomas. Overall, of 1,856 neoplastic polyps analyzed, pure villous tumors comprised 11.6% of the series. The villous adenoma occurs most commonly during the sixth decade of life and rarely occurs in patients under the age of 45.

HISTOLOGY.—Unlike tubular adenomas, the villous counterpart assumes a gross cauliflower-like appearance (Fig 46–7). These soft, smooth, velvety projections have frondlike processes. No appreciable extension of the muscularis mucosae into the villous process is detectable, and a sparse core of delicate connective tissue is identifiable (Fig 46–8). The pure villous lesion is usually confined to the sigmoid or rectum; only 15% originate in the proximal colon. The average diameter of these lesions is 3.7 cm (range 0.5–9.0 cm), much larger than their tubular counterparts.[2] Also, the villous adenoma has a much greater probability of harboring an *in situ* or invasive carcinoma. In the series by Muto et al.[4] and Day and Morson,[5] 53% of villous adenomas > 2 cm were histologically malignant (Table 46–4). These specimens were all removed surgically. In a more recent colonoscopic series,[8] 38% of villous adenomas > 2 cm contained carcinoma; the incidence fell to ≤ 5% for smaller lesions. This frequency repre-

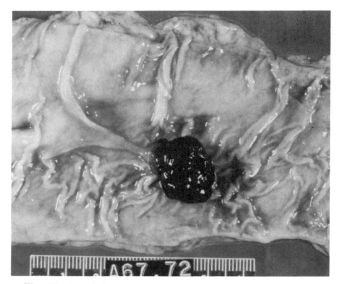

Fig 46–3.—A benign pedunculated tubular adenoma of the colon in which infarction of the head of the polyp has occurred. (Courtesy D.A. Franzini, Department of Pathology, University of Florida.)

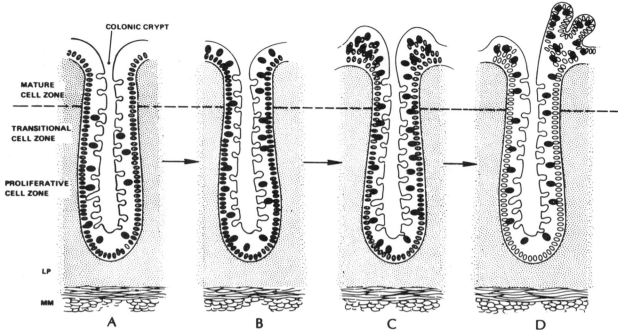

Fig 46–4.—Epithelial proliferation in colonic polyps. One sequence of events to account for the location of abnormally proliferating colonic epithelial cells before and during the formation of polypoid neoplasms in man. *A,* the location of proliferating and differentiating epithelial cells in the normal colonic crypt. Dark cells illustrate thymidine labeling in cells that are synthesizing DNA and preparing to undergo cell division. As cells pass from the proliferative zone through the transitional zone, DNA synthesis and mitosis are repressed, and migrating epithelial cells leave the proliferative cell cycle to undergo normal maturation before they reach the surface of the mucosa. *B,* the development of a phase 1 proliferative lesion in colonic epithelial cells as they fail to repress the incorporation of ^{3}H-thymidine into DNA and begin to develop an enhanced ability to proliferate. The mucosa is flat and the number of new cells born equals the number extruded, without an excess cell accumulation in the mucosa. *C,* the development of a phase 2 proliferative lesion in colonic epithelial cells. The cells incorporate ^{3}H-thymidine into DNA and also have developed additional properties that enable them to accumulate in the mucosa in increasing numbers. *D,* further development of abnormally retained, proliferating epithelial cells into pathologically defined, neoplastic lesions including tubular and villous adenomas. (From Lipkin M.: *Cancer* 34:878, 1974. Used by permission.)

sents an almost tenfold increase of the presence of malignancy in villous adenomas compared with the tubular lesion. Additionally, these data support the increased risk of malignancy developing in any villous adenoma (approximately 10%) with an increase in this frequency as the size of the lesion increases. Although histologic type and size are not independent of each other (see Table 46–4), a third factor, degree of dysplasia, contributes to the probability of malignant transformation (see Table 46–3).

CLINICAL PRESENTATION.—The large surface area of the villous tumor in contact with the fecal stream initiates discharge of mucus or blood from the anus. On occasion, the patient may present with tenesmus or the sensation of inadequate evacuation of rectal contents. Patients with large circumferential villous tumors may present with obstruction, constipation, and abdominal cramps. McKittrick and Wheelock[9] characterized the rare syndrome of profuse mucous diarrhea, electrolyte and water depletion with circulatory collapse associated with metabolic acidosis, and prerenal azotemia. This syndrome, which is perhaps mediated by the prostaglandin E_2 secretagogue from the villous tumor,[10] initiates secretion of large quantities (e.g., 2–3 L/day) of electrolyte-rich fluid into the colonic lumen. The concentration of sodium and chloride in this fluid is isotonic; however, the potassium concentration is 4- to 20-fold that of plasma. Thus, hypokalemia and hypochloremia are common, and, on occasion, hyponatremia is observed. Rapid resuscitation with replacement of this profound desalting water loss is necessary to obviate the cardiovascular events which follow potassium and intravascular depletion. Infusion of as great as 1,000 mEq of potassium chloride daily may be necessary to replace these inordinately severe losses.

In the great majority of villous adenomas, diagnosis is confirmed by direct visualization and biopsy of the villous neoplasm. Multiple biopsies from the tumor surface and the junc-

TABLE 46–2.—RELATIONSHIP OF SIZE AND HISTOLOGIC TYPE OF TUMOR (2,489 TUMORS)

TYPE OF TUMOR	SIZE, MM (%)		
	< 10 (n = 1479)	10–20 (n = 580)	> 20 (n = 430)
Tubular adenoma	76.6	19.7	3.7
Intermediate (tubulovillous)	24.7	46.8	28.5
Villous adenoma	14.0	25.7	60.3

Adapted from Muto T., Bussey H.J.R., Morson B.C.: The evolution of cancer of the colon and rectum. *Cancer* 36:2251–2270, 1975.

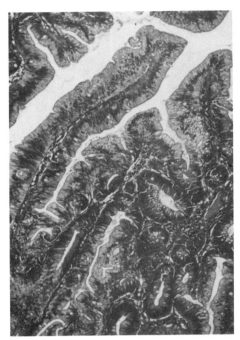

Fig 46–5.—Tubulovillous (villoglandular, mixed) adenoma. Typical tubular structures are admixed with slender villa, ×100. (Courtesy D.A. Franzini, Department of Pathology, University of Florida.)

ture of the lesions with presumably normal colorectal mucosa are advised to identify the coexistence of *in situ* or invasive carcinoma. The presence of villous tumors noted on air-contrast barium enema, proximal to the reach of the sigmoidoscope, necessitates colonoscopic inspection and biopsy. A diagnostic clue to a possible invasive cancer within a villous adenoma is "puckering" of the serosa beneath the adenoma as viewed on barium enema. This radiologic finding should elicit a strong suspicion of invasion within the polyp.

THE HYPOTHETICAL RELATIONSHIP OF THE NEOPLASTIC ADENOMA AND CARCINOMA

Until the late 1950s, all neoplastic polyps of the colorectum were considered premalignant tumors. As noted above, retrospective analyses suggested that the risk of these lesions' harboring invasive carcinoma directly correlated with size, his-

TABLE 46–3.—ADENOMATOUS POLYPS AND VILLOUS ADENOMAS: PERCENT OF CARCINOMA IN RELATION TO SIZE AND GRADE OF ATYPIA

| | SIZE | | |
GRADE OF ATYPIA	Under 1 cm	1–2 cm	Over 2 cm
Mild	0.3 (1,198)*	3.0 (329)	42.3 (196)
Moderate	2.0 (244)	14.4 (167)	50.0 (134)
Severe	27.0 (37)	24.1 (83)	48.0 (100)

*( ) = No. of specimens evaluated.
Adapted from Muto T., Bussey H.J.R., Morson B.C.: The evolution of cancer of the colon and rectum. *Cancer* 36:2251–2270, 1975.

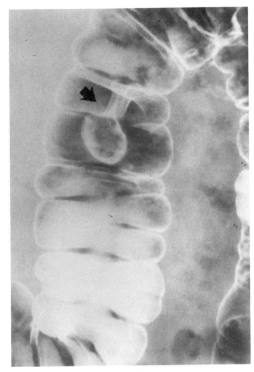

Fig 46–6.—Air-contrast barium enema spot view of stalked tubular (adenomatous) polyp of distal transverse colon. (Courtesy F. Clore, VA Medical Center, University of Florida.)

tologic cell type, and the presence of dysplasia or atypia within the polyp.[4, 5, 8] The observations of many investigators support the hypothesis that the majority of carcinomas of the colon arise in neoplastic epthelial adenomas that have undergone transformation from well-differentiated to poorly differentiated lesions over a considerable interval of time. Boland and Kim[11] noted that: (1) tiny, isolated colonic cancers are

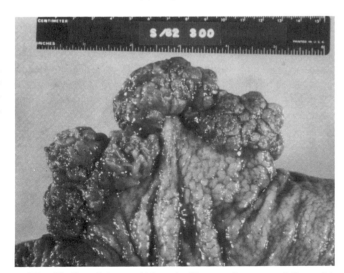

Fig 46–7.—A large (13-cm) villous adenoma of the mid- and terminal rectal mucosa. This extensive lesion presented with symptoms of partial obstruction.

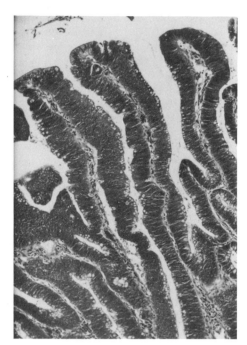

Fig 46–8.—Villous adenoma. Slender, finger-like villous projections within a delicate fibrovascular stalk; ×100. (Courtesy D.A. Franzini, Department of Pathology, University of Florida.)

rarely observed. Indeed, foci of carcinoma are usually found within tubular polyps; (2) patients who subsequently develop carcinoma often have had antecedent tubular polyps that predate the cancer by 10–15 years; and (3) both neoplastic adenomas and carcinomas have common epidemiologic and pathogenetic factors in their etiology. Additionally, in *multiple adenomatous polyposis syndromes*, these benign adenomas antedate the development of cancer by an average of 10–12 years. In the absence of multiple adenomatous polyposis, residual adenomatous tissue will be found surrounding the malignant neoplasm in the great majority of instances in which an early (*in situ* or invasive) cancer is observed.[12] As suggested by Correa and colleagues,[13] epidemiologic studies note that the patient group with the highest incidence of colonic neoplastic polyps is also the same group with the highest incidence of colon cancer. Further, the administration of colonic carcinogens to experimental animals initiates focal atypia and dysplasia to act as a carcinogenic substrate, which may

TABLE 46–4.—ADENOMATOUS POLYPS AND VILLOUS ADENOMAS: SIZE, HISTOLOGIC TYPE, AND PERCENT OF CARCINOMA

| | SIZE | | | |
TYPE OF TUMOR	Under 1 cm (n = 1,479)	1–2 cm (n = 580)	Over 2 cm (n = 430)	% Total
Tubular adenoma	1.0 (1,382)*	10.2 (392)	34.7 (101)	5
Intermediate type	3.9 (76)	7.4 (149)	45.8 (155)	23
Villous adenoma	9.5 (21)	10.3 (39)	52.9 (174)	41

*( ) = No. of specimens evaluated.
Adapted from Muto T., Bussey H.J.R., Morson B.C.: The evolution of cancer of the colon and rectum. *Cancer* 36:2251–2270, 1975.

induce the development of invasive carcinoma.[14]

Each of these observations supports the hypothesis that the majority of colon carcinomas originate within previously benign adenomas. This hypothesis of progressive stages of ontogeny, however, has its opponents. Spratt et al.[15] questioned the close correlation between the site and incidence of adenomatous polyps and carcinoma and advanced the alternative hypothesis that adenomas in the colon arise *de novo* and remain so or represent carcinomas *ab initio*. Berge et al.[16] and Ekelund and Lindström[17] reconfirmed the even distribution of neoplastic polyps throughout the colon yet observed that the maximal incidence of carcinoma was found in the sigmoid colon and rectum. Castleman and Krickstein[18] suggested that three histologic errors were responsible for the common assumption that tubular adenomas undergo malignant transformation: (1) polypoid carcinoma can arise *ab initio* with no evidence of origin from underlying benign polyps (these data were substantiated by Spratt and Ackerman,[19] who reported no evidence of origin of 20 small carcinomas of the colon (< 2 cm in diameter) from benign tubular polyps); (2) a common error of histologic distinction between adenomas and villous tumors exists, as the latter neoplasm has a much higher probability of malignant change; and (3) errors of interpretation exist among pathologists for the significance of apparent carcinomatous changes within adenomatous polyps. They further challenged the significance of foci of "atypism" for diagnosing *in situ* lesions when penetration of the lamina propria had not occurred. Castleman and Krickstein[18] suggest that if strict vigilance is exercised by the pathologist to discourage these errors, few circumstances of carcinomatous transformation will be demonstrable in tubular adenomas.

Grinnell and Lane[2] discovered histologic evidence of lymph node metastasis in one of 27 cases of tubular polyps with invasive carcinoma treated by colonic resection. Lockhart-Mummery and Dukes[20] followed 47 patients having malignant transformation in tubular polyps for 2–18 years after surgical polypectomy. No recurrences were observed in any patients with focal atypia or carcinoma *in situ*. However, 30% of the tubular polyps with coexisting invasive carcinoma developed recurrence in the colon wall. In an additional 10%, metastases developed in the regional, inguinal, and mesenteric lymphatics in the absence of local recurrence at the former site of the colonic polyps. Each of these observations indicates that malignant cells which penetrate the muscularis mucosae have metastatic potential.

The activity of hydrolytic, proteolytic, and respiratory enzymes in cells of normal colonic mucosa, tubular polyps, carcinoma *in situ*, and invasive adenocarcinomas suggests a trend toward the diminution of these enzymes with transformation to polyps and carcinoma.[21, 22] Phase I proliferative colonic epithelial cells that fail to repress incorporation of ^{3}H-thymidine into DNA develop an enhanced proliferative capability.[3] With the development of the phase II proliferative lesion, these same cells greatly accumulate in the mucosa. The final event for the phase II lesion was retention of these abnormal cells and the development of an identifiable neoplastic polyp. Although arguments for and against the polyp-carcinoma hypothesis can be formulated, we conclude from histochemical, pathologic, and clinical observations that invasive carcinoma can develop in benign adenomatous polyps. Goligher[23] acknowledges that the transformation of tubular polyps from a benign to a malignant state is probably rarer than has been previously suggested, and that they may be safely treated by conservative therapy. Tubular polyps indicate a diffusely abnormal state of the large bowel mucosa and render it more prone to genesis of additional epithelial tumors of benign or malignant cell types, the so-called neoplasm prone colon.

THE TREATMENT OF NEOPLASTIC POLYPS

The neoplastic polyp within reach of the rigid sigmoidoscope should be completely excised for pathologic analysis. The application of flexible fiberoptic colonoscopy has particular merit for lesions proximal to the range of visualization by sigmoidoscopy. These more proximal lesions are usually identified by air-contrast barium enema. The recent introduction of the flexible fiberoptic sigmoidoscope with 30-cm and 60-cm lengths allows accurate examination of the rectum and proximal sigmoid colon, with access to the distal descending colon. Thus, with this instrument direct visualization is possible of the colorectal mucosa where approximately 60%–70% of benign polyps and carcinomas originate.

Tubular or mixed tubulovillous polyps in the rectum or distal sigmoid within reach of the rigid or flexible sigmoidoscope can be directly visualized and totally excised. This may be accomplished by use of a diathermy snare. These polyps commonly have a distinct stalk which projects into the bowel lumen, facilitating total excision. Sessile polyps of any histology may be difficult to totally excise, especially if >1.5 cm. Sessile lesions 5–10 mm may be snared and fulgurated to control excessive blood loss. Retrieval of the polyp is critical to provide adequate pathologic study. Stools should be meticulously strained following loss of the polyp in the retrieval effort after excisional biopsy.

Simple polypectomy is considered adequate therapy for tubular or villous lesions which contain foci of *in situ* carcinoma; i.e., the muscularis mucosae has not been penetrated by malignant cells. It has been well established that metastases do not occur from polyps with *in situ* carcinoma, as no lymphatics have been identified in the epithelium above the muscularis mucosae. A therapeutic dilemma may be created by evidence of invasion of the head of the polyp with penetration of the muscularis mucosae and invasion of the submucosa. Identification of this pathologic finding should be sought diligently in all polyps. For *pedunculated* polyps, Shatney et al.[24] maintain that local removal via polypectomy is sufficient for polyps with foci of cancer limited to the head of the polyp. They believe that radical resection of the involved bowel should be done for all *pedunculated* polyps when: (1) the cancer is highly undifferentiated; (2) the blood or lymphatic vessels within the head of the polyp contain malignant cells; (3) the peduncle is extremely short, and malignant transformation extends to the neck of the adenoma; and (4) carcinoma extends to the base of the peduncle or the lesion represents a polypoid carcinoma (the entire polyp is malignant). For *sessile* lesions, standard radical resections are indicated when the muscularis mucosae is invaded by malignant cells. In this circumstance, lesser operations have a higher risk for local recurrence and distant metastatic spread. For villous tumors that present as broad-based sessile lesions (>1.5–2 cm), re-

section of the polyp with the contiguous bowel wall and mesentery is indicated. For *invasive* lesions in the rectal canal that are less than 7 cm above the dentate line, combined abdominoperineal resection is recommended. Villous adenomas harboring *atypia* (Fig 46–9) or carcinoma *in situ* require only local extirpation. These *noninvasive* lesions can be excised transanally or via posterior or lateral-transsacral approaches. Emphasis must be placed, however, on total excision of the lesion with a rim of normal mucosa.

Dilemmas may arise with the presentation of *nonfamilial polyposis*, tubular in type. Fiberoptic endoscopic polypectomy is recommended for the poor-risk patient, who then requires vigilant reexamination and air-contrast studies in follow-up. Serious consideration should be given to subtotal colectomy in the good-risk patient with nonfamilial polyposis, especially if these lesions are multiple and are larger than 1.5 cm in size. This approach is also indicated for subjects with associated villous tumors. In all circumstances, an aggressive approach is indicated when the risk of malignant invasion and of metastases outweigh the morbidity and mortality risk of operation. In frail patients, the most prudent therapeutic course is interval endoscopic polypectomy with reservation of colonic resection for invasive neoplasms.

HEREDITARY SYNDROMES

Familial Polyposis Coli (Multiple Familial Polyposis)

This familial disorder is inherited as a dominant mendelian trait which is not sex-linked. Familial polyposis coli (FPC) is

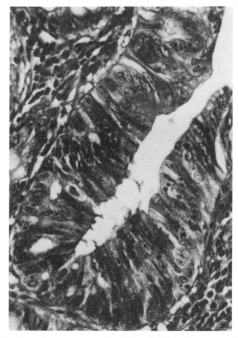

Fig 46–9.—Severe atypia (dysplasia) from section of a large villous adenoma of rectum. Microscopically, there is complete loss of cellular polarity. Identifiable are large, vesicular nuclei, prominent nucleoli, and numerous mitotic figures; ×200. (Courtesy D.A. Franzini, Department of Pathology, University of Florida.)

characterized by the development of hundreds of tubular adenomas (Fig 46–10) throughout the entire colon and rectum, and the development of associated intestinal cancer is an inevitable consequence of the natural history of FPC. The appearance of carcinoma postdates the onset of polyposis by some 10–15 years. The average number of tumors in the colon and rectum approaches 1,000 (range 150–5,000). The figure of 100 adenomas has been suggested as a convenient method to distinguish between FPC and the nonfamilial condition termed "multiple adenomas."

CLINICAL PRESENTATION.—The most common early symptoms are increasing bowel motility with the frequent passage of mucus and blood. Persons with FPC are usually asymptomatic until postadolescence, at which time polyps may appear. Winawer[25] noted the average age for the appearance of polyps and symptoms to be 25 years and 33 years, respectively. Average age for diagnosis of FPC was 36 years; of cancer, 39 years; and death from cancer, 42 years. The initial appearance of asymptomatic polyps antedates the clinical syndrome by eight to ten years. Intestinal cancer is estimated to occur in approximately two thirds of patients presenting for the first time. Cancer usually develops ten years following onset of symptoms from tubular adenoma.[25, 26] Predictably, the presence of large numbers of neoplastic polyps (Fig 46–11) enhances the probability of multiple, synchronous carcinomas of the colon and rectum. Bussey[26, 27] estimates that nearly one half of the polyposis patients with associated malignant disease have more than one carcinoma. These carcinomas are considered to have the same malignant virulence and a similar distribution within the colon as in the general population. Sex distribution of FPC is similar.

DISTINCTION OF FPC AND NONFAMILIAL MULTIPLE POLYPOSIS COLI SYNDROME.—Moertel and associates[28] were the first to recognize that patients with adenomatous polyposis coli of a nonfamilial type characteristically have absence of rectal involvement with polyposis. Additionally, the nonfamilial variant tends to have later onset of multiple polyposis and a bias toward the male sex of affected subjects. It is rare for rectal carcinoma to develop in the nonfamilial multiple polyposis syndromes.

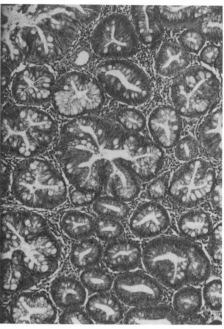

Fig 46–11.—Typical polyp of familial polyposis coli. Characteristic adenomatous polyp with tubular glands closely packed with crowded nuclei and variable amounts of mucin; ×100. (Courtesy D.A. Franzini, M.D., Department of Pathology, University of Florida.)

TREATMENT OF FAMILIAL POLYPOSIS COLI.—The presence of > 100 polyps on air-contrast barium enema (Fig 46–12) with visualization of tubular polyps via sigmoidoscopy or colonoscopy substantiates the working diagnosis. DeCosse et al.[29] described the efficacy of ascorbic acid to initiate regression of rectal polyposis. This approach would appear to have benefit for subjects with FPC who demand preservation of their rectum after colon resection. The most favored procedure for familial polyposis is total abdominal colectomy, proctectomy, and permanent ileostomy. The compliant patient who desires preservation of the rectal stump and who has an absence of rectal polyps may be treated with subtotal

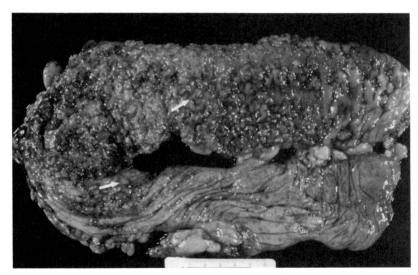

Fig 46–10.—Descending colon, sigmoid, and rectum in patient with familial polyposis coli following total abdominal colectomy and proctectomy. *Arrows* denote small tubular adenomas which occupy the mucosal surface of the entire abdominal colon. Note the abrupt disappearance of polypoid lesions in the terminal sigmoid with sparing of mucosal involvement of the rectum.

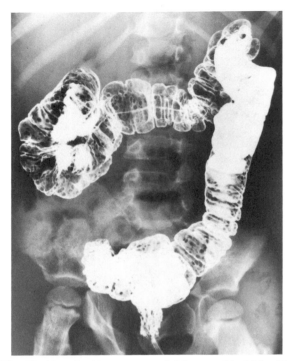

Fig 46–12.—Barium enema of 14-year-old child with familial polyposis coli. The entire colon and rectum have replacement of the mucosal surface with thousands of tubular adenomas. (Courtesy J. Williams, M.D., Department of Radiology, University of Florida.)

colectomy and ileorectal anastomosis. Follow-up sigmoidoscopy of the rectal stump is essential to remove developing polyps and to identify early carcinomatous transformation of these familial neoplastic polyps. Despite vigorous surveillance attempts to identify and fulgurate new polyps in the retained rectal segment, Moertel et al.[28] observed rectal cancer to develop in 22% of patients over a 5–23-year follow-up interval. Additionally, the prognosis for patients who subsequently developed carcinoma was poor (25% five-year survival) despite semi-annual sigmoidoscopic examinations. These data reinforce a more radical approach with total abdominal proctocolectomy and ileostomy. These authors advocate anorectal salvage only when patients have an absence of rectal polypoid lesions and insist on rectal preservation. This aggressive management approach was not supported by Stearns[30] and Morson and Dawson,[31] who observed a much lower frequency of carcinoma in the rectal stump. A conservative effort appeared justifiable so long as the patient returned for interval examination, and expeditious polypectomy could be done for lesions that were identified subsequently.

The discrepancy in the surgical literature over the exact incidence of subsequent rectal carcinoma in patients who undergo colectomy and ileorectal anastomosis was evaluated by Gingold and Jagelman.[32] On the basis of these authors' experience and the reported work of others, they identified five factors that potentially influence the development of carcinoma in the retained rectum in subjects with familial polyposis. These factors include: (1) the patient's *age* at the time of colectomy. They suggest that early surgical intervention, with

removal of the colon at an age before the natural history of the disease results in malignant degeneration, may reduce the risk of subsequent rectal cancer; (2) the *length of the retained colonic segment.* Data suggest that retention of part of the sigmoid colon may play a role in altering the environment of the rectum to enhance development of polyps and subsequent cancer; (3) the tendency of *spontaneous regression* of polyps in the retained rectum. This occurs more commonly with ileorectal than with ileosigmoid anastomosis; (4) the presence of carcinoma in the excised colon; and (5) the adequacy of patient follow-up in the postoperative period. This analysis provides some clarification on the apparent discrepancies in the aforementioned surgical series. We agree that the risk for development of rectal carcinoma following ileorectal anastomosis is real but, perhaps, overstated. The dogmatic approach of proctocolectomy for asymptomatic relatives with the disease initiates the concerns of permanent ileostomy, micturition dysfunction, and sexual impotence. For these reasons, we favor the more conservative total abdominal colectomy with ileorectal anastomosis combined with a formalized follow-up evaluation.

The recent technical refinements of *mucosal proctectomy* with *endorectal ileoanal anastomosis* for preservation of sphincteric function are encouraging. Beart et al.[33] reported good to excellent physiologic function and results in 77% of 39 evaluable patients with the ileoanal anastomosis performed for FPC, Crohn's, or ulcerative colitis. The description of the ileal pouch-anal anastomosis by Parks and Nicholls[34] has improved the clinical results following colectomy and mucosal proctectomy compared to the straight ileoanal anastomosis. This technical approach is appropriate for suitable patients desirous of preservation of sphincteric and sexual function, and in whom APR is advisable to obviate rectal mucosal polyps. Taylor et al.[35] evaluated anal sphincter resting pressures in straight and ileal pouch-anal anastomoses. Data suggest that the pouch-anal anastomosis increased distensibility of the neorectum and decreased its propulsive drive. This physiologic advantage allowed an improvement of clinical results.

Gardner's Syndrome

In 1951, Gardner described a syndrome of *intestinal polyposis* and *extracolonic abnormalities.*[36] The syndrome is inherited via an autosomal dominant, nonsex-linked gene of varying penetrance. The disorder begins with adenomatosis of the colon and rectum and invariably progresses to colonic carcinoma. Additionally, the entire small intestine is subject to neoplastic growth of these polyps with occasional involvement of the stomach. Lymphoid hyperplasia in the terminal ileum has also been reported with the syndrome.

The distinguishing feature of this variant of familial polyposis coli is the characteristic involvement of extracolonic sites: (1) bony and cartilaginous tissue tumors (osteomas and exostoses of the mandible, sinuses, and skull), (2) soft tissue tumors (sebaceous or epidermal inclusion cysts), (3) desmoid tumors, (4) dental abnormalities, (5) postoperative mesenteric fibromatosis, and (6) carcinoma of the adrenal and thyroid glands (Fig 46–13).

In contradistinction to FPC, the polyps in *Gardner's syndrome* characteristically are fewer, more diffuse throughout the entire gut, and do not occur until the third or fourth de-

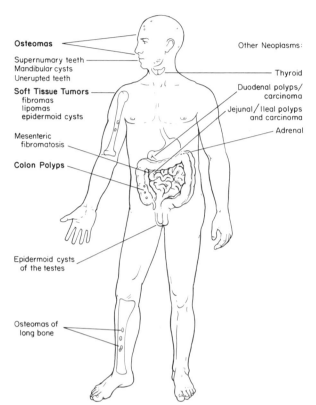

Fig 46–13.—Diagrammatic clinical presentation of Gardner's syndrome. Three primary components of the syndrome are illustrated: (1) GI polyposis, (2) osteomas of the mandible, skull, and long bones, and (3) benign soft tissue tumors (fibromas, lipomas, epidermoid cysts, and mesenteric fibromatosis). Tumors of the thyroid, small bowel, and adrenal glands may represent additional features of the syndrome.

cade of life, with the onset of carcinoma some 10–15 years later. FPC may also have extracolonic stigmas of *Gardner's syndrome,* especially occult osteomas of the mandible, which makes differentiation of the entities difficult.[37, 38] The treatment for *Gardner's syndrome* is essentially identical to that outlined above for FPC.

Therapy of Extracolonic Abnormalities of Gardner's Syndrome

OSTEOMAS.—These extracolonic abnormalities produce cosmetic and functional abnormalities. Their primary presentation is in the mandible, and symptoms may occur in this site prior to recognition of the clinical syndrome. Additional sites of presentation include the skull and long bones. Rarely do these exostoses cause pathologic fractures. Treatment is primarily initiated for cosmetic or functional abnormalities and requires excision of the bony prominence.

DERMOID OR SEBACEOUS CYSTS.—These unsightly cysts or tumors of epidermal origin can represent a major cosmetic or functional disfigurement for the exposed parts of the torso or face, and local excision is the treatment of choice.

DESMOID TUMORS.—These soft tissue lesions arise from the primitive mesenchyme of the musculoaponeurotic sheath

of the rectus abdominus muscle. Extra-abdominal sites include the region of the shoulder and thighs. Desmoids are considered benign lesions with no metastatic potential, yet they have a great propensity for local recurrence. Thus, wide radical excision, to include the musculoaponeurosis contiguous with the enlarging desmoid tumor, represents the treatment of choice. For very large lesions within the abdominal wall, reconstruction with polypropylene mesh and coverage of the tissue defect with musculocutaneous flaps may be required.

INTRA-ABDOMINAL DESMOIDS AND POSTOPERATIVE MESENTERIC FIBROMATOSIS.—Desmoids may originate in retroperitoneal tissues and infiltrate contiguous retroperitoneal and intra-abdominal visceral structures. These benign nonmetastasizing lesions most commonly arise in the small-bowel mesentery and are easily amenable to surgical resection when small. Unfortunately, these lesions often invade contiguous organs and the superior mesenteric vessels. The decision to initiate subtotal or total enterectomy necessitates the commitment to prolonged, continuous total parenteral nutritional (TPN) supplementation. Yet, in otherwise healthy patients, total enterectomy to remove mesenteric fibromatosis has relieved the symptoms of pain and obstruction. In at least three patients managed by one of us (E.M.C.), fibromas have not recurred in a 5–8-year follow-up, although all patients have required long-term TPN.

Additional evidence of the combinations with incomplete phenotypic expressions of *Gardner's syndrome* is the association of colonic polyposis and multiple epidermoid cysts (*Oldfield syndrome*). This variant of polyposis, which may present as diffuse polypoid involvement of the GI tract with a single extracolonic manifestation, suggests that the penetrance of these additional abnormalities is distinctly less than that of the colonic disease.[37]

Rarer Familial Adenomatous Polyposis Syndromes

Another variant of familial polyposis coli is associated with malignant gliomas of the CNS and was described by Turcot et al.[39, 40] in 1959. The mode of inheritance is unclear but has been postulated to be an autosomal recessive, nonsex-linked gene.

The association of familial colonic polyposis and colon cancer with *multiple skin tumors* has been characterized as *Muir's (Torre's) syndrome.* Typically, the skin tumors include basal cell and squamous carcinomas, keratoacanthomas, and sebaceous adenomas.[11, 41] Table 46–5 differentiates the familial and nonfamilial adenomatous polyposis syndromes.

Nonfamilial Adenomatous Polyposis Syndromes

In 1955, Cronkhite and Canada[42] described a syndrome characterized by the development of *diffuse GI polyposis* with associated extraintestinal abnormalities that include hyperpigmentation, nail atrophy, alopecia, hypoproteinemia, edema, cachexia, and depletion of serum potassium and calcium. Initial descriptions of generalized polyposis suggested these lesions were *adenomas.* However, subsequent reports[11, 43] confirm that these intestinal polyps are *inflammatory* with cystic dilatation of the glandular components. These inflammatory lesions may resemble juvenile (retention) polyps and usually

TABLE 46–5.—DIFFERENTIATION OF FAMILIAL AND NONFAMILIAL ADENOMATOUS
POLYPOSIS SYNDROMES

SYNDROME	AGE (DECADE) OF SYMPTOMS	ORGAN(S) INVOLVED	EXTRACOLONIC ABNORMALITIES
Familial			
Polyposis coli	Second-third	Colon	Dental abnormalities
		Rectum	Mandibular osteomas
		Duodenum	
		? Stomach	
Gardner's syndrome	Third-fourth	Colon	Osteomas
		Small bowel	Skull
		Stomach	Mandible
			Long bones
			Exostoses
			Epidermal cysts
			Desmoid tumors
			Mesenteric fibromatosis
			Dental abnormalities
			? Cancer thyroid/adrenals
Oldfield	Fifth	Diffuse GI	Sebaceous cysts
Turcot's syndrome	Third	Colon	Malignant CNS tumors
Muir's (Torre's) syndrome	Third	Colon	Multiple skin tumors
			Basal cell CA
			Squamous cell CA
			Keratoacanthoma
Nonfamilial			
Polyposis coli	Fifth	Colon only	None
Cronkhite-Canada	Sixth	Diffuse GI	Hyperpigmentation
			Alopecia
			Protein-losing enteropathy
			Onychatropy
			Disaccharidase deficiency bowel

affect females in the fifth and sixth decades of life. The condition often is fatal within 18–24 months of onset and is initiated by a chronic, protein-losing enteropathy with associated abnormalities of the integument. The malabsorption defect is progressive and requires vigorous nutritional replacement by the parenteral route. Total parenteral nutrition has been associated with sustained and complete remissions in symptomatic patients.[44] Also, complete remissions have been reported following enteral administration of appropriate nutritional requirements. The chronic diarrhea is, perhaps, initiated by a disaccharidase deficiency and an associated bacterial overgrowth in the small intestine. Antibiotics may be beneficial when superinfection contributes to malabsorption. The role of corticosteroids is controversial, and no available data support their ability to induce remissions.

Surgical resections are indicated when endoscopic excision of the inflammatory polyps cannot be accomplished.[43] Colorectal resections are also indicated for obvious neoplastic transformations in this distressing entity.

NONNEOPLASTIC POLYPS

The *nonneoplastic polyps* are represented by *hamartomas*. These lesions represent polyps composed of an abnormal mixture of primitive tissues normally found in the developing human embryo. Additionally, a predominance of a particular tissue type is often identified.

JUVENILE (MUCUS RETENTION) POLYPS.—These polyps are typically rounded and have a smooth surface with a coarsely lobulated appearance.[45] With endoscopic visualiza-

tion, they have a bright red surface interspersed with patches of cysts filled with mucin. These lesions appear pedunculated, with a very short and narrow stalk. The head of the polyp is rarely larger than 2 cm in diameter.

HISTOLOGY.—The presence of mucin-filled, cystic, glandular spaces separated by lamina propria has initiated the description of *mucus retention polyp* by pathologists (Fig 46–14). Microscopically, the surface of the typical juvenile polyp has a single layer of columnar epithelium interlaced with goblet cells. Epithelial tubules often appear widely separated and may show cystic dilatation and tortuosity. The substance of the polyp is composed primarily of lamina propria.

Juvenile polyps rarely are seen in the first 12 months of life, but are observed most frequently in the prepubertal age group, thus the term *juvenile*. The most prominent histologic feature in support of a hamartomatous theory of origin is the quantitative increase of the lamina propria in comparison with the glandular component of this polyp. These lesions are composed of essentially normal tissues which are abnormally arranged and may have superimposed secondary inflammation, ulceration, and infarction that modify the cytologic and histologic features.

CLINICAL FEATURES.—The great majority of these lesions are multiple and occur in patients who tend to remain asymptomatic. Symptoms are related primarily to ulceration, torsion, inflammation, and autoamputation following infarction. The most common symptomatic presentation is painless rectal bleeding that can be associated with the synchronous passage of the juvenile polyp in the stool. Juvenile polyps that

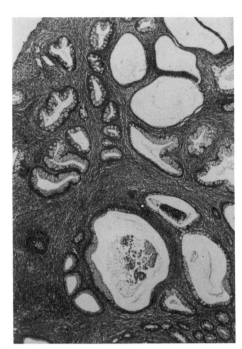

Fig 46–14.—Juvenile (retention) polyp. Microscopically, these hamartomas have cystically-dilated glands embedded in an inflamed stroma; × 40. (Courtesy D.A. Franzini, M.D., Department of Pathology, University of Florida.)

take origin in the anorectum may prolapse through the anus. Iron deficiency anemia may accompany the occult blood loss of multiple juvenile polyps. No evidence exists that isolated juvenile polyps undergo malignant transformation. Excision is curative and recurrence is unlikely.

Juvenile Polyposis Syndrome

This rare entity may be observed in infancy and early childhood (average age six to seven years). Although multiple cases of this syndrome have been reported, it is uncertain whether the entity is one disease with variable genetic penetrance or several different syndromes. Most of the reported cases can conveniently be grouped into one of three classifications: (1) *juvenile polyposis of infancy;* (2) *juvenile polyposis coli,* and (3) *generalized juvenile GI polyposis.*[38] *Juvenile polyposis of infancy* is associated with a high incidence of *congenital abnormalities* and the primary presentation is that of hemorrhage, severe anemia, hypoproteinemia, and failure to thrive. The number of polyps may be several dozen to hundreds. Bussey[27] estimates a familial incidence in approximately one third of the families investigated. While the infant variant is thought to be a recessive trait, the mode of inheritance is poorly documented. Approximately 30% of patients have congenital abnormalities which include malrotation of the bowel, cardiac defects, maldevelopment of the skull, Meckel's diverticulae, and undescended testis. The familial variant has a higher association with these congenital abnormalities. Both familial and nonfamilial variants of juvenile polyposis coli have polyp distribution principally in the rectum and large bowel, although a diffuse origin throughout the GI tract is recognized[38, 45, 46] (Fig 46–15). Thus, these polyps may initi-

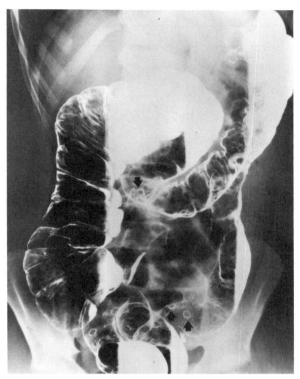

Fig 46–15.—Air-contrast barium enema of a 10-year-old child with familial variant of juvenile polyposis coli. These hamartomatous polyps have diffuse distribution in the mucosa of the entire colon and rectum. *Arrows* (sigmoid and transverse colon) depict the classic air-contrast radiographic appearance. (Courtesy J. Williams, M.D., Department of Radiology, University of Florida.)

ate the symptoms of upper or lower GI hemorrhage, obstruction, or intussusception. The potential risk of cancer for these nonneoplastic polyps is controversial. The association of the familial variant of this syndrome with the increased risk of carcinoma is best explained by the observation of synchronous adenomatous epithelium within the juvenile polyp.[11, 47–49]

The presentation of the polyposis syndrome represents a therapeutic challenge. Excision of the polyp(s) and the contiguous mucosa is required. Thorough inspection of the mucosal surface to identify polyps at proximal and distal sites is essential to abrogate recurrent symptoms of these nonneoplastic lesions. The documentation of an invasive neoplasm synchronous with diffuse juvenile polyposis of the large bowel is rare, yet requires radical resection when recognized. Table 46–6 differentiates the pathology, site of origin, and manifestations of the various *familial hamartomatous polyposis syndromes.*

Peutz-Jeghers Syndrome

This uncommon familial syndrome is inherited as a simple mendelian dominant, nonsex-linked type with variable penetrance. The original descriptions by Peutz in 1921 and Jeghers in 1949 identified an inheritable presentation of *GI polyposis* with the association of *mucocutaneous melanin pigmentation* distributed in the oral and pharyngeal mucosa, lips, palms of the hand, and soles of the feet. Additionally, there

TABLE 46–6.—FAMILIAL HAMARTOMATOUS POLYPOSIS SYNDROMES

SYNDROME	PATHOLOGY	LOCATION	OTHER MANIFESTATIONS
Juvenile polyposis	Juvenile polyps, also adenomatous and hyperplastic polyps	Colonic; also small intestine and stomach	Colon cancer in some families
Peutz-Jeghers syndrome	Hamartomas, with bands of smooth muscle in the lamina propria	Small intestine; also stomach and colon	Pigmented lesions of the mouth, hands, and feet; ovarian sex cord tumors (5%–12%); GI cancers (2%–3%)
Neurofibromatosis	Neurofibromas	Stomach and small intestine	Generalized neurofibromatosis
Cowden's syndrome (multiple hamartoma syndrome)	Hamartomas	Stomach and colon	Trichilemmomas and papillomas; breast cancer, multiple other hamartomas
Basal cell nevus syndrome	Hamartomas	Colon	Multiple basal cell carcinomas

Boland C.K., Kim Y.S.: Colonic polyps and the gastrointestinal polyposis syndromes in gastrointestinal disease, in Sleisenger M.H., Fordtran J.S. (eds.): *Gastrointestinal Disease: Pathophysiology, Diagnosis and Management.* Philadelphia, W.B. Saunders Co., 1983, 1196–1219. Used by permission.

may be similar mucocutaneous lesions in the genital and perianal areas. The differentiation of these melanin deposits from common freckles is essential. Classically, the Peutz-Jeghers pigmented lesion is greenish-black to brown and, with the exception of the buccal site, has the propensity to fade after puberty.

The hamartomatous polyps (Fig 46–16) are distributed throughout the entire GI tract, as well as extraintestinal sites such as the ureter and bronchus. The ileum and jejunum are the most frequently involved segments of the GI tract. The colon and rectum are involved in one third and the stomach in approximately one fourth of the cases.

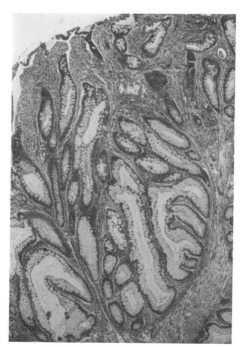

Fig 46–16.—Hamartomatous polyp of Peutz-Jeghers syndrome. Typical polyp is composed of large mucin-secreting glands admixed with bundles of smooth muscle; ×40. (Courtesy D.A. Franzini, M.D., Department of Pathology, University of Florida.)

Although rare, single-case reports of malignant tumors associated with this syndrome have been described. However, no documentation exists for malignant transformation of the hamartomatous Peutz-Jegher polyp. The most common presenting symptom is recurrent, colicky pain which is initiated by transient intussusception. Progression in size of the hamartoma may initiate colonic or rectal obstruction. Acute *GI hemorrhage* can take origin from polyps in the small intestine, colon, or rectum. Chronic anemia may be a presenting feature. Approximately 5% of females with this syndrome develop ovarian malignancies, 50% of which represent a granulosa cell (sex-cord) tumor unique to this entity. These sex-cord tumors may be hormonally active and malignant.[38, 50] Thus, presentation of Peutz-Jeghers polyposis in the adult female requires careful examination of the adnexa uteri. It would seem reasonable to perform prophylactic oophorectomy in older adult females being operated on for the intestinal complications of this entity. Surgical therapy is directed to the hamartomas that produce obstruction, intussusception, or bleeding and is dictated by the site of presentation. Only conservative procedures (e.g., polypectomy, sleeve resection) are necessary. The wide distribution and size of these hamartomatous polyps commonly preclude the ability to resect all lesions that may potentially initiate complicating symptoms in the future.

Neurofibromatosis (von Recklinghausen's Disease)

The presentation of multiple neurofibromas of the GI tract is occasionally reported in association with *von Recklinghausen's disease.* This entity may present as a *familial* or *nonfamilial* variant with *multiple neurofibromas of peripheral and central nerves, café-au-lait skin pigmentation, neurofibromas of the skin,* and *abnormalities of bone.* Additionally, *defective development of the CNS* may be apparent in some subjects. The peripheral tumors may vary from small elevations at the level of the skin to huge *pedunculated neurofibromas (pachydermatocele)* of skin and subcutaneous tissues.

Neurofibromas of the GI tract take origin from the submucosal primitive mesenchyme. Diagnosis of these lesions may be difficult with air-contrast barium studies or with direct visualization at colonoscopy. Donnelly et al.[51] have found multiple polyps in the large intestine that have proved to be a mixture of neurofibromas and juvenile polyps. Therapy is aimed at the symptoms of obstruction; mucosal ulceration with hemorrhage and abdominal pain. Conservative surgical therapy is indicated and usually requires resection with primary anastomosis.

Other Nonneoplastic Hamartomatous Polyposis Diseases

Lipomas, leiomyomas, and *hemangiomas* may present as polypoid hamartomatous lesions of the colon and rectum. *Lipomas* are benign neoplasms that most commonly present in the colon. Most often their origin is near the ileocecal valve, but they can be distributed throughout the colorectal submucosa. Lipomas may initiate symptoms of bleeding, incomplete obstruction, and intussusception. These lesions may be resected endoscopically; however, sleeve (segmental) resections are indicated for large lesions not amenable to endoscopic removal.

Leiomyomas (Fig 46–17,A to C) arise from the muscularis mucosae of the colon and rectum and are histologically interlaced with spindle cells. This rare neoplasm can present with clinical features similar to that of the lipoma. The recognition of a submucosal lesion and its subsequent biopsy through the mucosa should be performed carefully to obviate colonic perforation. On occasion, the differentiation of the benign leiomyoma from its malignant variant, *leiomyosarcoma* (Fig 46–18,A and B), is difficult. The histologically benign lesion may

be treated by conservative colonic resection, whereas the leiomyosarcoma requires radical colonic and mesenteric resection or abdominoperineal resection.

Hemangiomas are to be differentiated from the *angiodysplastic lesions* that represent localized vascular malformations occurring predominately in the cecum and ascending colon (chapter 48). Histologically, angiodysplasia consists of foci of ectatic veins or capillaries that occupy the submucosal position of the colon wall. The *hemangioma* is a true nonneoplastic, polypoid lesion which represents outgrowth of ectopic endothelium-lined, blood-containing spaces. Although small, the hemangioma may assume a sessile configuration and produce obstructive or hemorrhagic symptoms. Surgical therapy for colonic and rectal hemangiomas is similar to that for lipomas and leiomyomas. The polypoid hemangioma can bleed profusely if biopsied. Resection of the lesion and contiguous bowel will avoid such therapeutic complications.

Weinstock and Kawanishi[52] have described the association of *multiple hamartomatous polyps (Cowden's disease)* with orocutaneous hamartomas, colon carcinoma, and fibrocystic disease of the breast. Additionally, these multiple hamartomas in the colon and stomach may be associated with nontoxic thyroid goiter and thyroid carcinoma. The finding of colonic hamartomas in an individual with documented *basal cell nevus syndrome* is usually incidental as these patients are rarely symptomatic with these nonneoplastic polyps.[11, 53]

Inflammatory Polyps (Pseudopolyps)

The *inflammatory polyp (pseudopolyp)* arises from the islands of mucosa or granulation tissue occurring as a result of

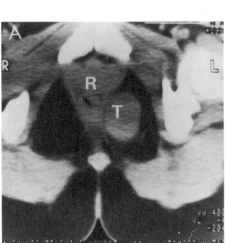
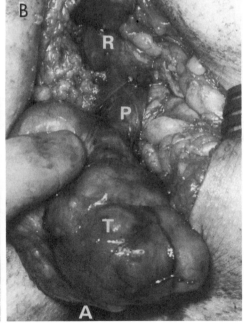
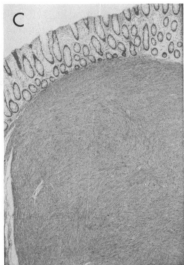

Fig 46–17.—Leiomyoma of submucosal rectal origin. **A,** CT scan of distal one third of rectum *(R)*. A large leiomyoma *(T)* with origin from the muscularis mucosae of the rectum is identifiable as a discrete homogeneous mass separate from the rectal wall. **B,** intraoperative appearance of large tumor mass exposed via ischiorectal fossa incision. The rectal wall *(R)* is identified. The tumor mass *(T)* has a discrete pedicle *(P)* attached to the submucosa of the rectum. **C,** microscopic appearance of submucosal leiomyoma with intact mucosa covering proliferation of uniform spindle cells arranged in interlacing fascicles, ×40.

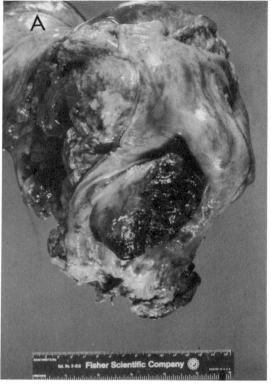

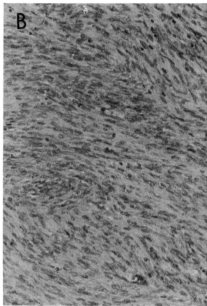

Fig 46–18.—A, gross specimen of rectal leiomyosarcoma with transmural extension and mucosal ulceration. **B,** microscopic high magnification (×200) of cellular tumor composed of interlacing fascicles of pleomorphic spindle cells with high mitotic rate. (Courtesy D.A. Franzini, M.D., Department of Pathology, University of Florida.)

the extensive mucosal disease in *ulcerative colitis, amebiasis, schistosomiasis, Crohn's colitis* or other nonspecific *rectal granulomatous diseases.* Following full-thickness ulceration of the colonic mucosa, a regenerative process is initiated, and the residual false polypoid masses are recognized as bizarre configurations. Often, the pseudopolyps have the appearance of a jagged mucosal strap or tag which is elevated beyond the previously existing mucosal surface. Inflammatory polyps are scattered, discrete, often confluent, and hyperplastic on visual inspection.

Diagnosis of *inflammatory* polyps is best made by excisional biopsy from several areas of the involved colorectum. The early, postinflammatory histologic features include a benign, but disorderly, inflammatory granulation response which tends to be more organized and reparative in the terminal phases of reepithelialization of the mucosa. The potential for malignant transformation of inflammatory polyps has remained conjectural, as the incidence of colonic carcinoma is approximately 30-fold for those with chronic ulcerative colitis compared to the general population. While no intrinsic predisposition of the inflammatory polyp to malignant transformation can be confirmed, the distinction of the pseudopolyp from an invasive neoplasm is necessary in intestinal mucosa at high-risk for development of colorectal carcinoma (ulcerative colitis, schistosomiasis).[11, 12, 54]

Benign lymphoid polyps (hyperplasia) may present as solitary submucosal nodules of the colon and rectum (Fig 46–19). Most commonly, these lesions present in the lower portion of the rectum. These nodules may vary from a few millimeters to 2 or 3 cm. Distinction of these nonneoplastic pseudopolyps in children from familial polyposis coli, multiple juvenile pol-

yps, and inflammatory pseudopolyposis associated with inflammatory changes of the colonic mucosa is necessary. These polypoid masses are usually identified at proctosigmoidoscopy or radiographic contrast studies performed for other reasons. No malignant potential exists for these lesions. Endoscopic or surgical excision is curative.

Colitis cystica represents a benign, mucus-filled lesion which may present superficial (*colitis cystica superficialis*) or deep (*colitis cystica profunda*) to the muscularis mucosae of the colonic wall. The superficialis variant most commonly presents with thousands of grey, minute blebs distributed throughout the entire colonic mucosal surface. Mucus can often be expressed from these blebs. *Colitis cystica profunda* (CCP) may present in three specific anatomical sites. The variance of site distribution has been recognized pathologically and includes: (1) the common localized form, which is usually restricted to the rectum; (2) a segmental form; and (3) the presence of cystica profunda lesions involving extensive areas of the colon and rectum.[55] The overlying intestinal mucosa appears grossly normal but may be umbilicated or ulcerative. Radiographically and endoscopically, the bowel wall is thickened, with a mass effect compressing the mucosa. This thickening is secondary to the submucosal cysts, which vary from 0.1–3.0 cm in diameter.[56] Microscopically, the surrounding mucosa has evidence of chronic fibrosis and inflammatory changes (Fig 46–20). A basophilic-staining mucoid material is present in the dilated cystic spaces that occupy the muscularis mucosa position and may penetrate it.

The pathogenesis of CCP is unsubstantiated but may be initiated by: (1) postinflammatory changes, (2) congenitally ectopic mucosa, or (3) submucosal herniation of mucosal epithe-

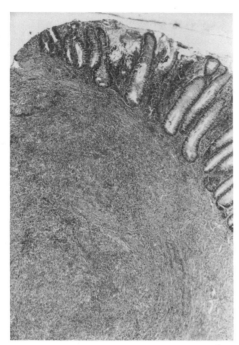

Fig 46–19.—Lymphoid polyp. Typical small polypoid nodule which is microscopically composed of mature lymphocytes in the lamina propria and submucosa. Overlying mucosa is intact; ×40. (Courtesy D.A. Franzini, M.D., Department of Pathology, University of Florida.)

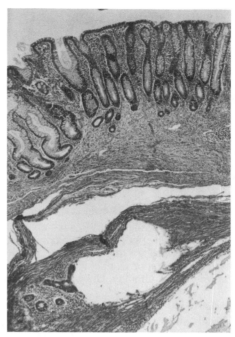

Fig 46–20.—Microscopic section of resected colonic segment with diffuse colitis cystica profunda. The submucosal area of the bowel is replaced by large mucin-filled cysts partially lined by colonic mucosa; ×40. (Courtesy D.A. Franzini, M.D., Department of Pathology, University of Florida.)

lium secondary to defects of the muscularis mucosae.[55, 56]

The lesions commonly present on rectal examination as compressible, smooth, firm masses that are mobile and nonadherent to contiguous rectal structures or the overlying mucosa. The lesions are usually present in the distal 12 cm of the anterior rectum,[57] but may occur in the descending, transverse, and ascending colon. Radiographic identification of the submucosal position of the colorectal lesions initiates an extensive differential diagnosis. Endoscopic submucosal biopsy rarely provides diagnosis. Confirmation of the CCP lesion is most commonly obtained with excisional biopsy or segmental resection of bulky lesions. The differentiation from colloid carcinoma is important to avoid inappropriate radical surgical resection. Rarely are recurrences identified in uninvolved portions of the colorectum following adequate primary resection. The excessive secretion of colonic mucus and bleeding from the CCP lesion may result in iron deficiency anemia, hypokalemia, and hypoalbuminemia.[58, 59]

ADDITIONAL UNCLASSIFIED POLYPOID LESIONS OF COLORECTAL ORIGIN

Hyperplastic (Metaplastic) Polyps

These polyps have only recently been recognized as distinct from tubular and other forms of polyps. Hyperplastic lesions are usually multiple and appear as minute, sessile, plaquelike excrescences which are typically 1–2 mm in diameter and are seldom larger than 5 mm. These polyps are seen most frequently arising from the mucosa of the colorectum. Lane et al.[60] observed that over 90% of the polypoid lesions of the

colon and rectum measuring < 3 mm in diameter were hyperplastic. With increasing size of the colorectal polyp, there is an inverse relationship to the incidence of hyperplastic lesions.[61] These lesions are found in all ages and can occur synchronously in normal bowel mucosa or in individuals harboring a cancer of the colon or rectum.

Microscopically, the metaplastic polyp has a structure that can clearly be differentiated from adenomas. There appears to be elongation of the mucosal tubules with a tendency to cystic dilatation. The epithelium appears serrated with patchy flattening of the well-differentiated goblet cells (Fig 46–21). The proportion of goblet cells is diminished, and the lamina propria reveals an increased number of lymphocytes and plasma cells. Mitoses and DNA synthesis are observed at the base of the crypts; orderly cell maturation is preserved; and cytologic atypia is absent.

Hyperplastic polyps rarely initiate clinical symptoms. They typically remain small and sessile with a diffuse distribution throughout the mucosa of the colorectum. Interval follow-up surveillance through colonoscopic or sigmoidoscopic visualization is adequate. These lesions are commonly biopsied at the time of endoscopic evaluation for symptomatic, noninvasive, and invasive neoplastic lesions.

Pneumatosis Cystoides Intestinalis

This relatively uncommon condition of the colorectum is characterized by the presence of multicentric, gas-filled cystic spaces in the wall of the large intestine. Additionally, the small bowel, stomach, mesentery, and omentum may be involved with pneumatosis cystoides intestinalis (PCI).

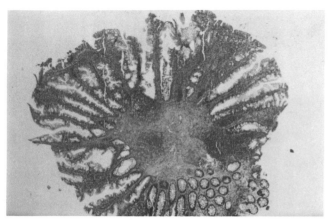

Fig 46–21.—Low-power (×40) cross-sectional view of hyperplastic (metaplastic) polyp which is composed of elongated glands with papillary infoldings and production of a characteristic serrated appearance. (Courtesy D.A. Franzini, M.D., Department of Pathology, University of Florida.)

Many of the cases of PCI are associated with chronic pulmonary or acute intestinal (pyloroduodenal) obstructive diseases, and in those who have had recent intestinal surgery. Feinberg and associates[62] noted 24 patients (6.0%) in a series of 402 jejunoileal bypass patients who had roentgenographic evidence for PCI on 28 separate occasions. These lesions primarily involved the right colon. Despite the radiographic evidence for these lesions, no specific clinical evidence of bypass enteritis was evident. Patients may develop colonic pneumatosis intestinalis following traumatic endoscopy, polypectomy, or mucosal biopsy.[53] Table 46–7 enumerates the GI conditions which are associated with this entity. Earnest[56] acknowledges three potential mechanisms that may be operative in the genesis of PCI: (1) disruption of the intestinal mucosa by surgery, traumatic endoscopy, or ruptured pulmonary blebs which dissect, under pressure, into the tissue spaces of the

bowel wall, mesentery, or omentum; (2) invasion and colonization of intestinal wall by gas-producing bacteria following mucosal disruption as a result of ischemia, trauma, or intestinal resection; and (3) excessive gas produced by bacterial fermentation of carbohydrate in the bowel lumen. The last theory presumes that the absorbed gas is trapped within the intestinal wall. Despite the plausibility of the three etiologic mechanisms above, precise documentation is lacking and all three mechanisms may be operative in the etiology of PCI.

The patient with PCI may be totally asymptomatic with discovery of diffuse colorectal involvement with pneumatosis at sigmoidoscopy or air-contrast barium enema studies. Diffuse involvement of the colorectum and small intestine may occur simultaneously. Progression of cystic lesions in the bowel wall (Fig 46–22) may initiate symptoms of abdominal cramps, tenesmus, rectal bleeding with mucoid discharge, or diarrhea. Mild steatorrhea has been observed.

Mechanical obstruction of the colorectum or small intestine may develop with large cysts or may result secondary to volvulus, intussusception, or adhesions. Marked dilatation of the cyst-filled bowel wall may initiate transmural ischemia with bleeding or bowel perforation. The presence of free air and abdominal pain associated with pneumatosis coli is suggestive of perforation and the necessity of emergency operation.

As many patients are asymptomatic with PCI, a physical examination may give no specific clue to the presence of this entity. On occasion, the presence of ballottable, nontender masses may be noted if the cysts are large. Typical grapelike masses may be palpable on rectal examination. Sigmoidoscopic or colonoscopic inspection of the mucosa reveals soft, distinct, gas-filled spaces which are pale or bluish in appearance. Roentgenographic examination is most revealing of this entity and shows air-filled spaces localized in the bowel wall, often arranged in clusters or in a linear fashion[63] (Fig 46–23). Gas may be seen between layers of the mesentery or in the free peritoneal cavity following iatrogenic or spontaneous cystic perforation. Barium examination of the large bowel dis-

TABLE 46–7.—GASTROINTESTINAL
CONDITIONS ASSOCIATED WITH
PNEUMATOSIS CYSTOIDES INTESTINALIS

Peptic ulcer disease
Intestinal obstruction
Postsurgical bowel anastomosis
Jejunoileal bypass for obesity
Mesenteric vascular occlusion
Acute necrotizing enterocolitis
Chronic inflammatory disease (regional enteritis,
　ulcerative colitis, tuberculosis)
Perforated diverticula
Collagen disorders (especially scleroderma)
Diabetic enteropathy
Whipple's disease
Abdominal trauma
Ingestion of caustic agents
Intestinal parasites and tuberculosis
Intestinal lymphosarcoma and leukemia

Earnest D.L.: Other diseases of the colon and rectum, in Sleisenger M.H., Fordtran J.S. (eds.): *Gastrointestinal Disease: Pathophysiology, Diagnosis and Management.* Philadelphia, W.B. Saunders Co., 1983, p. 1302. Used by permission.

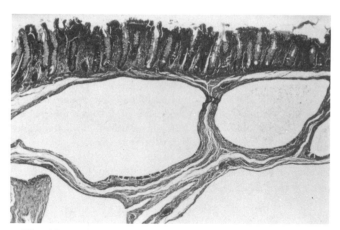

Fig 46–22.—Low-power (×40) microscopic section of colonic segment with extensive pneumatosis cystoides intestinalis. Enlarged, irregular submucosal cysts characteristically involve the entire colon and rectum. These submucosal cystic spaces are lined by histiocytes and giant cells. (Courtesy D.A. Franzini, M.D., Department of Pathology, University of Florida.)

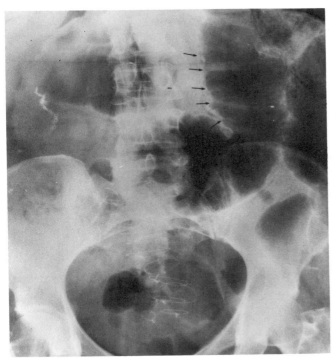

Fig 46–23.—Flat-plate abdominal radiograph of 31-year-old man two weeks status post-gunshot wound to abdomen. *Arrows* denote the irregular submucosal air-filled cystic spaces of pneumatosis cystoides intestinalis which diffusely involves the small and large bowel. (Courtesy F. Clore, M.D., VA Medical Center, University of Florida.)

closes radiolucent spaces which coalesce within the bowel wall to indent the barium column. The diffuse distribution and the smooth margin of the cystic-filled spaces differentiate this entity from neoplastic, polypoid, or carcinomatous growth. Skip areas may appear in multicentric sites.

Pneumatosis coli is asymptomatic in the majority of patients and therapy is directed to the underlying disease process. In this circumstance, resolution is usually spontaneous following correction of the primary disease. Individuals who present with colonic hemorrhage, pain, tenesmus, and incomplete obstruction may have initial management with medical measures. Conservative medical therapy is begun only if evidence of bowel ischemia or perforation is absent. Medical therapy is directed at reducing the available atmospheric nitrogen by breathing high concentrations of oxygen.[64, 65] These therapeutic efforts promote diffusion of hydrogen, methane, nitrogen, and other gases from the intestinal cyst into surrounding tissues. Hyperbaric oxygen has been successfully utilized by Masterson et al.[65] Optimal results were obtained when arterial oxygen tension was regularly monitored to assure a PaO_2 in the range of 200 mm Hg or above (2.5 atm absolute). Recurrence of the cystic lesions has been noted following cessation of the intensive hyperbaric therapy. A second course of hyperbaric oxygen may be attempted simultaneously with efforts to reduce the bacterial conversion of dietary carbohydrate to hydrogen.

Surgical intervention is indicated for the aforementioned complications of ischemia, perforation, obstruction, or hemorrhage. At times, colonic resections have been transiently successful, only to have recurrence of extensive pneumatosis in the proximal colonic or small bowel segments. For extensive recurrent pneumatosis, intensive medical therapy with elemental diets, antibiotics, and hyperbaric oxygen should be initiated in the medically stable patient.

Heterotopic Colorectal Lesions

Submucosal involvement with benign conditions may initiate motility and functional disturbances of the colorectum. Progressive involvement of the colonic or rectal wall with a benign process may initiate luminal obstruction which may be partial or complete. This event is observed typically in *endometriosis* and results from dense adhesive bands that develop following repeated shedding of endometrium and blood into the peritoneal cavity.

In the colon, especially the sigmoid, endometrial nodules may implant and proliferate to initiate complete obstruction. Ectopic endometrium in the cul-de-sac of Douglas may cause dense adherence of the anterior rectal wall to the posterior uterus. Colonic obstructive symptoms are rare, as the rectal diameter is large enough to obviate these symptoms. However, dyspareunia, tenesmus, or bowel irritability symptoms may be present. The severity of colorectal symptomatology poorly correlates with the extent and duration of involvement by the endometrial lesions. Typically, this presentation occurs in the reproductive age group and is rare in the postmenopausal patient. A prior history of dysmenorrhea and intermenstrual pelvic and low back pain are common. With progressive rectosigmoidal involvement, colicky abdominal pain is common, whereafter patients present with mild to severe tenesmus, diarrhea, constipation and partial obstructive symptoms. Hematochezia is uncommon for these submucosal implants.

Diagnosis is usually established by history and the classic symptoms of menstrual irregularity and exaggerated cyclic menstrual pain. The finding of tender endometrial nodules in the rectovaginal septum or the cul-de-sac in bimanual pelvic examination is classic. The presence of a solitary mass in the rectosigmoid and the absence of disease in the cul-de-sac makes the diagnosis of endometriosis dubious. A bluish, submucosal polypoid mass may be visualized sigmoidoscopically. Palpation of the mass initiates pain, characteristically absent in carcinomatous lesions. Submucosal biopsy should be attempted but may not be diagnostic when the endometrial implant occupies a deep submucosal or submuscularis position in the bowel wall. Laparoscopic examination is of value if uterine, pelvic, or peritoneal implants can be visualized and biopsied. An intramural submucosal lesion characterizes the *roentgenographic* appearance on air-contrast barium enema study (Fig 46–24). Differential diagnosis is extensive and includes pelvic and mesenteric tumors and cysts, granulomatous (Crohn's) and ulcerative colitis, ameboma, diverticular abscess, and carcinoma. The rare occurrence of endometrial adenocarcinoma of the rectovaginal septum with origin from endometrial tissue has been reported.[66]

Therapy is directed at control of the primary endometrial disease in consultation with a gynecologist. The identification of rectal endometrial implants by direct or needle biopsy is diagnostic. Treatment aimed at medical control of the estro-

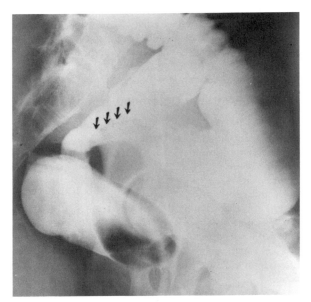

Fig 46–24.—Barium enema demonstrating heterotopic submucosal endometrioma of the rectosigmoid. *Arrows* identify the extent of compression of the barium column by this intramural submucosal lesion. (Courtesy F. Clore, M.D., VA Medical Center, University of Florida.)

gen-sensitive endometrial implants may initiate complete regression of the colorectal symptoms. Androgens and progestational agents have provided effective forms of hormonal therapy. The recent introduction of the antigonadotrophin compound danazol (Danocrine) has effectively controlled the pelvic and abdominal symptoms via feedback inhibition of the pituitary-ovarian stimuli common with cyclic proliferation of the endometriomas.[67] However, the side effects of this drug in the moderately high doses (400–800 mg twice daily for 3–6 months) that are necessary to control the symptoms represent a detracting feature for its usage. As patients approach the menopausal era, endometrial symptoms commonly begin to regress. Resolution of the pelvic and colonic symptoms may be complete following surgical castration. For individuals who fail hormonal medical therapy, or in whom previous surgical excision has been unsuccessful, limited surgical resection of the involved colorectal segment is indicated with restoration of intestinal continuity. Prior to surgical intervention, a conservative trial of medical treatment over several menstrual cycles is indicated to palliate the symptoms and potentially eliminate these benign heterotopic lesions.

REFERENCES

1. Mettlin C., Mittelman A., Natarajan N., et al.: Trends in the United States for the management of adenocarcinoma of the rectum. *Surg. Gynecol. Obstet.* 153:701, 1981.
2. Grinnell R.S., Lane N.: Benign and malignant adenomatous polyps and papillary adenomas of the colon and rectum. *Int. Abstr. Surg.* 106:519, 1958.
3. Lipkin M.: Phase 1 and Phase 2 proliferative lesions of colonic epithelial cells in diseases leading to colonic cancer. *Cancer* 34:878, 1974.
4. Muto T., Bussey H.J.R., Morson B.C.: The evolution of cancer of the colon and rectum. *Cancer* 36:2251, 1975.

5. Day D.W., Morson B.C.: Pathology of adenomas, in Morson B.C. (ed.): *The Pathogenesis of Colorectal Cancer*. Philadelphia, W.B. Saunders Co. 1978, pp. 43–57.
6. Blackshaw A.J. Bussey H.J.R., Morson B.C.: Pathology, in Thomson J.P.S., Nicholls R.J., Williams C.B. (eds.): *Colorectal Disease*. New York, Appleton-Century-Crofts, 1981, pp. 235–258.
7. Sherlock P. Lipkin M. Winawer S.J.: The prevention of colon cancer. *Am. J. Med.* 68:917, 1980.
8. Gillespie P.E., Chambers T.J., Chan K.W., et al.: Colonic adenoma—A colonoscopy survey. *Gut* 20:240, 1979.
9. McKittrick L.S., Wheelock F.C.: *Carcinoma of the Colon*, Springfield, Ill., Charles C Thomas Publisher 1954, pp. 61–63.
10. Steven K., Lange P., Bukhave K., et al.: Prostaglandin E₂-mediated secretory diarrhea in villous adenoma of rectum: Effect of treatment with indomethacin. *Gastroenterology* 80:1562, 1981.
11. Boland C.R., Kim Y.S.: Colonic polyps and the gastrointestinal polyposis syndromes, in, Sleisenger M.H., Fordtran J.S. (eds.): *Gastrointestinal Disease: Pathophysiology, Diagnosis and Management*. Philadelphia, W.B. Saunders Co., 1983, pp. 1196–1219.
12. Morson B.C.: Factors influencing the prognosis of early cancer of the rectum. *Proc. R. Soc. Med.* 59:607, 1966.
13. Correa P., Strong J.P., Reif A., et al.: The epidemiology of colorectal polyps. *Cancer* 39:2258, 1977.
14. LaMont J.T., O'Gorman T.A.: Experimental colon cancer. *Gastroenterology* 75:1157, 1978.
15. Spratt J.S. Jr., Ackerman L.V., Moyer C.A.: Relationship of polyps of the colon to colonic cancer. *Ann. Surg.* 148:682, 1958.
16. Berge T., Ekelund G., Mellner C., et al.: Carcinoma of the colon and rectum in a defined population. An epidemiological, clinical, and postmortem investigation of colorectal carcinoma and co-existing benign polyps in Malmö, Sweden. *Acta. Chir. Scand.* [Suppl.] 1–86, 1973.
17. Ekelund G., Lindström C.: Histopathological analysis of benign polyps in patients with carcinoma of the colon and rectum. *Gut* 15:654, 1974.
18. Castleman B., Krickstein H.I.: Do adenomatous polyps of the colon become malignant? *N. Engl. J. Med.* 267:469, 1962.
19. Spratt J.S., Jr., Ackerman L.V.: Small primary adenocarcinomas of the colon and rectum. *J.A.M.A.* 179:337, 1962.
20. Lockhart-Mummery H.E., Dukes C.E.: The surgical treatment of malignant rectal polyps, with notes on their pathology. Lancet 2:751, 1952.
21. Cole J.W., McKalen A.: Observations on the cytochemical composition of adenomas and carcinomas of the colon. *Ann. Surg.* 152:615, 1960.
22. Nachlas M.M., Hannibal M.J.: Histochemical observations on the polyp-carcinoma sequence. *Surg. Gynecol. Obstet.* 112:534, 1961.
23. Goligher J.C.: Benign polyps with particular reference to adenoma and papilloma of the colon, rectum and anus, in Goligher J.C. (ed.): *Surgery of the Anus, Rectum and Colon*. London, Bailliére Tindall, 1980, pp. 321–374.
24. Shatney C.H., Lober P.H., Gilbertsen V.A., et al.: The treatment of pedunculated adenomatous colorectal polyps with focal cancer. *Surg. Gynecol. Obstet.* 139:845, 1974.
25. Winawer S.J.: Colorectal cancer screening and early diagnosis, in: Brodie O.R. (ed.): *Screening and Early Detection of Colorectal Cancer*. Consensus Development Conference Proceedings. Washington, NIH Publication no. 80–2075, 1979.
26. Bussey H.J.R.: *Familial Polyposis Coli: Family Studies, Histopathology, Differential Diagnosis, and Results of Treatment*. Baltimore, Johns Hopkins University Press, 1975.
27. Bussey H.J.R.: Polyposis syndromes, in Morson B.C. (ed.): *The Pathogenesis of Colorectal Cancer*. Philadelphia, W.B. Saunders Co., 1978, pp. 81–94.
28. Moertel C.G., Hill J.R., Adson M.A.: Management of multiple polyposis of the large bowel. *Cancer* 28:160, 1971.
29. DeCosse J.J., Adams M.B., Kuzma J.F., et al.: Effect of ascorbic acid on rectal polyps of patients with familial polyposis. *Surgery* 78:608, 1975.
30. Stearns M.W. Jr.: Early and definitive surgical therapy for co-

lonic and rectal cancer, in Lipkin M., Good R.A. (eds.): *Gastrointestinal Tract Cancer*. New York, Plenum Medical Book Co., 1978, pp. 537–550.

31. Morson B.C., Dawson I.M.P.: *Gastrointestinal Pathology*. Oxford, London, Blackwell Scientific Publications, 1972, p. 535.

32. Gingold B.S., Jagelman D.G.: Sparing the rectum in familial polyposis: Causes for failure. *Surgery* 89:314, 1981.

33. Beart R.W. Jr., Dozois R.R., Kelly K.A.: Ileoanal anastomosis in the adult. *Surg. Gynecol. Obstet.* 154:826, 1982.

34. Parks A.G., Nicholls R.J.: Proctocolectomy without ileostomy for ulcerative colitis. *Br. Med. J.* 2:85, 1978.

35. Taylor B.M., Cranley B., Kelly K.A., et al.: A clinico-physiological comparison of ileal pouch-anal and straight ileoanal anastomoses. *Ann. Surg.* 198:462, 1983.

36. Gardner E.J.: A genetic and clinical study of intestinal polyposis, a predisposing factor for carcinoma of colon and rectum. *Am. J. Hum. Genet.* 3:167, 1951.

37. Utsunomiya J., Nakamura T.: The occult osteomatous changes in the mandible in patients with familial polyposis coli. *Br. J. Surg.* 62:45, 1975.

38. Sachatello C.R., Griffen W.O. Jr.: Hereditary polypoid diseases of the gastrointestinal tract: A working classification. *Am. J. Surg.* 129:198, 1975.

39. Turcot J., Després J.P., St. Pierre F.: Malignant tumors of the central nervous system associated with familial polyposis of the colon: Report of two cases. *Dis. Colon Rectum* 2:465, 1959.

40. Binder M.K., Zablen M.A., Fleischer D.E., et al.: Colon polyps, sebaceous cysts, gastric polyps, and malignant brain tumor in a family. *Am. J. Dig. Dis.* 23:460, 1978.

41. Anderson D.E.: An inherited form of large bowel cancer: Muir's syndrome. *Cancer* 45:1103, 1980.

42. Cronkhite L.W., Canada W.J.: Generalized gastrointestinal polyposis: An unusual syndrome of polyposis, pigmentation, alopecia, and onychotrophia. *N. Engl. J. Med.* 252:1011, 1955.

43. Rubin M., Tuthill R.J., Rosato E.F., et al.: Cronkhite-Canada syndrome: Report of an unusual case. *Gastroenterology* 79:737, 1980.

44. Daniel E.S., Ludwig S.L., Lewin K.J., et al.: The Cronkhite-Canada syndrome: An analysis of clinical and pathologic features and therapy in 55 patients. *Medicine* 61:293, 1982.

45. Gibbs N.M.: Juvenile and Peutz-Jeghers polyps, in Morson B.C. (ed.): *The Pathogenesis of Colorectal Cancer*. Philadelphia, W.B. Saunders Co., 1978, pp. 21–32.

46. Bussey H.J.R. Gastrointestinal polyposis. *Gut.* 11:970, 1970.

47. Watanabe A., Nagashima H., Motoi M., et al.: Familial juvenile polyposis of the stomach. *Gastroenterology* 77:148, 1979.

48. Beacham C.H., Shields H.M., Raffensperger E.C., et al.: Juvenile and adenomatous gastrointestinal polyposis. *Am. J. Dig. Dis.* 23:1137, 1978.

49. Goodman Z.D., Yardley J.H., Milligan F.D.: Pathogenesis of colonic polyps in multiple juvenile polyposis. *Cancer* 43:1906, 1979.

50. Scully R.E.: Sex cord and tumor with annular tubules: A distinctive ovarian tumor of the Peutz-Jeghers syndrome. *Cancer* 25:1107, 1970.

51. Donnelly W.H., Sieber W.K., Yunis E.J.: Polypoid ganglioneurofibromatosis of the large bowel. *Arch. Pathol.* 87:537, 1969.

52. Weinstock J.V., Kawanishi H.: Gastrointestinal polyposis with orocutaneous hamartomas (Cowden's disease). *Gastroenterology* 74:890, 1978.

53. Schwartz R.A.: Basal-cell-nevus syndrome and gastrointestinal polyposis. *N. Engl. J. Med.* 299:49, 1978.

54. Jackman R.J., Beahrs O.H.: Pseudopolyposis, in *Tumors of the Large Bowel: Major Problems in Clinical Surgery*. Philadelphia, W.B. Saunders Co., 1968, vol. 8, pp. 124–130.

55. Herman A.H. Nabseth D.C.: Colitis cystica profunda: Localized, segmental and diffuse. *Arch. Surg.* 106:337, 1973.

56. Earnest D.L.: Other diseases of the colon and rectum, in Sleisenger M.H., Fordtran J.S. (eds.).: *Gastrointestinal Disease: Pathophysiology, Diagnosis and Management*. Philadelphia, W.B. Saunders Co., 1983, pp. 1294–1323.

57. Magidson J.G., Lewin K.J.: Diffuse colitis cystica profunda: Report of a case. *Am. J. Surg. Pathol.* 5:393, 1981.

58. Martin J.K. Jr. Culp C.E., Weiland L.H.: Colitis cystica profunda. *Dis. Colon Rectum* 23:488, 1980.

59. Crane C.W.: Observations on the sodium and potassium content of mucus from the large intestine. *Gut* 6:439, 1965.

60. Lane N., Kaplan H., Pascal R.R.: Minute adenomatous and hyperplastic polyps of the colon: Divergent patterns of epithelial growth with specific associated mesenchymal changes. *Gastroenterology* 60:537, 1971.

61. Granqvist S., Gabrielsson N., Sundelin P.: Dimunitive colonic polyps—clinical significance and management. *Endoscopy* 11:36, 1979.

62. Feinberg S.B., Schwartz M.Z., Clifford S. et al.: Significance of pneumatosis cystoides intestinalis after jejunoileal bypass. *Am. J. Surg.* 133:149, 1977.

63. Marshak R.H., Linder A.E., Maklansky D.: Pneumatosis cystoides coli. *Gastrointest. Radiol.* 2:85, 1977.

64. Van DerLinden W., Marsel R.: Pneumatosis cystoides coli associated with high H_2 excretion. Treatment with an elemental diet. *Scand. J. Gastroenterol.* 14:173, 1979.

65. Masterson J.S.T., Fratkin L.B.,. Osler T.R., et al.: Treatment of pneumatosis cystoides intestinalis with hyperbaric oxygen. *Ann. Surg.* 187:245, 1978.

66. Young E.E., Gamble C.N.: Primary adenocarcinoma of the rectovaginal septum arising from endometriosis: Report of a case. *Cancer* 24:597, 1969.

67. Dmowski W.P., Cohen M.R.: Antigonadotropin (Danazol) in the treatment of endometriosis: Evaluation of posttreatment fertility and three-year follow-up data. *Am. J. Obstet. Gynecol.* 130:41, 1978.

47

Perianal Disease and Rectal Prolapse

STANLEY M. GOLDBERG, M.D.
JOHN G. BULS, M.D.

NORMAL ANATOMY AND PHYSIOLOGY

Anatomy

The rectum, the distal portion of the large intestine, measures 12–15 cm long, begins at the level of the third sacral vertebra and ends at the anal canal. While the junction between the rectum and distal sigmoid colon is not distinct, the rectum differs from the sigmoid in that it lacks haustra, teniae coli, and appendices epiploicae. The valves of Houston in the rectum represent folds of mucosa, submucosa, and circular muscle but contain no longitudinal muscle. The upper one third is covered by peritoneum anteriorly and laterally, while only the anterior portion of the middle third of the rectum is covered. The lower one third of the rectum is devoid of peritoneal covering. Anteriorly, the peritoneum reflects onto the back of the vagina or bladder. This reflection is 7.5–8.5 cm from the anal verge in a male, and in a female 5.0–7.5 cm. The posterior peritoneal reflection is usually 12–15 cm from the anal verge (Fig 47–1).[1]

The anal canal is the outlet of the rectum. It begins at the level of the anorectal ring and terminates at the anal verge. The length of the surgical anal canal varies but averages 4 cm.[2] The inner circular smooth muscle layer of the rectum continues downward and thickens to form the internal anal sphincter. The external anal sphincter, which is striated muscle, loops around the entire length of the anal canal. It has three distinct components: the subcutaneous, superficial, and deep portions. The puborectalis muscle is fused with the deep portion of the external sphincter.[3] The external sphincter muscle is intimately attached to the levator ani muscle. Between the internal and external sphincter is the downward continuation of the longitudinal smooth muscle of the rectum. This outer rectal muscle is supplemented with fibers from the levator ani and puborectalis muscles to constitute the conjoined longitudinal muscle. These thin muscle fibers pass downward and form a series of septa, which ultimately attach to the anal and perianal skin. Some of the septa traverse the internal sphincter to attach to the submucosa and are termed muscularis submucosa ani; other fibers traverse the external sphincter to constitute the transverse septum of the ischiorectal fossa (Fig 47–2). This longitudinal muscle fixes the anal canal and everts the anus during defecation.

The easily palpable anorectal ring is constituted from the puborectalis, the deep part of the external sphincter, the longitudinal muscle, and the upper part of the internal sphincter.[3]

Anal Sphincter Mechanism

The anal sphincter should be considered as being made up of three distinct "U"-shaped loops. Such a concept simplifies the understanding of its mechanism.[4–6]

The top loop consists of the deep portion of the external sphincter and the puborectalis fused, functioning as one muscle. This loop attaches to the lower part of the pubic symphysis and loops around the upper part of the anal canal with a downward inclination.

The intermediate loop is the superficial external sphincter arising from the tip of the coccyx as a tendon, with its strong muscle passing anteriorly to encircle the anal canal inferior to the top loop.

The base loop is the subcutaneous external sphincter. Its attachment is anteriorly to the perianal skin with the muscle fibers passing posteriorly with an upward inclination to encircle the lower part of the anal canal.

With voluntary anal sphincter contraction the three separate loops contract in the direction of their origin. The top and base loops, innervated by the inferior hemorrhoidal branch of the pudendal nerve, pull the posterior anal wall anteriorly. The intermediate loop, supplied by branches of the fourth sacral nerve, detracts the anal canal posteriorly. The complementary function of each loop acting separately maintains continence.

Surgical Anal Canal

The upper part of the anal canal is lined by rectal mucosa. The lower half of the anal canal is lined by special skin devoid of hair follicles and sweat glands. Anal crypts are in the upper part of the anoderm. The dentate line or pectinate line is the circumferential line at the level of the crypts. Above this line the rectal mucosa appears in a number of vertical folds, the columns of Morgani, which are the external lining of the internal hemorrhoids. Immediately above the dentate line is a zone measuring 0.5–1.0 cm, called the transitional zone, since it has elements of both anoderm and rectal mucosa.[1]

The dentate line is an important landmark for the surgeon. The epithelium above this line is innervated by sensory fibers

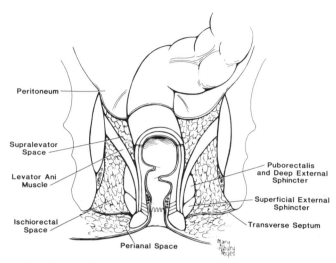

Fig 47–1.—The distal sigmoid colon, rectum, and anal canal illustrating the peritoneal reflection, anal sphincters, and major tissue spaces.

from the autonomic nervous system and therefore is insensitive to painful stimuli. The anoderm below this line is innervated by spinal nerves and has somatic pain sensation.

The anal glands are vestigial structures lined by stratified mucus-secreting columnar epithelium and squamous epithelium (see Fig 47–2).[7] Normally there are 6–10 glands in the circumference of the anus, although the largest number are situated posteriorly. Each gland has a short duct which drains into an anal crypt. In some instances the glands penetrate the internal sphincter as far as the conjoined longitudinal muscle. It is thought that infection originating in these glands is the most common cause of perianal abscess with subsequent fistula-in-ano.

Arterial Supply of the Rectum and Anal Canal (Fig 47–3)

The inferior mesenteric artery continues and terminates as the superior rectal artery, descending posteriorly to the rec-

tum and constituting the major arterial supply to the rectum and upper anal canal.[1] Middle rectal arteries are branches of the internal iliac artery on each side. These are usually small, several in number, and enter the lower portion of the rectum antrolaterally at the level of the levator ani muscles.[8] The terminal branches anastomose with the branches of the superior rectal artery. The inferior rectal arteries are terminal branches of the internal pudendal arteries which, in themselves, are branches of the internal iliac arteries and traverse the ischiorectal fossa to basically supply the anal sphincter muscles. The middle sacral artery does supply a small amount of blood to the lower portion of the posterior wall of the rectum. Its importance resides as a landmark in retrorectal dissection rather than its intrinsic blood supply.

Venous Drainage of the Rectum and Anal Canal

The blood from the anorectum returns via two separate systems, portal and systemic. The superior rectal vein, the counterpart of the artery, drains the upper part of the rectum and anal canal into the inferior mesenteric vein and hence into the portal system. The middle rectal veins drain the lower part of the rectum and upper portion of the anal canal. They terminate in the internal iliac veins. Likewise, the inferior rectal veins drain via the internal pudendal veins into the internal iliacs.[1]

Lymphatic Drainage of the Rectum and Anal Canal

Lymphatic channels from the upper and middle portion of rectum ascend along the superior rectal artery and vein and hence into the inferior mesenteric and para-aortic nodes (see Fig 47–3) The lower part of the rectum and upper anal canal drain lymph in the same direction; however, lymphatics do travel laterally in accompaniment with the middle rectal vessels and hence to the lateral pelvic walls. Lymph from below the dentate line usually drains to the inguinal nodes; however, it may also drain via the superior rectal or middle rectal channels. These modes of lymphatic drainage are usually distorted in the presence of lymphatic obstruction as in cases of metastatic malignancy to lymph nodes.[1]

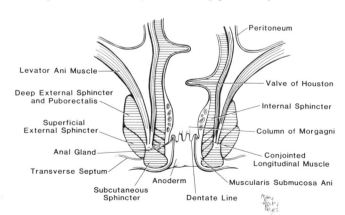

Fig 47–2.—The anal canal with the different components of the sphincter musculature, the dentate line, and the anal glands.

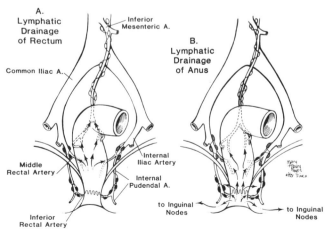

Fig 47–3.—The arterial supply and lymphatic drainage of the rectum and anal canal.

Anatomical Spaces (Fig 47–4)

Several potential spaces filled with connective tissue and/or fat are found around the anal canal. These may become sites of circumferential spread of perianal or perirectal sepsis. The supralevator space is found on each side of the rectum above the levator ani muscle. Superiorly it is limited by the pelvic peritoneum, laterally by the pelvic wall structures, and medially by the rectum itself. The spaces filled with fibroareolar tissue communicate posteriorly via the retrorectal space. The retrorectal space is limited inferiorly by Waldeyer's fascia, which is the continuation of the presacral fascia covering the front of the sacrum and coccyx (Fig 47–5). As it passes downward and forward, it attaches to the posterior wall of the rectum at the anorectal junction.[9] The ischiorectal space lies inferior to the levator ani muscle. It is limited superiorly by the levator ani, medially by the external anal sphincter, laterally by the ischium and obturator fascia of the pelvic wall, and inferiorly by the transverse septum of the ischiorectal fossa. This space, which contains the inferior rectal vessels and lymphatics, is filled with coarse fat. The space communicates posteriorly via the deep postanal space between the levator ani and the tendonous portion of the superficial external sphincter. The perianal space is confined superiorly by the transverse septum of the ischiorectal fossa and inferiorly by the perianal skin. The spaces on either side communicate posterior to the anal canal via the superficial postanal space. The intersphincteric space lies circumferentially within the conjoined longitudinal muscle between the internal and external anal sphincters.[1]

Anal Rectal Function

Functionally the anorectum consists of two embryologically distinct and functionally separate tubes.[10] The inner tube, composed of mucosa, submucosa, and smooth muscle of the rectum, ends as the internal sphincter of the anus and the

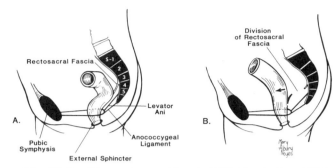

Fig 47–5.—The rectosacral fascia ("Waldyer's Fascia") is the continuation of the presacral fascia to attach to the posterior wall of the rectum. Division of the fascia enables upward and anterior displacement of the rectum.

longitudinal muscle. It is innervated by the autonomic nervous system, and therefore is not subject to voluntary control. The outer tube consists of the external sphincter muscles, puborectalis, and levator ani muscles. Its funnel shape constitutes the pelvic floor by wrapping around the inner tube.

Anal continence is a complex motor and sensory mechanism determined by the complementary but separate functions of the two muscular tubes.[11] It is also due in part to the spatial configuration of the whole anorectal mechanism. The external sphincters, especially the puborectalis, play a major role in maintaining rectal continence. The angle between the rectum and anal canal, usually 30–90° is produced largely by the action of the puborectalis. The internal sphincter functions in a continuous tonic state and is largely responsible for ensuring closure and hence continence of the resting anal canal. Stretch receptors are located in the pelvic floor muscles and, via a reflex arc, are able to activate a spinal nerve supply of the outer muscular tube. Through this reflex activity the outer muscular tube, although composed of skeletal muscle, is in effect contracting continuously even at rest. These muscles will respond according to increase in the intra-abdominal pressure such as with walking, coughing, and laughing. Intra-abdominal pressure itself also exerts forces from side to side at the level of the pelvic floor to aid in maintaining closure. The anal canal is in fact an anteroposterior slit, and the intra-abdominal pressure would thus tend to compress the canal as in a flutter valve. The near-90° angle between the rectum and anal canal, moreover, creates a flap-valve mechanism. Intra-abdominal pressure rises occlude the outlet by impinging the anterior rectal wall onto the anal canal.[11] The greater the abdominal pressure, the more secure the occlusive effect via this mechanism. During defecation, a rise in intrarectal pressure occurs to unlock this flap valve.

Any distention of the rectum or lower sigmoid colon produces an immediate relaxation of the internal sphincter muscle. Continence is maintained by a simultaneous contraction of the external sphincter. With defecation in a squatting or sitting position, the rectoanal angle is straightened to facilitate emptying the rectum. A Valsalva maneuver produces very high abdominal pressure, which in turn inhibits the pelvic floor muscles, allowing the pelvic floor to descend and the fecal bolus to pass.

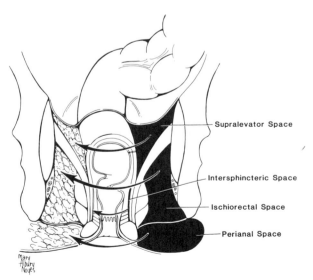

Fig 47–4.—The perirectal and perianal tissue spaces: supralevator, intersphincteric, ischiorectal, and perianal. Note that all are circumferential.

Anorectal Examination

All patients undergoing anorectal examination, even those with painful lesions, can be evaluated thoroughly but gently if they are informed of every step of the procedure.

All patients presenting for routine examination should undergo preparation consisting of a small-volume, disposable phosphate enema given one hour prior to the examination. If inflammatory bowel disease is likely, this step should be omitted because the enema may mask some of the more subtle early changes. Moreover, the enema may produce irritation of the lower rectal mucosa, simulating minimal inflammatory bowel disease. Proctoscopic examination should be carried out prior to any contemplated barium enema x-ray study. If biopsy or electrocoagulation is performed, the barium x-ray should be postponed for three to four weeks.

Proctoscopic Examination

The proctoscopic table which places the patient in an inverted position allows for rapid, comfortable, and easy examination with a proctoscope. The inverted position displaces the viscera, creating a negative pressure, and hence minimizes the need for air insufflation to distend the bowel. For the elderly, frail, or seriously ill patient who cannot tolerate the inverted position, the lateral or Sims' position is used. After turning the patient on the left side, the lower leg is extended while the upper leg is flexed at the knee and hip, in order to spread the buttocks and lend some stability to the patient. It is important to position the patient with the buttocks 10–12 cm over the edge of the bed or table to enable the complete rotation of the proctoscope.

A variety of proctoscopes is available: the proximally lighted, distally lighted, and fiberoptic. Makers of the proximally lighted scopes claim that the distally lighted scopes become coated with bowel contents or blood, obscuring visability. In contrast, advocates of the distally lighted scopes claim that better illumination is possible with this instrument. The instruments come in various sizes. The 19-mm scope with a 25-cm length is the most universally used instrument, especially for snaring of polyps, for biopsy, or for electrocoagulation. The 15-mm diameter scope is much more acceptable to patients and is the ideal size for general routine examination. The 11-mm diameter scope should be available for examining patients with anorectal strictures. As its name implies, the proctoscope is suitable only to examine the rectum.[12] To examine the anal canal, an anoscope should be used.

The flexible sigmoidoscope is a 60-cm long fiberoptic endoscope designed for examination of the rectum, sigmoid, and portions of the left colon.[13] Because of the increased range of examination, this instrument is superior to the rigid scope for detecting pathology.[14,15] Used in conjunction with the air-contrast barium enema, a complete large-bowel evaluation can be performed, since most polyps or cancers not detected by x-ray are in the sigmoid colon. Because of the change in distribution of large bowel cancer, with increasing incidence toward the right side, a flexible sigmoidoscopy alone is an inadequate examination for higher-risk patients.[16,17] The fiberoptic colonoscope is a 130–180-cm instrument. In experienced hands it is possible to pass the scope to the cecum

70%–90% of the time.[18] It is the ideal instrument for diagnostic procedures and is therapeutic in the presence of colonic polyps. A full mechanical preparation of the colon is required.

PRINCIPLES OF ANORECTAL SURGERY

Preoperative Preparation

Any patient who is to undergo an anorectal operation requires a thorough general evaluation. Proctoscopic examination should be carried out preoperatively and deferred only if the patient has an extremely painful condition, in which case it is carried out with anesthesia in the appropriate circumstances. The more proximal colon and possibly the small intestine require colonoscopy and/or contrast x-ray examination when neoplastic or inflammatory bowel diseases are suspected or likely. Any patient older than 40 years who presents with bright red rectal bleeding or a positive Hemoccult test while on a restricted diet requires a complete evaluation of the lower intestinal tract, even though anal pathology sufficient to account for the symptoms may be discovered. This is particularly so in the situation of bleeding in association with prolapsing hemorrhoids. Under such circumstances, it may be necessary to perform a barium enema x-ray and/or a total colonscopy. If the patient gives a history of diarrhea or other symptoms suggestive of inflammatory bowel disease, both the small and large intestine should be studied by x-ray techniques or endoscopically prior to the performance of any anorectal operation. Systemic disease such as leukemia, syphilis, or Crohn's disease may present with anal or rectal lesions. If these conditions are suspected, the patient requires a complete evaluation prior to any surgery on the anorectum.

The immediate preoperative preparation of the patient should take into consideration the specific anxieties related to rectal surgery. These usually include a fear of pain, incontinence, recurrence, and the possibility of malignancy. Preparation of the bowel for most anorectal operations requires a single, packaged, low-volume phosphate enema immediately prior to the operation,; the bowel is then completely evacuated. No antibiotic preparation is given except when inadvertent perforation of the bowel is a significant possibility; e.g., when sessile adenomas are excised from high in the rectum or a large polyp is snared from the sigmoid colon with electrocautery probe. Laxatives or stool softeners are not administered routinely. It is desirable to induce a spontaneous bowel movement by the second or third postoperative day; hence, special diets are not advocated. The long-standing tradition of shaving the perineal and perianal skin is at best uncomfortable and totally unnecessary. Regrowth of perianal hair adds to the postoperative irritation, and the presence of hair does not complicate the operation or the healing process in any way.

Anesthetic Technique (Fig 47–6)

Many of the common anorectal operations can be carried out on an outpatient basis. Anesthesia required to carry out anorectal operations can be varied to suit the individual patient's needs and the needs of the surgeon. In all cases, irre-

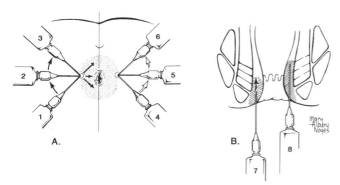

Fig 47–6.—Technique of infiltrating local anesthetic agents into the perianal tissues. **A,** Step 1: An intradermal wheal is raised. Steps 2–6: The subcutaneous tissues and lower anal sphincters are infiltrated circumferentially. **B,** Steps 7–8: The anoderm and submucosa are infiltrated.

spective of whether a regional field block, epidural anesthesia, spinal anesthesia, or general anesthesia with or without an endotracheal tube is used, local infiltration of a long-acting anesthetic agent combined with epinephrine solution (0.25% bupivacaine with epinephrine 1:200,000) to aid hemostasis and facilitate identification of anatomy is recommended.[1]

Technique

For any anorectal operation, proper exposure of the perineum is mandatory. This is best achieved with the patient being placed in the prone jack-knifed position. This affords the best exposure but adds to anesthetic problems, necessitating placement of an endotracheal tube for general anesthesia. The dorsal lithotomy position is not recommended for the majority of anorectal operations, since it affords a more difficult field of exposure. The left lateral position may be adopted in some instances where it is undesirable to have the patient in the prone position.[19] The operative technique should be characterized by minimal handling of the tissues, sharp dissection, and primary closure of wounds, when possible, using fine absorbable sutures without tension. In all circumstances normal skin must be conserved and unnecessary injury to the sphincter mechanism avoided.

Postoperative Care

Packing of the anal canal and rectum is an ineffective way of achieving hemostasis and rarely is necessary. Some surgeons use a small volume of oxydized cellulose topically to aid hemostasis. Bulky, painful dressings should be avoided to ensure patient comfort, to allow spontaneous voiding, and to minimize the need for urinary catheterization. A stool bulk-producing compound and a lubricant are administered orally starting on the day of operation. If the patient has not had a spontaneous bowel movement by the third postoperative day, a tap water enema is administered through a soft rubber catheter. Routine dilatations and irrigations of the anal canal are not used postoperatively. After most anorectal operations, the patient receives a regular diet, usually on the first postoperative day. Hospital discharge is indicated by the patient's com-

fort and ability to manage at home. A large percentage of anorectal operations can be performed on an outpatient basis or with only a short hospital stay. Should postoperative enemas be necessary, they can be administered in the office or on an outpatient basis. A psyllium seed bulk producer is prescribed, and the patient instructed to keep a cotton dressing in place to collect discharge and drainage. Sitz baths are encouraged for cleanness and comfort. Patients are seen postoperatively approximately ten days following hospital discharge and at regular intervals until complete healing has occurred. In all cases the patient is discharged with specific written instructions:

1. The following medicines or prescription will be sent home with you:
   a. Psyllium seed bulk agent evacuant.
     2 doses daily in full glass of water
   b. Analgesic pills—one or two tablets every 3–4 hours as needed for pain.
   c. Local anesthetic ointment or cream.
     Apply externally with cotton dressing after each bath and bowel movement.
2. Postoperative office visits are essential to ensure proper healing of your rectal wounds. Please call the office to make your first appointment as instructed.
3. Sitz baths, comfortably warm, should be taken three times a day, especially after bowel movements. Baths should last no longer than 20 minutes.
4. Some bloody discharge, especially after bowel movements, can be expected after rectal surgery. If there is prolonged or profuse bleeding, call us at once.
5. Bowel movements after rectal surgery are usually associated with some discomfort. This will diminish as the healing progresses. You should have a bowel movement at least every other day. If 2 days pass without a bowel movement, take an ounce of milk of magnesia and repeat in 6 hours if no results.
6. The use of dry toilet tissue should be avoided. After bowel movements, use wet facial tissue or cotton to clean yourself, or if possible take a sitz bath.
7. A general diet is recommended, including plenty of fruit and vegetables. Try to drink 6 to 8 glasses of water a day.
8. No strenuous exercise or heavy lifting should be attempted until healing is well under way. Climbing stairs, walking, and car riding may be done in moderation.
9. If you have any questions about your postoperative care, feel free to call the physician any time at home or the office.

Complications

Hemorrhage is one of the most common complications following anorectal surgery. Its occurrence can be reduced by the use of electrocautery or suture ligature technique at the time of the operation. In most instances immediate postoperative bleeding is related to ineffective hemostasis at the time of operation or to unnecessarily heavy packing of the anal canal. Corrective suture of the bleeder is the treatment of choice to control the postoperative hemorrhage occurring during the first 24 hours. Any patient who begins to bleed immediately postoperatively and does not respond to bed rest and spontaneous cessation of the bleeding should be taken back to the operating room where, with proper anesthesia with optimal exposure, the site of bleeding usually can easily be demonstrated and controlled. Secondary hemorrhage occurs in 1%–4% of patients undergoing hemorrhoidectomy.[20] This usually presents on the 7–10th postoperative day, when the absorbable sutures used for the operation have disintegrated. In most instances bleeding ceases spontaneously. In those patients in whom control cannot be achieved by conservative measures, return to the operating room for examination with anesthesia, evacuation of clots, and suture ligature of the bleeding point is necessary.

Postoperative Pain

Anorectal operations on the whole tend to produce situations of moderate to severe pain in the immediate postoperative period. Anxiety, particularly in the preoperative period, tends to magnify the problem. Abnormal pain accompanies a variety of complications related to anorectal surgery. The constant, pressure-like pain associated with fecal impaction must be differentiated from the usual postoperative pain related to the surgical procedure. This distressing complication can be avoided or treated with a simple tap water enema administered through a soft-tipped rubber catheter. The pain associated with perianal suppuration such as intersphincteric abscess is usually described as a "toothache" type of pain and characteristically appears on the 3rd–5th postoperative day. Unusually severe pain in the first 24–48 hours after anorectal surgery indicates fulminating sepsis, often of a synergistic type. The sharp, tearing pain of an anal fissure, which persists well into the healing phase following anorectal surgery, indicates the possibility of anal stenosis. The fissure usually occurs in the midline posteriorly or in one of the posterior lateral quadrants and rarely responds to conservative management; a second operation is generally indicated. Undiagnosed Crohn's disease should be suspected in patients presenting with such a fissure, suppurative process, or a slowly healing anorectal wound. In many patients with Crohn's disease, the initial symptom is related to problems occurring in the immediate postoperative period following anorectal surgery.[21]

Anal stricture is an infrequent complication of anal rectal operations utilizing minimal dissection techniques with primary wound closure. It is a dreaded problem, since treatment is difficult. Efforts are best directed at its prevention. Anal dilatation has been used for many years, but this is a painful, often unsuccessful procedure in the long term. The regular use of a bulk-producing agent such as a pysillium seed evacuant compound following anorectal surgery is the simplest and most physiologic method for dilating the anal canal. It is far superior to forceful, painful dilatation with a finger or anal dilator. If anal stricture persists and is painful and symptomatic, an anoplasty is indicated.

In certain anorectal operations, where the rectal mucosa is advanced to form a new dentate line, an ectropion may result. This condition occurs when the mucosa has been advanced beyond the anal verge, resulting in a continual mucous discharge and "wet anus." Such a complication is best treated by excision of the offending mucosa and repair by a sliding skin pedicle graft.

Incontinence from anorectal procedures can arise from several causes. The most common early problem is fecal impaction, resulting in bypass of liquid stool with continuous relaxation of the anal sphincter mechanism by the impacting bolus. This is best corrected with tap water enemas. Early in the postoperative period, fecal staining and the patient's inability to distinguish between flatus and stool are common and to be expected. This is invariably temporary, self-limiting, and due to the interference with the proprioceptive nerve endings of the anoderm. The use of large amounts of mineral oil compound to lubricate the stool following surgery results in a leakage of mineral oil, which may be interpreted as incontinence. Severe forms of incontinence generally are related to injury or division of the sphincter musculature. Partial internal sphincterotomy, commonly carried out for anal fissure, invariably results in immediate fecal spoilage of a slight degree. This is rarely permanent. In certain situations where large percentages of the sphincter mechanism require transection, as in extensive fistula surgery, incontinence may persist. Under such circumstances sphincter repair may be indicated. Preservation of the sphincteric mechanism is a most important consideration in the treatment of deep or high fistulas and when fistulas involve the anterior sphincter mechanism, especially in females.

Perianal irritation and discomfort are very common after anorectal surgery. This is partly due to the healing of the cutaneous wound plus minor degrees of soiling and discharge of blood and serum. It is usually self-limiting and requires no special therapy. Persistent anal pruritus may indicate anal fissure or a sensitivity to one of the topical anesthetic ointments commonly used following such surgery.

Urinary tract symptoms, particularly retention and infection, are minimized by ensuring decreased fluid administration during the operation and immediately postoperatively. It is also important to resort to catheterization only when the patient has distention and is in distress. Routine catheterization at a set period following surgery, even though the patient has not voided, is to be condemned.

Incontinence

"Anal incontinence" is a term which covers a broad spectrum of anal function impairment ranging from occasional perianal fecal staining to complete loss of sphincter tone with the involuntary passage of formed stool. Such total anal incontinence with the complete loss of sphincter muscle control is always due to physical injury or loss of muscle mass, sensory denervation, or CNS problems. Partial anal incontinence, which is far more common, is usually intermittent, resulting in involuntary soiling or passage of flatus. Such problems may occur if either the internal or the external sphincter muscle is defective. Trauma, obstetrical procedures, and anorectal surgery are three identifiable causes of partial incontinence. Inflammatory bowel disease, carcinoma of the rectum, or complete rectal prolapse may produce continence problems as the first manifestation of the problem. In many cases, particularly in older-age groups, no such identifiable causes exist, and one must postulate a degeneration of the neuromuscular components of the continence mechanism.[22]

Overflow anal incontinence accompanies a fecal impaction or chronic constipation with prolonged laxative use. Such patients are usually bedridden or chronically debilitated and often elderly. Similar problems may occur in young children with acquired constipation and/or megacolon. The sphincter musculature is intact, but a large bolus of feces distends the rectal ampula, causing reflex relaxation of the internal sphincter, and is responsible for loss of the defecation reflex. Correction consists of immediate evacuation of the impaction with enemas and occasionally manually. Prevention is achieved by dietary alteration, the use of bulk stool softeners, increased fluid intake, and reestablishment of regular bowel habits. This may require the regular use of enemas over a long period.

Treatment of Anal Incontinence

Therapy must be based on consideration of etiologic factors with judicious selection of patients for operative correction. Only patients with incontinence where there is a muscle defect secondary to trauma, obstetrical tear, or operative procedures should be considered for a direct operative repair of the anal sphincter. Such a sphincteroplasty involves mobilization of the divided sphincter muscle and reapproximation without tension (Fig 47–7).[23, 24] Success of such a procedure is dependent on an intact nerve supply to the sphincter muscle. In situations where extensive sphincter injury exists with or without denervation, gracilis muscle transfer with encirclement of the anus produces a circumferential physiologic sling, which may be trained to act as a sphincter.[25] In relatively young patients who have idiopathic anal incontinence, particularly associated with complete prolapse of the rectum, a postanal repair of the pelvic floor muscles performed through the intersphincteric plane has produced improvement in continence in a large percentage of patients (Fig 47–8).[10] Finally, if local operation is futile, an expertly sited and performed colostomy produces a situation which is far more easily cared for than the alternative, which is a perineal colostomy.

Prolapse of the Rectum

Prolapse or procidentia is a relatively uncommon condition whereby the full thickness of the rectal wall turns inside out and prolapses into or through the anal canal. Typically the extruded rectum, variable in length, is seen as concentric rings of mucosa. This distinguishes it from rectal mucosal prolapse, which is far more common and in which the radial folds of mucosa extrude a shorter distance through the anus. Al-

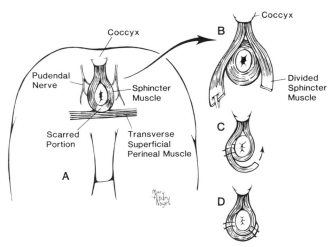

Fig 47–7.—Anal sphincteroplasty. **A,** the approach in prone position. **B,** the previously injured anal sphincter is dissected from perianal tissues preserving its nerve supply. The sphincter is divided through the scar. **C** and **D,** the sphincter is wrapped around the anal canal and sutured.

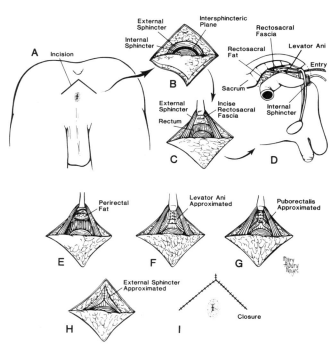

Fig 47–8.—Post anal repair via the intersphincteric plane. **A,** the prone position with the incision between the coccyx and anus. **B,** the flap is raised and the intersphincteric plane identified. **C** and **D,** the rectum is exposed and displaced anteriorly via the intersphincteric plane. Note this enables exposure of the superior surface of the levator ani muscles. The retrosacral fascia is incised from its inferior surface to enable complete anterior displacement of the rectum. **E,** the perirectal fat in the retrorectal space is visualized. **F,** the levator ani muscles are approximated loosely in the midline. **G,** the puborectalis muscle is approximated in the midline. **H,** the external sphincter muscles are approximated in the midline. **I,** the incision is closed.

though prolapse of the rectum can occur at any age, peak incidence is between 60 and 70 years of age, with a female-to-male ratio of 5:1.[26] The etiology of this problem remains unknown; however, with the more widespread use of cineradiography,[29] the mechanism of prolapse has been shown to be due to a rectorectal intussusception commencing circumferentially at 6–7 cm proximal to the anal verge.[27–30]

In many patients, few if any symptoms exist. The early symptoms are usually minor and include anorectal pain, discomfort during defecation, difficulty in initiating bowel movements, feeling of incomplete evacuation, and varying degrees of anal incontinence. Diagnosis is readily made if the prolapsing rectum comes through the anus. In early stages of prolapse, where the intussusception remains in the upper anal canal (hidden prolapse), the diagnosis can be extremely difficult. Anal incontinence, especially associated with inflammatory changes of the rectal mucosa anteriorly at the 6–7 cm level, may indicate presence of such a prolapse. Under such circumstances straining on a commode or at the time of cineradiography (defecatogram) may induce the prolapse to become evident.[28] In long-standing or advanced cases both fecal and urinary incontinence may be present. This has been shown to be the consequence of entrapment or stretching of the pudendal and perineal nerves. Surgical repair of hidden rectal prolapse therefore is essential to prevent ongoing neuromuscular damage and the ultimate development of incontinence.[22]

The etiology of a complete rectal prolapse remains unknown, however, certain anatomical defects which are in some way related but not necessarily the cause of the prolapse are well known (Fig 47–9). The levator muscles are diastased. The endopelvic fascia is loose. The normal horizontal position of the rectum is lost. The anterior rectovaginal or rectovesical pouch is unusually deep. The anal sphincter muscle is commonly weak.[1] Surgical treatment of rectal prolapse focuses on correction of one or several of these anatomical changes. As these are not the cause of the prolapse, not surprisingly surgical correction is not universally successful, having a relatively high incidence of recurrence.

Treatment of Complete Rectal Prolapse

A wide diversity of surgical repairs exists for patients with rectal prolapse. Each has its proponents. Current emphasis on surgery, however, is to remove the intussusception, prevent the intussusception, or both. On this basis operative treatment can be divided into five main subgroups.

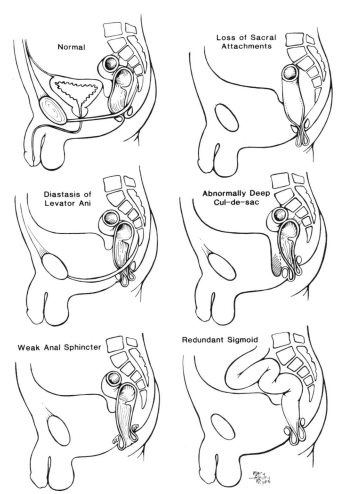

Fig 47–9.—The anatomical defects found in patients with complete rectal prolapse is shown. The normal anatomy is shown for comparison.

RECTAL SLING OPERATION.—Several variations on a main theme exist with this procedure (Fig 47–10). An abdominal approach is required, whereby the rectum with its mesentery is mobilized for varying degrees posteriorly. The partly or completely mobilized rectum is anchored to the front of the sacrum, utilizing a sling of Teflon or Marlex mesh.[31] If this type of technique is used, it is important to ensure that the sling be loose enough to allow easy passage of two fingers between it and the rectum to be suspended. If made too snug, fecal impaction above the level of the sling may occur.[32]

IVALON SPONGE WRAP AROUND OPERATION.—This technique involves an abdominal approach (Fig 47–11). Although not popular in this country, it has been widely utilized in the United Kingdom and Europe.[33, 26] The rectum with its mesentery is completely mobilized posteriorly. Polyvinyl alcohol sponge material is wrapped around the back of the rectum and then is attached to the persacral fascia and periosteum on the sacrum. In some instance Marlex or Teflon mesh is used in preference to the polyvinyl alcohol.

ANTERIOR RESECTION OF THE RECTUM.—Again, an abdominal approach is required, with the operative technique being similar to that for low anterior resection of the rectum for other reasons.[34] As the disease process is benign, radical clearance of perirectal tissues is not necessary. Dissection close to the rectal wall minimizes the chance of injury to the pelvic autonomic nerves. The rectum at or just above the anterior peritoneal reflection, which is the starting point of the intussusception, is resected. The proximal line of resection should be at a convenient level in the rectosigmoid or sigmoid colon so that any redundancy is removed without tension on the anastomosis.

TRANSABDOMINAL PROCTOPEXY.—As its names implies, this is an abdominal procedure whereby the rectum is fixed to the front of the sacrum without the necessity of using a foreign material (Fig 47–12).[35] This operation is our proce-

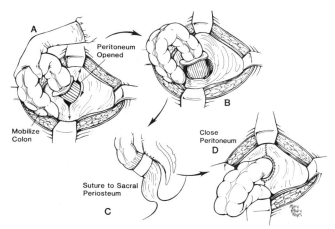

Fig 47–10.—The rectal sling operation for complete rectal prolapse is depicted. **A,** the sigmoid colon is mobilized. **B,** the rectum is mobilized out of the hollow of the sacrum. **C,** a sling is utilized to suspend the mobilized rectum to the front of the sacrum. **D,** the completed operation with pelvic peritoneum is closed, showing the isolated sling from the peritoneal cavity.

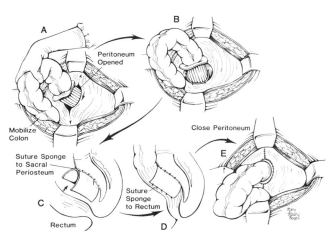

Fig 47–11.—The Ivalon® sponge wrap around operation for complete rectal prolapse. **A,** the sigmoid colon is mobilized. **B,** the rectum is mobilized out of the hollow of the sacrum. **C,** The Ivalon® sponge is sutured to the front of the sacrum to form a "cradle." **D,** the mobilized rectum is placed into the Ivalon® sponge "cradle" and sutured laterally. **E,** the completed operation with the pelvic peritoneum is closed, isolating the Ivalon® sponge from the peritoneal cavity.

dure of choice.[26, 36] Our preference is to use a low transverse abdominal incision. The rectum is fully mobilized posteriorly and laterally down to the pelvic floor. The lateral ligaments of the rectum are not divided. The mobilized rectum is drawn up toward the sacrum, and the peritoneum, including the endopelvic fascia of the lateral ligament on each side of the rectum is sutured to the presacral fascia and periosteum just below the promontory of the sacrum. One to three sutures of 2-0 silk on each side are all that is necessary. No attempt is made to obliterate the anterior cul-de-sac or to approximate the levator hiatus. In many instances rectosigmoid colon resection with a high end-to-end anastomosis is performed because of the concurrent presence of marked redundancy, predisposing to sigmoid volvulus.

PERINEAL RECTOSIGMOIDECTOMY.—Via a perineal approach, it is possible to resect the rectum and the rectosig-

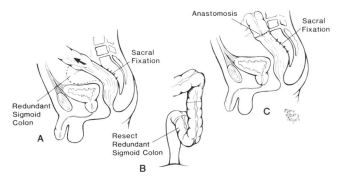

Fig 47–12.—Transabdominal proctopexy operation for complete rectal prolapse. **A,** the mobilized rectum is sutured to the front of the sacrum using sutures through the lateral ligaments of the rectum bilaterally. **B,** the redundant sigmoid colon is resected. **C,** a "high" anastomosis is made between the proximal sigmoid colon and the upper, mobilized colon.

moid colon via the prolapse itself.[37, 38] This procedure is well tolerated by all patients, especially the elderly or frail, and general, regional, or even local anesthesia can be used. The procedure may be performed in the lithotomy or prone jackknife positions. The prolapse is exteriorized and a circular incision is made at 2cm proximal to the dentate line. This is deepened so that the intussusception along with the redundant rectosigmoid and sigmoid colon can be resected and an end-to-end anastomosis performed perineally.[36]

Our choice of procedure has been the transabdominal proctopexy for all good-risk patients. For patients who are thought not to be suitable for a safe intra-abdominal procedure but who can withstand general or regional anesthesia, perineal rectosigmoidectomy is the method of choice. In the elderly and in those whose general medical condition preclude a definitve repair, a perineal rectosigmoidectomy can be performed using local anesthesia.[36] The Thiersch wire encirclement procedures are not recommended even in the poor-risk patient. Such procedures, although simple, produce an alarmingly high incidence of fecal impaction, which makes nursing more difficult. Under such circumstances it is probably better not to offer any surgical therapy at all.

The Delorme procedure likewise is a perineal operation. The technique is based on a submucosal resection, with reefing and plication of the lower rectal musculature to produce in effect an encirclement of the anal sphincters. It has the advantage, like the perineal rectosigmoidectomy, of avoiding an abdominal approach.[39]

ASSOCIATED ANAL INCONTINENCE.—Anal incontinence accompanies complete rectal prolapse in approximately 50% of the cases.[36] Definitive surgical repair of the prolapsing rectum usually results in resolution of or improvement in the continence problems in a large percentage of patients. In those patients in whom incontinence persists despite a successful repair of the prolapse, further operative intervention may become necessary. Under such circumstances extensive denervation of the sphincter muscle exists, precluding direct sphincteric repair. Increasing the anorectal angle by performing a postanal repair through the intersphincteric plane has been successful in some individuals with this problem (see Fig 47–8).[10]

Pruritus Ani

Itching of skin around the anus is a common symptom and one which is likely to be seen, usually in males, at times of stress and in hot weather when sweating is excessive. The skin of the perinanal area is sensitive, and any condition causing moisture or soiling can predispose to itching. In the vast majority of patients no underlying specific problem is found; hence, the condition is considered to be idiopathic.[40] It is important, however, to seek possible causal or aggravating factors in each patient. Surgically correctable conditions contributing to this symptom are prolapsing internal hemorrhoids, rectal mucosal prolapse, ectropion, anal fissure, fistula-in-ano, condyloma acuminatum, and neoplasms of the anal canal and perineal skin. Systemic problems including diabetes mellitus, eczema, chronic diarrhea, jaundice, uremia, and lymphoma should all be considered. Fungus infections are most commonly due to *Candida* and *Epidermophyton* organisms. These are mainly secondary invaders rather than initiating factors. In children, pinworm infestation is a common cause. Contact dermatitis caused by dyed or perfumed toilet tissue, soaps, powders, or clothing, as well as a variety of over-the-counter prescriptions. In the vast majority of patients, however, no such problems will be found. Under such circumstances poor perianal hygiene along with excessive perianal sweating and possibly minor degrees of fecal incontinence are the main causes.

There is no specific treatment for idiopathic pruritus ani; however, it is possible to alter poor perianal hygiene habits and to minimize the effects of sweating.[41] It is also important in all circumstances to ensure bowel habit regulation to prevent incomplete evacuation of the rectum with possible mucous or fecal leakage. Gentle cleansing of the perineal skin with moist tissue or warm water is the cornerstone of successful control. It is equally important to obtain dryness of the area by utilizing a gentle drying technique, perferably with a hair blow-dryer. Therapy is often supplemented with intermittent use of topical 1% hydrocortisone cream. It is important to stress that fluorinated steroid creams, although giving temporary relief, do cause skin atrophy and should not be used for long periods.

Direct operative therapy for idiopathic pruritus ani is to be condemned. Any pathology which may be thought to be contributing to the patient's symptoms should be treated on its merits, although very often such problems are an accompaniment rather than the cause of the pruritus ani. This is particularly so in patients with anal fissures where surgical treatment of the anal fissure may produce more minor incontinence, potentiating and worsening the pruritus ani. In all cases reassurance and persistence will produce relief of symptoms in all but a small percentage. If, after several weeks of strict adherence to the regimen outlined, the patient's symptoms persist, a dermatologic consultation is required.

Hemorrhoids

The upper anal canal is lined by normal rectal mucosa. At the level of the dentate line, this changes to modified skin. Beneath the upper anal lining are situated the tissues that are called hemorrhoids. These tissues are in fact localized, separate, bulky cushions of a specialized submucosal vascular tissue. The tissue is composed of a fibroelastic connective tissue containing smooth muscle fibers derived from the internal sphincter and conjoined longitudinal muscle. This stroma supports rich venous and arterial plexuses.[42,28] The concept that hemorrhoids are varicose veins is entirely incorrect. These tissues, as described, are normal anatomical features of the anal canal, and their presence does not constitute disease. These hemorrhoidal cushions or prominences are discrete and separated so that the anal canal lumen forms a tri-radiate slit. The stem of the "Y" so formed invariably approaches the midline posteriorly, so that its arms separate three cushions or bulges lying in constant sites—left lateral, right anterior, and right posterior. Secondary folds are present in each of these discrete cushions. Such an anatomical arrangement is remarkably constant; however, it bears no relationship, as previously thought, to the terminal branching of the superior rectal artery, which is inconstant.[43] That such an arrangement is the normal state is attested to by the fact that these anal cushions

or bulges are present in children and can be demonstrated in the fetus and even in the embryo. The function of hemorrhoids is not known. They may aid in anal continence by their sheer bulk. It is not uncommon for patient to complain of minor degrees of incontinence after radical hemorrhoidectomy. During the act of defecation, when with straining they become engorged, it is postulated that they cushion the anal canal and support its lining. Being separate structures rather than a continuous ring of vascular tissue allows the anal canal to dilate during defecation.

Hemorrhoidal Disease

Pathologic change in the anatomical situation as described above results in symptoms which, by common usage, have been termed "hemorrhoids." Many factors have been implicated in the cause of symptoms referable to the hemorrhoids. These include the erect position of the human being, the absence of venous valves in the portal venous system, obstruction of venous return, and hereditary weakness of the vessels. While such factors are no doubt important in the causation of varicose vein disease, this is not the situation in the hemorrhoid problem. Prolonged straining at defecation and the chronic passage of hard, small volumes of stool, however, result in repeated tense engorgement of the hemorrhoidal tissues. In the early stages of disease this may cause superficial injury to the rectal mucous membrane, resulting in painless, bright red bleeding from the capillaries of the lamina propria. With repeated straining and engorgement, the normal supports of the hemorrhoidal cushions are stretched and damaged, resulting in a tendency to prolapse downward and hence outside the anal canal.[43] Early in the evolution of the disease, such a prolapse occurs only with straining and resolves spontaneously. With repeated episodes, however, the situation becomes irreversible, so that manual replacement of prolapsed tissue is necessary. In the chronic state of the disease, the normally lax rectal mucosa above the hemorrhoid is eventually incorporated with the prolapsing anal cushion so that it adds to the bulk which now could be described as the classic prolapsing hemorrhoid. Occasionally such prolapsed hemorrhoids lying outside the normally contracted anal sphincter ring may become strangulated, with resulting thrombosis occurring in the vascular plexuses. This in turn may result in gangrene and sloughing of the tissues.

Currently epidemiologic studies implicate the low fiber-low residue Western diet as the cause of many of the common diseases of our society, including hemorrhoids. Strict alteration to a high-fiber type of diet, with the addition of bulk in the form of cereal fiber or bulk-forming compounds, can prevent hemorrhoidal disease and in many cases can reverse the symptoms of the early stages. Under such circumstances, although symptoms may disappear, the physical characteristics of the hemorrhoidal tissues remain unaltered, lending support to the concept that chronic straining plays the largest part in the causation of such problems.

Several states of hemorrhoidal disease can be defined.[1] Internal hemorrhoids are normally occurring, submucosal vascular cushions located above the dentate and covered by rectal mucosa. External hemorrhoids are normally occurring, subcutaneous venules and arterioles of the inferior hemorrhoidal plexus, located below the dentate line, and hence covered by squamous epithelium. A mixed hemorrhoid is a combination of both internal and external hemorrhoids. Prolapsing hemorrhoids are internal hemorrhoids which protrude beyond the dentate line or lie outside the anal canal. They are always associated with redundant prolapsing rectal mucosa. A thrombosed hemorrhoid is one in which the blood has clotted intravascularly and to some extent extravascularily. Perianal skin tag is an area of fibrous connective tissue covered by perianal skin, which is usually the result of a previously thrombosed external hemorrhoid or anal surgery.

CLINICAL MANIFESTATIONS.—External hemorrhoids are usually asymptomatic. Perianal irritation and pruritus do not result from external hemorrhoidal disease. Commonly such patients do have perianal skin tags, which make any perianal irritation or pruritus worse and much more difficult to treat. However, such skin tags are usually the result of previous external hemorrhoidal thrombosis. Swelling and edema of such skin tags are the result of perianal irritation and not the cause of it. The patient's awareness of an external hemorrhoid is usually the pain which accompanies acute thrombosis. Thrombosis may recur in the same or a different hemorrhoidal complex. Internal hemorrhoids most commonly are manifested by painless, bright red rectal bleeding at the time of defecation. The patient commonly describes the bleeding episode as "the blood drips into the toilet bowl." Prolapse of an internal hemorrhoid may be accompanied by a feeling of moisture in the anal region and palpation of the protruding rectal mucosa with underlying hemorrhoids. Early in its course, the prolapsed hemorrhoid reduces spontaneously. As the condition becomes chronic, permanent prolapse results in a situation frequently accompanied by irritation and possible thrombosis. Other sequelae of internal hemorrhoids—anemia, edema, suppuration, ulceration, fibrosis, strangulation, and, rarely, thrombophlebitis with gangrene. Pain is not a symptom of hemorrhoids unless associated with thrombosis, or it is indicative of other anal disease which may coexist with hemorrhoids such as perianal infection, anal fissure, proctalgia fugax, or occasionally anal carcinoma. Likewise, discharge or feeling of moisture with or without perianal irritation or pruritus is not a symptom of hemorrhoids unless chronic or recurring prolapse is present, but is indicative of other diseases such as fistula-in-ano, proctitis, rectal prolapse, and neoplasm.

Uncomplicated internal hemorrhoids usually are not palpable. Having the patient strain at the completion of a digital rectal examination will reveal a prolapse of rectal mucosa with internal hemorrhoid. The anoscope is particularly suitable for viewing internal hemorrhoids, but proctoscopy, fiberoptic sigmoidoscopy, barium enema, or colonoscopy may have to be performed in patients to rule out neoplastic or inflammatory bowel disease, which may present with similar symptoms. In patients with an atypical history or in the older-age group, such a complete colonic workup is mandatory even though obviously prolapsing hemorrhoids are present.

Treatment

THROMBOSED EXTERNAL HEMORRHOIDS.—In most instances the treatment of a painful external thrombosed hemorrhoid is an outpatient or office procedure. Anesthesia is readily achieved by subcutaneous injection of a 0.5%–1.0% solution of lidocaine or 0.25% solution of bupivacaine containing 1:200,000 epinephrine. Usually 3–5 ml are required. Injection is slightly uncomfortable and in some instances may be painful. This may be minimized by using a very fine-gauge needle, such as a 30-gauge dental needle, and warming the local anesthetic to body temperature prior to its injection.

Incision alone does not suffice. It is preferable to excise the entire thrombosed external hemorrhoid and to cauterize the bleeding points. Adequate treatment of a single thrombosed external hemorrhoid prevents further thrombosis in that area and usually obviates subsequent hemorrhoidectomy. If the thrombosed external hemorrhoid is unassociated with pain, nonoperative therapy is indicated.[20] Severe pain associated with such thrombosis lasts several days and as long as a week. Complete resolution, however, requires several weeks.

INTERNAL HEMORRHOIDS.—The vast majority of patients with symptoms referable to internal hemorrhoids are treated at least initially and usually definitively by nonoperative means. In all cases emphasis is placed on dietary modification to correct any underlying bowel disturbance contributed to by constipating foods, especially dairy foods, inadequate hydration, and lack of high fiber in the usual diet. This may be supplemented with the use of hydrophylic bulk-forming additives. In many instances these measures alone will relieve the patient of the hemorrhoidal symptoms, although there will be no noticeable change in the clinical appearance of the hemorrhoidal tissue. For ease of clarification of surgical therapy, hemorrhoidal symptoms are best thought of in four stages[20]: Stage 1: symptoms of painless bright red rectal bleeding at the time of defecation not due to any other anal, rectal, or colonic pathology. In appropriate circumstances this requires a complete colonic evaluation and in some instances scrutinization of the upper GI tract. Bleeding from otherwise asymptomatic internal hemorrhoids cannot be assumed until all other possible causes have been excluded. This is particularly so with the older-age groups in whom the likelihood of coexisting rectal and colonic neoplasms is increased. Stage 2 hemorrhoidal symptoms are those in which the patient has bleeding and prolapse at the time of defecation which spontaneously reduces. Again, bleeding cannot be assumed to be coming from such hemorrhoids unless other pathology has been excluded. Stage 3 disease produces symptoms of bleeding associated with prolapse which requires manual reduction after defecation. Stage 4 hemorrhoidal disease exists either as an acute phase, with prolapsed thrombosed internal/external hemorrhoids, or, rarely, as a chronic phase, where the internal hemorrhoids along with the prolapsing rectal mucosa are chronically prolapsed outside the anus.

Patients with hemorrhoids which have not responded to dietary measures are candidates for further manipulation. Injection therapy utilizing 5% phenol in a vegetable oil or other sclerosing agents is a useful technique particularly in patients with otherwise uncomplicated bleeding internal hemorrhoids with minimal or no prolapse.[44] One to 3 milliliters of the prescribed solution is injected into the submucosa at the level of the anorectal ring at the three commonly occurring sites of internal hemorrhoids. This is done without anesthesia and, apart from some rectal fullness, produces no posttreatment symptoms.

Internal rubberband ligation is an effective and simple procedure utilized in patients with early degrees of rectal mucosal or hemorrhoidal prolapse (Fig 47–13).[45] This is an office or outpatient procedure requiring no anesthesia in which a small constricting rubberband is placed at the level of the anorectal ring onto the most redundant portion of the rectal mucosa immediately above the prolapsing internal hemorrhoid.[46] The incorporated tissue sloughs in approximately four to seven days, leaving an area of ulceration and inflammation resulting in submucosal fibrosis and ultimate fixation of the prolapsing mucosa. Excessive discomfort at the time of banding indicates that the band has been placed in close proximity to the dentate line. This technique provides an alternative to injection therapy but with a precisely controlled loss of redundant mucosa.[47] Repeated applications may be carried out at four- to six-week intervals until the patient's symptoms are relieved. Occasionally two to three areas may be banded per visit. The procedure may be performed without incident on patients receiving anticoagulant therapy, although this is not encouraged. The contraindications are the same as those for surgical hemorrhoidectomy; namely, inflammatory bowel disease, leukemia, and portal hypertension.

Cryotherapy is a method of freezing the hemorrhoidal tissues through a probe which circulates liquid nitrogen, nitrous oxide, or carbon dioxide.[44, 48] Originally cryodestruction was thought to be painless and thus was advocated for an outpatient procedure. It has been found that this procedure does produce significant pain and results in profuse discharge from tissue necrosis and prolonged wound healing.[49] Improperly performed, the freezing can destroy the anal sphincter muscles, rendering the patient incontinent and producing an anal stricture. In experienced hands, however, the final results of such treatment have been shown to be excellent.[50] Similar results, however, can be achieved by less destructive, less painful means.

HEMORRHOIDECTOMY.—Hemorrhoidectomy is reserved for patients having severe symptoms related to grade 3 or 4 hemorrhoids which cannot be controlled by other methods. If the patient is having another anorectal operation, particularly one in which the anal sphincter is to be divided, and is found to have enlarged prolapsing but otherwise asymptomatic hemorrhoids, it is advisable that hemorrhoidectomy be done at the same time. Hemorrhoidectomy may be indicated in the immediate postpartum period in women who have had problems prior to pregnancy and in whom prolapse and thrombosis occur at the time of delivery. In most instances hemorrhoidal symptoms which appear to intensify during delivery resolve, but there is a small group of women whose problem is of such magnitude as to indicate an operation.

Although there are many variations, all hemorrhoid operations basically employ the ligature and excision technique. The method of handling the perianal skin differentiates the techniques. Principles for all operative procedures include removing all diseased tissues—that is, internal and external hemorrhoids and redundant rectal mucosa, leaving minimum scarring of the anal canal, avoiding interference with the sphincteric mechanisms, and leaving ample anal orifice for a normal bowel movement.

The technique of closed hemorrhoidectomy offers effective removal of diseased hemorrhoidal tissues, prompt healing of wounds, elimination of mucous drainage by ensuring a lining of the anal canal with stratified squamous epithelium, minimal inpatient and virtually no outpatient care, less postoperative discomfort, no loss of continence, and no need for anal dilatation.[20, 51] An adequate dissection-type closed hemorrhoidectomy may be carried out on the acute prolapsed thrombosed edematous hemorrhoids without fear of anal stenosis or stricture if meticulous dissection and preservation of anoderm are accomplished. This technique may be combined with any other operative procedures such as fistulotomy, internal anal sphincterotomy, or excision of hypertrophied anal papilla.

Operative Technique (Fig 47–14)

All patients are completely assessed as to operative risk. Thorough anorectal examination is undertaken to exclude rectal disease, particularly inflammatory bowel disease or malignancy. When the symptoms are atypical or the patient is older (particularly over 45 years), a complete colonic examination may be necessary. Under appropriate circumstances an air-contrast barium enema, colonoscopy, or both are indicated. Inflammatory bowel disease, especially Crohn's disease, portal hypertension, and bleeding tendencies, are relative contraindications to the procedure.

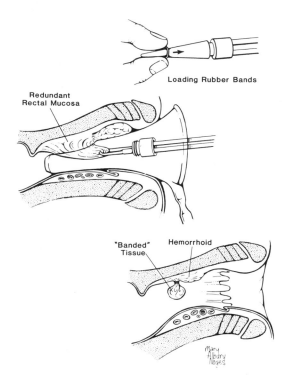

Fig 47–13.—Rubber band ligation of redundant rectal mucosa and internal hemorrhoids. The small rubber bands are "loaded," using a cone applicator. With a fenestrated anoscope in situ, the redundant rectal mucosa at the top of the internal hemorrhoid is grasped. The rubber band is placed around the tissue at the anorectal ring well above the dentate line. The "banded" tissue includes redundant rectal mucosa and only the top of the internal hemorrhoid.

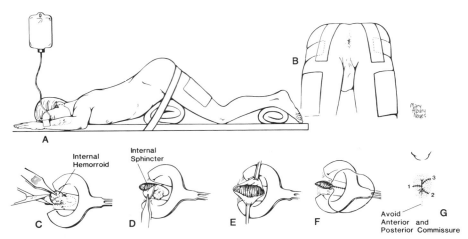

Fig 47–14.—The operative technique of closed hemorrhoidectomy. **A**, the prone position of a roll under the hips and ankles. **B**, the buttocks are taped apart and electrocautery grounding pads in situ. No shaving is performed. **C**, exposure of the operating field is accomplished using a Fansler, large fenestrated operating anoscope. Using a forceps and scissors, dissection is commenced on the perianal skin. **D**, a narrow elipse of skin, anoderm, prolapsing internal hemorrhoid, and prolapsing rectal mucosa are excised and dissected off the internal anal sphincter. **E**, flaps of rectal mucosa and anoderm are elevated and the secondary hemorrhoids excised from beneath them. **F**, the wound is closed with a running suture. **G**, the procedure is then repeated in two other sites, avoiding the midline.

Complete, honest explanation of the procedure will allay most unfounded fears of the patients. No purgatives or antibiotics are necessary. A small, disposable phosphate enema administered one hour before the operation is the only bowel preparation necessary.

The procedure is most adequately performed with the patient in the prone jack-knife position—the pelvis and chest supported on rolls.[52] The buttocks are taped apart for maximum exposure. Shaving is not undertaken, since it is totally unnecessary and markedly adds to the postoperative discomfort. Deliberate anal dilatation is unnecessary. An electrocoagulation grounding plate is placed on the patient, usually on the posterior aspect of the thigh.

General or regional anesthesia, either spinal or caudal, may be used. In all cases supplemental anesthesia is achieved by the use of 0.25% bupivacaine with epinephrine 1:200,000 solution (see Fig 47–5). In some instances local anesthesia may suffice, in which case 0.5% lidocaine with epinephrine 1:200,000 solution would be used. This may be supplemented with IV sedation.

Via a bivalved operating anal speculum, the prolapsing hemorrhoidal tissue and associated redundant rectal mucosa are demonstrated by grasping the loose mucosa with a tissue forceps. Although every case does not conform to the classic three-quadrant distribution, the most frequently involved quadrants are the left lateral, right anterior, and right posterior. It is not necessary to attempt to remove all hemorrhoidal tissue, since the symptoms are related only to the prolapse, not to the presence of this tissue.

Exposure is accomplished with the use of a large fenestrated operating Fansler anoscope. Dissection is started on the perianal skin using fine, sharp, pointed scissors. A narrow ellipse of the skin, anoderm, the prolapsing internal hemorrhoidal mass, and associated redundant rectal mucosa are dissected off the sphincteric mechanism. Care is taken not to injure the underlying internal sphincter muscle. This is best achieved by excising the mass using the heel of the scissors rather than the tips. The redundant rectal mucosa is excised as far as necessary above the anorectal ring to correct the redundancy, even as high as the distal rectal valve. The rectal mucosa and anoderm are then elevated, and the remaining hemorrhoidal tissue is dissected from beneath these flaps to remove any symptomatic secondary hemorrhoidal complexes. Hemostasis is achieved by electrocautery. In all cases the bleeding will be coming from the submucosa. This can easily be identified by elevating the flaps and point, coagulating any bleeding. Anoderm is preserved, and rectal mucosa is then approximated and sutured to the underlying internal sphincter with a running absorbable suture of 3–0 chromic catgut or 5–0 polyglycolic acid. The perianal skin is closed without tension after the edges have been trimmed to prevent excessive skin tag formation. The same procedure is then repeated in as many areas as is necessary. At the completion of the operation, the reconstituted anal canal should easily admit two fingers without stretching the suture lines. Intra-anal dressings are not required.

In the postoperative period patients are encouraged to restrict fluid intake until spontaneous voiding has occurred. By use of this regimen, the problem of postoperative retention of urine has been almost eliminated. Having voided or having been catheterized, the patients are allowed to take fluids and diet as desired and tolerated. Pain is managed by "on demand" IM injection of analgesics for the duration of the hospital stay, supplemented with an oral pain medication. Early activity is encouraged. Warm packs are applied to the perineum during the postoperative period. After 24 hours, patients are encouraged to take as many warm sitz baths as desired for comfort and cleanliness. A small cotton dressing is put in the perianal area to collect whatever drainage or discharge may be present. No other local treatment is carried out. Psyllium seed mucilloid and liquid paraffin-Irish moss emulsion are commenced immediately and are given twice daily. The liquid paraffin-Irish moss emulsion is discontinued after the first bowel movement, which usually occurs on the second or third postoperative day. If it does not, a tap water enema is given using a soft rubber catheter on the third postoperative day.

Routine anal dilatations are painful and unnecessary. Patients are usually discharged from the hospital when they are comfortable and have had a bowel movement, usually by the third or fourth day. In some instances the procedure can be done as an outpatient with very close follow-up in the immediate postoperative period. Patients are instructed to do no lifting or straining; however, they may return to work whenever they wish if no heavy lifting is involved. The discharge medications consist of psyllium hydrophylic mucilloid and oral analgesics to be used as necessary. Patients are reviewed in ten to 14 days, at which time digital examination is usually carried out. A follow-up at two-week intervals is maintained until complete healing has occurred.

Symptoms rarely reappear following an adequate hemorrhoidectomy. Reappearance of bleeding and prolapse is frequently related to inadequate removal of redundant rectal mucosa, rather than hemorrhoidal tissue itself. Concern regarding the possibility of infection and abscess formation with consequent pain and stenosis following such a closed operative technique is unfounded. Such complications occur rarely.[20]

Anal Fissure

An anal fissure is a split or tear in the modified skin or anoderm of the anal canal and as such is situated distal to the dentate line. It occurs in either sex and tends to occur mainly in the midline posteriorly or in the midline anteriorly. The relatively immobile skin of the posterior quadrant of the anal canal associated with angulation is the area that is traumatized by stool, particularly at the time of excess straining, to produce a split or a tear. An acute anal fissure is invariably superficial, is extremely painful, and develops quite precipitously. Edematous skin edges and induration are absent. Most of the acute fissures will heal with adjustment of bowel habits, with some stool softeners and laxatives. A chronic fissure is one that results from repeated or persistent trauma to the fissure-bearing area of the anal canal. It is usually deep, exposing the underlying circular fibers of the internal sphincter muscle. Such a chronic state may be due in part to an abnormality of the internal sphincter muscle. It has been shown that the resting tone of the anal canal in patients with a fissure is increased.[53–55] Very often a tight anal sphincter is observed in these patients.[56] It is assumed that defecation stimulates the sensitive fissure and causes a severe reflex spasm. This would result in drawing the anal canal proximally during anal contraction and the passage of stool, repeatedly traumatizing the already established fissure.

Diagnosis of an anal fissure usually presents no problem. History is one of pain during and immediately after defecation associated with bright red rectal bleeding, usually seen on the toilet tissue after the bowel movement. A fissure in the majority of the patients can be visualized readily on simple inspection of the anal canal after gently spreading the buttocks. This will be present in the midline posteriorly or anteriorly. Indolent-looking fissures or fissures located off the midline suggest some other problem, particularly inflammatory bowel disease, especially Crohn's disease.[57] Care should be taken to make the examination as painless as possible. It is not neces-

sary to perform an anoscopic or proctoscopic examination in all cases, since this is at best uncomfortable and may be extremely painful. If possible, this should be carried out gently. It may be necessary to defer this examination. On occasion it may be necessary to examine the patient using anesthesia to ensure that no other problem exists.

Differential diagnosis of anal fissure includes superficial abrasion of the anal canal induced by trauma (usually a particularly hard bowel movement). This invariably heals with conservative management and usually does not recur. Anal ulcers or fissures secondary to Crohn's disease or ulcerative colitis are usually situated off the midline and are frequently multiple and associated with obvious edema. In the early stages, epidermoid carcinoma of the anal canal may have the appearance of an anal fissure. Tuberculous ulcers are rare. Syphilitic fissure should be considered in appropriate circumstances. Patients with leukemia/lymphoma who develop neutropenia as a result of treatment may develop indolent anal fissures. Perianal fissuring, a problem of perianal skin usually in association with severe anal pruritus, is a manifestation of major skin damage and has no bearing on anal fissure as such.

Treatment

In most cases of superficial or acute fissures conservative therapy results in spontaneous healing. The patient is reassured and begins therapy with psyllium seed compounds to soften the stool, with symptomatic treatment consisting of warm baths and analgesics. In children an increased fluid intake with a decreased consumption of dairy products in an effort to correct constipation is usually all that is required. Operative treatment of anal fissure is considered if such conservative measures fail or if the situation is chronic. The concept of the treatment is to enlarge the skin-lined segment of the anal canal and to relieve spasm during and after defecation. A classic fissurectomy and posterior midline sphincterotomy should be avoided, since healing is prolonged.[58] A posterior sphincterotomy, moreover, is associated with a high incidence of persistent postoperative soiling from the resulting keyhole deformity. Anal sphincter stretching under anesthesia is effective in some instances; however, the disadvantage is that it is uncontrolled as to the amount of sphincter muscle that may be damaged or even disrupted. In all instances a general or at least regional anesthetic is required. Partial lateral, internal sphincterotomy performed as an open or subcutaneous technique is the treatment of choice (Figs 47–15 and 47–16). This procedure may be performed with local, regional, or general anesthetic depending on the individual circumstance. Properly performed, this operation results in healing of the fissure in the vast majority of cases with a very low recurrence rate. There is a high incidence of minor fecal soiling and inability to control flatus. This is in the majority of cases temporary but may last for several months.[1]

Perianal Suppuration

Introduction

Acute suppuration in the tissues of the perineum and perianal region is a common problem encountered in all phases of medical practice.[59] Its early recognition and proper management will, in most cases, lead to complete resolution with little chance of recurrence. In most cases, no preexisting le-

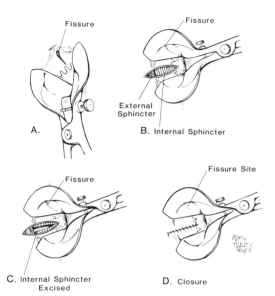

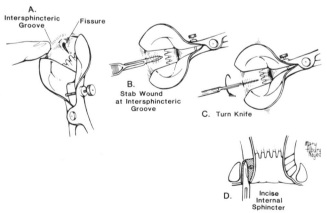

Fig 47–15.—Partial internal anal sphincterotomy is performed by the open technique. **A,** the anal fissure is exposed in the midline using a bi-valve operating anal speculum. **B,** the lateral aspect of the anal canal is exposed. A radial incision is made to expose the internal sphincter up to the level of the dentate line. Note the circumferential fibers of the exposed muscle. **C,** the lower half of the internal sphincter is divided. **D,** the wound is closed.

sion is present; however, it must be remembered that distinct suppurative lesions or unrelated lesions which can become secondarily infected do occur in this region. They must be differentiated from suppuration associated with anal gland infection, the commonly accepted cause of these problems.

Fig 47–16.—Partial internal sphincterotomy is performed by the closed technique. **A,** the anal fissure is exposed in the midline using a bi-valve operating anal speculum. With the blades of the anoscope spread, the lower edge of the anal sphincter and the intersphincteric groove are palpated at the lateral aspect. **B,** the lateral aspect of the anal canal is exposed. Using a fine blade, a stab wound has been made in the intersphincteric groove to enter the intersphincteric plane at the level of the dentate line. **C,** the knife blade is rotated. **D,** the lower half of the internal anal sphincter is divided by incising towards the lumen of the anal canal. The anoderm is not incised.

These specific suppurative conditions include: (1) pilonidal abscess, (2) hydradenitis suppurative of the perineal skin, (3) infected sebaceous cyst, (4) folliculitis, (5) periprostatic abscesses, (6) Bartholin's gland abscess, and (7) intra-abdominal disease (inflammatory or malignant) with extra-abdominal perforation leading to drainage in the perineum.

Specific Infections

Rarely, specific infections such as actinomycosis, tuberculosis, or syphilis may arise in the area. These must be always suspected in any case where the lesion present has unusual features or where resolution is delayed or prolonged. In proved cases, specific therapy is mandatory for a successful outcome.

Inflammatory Bowel Disease

It must also be remembered that perianal suppuration may be a manifestation of inflammatory bowel disease—notably, Crohn's disease.[60] In any case, where the features are atypical or the course is protracted with frequent recurrence, inflammatory bowel disease must always be considered and excluded. The perianal disease may be the initial manifestation of this condition in many patients and may precede bowel involvement by some time, even years.

Leukemia and Lymphoma

Patients with leukemia or lymphoma frequently have perianal problems. In many cases these are true abscesses arising as complications of the associated immunodeficiency. Local infiltration with tumor may also occur, which may present with features identical to those of an abscess. Because of leukopenia in these patients, pus may be scanty or absent. Necrotic tissue with a tendency to bleed may be all that is found in these "abscesses." Treatment should be expectant and symptomatic. Incisions under such circumstances usually bleed excessively and rarely heal.

Perirectal Abscess

The anal glands situated in the submucosa of the anal canal circumferentially at the level of the dentate line open via narrow ducts into the bases of anal crypts.[61] These glands penetrate for variable depths, as deep as the plane between the internal and external sphincter muscles (see Fig 47–2) Obstruction to the ducts can lead to infection and suppuration in the gland, with formation of an abscess in the area of the gland and hence in the intersphincteric space. From this origin the suppuration may spread downward, upward, circumferentially, or laterally to involve the various perianal and perirectal spaces (see Fig 47–4).

Diagnosis

Perirectal suppuration characteristically presents with: (1) pain—acute, throbbing pain in the perianal region aggravated by sitting, coughing, sneezing, and straining is classic; (2) palpable lump—a palpable inflammatory process is often but not invariably present; occasionally the only visible evidence is an area of cellulitis or tender induration of the skin; (3) pyrexia—fever is common, and patients often complain of sweats and shaking chills, especially at night.

Horseshoe Abscess

The horseshoe abscess is an uncommon but spectacular manifestation of perirectal suppuration.[62, 63] This arises as an infection in a posterior midline anal gland that spreads to involve both ischorectal spaces communicating through the deep postanal space. Patients have an obvious septic course associated with bilateral perineal findings. Frequently, acute urinary retention is also present and may, in fact, be the first manifestation of the problem.

Intersphincteric Abscess

This occurs infrequently and is often misdiagnosed, since the clinical features are not the same as in other perirectal abscesses. Patients complain of a dull aching in the rectum (likened to a toothache) rather than in the perianal region. There is no swelling or induraton of the perianal skin; however, tenderness or palpation of the perianal tissues can easily be elicited. Frequently, this tenderness is excessive, precluding further examination without anesthesia. Digital rectal examination reveals a soft, tender mass bulging into the lumen of the anus, which can often be accurately delineated by bidigital examination using a finger and thumb. If the abscess ruptures spontaneously, the patient will complain of passage of purulent material and blood per rectum. Examination in such a case will reveal pus in the rectum seen to be coming from an opening in the anal canal, usually at the level of the dentate line in the posterior midline.

Supralevator Abscess

This is an extremely rare occurrence which is difficult to diagnose accurately. Such abscesses usually arise as extensions of intra-abdominal suppuration but occasionally are the result of extensions of infralevator suppuration. In many cases it is the injudicious probing of infralevator suppuration or fistula-in-ano which causes a false passage in the previously uninvolved and uninfected supralevator space. Patients thus afflicted may present with fever of unknown origin and no history of anal or rectal pain. Rectal or vaginal examination may reveal tenderness in the pelvis, and signs of peritonitis may be present, suggesting an intra-abdominal process.

Two distinct conditions of the perineum should be highlighted at this stage, since they may be confused with true perirectal abscesses and treated as such, causing unnecessary damage to the normal underlying anal sphincter muscles.

Pilonidal Abscess

Pilonidal abscess arises as a secondary infection in a preexisting pilonidal cyst. The abscess may be the first indication of the disease to the patient, although most patients will have a prolonged history of recurrent discharge in this area. The abscess is situated in the midline, in the natal cleft, some distance cephalad from the anus. Secondary tracks which become infected may also be present; however, these usually spread laterally and proximally rather than caudally toward the anus and can be traced to their origin from the midline pilonidal cyst.

Hydradenitis Suppurativa

Hydradenitis suppurativa is a secondary infection of the skin and its appendages, notably the sweat glands. It can arise in any area of the skin where sweat glands are found in large numbers—the axilla, nape of the neck, groin, and the perineum. It is a disease of the skin alone and rarely involves the subcutaneous planes, although virulent infection may occur and extend as abscesses in the subcutaneous tissues; however, the origin is always in the skin.[7] Involvement of the skin in close proximity to the anus may simulate a fistula-in-ano, but the lack of disease in the anal canal and the superficial nature of the process can readily be established and the differentiation made.

Treatment

Incision and drainage form the standard treatment of perirectal suppuration. This should be performed even in the absence of evident fluctuation. Antibiotics should never represent principal therapy but may be used adjunctively with incision and drainage, especially in immunodeficient patients and in those prone to bacterial endocarditis.

Office Management

Most perianal abscesses can be drained in the office or in the emergency department using local anesthesia. This is achieved by subcutaneously injecting 1–3 ml of 1% lidocaine solution containing 1:200,000 epinephrine. After evacuation of the pus, the overhanging skin edges are trimmed and the wound inspected for bleeding. Hemostasis from the cut skin edges is readily achieved by electrocautery. In many cases primary healing will occur without formation of a fistula-in-ano.[64, 65] At least one third of the patients treated in this manner will have no further problem. Antibiotics are not generally prescribed, but the patients are instructed to take frequent sitz baths for comfort and cleanliness. Packing is at best uncomfortable and is not necessary for the resolution of the problem. A copy of instructions given to patients following incision and drainage of an abscess in the office includes: (1) avoid strenuous activity for eight hours after the procedure to prevent any excessive bleeding, (2) tub baths should be taken at least twice a day, (3) apply gauze or cotton dressing to wound at all times, (4) expect a bloody drainage for one to four days, (5) return to the office as directed by physician, and (6) do not hesitate to call if you have any problems.

Operating Room Management

Operating room management should be reserved for large ischiorectal abscesses, horseshoe abscesses, intersphincteric abscesses, supralevator abscesses, and immunodepressed patients with any evidence of perianal suppuration. In each case general or regional block anesthesia is necessary for the patient's comfort and to enable the surgeon adequately to examine, evaluate, and treat each problem.

Intersphincteric Abscess

Intersphincteric abscess may be an isolated problem or part of the more complex horseshoe abscess. The treatment is the same. The palpable bulging area in the anal canal is visualized using an operating anoscope, and an internal sphincterotomy is performed over the abscess. Subsequent to drainage, the cavity is palpated digitally to break down loculations. Invariably a cephalad extension is present which must be identified, since the internal sphincter muscle may need to be divided further to unroof this pocket. The cavity is then curetted and the edges marsupialized using an absorbable suture. Hemostasis is achieved by electrocautery, and the cavity is lightly covered with oxidized cellulose cotton.

Horseshoe Abscess

Horseshoe abscess requires incision and drainage of both ischiorectal fossae with breakdown of loculations and placement of soft drainage tubes (Penrose) (Fig 47–17).[63] A midline posterior intersphincteric abscess is also present, and this requires treatment as outlined above. Temporary catheter drainage of the bladder is commonly performed, since these patients have or invariably develop acute urinary retention. Antibiotics are usually administered, particularly if the patient is immunodeficient or has other problems which may potentiate infection, such as diabetes mellitus or valvular heart disease.

Supralevator Abscess

Supralevator abscess will frequently be a part of a more extensive intra-abdominal process and hence is treated by an abdominal procedure. In cases where this does not occur, it is preferable to drain the abscess directly into the rectum above the levator muscles. The abscess is localized by digital examination and then drained directly into the rectum. It is important that the aperture be enlarged to admit readily two fingers to ensure continued adequate drainage. If no continuing source of sepsis exists in the abdomen, such abscesses readily resolve.

Postoperative Care

Postoperative care consists of frequent sitz baths followed by a soft cotton dressing to the area to collect continuing dis-

charge and drainage. The patient is given a regular diet early in the postoperative period. A psyllium seed bulk laxative and a lubricant are prescribed from the day of surgery. If the patient has not had a spontaneous bowel movement by the third or fourth postoperative day, a tap water enema may be administered through a soft rubber catheter. Hospitalized patients are discharged as indicated following the first spontaneous bowel movement and when IM injections of analgesics are no longer necessary. Dilatations and irrigations of the anal canal are painful and unnecessary and are not employed postoperatively. The patient is seen postoperatively approximately ten days following discharge and at regular intervals until complete healing has occurred or a fistula-in-ano develops.

Fistula-in-ano

The fistula-in-ano is the chronic phase of perianal suppuration. It consists of an inflammatory tract with a secondary opening (external opening) on the perianal skin or perineum and a primary opening (internal opening) in the anal canal, usually at the level of the dentate line. The fistula is an end result of an abscess originating in the intersphincteric space. Goodsall's law relates the location of the internal opening to the external opening (Fig 47–18).[1] If the external opening is anterior to an imaginary line drawn across the midpoint of the anus, the fistula runs directly into the anal canal. If the external opening is posterior to that same line, the fistula usually will curve to the posterior midpoint of the anal canal. Exceptions to this rule includes situations where the external opening lies some distance from the anus, in which case even an anteriorly situated external opening may communicate with the midline posteriorly.

For clarity of surgical description, fistula-in-ano is classified based on the relationship to the sphincter muscle into four categories[66]: (1) intersphincteric, (2) trans-sphincteric, (3) suprasphincteric, and (4) extrasphincteric. It must be remembered that this concept is a two-dimensional one and that tracts do also take a circumferential route.

Most patients present with previous episodes of acute anorectal suppuration followed by intermittant drainage. Recurrent perianal abscesses suggest the presence of a fistula-in-ano. The external opening is usually visible as an elevation of granulation tissue with obvious purulent serosanguineous drainage. If the tract is superficial, often it can be palpated as

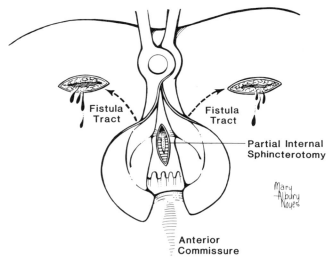

Fig 47–17.—The horseshoe abscess is treated by incision and drainage of the ischiorectal fossae bilaterally. The accompanying posterior midline intersphincteric abscess is drained by a partial internal anal sphincterotomy. A similar approach is adopted in cases of chronic horseshoe fistula-in-ano with coring out of the lateral tracts.

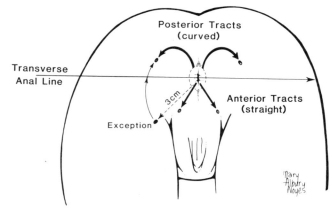

Fig 47–18.—"Goodsall's Law" relates the location of the internal opening to the external opening in the fistula-in-ano.

an indurated cord leading from the external opening to the anus. Deep, high, or horseshoe fistula tracts usually are not palpable.

Several disorders must be considered in the differential diagnosis of fistula-in-ano. In all cases it is important to rule out inflammatory bowel disease, particularly Crohn's disease, in which case one may refrain from the procedures for the fistula-in-ano because of poor secondary wound healing. It may be necessary to achieve this differential by proctoscopy, upper GI examination with small-bowel follow-through and barium enema, and colonoscopy. Diverticulitis of the sigmoid colon and rarely tumors of the colon with perforation may fistulize and drain to the perineum. Hydradenitis suppurativa is differentiated by the presence of multiple superficial perianal skin openings. Pilonidal sinus with perianal extension, although rare, and an infected perianal sebaceous cyst with chronic drainage must be considered. Rarely carcinomas, mostly low grade, may develop in a long-standing fistula. Rectal and anal carcinomas rarely present as a fistula in the perineum.

Treatment

The first step in the management of a fistula-in-ano is to identify the primary or internal opening. Approximately 50% of patients do not have clinically detectable internal openings. Positive identification is accomplished in the operating room using anesthesia. Bidigital palpation using the index finger and thumb delineates the indurated tract to the primary opening. Probing the tract from the external opening will be successful in a large percentage of cases, but care must be taken to avoid creating an artificial opening and thus running the risk of iatrogenic extension above and beyond the original fistula. Injections of methylene blue into the tract may be helpful, but more often than not result in the staining of normal tissues. An x-ray (fistulogram) using a water-soluable contrast solution is a valuable method to identify and manage high, complicated fistulas, particularly those that are recurrent or have unusual features. If definition of the primary opening is impossible at the time of operation, the crypt-bearing area suspected of harboring the infected duct and gland as outlined by Goodsall's law must be widely excised.

A fistula-in-ano is treated in the vast majority of cases by a fistulotomy rather than total excision of the tract. (Fig 47–19).[1] This includes unroofing all of the fistulous tract, eliminating the primary opening (infected source), and establishing adequate drainage. The fistulous tract is unroofed from the primary source at the dentate line through the secondary opening or openings by excising all overlying tissue, including anal sphincter muscle. Failure to unroof the entire tract and to divide the necessary amount of sphincter may lead to recurrence. The wound is allowed to heal by secondary intention. Marsupialization of the skin edges to the remaining fistula tract often decreases the size of the remaining wound and speeds eventual healing.

Occasionally the patient may present with an anal abscess associated with an obvious fistula-in-ano. Under such circumstances, drainage of the abscess by performing a primary fistulotomy is indicated. If the fistula is high in relation to the anorectal ring, a two-stage procedure may be indicated. In the first stage a seton of heavy black silk, silastic tubing, or

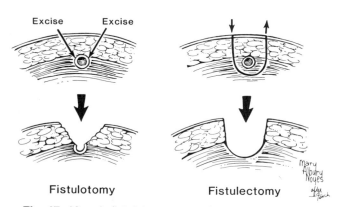

Fig 47–19.—A fistulotomy operation involves unroofing the fistula tract but retaining the base. A fistulectomy operation involves excising the entire fistula tract. In most patients this is not necessary.

rubber-band is placed loosely around the sphincter as a marker.[63] The external component of the fistula is treated by fistulotomy as already outlined. The seton stimulates fibrosis adjacent to the involved sphincter muscle so that when the second stage, which involves laying open the intersphincteric portion of the fistula tract, is completed, the sphincter will not gape. Incontinence is the most serious complication of operations for fistula. Concern about postoperative incontinence is the criterion for seton insertion.[67] This is most likely to occur in patients who are elderly or who have anteriorly situated fistulas, particularly in females or those in whom the fistula is considered to be extensive or high—that is, transsphincteric or suprasphincteric. Horseshoe fistula is an uncommon form of fistula-in-ano and is a direct extension of an intersphincteric abscess, commencing in the midline posteriorly and spreading through the deep post anal space. A direct total unroofing procedure is seldom necessary.[63] A posterior midline internal sphincterotomy, drainage of the intersphincteric space, and excision of the infected duct and gland associated with coring out of the lateral tracts is often effective.

Rectovaginal Fistula

The anterior rectal wall, for a distance of approximately 9 cm, is immediately adjacent to the posterior wall of the vagina. Depending on the underlying etiology, a rectovaginal fistula may appear at any site along this rectovaginal septum. For surgical convenience such fistulas are arbitrarily classified as low if they can be surgically corrected from a perineal approach, or high if they must be approached safely transabdominally. In most cases the opening of the fistula is small, being less than 2 cm in the majority. Rectovaginal fistula may result from congenital malformation or from several acquired disorders. The commonest etiology is obstetrical injury in cases where the fistula is benign. Inflammatory bowel disease, pelvic irradiation, neoplasms, and infections are the underlying cause in the remainder.[68]

Childbirth injuries of the perineum and obstetrical maneuvers such as episiotomies, especially when resulting in episioproctotomy, predispose to the development of rectovaginal fistula. Failure to recognize such an injury, failure to repair, or development of secondary infection in a repair would virtually ensure the development of a rectovaginal fistula. Operative trauma occasionally is responsible. Vaginal or rectal operative procedures, especially near the dentate line, may result in a fistula. Penetrating or blunt violence, such as impailment injury or forceful coitus, similarly may result in such a problem.

The likelihood of spontaneous or nonoperative healing of the rectovaginal fistula is primarily dependent on its etiology and to a lesser extent on its size. Approximately one half of the small fistulas secondary to trauma will heal spontaneously. Fistulas due to inflammatory bowel disease usually fail to heal or fail to remain healed, even with aggressive medical therapy. Operative repair, therefore, should not be attempted until the patient and the local tissues are in optimal condition. It is usually necessary to wait several months to allow the rectovaginal septum to return to its normal soft, pliable state. This is particularly so in cases resulting from obstetrical trauma.

Operative Approaches

Rectovaginal fistulas can be corrected by abdominal, rectal, vaginal, perineal, trans-sphincteric, and trans-sacral approaches, or by a combination of these methods. High rectovaginal fistulas can often only be approached safely transabdominally. Any of the other approaches may be suitable for low rectovaginal fistulas. The simplest approach is a transrectal one, since the primary opening is within the anorectal canal and not the vagina. The rectovaginal fistula joins the high-pressure system of the rectum (25–85 cm of water) with the low-pressure system of the vagina (atmospheric). A rectal approach therefore provides the local exposure of the high-pressure side of the fistula. An endorectal advancement of an anorectal flap consisting of mucosa, submucosa, and circular muscle is a simple technique which has provided excellent results (Fig 47–20).[58] Preoperatively, cleansing enemas are utilized, but a formal or aggressive bowel preparation is unnecessary. A colostomy is not used. After induction of general anesthesia, the patient is placed in a prone jack-knife position over a hip roll with buttocks spread by tape. In addition to a perianal field block, an IM injection of 0.25% bupivacaine with 1:200,000 epinephrine solution is made along the planned routes of dissection. Exposure is gained with a bi-valved operating anoscope, and the rectovaginal fistula is identified. The proposed rectal flap is then outlined around the fistula extending approximately 7–8 cm into the rectum. The base of the flap should be approximately two times the width of the apex of the flap to ensure adequate blood supply. The flap is raised from the apex to the base. The cut edges of the circular muscle are mobilized laterally so they may be approximated in the midline without tension. Hemostasis is achieved by point electrocautery. The perineal body and rectovaginal septum proximal to it are then reconstructed using interrupted 2–0 polyglycolic acid sutures, which are first placed and then tied serially. A final check for hemostasis is made before final advancement of the flap. Excess flap, including the rectovaginal fistula, is excised. The flap is sutured in place to restore the normal anatomy using 3–0 polyglycolic acid sutures at the apex and along each side of the flap. The vagina is left open for drainage. Postoperatively the patient is

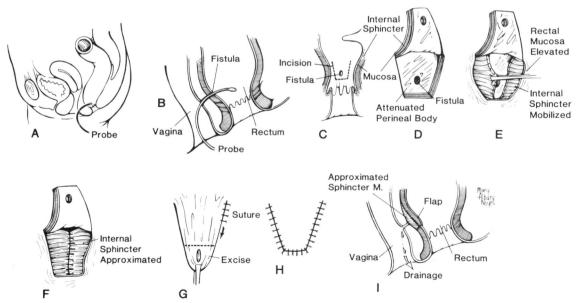

Fig 47–20.—The endorectal flap advancement operation for low recto-vaginal fistula. **A** and **B,** a probe demonstrates the fistula with the opening in the rectum being low, close to the dentate line. **C,** the proposed rectal wall flap is outlined on the anterior rectal wall. **D,** the full thickness of rectal wall is illustrated as the flap (base twice the width of the apex) is raised. The attenuated perineal body with the fistula into the lower vagina is seen. **E,** the divided circular muscle and internal sphincter are mobilized laterally. **F,** the perineal body and lower recto-vaginal septum are reconstructed by approximating the mobilized muscles. The fistula is obliterated. **G,** excess flap including the fistula is excised. **H,** the flap is sutured without tension to cover the reconstituted perineal body. **I,** the completed operation with the opening into the vagina left for drainage.

given analgesics and warm baths to control the pain and spasm, as well as bulk stool softeners to avoid constipation.

Sexually Transmitted Diseases of the Anorectum

Many factors have lead to a profound change in the types and prevalance of sexually transmitted diseases.[69] Gonorrhea and syphilis, the classic diseases, are still with us, but have been supplanted in importance by the much more common chlamydial infections (nonspecific genital infection, nongonococcal urethritis), which are harder to diagnose with specificity, and by diseases which have no cure, such as hepatitis and herpes. The latter may also have long-term consequences, such as chronic active hepatitis and hepatoma and cancer of the cervix and anus. Acquired immune deficiency syndrome (AIDS) is a newcomer whose etiology is unknown. Though of suspected viral origin, it is 50% fatal, and the incidence appears to be rapidly increasing.

The male homosexual is of most concern to the clinician. There are no physical characteristics which point to homosexual behavior, contrary to popular belief. Many sexual diseases mimic diseases of other etiology; i.e., ulcerative proctitis, Crohn's disease, and anal fissure. Frequently, multiple diseases are present in the homosexual person rather than a single one. The clinician must be alert to avoid mistakes.

Symptoms

Symptoms of anorectal venereal disease are protean and nonspecific, and, indeed, patients may frequently be asymptomatic. Gonorrhea is particularly problematic in the rectum and pharynx, pharyngeal gonorrhea being asymptomatic in up to 98% of patients. Rectal gonorrhea may be asymptomatic 60%–80% of the time in high-risk populations.[70] Non-lymphogranuloma venereum serotypes of *Chlamydia* are frequently associated with minimal or no symptoms.[71] Initial complaints from symptomatic individuals are nonspecific and include itching, soreness, burning, anorectal fullness, pain, purulent staining of clothes, profuse discharge, mucus in stools, bleeding, diarrhea with or without tenesmus, or a remotely plausible story of trauma. For AIDS, fatigue may be the only early symptom.

Diagnosis

The differential diagnosis of anorectal complaints should include all of the sexually transmitted diseases listed in Table 47–1. Certain of the groups are uncommon in the United States, but the diagnosis should be made by exclusion, since multiple infections are so common, particularly in homosexual patients. The term "gay bowel syndrome" has evolved because of the common association of gonorrhea and syphilis with enteric viral and protozoal infections and hepatitis.[72]

Nonlymphogranuloma chlamydial organisms have emerged from relative obscurity to be recognized as a major cause of urethritis (nonspecific or nongonorrheal urethritis), epididymitis, cervicitis, and pelvic inflammatory disease. Chlamydial infections are now the most prevalent sexually transmitted infections in the United States, and because of this are an increasingly important cause of proctitis in homosexual men and heterosexual women. Asymptomatic infections of the pharyngeal, urethral, and rectal mucosa occur. Part of the prevalence problem may be the relative reluctance of some physi-

TABLE 47–1.—MODERN LIST OF SEXUALLY TRANSMITTED DISEASES

Bacterial
  Nonspecific genital infection (*Chlamydia, Mycoplasma*)
  Gonorrhea
  Syphilis
  Chancroid (*Hemophilus ducreyi*)
  Lymphogranuloma venereum (serotype of *C. trachomatis*)
  Granuloma inguinale (*Calymmatobacterium granulomatis*)
  Salmonellosis
  Shigellosis
  Campylobacteriosis
  Candidiasis
Viral
  Herpes Types I + II
  Hepatitis B (A, non-A, non-B)
  Cytomegalovirus
  Genital warts (condyloma acuminatum)
  Molluscum contagiosum
  ? AIDS
Protozoal
  Trichomoniasis
  Amebiasis
  Giardiasis
Parasitic
  Scabies
  Pediculosis pubis

cians and clinics to treat when gonorrhea has not been diagnosed.[73] So called nonspecific genital infections we now know to be caused at least half of the time by *Chlamydia*, and should be treated on suspicion only. Lymphogranuloma (LGV) serotypes of *C. trachomatis* are generally implicated in the more severe forms of disease and almost always in the more severe forms of proctitis. The non-LGV serotypes are frequently involved in minor infections or asympmtomatic states.

The organism is an obligate, intracellular parasite which penetrates only columnar or transitional epithelium. The LGV types seem to be adapted to survive also in mononuclear cells, perhaps accounting for the prominent lymphadenopathy of LGV.

Diagnosis of chlamydial infection is based on suspicion, rising antibody titers, or preferably culture. Cultures are not generally available and are expensive, but with increasing demand are done by more and more laboratories with viral and tissue culture capabilities. Specimens should be collected on a swab by abrading mucosa to obtain surface cells and placed in a special transport medium. If immediate innoculation is not available, the specimen should be frozen at $-70°$ C for transport. This results in only partial loss of the innoculum.

The treatment of choice for chlamydial infection is tetracycline, 500 mg four times daily, for at least seven days (or doxycycline, 100 mg twice daily for seven days). An alternative regimen is erythromycin, 500 mg four times daily for seven days. Lymphogranuloma venereum should be treated for a minimum of three weeks.

Gonorrhea

The frequency of occult rectal *Neisseria gonorrhoeae* infections has already been alluded to. Presenting symptoms are often protean and nonspecific. The signs of gonorrhea are, likewise, nonspecific and reflect the entire differential diagnosis of proctitis (Table 47–2). "Mucopus," a thick, viscid, yellow exudate is the most suspicious finding and is almost diagnostic when coupled with cryptitis or proctitis confined to the lower rectum just above the dentate line. A sudden spurt of growth of condylomata, facilitated by moisture from anal discharge, should alert one to gonorrhea. Ulceration of the skin or mucosa, except nonspecific excoriations, is distinctly unusual. The usual appearance is one of intensely infected, friable mucosa, particularly the columns of Morgani and the anal crypts.

Diagnosis should be made by culture following immediate plating on Thayer Martin or Stuart's medium. Rapid transport for plating in special transport medium is also acceptable. Blindly obtained anorectal swabs inserted about 1.5 in. into the anus are probably as reliable as anoscopically obtained swabs, but the latter taken under direct vision are probably to be preferred, particularly when done for smear as well as cultures.

Treatment of rectal gonorrhea should be based on suspicion, because cultures are not 100% reliable and the consequences of untreated infection entail the serious complications of septic arthritis, meningitis, perihepatitis, and endocarditis, as well as dissemination to sexual partners. Patients who remain symptomatic or retain abnormal physical findings after treatment but have negative gonorrheal cultures are highly likely to have *Chlamydia* or *Mycoplasma* infections and should be further treated with tetracycline. All patients with positive cultures should have further cultures after treatment, since failure rates as high as 35% for rectal gonorrhea have been reported.[74] There are five accepted regimens for treatment of rectal (or pharyngeal) gonorrhea, outlined in Table 47–3. Note that the dose for rectal gonorrhea is twice that for urethritis. Probenecid is important for efficacy. Aqueous penicillin G is still the treatment of choice, because it is effective in a single parenteral dose and can abort syphilis. In the patient with suspected syphilis and gonorrhea, one should attempt to document the syphilis before treatment because dark field examination becomes negative as soon as four hours after treatment with penicillin. All patients with documented gonorrhea should have a serologic test for syphilis done three months after treatment to avoid missing masked or early syphilis.[75]

Syphilis

Primary anal syphilis is a disease of the homosexual.[76, 77] Seventy percent of syphilis cases now occur in the homosexual. The primary chancre, an irregular ulcer with a sloughing base, occurs at the anal margin or in the low anal canal. It is extremely rare for it to involve mucosa. In the anal area, the classic painless ulcer is unusual, and the disease may present as an anal fissure or multiple fissures with stenosis. These ulcers may be extremely painful but may also present as a trivial finding. Painless inguinal adenopathy is very common. Any odd or ulcerated cutaneous lesion should be treated as suspicious for syphilis. Pure proctitis due to syphilis has also been reported without concomitant anal or genital lesions.

The diagnosis may be established by the traditional dark field examination of scrapings from the cleansed ulcer. Be-

TABLE 47–2.—ETIOLOGY OF ACUTE PROCTITIS— DIFFERENTIAL DIAGNOSIS

Enteric infections (*Salmonella, Shigella, Campylobacter, Amoeba, Giardia*)
Veneral disease (gonorrhea, chlamydia, herpes, syphilis)
Idiopathic ulcerative proctitis and colitis
Crohn's disease
Antibiotics (*Clostridium difficile*)
Radiation
Miscellaneous, (chemical, lubricants, scents, enema, trauma)
Ischemia

cause this is less commonly available now, dried serum from the ulcer may be stained with fluorescent treponemal antibody. The specimen should be obtained free of any lubricant, and it is recommended that exudate be stimulated by cleansing of the ulcer with acetone or ether to remove debris and blood. Such manipulation may have to be done using anesthesia, because these rectal lesions are frequently painful. If the lesion is highly suspicious, examinations should be repeated daily for three days.

In untreated primary syphilis the VDRL or RPR is reactive in about 75% of cases, but in about 95% in early latent syphilis and 100% in the secondary stage. The antibody usually appears in the serum four to six weeks after the initial infection (one to three weeks after the chancre), so the serologic tests are not totally reliable unless repeated three months after the suspected primary infection.

The differential diagnosis of primary syphilis includes anal fissure, herpes, Crohn's disease, squamous cell carcinoma, and traumatic erosions.

The lesions of secondary syphilis, the disseminated stage, may be found on the skin (condyloma, rashes) or on the mucous membrane (mucous patches). Serologic tests are always positive in high titer, and scrapings of lesions always yield organisms. Oral scraping may be confusing due to the presence of commensal spirochetes.

The treatment of syphilis (in the absence of CNS involvement) is based on three regimens: (1) benzathine penicillin G, 2.4 million units as a single dose IM; (2) aqueous penicillin G, 600,000 units daily IM for ten days; this may be repeated every 14 days depending on the stage; and (3) erythromycin, 500 mg orally four times daily for 15 days, and tetracycline, 500 mg four times daily for 15 days, are alternative regimens but require strict compliance for success. Patients with syph-

TABLE 47–3.—TREATMENT OF ANORECTAL GONORRHEA

APPG, 4.8 million units IM; probenecid, 1.0 gm orally
Spectinomycin, 4.0 gm IM (high dose necessary to eliminate pharyngeal infection)
Kanamycin, 500 mg IM q 12 hr × 4 hours
Sulfamethoxazole-trimethoprim (*Septra*), iii orally TID × 3 days
Tetracycline, 500 mg orally QID × 10 days
Doxycycline, 100 mg orally BID × 10 days

From Fiumara.[88] Used by permission.

ilis must abstain from sexual relations until proved noninfective, and all contacts for the previous three months should be traced when dealing with primary syphilis, or all contacts for the previous year when dealing with secondary or disseminated stages. Follow-up should be every three months, with physical examination and serologic testing for two years.

Herpes

Anorectal herpes is almost always caused by herpes hominus virus, type II (HSV-2), the same organism implicated in genital herpes. The type I infection, though occasionally reported, is not nearly so common.

The prevalance of infections depends on socioeconomic group. Complement-fixing antibodies can be demonstrated in patients who have been infected previously but not imply active disease. These antibodies are found in almost 100% of older prostitutes, 20%–60% of lower socioeconomic groups, 10% of the upper socioeconomic group, but almost never in nuns.[78]

The clinical presentation usually begins with intense pruritus or paresthesia in the sacral distribution, which is followed by severe anal pain. This may be complicated by fecal impaction due to its intensity. Complete examination may not be possible initially, but can usually be done with gentle persuasion and topical anesthetic use. This may demonstrate lesions at various stages of development, the earliest being vesicles with a red areola which progress to rupture, leaving a superficial ulcer. These may be present on the perianal skin, in the anal canal, or may cause a proctitis, usually with punctate lesions and vesicles. Ulcerations in the anal canal may become confluent with secondary infections, resulting in a grayish ulcerating cryptitis with an erythematous border. Constitutional symptoms of fever and malaise occur one half of the time. Crusting of open lesions occurs in a few days, followed by healing at two weeks. A chronic, relapsing course is common, with sacral paresthesia or neuralgia-like symptoms preceding the recurrent lesions by a few days. The recurrent lesions are usually much less symptomatic than the initial infection and may be painless. Patients are infective while they have lesions and should abstain from sexual relations from the onset of the paresthesia until totally healed. Even after healing, use of a condom is recommended.

Diagnosis may be made by viral culture (highly sensitive with specimens tolerating transport in viral medium readily) or by the finding of intranuclear inclusion bodies in stained material from the base of a freshly ruptured vesicle. These dried preparations can be stained by Giemsa, hematoxylin-osin, or by Papanicolaou methods. The slides can be submitted as for Papanicolaou smear, with a specific query being made for evidence of herpes. Direct immunofluorescence staining is available. Less helpful is the complement-fixing antibody titer.

Treatment of herpes in the past has generally not been satisfactory. Approximately 20 treatments have been advocated but are either not proved by clinical trial or unavailable in the United States. None effects a cure. Systemic acyclovir promises to improve the treatment of acute episodes and may even prevent recurrent activation in certain high-risk situations, such as bone marrow transplantation; however, systemic treatment does not cure the disease in the sense that viral latency is not prevented, and recurrent episodes occur at the normal frequency. Acyclovir as a topical 5% ointment has been effective in reducing length of the symptomatic period, promoting healing of lesions and reducing the period of viral shedding.

Herpes proctitis is frequently a severe illness which may mimic Crohn's disease. It is characterized by signs of sacral nerve dysfunction (constipation; difficulty voiding; paresthesia of the posterior thigh, buttocks, and perineum), inguinal adenopathy, fever, severe anorectal pain and tenesmus, ulceration with pustular lesions in the distal third of the rectum, and perianal ulcerations. Pain is often out of proportion when compared with other forms of proctitis. Serologic studies suggest that patients with proctitis are often experiencing their first HSV-2 infection.

Condyloma Acuminata

The common anal wart is caused by a large papilloma virus and may be associated with active gonococcal proctitis. Transmission is most commonly through anal intercourse, and lesions may occur in the urethra, on the penis, perineum, and the rectal mucosa. The virus cannot be grown in vitro by present techniques, appears to be relatively scarce in the warty lesions, and has not met Koch's criteria, but there is little doubt or controversy about this being a transmissible, viral-induced disease. This group of papovaviruses, of which the papilloma virus is one, is a common cause of malignant tumors in some animal species but rarely in humans. Condylomata have been the site of squamous carcinoma. The incubation period is from one to six months, and the lesions are autoinnoculable, requiring their total destruction for control and frequent follow-up to ascertain cure. Overlooked lesions high in the transitional area of the anal canal, venereal reinfection, and failure of compliance with follow-up are common reasons for treatment failure.

Fifteen or more treatments have been advocated for the cure of viral warts. For practical purposes, application of freshly prepared 25% podophyllin in tincture of benzoin to each lesion has been successful and is preferred by many. The skin between lesions should be spared and may be protected by liberal sprinkling of talcum powder to the whole area before applying the podophyllin only to the warty excrescence. The podophyllin should be washed off four hours after application with soap and water. Topical podophyllin may cause histologic changes in the warts easily confused with squamous carcinoma. If there is any question of cancer or if lesions are to be submitted for pathologic examination, treatment with podophyllin should be delayed until the specimen has been obtained. The pathologist should be warned that there has been previous application of podophyllin.

Bichloracetic acid has also proved to be effective and is simple to use. This preparation has the additional advantage that it is immediately caustic, and one is able to assess the extent of destruction at the time of treatment. The lesions turn a frosty white almost immediately.

For more extensive lesions and those located high in the anal canal, fulguration with the electrocautery using anesthesia is the treatment of choice.

Refractory warts or extensive recurrences have been successfully treated with a vaccine prepared from 5 gm of warts removed from the patients.[82,83] Topical 5% fluorouracil and dinitrochlorobenzene (DNCB) have also been used with success.

A special form of giant condyloma, called a Buschke-Lowenstein tumor, may rarely involve the anus and is histologically benign but behaves in a locally malignant fashion and may degenerate into a verrucous carcinoma.[84]

Acquired Immune Deficiency Syndrome (AIDS)

AIDS is a disease of unknown cause, first described in male homosexuals in 1981.[85] The disease was first recognized because of clustering of *Pneumocystis carinii* pneumonia (usually found only in the immunosuppressed patient) and Kaposi's sarcoma (an extremely rare skin cancer) in Los Angeles homosexual men. Onset of disease is nonspecific, with fatigue, cough, generalized lymphadenopathy, weight loss, and fever, at which point pneumocystic pneumonia or other opportunistic infection occurs, and the patient may develop disseminated Kaposi's sarcoma. The usual course is one of uncontrolled infection, tumor growth, wasting debility, and finally death. Neurologic complication and unusual CNS tumors occur with alarming frequency.[86]

AIDS has epidemiologic characteristics that mimic hepatitis B and so far has been found in homosexual or bisexual men (71%), IV drug abusers (17%) of both sexes, hemophiliacs using pooled commercial plasma products (1%), and a few cases in Haitians, heterosexual partners of AIDS patients, and adults who have had blood transfusions. Evidence is very strong for a transmissible agent, and AIDS has been reported in infants after blood transfusion, in children of families at high risk for AIDS, and in infants born to promiscuous or drug-addicted mothers. Because of the hepatitis B-like pattern, it is thought that the disease may be transmitted by blood, tissue, semen, urine, and stool, and that isolation precautions similar to hepatitis B should be employed. No cases transmitted by casual contact have been seen.[87]

Diagnosis of AIDS may be suspected by the presence of fatigue, weight loss, fever, generalized adenopathy in patients at risk, or by recognition of opportunistic infection or unusual tumors. The diagnosis may be confirmed by an immune workup demonstrating cutaneous anergy, lymphopenia, defective killer cell function, and inversion of the T-helper/T-suppressor ratio.

Hospitalized patients should be isolated with enteric precautions and biohazard labels placed on specimens, which should be collected in waterproof containers. Gloves and gowns should be worn by workers in contact with excretions, body fluids, blood or fomites. Handwashing before and after contact is imperative. Contaminated environmental surfaces should be disinfected. Coughing patients should have respiratory isolation with masks, as for tuberculosis. Protective eyewear should be used when there is risk of splatter. Linen and fomites should be double-bagged and marked "contaminated."

There is some hope for at least partial treatment of AIDS. The helper T cells and natural killer cells appear in vitro to be deficient in ability to release the lymphokines, interleukin 2 (Il-2), and interferon. In vitro, addition of Il-2 appears to restore the ability of the cytotoxic cells to proliferate and function and enhances killer cell function.

Proctalgia Fugax

Severe, episodic, intrarectal pain with no association of abnormal findings is a condition known as proctalgia fugax.[89] This is thought to be due to intense spasm of the levator ani muscles.[90] The symptom usually occurs in a patient who is anxious and often overworked. The characteristic history is that of severe pain awakening the patient, usually described as being located in the midrectum and disappearing spontaneously without residual symptoms. Complete proctosigmoidoscopic examination is usually negative but must be performed to rule out anorectal disease. Therapy to relieve the spasm during an acute attack is unreliable, since the attack is usually short-lived and resolves spontaneously. Some patients find that hot baths or a heating pad applied to the perineum during an attack will cut it short. Many of these patients are anxious and have cancerphobia; hence, reassurance is an important aspect of therapy. Another group of patients have persisting pain in the anorectum and on examination exhibit tenderness of the levator ani muscle, usually on the left side. Digital massage at regular intervals or low-grade electrical stimulation may provide an effective long-term therapy.

Pilonidal Disease

The average patient with symptomatic disease is a moderately obese male in his second or third decade. Persons of either sex, any age, and any physical characteristics, however, can be affected. This has led to controversy in regard to the etiology of this condition. Currently, pilonidal sinus is thought to be an acquired lesion which results from hair penetrating the skin and subcutaneous tissue. There are, however, several aspects of the disease which are not fully explained by the acquired-lesion theory.

The main feature of a pilonidal sinus is the primary, midline tract, which may be lined with squamous epithelium. This tract extends into the subcutaneous tissue for a variable distance, usually 2–3 cm. There may be small abscess cavities or small branching tracts coming off this primary tract. These may rupture. The abscess cavity and secondary tract are usually lined with granulation tissue. Often hairs which are disconnected from the surrounding skin are seen projecting from the sinus opening. The pilonidal cavity is situated in the midline and has a longitudinal direction in most cases. It varies in length, 1–15 cm. The walls of the cavity are composed of dense, fibrous tissue. Secondary tracts may lead from the pilonidal opening into the subcutaneous tissue and may discharge onto the skin. These secondary tracts usually extend laterally in a cephalad direction and only occasionally toward the anus.

Pilonidal disease often presents for the first time as an acute abscess at the base of the spine. It may rupture spontaneously. Diagnosis is made quite easily, and it is treated simply by incision and drainage with local anesthesia by making a cruciate incision over the most fluctuant or tender area off the midline. Antibiotics are not a substitute for surgical drainage, but occasionally may be used to treat accompanying cellulitis or other conditions in selected patients (diabetes, valvular heart disease, or immunodeficiency). It is important to examine the patient frequently in the postoperative period to ensure healing of the wound and to perform shaving of the surrounding skin. After adequate healing of the abscess has taken place, definitive surgery on the chronically pilonidal sinus may be performed. Many of these abscesses may not require definitive surgery, since they heal per primum. The need for definitive surgery can generally be ascertained at one to two months after the initial onset.

Treatment of Chronic Pilonidal Sinus

No one method of treatment of pilonidal sinus has proved completely successful. Because of its simplicity and equal results when compared to other modalities, the preferential treatment is marsupialization.[1] This consists of excising the superficial portion of the sinus wall and the overlying skin (Fig 47–21). The cut edges of the remaining sinus and surrounding skin are sutured to decrease the size of the wound and to speed healing. Lateral tracts are followed to their termination and marsupialized in a similar fashion. Chromic catgut or polyglycolic sutures are utilized. Such a procedure in many instances can be performed with local anesthesia in the office or as an outpatient at the hospital. Complete excision of the sinus tract and various amounts of surrounding tissue is not required. Detailed postoperative care is vital to the successful healing of the operated pilonidal sinus. The patient is instructed to keep a fluffy gauze dressing in place and to keep the edges of the wound separated and the base as flat as possible. The dressings are maintained in position by the undergarments, which prevents skin irritation by frequent application of tape. Local hygiene is stressed, and it is important that the wound edges are pulled apart. The wound must be kept from bridging over. If it occurs, such bridging is broken down with a cotton applicator. If there is excessive hair in the area, frequent shaving is necessary. Excessive granulation tissue is removed either with a curet or silver nitrate application. The wound must be followed up regularly until complete healing has occurred. No antibiotics are necessary.

Occasionally a patient is left with an unhealed wound. This is best handled by frequent curettage in the office. The use of a Waterpik to ensure cleanliness is simple and practical.[91] Reverse bandaging to keep pressure on the wounds has in some instances worked to promote healing.[92]

Treatment of a recurrent pilonidal sinus should be similar to the primary operation that is, marsupialization. It is as effective as any other treatment and is very simple. No attempt needs to be made to reexcise totally a recurrent pilonidal sinus and close the defect by suture or flaps.

Hydradenitis Suppurativa

Hydradenitis suppurativa is an acute or chronic infection of the apocrine glands of the skin. It exists in its chronic state as an indolent inflammatory disease of the epidermis, dermis, and subcutaneuos tissues characterized by abscess and sinus formation. It is located where the apocrine sweat glands are found, particularly to axilla, inguinal, genital, perianal, and scalp regions. It is more prevalent in blacks. The organisms usually found in the area are *Staphlococcus aureus*, although hemolytic streptococcus and coliforms have been isolated. The disease may start insidiously, but as the inflammatory process develops, subcutaneous nodules with inflammation usually result, that slowly resolve or more commonly progress

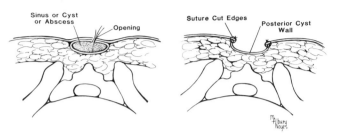

Fig 47–21.—Chronic pilonidal sinus is treated by unroofing and marsupulization. Note that the sinus base is left intact.

and coalesce to form a network of sinuses. Suppuration is usually slight, and only a few drops of pus may be evacuated from a nodule. Resolution with scarring and characteristic skin dimpling may occur, or a series of recurrences or remissions may ensue with the formation of considerable induration, abscesses, and deep sinus tracts. Discharge may persist, and in the later stages ulceration may occur. The symptoms are usually present for a long time, often years.

This chronic inflammatory condition affects the skin and subcutaneous tissues. The affected area often has a red, blotchy appearance and is thick and edematous with watery pus draining from multiple openings of sinus tracts. The chronic nature often leads to scarring with characteristic skin dimples and pits. Lesions may be localized or involve large areas of perianal skin and may extend into the buttocks and groin. Microscopic examination of excised specimens shows an inflammatory exudate consisting of plasma cells, lymphocytes, an occasional giant cell of foreign body type, with the formation of sinus tracts.[93] These tracts may become lined with squamous epithelium by downgrowth from the surface, and occasionally squamous cell carcinoma has been reported in long-standing cases.[94] The disease may be confused with fistula-in-ano, pilonidal disease, furunculosis, or Crohn's disease of the anal skin.

The surgical treatment of the acute phase of hydradenitis suppurativa is incision of drainage of any localized abscess. The chronic stage is treated in a variety of ways depending on the location and extent of involvement. In mild chronic cases simple unroofing of the area with curettage of the granulating tract may be all that is necessary. For extensive lesions wide excision along with split-thickness skin grafting may be required. Very localized lesions may be excised and primarily closed. In all situations a colostomy is generally unnecessary. Should it be thought to be necessary to obtain decreased bowel function during the healing phases, a full mechanical bowel preparation along with an elemental diet supplemented with obstipating medications will provide the desired results.[95]

Solitary Rectal Ulcer Syndrome

A benign-appearing ulcer situated on the anterior or anterolateral wall of the rectum some 4–10 cm from the anal verge, varying in size, may be present. This situation has been dubbed the solitary rectal ulcer syndrome and occurs equally in males and females, most commonly between the ages of 20 and 30. A variety of symptoms exists, but usually rectal bleeding associated with a feeling of rectal fullness, tenesmus, or unsatisfied defecation is very common. Most patients admit to chronic straining. The etiology is unknown, although in some instances a history of direct intrarectal trauma may be elicited. Ocassionally the patient will have an obvious or suspected rectal prolapse.[96] In the remainder of the patients, despite intensive investigation, no underlying pathology apart from the presence of the ulcer can be elicited. In all situations it is important to differentiate the ulcer from that due to Crohn's disease, ulcerative colitis, and neoplasm. This is usually simple on a rectal biopsy, since there are histologic changes characteristic of the solitary rectal ulcer syndrome. Superficial mucosal ulceration is common. Tubules show structural irregularity, and the epithelium is hyperplastic. The lamina propria is obliterated by fibrosis, and the muscular fibers of the muscularis mucosa grow toward the lumen of the bowel[7] It is possible that the solitary rectal ulcer is related to colitis cystica profunda.

Unfortunately, no local or systemic therapy has been shown to be reliably effective. Patients with few symptoms require no treatment. Tranquilizers may by effective, since some of these patients have a marked preoccupation with their bowels and worry endlessly about defecation. The difficulty is due to faulty bowel training and dietary education. The taking of increased amounts of dietary fiber may be helpful. The straining may be reduced by liquifying the stools and using glycerine suppositories. Should the ulceration be associated with rectal prolapse, a definitive repair should be performed. Sulfasalazine and local steroids have been used without any obvious lasting improvement.

Colitis Cystica Profunda

Colitis cystica profunda is a benign disease characterized by the presence of mucin-filled cysts of varying sizes located deep to the muscularis mucosae.[97, 98] The chief importance of this entity lies in its differentiation from colonic mucinous adenocarcinoma. Failure to recognize this benign condition may lead to an unnecessary radical operation. Its etiology remains unclear, however, it does appear to be involved with chronic inflammation which in some way results in its appearance.

Most cases involve only the anterior rectal wall between 5 and 10 cm from the anal verge.[99] This has implicated the solitary rectal ulcer as being the possible etiologic factor in the pathogenesis of colitis cystica profunda, which may in fact represent the healing phase of the ulcer. Patients usually present with a variety of symptoms consisting of tenesmus, passage of mucus and blood per rectum, and a feeling of rectal fullness and discomfort. Examination usually reveals an irregular area with nodularity usually situated on the anterior rectal wall, easily palpable with a finger.[5] The mucosa remains intact but mainly ulcerated, in which case it may resemble a carcinoma. Stenosis as well as rectal prolapse have been found in association with colitis cystica profunda.

It is important to differentiate this lesion from other inflammatory conditions, particularly Crohn's diesase, ulcerative colitis, ischemic colitis, or the unusual parasitic infestations. It is most important, however, to differentiate this from a mucinous secreting adenocarcinoma. Adequate biopsies will usually make the differentiation.

Treatment of choice is local excision to confirm the diagnosis. If any underlying bowel disease exists, this of course must be treated.

GUIDELINES FOR THE POSTOPERATIVE CARE OF PATIENTS UNDERGOING ANORECTAL SURGERY

The majority of the patients who are scheduled for anorectal surgery have an unjustified dread of the postoperative course, particularly with regard to pain. It is therefore important to reassure the patient before the operation and to emphasize the importance of both mental and physical relaxation. The patient can be assured that the pain that is to be expected will be no more than that after any other operation and that medication will be readily available. Although pain can be reduced by certain measures undertaken in the operating room, particularly the avoidance of packs and pressure dressings, the variation and degree of pain depends largely on the patient's emotional status. It is important to reassure that the prescribed pain medication, particularly the IM injections, are available in adequate dosage on demand and, if necessary, can be given as often as every two hours.

The bladder and rectum derive their nerve supply from the same segments of the spinal cord. In view of this, there is often temporary paralysis of the bladder musculature as well as failure of relaxation of the bladder sphincter. Over distention of the bladder during this period will trigger acute urinary retention. For this reason the patient receives only small volumes of water by mouth until spontaneous voiding has occurred. If the bladder is emptied prior to operation and fluids are restricted after operation, 18–20 hours may pass before bladder capacity is reached, and it may be longer before the bladder is significantly distended. It is therefore not unusual for the patient not to void for this period. If the patient remains comfortable and undistressed, no further action need be taken at this stage. The nervous, tense patient will have greater difficulty voiding. Questioning if voiding has occurred or threats of catheterization will only aggravate the difficulty. The patient is instructed to attempt to void only if the urge to do so is felt. If the patient is uncomfortable due to bladder distention and is unable to void, catheterization is necessary. If more than two catheterizations are necessary, prolonged drainage using a self-retaining catheter is recommended.

As a routine, all patients begin eating a regular diet within 24 hours of anorectal surgery. This is supplemented with a bulk-forming psyllium seed compound. A lubricant stimulant such as mineral oil with Irish moss emulsion is added immediately and can be discontinued after the first bowel movement. It is not unusual for the patient to forego a spontaneous bowel movement for 48 hours following anorectal surgery. If no spontaneous bowel movement has occurred by 72 hours, it is recommended that a tap water enema be given via a soft, well-lubricated rubber catheter. If the patient is at home, this can be administered at home or the patient may come to the physician's office.

In the vast majority of cases the necessary anorectal incisions will be closed by suture. A small amount of drainage therefore is to be expected. All that is required in the way of dressing is a small absorbent cotton pad to be worn on the exterior of the anus and held in place with the under clothing. The pad must be changed frequently and frequent warm water sitz baths encouraged.

The patient is instructed that bloody drainage will continue for several days and that there will be perianal swelling. This is usually accompanied with soreness, burning, itching, or dull aching. During a bowel movement, a mild, sharp pain will occur and may be accompanied with the passage of a small amount of bright-red rectal blood. Patients are instructed to report immediately should heavy, bright-red rectal bleeding with the passage of large amounts of clots occur. Extreme or worsening pain may indicate the presence of perianal sepsis. Under such circumstances the patient must be examined immediately and appropriate steps taken.

REFERENCES

1. Goldberg S.M., Gordon P.H., Nivatvongs S.: *Essentials of Anorectal Surgery.* Philadelphia, J.B. Lippincott Co., 1980.
2. Nivatvongs S., Stern H.S., Fryd D.S.: The length of the anal canal. *Dis. Colon Rectum* 24:600, 1982.
3. Oh C., Kark A.E.: Anatomy of the external anal sphincter. *Br. J. Surg.* 59:717, 1972.
4. Shafik A.: A new concept of the anatomy of the anal sphincter mechanism and the physiology of defecation—The external anal sphincter: A triple-loop system. *J. Urol.* 12:412, 1975.
5. Shafik A.: A new concept of the anatomy of the anal mechanism and the physiology of defecation: II. Anatomy of the levator ani muscle with special reference to puborectalis. *J. Urol.* 13:175, 1975.
6. Shafik A.: A new concept of the anatomy of the anal sphincter mechanism and the physiology of defecation: III. The longitudinal anal muscle: Anatomy and role in anal sphincter mechanism. *J. Urol.* 13:271, 1976.
7. Morson B.C., Dawson I.M.P.: *Gastorintestinal Pathology.* London, Blackwell Scientific Publications, 1979, p. 698.
8. Boxall T.A., Smart P.J.G., Griffiths J.D.: The blood supply of the distal segment of the rectum in anterior resection. *Br. J. Surg.* 50:399, 1962.
9. Crapp A.R., Cuthbartson A.M.: William Waldeyer and the retrosacral fascia. *Surg. Gynecol. Obstet.* 138:252, 1974.
10. Parks A.G.: Anorectal incontinence. *Proc. R. Soc. Med.* 68:681, 1975.
11. Duthie H.L.: Dynamics of the rectum and anus. *Clin. Gastroenterol.* 4:467, 1979.
12. Nivatvongs S., Fryd D.S.: How far does the proctosigmoidoscope reach? A prospective study of 1000 patients. *N. Engl. J. Med.* 303:380, 1982.
13. Christie J.P.: Flexible sigmoidoscopy—Why, where, and when. *Am. J. Gastroenterol.* 73:70, 1980.
14. Marks G., Boggs H.W., Castro A.F., et al.: Sigmoidoscopic examinations with rigid and flexible fiberoptic sigmoidoscopes in the surgeon's office: A comparative prospective study of effectiveness in 1,012 cases. *Dis. Colon Rectum* 22:162, 1979.
15. Tedesco F.J.: Flexible sigmoidoscopy—What is its role? *J. Clin. Gastroententerol.* 1:46, 1979.
16. Nivatvongs S., Gilbertsen V.A., Goldberg S.M., et al.: Distribution of large bowel cancers in asymptomatic patients detected by occult blood test. *Dis. Colon Rectum* 25:420, 1982.
17. Shinya H., Wolff W.I.: Morphology, anatomic distribution and cancer. Potential of colonic polyps: An analysis of 7000 polyps endoscopically removed. *Ann. Surg.* 190:697, 1979.
18. Shinya H.: *Colonoscopy—Diagnosis and Treatment of Colonic Disease.* New York, Igaku-Shoin, 1982.
19. Nivatvongs S.: Alternative positioning of patients for hemorrhoidectomy. *Dis. Colon Rectum* 23:308, 1980.
20. Buls J., Goldberg S.M.: Modern management of hemorrhoids. *Surg. Clin North Am.* 58:469, 1978.
21. Alexander-Williams J., Buchmann P.: Perianal Crohn's disease. *World J. Surg.* 4:203, 1980.
22. Parks A.G., Swash M., Urich H.: Sphincter denervation in anorectal incontinence and rectal prolapse. *Gut* 18:656, 1977.
23. Fang O.T., Nivatvongs S., Vermeulen F.D., et al.: Overlapping sphincteroplasty for acquired anal incontinence. *Dis. Colon Rectum* 27:720, 1984.
24. Slade M.S., Goldberg S.M., Schottler J.S., et al.: Sphincteroplasty for acquired anal incontinence. *Dis. Colon Rectum* 20:33, 1977.
25. Gorman M.L.: Management of fecal incontinence by gracilis muscle transposition. *Dis. Colon Rectum* 22:290, 1979.
26. Goldberg S.M., Gordon P.H.: Treatment of rectal prolapse. *Clin. Gastroenterol.* 4:489, 1975.
27. Broden B., Snellman B.: Procidentia of the rectum studies with cineradiograph: A contribution to the discussion of causative mechanism. *Dis. Colon Rectum* 11:330, 1968.
28. Haas P.A., Fox T.A. Jr., Haas G.P.: The pathogeneisis of hemorrhoids. *Dis. Colon Rectum* 27:442, 1984.
29. Hoffman M.J., Kodner I.J., Fry R.D.: Internal intussusception of the rectum: Diagnosis and surgical management. *Dis. Colon Rectum* 27:435, 1984.
30. Ihre T., Seligson U.: Intussusception of the rectum-internal procidentia: Treatment and results in 90 patients. *Dis. Colon Rectum* 18:391, 1975.
31. Ripstein C.B., Lanter B.: Etiology and surgical therapy of prolapse of the rectum. *Ann. Surg.* 157:259, 1963.
32. Gordon P.H., Hoexter B.: Complications of the Ripstein procedure. *Dis. Colon Rectum* 21:277, 1978.
33. Boulos P.B., Stryker S.J., Nicholls R.J.: The long term results of polyvinyl alcohol (Ivalon) sponge for rectal prolapse in young patients. *Br. J. Surg.* 71:213, 1984.
34. Theuerkauf F.J., Beahrs O.H., Hill J.R.: Rectal prolapse: causation and surgical treatment. *Ann. Surg.* 171:819, 1970.
35. Frykman H.M.: Abdominal proctopexy and primary sigmoid resection for rectal procidentia. *Am. J. Surg..* 90:780, 1955.
36. Watts J.D., Rothenberger D.A., Buls J.G., et al.: The management of procidentia—Thirty years experience. *Dis. Colon Rectum,* in press.
37. Altemeier W.A., Culbertson W.R., Schowendert C., et al.: Nineteen years' experience with the one-stage perineal repair of rectal prolapse. *Ann. Surg.* 173:993, 1971.
38. Gabriel W.B.: The treatment of complete prolapse of the rectum by rectosigmoidectomy. *Dis. Colon Rectum* 1:241, 1958.
39. Uhlig B.E., Sullivan E.S.: The modified Delorme operation: Its place in surgical treatment for massive rectal prolapse. *Dis. Colon Rectum* 22:513, 1979.
40. Alexander S.: Dermatological aspects of anorectal disease. *Clin. Gastroenterol.* 4:651, 1975.
41. Smith L.E., Henrichs D., McCullah R.D.: Prospective studies on the etiology and treatment of pruritis ani. *Dis. Colon Rectum* 25:358, 1982.
42. Bernstein W.C.: What are hemorrhoids and what is their relationship to the portal venous system? *Dis. Colon Rectum* 26:829, 1983.
43. Thomson W.H.F.: The nature of hemorrhoids. *Br. J. Surg.* 62:542, 1975.
44. Alexander-Williams J., Crapp A.R.: Conservative management of hemorrhoids, Part I: Injection, freezing and ligation. *Clin. Gastroenterol* 4:595, 1975.
45. Barron J.: Office ligation treatment of hemorrhoids. *Dis. Colon Rectum* 6:109, 1963.
46. Nivatvongs S., Goldberg S.M.: An improved techniques of rubber band ligation of hemorrhoids. *Am. J. Surg.* 144:379, 1982.
47. Wrobleski D.E., Corman M.L., Veidenheimer M.C., et al.: Long-term evaluation of rubber ring ligation in hemorrhoidal disease. *Dis. Colon Rectum* 23:478, 1980.
48. Goligher J.C.: Cryosurgery for hemorrhoids. *Dis. Colon Rectum* 19:213, 1976.
49. Smith L.E., Goodreau J.J., Fouty W.J.: Operative hemorrhoidectomy versus cryodestruction. *Dis. Colon Rectum* 22:10, 1979.
50. Oh C.: One thousand cyrohemorrhoidectomies: An overview. *Dis. Colon Rectum* 24:613, 1981.
51. Ferguson J.A., Mozier W.P., Canchrow M.I., et al.: The closed

technique of hemorrhoidectomy. *Surgery* 70:480, 1971.

52. Todd I.P., Fielding L.P.: *Operative Surgery. Alimentary Tract and Abdominal Wall.* part 3 *Colon, Rectum and Anus,* ed. 4. London, Butterworths, 1983.

53. Duthie H.J., Bennett R.C.: Anal sphincteric pressure in fissure-in-ano. *Surg. Gynecol. Obstet.* 119:19, 1964.

54. Northman B.J., Schuster M.M.: Internal anal sphincter derangement with anal fissures. *Gastroenterology* 67:216, 1974.

55. Hancock B.D.: The internal sphincter and anal fissure. *Br. J. Surg.* 64:92, 1977.

56. Crapp A.R., Alexander-Williams J.: Fissure-in-ano and anal stenosis. *Clin. Gastroenterol.* 4:619, 1975.

57. Homan W.P., Tang C., Thorbjarnarson B.: Anal lesions complicating Crohn's disease. *Arch. Surg.* 111:1333, 1976.

58. Abcarian H.: Surgical correction of chronic anal fissure: Results of lateral internal sphincterotomy vs fissurectomy—midline sphincterotomy. *Dis. Colon Rectum* 23:31, 1980.

59. Abcarian H.: Acute suppuration of the anorectum. *Surg. Annu.* 8:305, 1976.

60. Williams D.R., Coller J.A., Corman M.L., et al.: Anal complications of Crohn's disease. *Dis. Colon Rectum* 24:22, 1981.

61. McColl I.: The comparative anatomy and pathology of anal glands. *Ann. R. Coll. Surg.* 40:36, 1967.

62. Hanley P.H.: Anorectal abscess fistula. *Surg. Clin. North Am.* 58:487, 1978.

63. Hanley P.H., Ray J.E., Pennington E.E., et al.: Fistula-in-ano: A ten year follow-up study of horseshore abscess fistula-in-ano. *Dis. Colon Rectum* 19:507, 1976.

64. Scoma J.A., Salvati E.P., Rubin R.J.: Incidence of fistulae subsequent to anal abscesses. *Dis. Colon Rectum* 17:357, 1974.

65. Vasilevsky C.A., Gordon P.H.: The incidence of recurrent abscesses or fistula-in-ano following anorectal suppuration. *Dis. Colon Rectum* 27:126, 1984.

66. Parks A.G., Gordon P.H., Hardcastle J.D.: A classification of fistula-in-ano. *Br. J. Surg.* 63:1, 1976.

67. Parks A.G., Stitz R.W.: The treatment of high fistula-in-ano. *Dis. Colon Rectum* 19:487, 1976.

68. Rothenberger D.A., Goldberg S.M.: The management of rectovaginal fistulae. *Sug. Clin. North Am.* 63:61, 1983.

67. Hansfield H.H.: Sexually transmitted diseases. *Hosp. Pract.* 17:99, 1982.

70. Owen R.L., Hill J.L.: Rectal and pharyngeal gonorrhea in homosexual men. *J.A.M.A.* 220:1315, 1972.

71. Quinn T.C., Goodell S.C., Mkrtichian E., et al.: Chlamydia trachomatis proctitis. *N. Eng. J. Med.* 305:195, 1981.

72. Kasal H.L., Sohn N., Corrasco J.I., et al.: The gay bowel syndrome: Clinicopathological in 260 cases. *Ann. Clin. Lab. Sci.* 6:184, 1976.

73. Holmes K.: The chlamydia epidemic. *J.A.M.A.* 245:1718, 1981.

74. Klein E.J., Fisher L.S., Chow A.D., Guz L.B. et al.: Anorectal gonococcal infection, a clinical review. *Ann. Intern. Med.* 86:340, 1977.

75. Sands M.: Treatment of anorectal gonorrhea infections in men. *J.A.M.A.* 243:1143, 1980.

76. Catterall R.D.; Sexually transmitted diseases of the anus and rectum. *Clin. Gastroenterol.* 4:659, 1975.

77. Wilcox R.R.: The rectum viewed by the venereologist. *Br. J. Veher. Dis.* 57:1, 1981.

78. Corey L.: The diagnosis and treatment of genital herpes. *J.A.M.A.* 248:1041, 1982.

79. Byrson Y.J., Dillon M., Lovett M., et al.: Treatment of first episodes of genital herpes simplex virus infection with oral acylovir: A randomized trial in normal subjects. *N. Engl. J. Med.* 308:916, 1983.

80. Goodell S.E., Quinn T.C., Mkrtichian E. et al.: Herpes simplex proctitis in homosexual men: Clinical, sigmoidoscopic, and histopathologic features. *N. Engl. J. Med.* 308:868, 1983.

81. Thomson J.P.S., Grace R.H.: The treatment of perianal and anal condylomata acuminata: A new operative technique. *J.R. Soc. Med.* 71:180, 1978.

82. Abcarian H., Sharon N.: Long term effectiveness of the immunotherapy of anal condylomata accuminatum. *Dis. Colon Rectum* 25:648, 1982.

83. Eftahia M.S., Amshel A.L., Shonberg I.L., et al.: Giant and recurrent condyloma accuminatum. Appraisal of immunotherapy. *Dis. Colon Rectum* 25:136, 1982.

84. Eliott M.S., Werner I.D. Immelman E.J., et al.: Giant condyloma (Bushke-Loewenstein Tumor) of the anorectum. *Dis. Colon Rectum* 22:497, 1979.

85. Siegel F.P., Lopez C., Hammer G.S., et al.: Severe acquired immunodeficiency in male homosexuals manifested by chronic perinal ulcerative herpes simplex lesions. *N. Engl. J. Med.* 305:1439, 1981.

86. Gapen P.: Neurological complications now characterizing many AIDS victims. Medical News. *J.A.M.A.* 248:2941, 1982.

87. Curran J.W.: AIDS—Two years later (editorial). *N. Engl. J. Med.* 309:609, 1983.

88. Fiumara N.J.: The treatment of gonococcal proctitis: An evaluation of 173 patients treated with 4 g of Spectinomycin. *J.A.M.A.* 239:735, 1978.

89. Douthwaite A.H.: Proctologia fugax. *Br. J. Med.* 2:164, 1962.

90. Grant S.R., Salvati E.P., Rubin R.J.: Levator syndrome: Analysis of 316 cases. *Dis. Colon Rectum* 18:161, 1975.

48

Vascular Lesions of the Gut

EDWARD B. BORDEN, M.D.
SCOTT J. BOLEY, M.D.

INTESTINAL ISCHEMIA

Acute intestinal ischemia is defined as acute insufficiency of blood flow in the distribution of the superior mesenteric artery (SMA) involving portions or all of the small bowel and/or right half of the colon. Colonic ischemia is inadequate circulation to any part or all of the colon. These two disorders have different clinical manifestations and are managed in different fashions.

Acute Mesenteric Ischemia

During the past 30 years, there has been increasing recognition of the importance and frequency of acute mesenteric ischemia (AMI). This is due in part to an increase in its incidence, but, more important, it is also a result of the realization that many clinical syndromes have as their common etiology interference with intestinal blood flow.

Reduction in blood flow to the intestine may be a reflection of generalized poor perfusion, as in hypovolemic or cardiogenic shock, or it may result from either functional or local morphological changes. Narrowings of the major mesenteric vessels, emboli of atheromatous material or blood clot, thromboses, vasculitis as part of a systemic disease, and mesentric vasoconstriction all can lead to inadequate circulation at the cellular level. However, whatever the cause, intestinal ischemia has the same end results—a spectrum ranging from completely reversible functional alterations to total hemorrhagic necrosis of portions or all of the bowel.

History

Tiedenman's clinical case report in 1843 first stimulated interest in mesenteric thrombosis, but the first description of the problem is attributed to Antonio Beniviene of Florence in the 15th century. The first successful bowel resection for intestinal infarction was reported by Elliott in 1895. Eleven years later, Delbet suggested the possibility of revascularization for superior mesenteric artery obstruction.

Although Ryvlyn in 1943 and Blinov in 1950 described patients in whom superior mesenteric artery (SMA) embolectomy was unsuccessfully attempted, Klass is generally credited with establishing the feasibility of this operation. In 1951 he described two patients who underwent successful embolectomy, but died of cardiac causes postoperatively.[1] One year later, Stewart performed the first SMA embolectomy with

survival of the patient. Successful operative approaches to acute SMA thrombosis as well as chronic mesenteric ischemia were reported in the 1950s.

In 1958 Ende first described nonocclusive mesenteric ischemia (NOMI),[2] and during the 1960s various attempts to treat this condition using local and regional anesthetic blocks as well as systemic and intraarterial vasodilators were reported.

Incidence

The exact incidence of AMI is difficult to ascertain, but was 1/1,000 admissions to our large metropolitan medical center in the late 1970s. Recently, there appears to be a real increase in the occurrence as well as in the recognition of AMI. With this increased incidence, there has also been a change in the distribution of cases due to each of the different causes. Whereas in the past, mesenteric venous and arterial thrombosis were most common, in recent series arterial emboli and NOMI were responsible in 70%–80% of patients.

More recently we have noticed a decline in the incidence of nonocclusive ischemia, possibly due to the increasingly widespread use of vasodilators, such as calcium channel-blocking agents and IV nitrates in the treatment of ischemic heart disease. It may also be a result of the more common use of left ventricular assist devices in the treatment of cardiogenic shock, resulting in the less frequent occurrence of prolonged periods of hypotension after myocardial infarction.

Etiology

Emboli to the superior mesenteric artery are responsible for 40%–50% of episodes of AMI, and usually originate from a mural or atrial cardiac thrombus. In the past, such thrombi were most commonly associated with rheumatic valvular disease, but today arteriosclerotic heart disease is the most frequent cause. Many patients with AMI have a history of previous peripheral arterial embolism, and approximately 20% have synchronous emboli in other arteries. SMA emboli tend to lodge at points of normal anatomical narrowings, usually just distal to the origin of a major branch (Fig 48–1). In 10%–15% of patients the emboli are more peripheral in the SMA or in branch arteries. An embolus may completely occlude the artery, but more often it only partially obstructs blood flow. Mild to marked vasoconstriction is frequently present in

733

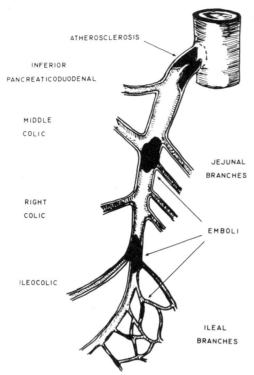

Fig 48–1.—Sites where SMA emboli commonly lodge. Thromboses most commonly occur near the origin of the artery. (From Boley S.J., Veith, in Hardy J.D. (ed.): *Hardy's Textbook of Surgery,* Philadelphia, J.B. Lippincott Co., 1983. Reproduced by permission.)

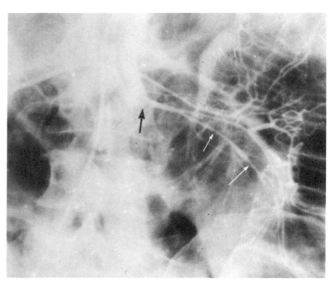

Fig 48–2.—Superior mesenteric artery angiogram of a patient with an embolus at the origin of the middle colic artery *(black arrow)* with vasospasm of the unobstructed arterial branches *(white arrows).* (From Brandt L.J., Boley S.J., in Maclean L.D. (ed.): *Advances in Surgery.* Chicago, Year Book Medical Publishers, 1981. Used by permission.)

arteries both proximal and distal to the embolus (Fig 48–2), and affects the retrograde filling of the SMA and its branches distal to the embolus.

Nonocclusive mesenteric ischemia was first described by Ende in 1958.[2] Following this initial description, the proportion of mesentric vascular accidents diagnosed as resulting from this entity rose from 12% to over 50% in the 1970s, but recently has been declining. NOMI is believed to result from splanchnic vasoconstriction occurring in response to a decrease in cardiac output, hypovolemia, dehydration, vasopressor agents, or hypotension. This vasoconstriction may persist even after the initiating cause has been corrected. Predisposing conditions include myocardial infarction, congestive heart failure, aortic insufficiency, renal and hepatic disease, or major abdominal or cardiac operations. In addition, a more immediate precipitating cause such as pulmonary edema, cardiac arrhythmia, or shock is usually present, although the intestinal ischemic episode may not become manifest until hours to days later.

The incidence of SMA thrombosis varies in different reports. While Ottinger[3] and Jackson[4] found thromboses to be almost as common as emboli, in most recent reports emboli were three to four times more frequent. SMA thrombosis is almost always superimposed on severe atherosclerotic narrowing, most often in the region of the origin of the SMA. Since the acute episode represents the end stage of a chronic problem, it is not surprising that 30%–50% of patients have had abdominal pain during the preceding weeks or months.

Most patients have severe diffuse atherosclerosis and a prior history of coronary, cerebral, or peripheral arterial ischemia.

Mesenteric venous thrombosis was considered the most frequent cause of intestinal infarction 58 years ago,[5] when infarction in the absence of arterial occlusion was interpreted as being the result of venous thrombosis. Today NOMI is recognized as the cause of most of these cases.

Pathophysiology

The intestines are protected from ischemic injury to a great extent by their abundant collateral circulation. Collateral pathways around occlusions of smaller mesenteric arterial branches are provided by the primary, secondary, and tertiary arcades in the mesentery of the small bowel, and the marginal arterial complex of Drummond in the mesocolon. Within the bowel wall itself, there is a network of communicating submucosal vessels which can maintain the viability of short segments of the intestine whose extramural arterial supply has been lost. There is good clinical evidence that during gradual occlusions of the major mesenteric arteries, and after acute occlusions when mesenteric vasoconstriction does not supervene, the collateral blood supply is adequate to maintain intestinal viability.

In response to the fall of arterial pressure distal to an obstruction, collateral pathways open immediately when a major vessel is occluded. Increased blood flow through the collateral circulation continues as long as the pressure in the vascular bed distal to an obstruction remains below the systemic arterial pressure. If vasoconstriction develops in the distal bed, raising arterial pressure distally, the pressure difference narrows and flow diminishes. Similarly, if normal blood flow is reconstituted, the distal pressure rises and flow through collateral channels ceases.

It has been postulated that vasoconstriction of the mesenteric vascular bed is the mechanism responsible for NOMI. Vasoconstriction has been demonstrated experimentally, angiographically, and intraoperatively in association with acute occlusions of the SMA. The occurrence of persistent or sustained vasoconstriction after the initiating cause is corrected, however, has only recently been identified. We have demonstrated such persistent vasoconstriction following a controlled decrease in mesenteric blood flow in a series of experiments performed on more than 200 anesthetized dogs.[6] The flow in the SMA was decreased 50% with a hydraulic occluder and maintained at this level, while alterations in cardiac output, intestinal perfusion, oxygen consumption, systemic and mesenteric arterial pressures, and blood flow through other arteries of the splanchnic circulation were measured.

Following acute diminution in SMA flow to 50% of control values, the mesenteric arterial pressure (MAP) in the peripheral bed immediately fell a mean of 49% (range 36%–71%), and in several instances the percentage decrease in MAP exceeded the decrease in blood flow. When SMA flow was maintained at 50%, the MAP returned to control levels within one to six hours, while celiac artery flow, which initially had increased, returned to normal. If the occluder was released when the MAP first returned to its control value, the SMA flow immediately rose to control levels. However, if the SMA occlusion was continued for intervals ranging from 30 minutes to four hours after MAP had returned to control, SMA flows remained at 30%–35% of control, even after removal of the occluder. These low SMA flows persisted for up to five hours of observation. However, in several of the experimental animals with persistent vasoconstriction, injection of papaverine into the SMA relieved the vasoconstriction and produced an immediate return of SMA flow to control levels. In other animals, when papaverine was infused continuously into the SMA (30%–60% mg/hour) while 50% flow was maintained in this vessel, the MAP remained low during the entire four hours of the experiment, and SMA flow returned to normal promptly on releasing the occluder. Thus, mesenteric vasoconstriction probably plays a significant role both during an acute occlusive or nonocclusive episode and for varying periods after correction of its cause.

In summary, low SMA flow initially produces mesenteric vascular responses that tend to maintain adequate intestinal flow, but if the diminished flow is prolonged, active vasoconstriction develops and may persist even after the primary cause of mesenteric ischemia is corrected. Such persistent vasoconstriction appears to violate the concept of autoregulatory escape but is not unique to the GI circulation. A similar potential for persistent vasoconstriction has been described in the kidney in man.

One of the puzzling characteristics of intestinal necrosis caused by "low-flow" states has been the frequent observation of a lag between correction of the primary systemic problem and the onset of abdominal symptoms and signs. The theory that the bowel is injured during an episode of diminished cardiac output or hypotension, and that correction of the primary problem returns mesenteric blood flow to normal does not explain the operative finding of persistent bowel ischemia without venous or arterial occlusion in patients whose cardiovascular problems have been corrected. The paradox can be explained, however, by our experimental observation that an episode of low mesenteric blood flow of as short as two hours' duration can produce mesenteric ischemia which may persist for many hours after correction of the primary problem.

Clinical Presentations

Early identification of acute mesenteric ischemia (AMI) depends upon recognition of those patients who are at risk of developing this catastrophe. AMI is most likely to develop in patients over 50 years of age with heart disease and long-standing congestive heart failure (especially with unsatisfactory control of digitalis therapy or prolonged use of diuretics), cardiac arrhythmias, recent myocardial infarctions, or in any patient with hypovolemia or hypotension due to such causes as burns, pancreatitis, or hemorrhage. The development of abdominal pain in a patient with one of these conditions should raise the suspicion of AMI. Previous or simultaneous arterial emboli increase the possibility of the intestinal ischemia being due to an SMA embolus.

Abdominal pain is present in 75%–98% of patients with intestinal ischemia, but varies in severity, nature, and location. Patients with acute SMA thrombosis commonly have had postprandial abdominal pain for several weeks or months preceding the acute episode. A characteristic early clinical feature of AMI is a disparity between the severity of the pain and the paucity of significant abdominal findings. Sudden, severe pain accompanied by forceful intestinal emptying is strongly suggestive of an acute arterial occlusion, especially when there are minimal or no abdominal findings. Mesenteric venous thrombosis is associated with abdominal pain, nausea, and vomiting which may be present for two to three weeks before abdominal signs develop.

Unexplained abdominal distention or GI bleeding may be the only indication of acute intestinal ischemia, since pain may be absent in up to 25% of patients, especially those with NOMI. Distention, while usually absent early in the course of mesenteric ischemia, may be the first sign of impending intestinal infarction. Lower GI bleeding may precede any other symptom of mesenteric ischemia, and stools contain occult blood in up to 75% of patients.

Early in the course of an ischemic episode there are no abdominal findings, but as infarction develops, increasing tenderness, rebound tenderness, and muscle guarding reflect the progressing intestinal changes. Significant abdominal findings are strong evidence for the presence of nonviable bowel. Nausea, vomiting, fever, rectal bleeding, hematemesis, intestinal obstruction, back pain, shock, and increasing abdominal distention are other late signs.

Diagnosis

Leukocytosis (above 15,000 cells/mm[3]) occurs in approximately 75% of patients with AMI, and metabolic acidosis is present in about 50%. Elevations of serum amylase and of peritoneal fluid intestinal alkaline phosphatase and inorganic phosphates have all been reported, but the sensitivity and specificity of these findings have not been established. Leukocytosis (especially out of proportion to the physical findings), elevated hematocrit, and blood-tinged peritoneal fluid, often with a high amylase content, are all signs of advanced intestinal necrosis.

Several potentially diagnostic radioisoptopic techniques utilizing technetium 99^m Tc pyrophosphate or diphosphonate 99^m Tc and sulfur colloid-labeled leukocytes[7] have been developed in animal studies. These are being evaluated clinically, but have not yet been proved reliable.

Laparoscopy is another diagnostic modality, especially useful for patients too ill to undergo angiography. This technique is potentially hazardous in the presence of AMI, however, since profound decreases in SMA flow occur with intraperitoneal pressures over 20mmHg. Lower pressures for brief periods produce only minimal alterations in flow. Unfortunately, laparoscopy enables visualization of only the serosal aspect of the bowel. Thus, while this modality is useful for identifying transmural ischemic changes, it is not reliable for diagnosing earlier stages of mucosal ischemia, when the serosa appears normal.

Angiography has been successfully employed to diagnose AMI, but until recently its role has been limited to identifying an embolus or acute thrombosis, both of which might be successfully treated by prompt operation. In 1974, we reported on a series of studies aimed at establishing criteria for the angiographic diagnosis of mesenteric vasoconstriction, the presence of which suggests nonocclusive mesenteric ischemia.[8] Mesenteric vasoconstriction was produced in dogs and the resulting angiographic abnormalities identified. Subsequently, selective superior mesenteric angiograms of a control group of 65 patients were examined to determine if the observed angiographic abnormalities occurred in the absence of vasoconstriction. The reliability of the angiographic signs of vasoconstriction was then evaluated in patients with AMI.

Based upon these studies, four reliable angiographic criteria for the diagnosis of mesenteric vasoconstriction were identified: (a) narrowing at the origins of multiple branches of the SMA, (b) irregularities in intestinal branches, (c) spasm of arcades, and (d) impaired filling of intramural vessels. While mesenteric vasoconstriction occurs with hemorrhage, pancreatitis, and other conditions, its presence in patients with suspected intestinal ischemia who are not in shock or receiving vasopressors is strong evidence for the presence of NOMI. Thus, if angiography is performed sufficiently early in their course, patients with both occlusive and nonocclusive AMI can be identified before bowel infarction occurs.

Plan for Diagnosis and Therapy

Patients over 50 years of age with any of the previously enumerated conditions predisposing to AMI, who develop sudden onset of abdominal pain lasting more than two or three hours, are started on the management protocol. Less absolute indications for an aggressive investigation are unexplained abdominal distention, GI bleeding, or metabolic acidosis. Broad-selection criteria are essential if early diagnosis and treatment are to be achieved, because the presence of more extensive and specific signs and symptoms usually signifies irreversible intestinal damage.

GENERAL PRINCIPLES.—Initial treatment is directed toward the correction of predisposing or precipitating causes of the mesenteric ischemia. Relief of acute congestive heart failure, and correction of hypotension, hypovolemia, and cardiac arrhythmias must precede any diagnostic studies. In general,

efforts to increase intestinal blood flow will be futile if low cardiac output, hypotension, or hypovolemia persist. Plain roentgenographic studies of the abdomen are then obtained and unless some other intra-abdominal condition is diagnosed on the plain film examination, abdominal angiography is then routinely performed. Based on the angiographic findings and the presence or absence of signs of peritoneal irritation on physical examination, the individual patient is then treated according to the schema outlined in Figures 48–3 and 48–4.

Even when a decision to operate has been made based on clinical grounds, an angiogram *must* be obtained to manage the patient properly at operation. Moreover, the relief of mesenteric vasoconstriction is an integral part of the therapy for emboli and thromboses, as well as the "low-flow" states, and can best be achieved by intra-arterial infusion of papaverine through an angiography catheter left in the SMA.

When papaverine is used, it is infused at a constant rate of 30–60 mg/hour using an infusion pump. Since these amounts of papaverine may have systemic effects, systemic arterial pressure and cardiac rate and rhythm must be monitored during the infusion. The duration of the infusion is dependent upon both the purpose for its use and the clinical and angiographic response of the patient.

Laparotomy is indicated during the course of AMI, either to restore intestinal arterial flow after an embolus or thrombosis or to resect irreparably damaged bowel. Revascularization should precede any evaluation of intestinal viability since bowel that initially appears infarcted may show surprising recovery after restoration of blood flow.

After revascularization, any short segments of bowel that are nonviable or questionably viable are resected. If extensive segments of bowel are involved, only the frankly necrotic bowel is resected, and a planned reexploration ("second-look") is performed within 12–24 hours.

A decision to perform a second look is made during the initial laparatomy if there is questionable viability of either a major portion or multiple segments of intestine. The purpose of the second look, as proposed by Shaw,[9] is "not just to allow a clear definition between dead and live bowel to take place, but also to allow time for the institution of supportive measures which may render more of the bowel viable."

The use of anticoagulants in the management of AMI is controversial. We do not employ heparin anticoagulation in the immediate perioperative period, except for cases of venous thrombosis, because of the danger of intestinal hemorrhage. Thromboses late in the postoperative period, however, have prompted us to start anticoagulation 48 hours postoperatively following embolectomy or arterial reconstruction.

The value of both systemic and locally administered antibiotics to improve the viability of compromised bowel is well accepted. For this reason, and because of the high incidence of positive blood cultures in patients with AMI, systemic antibiotics are started as soon as the diagnosis is established.

SPECIFIC MANAGEMENT.—*Superior Mesenteric Artery Embolus (SMAE):* If an embolus is identified on the angiogram, a papaverine infusion is begun through the angiographic SMA catheter, which is secured in place. The patient is then managed according to the schema in Figure 48–4 based on the site of the embolus, the presence or absence of

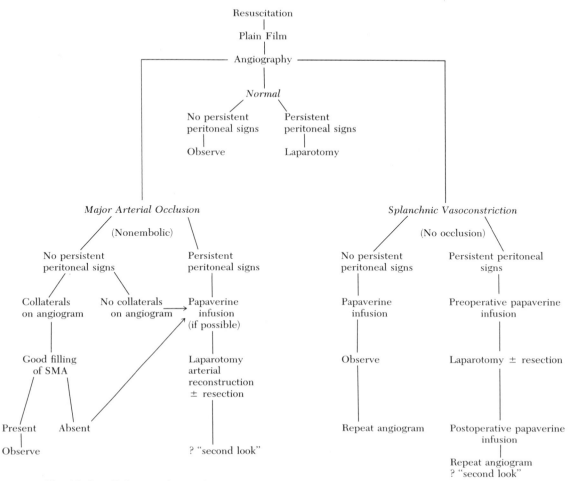

Fig 48–3.—Schema of plan for diagnosis and treatment of acute mesenteric ischemia.

peritoneal signs, and the state of perfusion of the vascular bed distal to the embolus as determined from a repeated angiogram after an intra-arterial bolus of 25 mg of tolazoline.

Minor emboli are defined as those limited to branches of the SMA or to the SMA distal to the origin of the ileocolic artery. Patients with major emboli who also have compelling medical reasons for avoiding operation, no peritoneal signs, and angiographically demonstrated good perfusion of the vascular bed distal to the embolus after the bolus dose of tolazoline are selected for nonoperative management, using only papaverine infusions. Thrombolytic agents infused through the angiographic catheters have been employed successfully in a few patients with SMA emboli, but this approach is still experimental.

Embolectomy is performed before assessing intestinal viability. We prefer to approach the embolus directly, or, less optimally, through a proximal arteriotomy. The proximal SMA is exposed by drawing the transverse colon superiorly and anteriorly, and packing off the small intestine inferiorly. The inferior leaf of the transverse mesocolon is incised and the proximal SMA is identified by dissection between the pancreas and duodenum. The origin of the middle colic artery is identified and isolated, and the main SMA is freed for a

distance of 2–3 cm proximal and distal to the origin of this branch. After identifying the site of the embolus, the vessel is occluded proximally and distally with double-looped tapes, gentle vascular clamps, or bulldog clamps (Fig 48–5). A longitudinal arteriotomy is made over the embolus or just proximal to it. The embolus is removed and the proximal and distal occlusions released to flush out retained fragments of clots. A Fogarty balloon catheter is then passed proximally and distally to remove all residual clots. The arteriotomy is closed with or without a vein patch as necessary.

Following embolectomy, if no second look is planned, the papaverine infusion is continued for 12–24 hours, and an angiogram is obtained immediately prior to removing the catheter. If a second look is scheduled, the infusion is maintained until that procedure is completed.

Nonocclusive Mesenteric Ischemia (NOMI): Angiographically, NOMI is diagnosed when the signs of mesenteric vasoconstriction are seen in a patient who has a clinical picture suggestive of intestinal ischemia, but who is neither in shock nor receiving vasopressors. The angiographic findings may vary from localized spasm to a "pruned" appearance of the entire mesenteric tree.

A papaverine infusion is begun on all patients with NOMI as soon as the diagnosis is made (see Fig 48–3), and in pa-

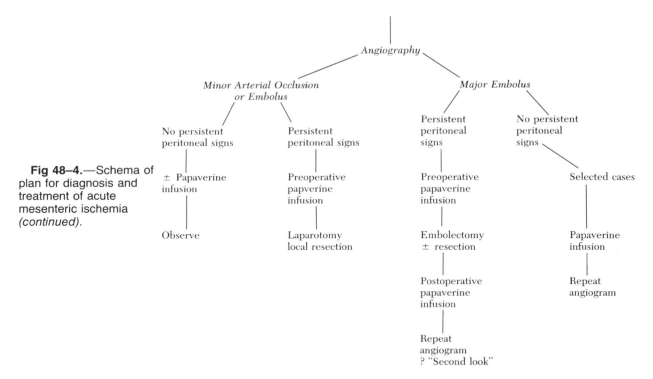

Fig 48–4.—Schema of plan for diagnosis and treatment of acute mesenteric ischemia *(continued).*

tients with persistent peritoneal signs, the infusion is continued during and after laparotomy.

At operation, manipulation of the SMA is kept to a minimum. Bowel that is obviously necrotic is resected, and a primary anastomosis is performed. If bowel of questionable via-

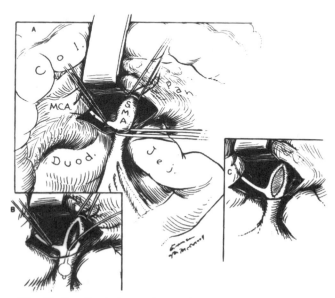

Fig 48–5.—Technique of superior mesenteric artery embolectomy. **A,** the artery has been isolated at the base of the transverse mesocolon and controlled with tapes. **B,** longitudinal arteriotomy placed proximal to the origin of the middle colic artery. A Fogarty catheter has been passed distally. **C,** the arteriotomy closure using a vein patch. The patch is usually not required. (From Boley S.J. et al., in Nyhus L.M. (ed.): *Surgery Annual.* 1973. By permission of Appleton-Century Crofts.)

bility is left behind, a second look is scheduled. It is better to leave bowel of doubtful viability than to perform a massive small-bowel resection, for in many instances the circulation will have improved by the time of the second exploration.

When papaverine infusion is used as the primary treatment for NOMI, it is continued for approximately 24 hours. A repeated angiogram is then performed 30 minutes after changing the infusion to isotonic saline without papaverine (Fig 48–6). Based on the clinical course of the patient and the response of the vasoconstriction to therapy as noted on the angiogram, the infusion is either discontinued or maintained for another 24 hours, at which time the patient is reevaluated. Infusions usually can be stopped after 24 hours, but have been continued for as long as five days. When papaverine is used in conjunction with laparotomy for nonocclusive disease, a second look is frequently necessary. In such cases the infusion is continued, as described previously for second-look operations following embolectomy. The papaverine infusion is discontinued when no signs of vasoconstriction remain on an angiogram obtained 30 minutes after the vasodilator infusate is replaced by saline alone. The SMA catheter is removed promptly when the intra-arterial infusion is stopped.

Acute Superior Mesenteric Artery Thrombosis (SMAT): Identification of SMAT is usually made from the flush aortogram, which most often shows total occlusion of the SMA within 1–2 cm of its origin. Some filling of the artery distal to the obstruction is almost always present because of collateral circulation. Branches both proximal and distal to the occlusion may show local spasm or diffuse vasoconstriction. Angiographic differentiation between thrombosis and an old embolus may be difficult; in such instances the patients are treated initially as if they have emboli. A more difficult problem arises when total occlusion of the SMA is demonstrated by angiography in a patient with abdominal pain but no ab-

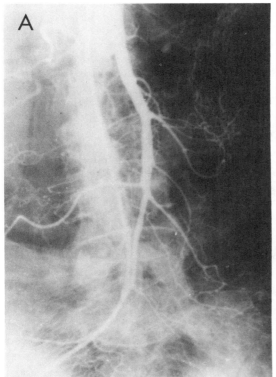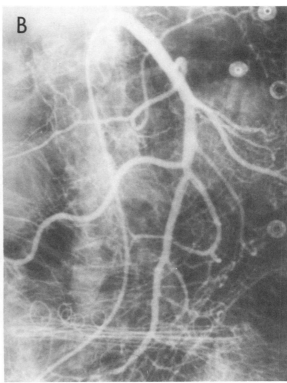

Fig 48–6.—Patient with nonocclusive mesenteric ischemia managed with papaverine infusion for three days. **A,** initial angiogram showing spasm of main superior mesenteric artery, origins of branches and intestinal arcades. **B,** angiogram after 36 hours of papaverine infusion. Study was obtained 30 minutes after papaverine was replaced with saline. At this time the patient's abdominal symptoms and signs were gone. (From Boley, S.J., Brandt L.J., Veith, (in Ravitch M.M. (ed.): *Curr. Prob. Surg.* 1978. By permission of Year Book Medical Publishers.)

dominal findings. In such cases, it is important to be able to differentiate an acute occlusion from a long-standing one, as the latter may be coincidental to an unrelated present illness. The presence or absence of prominent collaterals between the superior mesenteric and the celiac and/or inferior mesenteric circulation is the most helpful finding. If large collaterals are demonstrated on the angiogram, chronic occlusion is most likely, and is confirmed by good filling of the SMA in late films. In the absence of any peritoneal signs, such patients are treated expectantly. The absence of collaterals indicates acute occlusion, and prompt intervention is indicated whether or not peritoneal signs are present.

If the position of the angiographic catheter permits, papaverine infusion is started preoperatively and maintained during and after the arterial reconstruction.

Revascularization procedures for SMAT are similar to those used for chronic mesenteric ischemia, in which thrombectomy and endarterectomy, or some form of bypass graft to the SMA distal to the obstruction are employed. While a short graft from the aorta to the SMA is the easiest and most satisfactory operation in our opinion, extensive aortic disease may make this impossible. Often a common or external iliac artery may be the best source of inflow, and we have had success with prosthetic grafts from either to the SMA.

Acute Mesenteric Venous Thrombosis (AMVT): Mesenteric venous thrombosis may be primary ("agnogenic") or secondary to a variety of conditions, including hematologic disorders, hypercoagulable states, intra-abdominal sepsis, local venous stasis, and abdominal trauma. Recently there has been a spate of reports of minor and major mesenteric venous thromboses in patients taking oral contraceptives. The angiographic diagnosis of AMVT has only rarely been made in the clinical setting.

Mesenteric venous thrombosis is most often diagnosed at laparotomy. Angiography is usually nondiagnostic, and laparotomy is performed because of the presence of peritoneal signs. The thrombosis may involve the superior mesenteric vein (SMV) and portal vein, but more frequently involves a segmental jejunal or ileal vein. At operation the diagnosis can be confirmed by mesenteric venous angiography and by pressure measurements performed through a peripheral venous branch.

Localized segments of infarcted intestine are resected and primary anastomoses performed. When most of the small bowel is ischemic but not frankly infarcted, a thrombectomy should be attempted. If thrombosis of the SMV and/or portal vein is identified, the SMV is dissected out just below the pancreas and proximal and distal control obtained. Through a transverse venotomy in the SMV, a Fogarty catheter is passed up to the liver and clot from the portal vein removed. Clot from the intestinal side of the venotomy is removed by massaging the intestines and mesentery and by passage of a small Fogarty catheter. Good blood flow must be obtained from both the portal and peripheral ends of the venotomy. The venotomy is closed with simple interrupted sutures without a patch graft.[10] AMVT is the one condition for which anticoagulants are used routinely postoperatively to prevent the frequent recurrence of venous thromboses.

Summary of Key Points in Treatment

1. Always obtain an angiogram even when laparotomy is already scheduled and leave the catheter in place in the SMA:
   —establishes diagnosis of AMI and its cause;
   —provides a "road map" for revascularization; and
   —catheter provides access for intraarterial infusion of vasodilators.
2. Always revascularize when there is occlusion of the SMA above the origin of the ileocolic artery, unless all of the small bowel is necrotic. This rule applies even if all the bowel appears viable at laparotomy.
3. Postoperative infusions of papaverine should be employed following revascularization procedures and for NOMI when laparotomy is performed for resection of infarcted intestine.
4. When short segments of bowel are of questionable viability after revascularization or with NOMI, resection is advisable, but when a major portion of the small bowel is involved a second look is preferable. Every attempt to prevent a short-bowel syndrome is worthwhile.

Prognosis

Although mortalities of 70%–90% have been reported through 1980 using traditional methods of diagnosis and therapy, the aggressive approach described above can reduce these catastrophic figures.[11] Of the first 50 patients managed by this approach, 35 (70%) proved to have AMI. Of these, 33 had angiographic signs of ischemia. The remaining two patients had normal angiograms. Nineteen (54%) of the patients with AMI survived, including 9 of 15 patients with NOMI, 7 of 16 with SMAE, 2 of 3 patients with SMAT, and 1 patient with AMVT. Seventeen of the 19 survivors lost no bowel or less than three feet of small intestine.

In a more recent review of 47 patients with intestinal ischemia resulting from SMA emboli,[12] a survival rate of 55% was achieved in patients managed according to our aggressive protocol, whereas only 20% of those treated by traditional methods survived. Intra-arterial papaverine as the primary treatment was successful in four patients; two were not operated on, and the other two had normal intestine at the time of delayed laparotomy.

The complications due to angiographic studies and prolonged infusions of vasodilator drugs have not been excessive. Three of our first 50 patients developed transient acute tubular necrosis following angiography and treatment of mesenteric ischemia. One patient developed arterial occlusions in both lower extremities during a papaverine infusion for an SMA embolus, probably representing other emboli from his primary source of embolization. However, the SMA catheter could not be excluded as a factor. Several patients developed local hematomas at arterial puncture sites, but no major problems were encountered with blood flow to the lower extremities.

Problems due to prolonged papaverine infusions have been minimal. Infusions for more than five days have been used without significant systemic effects. Fibrin clots on the arterial catheter have been observed commonly, but have not caused any difficulty. Three catheters clotted and had to be removed, but this complication can be avoided by use of a continuous infusion pump. Catheter dislodgment requiring replacement occurred several times.

Ninety percent of patients with AMI who had angiography but no physical signs of peritonitis have survived, demonstrating the potential value of early diagnosis. Ideally all patients with AMI should be studied at a time when the plain films of the abdomen are normal, before physical signs develop.

Future Trends

Research efforts at present are focusing on three areas: (1) methods of earlier diagnosis, (2) means for evaluating the viability of ischemic bowel at operation, and (3) pharmacologic means of improving survival of ischemic bowel. While no good serum marker has as yet been found, the identification of one or a group of markers with a high degree of specificity and sensitivity is possible. Quantitative fluorescein fluorescence has been shown to be extremely accurate in evaluating intestinal viability in dogs and is now being employed clinically. A number of drugs directed at neutralizing the deleterious effects of reperfusion are being investigated.

COLONIC ISCHEMIA

Since the identification in the early 1960s of the noncatastrophic forms of colonic ischemia, this condition has been recognized as one of the commonest diseases of the large bowel in the elderly. When compared with acute mesenteric ischemia, CI usually produces milder symptoms, fewer physical findings, and far fewer systemic derangements. For the most part, colonic ischemia is diagnosed only after the ischemic episode is over and, the circulation has returned to normal. Thus, AMI and colonic ischemia are generally very different problems; AMI is a catastrophic emergency with a high mortality, while CI is usually noncatastrophic and does not require prompt intervention.

Many names have been applied to the various clinical forms of CI. Most characterize only one aspect of the condition, and often an overlap of the pathologic changes signified by different terms has created confusion. Moreover, as understanding of the nature of colonic ischemia has increased, it has become apparent that some of the names used are inaccurate. For example, our original term, "reversible vascular occlusion of the colon," to describe the transient manifestations of CI is not completely correct, since it is the effect of an occlusion rather than the occlusion itself which is reversible and, in fact, there may not be a demonstrable occlusion responsible for the ischemia. Similarly, the terms "ischemic colitis" and "colonic infarction" are suitable for only parts of the spectrum of CI, for the milder reversible ischemic episodes are not inflammatory but hemorrhagic, and coagulation necrosis, i.e., true infarction, is often absent. Colonic ischemia is an appropriate overall appellation to describe both reversible and irreversible lesions. Specific forms of ischemic damage can then be further classified pathologically and clinically as: (1) reversible ischemic lesions of the colon or reversible ischemic colopathy; (2) reversible or transient ischemic colitis; (3) chronic ischemic colitis; (4) ischemic colonic stricture; or (5) ischemic colonic gangrene. The adoption of this terminology and elimination of nonspecific names would enable the experience of many clinicians to be combined and uniformly compared, broadening our understanding of these entities.

History

Prior to the late 1950s most reports of intestinal vascular disease described catastrophic mesenteric vascular accidents involving the small and, only rarely, the large intestine. Lauenstein[13] in 1882 described gangrene of the transverse colon following ligation of the middle colic artery during a gastrectomy. Only sporadic cases were reported until the 1950s, when the increasing number of operations for aortic aneurysms and the introduction of ligation of the inferior mesenteric artery (IMA) during resections of colonic carcinomas resulted in numerous instances of large-bowel ischemia, resulting in gangrene, stricture, and colitis. Experimental and clinical studies during the past 25 years have led to the recognition of both the full gamut of pathologic changes produced by intestinal ischemia and the protean clinical manifestations with which it may present. In 1963, based on a series of laboratory and clinical investigations, Boley and coworkers[14,15] first identified the spontaneous and reversible nature of some episodes of CI and described the radiologic criteria for their early diagnosis. The ability to diagnose CI in its early stages enabled those investigators to observe the natural history and late results of acute ischemic insults and led to their emphasis of the vascular origin of segmental colitis in the elderly, nonspecific colonic ulcers, and colonic strictures.[16] In 1966 Marston and associates[17] coined the term "ischaemic colitis" to describe a series of 16 patients and categorized them into gangrenous, stricturing, and transient forms.

Incidence

An accurate determination of the incidence of colonic ischemia is impossible because the various clinical manifestations of the disorder have only recently been recognized. Also, since barium enemas are not always performed early, many cases of transient, or reversible, ischemic lesions are probably missed. However, based on our experience with more than 200 cases, as well as numerous other cases reported since our original paper in 1963, ischemic lesions appear to be more common in the colon than in the small bowel. As awareness by clinicians and radiologists is increasing, and as emphasis is being placed on the performance of barium enemas early in the evaluation of patients with rectal bleeding, colonic ischemia is becoming recognized as one of the more common colonic disorders.

In a review of 150 cases of colonic ischemia in 148 patients, 53% occurred in females and 47% in males. Although the patients ranged in age from 1 to 87 years, 91% of those whose lesions were not iatrogenic were in the seventh decade or older. This prevalence in the older age group is confirmed by other reports and is to be expected in view of the general deterioration of the vascular tree that accompanies aging.

Ischemia may involve any portion of the colon, but most commonly involves the splenic flexure, descending colon and sigmoid colon (Fig 48–7). Although the distribution and pattern of involvement do not bear any relationship to the severity of the ischemia, specific causes of ischemia do appear to

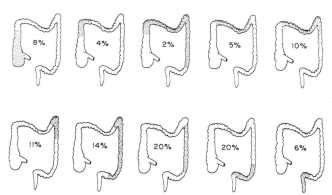

Fig 48–7.—Distribution and length of involvement in 150 cases of colonic ischemia. More frequent involvement of left half of colon is apparent. (From Boley S.J., Brandt L.J., Veith, in Ravitch M.M. (ed.): *Curr. Probl. Surg.* 1978. By permission of Year Book Medical Publishers.)

more commonly affect certain areas. Iatrogenic ischemia resulting from ligation of the IMA usually produces changes in the sigmoid colon, while low-flow states show a predilection for involving the splenic flexure. Similarly, the length of bowel involved varies with the cause, e.g., atheromatous emboli often result in short segment changes and low-flow states usually involve much longer ones.

British authors initially considered rectal involvement to be rare or nonexistent.[17] However, in our experience and that of others, it is a relatively frequent finding. Farman[18] found that rectal ischemic disease was always accompanied by involvement of the sigmoid colon, but we have seen several instances of isolated rectal changes, including one patient who developed a short rectal stricture with normal bowel proximally. The wide variation in the site and degree of ischemic changes is understandable in view of the many causes of colonic vascular insufficiency. We have documented second episodes of ischemia in only three of more than 200 patients, but recurrences probably are more frequent.

Etiology

In the colon, ischemia results from many causes. These may be broadly classified as being iatrogenic or noniatrogenic, occlusive or nonocclusive, and systemic or local (Table 48–1). Although a cause of the colonic ischemia or a site of occlusion is often recognized, no specific cause or occlusion can be identified in the majority of cases. The "spontaneous" epi-

TABLE 48–1.—CAUSES OF COLONIC ISCHEMIA

1. Inferior mesenteric artery thrombosis	10. Rheumatoid arthritis
2. Arterial embolus	11. Necrotizing arteritis
3. Cholesterol emboli	12. Thromboangiitis obliterans
4. Cardiac failure or arrhythmias	13. Strangulated hernia
5. Shock	14. Oral contraceptives
6. Digitalis toxicity	15. Polycythemia vera
7. Volvulus	16. Parasitic infestation
8. Periarteritis nodosa	17. Allergy
9. Systemic lupus erythematosus	18. Trauma—blunt and penetrating
	19. Ruptured ectopic pregnancy

20. Iatrogenic Causes
    a. Aneurysmectomy
    b. Aortoiliac reconstruction
    c. Gynecologic operations
    d. Exchange transfusions
    e. Colon bypass
    f. Lumbar aortography
    g. Colectomy with inferior mesenteric artery ligation

sodes (generally classified as being NOMI) have been attributed to low-flow states, small-vessel disease, or both in concert. While low flow certainly can be implicated in those patients with congestive heart failure, digitalis toxicity, or cardiac arrhythmias, these conditions are usually not present.

The frequency of colonic ischemic lesions in the elderly suggests a relationship to degenerative vascular changes. While angiography in these disorders has only rarely demonstrated a significant occlusion or abnormality, present techniques have limitations in evaluating smaller vessels. Narrowing of small arteries, arterioles and veins is probably a factor in nonocclusive mesenteric ischemia, and certainly this term does not imply that the mesenteric vessels are normal. Histologic evidence of narrowing in the small colonic vessels has been demonstrated and indicates the probable existence of increased resistance and restriction of free blood flow prior to the acute insult. What finally triggers an ischemic episode is still conjectural in most instances; whether increased demand by the colonic tissues is superimposed on an already borderline flow or whether flow itself is acutely diminished has yet to be determined.

One possible factor predisposing the colon to ischemia is an inherently lower blood flow than that of the small intestine. Geber, using an electromagnetic flowmeter, found normal colonic blood flow to be 73 ml/minute/100 gm, the lowest of any intestinal segment. Others, using indicator fractionation techniques, have reported conflicting values, both higher and lower, but most investigators agree that the large bowel has a lower flow than the other areas of the GI tract. Of even greater importance is experimental evidence that functional motor activity of the colon is accompanied by a decrease in blood flow. This is contrary to the increase in small intestinal blood during periods of digestion and increased peristalsis. Geber has postulated that "the combination of normally low blood flow and decreased blood flow during functional activity would seem to make the colon (1) rather unique among all areas of the body where increased functional activity is usually accompanied by an increased blood flow and (2) more susceptible to pathology." Furthermore, the more pronounced effect of "straining" on systemic arterial and venous pressure in constipated, as compared to normal, patients provides indirect evidence that constipation may accentuate the circulatory effects of defecation.

Colonic blood flow also has been shown to be responsive to changes in environment, eating a meal, and emotionally stressful situations. These conditions may either place greater demands on a restricted blood inflow or further decrease an already compromised circulation. In addition, recent experimental studies of the hypothalamic influence on GI blood flow in the awake cat suggest that "of the entire gastrointestinal tract, the colon blood flow is most affected by autonomic stimulation."

Pathophysiology

Regardless of its cause, bowel ischemia produces a spectrum of pathologic, clinical, and radiologic manifestations. The pathologic changes evoked by ischemia range from simple submucosal edema to infarction and necrosis. Between these extremes are gradations of tissue damage which form the basis for the diverse clinical courses that individual epi-

sodes of CI may take (Fig 48–8), varying with the severity of the episode. Mild ischemia produces morphological changes which regress and ultimately disappear or heal, a sequence of events reflected clinically and radiologically by transient or reversible colonic findings. More severe ischemia may result in irreparable damage, with gangrene, perforation, or persistent colitis; if healing occurs, it does so with scarring, fibrosis, and resultant stricture.

The ultimate outcome of an episode of CI depends on many factors. Among these are: (1) the cause, i.e., occlusion or low flow; (2) the level of the occlusion; (3) the duration and degree of the ischemia; (4) the rapidity of onset of the ischemic process; (5) the adequacy of the collateral circulation; (6) the state of the general circulation; (7) the metabolic requirements of the affected bowel; (8) the presence of bacteria within the lumen; and (9) the presence of associated conditions, such as colonic distention. While the end results of the interaction of all these factors are obviously multifold, the initial response to ischemia may be the same regardless of its severity. *It is, therefore, impossible to predict the progression of the ischemic process based on the initial physical, radiologic, or sigmoidoscopic evaluation.*

Symptoms and Signs

Most episodes of CI produce clinical, radiologic, and pathologic changes that are completely reversible. Recognition of the nature and reversibility of these lesions will prevent unnecessary operations and the use of improper medical therapy that may aggravate an otherwise self-limited condition. Irreversible damage resulting in gangrene, perforation, stricture, or chronic colitis may have the same clinical onset as reversible episodes, but the greater severity of the lesion soon becomes apparent.

Typically, CI presents with sudden onset of mild lower abdominal pain, usually crampy and localized to the left side. The pain is frequently accompanied by tenesmus and is followed within 24 hours by passage of dark or bright red blood per rectum or by bloody diarrhea. Less commonly, especially with irreversible lesions, the pain is severe. In other patients, pain may be minimal or absent. Characteristically, the blood loss is minimal. Although massive bleeding has resulted from CI, its presence militates against this diagnosis.

Diagnosis

Initially, the only physical finding is abdominal tenderness over the area of the involved colon, most commonly on the left side. Signs of peritoneal irritation have been noted with

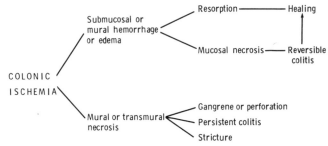

Fig 48–8.—Various end results of colonic ischemia.

ultimately reversible lesions, but if these persist for more than a few hours, they should be considered evidence of irreparable tissue damage. Fever and leukocytosis are usually present and, together with the physical findings, are parameters to be followed in assessing the progress of ischemic lesions. Early and serial barium enema studies are the keys to diagnosing CI. Colonoscopy is being employed with increasing frequency, but when colonoscopy is used extreme care is necessary, since high intraluminal pressures may lead to further ischemia or perforation of already damaged colon.

Treatment

Proper treatment of ischemic lesions of the colon is based on early diagnosis, prompt recognition of irreversible ischemic damage, continued monitoring of the patient, and on the radiologic or endoscopic appearance of the colon. If a presumptive diagnosis of CI is made, and the physical findings do not suggest intestinal gangrene or perforation, the patient is observed for fever, a rising WBC count, or changes in his abdominal signs. Systemic antibiotics are administered and blood and fluids replaced when indicated. In the early stages of the disease it is best to place the bowel at rest and provide IV fluids. If the colon appears distended, it is decompressed with a rectal tube and careful saline irrigations, since increased intraluminal pressure may further compromise the intestinal blood supply. Contrary to their efficacy in ulcerative colitis, systemic corticosteroids are not only of no value but may be harmful, since they increase the possibility of intestinal perforation and secondary infection.

Serial barium studies or endoscopy of the colon are an essential part of the therapy, since they definitely establish the diagnosis of ischemia and either will verify the reversibility of the colonic damage or demonstrate progression to an ischemic colitis or stricture.

If deterioration in the clinical course is suggested by worsening abdominal signs and increasing fever and leukocytosis, or if diarrhea or bleeding persist for more than two weeks, irreversible damage almost certainly has occurred, and surgical intervention is indicated. Reversible lesions usually improve within seven to ten days, and continued symptoms beyond this period warrant a change from a very conservative therapeutic approach to a very aggressive one. In our experience, patients with persistence of diarrhea and bleeding have often developed perforation and peritonitis.

Unless symptoms of obstruction are present, a patient with a stricture should be observed, as strictures may improve spontaneously after several months. When symptoms of obstruction occur, however, surgical intervention is necessary.

The operative treatment of irreversible ischemic lesions of the colon is local resection of only the involved area with restitution of intestinal continuity by primary anastomosis. The specimen should be opened immediately by the surgeon or by the pathologist to be certain that all of the involved colon has been removed. Bowel with mucosal damage should be excised, even though it may have a normal external appearance, since anastomoses of such bowel are likely to leak or go on to stricture.

Thus, the treatment of CI consists of early identification and continued surveillance, an ultraconservative approach

where reversibility is probable, and a very aggressive surgical approach where permanent ischemic damage is likely to have occurred.

Prognosis

The outlook for patients with colonic ischemia is generally good. Recurrent episodes probably occur in fewer than 5%, and we have not seen late sequelae in patients whose initial clinical complaints and roentgenographic abnormalities have subsided. Areas of ischemic colitis and even apparent strictures sometimes resolve without treatment after many months. The high risk of developing a stricture projected by Marcuson[19] is contrary to our experience with over 200 patients, only a small fraction of whom have required an operation.

VASCULAR LESIONS OF THE INTESTINES PRODUCING BLEEDING

During the past decade, vascular lesions of the small and especially the large bowel have been recognized as a major cause of lower intestinal bleeding, particularly in the elderly. However, a great deal of confusion and controversy has resulted from the application of different terms to the same morphological abnormality, and, conversely, from the use of one term to describe many different histologic lesions. Although many reports have lumped them together, several histologically and clinically distinct vascular lesions can be identified. Moreover, the nature, etiology, natural history, and treatment can vary depending on the type of lesion.

Vascular Ectasias

Definition

Vascular ectasias of the right side of the colon, also referred to as angiodysplasias, arteriovenous malformations, and angiomas, are by far the most common vascular abnormalities seen in the intestines and are probably the most frequent cause of recurrent lower intestinal bleeding after 60 years of age.[20] They are a distinct clinical and pathologic entity,[21, 22] and are degenerative lesions associated with aging. In contrast with congenital or neoplastic vascular lesions that occur throughout the GI tract in various age groups, vascular ectasias are not associated with angiomatous lesions of the skin or other viscera, almost always occur in the cecum or proximal part of the ascending colon, are usually multiple rather than single, are usually less than 5 mm in diameter, rarely can be identified by the surgeon at operation or by the pathologist in the laboratory using standard techniques, and usually can be diagnosed clinically by angiography or colonoscopy.

Historical Background

Prevailing concepts of the causes of lower intestinal bleeding in patients over 60 years of age have been continually changing since the 1920s, when neoplasms were considered the most frequent cause of significant bleeding. By the late 1940s and early 1950s, hemorrhage attributed to diverticulitis was being reported commonly. In the late 1950s and early 1960s a clear differentiation was made between the frequent occurrence of hemorrhage complicating diverticulosis and the much less common association of bleeding with diverticulitis. During the latter period, a predominant etiologic role for diverticulosis in massive lower intestinal bleeding was postulated and widely accepted, based on the acceptance of "diagnosis by exclusion"; i.e., failure to identify another cause of bleeding in patients with diverticulosis. This approach was exemplified by the criteria established by Quinn and Ochsner[23]: (1) the passage of considerable volumes of bright red or maroon blood via the rectum; (2) radiographic evidence of diverticula; (3) no other demonstrable cause of hemorrhage on barium enema or sigmoidoscopy; (4) no blood in the gastric aspirate and/or no abnormality on upper GI series; and (5) normal blood coagulation studies.

In 1961, using operative angiography, Margulis, Heinbecker, and Bernard, identified a "vascular malformation" of the cecum as the cause of massive bleeding in a 69-year-old woman. Since that time, and especially after the introduction by Baum et al. of selective angiography for identifying the source of intestinal bleeding, there have been numerous reports of bleeding from small cecal vascular abnormalities. Our experience and that of others suggest that these cecal vascular ectasias, or angiodysplasias, are at least as important a cause of lower intestinal hemorrhage in the elderly as diverticular disease.[20] Welch and co-workers[24] reviewed the records of all patients in whom a diagnosis of either angiodysplasia (vascular ectasia) or diverticular bleeding was made at the Massachusetts General Hospital. They found that 43 of 72 patients had angiodysplasias, and the other 29 had diverticular bleeding.

We reviewed the records of all patients over 60 years of age with lower intestinal bleeding admitted to the Montefiore Medical Center between 1971 and 1976.[20] Ninety-nine patients had 100 episodes of major bleeding, 43 of which were diagnosed as being diverticular bleeding and 20 bleeding from vascular ectasias. In 11 episodes the source of bleeding was not determined; there were 9 due to colonic carcinomas or polyps, 6 due to radiation proctitis, and 2 to ischemic colitis. The other 9 episodes were ascribed to miscellaneous causes.

All patients with ectasias had angiographic demonstration of these lesions in the right colon. However, only eight of the 43 patients diagnosed as having diverticular bleeding had angiographic demonstration of extravasation of contrast material into a colonic diverticulum; four were on the left side and four were on the right. In the remaining 35 patients, the diagnosis was based solely upon the presence of diverticulosis and failure to identify another definite cause of bleeding. None of these patients fulfilled all five of Quinn and Ochsner's proposed criteria for the diagnosis of diverticular bleeding, and only 19 patients fulfilled four of the five criteria. Surprisingly, 11 patients had other possible sources of bleeding identified, but were still discharged with the diagnosis of diverticular bleeding. Angiography performed in 15 of the 35 patients was normal.

These studies reflect both the changing pattern of the causes believed responsible for the bleeding and the inexact nature of the criteria on which these beliefs are based. Although diverticular bleeding was the most frequent discharge diagnosis in our study, it is obvious that in most cases there was insufficient evidence to support this conclusion. Even the minimal criteria established by Quinn and Ochsner to diagnose diverticular bleeding by the exclusion of other causes

were not fulfilled in any of the patients in our study. On the other hand, it must be recognized that, although vascular ectasias were identified by angiography in 20 patients, in only two of these was bleeding from the ectasias proved by extravasation of contrast material.

Incidence and Associated Conditions

There does not appear to be any sex predilection for vascular ectasias. Most patients have been over 50 years of age; all but one of ours were older than 55 years, and two thirds were over 70 years of age. There have been reports of angiodysplasias in adolescents, in one report in association with Meckel's diverticula, but none of these reports included corroborating histologic findings. If investigators are to establish the occurrence of vascular ectasias in younger patients, or in the GI tract in areas other than the right colon, histologic proof of the nature of these lesions is mandatory. We have reviewed tissue sections from lesions in the left colon, originally reported as ectasias or angiodysplasias, and found totally different changes from those seen with ectasias.

Approximately one half of the patients with ectasias have a history or clinical diagnosis of cardiac disease, and approximately half of the patients in this group have aortic stenosis.[21, 25] While some consider the ectasias and cardiac disease to be related congenital lesions, others ascribe a causative role to the aortic stenosis. We do not believe the low perfusion pressure and low pulse pressure produced by aortic stenosis contribute to the development of vascular ectasias, but that they increase the chance of bleeding in individuals who have ectasias. The low perfusion pressure might well cause ischemic necrosis of the single layer of endothelium which often separates ectatic vessels from the colonic lumen. Since our studies show that a substantial portion of the elderly population probably have ectasias, the increased incidence of intestinal bleeding in older patients with aortic stenosis is not surprising. The low perfusion pressure seen with aortic stenosis would then be a factor in producing bleeding in patients who also have vascular ectasias.

Etiology and Pathophysiology

Vascular ectasias are degenerative lesions associated with aging and represent a unique entity distinct from previously described intestinal vascular abnormalities.[26] We believe they are caused by repeated, partial, intermittent, low-grade obstruction of the submucosal veins, especially where they pierce the muscle layers of the colon. This obstruction, repeated for many years during muscular contraction and distension of the colon, results in dilatation and tortuosity, initially of the submucosal veins, and then, in a retrograde manner, of the venules of the arteriolar-capillary-venular units draining into them. Ultimately, the capillary rings surrounding the crypts dilate, and the competency of the precapillary sphincters is lost, thus producing a small arteriovenous communication (Fig 48–9). The prevalence of these degenerative lesions in the right colon can be attributed to the greater tension in the cecal wall as compared to the other parts of the colon, according to LaPlace's principle.

The angiographic identification of colonic ectasias in a few patients who had no bleeding and the concept that ectasias

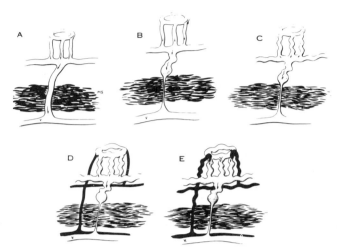

Fig 48–9.—Diagrammatic illustration of proposed concept of the development of cecal vascular ectasias. **A,** normal state of vein perforating muscular layers. **B,** with muscular contraction or increased intraluminal pressure, the vein is partially obstructed. **C,** after repeated episodes over many years, the submucosal vein becomes dilated and tortuous. **D,** later the veins and venules draining into the abnormal submucosal vein become similarly involved. **E,** ultimately, the capillary ring becomes dilated, the precapillary sphincter becomes incompetent, and a small arteriovenous communication is present through the ectasia. (From Boley S.J., et al.: On the nature and etiology of vascular ectasias of the colon: Degenerative lesions of aging. *Gastroenterology* 72:650, 1977. Reproduced by permission.)

are degenerative lesions of aging suggest that they should be present in many asymptomatic older persons. To determine this, we studied the colons resected from a control group of patients older than 60 years of age with carcinoma of the colon and no history of GI bleeding or obstruction of the large intestine.[26] In no instance did the tumor of the colon involve the cecum. Using our injection and clearing technique, mucosal ectasias were found in four of 15 colons, and ectatic sub-

mucosal veins in eight of the 15 colons. All of the colons with mucosal ectasias also contained ectatic submucosal veins. While these patients are not a normal control group in the usual sense of the term, the presence of ectasias in such a high percentage of patients support our belief that they are acquired lesions associated with aging.

Histologic identification of vascular ectasias is difficult without special techniques, as demonstrated by our own experience. In seven colons resected from patients with angiographically demonstrated ectasias and studied only by routine gross examination and by microscopic study of random or selected sections, a mucosal ectasia could be identified in only two.

Our present technique for the localization and identification of vascular ectasias consists of the injection of a silicone rubber compound, Microfil, through catheters placed in one or more of the arteries supplying the colon. Specimens are then dehydrated in increasing concentrations of ethyl alcohol and cleared with methyl salicylate. This produces a transparent specimen with a filled vascular bed, which is studied by dissecting microscopy, using direct light as well as transillumination.

We have utilized this method in 24 colons[22] and one or more mucosal ectasias, measuring 1 mm to 1 cm in diameter, were identified in all of the specimens (Fig 48–10). Seven colons contained two such lesions, and 11 colons had three or more. The ectasias were all located within the cecum and the proximal part of the ascending colon; the most distal one was 23 cm from the ileocecal valve.

All of the cleared specimens had prominent dilated and tortuous submucosal veins present beneath the ectasias and also in areas where the mucosal vessels appeared normal (Fig 48–11). The colon from the oldest patient, an 88-year-old man, contained approximately 50 mucosal ectasias of varying sizes.

Microscopically, vascular ectasias consist of dilated, distorted, thin-walled vessels, mostly lined only by endothelium and, less frequently, by a small amount of smooth muscle. Structurally, they appear to be ectatic veins, venules, and capillaries. The degree of distortion of the normal vascular

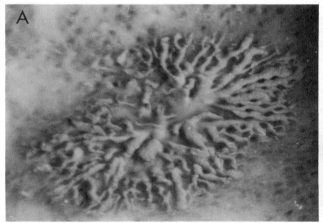
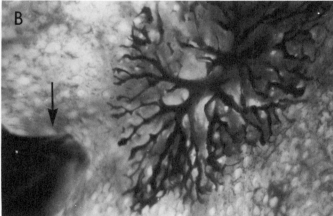

Fig 48–10.—**A,** "coral reef" appearance of an ectasia in an injected but not cleared colon. Normal crypts are seen surrounding the ectasia. (From Mitsudo S., et al.: Vascular ectasias of the colon. *Hum. Pathol.* 10:585, 1979. Reproduced by permission.) **B,** transilluminated, cleared colon showing an ectasia involving the mucosal capillaries and venules. Pinhead shown for size comparison *(arrow).* (From Sprayregen S., et al.: Vascular ectasias of the colon. *J.A.M.A.* 239:962, 1978. Reproduced by permission.)

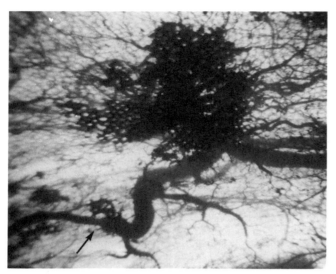

Fig 48–11.—Transilluminated, cleared colon showing a mucosal ectasia surrounded by normal crypts with ectatic venules leading to a large, distended, tortuous, underlying submucosal vein. A sharp constriction *(arrow)* can be seen where the vein traverses the muscle layers. (From Boley S.J., Brandt L.J., Mitsudo S., in Stollerman G.H. (ed.): *Advances in Internal Medicine.* 1984. vol. 29. By permission of Year Book Medical Publishers.)

architecture varies in different lesions, but the most consistent, and apparently the earliest, abnormality noted in all of the lesions we have studied is the presence of dilated, often huge, submucosal veins (Fig 48–12,A). Progressively more extensive lesions show increasing numbers of dilated and deformed vessels traversing the muscularis mucosa and involving the mucosa until, in the most severe lesions, the mucosa is replaced by a maze of distorted, dilated vascular channels (Fig 48–12,B).

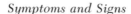
Symptoms and Signs

Recurrent lower intestinal bleeding in a patient over the age of 50 should arouse the suspicion of the presence of vascular ectasias of the colon. Bleeding from ectasias is most often recurrent and low grade, although approximately 15% of patients present with acute massive hemorrhage, some of whom are in shock. The nature and degree of bleeding frequently varies in the same patient with different episodes, and patients may have bright red blood, maroon-colored stools, and melena on separate occasions. In 20%–25% of episodes, only tarry stools are passed, and in 10%–15% of patients bleeding is evidenced by iron-deficiency anemia and stools that intermittently contain occult blood. This spectrum reflects the varied rate of bleeding from the ectatic capillaries, venules and, in advanced lesions, arteriovenous communications. In more than 90% of patients the bleeding stops spontaneously.

As many as 30% of patients reported with vascular ectasias have had previous operations for other suspected sources of intestinal bleeding, including partial gastrectomy, vagotomy with antrectomy or pyloroplasty, and left colon resection for supposed diverticular bleeding. None of the patients in our series who had left colectomy had angiographic or histologic documentation of a bleeding site at the time of the prior operations. More recently, the percentage of patients having had previous operations has decreased as the diagnosis is established earlier and physicians have been more willing to refer patients for operation before repeated episodes of bleeding occur.

The problem of attributing bleeding to a vascular ectasia or to diverticulosis when bleeding from the lesion is not demonstrated either endoscopically or by extravasation of contrast material on angiography is compounded by the frequent occurrence of these lesions without bleeding in people over 60 years of age. Diverticulosis has been estimated to occur in up to 50% of the population older than 60 years, and we previ-

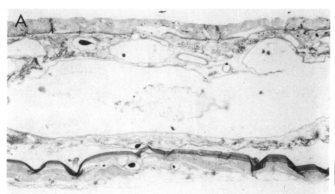
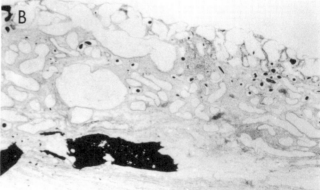

Fig 48–12.—**A,** a large distended vein completely filling the submucosa with a few dilated venules in the overlying mucosa. This is the hallmark of an early ectasia (H&E, ×50). (From Boley S.J., et al.: On the nature and etiology of vascular ectasias of the colon: Degenerative lesions of aging. *Gastroenterology* 72:650, 1977. Reproduced by permission.) **B,** advanced lesion showing total disruption of the mucosa with replacement by ectatic vessels. Only one layer of endothelium separates the lumen of the cecum from those of the dilated vessels (H&E ×50). (From Boley S.J., Brandt L.J., Mitsudo S., in Stollerman G.H. (ed.): *Advances in Internal Medicine.* 1984. vol. 29. By permission of Year Book Medical Publishers.)

ously have shown that mucosal vascular ectasias of the right colon can be found in more than one quarter of people of the same age with no evidence of bleeding.[26] Therefore, in the absence of a demonstrated site of hemorrhage, the only basis for determining if identified ectasias or diverticulosis are responsible for bleeding is the indirect evidence provided by the course of the patient after resection of the suspected lesion.

Diagnosis

The diagnostic approach we employ for all lower intestinal bleeding (Fig 48–13)[27] varies with the age of the patient and the presence or absence of active bleeding. Aspiration of gastric contents is the initial procedure in all patients, since the absence of blood and the presence of bile in the aspirate virtually exclude a source of bleeding proximal to the ligament of Treitz. A clear nonbilious aspirate eliminates the possibility of an actively bleeding lesion in the esophagus or stomach, but does not exclude the possibility of one in the duodenum, since the pylorus may be obstructed. Therefore, a nonbloody, nonbilious aspirate is an indication for upper GI endoscopy prior to colonoscopy or angiography in actively bleeding patients. A BUN level greater than 30 mg/dl, which occurs in approximately two thirds of patients with major upper GI hemorrhage, strongly suggests a bleeding site proximal to the colon. Standard proctosigmoidoscopic examination is done to exclude the presence of anorectal pathology, and coagulation studies, including a platelet count, prothrombin time, and partial thromboplastin time are performed to rule out any underlying coagulopathy.

In patients who are thought to be actively bleeding, the next diagnostic step is to attempt colonoscopy. Different investigators have reported varying success in visualizing the colon in the presence of severe hemorrhage because of the difficulty in suctioning large amounts of blood through a standard colonoscope. However, newly developed operating endoscopes with a larger suction capacity obviate this difficulty.

If endoscopy does not reveal the source of bleeding, scintigraphy may be useful. When a radioactive agent is injected IV into a patient who is actively bleeding, a fraction of the injected material will be extravasated at a bleeding site. Each time the blood recirculates, another small fraction of the radionuclide extravasates at the site. Ideally, the radionuclide used should be actively cleared by a specific target organ out of the scanning field, allowing a contrast to be seen between the site of bleeding and the surrounding background.

Abdominal scintigraphy obtained after injection of ^{99m}Tc sulfur colloid or RBCs has been successfully employed to identify the site of lower intestinal bleeding. It has also been used to determine if bleeding has stopped after an intravenous infusion of vasopressin.[28] Using ^{99m}Tc sulfur colloid, rates of bleeding as low as 0.1 ml/minute have been detected experimentally as this agent is rapidly cleared by the reticuloendothelial system. Unfortunately, the ^{99m}Tc sulfur colloid is concentrated in the liver and spleen and hence may obscure bleeding from the area of the hepatic or splenic flexure of the colon. With their longer half-life in blood, ^{99m}Tc-tagged RBCs are not as accurate as ^{99m}Tc sulfur colloid for detecting active bleeding. However, they are superior for detecting the site of intermittent bleeding, since scintigraphy may be repeated at intervals over a 24-hour period. It may be that the ideal scintigraphic approach would be a study with ^{99m}Tc-tagged RBCs if an initial study with ^{99m}Tc sulfur colloid does not reveal an actively bleeding site.

If colonoscopy is unsuccessful in identifying a source of hemorrhage and the scintiscan indicates active bleeding, or if both colonoscopy and scintigraphy are negative but arterial bleeding continues or reoccurs, emergency angiography is performed. Selective angiograms of the superior mesenteric artery, inferior mesenteric artery, and celiac axis are obtained, in that order. Extravasation of contrast medium identifies the site of bleeding while angiographic signs of tumors, arteriovenous malformations, or vascular ectasias may identify both the location and cause.

The efficacy of selective arteriography in locating the sites of acute GI bleeding has been well established in the last decade. Nusbaum and Baum[29] showed that rates of bleeding of as low as 0.5 ml/minute could be detected in laboratory animals. However, intermittent bleeding, cessation of bleeding prior to the study, or a slower rate of hemorrhage may limit successful angiographic detection.

Angiography is successful in identifying the source of massive lower intestinal bleeding in approximately two thirds of patients. Pooling of extravasated contrast material in a diverticulum is the angiographic sign of diverticular bleeding and was present in 75% of patients with diverticular bleeding in the series of Welch et al.[24]

In contradistinction, extravasation has been shown in only 10%–20% of patients bleeding from vascular ectasias of the colon, since the bleeding is usually episodic. However, the presence of other angiographic signs enables the diagnosis of colonic ectasias or other vascular lesions of the small and large bowel to be made even in the absence of bleeding. There are three major angiographic signs of ectasias (Fig 48–14). The earliest and most frequent sign is a densely opacified, dilated, tortuous, slowly emptying intramural vein which reflects ectatic changes in a submucosal vein and is present in more than 90% of patients with ectasias. A vascular tuft, present in 70%–80% of patients, represents a more advanced lesion and corresponds to extension of the degenerative process to mu-

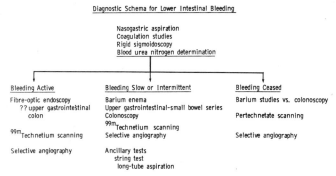

Fig 48–13.—Schema of plan for diagnosis of lower intestinal bleeding. (From Boley S.J., Brandt L.J., and Mitsudo S., in Stollerman G.H. (ed.): *Advances in Internal Medicine.* 1984. vol. 29. By permission of Year Book Medical Publishers.)

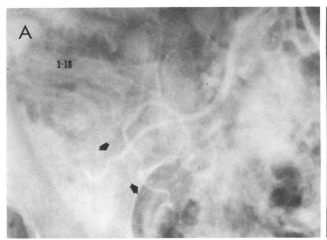

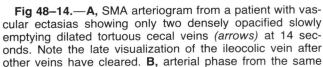

Fig 48–14.—**A,** SMA arteriogram from a patient with vascular ectasias showing only two densely opacified slowly emptying dilated tortuous cecal veins *(arrows)* at 14 seconds. Note the late visualization of the ileocolic vein after other veins have cleared. **B,** arterial phase from the same arteriogram showing two vascular tufts *(large arrows)* and two early filling veins *(small arrows)* at six seconds. (From Boley S.J., et al.: The pathophysiologic basis for the angiographic signs of vascular ectasias of the colon. *Radiology* 125:615, 1977. Reproduced by permission.)

cosal venules. An early filling vein is a sign of an even more advanced disease and reflects an arteriovenous communication through a dilated arteriolar-capillary-venular unit—i.e., a mucosal ectasia. It is a late sign, present in only 60%–70% of the patients. All three angiographic signs are present in more than one half of the patients with bleeding ectasias. Intraluminal extravasation of contrast material alone is inadequate to diagnose an ectasia, but when seen in conjunction with at least one of the three signs of ectasias is indicative of a ruptured mucosal ectasia.

In patients whose bleeding has stopped, gastric aspiration, coagulation studies, and colonoscopy are followed by barium enema and upper GI and small-bowel series. If these are all normal, elective mesenteric angiography is performed primarily for the identification of a vascular lesion. On rare occasions, the use of a GI string test has been helpful to localize the level of bleeding.

The colonoscopic diagnosis of ectasias in a patient not actively bleeding was reported first by Skibba et al.[30] and by others since then. Unfortunately, only a few of the lesions purported to be ectasias have been documented by tissue examination. A number of lesions thought to be ectasias by an endoscopist have proved to be otherwise when biopsies were obtained. We believe that if a colonoscopic identification is to be the basis either for a definitive diagnosis or for treatment of a vascular ectasia a confirmatory biopsy is necessary. This can be obtained with a "hot biopsy" forceps, which can also be used to electrodessicate the lesion. However, this technique has a risk of hemorrhage and perforation and should only be performed by skilled endoscopists with surgical backup available.

Treatment

The probable presence of vascular ectasias of the right colon in many elderly patients with or without bleeding raises questions as to the proper management of these lesions when demonstrated angiographically or by colonoscopy. At present there is no indication for any treatment if the patient has not had bleeding and is not anemic from chronic blood loss. However, in a person who has bled or who is chronically anemic and in whom all findings are normal except for an angiogram showing an ectasia in the right colon, the ectasia can be considered to be the likely source of bleeding. Bleeding from ectasias usually stops spontaneously, but if bleeding persists, it may be controlled by the infusion of vasoconstrictors through an angiography catheter left in the superior mesenteric artery.

When no other source of bleeding is found, an ectasia of the right colon is, at present, an indication for right hemicolectomy, and 80%–90% of patients will have no further bleeding after that operation. It is important that the entire right half of the colon be removed to ensure that no ectasias are left behind. The presence of diverticula in the left side of the colon does not alter the decision to perform a right hemicolectomy; since up to 80% of bleeding diverticula are located in the right side of the colon, the risks of leaving the left colon are far outweighed by the increased morbidity and mortality of subtotal colectomy in this age group. If an emergency operation is necessitated by uncontrolled bleeding in a patient with an angiographically identified ectasia of the right colon, a right hemicolectomy is still the procedure of choice, regardless of the presence of diverticulosis of the left colon.

A suggested alternative to resection, especially attractive in elderly patients, is colonoscopic electrocoagulation or laser coagulation of the ectasias. Several reports have claimed success with electrocoagulation, but the number of patients involved is small, and in most instances the diagnoses have not been established histologically. Electrocoagulation would appear to be most practical as the lesion can be destroyed at the time a "hot biopsy" is obtained. Instances of cecal perforation or bleeding have occurred with both this technique and laser coagulation, thus they must be performed carefully. Before a nonresectional approach can be recommended as the standard therapy for ectasias, studies with biopsy confirmation of all lesions, and careful follow-up observations to establish the incidence of rebleeding will have to be made. Until then, these methods are an option in the management of patients in whom operation carries a high risk.

Hemangiomas

The second most common vascular lesions of the colon are hemangiomas. While these lesions are considered by some to be true neoplasms, they are generally thought to be hamartomas because of their presence at birth in most cases. Colonic hemangiomas may occur as solitary lesions, as multiple growths limited to the colon, or as part of diffuse GI or multisystem angiomatoses. Individual hemangiomas may be broadly classified as cavernous, capillary, or mixed types. Most hemangiomas are small, ranging from a few millimeters to 2 cm. Larger lesions do occur, however, especially in the rectum.

Clinically, bleeding from colonic hemangiomas is usually slow, producing occult blood loss with anemia or melena. Hematochezia is less common, except in the case of large cavernous hemangiomas of the rectum which cause massive hemorrhage. The diagnosis is best established by colonoscopy, since roentgenologic studies including angiography may be normal. In the presence of GI bleeding, hemangiomas of the skin or mucus membranes should suggest the possibility of associated bowel lesions.

Hemangiomas are well circumscribed but not encapsulated. Grossly, cavernous hemangiomas are polypoid or mound-like, reddish purple lesions on the mucosa. Sectioning of the lesion reveals numerous dilated, irregular blood filled spaces within the mucosa and submucosa, sometimes extending through the muscular wall to the serosal surface. The vascular channels are lined by flat endothelial cells with flat or plump nuclei. Their walls do not contain smooth muscle fibers, but are composed of fibrous tissue of varying thickness (Fig 48–15,A). Capillary hemangiomas are plaque-like or mound-like, reddish purple lesions composed of a proliferation of fine, closely packed, newly formed capillaries separated by very little edematous stroma. The endothelial lining cells are large, usually hypertrophic, and in some areas may form solid cords or nodules with ill-defined capillary spaces. There is little or no pleomorphism or hyperchromasia. Small hemangiomas that are either solitary or few in number can be treated by colonoscopic laser coagulation. Large or multiple lesions usually require resection of either the hemangioma alone or the involved segment of colon.

Cavernous Hemangiomas of the Rectum

A distinct form of colonic hemangioma is the cavernous hemangioma of the rectum. These lesions are usually not associated with other GI hemangiomas and are extensive, involving the entire rectum or portions of the rectosigmoid. They cause massive, sometimes uncontrollable hemorrhage. The diagnosis can often be suggested on plain films of the abdomen by the presence of phleboliths and by displacement or distortion of the rectal air column. A barium enema study showing narrowing and rigidity of the rectal lumen, scalloping of the rectal wall, and an increase in the size of the presacral space further supports the diagnosis. Endoscopically, elevated nodules or vascular congestion causing a plum-red coloration are seen. Ulcers and signs of proctitis may be evident. Angiography can be used to demonstrate these lesions but is rarely necessary to establish the diagnosis.

The massive bleeding resulting from these rectal hemangiomas often necessitates excision of the rectum by either abdominal perineal or low anterior resection. Ligation and embolization of major feeding vessels have been employed. Attempts at local measures to control bleeding have been of value in some instances, but are usually only temporarily effective.

Colonic and Extracolonic Involvement

The association of skin or subcutaneous hemangiomas with hemangiomas in the colon has been mentioned, and heman-

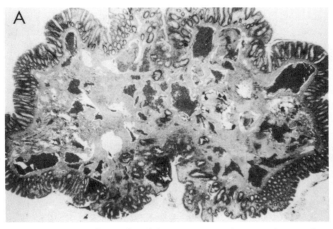
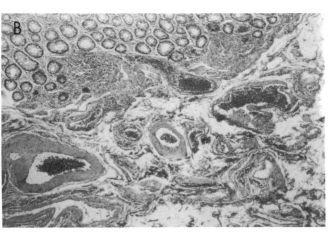

Fig 48–15.—A, polypoid cavernous hemangioma, located in the submucosa with focal extension into the mucosa. Note the large, irregular vascular channels with fibrous walls of varying thickness (H&E ×20). **B,** arteriovenous malformation with tortuous veins, having sclerotic intima and hypertrophied smooth muscle, and thick walled sclerotic arteries (H&E ×100). (From Boley S.J., Brandt L.J., Mitsudo S., in Stollerman G.H. (ed.): *Advances in Internal Medicine.* 1984. vol. 29. By permission of Year Book Medical Publishers.)

giomas of the liver are also not uncommonly present. Several disorders embodying multiple GI hemangiomas have been described.

DIFFUSE INTESTINAL HEMANGIOMATOSIS.—This connotes numerous, as many as 50–100, lesions involving the stomach, small bowel, and colon. Bleeding or anemia usually leads to the diagnosis in childhood. Hemangiomas of the skin or soft tissues of the head and neck are frequently present. Continuous slow but pernicious bleeding requiring transfusions or an intussusception led by one of the lesions may necessitate surgical intervention. The diagnosis may be made by endoscopy and barium studies; angiography can be normal in spite of numerous lesions. The hemangiomas are similar in appearance to solitary lesions and are usually cavernous, although some have the histologic appearance of hemangioendotheliomas (benign lesions in children). At operation all identifiable lesions should be excised either through enterotomies or by limited bowel resections. Transillumination and compression of the bowel wall are helpful in finding small lesions. Repeated operations may be necessary to control blood loss.

Universal (miliary) hemangiomatosis is usually fatal in infancy. It is, fortunately, a rare condition in which there are hundreds of hemangiomas involving the skin, brain, lung, and abdominal viscera. Death results from congestive heart failure due to large arteriovenous shunts or may be a result of the local effects of the lesions. Colonic lesions rarely are of significance.

BLUE-RUBBER-BLEB NEVUS SYNDROME (CUTANEOUS AND INTESTINAL CAVERNOUS HEMANGIOMAS).—In 1860, Gascoyen reported an association between cutaneous vascular nevi, intestinal lesions, and GI bleeding. Bean later coined the name "blue-rubber-bleb syndrome" and distinguished it from other cutaneous vascular lesions. A familial history is infrequent, although a few cases of transmission in an autosomal dominant pattern have been reported.

The lesions in this syndrome are distinctive. They vary in size from 0.1 to 5.0 cm, are blue and raised, and have a wrinkled surface. Characteristically, the contained blood can be emptied by direct pressure leaving a wrinkled sac. The hemangiomas may be single or innumerable and are usually found on the trunk, extremities, and face but not on mucous membranes. They may be present in any portion of the GI tract but are most common in the small bowel. In the colon they occur more commonly on the left side and in the rectum. They are infrequently seen by barium opacification or angiographic studies and are detected best by endoscopy if they are proximal to the ligament of Treitz or in the colon. Microscopically, they are cavernous hemangiomas composed of clusters of dilated capillary spaces lined by cuboidal or flattened endothelium with connective tissue stroma. In the bowel they are located in the submucosa. Resection of the involved segment of bowel is recommended for recurrent hemorrhage, although endoscopic laser coagulation is an attractive therapeutic option.

Other Less Common Vascular Lesions

Congenital Arteriovenous Malformations (AVMS)

These lesions are embryonic growth defects and are considered to be developmental anomalies. While they are found mainly in the extremities, they occur anywhere in the vascular tree. In the colon they may be small, similar to ectasias, or they may involve a long segment of bowel. The more extensive lesions are most often seen in the rectum and sigmoid.

Histologically, AVMs are persistent communications between arteries and veins located primarily in the submucosa. Characteristically there is "arterialization" of the veins; i.e., tortuosity, dilatation and thick walls with smooth muscle hypertrophy and intimal thickening and sclerosis (Fig 48–15,B). In long-standing AVMs the arteries are dilated with atrophic and sclerotic degeneration.

Angiography is the primary means of diagnosis. Early filling veins in small lesions, and extensive dilatation of arteries and veins in large lesions (Fig 48–16) are pathognomonic of arteriovenous malformations. Patients with significant bleeding should have resection of the involved segment of colon.

Colonic Varices

Varices of the colon are very rare, but may be a cause of hematochezia or melena. In most cases the varices are located in the rectosigmoid and are found progressively less often in the more proximal colon. The most common cause of colonic varices is portal hypertension; congenital anomalies, mesenteric vein obstruction, congestive heart failure and pancreatitis account for the others. Why varices form so rarely in the colon and why they bleed is unclear. Varices are easily diagnosed by proctosigmoidoscopy, colonoscopy, or angiography and may even be seen on conventional barium studies of the colon. Therapy consists of segmental colonic resection, portocaval shunting or local ligation or sclerosis.

Hereditary Hemorrhagic Telangiectasis (Osler-Weber-Rendu Disease)

This is a familial disorder characterized by telangiectasias of the skin and mucous membranes and recurrent GI bleeding. Lesions are noticed frequently in the first few years of life and recurrent epistaxis in childhood is characteristic of the disease. By age 10, about one half of patients will have had some bleeding, but severe hemorrhage is unusual before the fourth decade of life and occurs with a peak incidence in the sixth decade. In almost all patients, bleeding presents as melena, while epistaxis and hematemesis are less frequent. Bleeding may be quite severe and patients not uncommonly receive more than fifty transfusions in a lifetime. A family history of disease has been reported in 80% of patients with the disorder, have less commonly in those with bleeding, especially when the bleeding occurs later in life.

Telangiectasias are almost always present on the lips, oral and nasopharyngeal membranes, tongue, or hand; lack of involvement of these sites casts suspicion on the diagnosis. Lesions on the lips are more common in patients with GI bleeding than in those without. Telangiectasias occur in the colon but are far more common in the stomach and small bowel. Upper GI lesions are more apt to cause significant bleeding.

The telangiectasias are not demonstrable on barium enema examination but are easily seen on endoscopy. Occasionally, in the presence of severe anemia and blood loss, they transiently become less visible, but with blood replacement they again increase in prominence. Angiography is usually normal

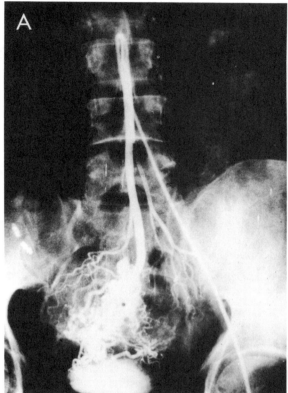 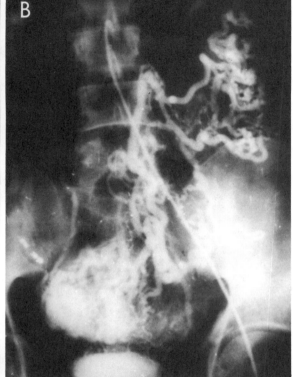

Fig 48–16.—A, arterial phase of inferior mesenteric arteriogram from a patient with a congenital arteriovenous malformation showing multiple dilated arteries going to a large segment of the rectosigmoid. **B,** venous phase of the same arteriogram showing dilated tortuous vessels to the same segment as well as other more proximal areas. (From Boley S.J., Brandt L.J., Mitsudo S., in Stollerman G.H. (ed.): *Advances in Internal Medicine,* 1984, vol. 29. By permission of Year Book Medical Publishers.)

but may demonstrate arteriovenous communications or small clusters of abnormal vessels.

Grossly, and at endoscopy, the telangiectasias are millet-seed sized and appear as cherry-red, smooth hillocks or as ordinary spider angiomas. Pathologically, the major changes involve the capillaries and venules, but arterioles may also be affected. The lesions consist of irregular ectatic tortuous blood spaces lined by a delicate single layer of endothelial cells and supported by a fine layer of fibrous connective tissue. No elastic lamina or muscular tissue is present in these vessels. The arterioles show some intimal proliferation and often have thrombi in them suggesting vascular stasis, but the most conspicuous findings are in the venules. In contrast to those in vascular ectasias, these venules are abnormally thick and have very prominent, well-developed longitudinal muscles. Apparently these abnormal venules play the major role in regulating blood flow to the telangiectasia.

Many treatments have been recommended including estrogens and multiple resections of involved bowel. At present, endoscopic electrosurgery or laser coagulation appear most promising and may be performed during active bleeding or between bleeding episodes. While endoscopic therapy has diminished the need for resecting bowel in some cases, long-term, follow-up studies are needed to evaluate the ultimate course of patients so treated.

Klippel-Trenaunay-Weber Syndrome

An ill-defined and uncommon vascular lesion of the rectum and rectosigmoid has been described in association with the Klippel-Trenaunay-Weber syndrome. The latter refers to unilateral congenital lesions of the lower extremities characterized by: (a) superficial angiomas, usually of the flat, diffuse capillary type, (b) varicose veins dating from childhood, and (c) bony elongation. The cause of the syndrome has been variously ascribed to congenital arteriovenous fistulas or to aplasia or obstruction of the deep venous system. The rectal lesions usually have caused bleeding during childhood, and have been described by some authors as being cavernous (with reported biopsy documentation), or as varicosities of the rectal veins by Servelle (based upon venography).

Severe rectal or bladder bleeding has occurred in a few children, with one reported mortality. Ligation of bleeding hemorrhoids or sclerosis of rectal veins is at least temporarily effective, but rectal resection may be necessary in isolated instances.

REFERENCES

1. Klass A.A.: Embolectomy in acute mesenteric occlusion. *Ann. Surg.* 134:913, 1951.

2. Ende N.: Infarction of the bowel in cardiac failure. *N. Engl. J. Med.* 258:879, 1958.

3. Ottinger L.W.: The surgical management of acute occlusion of the superior mesenteric artery. *Ann. Surg.* 188:721, 1978.

4. Jackson B.B.: Occlusion of the superior mesenteric artery. Monograph in *American Lectures in Surgery.* Springfield, Ill.: Charles C Thomas Publisher, 1963.

5. Cokkinis A.J.: *Mesenteric Vascular Occlusion.* London, Bailliere, Tindall & Cox, 1926.

6. Boley S.J., Regan J.A., Tunick P.A., et al.: Persistent vasoconstriction—a major factor in non-occlusive mesenteric ischemia. *Curr. Top. Surg. Res.* 3:425, 1971.

7. Bardfeld P.A., Boley S.J., Sammartano R.J., et al.: Scintigraphic diagnosis of ischemic intestine with technetium 99m sulfur colloid labelled leukocytes. *Radiology* 112:553, 1974.

8. Siegelman S.S., Sprayregen S., Boley S.J.: Angiographic diagnosis of mesenteric arterial vasoconstriction. *Radiology* 122:533, 1974.

9. Shaw R.S.: The "second look" after superior mesenteric arterial embolectomy or reconstruction for mesenteric infarction, in Ellison E.H., Friesen S.R., Mulholland J.H. (eds.): *Current Surgical Management.* Philadelphia, W.B. Saunders Co., 1965, p. 509.

10. Inhara T.: Acute superior mesenteric venous thrombosis: Treatment by thrombectomy. *Ann. Surg.* 74:956, 1971.

11. Boley S.J., Sprayregen S., Siegelman S.S., et al.: Initial results from an aggressive roentgenological and surgical approach to acute mesenteric ischemia. *Surgery* 82:848, 1977.

12. Boley S.J., Feinstein F.R., Sammartano R.J., et al.: New concepts of management of superior mesenteric artery emboli. *Surg. Gynecol. Obstet.* 153:4, 1981.

13. Lauenstein C.: Ein unerwartetes Ereignis nach der Pylorusresektion. *Zentralblatt Chir.* 9:137, 1882.

14. Boley S.J., Schwartz S., Lash J., et al.: Reversible vascular occlusion of the colon. *Surg. Gynecol. Obstet.* 116:53, 1963.

15. Schwartz S., Boley S.J., Lash J., et al.: Roentgenologic aspects of reversible vascular occlusion of the colon and its relationship to ulcerative colitis. *Radiology* 80:625, 1963.

16. Boley S.J., Schwartz S., Krieger H., et al.: Further observations on reversible vascular occlusion of the colon. *Am. J. Gastroenterol.* 44:260, 1965.

17. Marston A., Pheils M., Thomas M.C., et al.: Ischaemic colitis. *Gut* 7:1, 1966.

18. Farman J.: The radiologic features of colonic vascular disease, in Boley S.J., Schwartz S.S., Williams L.F. (eds.): *Vascular Disorders of the Intestine.* New York, Appleton-Century-Crofts, 1971, p. 229.

19. Marcuson R.W.: Ischaemic colitis. *Clin. Gastroenterol.* 1:745, 1972.

20. Boley S.J., Dibiase A., Brandt L.J., et al.: Lower intestinal bleeding in the elderly. *Am. J. Surg.* 137:57, 1979.

21. Boley S.J., Sammartano R.J., Brandt L.J., et al.: Vascular ectasias of the colon. *Surg. Gynecol. Obstet.* 149:353, 1979.

22. Mitsudo S., Boley S.J., Brandt L.J., et al.: Vascular ectasias of the right colon in the elderly: A distinct pathologic entity. *Hum. Pathol.* 10:585, 1979.

23. Quinn W.C., Ochsner A.: Bleeding as a complication of diverticulosis or diverticulitis of the colon. *Am. Surg.* 19:397, 1953.

24. Welch C.E., Athanasoulis C.A., Galdabini J.J.: Hemorrhage from the large bowel with special reference to angiodysplasia and diverticular disease. *World J. Surg.* 2:73, 1978.

25. Athanasoulis C.A., Galdabini J.J., Waltman A.C., et al.: Angiodysplasia of the colon; a cause of rectal bleeding. *Cardiovasc. Radiol.* 1:3, 1978.

26. Boley S.J., Sammartano R.J., Adams A., et al.: On the nature and etiology of vascular ectasias of the colon: Degenerative lesions of aging. *Gastroenterology* 72:650, 1977.

27. Boley S.J., Brandt L.J., Frank M.S.: Severe lower intestinal bleeding: Diagnosis and treatment. *Clin. Gastroenterol.* 10:65, 1981.

28. Alavi A., Dann R.W., Baum S., et al.: Scintigraphic detection of acute gastrointestinal bleeding. *Radiology* 124:753, 1977.

29. Nusbaum M.H., Baum S.: Radiographic demonstration of unknown sites of gastrointestinal bleeding. *Surg. Forum* 14:374, 1963.

30. Skibba R.M., Hartong W.A., Mantz F.A., et al.: Angiodysplasias of the cecum; colonoscopic diagnosis. *Gastrointest. Endosc.* 22:177, 1976.

49

Intestinal Malabsorption Syndromes

HARRY M. RICHTER III, M.D.
KEITH A. KELLY, M.D.

THE HEALTHY HUMAN GI tract accomplishes the digestion and absorption of food with remarkable efficiency and completeness. Through the well-ordered cooperation of mechanical, chemical, enzymatic, and transport processes, the alimentary tract regularly reduces an enormous range of dietary input to a fairly constant residue of negligible nutrient content. The component digestive viscera each possesses enough functional reserve that often a mild or localized disease or partial surgical loss will produce no detectable impairment. Thus, hepatic lobectomy, distal pancreatectomy, jejunectomy, and left hemicolectomy are usually attended by no overt change in GI function. When disease causes more generalized organ dysfunction or when more substantial or strategic resections are required, the resulting loss of digestive capacity may produce malabsorption. Of the long list of conditions causing malabsorption, this chapter is concerned with three of particular importance to surgeons; the short-bowel syndrome, the bacterial overgrowth syndrome, and radiation enteritis. Malabsorption syndromes appearing after gastric surgery and from intestinal ischemia, biliopancreatic insufficiency, intestinal pseudo-obstruction, and gastric and intestinal bypass are covered in other chapters of this book.

SHORT-BOWEL SYNDROME

The short-bowel syndrome is caused by extensive or repeated intestinal resection of sufficient magnitude to produce chronic malnutrition, diarrhea, and steatorrhea (Fig 49–1). Historically, the common causes were mesenteric arterial embolism or thrombosis, midgut volvulus, strangulation-obstruction, and complex congenital atresias. Crohn's disease, radiation enteritis, and nonocclusive intestinal ischemia now also figure prominently as causative diseases. As surgical and supportive techniques improve, more patients are able to survive catastrophic loss of intestine, making the short-bowel patient an increasingly frequent challenge.

Pathogenesis and Pathophysiology

It is axiomatic that the nutritional and functional consequence of extensive intestinal resection depends on the length, site, and health of the remaining gut. One can predict the effect of a given resection based on an understanding of the functions of several specialized regions of the alimentary tract.

JEJUNUM.—Defined arbitrarily as the orad two fifths of the mesenteric small bowel, the jejunum in health absorbs nearly the entire fat, carbohydrate, and protein content of a meal.[1] Also, the proximal jejunum (and duodenum) preferentially absorbs iron, calcium, and magnesium. Because the ileum also shares the digestive and transport properties required for efficient absorption of these nutrients, the jejunum can be sacrificed without incurring malabsorption.

ILEUM.—In addition to the absorptive capabilities shared with the jejunum, two important specialized active transport systems are located in the ileum—those responsible for the absorption of bile salts and vitamin B_{12}. Ileal loss interrupts the enterohepatic circulation of bile salts, reducing the bile salt pool. Resection of less than 100 cm of ileum will cause bile salt malabsorption, but the liver is able to compensate with increased synthesis from the precursor cholesterol, maintaining a nearly normal bile salt pool and enteric luminal bile salt concentration. Micelle formation is adequate, and little or no fat malabsorption occurs.[2, 3] Nonetheless, nonabsorbed bile salts pass into the colon and may cause "cholerheic diarrhea" by stimulating colonic water and electrolyte secretion.[4] Resections of greater than 100 cm of ileum cause bile salt malabsorption of such an extent the liver can no longer make up for the large bile salt loss. Reduced luminal bile salt concentration results in impaired micelle formation and steatorrhea.[2, 3] Malabsorption of the fat-soluble vitamins A, D, E, and K may accompany the steatorrhea. Nonabsorbed free fatty acids enter the colon, where they are subject to hydroxylation by colonic bacteria. In this form they inhibit colonic water and electrolyte absorption, leading to "steatorrheic diarrhea."[5]

Gallstones and calcium oxalate kidney stones are both common after extensive ileal resection or bypass. Decreased concentrations of bile salts in the bile reduce the solubility of cholesterol in bile, predisposing to supersaturation of that molecule and subsequent gallstone formation. Oxalate kidney stones result in part from increased urinary oxalate concentration, a condition called "enteric hyperoxaluria."[6, 7] In health, enteric luminal oxalate is complexed to calcium ions. The calcium-oxalate complex precipitates and is not absorbed. Moreover, the healthy intestinal mucosa is relatively impermeable to oxalate. Following ileal resection or in the presence of extensive ileal disease, malabsorbed free fatty acids chelate lu-

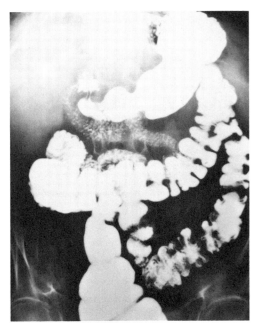

Fig 49–1.—Short-bowel syndrome following extensive small-bowel and right colon resection for superior mesenteric artery embolism. Remaining small bowel and colon fill rapidly after ingestion of contrast medium.

minal calcium, liberating soluble oxalate. In addition, the free fatty acids and bile acids alter colonic mucosa, rendering it abnormally permeable to oxalate. The net result is the markedly enhanced absorption of oxalate by the colon and subsequent excretion of the oxalate in the urine. Urinary volume is often low in these patients because of excessive loss of water from the GI tract. The low volume favors the precipitation of urinary stones. A low-oxalate diet may reduce urinary oxalate excretion, but apparently not all of the absorbed oxalate is of dietary origin.[7] The colon must be in enteric continuity for hyperoxaluria to occur; patients with ileostomy are not at risk for enteric hyperoxaluria.

Malabsorption of vitamin B_{12} follows a pattern similar to that of the bile salts; that is, ileal resection of less than 100 cm may not lead to a deficiency, whereas resections greater than 100 cm will probably necessitate regular parenteral replacement.

ILEOCECAL JUNCTION.—The ileocecal junctional area appears to serve two functions—the regulation of gastric emptying and of small intestinal emptying into the colon and the prevention of reflux of colonic content into the small bowel. In health, the distal ileum, ileocecal junction, and right colon probably function as a unit to slow gastric emptying and small-bowel transit. Resection of the ileum, the junction, and the right colon speed gastric emptying and hasten small-bowel transit. The bacterial population of the cecum is several orders of magnitude greater than that of the terminal ileum. Resection or bypass of the ileocecal junction results in bacterial proliferation within the small bowel.[8, 9] This suggests that the junctional area ordinarily maintains the bacterial gradient. The specific contribution of the ileocecal junction itself has

been difficult to dissect. Whether the anatomical ileocecal junction per se is a true valve or sphincter is uncertain.

COLON.—The colon is an important site of fluid and electrolyte absorption. In healthy subjects, an estimated average of 1,500 ml of water pass into the colon daily.[10] All but about 150 ml of this water is absorbed. Experimentally, the human colon can absorb up to 5 L/day.[11] After partial ileocolonic resections, the volume of diarrhea depends more on the amount of remaining colon than remaining ileum, emphasizing the important role of the colon in water absorption.[12, 13]

Experimental and clinical studies of massive bowel resection or bypass demonstrate the relative importance of the specialized regions of the intestinal tract and the limits of tolerable loss. Dogs remain healthy without weight loss after 50% or 70% proximal small-bowel bypass.[14] A 50% or 70% distal resection or bypass is also well tolerated (although fat malabsorption and weight loss occur) if the ileocecal junction remains intact, but not if this structure is also lost.[14, 15] The contribution of the ileocecal junction itself (whether functioning as a valve, or sphincter, or both) can be experimentally discriminated from that of the adjacent small and large intestine by selectively ablating its function through a "valvotomy" or "sphincteroplasty" procedure without resection or bypass. When puppies were subjected to massive enterectomy with or without concomitant ileocolonic "valvotomy," those in the former group suffered progressive weight loss and eventual death, while those in the latter eventually recovered their weight loss and survived.[16]

The response of the human to extensive bowel resection or bypass parallels that of the experimental animal.[17] Proximal resections are better tolerated than distal.[18, 19] Retention of the ileocecal junction appears important,[18–20] but clinically, sacrifice of this structure is always accompanied by ileal and partial colon resection, making it impossible to determine selectively the exact role of the junction. The evolution of the intestinal bypass operations for hypercholesterolemia and morbid obesity sheds light on the minimal intestinal requirement for adequate nutrition. Bypass of the distal 200 cm of ileum and the ileocecal valve causes fat and vitamin B_{12} malabsorption and diarrhea, but not weight loss or other nutritional deficits.[21] An early antiobesity operation, joining the proximal 15 cm of jejunum to the transverse colon, caused intolerably excessive malabsorption and required surgical reversal. Successive variants of jejunoileal shunt were then explored. The 30-cm jejunum to 30-cm ileum shunt resulted in early weight loss, but most patients subsequently regained weight unacceptably. Satisfactory revisions eventually developed include the the the 30-cm jejunum to 15-cm or 20-cm ileum and 40-cm jejunum to 4-cm ileum end-to-end shunts, and the 14-in. jejunum to 4-in. ileum end-to-side shunt. These operations produce a controlled short-bowel syndrome, which is usually compatible with adequate long-term oral nutrition. When the large intestine and the ileocolic valve are resected or bypassed, at least 100 cm of jejunoileum must remain intact to prevent development of the short bowel syndrome.

CHANGES IN GI MOTILITY.—Disappointingly little exact information is available concerning gut motility and transit in the short-bowel patient. Gastrointestinal contrast radiographic studies indicate that intestinal transit is accelerated, particularly after ileal and ileocecal resections. Similar radiographic findings can be demonstrated in the dog. Several experiments using the rat model showed that a small or large distal resection accelerates small-bowel transit, at least initially; large proximal resections hasten transit as well, but lesser proximal resections have the opposite effect.[22, 23] The fasting small-bowel manometric pattern in short-bowel patients differs from controls only in that the interdigestive cycle length is shorter because of a shortened phase II. The motor response to feeding, however, is identical to controls.[24] Gastric emptying, at least of liquids, is normal in short-bowel patients[24] and in monkeys with 50% distal bowel resection.[25] Murine experiments on the short-bowel syndrome are largely consistent with these findings. In summary, gastric emptying appears normal, but small-bowel transit is hastened, at least in the early postoperative period, particularly after major distal small-bowel resections.

INTESTINAL ADAPTATION.—It has long been known that a gradual improvement in the absorptive function of remaining intestine follows extensive bowel resection. Patients with a seemingly inadequate length of intestine may, over the course of months, improve to the point that oral alimentation alone will maintain satisfactory nutrition. This enhanced absorption is the result of a compensatory adaptation of the remaining gut, manifested grossly by intestinal lengthening and dilatation, and microscopically by increased villus height, crypt depth, and number of enterocytes per villus.[26, 27] The mechanism of postresectional hyperplasia appears multifactorial. Luminal nutrients are necessary, for short-bowel animals maintained on parenteral nutrition do not manifest adaptive hyperplasia.[26] Bile, pancreatic juice, and GI hormones probably play a role as well. The ileum is capable of greater adaptive response to jejunal loss than is the jejunum to ileal loss.[26]

GASTRIC HYPERSECRETION.—Massive intestinal resection causes both gastric acid hypersecretion and hypergastrinemia in humans and experimental animals.[28] It appears that the gastric hyperacidity results from excessive gastrin secretion, because antrectomy will abolish both.[29] The mechanism of the hypergastrinemia remains uncertain; probably removal of small intestine also removes or suppresses secretion of an unknown inhibitor of gastrin release. The small intestine may also catabolize gastrin; after resection, the catabolism is impaired. In man, this hypersecretory state seems to be transitory, lasting roughly for the duration of the postresectional adaptation response. The effects of gastric hypersecretion superimposed on an extensive bowel resection can be particularly detrimental. Peptic ulcer, inactivation of pH-sensitive pancreatic enzymes, precipitation of bile salts, acid-peptic enteritis with damage to brush-border enzymes, accelerated intestinal transit, and increased luminal water and solute load can result from the acid hypersecretion.

Clinical Features and Diagnosis

The short-bowel syndrome presents in one of two ways: in the immediate postoperative period following massive resection, or, more insidiously, weeks or months after apparent recovery from operation. The diagnosis in the first instance is obvious. Voluminous diarrhea will be present, but dehydra-

tion and malnutrition may have been avoided by appropriate perioperative IV therapy. Patients in the second category, who have suffered a less catastrophic intestinal loss, present a picture of chronic diarrhea and weight loss. They may require occasional hospitalization for episodic dehydration. There might be overt signs of specific vitamin or mineral deficiency (e.g., night blindness, dermatitis, microcytic or macrocytic anemia, tetany). The diagnosis is suggested by an appropriate history of intestinal resection. It is necessary in this case to rule out both recurrence of the original condition (Crohn's disease, radiation enteritis) and postoperative mechanical complications (partial obstruction, fistula, blind loop) to establish the diagnosis of short-bowel syndrome. Gastrointestinal contrast radiographs supplemented by appropriate endoscopy should suffice to clarify the issue, although a more complete malabsorption workup may sometimes be indicated.

Overall Management

PHASES OF TREATMENT.—Three phases of recovery from massive bowel resection are recognized; phase I—severe diarrhea, large parenteral fluid and electrolyte requirement, nothing by mouth; phase II—moderately severe diarrhea, less parenteral fluid needed, initiation and progression of oral diet; phase III—moderate or modest diarrhea, no parenteral fluids needed, stabilization on oral alimentation.

PHASE I.—The goal during the first phase of recovery is to maintain fluid and electrolyte homeostasis by accurate replacement of diarrheal loss and to initiate total parenteral nutrition. Oral intake is prohibited, as this would only further stimulate GI secretions and worsen the diarrhea. Central venous access is secured via percutaneous subclavian venous catheterization or, when at least several months of parenteral alimentation are anticipated, by operative placement of a permanent right atrial (Hickman) catheter. The volume of diarrhea gradually declines as intestinal adaptation progresses. Usually by several weeks the output reaches 2 L/day, and oral intake can begin.

PHASE II.—Oral feeding must start with small quantities of a simple hyposomolar liquid diet, emphasizing carbohydrate and restricting fat. Initially, an increase in stool volume is expected. Antidiarrheal medications, such as coedine sulfate or loperamide hydrochloride, should be given. Once the GI tract tolerates this simple intake, the diet may be slowly and progressively increased in consistency and complexity, incorporating protein (as lean meat) and finally small quantities of fats. This is a period of trial and error; experimentation and patience are required while progress is slowly made. Intestinal adaptation continues to increase the absorptive capacity of the remaining gut. Meanwhile, parenteral hyperalimentation is essential to maintain the weight, energy, and defense mechanisms of the patient.

PHASE III.—When positive fluid, electrolyte, and caloric balance can be maintained by oral intake, parenteral alimentation is gradually weaned and discontinued. Antidiarrheal medications are continued as needed. Oral vitamin supplements are standard, as is parenteral vitamin B_{12}, unless a substantial amount of ileum was spared. Dietary experimentation and ongoing intestinal adaptation leads to progressive improvement for up to one year or even two years after resection. Further details of management are found in several recent reviews.[30–32]

Surgical Treatment

GENERAL PRINCIPLES.—Operative intervention in the short-bowel syndrome may be indicated to deal with mechanical complications, to restore intestinal continuity, or to attempt to improve the absorptive capacity of the remaining gut. Extensive bowel resection is usually undertaken in a setting which predisposes to operative complications. For example, mesenteric vascular occlusion or strangulation-obstruction presents as a surgical emergency, in which peritoneal contamination is likely. Similarly, patients requiring repeated or extensive resection for Crohn's disease or radiation enteritis often suffer preoperatively from malnutrition, partial bowel obstruction, and enteric fistulas. Occasionally, bowel of uncertain viability is conserved in the hope of avoiding the creation of the short-bowel syndrome. Thus, postoperative peritonitis, abscess, fistula, bowel obstruction, and wound infection or dehiscence may complicate the recovery of the short-bowel patient. Treatment of such mechanical complications is guided by standard surgical principles, bearing in mind the danger of further loss of bowel.

Following certain resections when primary anastomosis is contraindicated, the divided ends are exteriorized, leaving a length of intestine unused and out of the enteric stream. Subsequent restoration of alimentary continuity may be of nutritional as well as esthetic benefit. This should be true if at least half of the colon remains, and even more so if the excluded distal segment includes ileum and the ileocecal valve. Conversely, little if any gain would be expected from, for example, reanastomosis of jejunum to rectum; the diarrhea so produced likely would prove more disturbing than a well-functioning abdominal stoma.

During the decade prior to the development of practical IV alimentation, an increasing number of patients were able to withstand the insult of massive intestinal resection, only to then fall prey to chronic fluid, mineral, and caloric depletion, frequently with fatal outcome. This situation stimulated the investigation and clinical application of surgical techniques designed to increase absorption from the residual intestine. The aim was to delay intestinal transit, prolonging the duration of contact between luminal content and intestinal mucosa. The methods used included vagotomy, reversed (antiperistaltic) intestinal segments, recirculating loops, and artificial valves or sphincters. In addition, several experimental procedures show promise for future application, including intestinal transplantation, retrograde electrical pacing of the gut, and the growth of intestinal neomucosa on adjacent serosal or muscular surfaces. The surgical treatment of the short-bowel syndrome has been detailed in several recent reviews.[32–35]

VAGOTOMY.—The aim of vagotomy in the treatment of the short-bowel syndrome is twofold; first, to reduce gastric acid secretion (and the associated adverse sequelae), and second, to produce a delay in small-bowel transit. Past clinical and experimental observations indicated that truncal or selective gastric vagotomy and pyloroplasty was of some benefit in selected short-bowel cases.[36, 37] However, truncal vagotomy also impairs pancreatic and biliary secretion, while pyloroplasty speeds gastric emptying. Moreover, vagotomy does not reliably slow intestinal transit, and in fact may itself cause diarrhea. Both the risks and adverse consequences of vagotomy and drainage can be avoided, now that effective medical control of gastric hypersecretion is possible. The H_2-receptor antagonist cimetidine, has proved effective in clinical experience with short-bowel patients.[38, 39] Because acid hypersecretion appears to be temporary following resection, the drug is continued only as long as necessary. Vagotomy is now reserved for those patients with the short-bowel syndrome who develop complicated peptic ulcer resistant to medical therapy. Proximal gastric vagotomy produces the least functional and metabolic derangement of the anti-ulcer operations, and hence is the operation preferred.[40]

REVERSED INTESTINAL SEGMENTS.—A segment of small bowel isolated from the intestinal tract retains its functional orad-aborad orientation, and thus its overall direction of propulsion as well.[41, 42] When such a segment is isolated and reinserted in reversed direction it functions as a fixed brake on antegrade luminal transit. As early as 1887, Mall[43] investigated the effects of intestinal reversal in dogs operated by Halsted. The reversed segments were quite long, producing chronic obstruction and leading to progressive inanition. Further experimentation, however, demonstrated that reversal of shorter segments was compatible with life. When applied to dogs with experimental short-bowel syndrome, reversed segments of appropriate length delayed transit, increased apsorption, and prevented intractable weight loss and ultimate death.[41, 44–46] In 1962, Gibson et al.[47] reported the first clinical application of a reversed intestinal loop. In an 84-year-old woman, massive intestinal resection for mesenteric vascular occlusion was accompanied by reversal of a 7.5-cm, small-intestinal segment. This patient demonstrated diarrhea and malabsorption in the early postoperative period, but follow-up more than one year later revealed that the patient was well nourished, with healthy bowel habits.

Enthusiasm for the use of reversed segments grew as further reported cases seemed successful. The accumulated experience yielded conclusions regarding the technique and timing of the operation. Because most patients ultimately recover from massive resection without needing additional treatment, reversal of a segment should not be undertaken at the initial operation. The decision to proceed is made only after a minimum of six months of careful medical management demonstrates an absolute failure of satisfactory oral alimentation. The length of the reversed segment is critical; if it is too long, it will cause intolerable obstruction, while if too short, it will be ineffective. In adult humans, a 10–12-cm length achieves the best results, whereas in infants and children, a shorter length is appropriate. A site in the most distal remaining small bowel is traditionally reversed in treating the short-bowel syndrome. Reversal of a proximal segment, however, might also delay gastric emptying, improve nutrient mixing with bile and pancreatic juice, and avoid rapid saturation of distal mucosal transport sites. This theoretically attractive alternative has not been studied. Prejejunal transposition of a segment of colon is beneficial, probably due to a similar mechanism.

Simple reversal of an intestinal loop produces a 180° torsion of its mesenteric pedicle. Rygick and Nasarov[48] described a method of anastomosis of the reversed loop which avoids twisting the loop's mesentery and the attendant risk of infarction. In this method, the distal cut end of the isolated segment is anastomosed to the proximal cut end of the main tract. The distal cut end of the main tract is then brought through a defect in the mesentery of the proximal tract and anastomosed to the proximal cut end of the segment (Fig 49–2).

Undoubtedly, the majority of reports of reversed intestinal segments for the short-bowel syndrome are favorable (Table 49–1). However, a prospective, controlled clinical trial providing standardized operative treatment, objective documentation of results, and long-term follow-up of all cases is lacking. Until such a study is completed, the results of intestinal reversal remain unproved.

RECIRCULATING LOOPS.—Construction of a circular intestinal loop might permit intestinal content to recirculate several times over the same mucosal surface, promoting increased nutrient absorption.[57] In practice, this goal is difficult

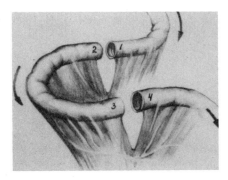

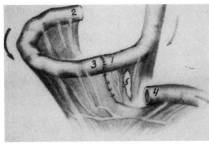

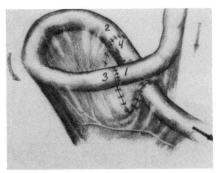

Fig 49–2.—Method of constructing a reversed intestinal segment, after Rygick and Nasarov.[48]

to achieve. Experimental comparison with a simple reversed segment showed the recirculating loop to give inferior results.[58] In addition, construction of a recirculating loop entails the risk of multiple anastomoses, provides the potential setting for stasis and bacterial overgrowth, and runs the risk of short-circuiting of remaining gut. This operation has no place in the treatment of the short-bowel syndrome at this time.

ARTIFICIAL ENTERIC SPHINCTERS.—Loss of the ileocolonic sphincter increases the morbidity and mortality of massive intestinal resection. This may be due to bacterial proliferation in the small bowel, loss of a braking mechanism causing hastened intestinal transit, or both. Several methods of surgically reconstructing an ileocolonic valve or sphincter have been explored, mostly in dogs. Perhaps the most promising is the antegrade intussuscepting jejunocolonic anastomosis described by Ricotta et al.[59] In dogs, following 80% distal enterectomy, the distal jejunum is everted back on itself for a length of 4 cm. The everted bowel is then invaginated into the colon to produce a new enterocolonic valve. Canine experiments showed that, compared to controls without the valve, bacterial contamination of the small bowel was diminished, intestinal transit was slowed, and survival enhanced. This group has used the valve once, with evident success, in a patient with 75 cm of residual small bowel. Other clinical reports of valve reconstruction are anecdotal, and do not form the basis for recommending their present use.

INTESTINAL TRANSPLANTATION.—Intestinal transplantation holds promise as the optimal surgical treatment of the short bowel syndrome. The technical features of the operation are now straightforward, with venous drainage into the portal system preferred. Improved immunosuppression with cyclosporine has produced survival with good function for over 200 days in dogs with near-total orthotopic jejunoileal grafts.[60] Late or chronic rejection could still lead to graft failure. Ready methods of monitoring function are needed. A living-related donor could sacrifice several feet of small bowel without difficulty. Alternatively, longer lengths could be harvested from brain-dead cadavers that are deemed suitable donors. Graft vs. host disease due to the large population of transplanted intestinal and mesenteric lymphoid tissue remains a potential problem.

GROWING INTESTINAL NEOMUCOSA.—When the small intestine is opened longitudinally and the defect closed with a patch of viable tissue, such as adjacent bowel serosa or abdominal wall, the luminal surface of the patch will rapidly become covered with intestinal mucosa. This new mucosal surface has histologic and functional characteristics resembling normal intestinal mucosa, including brush border enzymatic and transport activity. This method of increasing mucosal surface area has proved beneficial in pigs with the short-bowel syndrome but has not yet been tried in man.[33]

RETROGRADE INTESTINAL PACING.—A method that delays intestinal transit and prolongs contact between nutrients and gut mucosa should improve absorption and ameliorate the short-bowel syndrome. Use of the reversed intestinal segment is an attempt to achieve this result, but the reversed segment produces a fixed partial obstruction, risks further loss of

TABLE 49–1.—RECENT REPORTS OF REVERSED INTESTINAL SEGMENTS
FOR THE SHORT-BOWEL SYNDROME

FIRST AUTHOR	PATIENT'S AGE	LENGTH OF SEGMENT, CM	FOLLOW-UP	RESULT
Fink	49 yr	17	1 yr	Improved
	23 yr	10	6 mo.	Improved
	65 yr	7	18 mo.	Improved, then worsened
		10	2 mo.	Improved
	66 yr	10	≤1 mo.	Improved
Venables	58 yr	7.5	<1 mo.	Improved
Simons	Adult	15	7.5 yr	Improved
Perlman	25 yr	9	1 yr	Improved
Pertsemlidis	33 yr	14	2 yr	Improved
Hakami	56 yr	9	3 mo.	Improved
	26 yr	9	≤1 mo.	Improved
Wilmore	52 yr	10	1 yr	Improved at 1 mo., returned to preoperative condition at 10 mo.
Warden	6 wk	3	3 mo.	Improved
	14 wk	3	4 yr	Improved
	7 wk	3		Improved
	5 mo.	2.5	<1 mo.	Improved
	9 mo.	3	1 yr	Improved

bowel, and is accompanied by uncertain short-term and long-term results. Electrical pacing of the gut is a new technique designed to provide flexible extrinsic control of intestinal motility.

The electrical activity of the small intestine is characterized by a periodic wave of depolarization originating in the proximal duodenum and propagating via the tunica muscularis throughout the length of the small bowel. This periodic depolarization is known variously as the pacesetter potential, the intestinal slow wave, the basic electrical rhythm, or the electrical control activity. The frequency of the pacesetter potential, determined by the duodenal "pacemaker," is 19 cycles per minute (cpm) in the dog and about 12 cpm in man. The pacesetter potentials themselves are accompanied by little, if any, muscular contractions. In the presence of sufficient stimulation, such as the eating of a meal, many or all of the pacesetter potentials will be accompanied by a further burst of depolarizations, known as action potentials or spike potentials. The action potentials trigger muscular contractions. Thus, the pacesetter potentials are central to the coordination of gut motility and transit.

Canine experiments show that the application of an appropriate electrical impulse at a frequency greater than the native pacesetter potential frequency will "entrain" the intestinal pacesetter potentials to the exogenous rate.[61] The pacesetter potentials propagate both aborally and orally from the locus of stimulation. Orally propagating pacesetter potentials will, in turn, phase the onset of orally moving contractions. This retrograde pacing will slow the antegrade transit or even reverse the direction of transit of fluid chyme within the paced bowel.[62] Water, glucose, and electrolyte absorption from an isolated bowel segment can be enhanced by retrograde electrical pacing.[63] When applied to dogs with the experimental short-bowel syndrome, absorption was improved (Fig 49–3) and weight loss blunted or even reversed by daily periods of postcibal retrograde pacing.[64–66]

A totally implantable adjustable-rate intestinal pacemaker has been developed for clinical trial. The flexibility of inter-

mittent intestinal pacing allows for a controlled delay in intestinal transit for several hours after a meal. The unit may then be turned off to allow undigestable residue and debris to be cleared from the intestine.

Summary

The short-bowel patient can now be sustained indefinitely by total parenteral nutrition, allowing maximal adaptation of the remaining gut. With the aid of careful dietary and medical management, few patients will remain permanently incapable of oral sustenance alone. For these few, the choice now lies between permanent, parenteral home alimentation and an attempt at surgical improvement of intestinal absorption. In spite of its admitted drawbacks, home parenteral alimentation appears the preferable approach at present. Perhaps intestinal transplantation or pacing will eventually offer a more satisfactory life-style for these patients.

BLIND LOOP SYNDROME

The blind loop syndrome, or small-bowel bacterial overgrowth syndrome, is an uncommon syndrome characterized

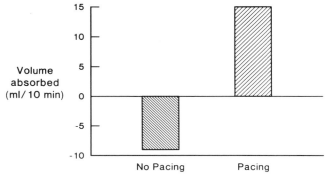

Fig 49–3.—Pacing changes the absorption pattern in the canine short-bowel syndrome from a net loss of fluid to a net gain of fluid.[64]

clinically by a variable combination of weight loss, steatorrhea, diarrhea, and vitamin B_{12} deficiency anemia. Abnormally high populations of bacteria within the small intestine compete for nutrients, alter the luminal milieu, and cause damage to the gut mucosa, producing malabsorption. Factors predisposing to bacterial overgrowth may be mechanical, such as an intestinal stricture or diverticulum, or functional, as in chronic idiopathic intestinal pseudo-obstruction (chapter 30). The surgeon is sometimes responsible for the cause of the blind loop syndrome (e.g., a partial afferent limb obstruction after gastrectomy), but likewise may also effect its cure.

Pathogenesis

NORMAL GI FLORA.—In health, the stomach and proximal small intestine harbor a scant bacterial population consisting mainly of swallowed salivary aerobic cocci (Table 49–2).[67] Progressing distally down the small bowel, a denser growth is apparent. Colonic gram-negative aerobes supersede the oral species, and anaerobes are also found. Bacterial density increases markedly on crossing the ileocecal junction, with anaerobes outnumbering aerobes by several orders of magnitude.

The relative sterility of the stomach, duodenum, and jejunum, and the increasing aboral gradient of bacterial density is a function of three principal control mechanisms. Gastric acidity destroys the majority of swallowed oral organisms and nonresident bacterial enteric pathogens. Thus, many (but not all) subjects with spontaneous, surgical, or medically induced achlorhydria will demonstrate bacterial proliferation in the stomach and/or upper small bowel. At the other end of the small bowel, the ileocecal junction may be valuable in preventing reflux of bacteria-rich colonic content into the ileum. Several experimental studies demonstrate that ileocecal resection promotes small-bowel bacterial proliferation. However, studies of jejunal flora in patients following ileocecal resection do not regularly reveal overgrowth.[68–70]

The third important mechanism limiting bacterial concentration is the normal interdigestive motility pattern of the small bowel. Beginning several hours after a meal, a cyclically recurring pattern of intense migrating contractions occurs and lasts until interrupted by the next meal. Each cycle consists of a burst of contractions originating in the stomach and duodenum and slowly (over 60–120 minutes in man) migrating the length of the small intestine. This migrating "activity front" is propulsive, clearing luminal debris and presumably bacteria as it goes. When one cycle reaches the terminal ileum, another is beginning in the stomach. This normal fasting motility pattern has been dubbed the "interdigestive housekeeper" because of its function in preventing intraluminal accumulation of debris between meals. Defects in the interdigestive pattern have been associated with bacterial overgrowth[71]; however, it remains to be determined which one of these abnormalities actually causes the other.

CONDITIONS ASSOCIATED WITH BACTERIAL OVERGROWTH.—As is true in any organ system, intestinal bacteria are bound to proliferate in the presence of stasis or obstruction. Stasis due to impaired motility of the intestinal tract occurs in pseudo-obstruction, diabetic enteropathy, systemic sclerosis, and perhaps other conditions. Stasis will result within a blind loop, which may occur spontaneously, as a solitary duodenal diverticulum, a Meckel's diverticulum, multiple jejunal diverticulosis (Fig 49–4), or postoperatively. The last may complicate the bypass of diseased intestine, an ill-constructed side-to-side or side-to-end anastomosis, or the afferent limb of a gastrojejunal anastomosis. Finally, chronic partial mechanical small-bowel obstruction causes bacterial proliferation proximal to the lesion. Occasionally, perhaps usually, this overgrowth contributes to the pathophysiology of the obstruction itself.[72]

MUCOSAL CHANGES.—While frank invasion of the intestinal mucosa by bacteria does not occur in the bacterial overgrowth syndrome, it is now believed that some degree of morphological and functional damage to the epithelium is present.[73] Activity of brush border enzymes is diminished, and blood and protein may be lost into the gut. These changes are at least partly reversible with antibiotic therapy. It is possible that bacterial toxins or toxic bacterial catabolites are responsible. This mucosal disturbance may be considered an additive factor to other established mechanisms of malabsorption.

STEATORRHEA.—The primary bile acids, cholic and chenodeoxycholic acid, are conjugated to glycine or taurine in the liver, and secreted in the bile in that form. Conjugated bile salts participate in the formation of micelles with monoglyceride and free fatty acids (the product of pancreatic lipase acting on dietary fat). In micellar form, fatty acids are soluble and are readily absorbed in the proximal small bowel. Certain anaerobic bacteria (particularly *Bacteroides*) possess the enzymatic capacity to deconjugate bile salts within the gut lumen.[74, 75] Deconjugated bile salts do not participate in micelle formation; instead, they tend to be passively absorbed or to precipitate due to their low solubility at the pH of jejunal content. When bacterial deconjugation is excessive, the luminal concentration of conjugated bile salts falls below the critical micellar concentration. Fatty acids then remain insoluble and hence are poorly absorbed. Steatorrhea occurs only when bacterial overgrowth is present in the proximal small bowel, the site of maximum fat absorption. Bacterial deconjugation of bile salts at a more distal site would not greatly affect luminal micellar concentration in the proximal gut.

TABLE 49–2.—THE GASTROINTESTINAL FLORA OF HUMANS[67]

ORGANISMS	STOMACH	JEJUNUM	ILEUM	FECES
Total bacterial count	$0–10^3$	$0–10^5$	$10^3–10^7$	$10^{10}–10^{12}$
Aerobic or facultative anaerobic bacteria				
Enterobacteria	$0–10^2$	$0–10^3$	$10^2–10^6$	$10^4–10^{10}$
Streptococci	$0–10^3$	$0–10^4$	$10^2–10^6$	$10^5–10^{10}$
Staphylococci	$0–10^2$	$0–10^3$	$10^2–10^5$	$10^4–10^7$
Lactobacilli	$0–10^3$	$0–10^4$	$10^2–10^5$	$10^6–10^{10}$
Fungi	$0–10^2$	$0–10^2$	$10^2–10^3$	$10^2–10^6$
Anaerobic bacteria				
Bacteroides	Rare	$0–10^2$	$10^3–10^7$	$10^{10}–10^{12}$
Bifidobacteria	Rare	$0–10^3$	$10^3–10^5$	$10^8–10^{12}$
Gram-positive cocci*	Rare	$0–10^3$	$10^2–10^5$	$10^8–10^{11}$
Clostridia	Rare	Rare	$10^2–10^4$	$10^6–10^{11}$
Eubacteria	Rare	Rare	Rare	$10^9–10^{12}$

*Includes *Peptostreptococcus* and *Peptococcus*.

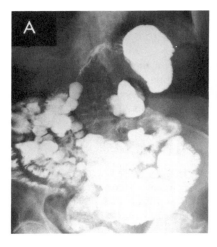
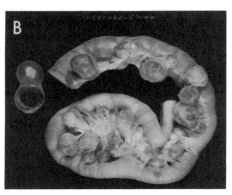

Fig 49–4.—Jejunal diverticulosis. **A,** contrast roentgenographic appearance. **B,** surgical specimen.

VITAMIN B$_{12}$ MALABSORPTION.—Vitamin B$_{12}$ and intrinsic factor-vitamin B$_{12}$ complex are competitively bound and internalized by intestinal bacteria.[75] Once taken up by bacteria, the vitamin may be metabolized to an inactive form; in any case it is no longer available for host absorption. As with steatorrhea, overgrowth of anaerobic bacteria, in particular *Bacteroides*, appears to be most capable of producing vitamin B$_{12}$ deficiency. Unlike fat malabsorption, however, the anemia of vitamin B$_{12}$ deficiency may arise from overgrowth in the distal small bowel, because the vitamin is only absorbed in the terminal ileum.

CARBOHYDRATE AND PROTEIN MALABSORPTION.— While not classically included among the features of the blind loop syndrome, malabsorption of carbohydrate and protein does occur.[73] Damage to gut mucosa may impair brush-border digestion and absorption of these nutrients and promote intestinal loss of protein as well. Bacterial catabolism of luminal carbohydrate is a further established mechanism of malabsorption.

Clinical Features

The clinical features of small-bowel bacterial overgrowth are variable, the overall symptom complex depending on the cause of the overgrowth and the duration and extent of the resulting malabsorption. Weight loss accompanied by steatorrhea and diarrhea forms the clinical hallmark of the syndrome. Abdominal discomfort, cramping pain, and bloating are common subjective complaints that may be due to the underlying disorder rather than bacterial overgrowth per se. Anemia and other secondary clinical signs of malabsorption of specific nutrients can occur.

Diagnosis

Bacterial overgrowth must be suspected in a patient with malabsorption whose history suggests a possible predisposing cause, such as gastric resection or intestinal pseudo-obstruction. The sine qua non is a bacterial culture of fasting jejunal aspirate revealing at least 10^7 organisms/ml. Because the intestinal intubation and culture techniques are cumbersome and demanding, several noninvasive tests have been developed. These include the ^{14}C-glycocholate breath test (bile acid breath test), ^{14}C-xylose test, and the hydrogen breath

test. Each of these tests measures the abnormal respiratory excretion of a product of bacterial metabolism within the small bowel in patients with bacterial overgrowth. The three-stage Schilling test in patients with the blind loop syndrome demonstrates malabsorption of oral vitamin B$_{12}$ and of vitamin B$_{12}$ and intrinsic factor given together, but normal vitamin B$_{12}$ absorption following a five-day course of oral antibiotics (usually tetracycline). Appropriate abdominal x-rays and GI contrast studies may then help to delineate the responsible pathologic anatomy or physiology.

Treatment

In a minority of cases of small-bowel bacterial overgrowth, a surgically correctable lesion will be found. Appropriate resection of diverticula, strictures, and blind loops or improved drainage of an afferent jejunal loop is curative. A course of preoperative oral antibiotics in addition to appropriate nutritional replenishment is probably wise to minimize the risk of septic postoperative complications.

When bacterial overgrowth complicates a generalized motility disorder of the intestine, surgery has little to offer. Treatment with oral antibiotics is usually effective in correcting the malabsorption due to bacterial proliferation. Tetracycline has been a standard first-line drug, but other drugs active against anaerobic species, such as metronidazole, are also effective. Usually one week of treatment with a single agent will suffice for weeks or months. The regimen may be repeated at regular intervals as needed, but sometimes continuous therapy is necessary. When one antibiotic no longer induces improvement, another is tried. Serial jejunal cultures to determine the predominant pathogenic strain and antibiotic sensitivity are probably not a useful adjunct to the trial-and-error method.[76]

Summary

Proliferation of bacteria within the lumen of the small intestine damages enterocytes and deconjugates bile salts. The bacteria compete for luminal vitamin B$_{12}$ and other nutrients. Fat malabsorption, macrocytic anemia, weight loss, and malnutrition ensue. Surgical correction of a mechanical cause is curative, while oral antibiotic treatment is effective when no surgically remediable lesion exists.

RADIATION ENTERITIS

The role of radiation therapy in the control of abdominal and pelvic cancers is large and increasing. Curative radiation therapy is now the definitive treatment for a number of tumors, especially those of the uterine cervix and corpus. Radiation is frequently employed as an adjunct to surgical excision, to assist in local and regional tumor control, or to palliate unresectable cancers. The conventional modes of administration include supravoltage (>1 meV) external beam radiation and internal or intracavitary radium or cesium implantation. For cervical or uterine carcinoma these methods are often used in combination. Effective tumor control generally requires a radiation dose close to that which predictably causes permanent injury to the bowel within the field of treatment. Radiation damage to the gut is, therefore, quite common, and likely will occur with increasing frequency.

This section deals with the problem of radiation injury to the small bowel, often called "radiation enteritis." Injuries to the colon and rectum usually coexist, however, because both large bowel and small bowel are usually within the same radiation field.

Pathology and Pathogenesis

Intestine exposed to radiation exhibits a characteristic early injury.[77–78] The principal immediate effect is to damage the dividing cells within the intestinal crypts, the cells which are responsible for the continuous repopulation of the mucosal epithelium. Fractionation of the total radiation dose into smaller daily exposures permits some repair and recovery of the cells between each dose, permitting a larger tolerable dose of radiation. The temporary impairment in crypt cell production leads to villus blunting and atrophy. The surface epithelial cells spread themselves out to maintain surface coverage. Thus, sufficient cell replication continues, so that mucosal ulceration generally does not occur. This acute phase injury is associated with transient mucosal dysfunction, which leads to malabsorption, as shown by abnormal bile acid breath tests and xylose excretion tests. While the acute radiation injury may produce troublesome symptoms and require medical and dietary treatment, spontaneous resolution is the rule.

Approximately 3%–10% of patients subjected to therapeutic abdominopelvic radiation will develop the progressive late changes of radiation enteritis. The gross pathologic features include a greyish white, opaque appearance of the bowel, with fibrinous or fibrous adhesions gluing the injured loops of bowel to themselves and to the adjacent abdominal wall. The affected bowel is edematous, thickened, fibrotic, and usually stenotic. Focal superficial ulceration is frequent, and deeper or transmural ulcers may occur. The chief histologic changes are submucosal fibrosis, with abundant collagen deposition and fibroblastic proliferation, and an obliterative vascular injury, consisting of hyalinization, intimal proliferation, and fibrin thrombi.[78] The vascular injury produces ischemia of the affected intestine, a feature which appears central to both the pathogenesis of the complications of radiation enteritis and the hazards of operative manipulation of the bowel.

The progressive ischemia, fibrosis, stenosis and ulceration that characterize chronic radiation injury eventually produce a symptomatic mechanical complication. This may be, in or-

der of likelihood, chronic partial intestinal obstruction, internal or external intestinal fistula, enteric necrosis with perforation and abscess, or intestinal bleeding. The complications may occur singly or in combination. The late radiation injury usually becomes clinically manifest within several years of treatment. However, a longer interval of apparent good health between the injury and the onset of symptoms is not uncommon. Furthermore, the pathologic process is progressive, so that successful treatment of one complication may be followed years later by further complications originating in the bowel that had earlier appeared normal.

Clinical Features

Radiation enteritis may follow therapeutic radiation for any cancer within the pelvis or abdomen. Treatment of cervical carcinoma produces the largest number of patients with this complication. Curative or adjuvant radiation for endometrial, bladder, rectal, testicular, ovarian, or prostatic cancer, or for lymphoma and other sarcomas, account for most of the remainder. The likelihood that chronic intestinal injury will follow a course of radiation depends on the total dose of radiation and the volume of bowel within the field of treatment.[77] Because most often radiation therapy is directed at a pelvic malignancy, the rectum, sigmoid colon, and terminal ileum sustain the greatest radiation exposure and are the most commonly injured viscera. During a course of radiation treatment, the normally mobile mesenteric small and large bowel may be sometimes within and sometimes outside of the treatment field. Such mobile segments, thus, are not exposed to the total radiation dose. In contrast, at regions of anatomical fixation, such as the rectum, ileocecal junction, duodenum, and duodenojejunal flexure, the bowel cannot escape exposure to the total radiation dose if it is within the treatment field. These areas are at particular risk for radiation injury.

A number of clinical factors appear to predispose the patient to the development of radiation enteritis, although none has been proved to the satisfaction of all investigators.[77] Radiation injury is probably more likely in patients who have been subjected to prior celiotomy, particularly a pelvic operation.[79, 80] The hypothesis is that postoperative adhesions fix loops of bowel within the pelvis, preventing their intermittent escape from subsequent radiation exposure. Patients with diabetes mellitus or hypertension may also be at greater risk. Presumably, the small-vessel occlusive disease frequently associated with these conditions compounds the ischemic changes of radiation enteropathy.[80] The development of congestive cardiac failure might precipitate overt intestinal manifestations in a previously irradiated individual by a similar mechanism. Finally, thin persons may suffer radiation injury more readily than their full-bodied counterparts.[81]

Several investigational methods could prove beneficial in limiting radiation damage to the small bowel. During an abdominal operation, if postoperative pelvic irradiation is anticipated, an attempt to exclude the small bowel from the pelvis should be considered. This may be accomplished by suturing the uterus to the posterior pelvic wall, by construction of a polyglycolic acid mesh barrier across the pelvic inlet,[82] or by filling the pelvic space with a silastic mammary prosthesis.[83] Prior to beginning radiation therapy, upper and lower GI roentgenographic contrast studies will determine the extent to which the bowel is fixed within the pelvis. The fraction of small bowel lying within the pelvis in the supine and prone positions should be noted, so that appropriate positioning during therapy can minimize intestinal radiation exposure.[84] Pharmacologic methods of radioprotection are being investigated, but as yet none is conclusively beneficial.

Diagnosis

Diagnosis of chronic small intestinal radiation damage is usually established by contrast radiography (Figs 49–5 and 49–6). The involved bowel appears thickened, rigid, and narrowed. It has diminished contractility and shows increased space between bowel loops on small-bowel x-ray examinations. The possibility of recurrent intra-abdominal malignancy may be assessed by ultrasound, CAT scans, or other imaging techniques.

Surgical Treatment

Surgical treatment of radiation enteritis, as with other inflammatory bowel diseases, is reserved for the complications of the disease. The most common manifestation, chronic small-bowel obstruction, is often managed nonoperatively for long periods. This entails dietary manipulation, pharmacologic measures, and occasional hospitalization with nasointestinal intubation and decompression. Progression to high-grade obstruction or persistence of incapacitating obstructive symptoms will ultimately require surgical relief. A fistula between bowel and skin, vagina, bladder, or another bowel segment is generally an indication for operative intervention. Intestinal necrosis with free perforation and/or abscess clearly requires operation. Acute massive and chronic low-grade bleeding are rarer indications for operation.

Once the decision to operate electively for obstruction or fistula has been made, thorough preoperative investigation is mandatory. Radiation injury to the small bowel is often accompanied by a similar injury to the large bowel, rectum, or urinary tract. Recognition of additional sites of damage is important. For example, a subclinical rectal stenosis will jeopardize the safety and success of a small-bowel resection for chronic obstruction. Complete GI contrast studies, excretory urography, proctoscopy, and cystoscopy are therefore recommended to help plan the elective operation. Intravenous hyperalimentation during the period of investigation is wise, since the nutritional depletion of these patients may be chronic and profound.

When operating on the irradiated abdomen, the incision is best placed outside the field of irradiation, provided this will permit adequate exposure. Typically, a large mass of adherent bowel is encountered, posing a challenge to safe mobilization and dissection. Traditional teaching holds that the diseased bowel should be manipulated as little as possible to avoid inadvertent damage. Some surgeons now believe, however, that with careful technique, a complete small-bowel mobilization is safe and even advisable to avoid overlooking diseased and prenecrotic lesions.[85, 86]

Debate continues as to whether resection[85, 87, 88] or bypass[89–92] should be used for intestinal obstruction produced by radiation injury. Bypass is achieved in one of two ways—by side-to-side anastomosis (nonexclusion bypass) or by dividing the bowel proximal to the obstruction, closing or venting as a mucous fistula the distal end cut, and anastomosing the proximal cut end to healthy bowel distal to the obstructing lesion (exclusion bypass). The argument in favor of bypass is, first, that dangerous mobilization of the mass of diseased bowel is avoided, and second, that a side-to-side anastomosis should interfere less with blood supply, and be more secure in radiated bowel than an end-to-end anastomosis. Proponents of resection counter that intestinal bypass may produce a blind loop syndrome, that disease in the bypassed segment may progress to necrosis and perforation or fistulization, and that a properly performed end-to-end anastomosis is as safe as any other. A definitive resolution in favor of one method or the other cannot at present be made on the basis of the data in the literature, and the choice still depends on judgment made at the operating table (Table 49–3).[80, 93, 94]

Important conclusions can be drawn from the accumulated

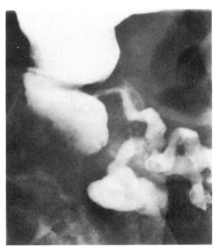

Fig 49–6.—Lower GI contrast roentgenogram demonstrating nondistensible cecum and narrowed, thickened, rigid terminal ileum due to radiation injury.

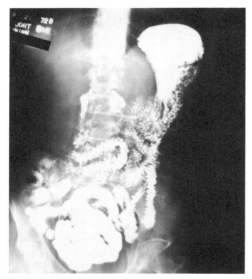

Fig 49–5.—Abdominal roentgenogram using BaSO₄ showing narrowed, thick-walled loops of small intestine secondary to radiation enteritis.

TABLE 49–3.—RESULTS OF OPERATION FOR RADIATION ENTERITIS

FIRST AUTHOR	RESECTION			BYPASS		
	No. of Patients	% Septic Complications	% Mortality	No. of Patients	% Septic Complications	% Mortality
Schmitt	65	15	8	20	0	5
Lillemoe	6	50	17	11	9	0
Wobbles	7	57	57	20	5	10
Localio	7	NA*	0	0	0	0
Palmer	10	NA	0	2	NA	0
Russell	17	35	NA	13	31	NA
DeCosse	16	6	12	2	NA	50
Cochrane	8	63	63	1	0	0
Galland	18	50	44	2	0	0
Deveney	20	10	NA	5	0	0

*NA = not available.

experience, however, to increase the safety of either approach. First, the potential metabolic and septic complications arising from bypassed bowel have only rarely been reported; this theoretical risk may be overstated. Second, any resection should be extremely generous, because it is crucial to perform an anastomosis with relatively healthy bowel. The intestine close to a lesion may appear grossly satisfactory and yet be microscopically diseased and relatively ischemic. Resection of ileal disease should routinely include the ileocecal junction and right colon, as these structures have usually been irradiated as well. The colon at the hepatic flexure, relatively fixed outside of the standard pelvic radiation field, is almost always suitable for anastomosis.[85] Microscopic evaluation of a frozen section of the resected margins should help determine the limits of resection. Finally, the surgeon should maintain a low threshold for temporary exteriorization of the bowel in preference to the construction of an insecure anastomosis.

Massive intestinal bleeding or perforation mandates resection of the involved bowel. Elective management of a fistula poses greater difficulties. The direct approach of intestinal resection is usually successful. In some reports, however, resection and primary anstomosis have been attended by an unacceptably large rate of intraperitoneal sepsis. An alternative is to isolate the involved segment, exteriorizing both of its ends, leaving the bowel in situ. An anastomosis is done between the proximal and distal cut ends of the remaining healthy bowel. Again, in patients in whom peritoneal soilage has occurred, an abdominal stoma to defunctionalize the anastomosis must be strongly considered.

Summary

Complications of radiation injury of the small intestine, such as obstruction, perforation, fistula, abscess, and bleeding, often require operative treatment. An elective operation should follow complete preoperative investigation and intensive nutritional replenishment. Wide intestinal resection with primary anastomosis for obstructing and bleeding lesions can be safely accomplished in most patients in whom the disease bowel is relatively mobile. When adhesions glue the diseased bowel firmly to itself or to the abdominal wall, a bypass is a safe, satisfactory alternative to resection. Resection with anastomosis for small-bowel perforation, fistula, or abscess carries

a greater risk of postoperative sepsis. In these patients, resection with temporary enterostomy or exclusion-bypass may be a better choice than resection and anastomosis.

REFERENCES

1. Borgstrom B., Dahlquist A., Lundh G., et al.: Studies of intestinal digestion and absorption in the human. *J. Clin. Invest.* 36:1521, 1957.
2. Hofmann A.F., Danzinger R.G.: Physiologic and clinical significance of ileal resection. *Surg. Annu.* 4:305–325, 1972.
3. Hofmann A.F., Poley J.R.: Role of bile acid malabsorption in pathogenesis of diarrhea and steatorrhea in patients with ileal resection: I. Response to cholestyramine or replacement of dietary long chain triglyceride by medium chain triglyceride. *Gastroenterology* 62:918, 1972.
4. Mekhjian H.S., Phillips S.F., Hoffman A.F.: Colonic secretion of water and electrolytes induced by bile acids: Perfusion studies in man. *J. Clin. Invest.* 50:1569, 1971.
5. Ammon H.V., Phillips S.F.: Inhibition of colonic water and electrolyte absorption by fatty acids in man. *J. Clin. Invest.* 65:744, 1973.
6. Sitrin M.D.: Nutritional and metabolic complications in a patient with Crohn's disease and ileal resection. *Gastroenterology* 78:1069, 1980.
7. Hofmann A.F., Laken M.F., Dharmsathaphorn K.: Complex pathogenesis of hyperoxaluria after jejunoileal bypass surgery. *Gastroenterology* 84:293, 1983.
8. Gazet J.-C., Kopp J.: The surgical significance of the ileocecal junction. *Surgery* 56:565, 1964.
9. Griffen W.O. Jr., Richardson J.D., Medley E.S.: Prevention of small bowel contamination by ileocecal valve. *South Med. J.* 64:1056, 1971.
10. Kerlin P., Phillips S.: Absorption and secretion of electrolytes by the human colon, in Bustos-Fernandez L. (ed.): *Colon Structure and Function.* New York, Plenum Medical Book Co., 1983, pp. 17–44.
11. Debongnie J.C., Phillips S.F.: Capacity of the human colon to absorb fluid. *Gastroenterology* 74:698, 1978.
12. Mitchell J.E., Breuer R.I., Zuckerman L., et al.: The colon influences ileal resection diarrhea. *Dig. Dis. Sci.* 25:33, 1980.
13. Cummings J.H., James W.P.T., Wiggins H.S.: Role of the colon in ileal-resection diarrhea. *Lancet* 1:344, 1973.
14. Kremen A.J., Linner J.H., Nelson C.H.: An experimental evaluation of the nutritional importance of proximal and distal small intestine. *Ann. Surg.* 140:439, 1954.
15. Singleton A.O., Redmond D.C. II, McMurray J.E.: Ileocecal resection and small bowel transit and absorption. *Ann. Surg.* 159:690, 1964.
16. Reid I.S.: The significance of the ileocecal valve in massive resection of the gut in puppies. *J. Pediatr. Surg.* 10:507, 1975.
17. Haymond H.E.: Massive resection of the small intestine: An

analysis of 257 collected cases. *Surg. Gynecol. Obstet.* 61:693, 1935.

18. Kalser M.H., Roth J.L.A., Tumen H., et al.: Relation of small bowel resection to nutrition in man. *Gastroenterology* 38:605, 1960.

19. Chen K.: Massive resection of the small intestine. *Surgery* 65:931, 1969.

20. Wilmore D.W.: Factors correlating with a succesful outcome following extensive intestinal resection in newborn infants. *J. Pediatr.* 80:88, 1972.

21. Buchwald H., Moore R.B., Varco R.L.: Partial ileal bypass for control of hyperlipidemia and atherosclerosis, in Sabiston D.C. Jr., Spencer F.C. (eds.): *Gibbons Surgery of the Chest.* Philadelphia, W.B. Saunders Co., 1983, pp. 1515–1534.

22. Reynell P.C., Spray G.H.: Small intestinal function in the rat after massive resections. *Gastroenterology* 31:361, 1956.

23. Nylander G.: Gastric evacuation and propulsive intestinal motility following resection of the small intestine in the rat. *Acta Chir. Scand.* 133:131, 1967.

24. Remington M., Malagelada J.-R., Zinsmeister A., et al.: Abnormalities in gastrointestinal motor activity in patients with short bowels: Effect of a synthetic opiate. *Gastroenterology* 85:629, 1983.

25. Hall A.W., Moossa A.R., Skinner D.B.: Effect of 50% distal small bowel resection on gastric emptying in rhesus monkeys. *Ann. Surg.* 185:214, 1977.

26. Weser E.: Nutritional aspects of malabsorption: Short gut adaptation, in Schlesinger M.H. (ed.): *Clinics in Gastroenterology.* Philadelphia, W.B. Saunders Co., 1983, vol. 12, pp. 443–460.

27. Williamson R.C.N.: Intestinal adaptation. *N. Engl. J. Med.* 298:1393–1402; 1444–1450, 1978.

28. Meyers W.C., Jones R.S.: Hyperacidity and hypergastrinemia following extensive intestinal resection. *World J. Surg.* 3:539, 1979.

29. Hall A.W., Moossa A.R., Wood R.A.B., et al.: Effect of antrectomy on gastric hypersecretion induced by distal small bowel resection. *Ann. Surg.* 186:83, 1977.

30. Flemming C.R., Remington M.: Intestinal failure, in Hill G.L. (ed.): *Nutrition and the Surgical Patient.* Edinburgh, Churchill Livingston, 1981, pp. 219–235.

31. Weser E., Fletcher J.T., Urban E.: Short bowel syndrome. *Gastroenterology* 77:572, 1979.

32. Wright H.K., Tilson M.D.: The short gut syndrome. *Curr. Probl. Surg.* 1971, pp. 1–51.

33. Thompson J.S.: Surgical therapy for the short bowel syndrome. *J. Surg. Res.* In press.

34. Mitchell A., Watkins R.M., Collin J.: Surgical treatment of the short bowel syndrome. *Br. J. Surg.* 71:329, 1984.

35. Richter H.M. III, Kelly K.A.: Surgical management of the short gut syndrome, in Cuschieri A., Skinner D.B. (eds.): *Reconstruction of the Gastrointestinal Tract.* London, Butterworth & Co. In press.

36. Leonard A.S., Levine A.S., Wittner R., et al.: Massive small-bowel resections. *Arch. Surg.* 95:429, 1967.

37. Albo R.J., Angotti D., Sorenson D., et al.: Value of selective and truncal vagotomy in massive bowel resection. *Am. J. Surg.* 128:234, 1974.

38. Cortot A., Flemming C.R., Malagelada J.-R.: Improved nutrient absorption after cimetidine in short-bowel syndrome with gastric hypersecretion. *N. Engl. J. Med.* 300:79, 1979.

39. Murphy J.P. Jr., King D.R., Dubois A.: Treatment of gastric hypersecretion with cimetidine in the short bowel syndrome. *N. Engl. J. Med.* 300:80, 1979.

40. Wolf S.A., Telander R.L., Go V.L.W., et al.: Effect of proximal gastric vagotomy and truncal vagotomy and pyloroplasty on gastric functions and growth in puppies after massive small bowel resection. *J. Pediatr. Surg.* 14:441, 1979.

41. Stahlgren L.H., Umana G., Ray R., et al.: A study of intestinal absorption in dogs following massive small intestinal resection and insertion of an antiperistaltic segment. *Ann. Surg.* 156:483, 1962.

42. Tanner W.A., O'Leary J.F., Byrne P.J., et al.: The effect of reversed jejunal segments on the myoelectrical activity of the small bowel. *Br. J. Surg.* 65:567, 1978.

43. Mall F.: Reversal of the intestines. *Johns Hopkins Med. J.* 1:93, 1896.

44. Hammer J.M., Seay P.H., Hill E.J., et al.: Intestinal segments as intestinal pedicle grafts. *Arch. Surg.* 71:625, 1955.

45. Hammer J.M., Seay P.H., Johnston R.L., et al.: The effect of antiperistaltic bowel segments on intestinal emptying time. *Arch. Surg.* 79:537, 1959.

46. Baldwin-Price H.K., Singleton A.O. Jr.: Reversed intestinal segments in the management of anenteric malabsorption syndrome. *Ann. Surg.* 161:225, 1965.

47. Gibson L.D., Carter R. Hinshaw D.B.: Segmental reversal of small intestine after massive bowel resection. *J.A.M.A.* 182:952, 1962.

48. Rygick A.N., Nasarov L.V.: Antiperistaltic displacement of an ileal loop without twisting its mesentery. *Dis. Colon Rectum* 12:409, 1969.

49. Fink W.J., Olson J.D.: The massive bowel resection syndrome. *Arch. Surg.* 94:700, 1966.

50. Venables C.W., Ellis H., Smith A.D.M.: Antiperistaltic segments after massive intestinal resection. *Lancet* 2:1390, 1966.

51. Simons B.E., Jordan G.L. Jr.: Massive bowel resection. *Am. J. Surg.* 118:953, 1969.

52. Perlman M.M., Stein A., Schamroth L.: Reversal of an intestinal segment in the long-term management of the short-bowel syndrome. *S. Afr. Med. J.* 46:1730, 1972.

53. Pertsemlidis D., Kark A.E.: Antiperistaltic segments for the treatment of short bowel syndrome. *Am. J. Gastroenterol.* 62:526, 1974.

54. Hakami H., Moslehy A., Mosavy S.H.: Reversed jejunal segment used to treat the short bowel syndrome. *Am. Surg.* 41:432, 1975.

55. Wilmore D.W., Johnson C.J.: Metabolic effects of small bowel reversal in treatment of the short bowel syndrome. *Arch. Surg.* 97:784, 1968.

56. Warden M.J., Wesley J.R.: Small bowel reversal procedure for treatment of the "short gut" baby. *J. Pediatr. Surg.* 13:321, 1978.

57. Mackby M.J., Richardt V., Gilfillan R.S., et al.: Methods of increasing the efficiency of residual small bowel segments. *Am. J. Surg.* 109:32, 1965.

58. Budding J., Smith C.C.: Role of recirculating loops in the management of massive resection of the small intestine. *Surg. Gynecol. Obstet.* 125:243, 1967.

59. Ricotta J., Zuidema G.D., Gadacz T.R., et al.: Construction of an ileocecal valve and its role in massive resection of the small intestine. *Surg. Gynecol. Obstet.* 152:310, 1981.

60. Reznick R.K., Craddock G.N., Langer B., et al.: Structure and function of small bowel allografts in the dog: Immunosuppression with cyclosporin A. *Can. J. Surg.* 25:51, 1982.

61. Akwari O.E., Kelly K.A., Steinbach J.H., et al.: Electrical pacing of intact and transected canine small intestine and its computer model. *Am. J. Physiol.* 229:1188, 1975.

62. Sarr M.G., Kelly K.A., Gladen H.E.: Electrical control of canine jejunal propulsion. *Am. J. Physiol.* 240:G355, 1981.

63. Collin J., Kelly K.A., Phillips S.F.: Enhancement of absorption from the intact and transected canine small bowel by electrical pacing. *Gastroenterology* 76:1422, 1979.

64. Gladen H.E., Kelly K.A.: Enhancing absorption in the canine short bowel syndrome by intestinal pacing. *Surgery* 88:281, 1980.

65. Gladen H.E., Kelly K.A.: Electrical pacing for short bowel syndrome. *Surg. Gynecol. Obstet.* 153:697, 1981.

66. Layzell T., Collin J.: Retrograde electrical pacing of the small intestine—a new treatment for the short bowel syndrome? *Br. J. Surg.* 68:711, 1981.

67. Simon G.L., Gorbach S.L.: Intestinal flora in health and disease. *Gastroenterology* 86:174, 1984.

68. Belken W.L., Kanich R.E.: Microbial flora of the upper small bowel in Crohn's disease. *Gastroenterology* 65:390, 1973.

69. Drasar B.S., Shiner M.: Studies on the intestinal flora: Part II. Bacterial flora of the small intestine in patients with gastrointestinal disorders. *Gut* 10:812, 1969.

70. Gorbach S.L., Tabaqchiaili S.: Bacteria, bile and the small bowel. *Gut* 10:963, 1969.

71. Vantrappen G., Janssens J., Hellemans J., et al.: The interdigestive motor complex of normal subjects and patients with bacterial overgrowth of the small intestine. *J. Clin. Invest.* 59:1158, 1977.

72. Banwell J.G.: Small intestinal bacterial overgrowth syndrome. *Gastroenterology* 80:834, 1981.

73. King C.E., Toskes P.P.: Small intestine bacterial overgrowth. *Gastroenterology* 76:1035, 1979.

74. Rosenberg I.H.: influence of intestinal bacteria on bile acid metabolsim and fat absorption: Contributions from studies of blind-loop syndrome. *Am. J. Clin. Nutr.* 22:284, 1969.

75. Donaldson R.M. Jr.: Small bowel bacterial overgrowth, in Stollerman G.H. (ed.): *Advances in Internal Medicine*. Chicago, Year Book Medical Publishers, 1970, pp. 191–212.

76. Isaacs P.E., Kim Y.S.: Blind loop syndrome and small bowel bacterial contamination, in Schlesinger M.H. (ed.): *Clinics in Gastroenterology*. Philadelphia, W.B. Saunders Company, 1983, vol. 12, pp. 395–414.

77. Kinsella T.J., Bloomer W.D.: Tolerance of the intestine to radiation therapy. *Surg. Gynecol. Obstet.* 151:273, 1980.

78. Berthrong M., Fajardo L.F.: Radiation injury in surgical pathology: Part II. Alimentary tract. *Am. J. Surg. Pathol.* 5:153, 1981.

79. LoIudice T., Baxter D., Balint J.: Effects of abdominal surgery on the development of radiation enteropathy. *Gastroenterology* 3:1093, 1977.

80. DeCosse J.J., Rhodes R.S., Wentz W.B., et al.: The natural history and management of radiation induced injury of the gastrointestinal tract. *Ann. Surg.* 170:369, 1969.

81. Patish R.A.: Importance of predisposing factors in the development of enteric damage. *Am. J. Clin. Oncol.* 5:189, 1982.

82. Devereux D.E., Kavanah M.T., Feldman M.I., et al.: Small bowel exclusion from the pelvis by a polyglycolic acid mesh sling. *J. Surg. Oncol.* 26:107, 1984.

83. Sugarbaker P.H.: Intrapelvic prosthesis to prevent injury of the small intestine with high dosage pelvic irradiation. *Surg. Gynecol. Obstet.* 157:269, 1983.

84. Green N., Iba G., Smith W.R.: Measures to minimize small intestine injury in the irradiated pelvis. *Cancer* 35:1633, 1975.

85. Marks G., Mohindden M.: The surgical management of the radiation-injured intestine. *Surg. Clin. North Am.* 63:81, 1983.

86. Grage T.B., Reed K.: Surgical management of radiation injury to the gastrointestinal tract, in Najarian J.S., Delaney J.P. (eds.): *Advances in Gastrointestinal Surgery*. Chicago, Year Book Medical Publishers, 1984, pp. 373–384.

87. Localio S.A., Patcher H.L., Gouge T.H.: The radiation-injured bowel. *Surg. Ann.* 11:181–205, 1979.

88. Palmer J.A., Bush R.S.: Radiation injuries to the bowel associated with the treatment of carcinoma of the cervix. *Surgery* 80:458, 1976.

89. Lillemoe K.D., Brigham R.A., Harmon J.W.: Surgical management of small-bowel radiation enteritis. *Arch. Surg.* 118:905, 1983.

90. Galland R.B., Spencer J.: Surgical aspects of radiation injury to the intestine. *Br. J. Surg.* 66:135, 1979.

91. Swan R.W., Fowler W.C. Jr., Boronow R.C.: Surgical management of radiation injury to the small intestine. *Surg. Gynecol. Obstet.* 142:325, 1976.

92. Wobbes T., Verschueren R.C.J., Lubbers E.C.: Surgical aspects of radiation enteritis of the small bowel. *Dis. Colon Rectum* 27:89, 1984.

93. Schmitt E.H. III, Symmonds R.E.: Surgical treatment of radiation induced injuries of the intestine. *Surg. Gynecol. Obstet.* 153:896, 1981.

94. Russell J.C., Welch J.P.: Operative managment of radiation injuries of the intestinal tract. *Am. J. Surg.* 137:433, 1979.

50

Mechanical Obstruction of the Small and Large Intestines

JOHN P. WELCH, M.D.

INTESTINAL OBSTRUCTION represents an ongoing problem that has challenged the diagnostic and therapeutic abilities of gastroenterologists and GI surgeons for decades. "Surgical judgment" and an understanding of the pathophysiologic mechanisms continue to represent integral aspects of patient management. Despite advances in perioperative supportive care and a progressive fall in hospital mortality, few recent major advances have emerged from the laboratory. Several major areas of controversy remain, including the differentiation of simple and strangulating small-bowel obstruction (both in the preoperative period and at the operating table); the differentiation of mechanical obstruction and paralytic ileus; and the choice of the proper operation for acute large-bowel obstruction, with or without associated perforation. The purpose of this chapter is to discuss *mechanical obstruction in adults*, where the actual passage of intestinal contents is hindered by abnormalities originating either within or extrinsic to the bowel.

TERMINOLOGY

In *simple obstruction* the intestinal lumen is partially or totally occluded in the presence of an adequate blood supply. This is contrasted with *strangulation obstruction*, where the blood supply to the obstructed segment is inadequate. A *closed loop* is an isolated segment of intestine that is occluded at either end, thus preventing decompression in either an antegrade or retrograde direction. In *obturation obstruction* there is intraluminal obstruction by a foreign body such as a gallstone. In *partial obstruction* some intestinal content passes through the narrowed segment, while there is total occlusion in *complete obstruction*. A *high small-bowel obstruction* lies in the proximal small bowel and a *low small-bowel obstruction* in the distal bowel.

SMALL-BOWEL OBSTRUCTION

Small-bowel obstruction is more common than large-bowel obstruction, representing about two thirds of cases in recent major series.[1, 2] Table 50–1 outlines the numerous factors responsible for mechanical obstruction, and Table 50–2 places the most common problems in perspective based on recent clinical series. The mortality accompanying simple obstruc-

tion has fallen to levels of 0%–6%,[3, 4] but it continues as high as 15%–30%[5–7] in the presence of strangulation.

Pathophysiology

Once the bowel lumen is occluded, air and fluid begin to collect proximal to the point of obstruction, leading to dilatation of the bowel. Nearly 75% of the intestinal air seen in simple mechanical obstruction follows air swallowing. Experimental animals with a cervical esophagostomy (for venting swallowed air) do not develop intestinal distention despite complete occlusion of the terminal ileum.[8] Other sources of intestinal gas are sugar fermentation, blood diffusion, and CO_2 produced by interaction of gastric acid and carbonates from biliary and pancreatic secretions. Approximately 8 L of fluid is delivered to the small bowel daily in the form of salivary and gastric juice, biliary and pancreatic secretions, and succus entericus. Much of this fluid is reabsorbed by the normal small bowel.

If small-bowel distention develops, fluid absorption is hindered, and secretion into the lumen is increased.[9] Rapid infusion of IV fluids also increases secretion.[10] Absorption in the human ileum drops rapidly at intraluminal pressures greater than 20 cm of water.[11] Intraluminal pressure increases to the range of 10–14 cm of water. The capillary system in the bowel wall is gradually compromised by the increased wall tension.

Transudation of fluids into the peritoneal cavity together with the above abnormalities causes a gradual shrinkage of the extracellular fluid volume and a dilutional hyponatremia. Since the intestinal fluid has similar tonicity and electrolyte concentrations as the extracellular fluid, electrolyte and acid-base abnormalities are not common. A notable exception is chronic duodenal obstruction that leads to a hypokalemic alkalosis. Patients may develop signs of hypovolemia such as oliguria and a low central venous pressure from the extracellular fluid contraction, but shock and its complications do not occur frequently (except in strangulation obstructions).

When strangulation obstruction occurs, there is necrosis of tissue and proliferation of bacteria in the affected segment. Eventually bacteria enter the peritoneal cavity transmurally. The bacterial count increases in the more distal small intestine, and the terminal ileum contains more coliforms and anaerobes. Hence, the complications of strangulation obstruc-

Intrinsic defects of intestine
  Congenital
  Inflammatory
    Crohn's disease
    Diverticulitis
  Neoplasms
  Trauma
  Intussusception
  Radiation strictures
  Endometriosis
  Pneumatosis intestinalis
Obturation obstruction
  Gallstones
  Bezoars
  Foreign bodies
  Enteroliths
  Worms
  Intestinal tube balloons
Volvulus
  Primary
  Secondary
Extraintestinal lesions
  Adhesions
  Hernias
  External
  Internal
Compression by mass
  Carcinomatosis
  Abscess or tumor
  Pregnancy
  Foreign body
  Superior mesenteric artery syndrome
  Annular pancreas
Postoperative (other than adhesions)
  Abscess
  Wound dehiscence
  Anastomotic leak, obstruction
  Obstructed external stoma
  Hernia through peritoneal defect or trap
  Volvulus

*Adapted from Colcock and Braasch.[54]

tion (such as contraction of the extracellular fluid volume) are greater when the distal small bowel is involved and the affected segment is longer.[12–14] A dark peritoneal fluid is produced which is toxic when injected into normal animals,[13, 15] perhaps due to substances such as clostridial exotoxins and coliform endotoxins. Patients are prone to develop rapid accumulations of fluid and colloid in the affected bowel and peritoneal cavity, and vomiting contributes to rapid depletion of extracellular volume. Hypotension and attendant cardiac and renal complications may follow.

Clinical Features

There are several characteristics of mechanical small-bowel obstruction: (1) abdominal pain; (2) vomiting; (3) abdominal distention; and (4) obstipation. The symptoms are variable, depending on the *anatomical level* (proximal or distal) and on the *degree* (partial or complete) of the obstruction.

The pain is typically intermittent and of variable severity, located in the periumbilical or epigastric regions. In the case of closed loop obstruction, the pain may be severe. Nausea and vomiting occur early and frequently with high, small-bowel obstructions and late with distal obstructions. Feculent vomiting, caused by bacterial overgrowth in the bowel, is characteristic of more distal obstructions. Bilious vomiting suggests a proximal small-bowel obstruction. Abdominal distention is variable and is most pronounced with ileal obstructions. Flatus or stool may be passed after the onset of pain as the distal bowel empties, but obstipation suggests complete obstruction.

Reduction in extracellular volume commonly results in dehydration and tachycardia, but frank hypotension is rare, except in some cases of strangulation obstruction. Fever is usually low-grade, unless an intra-abdominal abscess is present. In early stages of obstruction, peristaltic waves are sometimes visible and palpable on the abdominal wall during waves of colicky pain. An abdominal mass is rarely present. Tenderness is absent in early cases of simple obstruction; therefore, a "surgical abdomen" does not require tenderness. The bowel sounds are hyperactive, with tinkles and loud rushes as peristaltic waves attempt to overcome the point of the obstruction. The frequency of peristaltic rushes is lower when the obstruction is more distal. If persistent obstruction is observed, the peristaltic activity decreases and abdominal distention increases. In late neglected cases the abdomen is distended, silent, and tender.

Unfortunately, it is impossible to differentiate reliably simple from strangulation obstruction short of laparotomy. Fever, shock, tachycardia, abdominal tenderness, and guarding or a palpable mass are suggestive of strangulation, but simple obstruction can also precipitate these findings.[16] Operation is favored over "watchful waiting" if there is any uncertainty about the diagnosis or the presence of strangulation.

Furthermore, nonoperative conditions (e.g., pancreatitis, viral gastroenteritis, biliary or ureteral colic, food poisoning, porphyria, hemolytic crises, or diabetic ketoacidosis) may

TABLE 50–2.—SMALL-BOWEL OBSTRUCTION: MAJOR ETIOLOGIC FACTORS

CAUSE	LAWS AND ALDRETE (1976)[34]	KUDCHADKAR ET AL. (1979)[2]	SUFIAN AND MATSUMOTO (1975)[1]	AVERAGE
No. of cases	465	118	115	
Adhesion, %	69	51	48	56
External hernia, %	8	24	23	18
Carcinoma, %	10	14	12	12
Internal hernia, %	—	4	6	3
Intussusception, %	1	2	2	2
Vovulus, %	—	2	1	1

mimic small-bowel obstruction, and operation may be avoided inappropriately, especially in elderly patients where the physical findings accompanying peritonitis can be mild. Pancreatitis is suggested by a steady epigastric pain radiating to the back, accompanied by elevated serum amylase and lipase levels. Cramps and vomiting commonly accompany gastroenteritis, but diarrhea, a scaphoid abdomen, and normal abdominal radiograms suggest the diagnosis.

Diagnostic Adjuncts

Just as is the case with physical findings, laboratory tests do not reliably determine the presence of strangulation obstruction. Mild leukocytosis is common, but WBC counts of more than 15,000/mm^3 or a marked left shift should raise the suspicion of bowel ischemia. Elderly debilitated patients may not be able to mount a leukocytosis in this setting. Hyperamylasemia can accompany bowel distention or infarction, with leakage of intestinal amylase into the peritoneal cavity and later peritoneal absorption. Metabolic acidosis suggests the presence of bowel ischemia.

The most important early diagnostic tests are the supine and upright or lateral decubitus radiograms. Small-bowel obstruction is usually recognized by proximal distention and distal collapse (Fig 50–1). The distribution of air in the small and large bowel is very important. If obstruction is incomplete, the small bowel is distended and some air is present in the colon. In complete obstruction, little or no air is seen in the colorectum. With proximal obstruction, there is little small-bowel distention; a "stepladder" pattern of bowel loops from the left upper quadrant to the right lower quadrant characterizes ileal obstruction. Valvulae conniventes (best seen in the jejunum rather than the ileum) line up across the lumen like a stack of coins; these contrast with colonic haustrations that are large, deep, and more irregular. *Air-fluid levels* are also seen on upright or decubitus films, depending on the relative distribution of fluid and gas in the distended intestine. The presence of more than two air-fluid levels is probably abnormal, but differentiation of mechanical obstruction and adynamic ileus may be difficult[17] (Fig 50–2). With mechanical obstruction and peristalsis, differences between serial films are useful in evaluating resolution or progression of the obstruction. Considerable air may pass the suspected point of obstruction, or, conversely, distal gas may evacuate, leaving a gasless distal bowel.

Certain findings suggest strangulation obstruction. Edema or thickening of the bowel wall, thumbprinting and loss of mucosal pattern may be seen,[18] as well as intramural air and air within the intrahepatic portal veins. Free air suggests perforation complicating strangulation obstruction. Fixation of a bowel loop, together with loss of the valvulae conniventes, is highly suggestive of strangulation.[19] The "coffee bean" sign describes a bean-shaped distended loop with thick walls that tend to separate the walls of the loop.[20]

In about 6% of cases, distended bowel loops are filled with

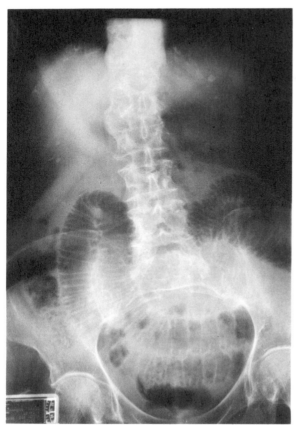

Fig 50–1.—Abdominal radiogram of mechanical small-bowel obstruction. Distended loops of small bowel containing valvulae conniventes.

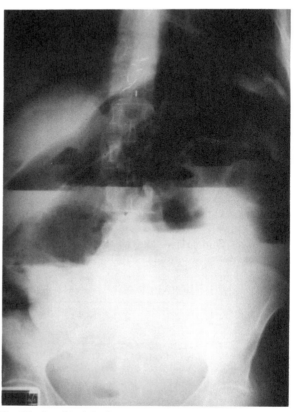

Fig 50–2.—Upright film of small-bowel obstruction. Multiple air-fluid levels at different levels.

fluid rather than air.[21] As a result, the film may appear normal to the unsuspecting clinician.[16] Particularly dangerous is that the incidence of strangulation is increased when there is fluid-filled obstruction.[21] A normal radiogram should never override clinical suspicion of strangulation obstruction (Fig 50–3). Ultrasound may demonstrate isolated small-bowel distention following normal x-rays.

Contrast studies are of use, especially if the diagnosis of intestinal obstruction is unclear from the plain films (Fig 50–4).[22] Occasionally, the tests help to decide which patients have a reasonable chance of resolving the obstruction without operation.[23] However, patients scheduled for early operation should never undergo the unnecessary delay needed for contrast examinations. A variety of techniques is available, including the standard small-bowel series, where barium or Gastrografin is given by mouth; the barium enema per rectum; or enteroclysis (the small-bowel enema),[24] in which contrast is provided by a tube introduced into the duodenum. Enteroclysis is more accurate than small-bowel series because there are fewer false negative results: in the latter, interruption of the passage of contrast prevents an adequate distention of the small bowel, and serial films may overlook discrete lesions in isolated locations.[25] In enteroclysis, contrast is followed fluoroscopically as it is introduced into the duodenum and then into the dilated small-bowel loops. If a long tube is situated above a point of obstruction, injection through the tube defines the anatomy and avoids unnecessary operative delay. Barium enemas are useful if the ileocecal valve is in-

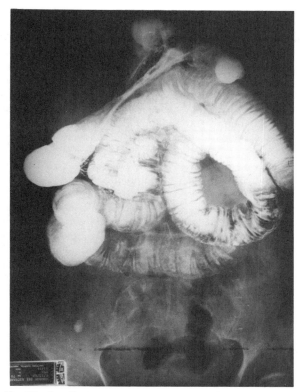

Fig 50–4.—Barium contrast study of small-bowel obstruction demonstrates distended bowel loops.

competent, allowing visualization of collapsed distal small-bowel loops.

Barium is the agent of choice in this setting. It is inert, and because of the fluid small-bowel contents, it remains liquefied. Partial small-bowel obstruction is not converted to complete obstruction by barium instillation,[26, 27] unless there is colonic obstruction, where formation of barium concretions is a risk. Water-soluble agents such as Gastrografin are more dilute, and with absorption and dilution by the small-bowel contents, little detail can be seen in the more distal small bowel. The hyperosmolar effect of these agents causes increased pooling of fluid in the bowel lumen, with possible decreases in intravascular volume and hypotension. Electrolyte imbalance can also be precipitated.

Medical Treatment

Therapy for patients with suspected mechanical obstruction is directed toward diagnosis and preparation for operation. Electrolyte and fluid disorders are corrected, and intestinal decompression is begun immediately. The complexity of patient preparation depends on multiple factors, such as the site and the chronicity of the obstruction, the nature of accompanying medical illnesses, and the presence or absence of strangulation.

Physical examination and a detailed history provide rapid clues to the degree of dehydration. Elderly or severely ill patients require careful monitoring, including blood pressure, pulse rate, temperature, central venous pressure, and hourly urine outputs. Younger patients with an acute history have

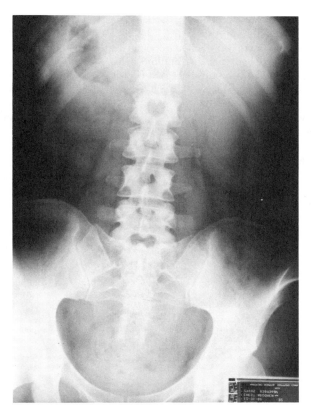

Fig 50–3.—Plain film, strangulation obstruction (adhesion-induced volvulus of small bowel). No obvious distended small-bowel loops.

fluid deficits in the range of 2 L, whereas dehydrated patients with a several-days' history of vomiting and obvious evidence of dehydration may have a 6-L deficit. A CBC and determinations of serum electrolytes, amylase, BUN, and creatinine should be obtained. Frequently the hematocrit is greater than 50; rapid hydration with Ringer's lactate lowers the value into the normal range. If chronic vomiting has occurred with high small-bowel obstruction, deficits of sodium, potassium, and chloride may be present. Sodium chloride (0.9%) is given IV, and potassium chloride is added once a satisfactory urine output has been established. In advanced cases with postural hypotension and acidosis, colloid in forms such as albumin is given rapidly. Wide-spectrum antibiotic therapy (e.g., a second-generation cephalosporin or an aminoglycoside together with an agent effective against anaerobes) is begun if strangulation is suspected. Antibiotics alone will not overcome the toxic effects of dead gut. The role of antibiotic usage is more controversial in simple mechanical obstruction. Adequate repletion of fluids will generally take 2–12 hours. Ideally, if operation is required, the hematocrit, urine output, and central venous pressure will be in normal ranges.

Intestinal Intubation

Intestinal intubation is a valuable adjunct in the management of mechanical small-bowel obstruction in certain settings. However, operation rather than intestinal intubation is the mainstay of therapy.

Nasogastric intubation is performed early in the course of treatment, providing two functions: (1) to decompress the stomach of excess gas and fluid, thus lessening the danger of vomiting and possible aspiration, and (2) to remove swallowed air from the stomach and thus reduce the amount of gas entering the distended small intestine. We prefer a large-bore (18 French) Salem sump tube because of its efficiency. Although serious complications are rare with these tubes, prolonged use causes pharyngeal discomfort and difficulty with swallowing.[28] Tubes also predispose debilitated postoperative patients to atelectasis and pneumonia.[29]

The role of the long intestinal tubes is more controversial. While it is difficult to determine whether nasointestinal or nasogastric tubes are more effective,[4] the former are associated with more frequent complications, a longer hospital stay (for both operative and nonoperative patients), and a longer period of postoperative ileus.[30, 31] In certain settings, long tubes occasionally provide an alternative to laparotomy in the first 12–48 hours of hospitalization:

1. in the *postoperative period,* when a combination of ileus and mechanical obstruction occurs frequently;

2. in patients who have had *multiple laparotomies* for adhesive obstruction;

3. in some patients with *partial small-bowel obstruction,*[32] the most frequent setting for primary intestinal intubation therapy;

4. during acute exacerbations of *Crohn's ileitis;* and

5. in patients with *abdominal carcinomatosis.*

As long as strangulation appears unlikely, patients can be observed for improvement; i.e., return of normal peristalsis as fluid deficits are replenished. If no improvement occurs within 12–24 hours, operation should be carried out. *Long tubes are no substitute for operation in cases of complete small-bowel obstruction.* Delay of a necessary operation can have grave consequences.[16, 33–35]

All patients who have had long tubes inserted should be carefully monitored for development of complications. Notable problems include intussusception,[36] tube knotting,[37] endobronchial inhalation of mercury, intestinal obstruction by a distended balloon,[38] and failure of the tube to pass beyond the ligament of Treitz. The balloons of single-lumen tubes should be deflated before insertion with a 21-gauge needle to allow escape of gas (as opposed to mercury) from the balloon (Fig 50–5). If a distended balloon (usually in place ten days or more) causes bowel obstruction, it can be deflated by techniques such as percutaneous needle puncture under fluoroscopy,[39] hyperbaric pressure,[40] or division of the tube to allow passage per rectum.[41] Progression of the tube through the small bowel is monitored with serial radiograms. If the distended bowel is atonic, passage into the jejunum is unlikely to be successful, and a nasogastric tube should be used in its place. Rapid intubation of the duodenum with endoscopes has been described but is not widely practiced. If peristalsis is active, the tube will usually enter the duodenum after the patient lies on the right side for several hours. *Changes in the physical examination at any time may herald the development of intestinal strangulation.*

Surgical Principles

Laparotomy and wide abdominal exploration using general anesthesia are necessary in most cases of mechanical small-bowel obstruction. The approach to external hernias is somewhat different (see below). Particular attention must be paid to gastric decompression prior to intubation because of the danger of massive tracheobronchial aspiration of gastric or small-bowel contents.[42] A midline incision is preferred, since it allows relatively rapid access to most recesses of the abdomen and strong closure. Usually the initial incision is placed on either side of the umbilicus and extended upward or downward as needed. If a previous midline scar is present, it should be excised and extended, if possible, to allow entry through unoperated abdominal wall. The peritoneum is opened with great care beneath an old incision because of the risk of underlying tightly adherent bowel. Adhesions to the abdominal wall are lysed with scissors, using gentle traction by the surgeon and countertraction by the assistant. Frequently adhesions are thin, and the surgeon's index finger can

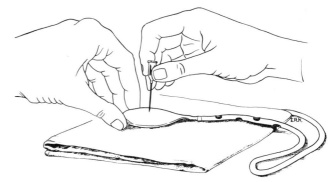

Fig 50–5.—Puncturing of long tube balloon prior to intubation to allow escape of gases within balloon.

be seen through them, allowing safe lysis (Fig 50–6). Small defects in the seromuscular layer caused by tearing are repaired with interrupted 3-0 silk sutures. Any open enterotomy should be closed in two layers using 3-0 or 4-0 Vicryl in the inner layer and 3-0 silk in the outer layer. Collapsed bowel is followed into the point of obstruction (Fig 50–7). If this is not possible, adhesions must be lysed gradually, until the bowel loops are eviscerated and the point of obstruction located (Fig 50–8). If the bowel is obstructed internally, the offending agent (e.g., a bolus of food or a gallstone) is removed through an enterotomy or by resection (e.g., small-bowel tumor).

Decompression of the bowel facilitates its handling, especially if resection is planned, and abdominal closure is simpler. However, there is no evidence that this maneuver shortens the period required for the bowel to regain its normal motility. If possible, retrograde decompression is done by stripping the bowel between the second and third fingers back to the duodenum and stomach, where the fluid is aspirated through a nasogastric tube. Tube gastrostomy should be considered in patients with chronic obstructive pulmonary disease, especially if a long period of decompression is anticipated.[43]

Alternatively, a long tube,[44] introduced through the nose, stomach, or cecum,[45] is advanced by the surgeon through the small bowel as it is aspirated. If possible, the bowel should not be intubated through the jejunum because of the high incidence of associated complications such as obstruction and leakage.[46] Long tube intubation may lengthen the period of postoperative ileus, and when only moderate small-bowel distention is present, decompression with a needle or catheter may be preferable.[47] These techniques may be compared to trocar decompression (Fig 50–9)[48, 49] through an enterotomy; the once-popular technique of threading the bowel over the tube is effective, but there is risk of peritoneal contamination and wound infection whenever an enterotomy is made.

It is important to determine the viability of the bowel intraoperatively and to carry out resection if appropriate (Fig 50–10). The antemesenteric border should be examined particularly carefully. Anastomoses must be made in viable segments of bowel. If the perfused state of the small bowel is

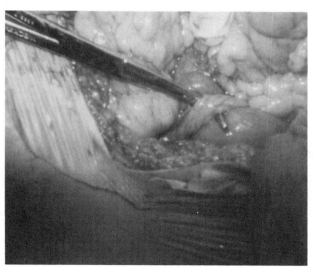

Fig 50–7.—Dense adhesion that caused mechanical small-bowel obstruction.

unclear, a "second-look" laparotomy may be indicated, especially if a long segment of bowel is involved. Standard parameters of small-bowel viability include: (1) color and luster of the bowel wall; (2) peristaltic activity; and (3) mesenteric pulsations. The bowel should appear pink and glistening beneath the operating room lights; a dusky, bluish bowel with little luster suggests ischemia. Peristalsis should generally be observed; if ileus is present, other criteria should be used. Pulsations should be present in the small vessels near the mesenteric border. Surgeons tend to err on the side of resection if these criteria are used.[50]

Several other techniques have been developed to assess bowel viability, but most are cumbersome and not applicable in most operating rooms. Two of the most useful methods include use of the gas-sterilized Doppler ultrasonic flow probe and study of the fluorescent pattern of blood supply under a Woods lamp after sodium fluorescein is injected.[51] Doppler probes are applied lightly over gel on the antemesenteric bor-

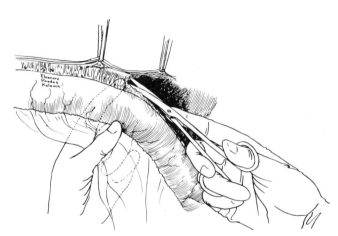

Fig 50–6.—Technique of lysis of adhesions to abdominal wall in region of laparotomy incision.

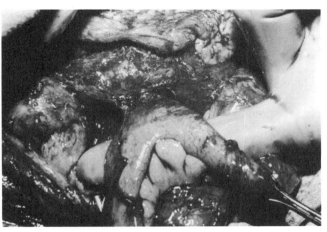

Fig 50–8.—Small-bowel obstruction caused by adhesion of small bowel to granulomatous colitis of right colon. (From Welch and Warshaw.[123] Used by permission.)

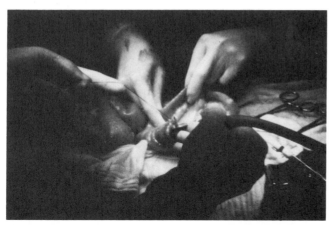

Fig 50–9.—Trocar decompression of small intestine. Wound protected by gauze pads and purse-string suture avoids contamination on trocar removal.

der. Audible flow signals are heard if there is blood supply to the bowel. In the laboratory, anastomoses carried out within 1 cm of a Doppler signal survive.[52, 53] In a prospective study the fluorescein pattern was significantly more accurate in predicting intestinal viability than either the Doppler method or standard clinical judgment.[50]

SPECIAL FORMS OF SMALL-BOWEL OBSTRUCTION

External Hernias

Hernias of many types are associated with intestinal obstruction, especially in economically impoverished parts of the world. They are second only to adhesions as a cause of small-bowel obstruction in the United States. External hernias are protrusions of a part of the abdominal cavity within a peritoneal sac into an extra-abdominal space (Fig 50–11). If

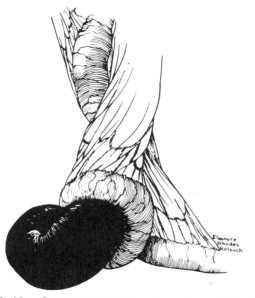

Fig 50–10.—Strangulation obstruction of small intestine.

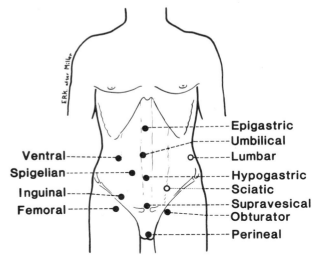

Fig 50–11.—Sites of external hernias, all of which predispose to mechanical small-bowel obstruction. (After Welch.[113] Used by permission.)

incarceration occurs within the hernial ring, simple or strangulation obstruction may result. All patients with acute small-bowel obstruction should be carefully examined for external hernias. Groin hernias can be confused with a variety of conditions, including lymphadenopathy, tumors, or thrombophlebitis. Lateral radiograms may show gas-containing bowel within the hernia sac (Fig 50–12). At operation the hernia sac, its neck, and the hernial contents must be exposed. If nonviable bowel is present, it is resected prior to repair of the hernia defect.

Richter's hernia describes a variant in which only a portion of the bowel circumference is incarcerated in the hernia sac (Fig 50–13). The most frequent sites of involvement are in the femoral and inguinal regions. Complete intestinal obstruction develops if more than two thirds of the wall is incarcerated.

Inguinal hernias usually incarcerate in the region of the internal ring. If strangulation is not suspected, the hernia can be reduced with analgesics and bed rest. If the hernia is reduced en masse, obstruction rarely will remain at the neck of

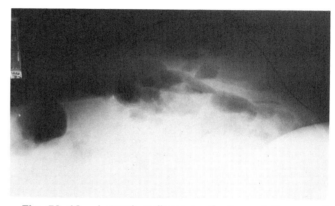

Fig 50–12.—Lateral radiogram of strangulating small bowel obstruction in ventral hernia.

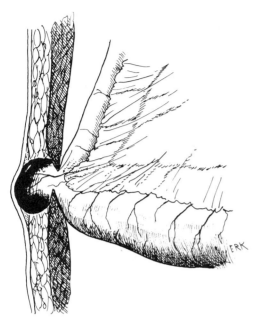

Fig 50–13.—Richter's hernia causing partial small-bowel obstruction.

the reduced sac in the preperitoneal space, and emergency operation is necessary. Forceful reduction can precipitate rupture of loops of bowel.[54] At operation the neck of the sac is separated from the inferior epigastric vessels, as the bowel is held to prevent retraction into the abdominal cavity.

Femoral hernias represent 5% of hernias.[55] Of importance, 20% incarcerate[56] because of the narrow neck of the hernia sac and the small size of the femoral canal.[57] The diagnosis can be confusing if there is no local groin tenderness or if signs of intestinal obstruction are subtle, as with a Richter's hernia. In obese patients there may be no palpable femoral mass. A standard incision is made above the inguinal ligament, and the sac is dissected free both above and below the inguinal ligament. If gangrenous bowel is suspected, it can be approached either intra-abdominally through a line deep to the inguinal incision[58] or through the opened sac, although there is greater risk of wound contamination in the latter case. The hernia repair uses Cooper's ligament as described by McVay.[59]

Umbilical hernias sometimes incarcerate in adults, especially in the obese, multiparous woman. Patients with ascites are at risk of hernia rupture, strangulation, ulceration, and infected ascites; operation should be done early in this population.[60] Large defects under any tension are closed with synthetic mesh.

Obturator hernias are unusual, but they cause intestinal obstruction 90% of the time.[61] Elderly thin women are usually affected, and the hernias can be bilateral. Strangulation is likely to occur because of the unyielding nature of the obturator canal.[62] Since the hernia contents press on the femoral nerve, pain or paresthesias running down the anteromedial aspect of the thigh (Howship-Romberg sign) are characteristic. A tender mass is palpable by rectal or vaginal examination. The diagnosis is only considered by the examiner in one quarter of the cases. Of the many surgical approaches, the

abdominal is preferable, since it allows excellent exposure of the obturator ring in the ischiopubic area. The ring is incised under direct vision. Following extraction of the small bowel, the base of the sac can be sutured over the obturator foramen orifice. Synthetic mesh is used if the defect is large.

Fewer than 2% of anterior abdominal wall hernias are *spigelian hernias*. Approximately 20% incarcerate because of the narrow, firm hernia neck.[63] They usually occur below the umbilicus in the "semilunar zone" between the muscular fibers and the aponeurosis of the transversus abdominis muscle.[64] The differential diagnosis includes rectus sheath hematomas and abdominal wall tumors. The diagnosis can be made with ultrasound of the abdominal wall.[65] The hernia sac is exposed by splitting the fibers of the external oblique muscle, and the successive abdominal layers are closed. Frequently the condition is confused with a direct inguinal hernia.

Parastomal hernias occur adjacent to stomas such as colostomies and ileostomies. Herniation occurs in the early postoperative period if the fascial defect is large. More commonly, hernias develop gradually with increased abdominal pressure from factors such as obesity or coughing, especially if the stoma exits lateral to the rectus sheath.[66] If intestinal obstruction occurs, the incarcerated bowel is freed, and frequently the stoma is moved to a new location.[66, 67] If the stoma is not moved, the stoma can emerge through mesh placed over the defect;[68] this approach is not favored unless there are multiple abdominal incisions.

Intestinal obstruction is a dreaded complication of *ambulatory peritoneal dialysis*. Increased intraperitoneal pressure from repeated infusion of dialysate and poor wound healing are associated with hernias in 10%–20% of this population[69] and intestinal obstruction in 4%–8%.[70] All such patients should be screened for hernias, and wound closure should be meticulous when dialysis catheters are inserted. In particular, a nonabsorbable monofilament suture is placed in a purse-string fashion around the dialysis catheter. Abdominal pain in these patients warrants careful examination for external hernias.

Internal Hernias

A viscus can protrude through a number of apertures within the abdomen to create internal hernias (Fig 50–14). At

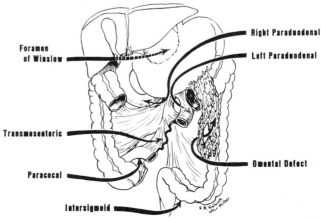

Fig 50–14.—Sites of internal hernias. (After Welch.[113] Used by permission.)

times the source of intermittent abdominal pain and nausea or full-blown episodes of mechanical obstruction, internal hernias should be suspected in patients who have no history of abdominal surgery or findings of external hernias. Contrast studies are of particular diagnostic value in the following circumstances: (1) inseparable loops of small bowel are seen crowded in the hernia sac; (2) the configuration and location of the small bowel are abnormal; or (3) there is abnormal stasis in the affected loops.[71] The relative incidence of the various types include paraduodenal (53%), paracecal (13%), foramen of Winslow (8%), transmesenteric (8%), pelvic and supravesical (7%), and intersigmoid (6%).[72]

Paraduodenal hernias occur on the left side 75% of the time, when the small bowel enters a sac behind the inferior mesenteric vein, where the fourth portion of the duodenum emerges from the retroperitoneum. Right paraduodenal hernias extend downward to the right behind the superior mesenteric artery. Contrast studies show the closely apposed loops passing through the hernia orifice; retroperitoneal protrusion is evident on lateral films.[73] Treatment is surgical. The hernia contents are reduced, and the hernia sac is either closed or opened widely. The inferior mesenteric vessels near the neck of the sac must be preserved when reducing left-sided hernias.[74] Several methods have been described to reduce incarcerated right paraduodenal hernias.[75] Division of the lateral attachments of the ascending colon allows transposition of the colon to the left side of the abdomen, and the right paraduodenal hernia sac becomes part of the peritoneal cavity.[75, 76]

Foramen of Winslow hernias may occur when mobile small-bowel loops on a long mesentery herniate through an enlarged foramen. In plain films, gas-containing loops of small bowel are seen medial and posterior to the stomach, together with small-bowel obstruction.[77] Simple reduction has not been followed by recurrence.[78] If closure of the foramen is attempted, extreme care must be taken to avoid damage to vital structures in the hepatoduodenal ligament and retroperitoneum. *Paracecal* hernias usually involve herniation of the ileum through the cecal mesentery into the right paracolic gutter. The treatment is surgical once the diagnosis is made.[79] Most *mesenteric* hernias in adults are related to inflammatory processes, previous trauma, or operation. Volvulus, closed loop obstruction, and strangulation may follow rapidly.[80] *Retroanastomotic* hernias rarely complicate gastrojejunostomies; they can involve the efferent (more commonly) or afferent loops. Half of the cases occur within a month of operation, and most are emergencies, with complete obstruction of the loop(s).[81] The disease is treacherous in the early postoperative period because of delay in diagnosis. Contrast studies are important in establishing the diagnosis, and hyperamylasemia is common. The hernia is reduced, and the retroanastomotic space is closed to prevent recurrence; a long afferent loop is shortened.

Postoperative Bowel Obstruction

Diagnosis and treatment of small-bowel obstruction in the early postoperative period (e.g., within two weeks of operation) may be exceedingly difficult. Common sequelae of abdominal operations, such as ileus related to sepsis or other factors, incisional tenderness, the use of analgesics, nausea,

or abdominal distention, tend to confuse the issue. The disease tends to follow colorectal or pelvic operations or appendectomies for acute appendicitis. Abdominoperineal resections are of particular concern, and trapping of the small bowel in the empty nonreperitonealized pelvis may be important.[82] Construction of an ileostomy following resection for inflammatory bowel disease is also associated with obstructive complications.[83] Intra-abdominal sepsis or adhesions are frequent causative factors.[84, 85] The operative mortality is considerable, in the range of 17%,[84] related to delay in diagnosis and general patient debility.[85]

All patients have abdominal distention, and most have colicky pain. However, vomiting is inconstant, since nasogastric tubes are frequently passed early.[84] Bowel sounds and bowel habits are variable, but the development of obstipation following a period of normal intestinal activity is worrisome. Differentiation of paralytic ileus and mechanical obstruction with plain films alone may be difficult.[86] If distended loops of small bowel are seen with little colonic gas, a mechanical source should be suspected. The use of enemas usually leads to the presence of air in the colon.

Initial treatment should include decompression with a long or short intestinal tube. If ileus or partial obstruction is suspected, this therapy may be continued for 24–72 hours safely if there is evidence of clinical improvement. The clinical tendency is to delay in this setting, given the known difficulty of relaparotomy in an already acutely ill patient.[87] However, with time, the affected bowel becomes more distended, thin-walled, and adherent.[83] The passage of flatus or stool should not be reassuring if the patient has other signs of intestinal obstruction.[86] Suspected high-grade obstruction requires prompt reoperation.

Gallstone Ileus

This condition, one of the many forms of obturation obstruction, is notoriously insidious in onset and difficult to diagnose. Primarily a disease of elderly women with past symptoms suggestive of chronic cholecystitis, it should be suspected in patients who have not had abdominal surgery. Gallstones obstructing the GI tract (typically in the terminal ileum)[88] are usually greater than 2.5 cm in diameter. The offending calculi usually travel into the duodenum through a fistulous connection with the inflamed gallbladder (Fig 50–15).

Symptoms of gallstone ileus tend to be intermittent ("tumbling obstruction") as the gallstone passes down the GI tract. "Classic" plain abdominal films show air in the biliary tree, distended small-bowel loops, and an opaque gallstone.[89] The calculus is also demonstrated with contrast studies.

Once the patient is hydrated, laparotomy is necessary. If the small bowel is viable, a longitudinal incision is made on the antemesenteric border proximal to the stone, which is milked proximally to the enterotomy site in dilated bowel (Fig 50–16). If there is firm impaction, the enterotomy is done directly at the point of obstruction. If bowel viability is in question, it is resected. The calculus can also be milked into the colon, although there is the theoretical danger of later colonic obstruction at a site of narrowing.[90] If the extracted gallstone is faceted, the entire large and small bowel should be examined for further gallstones. About 5% of patients de-

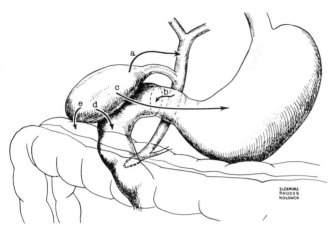

Fig 50–15.—Routes followed by biliary-enteric fistulas. The most common pathway is cholecystoduodenal. (From Welch.[88] Used by permission.)

velop recurrent gallstone ileus, usually attributable to retention of stones in the bowel proximal to the point of obstruction or to retained stones in the gallbladder.

The operative mortality has fallen to 5% from previous high levels. The issue of concomitant cholecystectomy revolves around the medical condition of the patient. A high-risk individual should have relief of the obstruction only. Other patients may have simultaneous cholecystostomy and later cholecystectomy if biliary symptoms persist. Low-risk patients tolerate cholecystectomy and fistula closure at the original operation well,[91] but morbidity may be associated with the extended operation, duodenal leakage, or other factors.

Recurrent Obstruction

A small proportion of patients develop dense, widespread adhesions requiring multiple operations. Complex adhesions are occasionally found at the first operation for mechanical

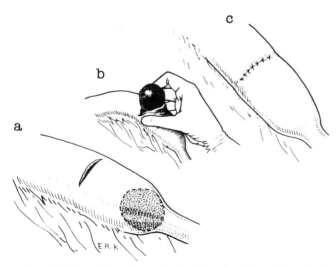

Fig 50–16.—Obturation obstruction (gallstone ileus): *(a)* enterotomy made in dilated proximal bowel; *(b)* calculus withdrawn through enterotomy; *(c)* final appearance of small intestine. (From Welch.[88] Used by permission.)

obstruction or in the presence of peritonitis. The surgeon finds himself mired in a difficult, time-consuming procedure in which there is considerable risk of creating inadvertent enterotomies. Several operations have been advocated for this setting. In 1937 the Noble plication procedure was introduced; multiple loops of adjacent bowel were sutured together in the hope of preventing further kinks and obstruction.[92] This time-consuming technique has been largely abandoned because of postoperative morbidity, including prolonged ileus, chronic abdominal pain, mesenteric strangulation, and a high incidence of internal fistula formation.[93] In the Childs-Phillips procedure, the small bowel is plicated with transmesenteric mattress sutures passed on long needles.[94] The procedure is not time-consuming, and the morbidity is lower than that following the Noble plication.[95] There is some risk of injuring the mesenteric vessels.

Today the intraluminal long tube stents popularized by Baker[96] for patients with complex adhesions are popular because of the relative safety and simplicity of tube insertion and positioning. Modifications of the Baker tube have been helpful in this regard.[44] The rationale for internal stenting together with lysis of adhesions is to control formation of adhesions in the early postoperative period, since the bowel is fixed in gentle curves rather than in acute angles by the stent. Introduced through one of several sites (e.g., nose, stomach, jejunum, cecum),[97, 98] the tube is not removed before the tenth postoperative day, by which time significant adhesions have formed.[99] Radiograms give an indication of the positioning of the bowel loops.

Complications of tube stenting include intraperitoneal contamination from enterotomy sites, prolonged ileus, difficulties with tube removal, or obstruction at the site of introduction (if the jejunum is used) or at a more distal site.[100] There are controversial data concerning the relative effectiveness of simple lysis of adhesions vs. lysis combined with internal stenting in lowering the reoperation rate for recurrent adhesions.[101, 102] Prospective randomized trials have not been done. The rate of recurrent obstruction in patients having internal stent procedures is in the range of 5%–10%.[96, 100, 103]

Miscellaneous Problems

Small-bowel obstruction in patients with a history of abdominal cancer should be treated aggressively with early operation, since benign disease or unrelated malignant disease may be present.[104] Treatment of the patient with known *carcinomatosis* is controversial. Obstruction in this setting is frequently incomplete, and strangulation obstruction is uncommon. The operative mortality is high because of poor nutrition and widespread carcinoma;[34, 105] yet, the alternative of continuous nasogastric suction and IV fluids is unsatisfactory for the patient and his family. In one study only 44% received palliation by surgery, for an average of two months.[106] When the colon was the site of obstruction, the palliation afforded by surgery was better.[106] Accurate determination of the cause of obstruction may be impossible short of operation. The gradual onset of obstruction in patients with malignant ascites without a specific radiological point of obstruction suggests carcinomatosis. Several factors such as patient age, tumor spread, and type and amount of prior therapy correlate well with prognosis in metastatic ovarian cancer.[107] Conservative measures with intubation should be attempted initially[108] and operation performed if improvement does not occur within several days. If multiple points of obstruction are encountered, enteroenterostomies or enterocolostomies should be attempted.[109] In the case of reobstruction, patient survival is short, and any benefit from surgery is unlikely.[110]

Malrotation of the intestinal tract may cause mechanical obstruction in adults. Anatomically the midgut rotation is arrested somewhere in its course.[111] Volvulus and gangrene of the small bowel may result when the entire jejunum and ileum hang by the long pedicle of the superior mesenteric vessels.[112] In the pregnant patient, crampy abdominal pain from this condition may be mistaken for labor pains; the outcome can be disastrous unless early operation is carried out.[113]

The management of *intussusception* in adults has been controversial, although traditionally it has been surgical.[114] In infants hydrostatic reduction alone serves as definitive treatment in many cases. Nagorney and colleagues[115] found that two thirds of colonic intussusceptions were associated with carcinoma of the colon (Fig 50–17); only one third of small-bowel malignancies were attributed to malignancy, and many of these were metastatic. Intestinal obstruction was incomplete in 80% of the cases. They concluded that colon intussusceptions should be resected without attempts at reduction, while small-bowel lesions should be reduced, followed by limited surgical resection. Occasionally, ileocecal intussusceptions in young adults are treated by simple reduction with intestinopexy of the cecum and terminal ileum if no intraluminal disease is palpable. Postoperative intussusception is a dif-

ferent entity, related to adhesions, suture lines, long intestinal tubes, or abnormal peristalsis of the bowel.[116] Reduction and lysis of adhesions is usually sufficient treatment. In the event of nonviability or an inability to reduce the intussusception, resection is necessary.

LARGE-BOWEL OBSTRUCTION

Mechanical large-bowel obstruction differs significantly from small-bowel obstruction in many respects, including the etiology, pathophysiology, and basic treatment approaches. At least 80% of colonic obstruction is attributed to colorectal cancer, and most of the remaining cases to volvulus, diverticulitis, and fecal impaction (Table 50–3).

Pathophysiology

Frequently, colonic obstruction related to diverticulitis or cancer is subacute or chronic, although impaction of feces in the narrowed portion can precipitate acute total obstruction. When swallowed air enters the colon proximal to a point of obstruction, dilatation occurs, but the early intraluminal fluid pooling and extracellular fluid deficits characteristic of acute small-bowel obstruction are not seen. In neglected cases, however, there can be large intraluminal fluid sequestrations,

TABLE 50–3.—CAUSES OF
MECHANICAL LARGE-BOWEL
OBSTRUCTION*

Intrinsic defects
  Congenital
  Inflammatory
    Diverticulitis
    Ulcerative and granulomatous colitis
    Miscellaneous
  Neoplastic
  Traumatic
  Intussusception
  Radiation strictures
  Peumatosis intestinalis
Obturation obstruction
  Gallstone
  Bezoar
  Foreign body
  Enterolith
  Fecal impaction
Volvulus
Extracolonic lesions
  Adhesions
  Herhias
    External
    Internal
  Compression by mass
    Carcinomatosis
    Abscess or tumor
    Pregnancy
    Foreign body
    Distended bladder
Postoperative
  Abscess
  Wound dehiscence
  Anastomotic leak, obstruction
  Obstructed external stoma
  Hernia through peritoneal defect or trap
  Volvulus

*Adapted from Love.[125]

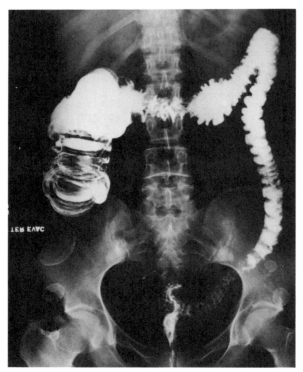

Fig 50–17.—Intussusception in proximal colon (barium enema view).

hypovolemia, oliguria, and hemoconcentration. Strangulation obstruction rarely occurs, except in occasional cases of colonic volvulus.

The response of the colon to mechanical obstruction varies depending on the "competency" of the ileocecal valve. If the valve is incompetent (in 50% of cases during barium enema examinations),[117] the small intestine serves to decompress the large bowel. In the case of a competent valve, the colon cannot decompress in a retrograde fashion, and a closed loop obstruction develops, with attendant dangers (Fig 50–18). Since the cecum has the widest diameter of the colon, its wall develops the highest pressures according to LaPlace's law, where the intraluminal pressure multiplied by the diameter of the particular segment of colon equals the tension on the colon wall at that point.[118] As a result, progressive colonic dilatation ultimately can cause cecal "diastatic" perforation. Studies suggest that the colon perforates when the intraluminal pressure increases to a range of 20–55 mm Hg.[119] Once the cecum reaches a diameter of 9–12 cm, the risk of perforation is significant.[120, 121] A variety of factors, including ischemia, bacterial overgrowth, and mechanical tearing of the bowel wall (not infrequently observed at operation), probably cause cecal perforation.[122]

Clinical Features

The most common symptoms of high-grade colonic obstruction are abdominal pain and distention, vomiting, and obstipation.[121] These symptoms may be superimposed on vague complaints related to the developing obstruction; e.g., flatulence, diarrhea, and variable degrees of abdominal distention. Most patients are elderly, since colorectal cancer predominates in this population. The disease presentation may be particularly insidious when lesions are situated in the right colon, where the lumen is wide and the contents similiquid. The onset of symptoms may be rapid if the lesion causes ileocolic intussusception or mechanical obstruction at the ileocecal valve, since acute small-bowel obstruction ensues.[123] Lesions in the left colon cause progressive constipation and finally obstipation, abdominal distention, and abdominal pain.

If an incompetent ileocecal valve allows retrograde decompression, the onset of distention may be gradual, with eventual development of feculent vomiting. In cases of volvulus, pain and abdominal distention occur rapidly if a closed loop obstruction and bowel ischemia are present.

Since abdominal distention is usually seen, it is difficult to

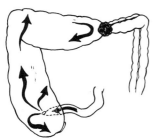 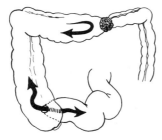

COMPETENT   INCOMPETENT

Fig 50–18.—Relationship of ileocecal valve to closed loop obstruction of the colon. Competent valve prevents reflux into small bowel.

localize specific areas of abdominal tenderness. Distention may be most marked in one region, e.g., the left upper quadrant in cecal volvulus. An abdominal mass is sometimes palpable if an advanced carcinoma (especially on the right side) is present. Hyperactive bowel sounds are common, especially if there is superimposed small-bowel obstruction. An empty rectal vault is suggestive of proximal obstruction, and blood on the examining finger indicates a distal lesion. Marked tenderness or rebound suggests the possibility of colonic perforation or strangulation.

Establishing the Diagnosis

Basic laboratory determinations are of little diagnostic import, but they are valuable in guiding later management. Anemia suggests poor nutrition or carcinoma, while leukocytosis is seen with dehydration, ischemia, and sepsis. Depending on the state of nutrition and disease severity, hypoalbuminemia, hemoconcentration, and azotemia are seen.

Radiologic studies are the most important diagnostic tools used in establishing the presence and level of obstruction. Plain and upright or decubitus films are obtained initially. Unfortunately, the films are sometimes difficult to evaluate, since the colon is prone to develop ileus or distention even in the absence of mechanical obstruction. In colonic ileus, the bowel is more likely to have thin, clear septa, a smooth inner contour, regular haustrations, and little intraluminal fluid. With chronic obstruction (e.g., carcinoma of the sigmoid colon), films show irregular septa, a ragged inner contour, irregular, thickened haustrations, a fluid-filled right colon, and considerable retained feces.[124]

Love[125] described three radiologic patterns of colon obstruction: (1) markedly dilated colon down to the point of obstruction, with little or no small-bowel dilatation (closed loop obstruction, Fig 50–19); (2) similar to 1, with the addition of severe small-bowel distention (closed loop with secondary small-bowel obstruction); (3) distention of the colon and small bowel, but the cecum is thick-walled and less distended than in 2 (incompetent ileocecal valve). However, factors other than an incompetent ileocecal valve may cause small-bowel distention, including simultaneous small-bowel obstruction caused by adherence to the colonic disease or secondary reflux ileus in response to colonic perforation.[122] In one review of large-bowel obstruction due to cancer, radiograms showed isolated large-bowel distention in 26%, combined large- and small-bowel distention in 58%, and isolated small-bowel distention in 16%[121] (Fig 50–20).

When x-rays suggest large-bowel obstruction, flexible or rigid sigmoidoscopy should be done to confirm the presence of a distal lesion. Careful pelvic and rectal examinations are necessary, because rectal lesions can be missed by endoscopic studies alone. Gentle insufflation of barium confirms the diagnosis of mechanical obstruction, whereas pseudo-obstruction is ruled out in most cases. Barium should not be refluxed above the point of obstruction because of the dangers of impaction. Diverticulitis is suggested by haustral thickening, a long length of involvement with preservation of the mucosa, and the presence of diverticula. With carcinoma, the involved segment tends to be shorter and the mucosa is destroyed. A "bird's beak" at the point of obstruction suggests volvulus (Fig 50–21). If there is suspicion of colonic perforation, a water-

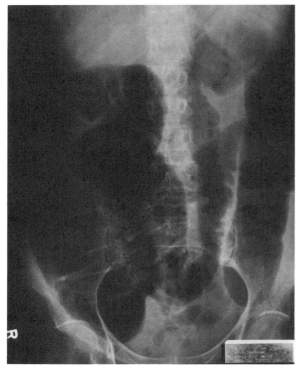

Fig 50–19.—Plain film demonstrating cut-off of colon gas in sigmoid colon by carcinoma. (From Welch and Welch.[128])

soluble contrast agent, rather than barium, should be used because of the morbidity associated with leakage of stool and barium into the peritoneal cavity.

Plan of Management

Intubation and infusion of fluids are begun immediately. Usually a nasogastric tube suffices, but a long tube may be

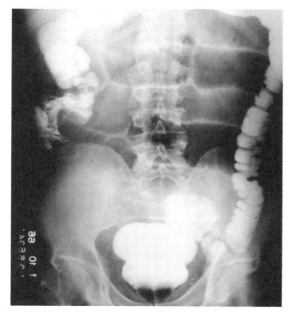

Fig 50–20.—Mechanical small-bowel obstruction caused by colon carcinoma at the ileocecal valve (From Welch and Warshaw.[123] Used by permission.)

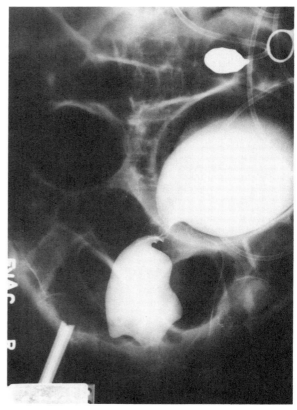

Fig 50–21.—Sigmoid volvulus. Barium enema shows characteristic "bird's beak" at point of obstruction.

passed if there is considerable small-bowel distention and evidence of peristalsis. The stomach must be emptied prior to induction of anesthesia. Monitoring of central venous pressure and urinary output are important in patients with marked distention. If a fecal impaction is suspected, this should be removed from below by manual means or enemas, if possible. In the case of sigmoid volvulus, passage of a soft rubber tube through a rigid sigmoidoscope relieves the obstruction and allows preparation for laparotomy on a less urgent basis. Cecal volvulus has been detorsed by barium enema[126] and by colonoscopy[127] as a temporizing measure.

Surgical intervention usually follows. The degree of obstruction and colonic dilatation influence the urgency of the procedure. Occasionally, a partially obstructing lesion will allow sufficient time preoperatively to prepare the colon mechanically for resection. The majority of patients, however, are prepared for early operation once the intravascular deficiencies are replaced and wide-spectrum antibiotics are administered. When complete colonic obstruction is present, the cecal diameter and degree of tenderness in the right lower quadrant provide further information concerning the risk of impending cecal perforation.

Surgical Approaches

A variety of operations can be broadly classified as: (1) decompressive procedures without resection, and (2) resections with or without anastomosis. The most common decompressive operations used are tube cecostomy and transverse colostomy.[128] Generally intended to provide temporary decompression as part of a "staged" procedure, they are closed once the primary disease has been treated or resected. Following surgical decompression, the colon is prepared adequately to allow resection and anastomosis under much safer conditions. If the underlying disease is incurable or unresectable, decompression can provide long-term relief from obstructive symptoms.

Tube cecostomy (Figs 50–22 and 50–23) is useful in fragile patients with carcinomas proximal to the splenic flexure, since it can be done using local anesthesia through a McBurney incision. It allows direct assessment of the cecal wall, and the fecal fistula closes after the tube is removed if there is no distal obstruction.[129] Mechanical preparation of the colon is not satisfactory unless a large-bore (e.g., 38 F) rubber catheter is passed into the ascending colon, which is irrigated frequently with several hundred milliliters of fluid. Wound sepsis is common, and intra-abdominal sepsis usually can be prevented by perioperative antibiotic use and protection of the wound and abdomen by gauze packs. Tube cecostomy is a valuable adjunct to detorsion in the treatment and prevention of further episodes of cecal volvulus. Together with colonoscopy, tube cecostomy has been useful for decompressing the cecum in acute colonic pseudo-obstruction.[130]

Transverse colostomies are of two major types: the "loop" colostomy and the divided stoma. In the former, a supporting bridge is passed through the transverse mesocolon (Figs 50–24 and 50–25). The divided stomas are usually matured to the abdominal wall, simplifying application of drainage bags and allowing complete diversion. Similar techniques are used in constructing sigmoid colostomies, although mobilization of this segment of the colon can be more difficult.

Transverse colostomy is used more widely than tube cecostomy for acute large-bowel obstruction, since it provides better decompression and complete defunctionalization. Wound contamination is less common, and there is no risk of erosion by an inlying tube. The procedure can be difficult in obese patients with distended abdomens, in which case general anesthesia is preferred. The colostomy also requires formal closure, exposing patients to an additional operation. Significant morbidity, such as prolapse (Fig 50–26), paracolostomy hernia, retraction, or stenosis, occurs 10%–20% of the time, and the direct mortality of the procedure is about 1%.[131] The eventual colostomy closure cannot be taken lightly, either,

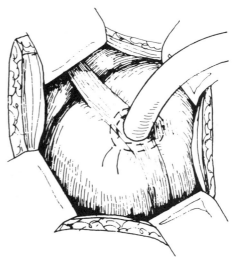

Fig 50–23.—Insertion of cecostomy tube into distended cecum. (From Welch and Welch.[128] Used by permission.)

since the risk of complications in one literature review was 28%, including wound infections (16%) and fecal fistulas (6%). The mortality was 1%.[132]

Bypass procedures provide relief of obstructive symptoms in patients with widespread incurable cancer. They also spare patients the morbidity and unpleasantness of a stoma. Closed loop obstruction may develop despite the bypass if the ileocecal valve is competent, and patients continue to have episodes of crampy pain. *Detorsion* is used in treatment of volvulus of the colon. In cecal volvulus, detorsion is followed by fixation with a tube cecostomy,[133] although some have favored cecopexy.[134] Since sigmoid volvulus is usually reduced by sigmoidoscopy alone, operative detorsion is rarely necessary.

Primary resection is well established as the operation of choice for perforating lesions of the colon. The ideal procedure in the presence of obstruction, especially of the left colon, is less clear.[135] Fecal loading and a distended, thin-walled colon are formidable obstacles for the surgeon, since it is established that manipulation or suturing of the distended colon

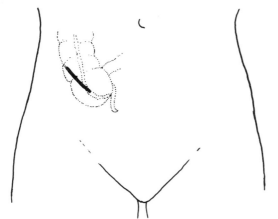

Fig 50–22.—Tube cecostomy incision. (From Welch and Welch.[128] Used by permission.)

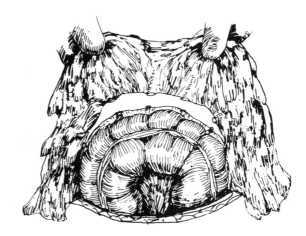

Fig 50–24.—Transverse colostomy. Omentum is separated from the transverse colon. (From Welch and Welch.[128] Used by permission.)

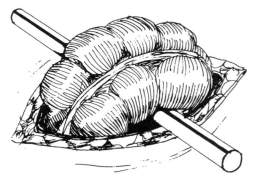

Fig 50–25.—Appearance of loop colostomy on abdominal wall. (From Welch and Welch.[128])

risks leakage and intra-abdominal contamination.[136] On the other hand, primary resection has the advantage of removing a colon cancer at the first operation and of lessening the number of operative procedures and the length of hospitalization.

If a primary resection is to be done safely, there must be no anastomotic tension or ischemia, and the united ends should be free of edema (Figs 50–27 to 50–29). The proximal segment should be free of large fecal fragments. Spillage of bowel contents must be avoided, and careful aseptic technique should include use of topical and systemic antibiotics. Gregg[137] has outlined several situations in which these objectives can be met: (1) when the entire obstructed segment can be removed, even with closed loop obstruction; (2) when the ileocecal valve is incompetent; and (3) when the bowel can be decompressed to a normal size intraoperatively, without vascular compromise. Following resection, the surgeon has the option of anastomosis or exteriorization of the cut ends. The anastomosis can be protected with a diverting colostomy.

Primary resection and anastomosis is the operation of choice for obstructing cancers of the right and transverse colon. The ileum and transverse colon are united by end-to-end

or side-to-end anastomosis (Fig 50–30), depending on the relative caliber of the bowel ends. Exposure is satisfactory, allowing a wide mesenteric resection. The cecum and ileum can be decompressed by a suction catheter placed into the portion of the ileum that is to be resected. Alternative procedures are used in two settings. For the very fragile patient, a preliminary cecostomy (for lesions distal to the cecum) or ileostomy (for lesions near the ileocecal valve) may be substituted. In the presence of established peritonitis, the risk of anastomotic leakage is increased,[138] and the bowel ends can be exteriorized (ileostomy and mucous fistula).

A variety of innovative techniques employing primary resection has been described for obstruction originating in the left colon.[139–144] Valerio and Jones[139] decompressed the colon with a Foley catheter, performed resection and anastomosis, and concluded with a protective colostomy. Subtotal colectomy allows anastomosis of small bowel and normal distal colon, which can be cleansed just prior to operation with Betadine enemas.[140, 141] Segmental left colectomy is possible following colon washout, using an irrigating catheter in the cecum and drainage tubing more distally.[144] Intraoperative rectal colonic irrigations can be used before and after the anastomosis to clear the distal colon of stool, to decompress the proximal bowel, and to demonstrate that the anastomosis is watertight.[143]

While several of the above reports have been notable, the fact remains that the leakage rate can be high following resection and anastomosis of the obstructed left colon, with mortalities as high as 50%.[145] Randomized prospective studies comparing primary resection and staged procedures in comparable groups of patients do not exist to my knowledge. At present, I prefer initial decompressive procedures in the presence of complete colonic obstruction with marked colonic (and at times small-bowel) distention. On occasion, with partial obstruction and minor colonic distention, a primary resection with exteriorization of the cut ends, or the Hartmann procedure, is favored. Primary resection and anastomosis is reserved for instances of low-grade obstruction without asso-

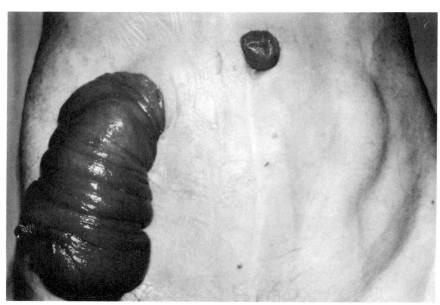

Fig 50–26.—Prolapse of transverse colostomy stoma.

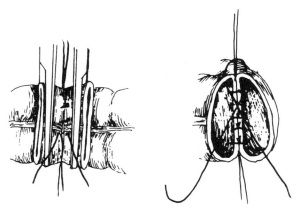

Fig 50–27.—End-to-end colocolic anastomosis. After posterior seromuscular row of 3-0 silk sutures *(left)* is completed, inner row of 3-0 chromic or Vicryl is begun *(right)*. (From Welch and Welch.[128])

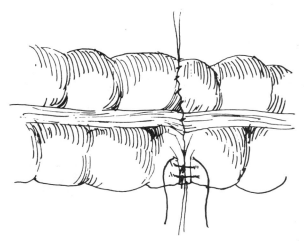

Fig 50–29.—Colocolic anastomosis. Outer layer of seromuscular sutures is created. (From Welch and Welch.[128])

ciated sepsis, where preoperative mechanical and antibiotic bowel preparation have been accomplished.

Major Types of Colon Obstruction

Eighty percent of acute large-bowel obstruction is attributable to *carcinoma*, and the principles discussed above apply primarily to this disease. Approximately 20% of colon cancers are complicated by some form of obstruction and 5%–10% by complete obstruction requiring emergency surgical intervention. Most cases involve the left colon, but the percentage of obstructing carcinomas is similar on both the left and right sides of the colon.[146] In recent years the percentage of cancers residing in the right colon has increased to 25%; the clinician should be alert to subtle signs of obstruction in these patients.

The hospital mortality rate remains high, in the range of 15%–30%,[121, 147–149] even when the offending carcinoma is situated in the right colon. If concurrent perforation exists, mortality rates are higher, and primary resection should be performed, if possible. Left-sided carcinoma with diastatic cecal perforation has been treated by cecostomy[150] and by subtotal colectomy;[137] the mortality is 18%.[121] The high mortality rates are attributable to the elderly patient population in a setting

of malnutrition, sepsis, and surgical stress. The overall five-year survival is only 15%–30%, reflecting high operative mortality and a high percentage of disseminated disease at the initial operation.[148, 149, 151]

Volvulus of the colon occurs in the cecum (25%–40%), in the transverse colon (0%–10%), and in the sigmoid. The symptoms of *cecal volvulus,* produced by at least a 180° twist of the mobile cecum, resemble those of acute small-bowel obstruction. Any factor distending the cecum (e.g., adhesions, colon cancer, pregnancy) can precipitate volvulus. Radiographically, the distended cecum is usually situated in the left upper quadrant (Fig 50–31), but the diagnosis can be confused with conditions such as sigmoid volvulus, ileus, or small-bowel obstruction. A gentle barium enema allows rapid diagnosis, when a "beaking" and sharply defined smooth arrest of contrast is seen. Operation is usually emergent (gangrene is seen in 25%–30%),[152] but mild, intermittent symptoms may allow elective intervention. Resection is necessary if gangrene is found. Recurrence rates following detorsion and cecopexy have ranged from 0% to 100%. The most important correlation with mortality (10%) is cecal gangrene.[153]

Transverse colon volvulus is unusual, and radiograms are

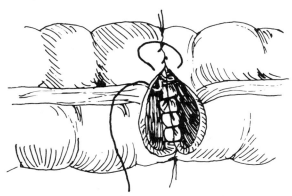

Fig 50–28.—Colocolic anastomosis. Completion of inner row. (From Welch and Welch.[128])

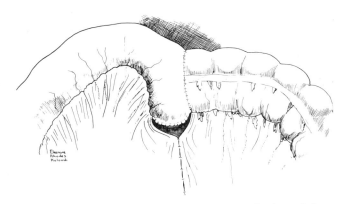

Fig 50–30.—Side-to-end ileotransverse colostomy following right hemicolectomy.

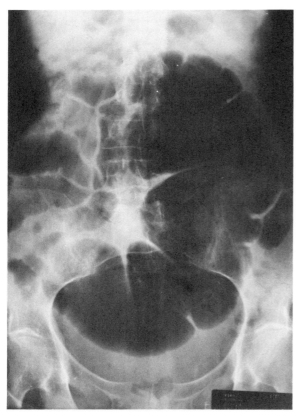

Fig 50–31.—Cecal volvulus. Plain film shows large distended bowel loop in left upper quadrant.

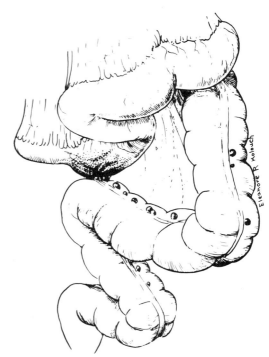

Fig 50–32.—Inflammatory small-bowel obstruction caused by adherence of small-bowel loop to area of diverticulitis.

suggestive of sigmoid volvulus. The point of obstruction is defined by barium enema. Resection is preferred to detorsion because of the high recurrence rate.[154] Colonoscopy is technically difficult, but it can detorse the bowel.[155] The operative mortality is as high as 33%.

Sigmoid volvulus accounts for 3%–5% of all cases of intestinal obstruction.[156] The sigmoid torses along a narrow mesenteric attachment. The disease typically occurs in elderly men; at least 15% have associated psychiatric disorders. Symptoms may be intermittent and mild (more common) or sudden and severe (seen in younger patients and associated with a high incidence of gangrene).[157] The affected loop resembles a "bent inner tube," and the characteristic "bird's beak" is apparent by barium enema. The volvulus can be detorsed 90% of the time with sigmoidoscopy;[158, 159] perforation by the sigmoidoscope is very rare.[160] If ischemic tissue is seen, immediate laparotomy is necessary. The recurrence rate is more than 50%.[159] The operative mortality ranges from 15% to 42%, and gangrene is seen 5%–10% of the time. Elective resection is best reserved for younger patients, since the mortality is as high as 15% in elderly patients having elective surgery.[158] Definitive treatment requires resection, and the Hartmann procedure has been quite effective.

Diverticulitis of the colon is associated with obstruction in 11% of patients, and the operative mortality is 2.6%.[161] Frequently, obstruction is subacute, and following a period of nasogastric suction and antibiotic administration, it resolves to

the point that bowel preparation is possible. A one-stage resection and anastomosis is feasible in this setting. If an intra-abdominal abscess is suggested by fever, leukocytosis, and an abdominal mass, early intervention is needed, usually consisting of abscess drainage and a completely diverting transverse colostomy. The small bowel may be adherent to the inflamed colon, causing a concomitant small-bowel obstruction that is relieved by a lysis of adhesions (Fig 50–32). Resection of a pelvic mass or distended colon may be difficult and hazardous. If a purely obstructive lesion, without evidence of perforation, is encountered, usually on the basis of circumferential pericolic fibrosis or of edema superimposed on chronic partial obstruction,[162] similar principles such as those outlined in the treatment of left colon cancer are followed.

REFERENCES

1. Sufian S., Matsumoto T.: Intestinal obstruction. *Am. J. Surg.* 130:9, 1975.
2. Kudchadkar A., Pauwaa M.C., Wilder J.R.: Acute intestinal obstruction. *Mt. Sinai J. Med.* (N.Y.) 46:247, 1979.
3. Shatila A.H., Chamberlain B.E., Webb W.R.: Current status of diagnosis and management of strangulation obstruction of the small bowel. *Am. J. Surg.* 132:299, 1976.
4. Bizer L.S., Liebling R.W., Delany H.M., et al.: Small bowel obstruction: the role of nonoperative treatment in simple intestinal obstruction and predictive criteria for strangulation obstruction. *Surgery* 89:407, 1981.
5. Barnett W.O., Petro A.B., Williamson J.W.: A current appraisal of problems with gangrenous bowel. *Ann. Surg.* 183:653, 1976.
6. Leffall L.D., Syphax B.: Clinical aids in strangulation intestinal obstruction. *Am. J. Surg.* 120:756, 1970.
7. VerSteeg K.R., Broders C.W.: Gangrene of the bowel. *Surg. Clin. North Am.* 59:869, 1979.

8. Wangensteen O.H.: The distention factor in simple intestinal obstruction. *Surgery* 5:32, 1939.
9. Herrin R.C., Meek W.J.: Distention as a factor in intestinal obstruction. *Arch. Intern. Med.* 51:152, 1933.
10. Sung D.T.W., Williams L.F. Jr.: Intestinal secretion after intravenous infusion in small bowel obstruction. *Am. J. Surg.* 121:91, 1971.
11. Wright H.K., O'Brien J.J., Tilson M.D.: Water absorption in experimental closed segment obstruction of the ileum in man. *Am. J. Surg.* 121:96, 1971.
12. Doyle R., Barnett W.O.: Toxicity of peritoneal fluid resulting from strangulation of various segments of the gastrointestinal tract. *Surg. Forum* 9:565, 1959.
13. Barnett W.O.: Experimental strangulated intestinal obstruction: a review. *Gastroenterology* 39:34, 1960.
14. Aird I.: Morbid influences in intestinal obstruction and strangulation. *Ann. Surg.* 114:385, 1941.
15. Cohn I., Hawthorne H.R.: Role of *Clostridium welchii* in strangulation obstruction. *Ann. Surg.* 134:999, 1951.
16. Silen W., Hein M.F., Goldman L.: Strangulation obstruction of the small intestine. *Arch. Surg.* 85:137, 1962.
17. Gammill S.L., Nice C.M. Jr.: Air-fluid levels: their occurrence in normal patients and their role in the analysis of ileus. *Surgery* 71:771, 1972.
18. Scott J.R., Miller W.T., Urso M., et al.: Acute mesenteric infarction. *A.J.R.* 113:269, 1971.
19. Levin B.: Mechanical small bowel obstruction. *Semin. Roentgenol.* 8:281, 1973.
20. Mellins H.Z., Rigler L.G.: The roentgen findings in strangulating obstructions of the small intestine. *A.J.R.* 71:404, 1954.
21. Williams J.L.: Fluid-filled loops in intestinal obstruction. *A.J.R.* 88:677, 1962.
22. Tibblin S.: Diagnosis of intestinal obstruction with special regard to plain roentgen examination of the abdomen. *Acta Chir. Scand.* 135:249, 1969.
23. Dunn J.T., Halls J.M., Berne T.V.: Roentgenographic contrast studies in acute small-bowel obstruction. *Arch. Surg.* 119:1305, 1984.
24. Sellink J.L.: Radiologic examination of the small intestine by duodenal intubation. *Acta Radiol.* 15:318, 1974.
25. Gurian L., Jendrzejewski J., Katon R., et al.: Small-bowel enema: an underutilized method of small-bowel examination. *Dig. Dis. Sci.* 27:1101, 1982.
26. Nelson S.W., Christoforidis A.J., Roenigk W.J.: Dangers and fallabilities of iodinated radiopaque media in obstruction of the small bowel. *Am. J. Surg.* 109:546, 1965.
27. Dixon J.A.: Barium sulfate and the obstructed small intestine. *Surg. Gynecol. Obstet.* 124:838, 1967.
28. Hanselman R.C., Mayer R.H.: Complications of gastrointestinal intubations: collective review. *Surg. Gynecol. Obstet.* 114:207, 1962.
29. Nagler R., Spiro H.M.: Persistent gastro-esophageal reflux induced during prolonged gastric intubation. *N. Engl. J. Med.* 269:495, 1963.
30. Brolin R.E.: The role of gastrointestinal tube decompression in the treatment of mechanical intestinal obstruction. *Am. Surg.* 49:131, 1983.
31. Hofstetter S.R.: Acute adhesive obstruction of the small intestine. *Surg. Gynecol. Obstet.* 152:141, 1981.
32. Peetz D.J. Jr., Gamelli R.L., Pilcher D.B.: Intestinal intubation in acute, mechanical small-bowel obstruction. *Arch. Surg.* 117:334, 1982.
33. Becker W.F.: Acute adhesive ileus: a study of 412 cases with particular reference to the abuse of tube decompression in treatment. *Surg. Gynecol. Obstet.* 95:472, 1952.
34. Laws H.L., Aldrete J.S.: Small bowel obstruction: a review of 465 cases. *South. Med. J.* 69:733, 1976.
35. Turner D.M., Croom R.D. III: Acute adhesive obstruction of the small intestine. *Am. Surg.* 49:126, 1983.
36. Shub H.A., Rubin R.J., Salvati E.P.: Intussusception complicating intestinal intubation with long Cantor tube: report of four cases. *Dis. Colon Rectum* 21:130, 1978.

37. Hafner C.D., Wylie J.H. Jr., Brush B.E.: Complications of gastrointestinal intubation. *Arch. Surg.* 83:147, 1961.
38. Smoger B.R., Rosen R.J., Teplick S.K., et al.: Small bowel obstruction caused by gaseous distention of the Cantor tube balloon. *A.J.R.* 135:612, 1980.
39. Coleman S.L., Miller W.E., Stroehlein J.R., et al.: Nonoperative retrieval of an impacted long intestinal tube. *Am. J. Dig. Dis.* 22:462, 1977.
40. Kulak R.G., Friedman B., Gelernt I.M., et al.: The entrapped intestinal balloon: deflation by hyperbaric therapy. *Ann. Surg.* 187:309, 1978.
41. Rozanski J., Kleinfeld M.: A complication of prolonged intestinal intubation: distention of the terminal balloon. *Dig. Dis. Sci.* 20:1067, 1975.
42. Stevens J.H.: Anesthetic problems of intestinal obstruction in adults. *Br. J. Anesth.* 36:438, 1964.
43. Shellito P.C., Malt R.A.: Tube gastrostomy: techniques and complications. *Ann. Surg.* 201:180, 1985.
44. Nelson R.L., Nyhus L.M.: A new long intestinal tube. *Surg. Gynecol. Obstet.* 149:581, 1979.
45. Jacobson Y.G.: Retrograde transcecal small-intestinal decompression in intestinal obstruction. *Dis. Colon Rectum* 16:110, 1973.
46. Chilimindris C.P., Stonesifer G.L. Jr.: Complications associated with the Baker tube jejunostomy. *Am. Surg.* 44:707, 1978.
47. Wickstrom P., Haglin J.J., Hitchcock C.R.: Intraoperative decompression of the obstructed small bowel. *Surgery* 73:212, 1973.
48. Barnes J.P.: Trocar decompression in acute small bowel obstruction. *Surgery* 37:542, 1955.
49. Williams C., Williams C. Jr.: Surgical aspiration of the bowel in advanced obstruction. *Ann. Surg.* 131:846, 1950.
50. Bulkley G.B., Zuidema G.D., Hamilton S.R., et al.: Intraoperative determination of small intestinal viability following ischemic injury. *Ann. Surg.* 193:628, 1981.
51. Mann A., Fazio V.W., Lucas F.V.: A comparative study of the use of fluorescein and the Doppler device in the determination of intestinal viability. *Surg. Gynecol. Obstet.* 154:53, 1982.
52. Cooperman M., Pace W.G., Martin E.W., et al.: Determination of viability of ischemic intestine by Doppler ultrasound. *Surgery* 83:705, 1978.
53. Wright C.B., Hobson R.W.: Prediction of intestinal viability using Doppler ultrasound techniques. *Am. J. Surg.* 129:642, 1975.
54. Colcock B.P., Braasch J.W.: Surgery of the small intestine in the adult, in Dunphy J.E. (ed.): *Major Problems in Clinical Surgery.* Philadelphia, W.B. Saunders Co., 1968, vol. 7, p. 220.
55. Ponka J.L., Brush B.E.: Problem of femoral hernia. *Arch. Surg.* 102:417, 1971.
56. Condon R.E., Nyhus L.M.: Complications of groin hernia, in Nyhus L.M., Condon R.E. (eds.): *Hernia.* Philadelphia, J.B. Lippincott Co., 1978, pp. 264–275.
57. McNealy R.W., Lichtenstein M.E., Todd M.A.: Diagnosis and management of incarcerated and strangulated femoral hernia. *Surg. Gynecol. Obstet.* 74:1005, 1942.
58. Dennis C., Varco R.L.: Femoral hernia with gangrenous bowel. *Surgery* 22:312, 1949.
59. McVay C.B.: The anatomic basis for inguinal and femoral hernioplasty. *Surg. Gynecol. Obstet.* 139:931, 1974.
60. O'Hara E.T., Lliai A., Patek A.J. Jr., et al.: Management of umbilical hernia associated with hepatic cirrhosis and ascites. *Ann. Surg.* 181:85, 1975.
61. Gray S.W., Skandalakis J.E.: Strangulated obturator hernia, in Nyhus L.M., Condon R.E. (ed.): *Hernia.* Philadelphia, J.B. Lippincott Co., 1978, pp. 427–442.
62. Joseph W.L., Kipen C.S., Longmire W.P. Jr.: Obturator hernia as a cause of acute intestinal obstruction. *Am. J. Surg.* 115:301, 1968.
63. Spangel L.: Spigelian hernia. *Surg. Clin. North Am.* 64:351, 1984.
64. Skandalakis J.E., Gray S.W., Akin J.T. Jr.: A surgical anatomy of hernia rings. *Surg. Clin. North Am.* 54:1227, 1974.
65. Gullmo A., Broome A., Smedberg S.: Herniography. *Surg. Clin. North Am.* 64:229, 1984.

66. Prian G.W., Sawyer R.B., Sawyer K.C.: Repair of peristomal colostomy hernias. *Am. J. Surg.* 130:694, 1975.
67. Cuthbertson A.M., Collins J.P.: Strangulated para-ileostomy hernia. *Aust. N.Z. J. Surg.* 47:86, 1977.
68. Leslie D.: The parastomal hernia. *Surg. Clin. North Am.* 64:407, 1984.
69. Engeset J., Youngson G.G.: Ambulatory peritoneal dialysis and hernial complications. *Surg. Clin. North Am.* 64:385, 1984.
70. Rubin J., Rajn S., Teal N., et al.: Abdominal hernia in patients undergoing continuous ambulatory peritoneal dialysis. *Arch. Intern. Med.* 142:1453, 1982.
71. Williams A.J.: Roentgen diagnosis of intra-abdominal hernia: an evaluation of the roentgen findings. *Radiology* 59:817, 1952.
72. Ghahremani G.G.: Internal abdominal hernias. *Surg. Clin. North Am.* 64:393, 1984.
73. Meyers M.A.: Paraduodenal hernias: radiologic and arteriographic diagnosis. *Radiology* 95:29, 1970.
74. Brigham R.A., Fallon W.F., Saunders J.R., et al.: Paraduodenal hernia: diagnosis and surgical management. *Surgery* 96:498, 1984.
75. Berardi R.: Paraduodenal hernias. *Surg. Gynecol. Obstet.* 152:99, 1984.
76. Bartlett M.K., Wang C., Williams W.H.: The surgical management of paraduodenal hernia. *Ann. Surg.* 168:249, 1968.
77. Erskine J.M.: Hernia through the foramen of Winslow. *Surg. Gynecol. Obstet.* 125:1093, 1967.
78. Schneider W.F., Hauck A.E., Stone H.H.: Hernia through the foramen of Winslow, in Nyhus L.M., Condon R.E. (eds.), *Hernia.* Philadelphia, J.B. Lippincott Co., 1978, pp. 494–498.
79. Bass J. Jr.: Paracecal hernia: case report and review of the literature. *Am. Surg.* 42:278, 1976.
80. Janin Y., Stone A.M., Wise L.: Mesenteric hernia. *Surg. Gynecol. Obstet.* 150:747, 1980.
81. Rutledge R.H.: Retroanastomotic hernias, in Nyhus L.M., Condon R.E. (eds.), *Hernia.* Philadelphia, J.B. Lippincott Co., 1978, pp. 499–506.
82. Hamer-Hodges D., Matheson N.A.: Intestinal obstruction after excision of the rectum. *Br. J. Surg.* 64:508, 1977.
83. Hughes E.S.R., McDermott F.T., Masterton J.P.: Intestinal obstruction following operation for inflammatory disease of the bowel. *Dis. Colon Rectum* 22:469, 1979.
84. Sykes P.A., Schofield P.F.: Early postoperative small bowel obstruction. *Br. J. Surg.* 61:594, 1974.
85. Coletti L., Bossart P.A.: Intestinal obstruction during the early postoperative period. *Arch. Surg.* 88:774, 1964.
86. Quatromoni J.C., Rosoff L. Sr., Halls J.M., et al.: Early postoperative small bowel obstruction. *Ann. Surg.* 191:72, 1980.
87. Harbrecht P.J., Garrison N., Fry D.E.: Early urgent laparotomy. *Arch. Surg.* 119:369, 1984.
88. Welch J.P.: Duodenal, gastric and biliary fistulas, in Schwartz S.I., Ellis H. (eds.): *Maingot's Abdominal Operations*, ed. 8. Norwalk, Appleton-Century-Crofts, 1985, pp. 701–739.
89. Rigler L.J., Borman C.N., Noble J.F.: Gallstone obstruction (pathogenesis and roentgen manifestations). *J.A.M.A.* 117:1753, 1941.
90. Holm-Nielsen P., Linnete-Jepsen P.: Colon obstruction caused by gallstones. *Acta Chir. Scand.* 107:31, 1954.
91. Day E.A., Marks C.: Gallstone ileus: review of literature and presentation of 34 new cases. *Am. J. Surg.* 129:552, 1975.
92. Noble T.B. Jr.: Plication of small intestine as prophylaxis against adhesions. *Am. J. Surg.* 35:41, 1937.
93. Wilson N.D.: Complications of the Noble procedure. *Am. J. Surg.* 108:264, 1964.
94. Childs W.A., Phillips R.B.: Experience with intestinal plication and a proposed modification. *Ann. Surg.* 152:258, 1960.
95. McCarthy J.D.: Further experience with the Childs-Phillips plication operation. *Am. J. Surg.* 130:15, 1975.
96. Baker J.W.: Stitchless plication for recurring obstruction of the small bowel. *Am. J. Surg.* 116:316, 1968.
97. Sanderson E.R.: Decompression of the small intestine by retrograde intubation. *Surg. Gynecol. Obstet.* 132:1073, 1971.
98. Robbins R.D., Hayes S.R., Thow G.B.: Long-tube gastrostomy with internal intestinal splinting: ten-year experience. *Dis. Colon Rectum* 23:10, 1980.
99. Heydinger D.K., Taylor P.H., Roettig L.C.: Recurrent intestinal obstruction. *Arch. Surg.* 80:670, 1960.
100. Weigelt J.A., Snyder W.H. III, Norman J.L.: Complications and results of 160 Baker tube plications. *Am. J. Surg.* 140:810, 1980.
101. Close M.B., Christensen N.M.: Transmesenteric small bowel plication or intraluminal tube stenting. *Am. J. Surg.* 138:89, 1979.
102. Brightwell N.L., McFee A.S., Aust J.B.: Bowel obstruction and the long tube stent. *Arch. Surg.* 112:505, 1977.
103. Munro A., Jones P.F.: Operative intubation in the treatment of complicated small bowel obstruction. *Br. J. Surg.* 65:123, 1978.
104. Pathak V., Swaminathan A.P., Ghuman S.S., et al.: Intestinal obstruction in carcinomatosis. *Am. Surg.* 46:691, 1980.
105. Ketcham A.S., Hoye R.C., Pilch Y.H., et al.: Delayed intestinal obstruction following treatment for cancer. *Cancer* 25:406, 1970.
106. Aabo K., Pedersen H., Bach F., et al.: Surgical management of intestinal obstruction in the late course of malignant disease. *Acta Chir. Scand.* 150:173, 1984.
107. Krebs H., Goplerud D.R.: The role of intestinal intubation in obstruction of the small intestine due to carcinoma of the ovary. *Surg. Gynecol. Obstet.* 158:467, 1984.
108. Glass R.L., LeDuc R.J.: Small intestinal obstruction from peritoneal carcinomatosis. *Am. J. Surg.* 125:316, 1973.
109. Sise J.G., Crichlow R.W.: Obstruction due to malignant tumors. *Semin. Oncol.* 5:213, 1978.
110. Osteen R.T., Guyton S., Steele G. Jr., et al.: Malignant intestinal obstruction. *Surgery* 87:611, 1980.
111. Wang C., Welch C.E.: Anomalies of intestinal rotation in adolescents and adults. *Surgery* 54:839, 1963.
112. Ripstein C.B., Miller G.G.: Volvulus of small intestine. *Surgery* 27:506, 1950.
113. Welch C.E.: *Intestinal Obstruction.* Chicago, Year Book Medical Publishers, 1958.
114. Weilbaecher D., Bolin J.A., Hearn D., et al.: Intussusception in adults: review of 160 cases. *Am. J. Surg.* 121:531, 1971.
115. Nagorney D.M., Sarr M.G., McIlrath D.C.: Surgical management of intussusception in the adult. *Ann. Surg.* 193:230, 1981.
116. Sarr M.G., Nagorney D.M., McIlrath D.C.: Postoperative intussusception in the adult. *Arch. Surg.* 116:144, 1981.
117. Ravid J.M.: Diastasis and diastatic perforation of the gastrointestinal tract. *Am. J. Pathol.* 27:33, 1951.
118. Stillwell G.K.: The law of LaPlace: some clinical applications. *Mayo Clin. Proc.* 48:863, 1973.
119. Novy S., Rogers L.F., Kirkpatrick W.: Diastatic rupture of the cecum in obstructing carcinoma of the left colon. *A.J.R.* 123:281, 1975.
120. Lowman R.M., Davis L.: Roentgen criteria of impending perforation of the cecum. *Radiology* 68:543, 1957.
121. Welch J.P., Donaldson G.A.: Management of severe obstruction of the large bowel due to malignant disease. *Am. J. Surg.* 127:492, 1974.
122. Greenlee H.B.: Acute large bowel obstruction: an update. *Surg. Annu.* 14:253, 1982.
123. Welch J.P., Warshaw A.L.: Isolated small bowel obstruction as the presenting feature of colonic disease. *Arch. Surg.* 112:809, 1977.
124. Bryk D., Soonuy K.Y.: Colonic ileus and its differential roentgen diagnosis. *Am. J. Roentgenol. Radium. Ther. Nucl. Med.* 101:329, 1967.
125. Love L.: Large bowel obstruction. *Semin. Roentgenol.* 8:299, 1973.
126. Meyers J.R., Heifetz C.G., Baue A.E.: Cecal volvulus: a lesion requiring resection. *Arch. Surg.* 104:594, 1972.
127. Anderson M.J., Okike N., Spencer R.J.: The colonoscope in cecal volvulus: a report of three cases. *Dis. Colon Rectum* 21:71, 1978.
128. Welch J.P., Welch C.E.: Operative management of cancer of the colon, in Maingot R. (ed.): *Abdominal Operations*, ed. 7.

New York, Appleton-Century-Crofts, 1980, pp. 2103–2150.

129. Stainback W.C., Christiansen K.H., Salva J.B.: Complementary tube cecostomy. *Surg. Clin. North Am.* 53:593, 1973.
130. Sterling J.R.: Treatment of nontoxic megacolon by colonoscopy. *Surgery* 94:677, 1983.
131. Hines J.R., Harris G.D.: Colostomy and colostomy closure. *Surg. Clin. North Am.* 57:1379, 1977.
132. Bozzetti F., Nava M., Bufalino R., et al.: Early local complications following colostomy closure in cancer patients. *Dis. Colon Rectum* 26:25, 1983.
133. Todd G.J., Forde K.A.: Volvulus of the cecum: choice of operation. *Am. J. Surg.* 138:632, 1979.
134. Howard R.S., Catto J.: Cecal volvulus: a case for nonresectional therapy. *Arch. Surg.* 115:273, 1980.
135. Carson S.N., Poticha S.M., Shields T.W.: Carcinoma obstructing the left side of the colon. *Arch. Surg.* 112:523, 1977.
136. Atik M., Castleberry J.W., Werner J.C., et al.: An experimental study of primary anastomosis of the obstructed colon. *Surg. Gynecol. Obstet.* 110:697, 1960.
137. Gregg R.O.: The place of emergency resection in the management of obstructing and perforating lesions of the colon. *Surgery* 37:754, 1955.
138. Debas H.T., Thompson F.B.: Mortality in emergency right hemicolectomy. *Can. J. Surg.* 16:399, 1973.
139. Valerio D., Jones P.F.: Immediate resection in the treatment of large bowel emergencies. *Br. J. Surg.* 65:712, 1978.
140. Deutsch A.A., Zelikovski A., Sternberg A., et al.: One-stage subtotal colectomy with anastomosis for obstructing carcinoma of the left colon. *Dis. Colon Rectum* 26:227, 1983.
141. Glass R.L., Smith L.E., Cochran R.C.: Subtotal colectomy for obstructing carcinoma of the left colon. *Am. J. Surg.* 145:335, 1983.
142. Fielding L.P., Wells B.W.: Survival after primary and after staged resection for large bowel obstruction caused by cancer. *Br. J. Surg.* 61:16, 1974.
143. Thow G.B.: Emergency left colon resection with primary anastomosis. *Dis. Colon Rectum* 23:17, 1980.
144. Dudley H.A.F., Radcliffe A.G., McGeehan D.: Intraoperative irrigation of the colon to permit primary anastomosis. *Br. J. Surg.* 67:80, 1980.
145. Irvin T.T., Greaney M.G.: The treating of colonic cancer presenting with intestinal obstruction. *Br. J. Surg.* 64:741, 1977.
146. Goligher J.C., Smiddy F.G.: The treatment of acute obstruction or perforation with carcinoma of the colon and rectum. *Br. J. Surg.* 45:270, 1957.
147. Clark J., Hall A.W., Moossa A.R.: Treatment of obstructing cancer of the colon and rectum. *Surg. Gynecol. Obstet.* 141:541, 1975.
148. Sugarbaker P.H.: Carcinoma of the colon-prognosis and operative choice. *Curr. Probl. Surg.* 18:754, 1981.
149. Umpleby H.C., Williamson R.C.N.: Survival in acute obstructing colorectal carcinoma. *Dis. Colon Rectum* 27:299, 1984.
150. Rack F.J.: Obstructive perforation of the cecum. *Am. J. Surg.* 84:527, 1952.
151. Willett C., Tepper J.E., Cohen A., et al.: Obstructive and perforative colonic carcinoma: patterns of failure. *J. Clin. Oncol.* 3:379, 1985.
152. Krippaehne W.K., Vetto R.N., Jenkins C.C.: Volvulus of the ascending colon: a report of 22 cases. *Am. J. Surg.* 114:323, 1967.
153. O'Mara C.S., Wilson T.H., Stonesifer G.L., et al.: Cecal volvulus: an analysis of 50 patients with long-term follow-up. *Ann. Surg.* 189:724, 1979.
154. Zinken L.D., Katz L.D., Rosin J.D.: Volvulus of the transverse colon: report of a case and review of the literature. *Dis. Colon Rectum* 22:492, 1979.
155. Jorgensen K., Kronborg O.: The colonoscope in volvulus of the transverse colon. *Dis. Colon Rectum* 23:357, 1980.
156. Anderson J.R., Lee D., Taylor T.V., et al.: Volvulus of the transverse colon. *Br. J. Surg.* 68:179, 1981.
157. Hinshaw D.B., Carter R.: Surgical management of acute volvulus of the sigmoid colon: a study of 55 cases. *Ann. Surg.* 146:52, 1967.
158. Drapanas T., Stewart J.D.: Acute sigmoid volvulus: concepts in surgical treatment. *Am. J. Surg.* 101:70, 1961.
159. Wertkin M.G., Aufses A.H. Jr.: Management of volvulus of the colon. *Dis. Colon Rectum* 21:40, 1978.
160. Arnold G.J., Nance F.C.: Volvulus of the sigmoid colon. *Ann. Surg.* 177:527, 1973.
161. Rodkey G.V., Welch C.E.: Changing patterns in the surgical treatment of diverticular disease. *Ann. Surg.* 200:466, 1984.
162. Hughes L.E.: Complications of diverticular disease: inflammation, obstruction and bleeding. *Clin. Gastroenterol.* 4:147, 1975.

PART VIII

Invited Commentaries

Esophageal Surgery

RONALD BELSEY, M.B., F.R.C.S.

ESOPHAGEAL SURGERY is currently passing through a stage of transition. The potential for cure of both benign and malignant disease has been demonstrated, but general acceptance of the principles involved remains elusive. The esophageal function laboratory has revealed a whole new spectrum of physiologic disorders of unknown etiology, frequently incurable but amenable to surgical palliation when diagnosed on objective evidence. The lower sphincter has attracted more attention than it deserves, and manometry has contributed little to the planning of the surgical control of reflux. Investigation of the efficiency of the esophageal pump and of gastric emptying has contributed more relevant information. However, the 24-hour pH study has been fully vindicated as the most reliable objective indication of pathologic reflux.

The variety of surgical antireflux procedures currently practiced, often based on unacceptable indications, suggests a persisting lack of comprehension of the basic principles involved in the control of reflux. The current spate of "modifications" of established techniques implies that former enthusiastic claims for their success were premature and certainly unsupported by the increasing incidence of recurrent reflux and failed antireflux surgery. Regrettably, the long-term results, as revealed in the harsh and unforgiving light of the follow-up clinic, continue to escape documentation: completely ignored or reported with a brevity designed to conceal the disillusionment. The opinions of gastroenterologists on the results continue to conflict dramatically with the complacency of the operating surgeons.

There is no "best" antireflux procedure. The operation of choice is that which, in the hands of an individual surgeon, satisfies all or most of the strict criteria demanded of any technique—complete and permanent relief of symptoms and complications; confirmation by objective evidence; applicability to infants and children, to cases of recurrent reflux, and to cases complicated by functional anomalies of the esophageal pump.

The more important role of manometry has emerged in the diagnosis of the complex functional disorders of the esophagus and in demonstrating the interrelationship of anomalies formerly considered to be confined to one section of the organ. In spite of the objective evidence now available, disagreement persists on the optimal surgical management of functional disorders. Fortunately, more attention is now directed to the underlying anomalies than to the pathologic sequelae that formerly monopolized the "state of play" in this intriguing field.

The prognosis of esophageal cancer remains, for the majority of patients, as depressing as ever. Skinner has demonstrated that the prospect for cure of a few early stage I tumors can be enhanced by a radical surgical approach enlisting the principles of cancer surgery demanded elsewhere in the body, within the limitations of the anatomical factors specific to the mediastinum. Skinner's contention is supported by the published evidence from China, but it is inconceivable that their methods of early detection will ever become economically or psychologically acceptable in the Western hemisphere. The futility of advocating early diagnosis is emphasized by the stage III status of 75% of patients admitted to hospital with symptoms. The rare early diagnosis is often frustrated by delay in definitive treatment, by preoperative radiation therapy now recognized as unhelpful, or by chemotherapy that seduces the oncologist by a sometimes dramatic response in the primary tumor, while metastases continue to disseminate inexorably. Until improvements in the efficacy of adjuvant therapy can be convincingly demonstrated, with less toxicity and fewer lethal complications, surgical excision at the earliest possible moment will continue to be the main line of attack.

The possibility for cure has introduced a further dimension, the long-term functional results of reconstruction following excision. Apparent cure may be thwarted by the late non-malignant complications peculiar to the technique employed. The technically easy reconstruction may not be in the best interest of the patient who has the chance of survival.

There is still a place for palliative surgery to relieve temporarily the suffering of the 75% of patients not amenable to curative resection. The quality of survival is of more concern to the patient than the duration, but symptomatic relief must be complete to justify "palliation." In this context, the technique of palliative resection is as important as that demanded of curative resection. The immediate and major problem in cancer surgery is the reduction of operative mortality and morbidity.

The management of esophageal trauma, and of corrosive burns in particular, remains highly controversial. There is no consensus on the indications for radiology and endoscopy in the early diagnosis of corrosive burns, nor on the emergency treatment. It is improbable that attempts to stage esophageal burns by superficial endoscopic examination will prove any more effective as a guide to treatment and prognosis than the superficial examination of a thermal burn of the skin. The overriding principle in the management of esophageal trauma is not to make the situation worse by ill-advised interference, including the proved trauma of endoscopy, jeopardizing the natural healing process. The majority of surgeons with experience in this field now accept the fact that no emergency treatment is likely to influence the prognosis or subsequent stenosis. The indications for emergency thoracotomy or laparotomy are clinical and radiologic evidence of perforation, rarely encountered. The time when endoscopy will prove informative and least dangerous is at three weeks following the trauma, when healing is in progress and dysphagia is increasing.

The majority of postcorrosive strictures can be treated by dilatation. Undilatable strictures call for resection, preferably, and reconstruction. Bypass does not eliminate the risk of subsequent malignancy. The type of reconstructive technique is dictated by the long-term survival of the patient; isoperistaltic interposition procedures are mandatory.

The attention paid to esophageal trauma secondary to penetrating chest wounds is timely and welcome. With a mortality rate of 50% from delayed diagnosis and treatment, a radiopaque esophagogram should now become a routine step in the early investigation of every penetrating wound and is mandatory on the most slender suspicion of an instrumental perforation or spontaneous rupture. In the latter situation, instruction in the clinical diagnosis must stress the 12-hour "stay of execution" allowed the surgeon with any hope of salvage by primary repair. A regrettable contemporary trend in surgery is the delay in definitive emergency treatment caused by irrelevant and frivolous investigations, probably prompted by the instinct of self-preservation in the face of possible medicolegal complications.

Gastroduodenal Disease

Jonathan E. Rhoads, M.D.

The section on "Gastroduodenal Disease" consists of an introduction by Frank G. Moody and seven chapters covering the pathogenesis of acid-peptic disease, stress erosive gastritis, duodenal ulcers, gastric ulcers, gastric cancer, postgastrectomy syndromes, and gastric procedures for morbid obesity. Each chapter is beautifully done, with lavish documentation providing complete catalogue of both historical and recent information in each field and a valuable index to both classic and modern, original papers.

An impressive amount of information has been compiled on the physiology and pathophysiology of diseases of the stomach and duodenum that somehow falls short of a complete, convincing picture. This is perhaps most apparent in the chapter on pathogenesis of acid-peptic disease. The evidence from epidemiologic, genetic, psychologic, and physiologic studies is presented. Acid remains clearly central to the ulcer problem: its exaggerated production resulting from excessive gastrin formation in the Zollinger-Ellison syndrome seems definitive. Evaluating nonphysiologic evidence in general is difficult. The authors' critical, perceptive review of these areas shows how little of the information developed can pass critical tests of statistical analysis. This is not to dismiss all such studies, since they propose relationships basic for future examination. The sections on gastric and duodenal ulcer in conjunction with the chapter on pathogenesis present an amazing picture: despite the gaps in our knowledge of the pathogenesis, surgeons have developed effective means of dealing with those gastric and duodenal ulcers that do not respond adequately to medical therapy.

It is the impression of most surgeons with whom I exchange information that the incidence of peptic ulcer surgery has declined materially. This may be due to reclassification of cases, but I find this explanation hard to accept. It is difficult to be sure whether the actual incidence of ulcer disease is declining or only that fraction that requires surgical intervention. The H_2 blockers—cimetidine and ranitidine are the best known—have been strikingly effective on a short-term basis, although the recurrence rate is high when their use is discontinued. Their ultimate role will evolve with longer experience, but frequently they can allay symptoms and lead to the healing of peptic ulcers during a course of treatment. Similar blockers with even a lower incidence of side effects may be developed for a longer term use.

In pernicious anemia the incidence of gastric cancer is higher, a relationship usually explained by the decrease in acid. There is apparently objective evidence that with the decrease in acid caused by H_2 blockers, microbiological activity in the stomach is increased, with the potential production of more nitroso compounds.

Stress ulcers were indeed rare 50 years ago, before the development of blood banks, probably because persons in deep shock tended to die. As blood banking and the free use of transfusions were developed, more patients close to fatal shock were kept alive. Stress ulcers became common, although the form associated with extensive burns described by Curling was not frequent. The more recent improvement in the incidence of these ulcers and in the outcome, both owing to better support of the circulation and to the use of H_2 blockers, is noteworthy, and I think constitutes a significant advance in the care of patients.

In the chapter on gastric cancer, I had hoped to find more information on the sharp decrease in the mortality of gastric cancer in this country—among the more striking phenomena of our time, followed only by the enormous rise in the incidence of lung cancer. It remains a mystery. The increase in mechanical refrigeration is often cited as one contributory factor to survival; the remainder are still unknown. Furthermore, since in this country the results of surgical treatment of gastric cancer have improved so little, this decrease in gastric cancer deaths must reflect an overall decrease in the incidence of gastric cancer of almost as great an extent.

In Japan, at least until recently, gastric cancer has accounted for nearly half of all the cancer deaths, much of which has been attributed to environmental factors—presumably food and its preparation (smoked fish; cooking over open charcoal braziers). Studies by Dr. Sugimura have identified a variety of mutagenic materials in the Japanese diet. The belief is that some of these are carcinogenic, since Japanese migrating to Hawaii have a reduced incidence of gastric cancer (studies designed largely by Haenszel). It behooves us to discover these cancer-producing factors, but definitive evidence is not yet at hand.

One chapter covered gastric procedures for morbid obesity, which has by now supplanted the jejunoileal bypass. It has undergone several modifications, the more recent of which, as pointed out by Dr. Griffin, have not been in use long enough for long-term evaluation. They seem remarkably successful and are quite likely to undergo further modification aimed at decreasing the number of patients who lose too little or gain too much weight after two to four years.

As with nearly all surgical endeavors, a fringe of poor results is associated with various forms of gastrectomy as related in the chapter on the postgastrectomy syndromes. Explanations are lacking of why patients react so differently to procedures that seem standardized. The experience and the current methods of affording patients' relief are well presented by Dr. Ritchie.

One cannot help being impressed with the enormous increase in knowledge over the past 50 years. When I was a house officer, histamine and gastrin were the only well-recognized hormones affecting the stomach. Secretin and cholecystokinin were then on the horizon, but now many active agents appear to be produced in the GI tract or elsewhere in the body to affect the GI tract. The surgical procedures have gone from hazardous gastrectomies for cancer, with timid gastroenterostomies for ulcer, up to 80% gastrectomies for ulcer, and back to pyloroplasty and vagotomy or antrectomy and vagotomy, or, as another alternative, selective vagotomy.

It is a privilege to have all of this information in one place and presented by acknowledged authorities in the several fields.

Gallbladder-Biliary Tract Disease

ROBERT E. HERMANN, M.D.

THE DIAGNOSIS AND MANAGEMENT of gallstones and of biliary tract disease have undergone many changes recently. Our understanding of why gallstones form, the solubility of bile, normal mechanisms of cholesterol and bile acid secretion, reabsorption in the intestine, and the relationship of these normal mechanisms to sex, hormonal changes, the aging process, fasting, and changes in dietary habits all are being actively investigated in many institutions. From studies in the Orient as well as in this country, it is recognized that bile stasis and primary bile duct stones in the intrahepatic and extrahepatic bile ducts occur with some frequency in certain disease conditions in which chronic infection or chronic bile stasis exist.

Attempts to prevent or dissolve gallstones and bile duct stones by medical means, by medications either taken orally or infused directly into the gallbladder or bile ducts, have been disappointing. Other attempts are under way in Germany to fragment gallstones using ultrasonic waves, with the hope that the small stone particles will pass through the bile duct into the intestine, with or without the help of endoscopic sphincterotomy.

Several diagnostic techniques have become available during the past ten years to aid in the diagnosis of biliary tract disease. These include ultrasound (US) scans of the gallbladder and bile ducts, computed tomography (CT) scans, endoscopic retrograde cholangiopancreatography (ERCP), percutaneous transhepatic cholangiography (PTC), and radionuclide scans using technetium 99 (HIDA, DISIDA, and PIPIDA). The oral cholecystogram is no longer routinely used for the diagnosis of acute cholecystitis but continues to be used for the diagnosis of chronic cholecystitis. Intravenous cholangiography has been generally abandoned with improvement in the methods of direct visualization of the biliary system.

Upper gastrointestinal (GI) endoscopy has contributed significantly to our diagnostic capabilities in biliary tract disease, becoming increasingly significant in the therapy for retained and recurrent bile duct stones. Endoscopic techniques permit the placement of small balloon catheters into the distal bile duct for manometric studies of the choledochal sphincter and for dilatation of bile duct strictures and areas of stenosis. Working through a matured T-tube tract, radiologists can extract retained stones from the bile duct, and endoscopists can pass small fiberoptic cholangioscopes into the biliary system directly to observe or biopsy intrabiliary ductal changes.

Gallstones continue to be identified in a presymptomatic stage in significant numbers of patients. The controversy about when to recommend prophylactic cholecystectomy for patients with asymptomatic gallstones continues. Individualizing this decision is probably the best recommendation that can be given. Guidelines

793

include the fact that from 20% to 30% of patients with silent gallstones will develop symptoms during a follow-up observation period of up to 20 years, and elective cholecystectomy is extraordinarily safe, whereas a semiurgent cholecystectomy for acute cholecystitis carries a significantly higher risk. When biliary disease presents symptomatically in the older patient, aged 65 years or older, it is more likely to be complicated by a high incidence of bile duct stones and a significantly higher morbidity and mortality. Cholecystectomy is advised by many surgeons as a prophylactic procedure for young, asymptomatic patients.

The technical aspects of performing cholecystectomy continue to be emphasized. Since this operation is performed so frequently, it must be performed safely. Bile duct injuries and overlooked common bile duct stones or other missed pathology of the bile ducts and liver, especially tumors, sclerosing cholangitis, and congenital anomalies of the biliary system, are still unacceptably common. A carefully performed cholecystectomy, accompanied routinely by intraoperative cholangiography and by intraoperative choledochoscopy whenever findings indicate a dilated bile duct, multiple stones in the duct, or any other unusual result, all will improve the safety and effectiveness of cholecystectomy and common bile duct exploration.

Antibiotic prophylaxis to cover the operative period is routinely performed for patients undergoing cholecystectomy for acute cholecystitis. Its use for patients undergoing elective cholecystectomy for chronic cholecystitis remains controversial, although several surgeons emphasize its value if common bile duct stones unexpectedly are found during the course of surgery. Since antibiotic prophylaxis for all patients undergoing cholecystectomy is safe and not expensive, there is a good argument for its use in all patients, even those without evidence of active biliary infection. Drains are no longer used routinely after cholecystectomy or other operations on the biliary tract. Many patients having elective operations on the biliary system are now admitted on the morning of the operative procedure and are discharged as early as two to five days postoperatively.

In my opinion the incidence of postcholecystectomy complications and recurrent pain after cholecystectomy, or the postcholecystectomy syndrome, can be minimized by careful, accurate preoperative diagnostic studies, so that cholecystectomy is performed for biliary symptoms and not for symptoms of other upper GI problems, and by careful performance of the operative procedure, so that other lesions are not missed and injury to other structures is not created. A small group of patients will continue to have symptoms. Further diagnostic efforts now frequently include endoscopic evaluation with ERCP and endoscopic manometric studies of the sphincter of Oddi; endoscopic sphincterotomy may sometimes be helpful. The role of operative sphincteroplasty with pancreatic duct sphincterotomy or septoplasty is controversial but has clearly provided relief for some patients. Selection of appropriate patients for this procedure is obviously the key to good results.

The incidence of strictures of the bile duct has continued to decrease during the past ten years, probably because of more careful performance of biliary surgery in the United States, the increased number of well-trained surgeons generally available, and, I believe, because of the increasingly routine use of intraoperative cholangiography to identify the bile duct and bile duct anomalies. When a bile duct injury occurs, it should be carefully repaired, using fine chromic catgut sutures over a T-tube stent. If it cannot be primarily repaired, it should be reconstructed by means of a choledochojejunostomy using a Roux-en-Y segment of jejunum. Late and recurrent strictures can be repaired with a high incidence of success, in the range of 80%, using careful techniques of choledochoduodenostomy or choledochojejunostomy.

The management of recurrent bile duct stones that occur after a previous cholecystectomy or common bile duct exploration is now, in most major centers, achieved primarily by means of endoscopic sphincterotomy. When large stones (2 cm or larger) are seen on a cholangiogram, when multiple stones (more than five) are found, when there is a significant degree of distal bile duct stenosis and proximal bile duct dilation, or when there are anatomical findings around the papilla of Vater, such as a periampullary diverticulum, which makes endoscopic sphincterotomy dangerous, then open operative exploration of the bile duct with removal of the stones should be undertaken. At operation, the surgeon is faced with deciding whether to explore the bile duct, remove the stones, and close the bile duct primarily with a T tube or whether to add a drainage procedure, choledochoduodenostomy or choledochojejunostomy. This decision is difficult. We add a drainage procedure selectively for patients with multiple bile duct stones, with stasis stones, and those with a dilated bile duct and relative stenosis of the distal duct.

Bile duct cysts are being identified with increasing frequency in the United States, paralleling the experience in the Orient, where they are seen much more frequently. Although the majority of these cystic problems are seen in children and teenagers, they can be seen in all age groups, including adults, with a much higher frequency in women. It is now generally agreed that in patients with cysts, there is frequently an anomalous communication of the distal bile duct with the pancreatic duct system and that the etiology includes stenosis of the distal bile duct. Reflex of pancreatic juice into the choledochal cyst, chronic bile stasis, and the formation of bile duct stones are thought to be the major reasons why cancers of the bile duct are found with increasing frequency in patients with bile duct cysts. Whenever possible, bile duct cysts should be excised up to the bifurcation of the right and left hepatic ducts or the common hepatic duct and a choledochojejunostomy, Roux-en-Y, constructed. The treatment of multiple intrahepatic biliary cysts within the liver, Caroli's disease, remains controversial and difficult. Occasionally, these cysts can be opened longitudinally for drainage into a segment of jejunum; occasionally, hepatic lobectomy or total excision of the liver with hepatic transplantation may be necessary.

Cancer of the bile ducts appears to have increased in the United States during the past ten years. During that same period, the incidence of cancer of the gallbladder has remained relatively stable. Its treatment remains dismal, a high percentage of patients being found at operation to have unresectable tumors. Cure is achieved apparently only when the cancer is confined to the mucosa and submucosal layers of the gallbladder. If there is penetration of the full thickness of the gallbladder wall extension of the tumor beyond the gallbladder into the liver, cystic duct, or bile duct lymph nodes, cure is unlikely.

The treatment of cancer of the gallbladder is still controversial. Most surgeons recommend an extended cholecystectomy if the disease is recognized and is confined to the wall of the gallbladder. Unfortunately, the tumor is not always recognized, often found only after the operative procedure has been terminated, when the pathologist examines the gallbladder specimen. The disputed issue as to whether operative reexploration of the porta hepatis should be undertaken for delayed wedge excision of the liver bed and lymph node dissection of the porta hepatis is not settled. My own belief is that cure is determined by the stage of the disease found at surgery. Only rarely would I recommend reexploration of a patient who has had a cholecystectomy to remove more tissue in the area.

Cancer of the bile duct is being identified more frequently by means of US, ERCP, or PTC. When the tumor is in the distal bile duct, pancreatoduodenectomy is potentially curative. If advanced disease is found, an upper bile duct-intestinal bypass procedure is almost always possible. If a midbile duct tumor is found, resection is less often possible, but should be attempted whenever possible. A biliary-intestinal bypass for unresectable tumors, again, is almost always possible. The real problem occurs with upper bile duct cancers, the Klatskin or bifurcation tumor: these tumors are rarely resectable. They should be resected whenever possible, but to perform a heroic resection that often includes a segment or lobe of the liver as advocated by several surgeons, only to find cancer at the cut margin of the intrahepatic bile duct, makes no sense in my opinion. I do exploration with the hope of performing resection. If the area above the tumor is inaccessible, I believe that the treatment of choice is a palliative bypass to a dilated intrahepatic bile duct or a common bile duct exploration below the tumor with dilation and intubation of the proximal bile duct through the tumor and placement of transhepatic tubes.

I have found bile duct tumors to be sensitive to radiation therapy. I have had one seven-year survivor and several two- and three-year survivors who had radiation therapy to an unresectable bile duct cancer with total relief of jaundice until the development of recurrent, diffuse intrahepatic disease. Although total excision of the extrahepatic and intrahepatic bile ducts, total resection of the liver, and hepatic transplantation seem to be the optimal treatment of choice for these patients, who have such slow-growing tumors and rarely have distant metastases, unfortunately, recurrence in the transplanted liver has been so common that hepatic transplantation, at the current stage of immunosuppressive therapy, is not recommended.

Liver and Portal Hypertension

W. DEAN WARREN, M.D.

HEPATIC SURGERY AND SURGERY for the complications of portal hypertension have undergone remarkable changes in the last decade. This complex field is presented lucidly and with little ambiguity by four outstanding authorities. The material is divided into four sections that facilitate a clear understanding of the pathophysiology of and therapy for the diverse diseases of surgical importance.

The first section deals with the common problem of a mass in the liver, often discovered by an imaging procedure. An effective, simple approach is to consider the lesions as solid tumors, cysts, or abscesses. This chapter is particularly helpful in the differential diagnosis and management of relatively uncommon problems such as liver cysts and benign tumors. Scott Jones's approach is clear and effective. Amoebic abscess, hydatid cyst, and pyogenic abscess require entirely different therapy; their differential diagnosis is crucial. While simple, nonoperative therapy for amoebic abscess (metronidazole) is effective, pyogenic liver abscess usually requires some type of drainage. Percutaneous catheter drainage with appropriate antibiotic therapy is often effective, and I have been impressed by the obviation of open drainage in a large percentage of patients. The evolving roles of catheter drainage and open surgical drainage should be watched carefully during the next few years.

Surgery for hepatic neoplasm is also being clarified. For primary hepatoma the problem is straightforward: if the patient is free of metastases and the tumor localized and resectable, excision should be accomplished. Only a small fraction of patients fit into this favorable group, and palliation, as always, is a much more severe test of judgment. The conflicting reports concerning hepatic arterial infusion of chemotherapeutic agents have been noted. However, some attempt at palliation is usually recommended, which should include the liberal use of narcotics. Another difficult decision arises in the occasional patient with an apparently solitary, late metastatic lesion to the liver, usually from the colon. As emphasized by the author, candid discussion with the patient is essential, and occasionally resection of such lesions is performed. There are no randomized data available to enhance decision making in this area.

Trauma is the facet of liver disease that will involve most surgeons. The evolution of care of the patient with an injured liver is carefully analyzed and thoughtfully presented by Dr. Walt, whose long-standing interest in the field brings an extensive experience to the reader. There are few revolutionary concepts at this time, but a thorough grasp of fundamentals is vital for success: control of hemorrhage, debridement resection, drainage of bile, and aggressive control of sepsis. Some readers will be surprised at the renewed interest in packs as an adjunct for the control of bleeding. When used properly (as in the management of pancreatic abscess), packing is valuable for the optimal management of a severely injured liver. Formal hepatic lobectomy is seldom used, and mortality has been decreased by more conservative resection. Walt again emphasizes, properly, that drainage of the common bile duct is deleterious unless there has been injury to the extrahepatic ducts.

Management of portal hypertension is changing rapidly, with improved patient care already evident. Layton Rikkers, a major authority in this field, presents the historical background necessary for a real understanding of the current approaches. Simply put, the major problem is control of variceal hemorrhage while protecting liver function as far as possible. Rikkers points out that randomized, controlled trials of therapy are prominent in this field of surgery. First were the trials of elective portacaval shunt vs. medical therapy (before sclerotherapy). They confirmed excellent control of bleeding by the shunt but little increased survival, which was negated by a high rate of morbidity (encephalopathy). If shunts were performed prior to the onset of bleeding, the so-called prophylactic shunt, surgery actually shortened survival. In the late 1960s, the selective shunt concept was introduced, and shortly thereafter interposition shunts were touted as achieving the same goals —selective decompression of varices while maintaining portal perfusion of the liver. Additional controlled trials were undertaken to evaluate these surgical procedures. Long-term studies from Atlanta, Toronto, and elsewhere confirmed the superiority of selective shunts over those that divert the portal flow completely. However, a major problem, the acute control of variceal bleeding, continued to elude a sound solution. The immediate portacaval shunt was tried and abandoned by all but one group. In the mid-1970s an old technique, endoscopic sclerotherapy, was reinstituted in Belfast. Sclerotherapy controlled bleeding, at least for short periods, in a high percentage of cases; long-term sclerotherapy resulted in significantly better long-term control of bleeding. This technique is now being studied intensively and is the primary therapy for most patients with acute bleeding.

Long-term sclerotherapy is considered the first approach for long-term therapy in many centers. When sclerotherapy fails, surgical procedures should be used promptly; good long-term results are anticipated from the combined approach. Thus, we are seeing a profound change in the treatment of one of our most difficult problems. From this change, a definitive improvement in patient care should result.

The section on liver transplantation is presented with both enthusiasm and clarity by Dr. Shaw. The recapitulation of the sequence of events leading to our current expertise in hepatic transplantation correctly emphasizes the unique role of Thomas Starzl. The contributions of others, often overlooked, are also documented. Although the actual transplantation of liver will undoubtedly be limited to relatively few centers for the foreseeable future, the general reader should understand the proper selection of recipient patients as well as the crucial importance of organ donation. At this time, the potential recipients far outnumber the donors, particularly among children. Improved understanding by the medical community is needed to increase greatly the number of organ donors. Although the statistical manipulations in this section are perplexing, it is clear that early survival has improved owing to several factors. Long-term survival has been disappointing in certain cancer patients and in those with viral or alcoholic cirrhosis; patients with diseases related to primary failure of hepatic mechanisms, such as biliary atresia and genetic metabolic abnormalities, have fared much better.

The complex operative techniques are well presented; when added to the general problems of organ procurement, organ preservation and transport, and recipient selection, the whole procedure assumes herculean proportions. This is an exciting era in the history of surgery, and the nontransplanting surgeon should learn much and enjoy greatly this presentation.

Surgery of the Pancreas

JOHN M. HOWARD, M.D.

ACUTE PANCREATITIS

Acute pancreatitis apparently consists of scores of disease entities. Mechanical obstruction, chemical or pharmacologic intoxication ischemia, hereditary predisposition, metabolic or nutritional alterations, viral infections, and occasionally bacterial infections are known to cause pancreatitis, obviously requiring varying approaches to therapy.

In the majority of recognized cases of acute pancreatitis, the basic process appears initially to be nonbacterial. Most patients have pancreatic inflammation marked by edema and capillary engorgement, and in some, surrounding areas of fat necrosis develop. Patients with more severe forms of the disease may experience ischemic necrosis or ischemic gangrene of the pancreas and retroperitoneal tissues, which can remain relatively indolent over the ensuing weeks or even months. Laparotomy five or six months later may show only a necrotic cavity without a fibrous inner lining. Peripheral necrosis of the gland may result in collections of pancreatic juice that more rapidly become encapsulated and assume the characteristics of the pseudocyst. Still other areas of edema, necrosis, or collections of juice or exudate may heal, with no long-term pseudocyst or ischemic necrosis. Early changes in blood volume are seldom, if ever, the result of hemorrhage. Only fat necrosis seems to be specific for acute pancreatitis; pancreatic enzymes can digest only dead tissue—not living cells, so fat necrosis indicates dead tissue and probably severe pancreatitis.

The diagnosis of acute pancreatitis rests on the clinical syndrome of constant upper abdominal pain, nausea, vomiting, and paralytic ileus. It is supported by the finding of a high serum amylase or lipase level and confirmed as the primary clinical problem when acute cholecystitis, perforated peptic ulcer, intestinal obstruction, and gangrene have been eliminated. In my experience many patients with blunt trauma have a serum amylase level of 200–250 Somogyi units/dl (normal 80–180) at the time of hospitalization. Diagnosis of pancreatic injury is seldom delineated in these patients, whose pancreatic convalescence is uneventful.

Review of the literature shows a striking similarity to the approaches used in therapy for thermal burns. A burn toxin would have explained early peripheral vascular collapse, renal failure, and death. Gradually, it became clear that the early cause of death was fluid translocation, resulting in reduced capillary perfusion, and later deaths were due to infection of the necrotic burn tissue. The entire concept of the toxicity of dead tissue, in contradistinction to the toxicity of secondary bacterial invasion of dead tissue, requires reevaluation. Scores of studies have sought unsuccessfully to demonstrate the toxicity of various pancreatic enzymes. The exudate of acute pancreatitis, however, may be toxic; its products have tentatively been incriminated in increased capillary permeability, pain, fat necrosis, and hypocalcemia. This has led to the trial of peritoneal lavage as an adjunct to therapy. Any beneficial effects of peritoneal lavage remain controversial.

Ransom has made significant contributions to clinical investigation by his internationally recognized studies of indices of prognosis. Perhaps "indices of severity" might be preferable, since prognosis depends on treatment as well as severity.

The criteria of severity that I consider most reliable are based on finding a low serum calcium concentration, an elevated hematocrit, the vital signs (including the urinary output) indicative of hypovolemia, and, over the first few days, (a) the deterioration of ventilatory function as monitored by sequential measurements of arterial oxygen, and (b) the relatively great volume of crystalloid and colloid required to maintain renal capillary perfusion. The age of the patient is obviously important. The magnitude of the rise in the serum amylase level does not seem to reflect the severity of the inflammatory process. A very high serum amylase level may indicate only that the exocrine cells were healthy, constituting a rich storehouse of enzymes before their damage.

Postoperative pancreatitis and drug-induced pancreatitis usually follow complicated operations or disease states in which the pancreatitis may play a limited role. They should probably be excluded from the effort to establish basic principles in treatment of acute pancreatitis. With these exclusions, the mortality of acute pancreatitis today should approach zero. I believe it to be achievable. Marked reduction in mortality has been achieved by intensive, supportive care with the prevention of acute renal failure; the avoidance of laparotomy and introduction of bacteria into an essentially sterile environment; the recognition of ischemic necrosis of tissue; the prevention of early secondary infection; the monitoring of the disease process by clinical observation and radiologic investigation; and appropriately delayed operative intervention to treat life-threatening complications such as secondary infection. The timing of laparotomy in acute gallstone pancreatitis has not been clearly delineated. Cholangitis and septicemia secondary to choledocholithiasis and associated pancreatitis may prove to be an indication for laparotomy.

Early operation results in increased mortality, with no clear demonstration that the drainage of pancreatic juice or exudate is beneficial. As a result, it seems that investigation of continued early resection should be restricted to one or two sophisticated clinics.

The treatment of acute pancreatitis now rests on the principles of restoring capillary perfusion by administration of adequate volumes of crystalloids and colloids, the maintenance of adequate oxygenation, the provision of adequate nutrition, and the continued monitoring for evidence of life-threatening intra-abdominal complications that may require delayed laparotomy. Prevention of acute renal failure is an essential, initial goal.

Acosta, Stone, and Kelly have clearly demonstrated that acute pancreatitis may result from the migration of a gallstone into and through the ampulla of Vater. Studies of emergency laparotomy in the treatment of gallstone pancreatitis have demonstrated an increased incidence of stones in the ampulla, that the pancreatic juice may be under increased pressure, and that the common bile duct may be obstructed. Such studies have resulted in a reduced incidence of recurrent attacks. The degree of severity of evolving pancreatitis might be reduced by the early removal of the obstructing stone. The authors have not, however, demonstrated a reduced mortality rate. Careful review of recent reports indicates a lower mortality when operative intervention is withheld until the patient is hemodynamically stable and the pancreatitis has clinically subsided. Most surgeons today delay removal of the gallstones during the initial hospitalization unless the patient has had a life-threatening attack of acute pancreatitis. In the latter instance, the patient should later have elective exploration of the biliary tract.

The studies of emergency endoscopic sphincterotomy as outlined by Saffrani and others have demonstrated that gallstones may be seen endoscopically to bulge through the ampulla of Vater, permitting the endoscopist to perform sphincterotomy and to remove the gallstone. They have not shown a reduced mortality rate. Most such patients would still require subsequent laparotomy for the removal of other gallstones.

Many outstanding students of pancreatitis in the United States have had their clinical base at a publicly supported hospital that cares for patients of a lower socio-economic status, with alcohol abuse rates disproportionately high. Gallstone pancreatitis has been indicted as causing mortality twice as high as that of alcoholic pancreatitis: most patients who die of acute pancreatitis die of their first attack. Gallstone pancreatitis is usually recognized and its natural history interrupted by definitive surgery. Alcoholic pancreatitis results in repetitive hospitalizations and mortality seems to decrease with each recurring attack.

CHRONIC PANCREATITIS

More and more young patients in temperate as well as tropical climates are being recognized to have recurrent episodes of pancreatitis, which, after years, become chronic. In those aged 18 to 30 years, neither alcohol nor obstruction is frequently a factor.

Greenlee presented fairly the advantages and disadvantages of drainage of the pancreatic duct vs. resection of the pancreas for the control of pain from chronic pancreatitis. Those experienced in resection of the pancreas for treatment of pancreatitis generally are resecting the right side of the pancreas rather than the left (i.e., Whipple or extended Whipple resection). Many patients present in the early stages of chronic pancreatitis, with the disease grossly limited to the head of the pancreas. In my experience, disease clearly limited to the left side is less frequent.

Chronic pancreatitis almost always reflects an atrophic, fibrotic, exocrine pancreas. Seldom can any operative procedure restore its physiologic function.

To achieve rapid progress in the treatment of chronic pancreatitis, the surgeon must describe the anatomical and pathological characteristics of the gland. Reports must be based on standard follow-up durations: 5-, 10-, or 20-year follow-up, not "*average* follow-up of three years." A recent review of the literature shows a growing need for comparative data.

PANCREATIC TUMORS

The advances in the diagnosis of pancreatic disease have been tremendous during the past few decades. Serum enzyme determinations are now almost routine for patients with acute abdominal pain. In addition, the immunoassay (particularly for the islet cell hormones), ERCP, percutaneous transhepatic cholangiograms, CT scans of the pancreas, ultrasonography, pancreatic arteriography, and fiberoptic examination of the duodenum have resulted in rapid progress in localization and characterization of pancreatic tumors.

Fitzgerald and Cubilla, as pointed out by Moossa, have made a significant contribution to the field of pancreatic cancer by their description of the multiple subtypes of carcinoma of the pancreas. Their contribution was not widely utilized by most pathologists until recently. Only by careful pathologic characterization and correlation with the patient's clinical course can the natural history of the various pancreatic cancers be elucidated. Additional effort is also needed from our colleagues in pathology as to the staging of pancreatic cancers. The surgeon must describe the extent of the tumor, but the pathologist must perform adequate dissections of the location of the tumor, its relationship to the duct and blood vessels, an adequate lymph node dissection, and adequate sections of the pancreas, while searching for spread or multicentric origin of the tumor.

Several authors have emphasized that the mortality in pancreatic surgery, perhaps as much as in any type of surgery performed today, has strikingly diminished as individual surgeons gained experience. This has certainly proved true of resection for pancreatic cancer. The need for centralization of such patients in specialty centers becomes apparent, at least until management principles are further refined and the centers have trained additional staff.

The mortality for resection of pancreatic cancer today should not exceed 5%. Experienced surgeons, dedicated housestaff, and high-quality intensive care unit nurses have made this possible. Nevertheless, the end results of treating cancer of the exocrine pancreas remain disappointing. Total vs. partial pancreatectomy does not appear to be a vital issue. The role of intraoperative radiotherapy remains uncertain, and chemotherapy has generally not proved helpful. Resection may prove clearly helpful to individual patients with five-year postresection survivals approximating 10% for cancer of the head of the pancreas and 30%–40% for cancer of the ampulla of Vater.

Despite the current limitations of cure, the ability to localize pancreatic-related cancers preoperatively has much improved, and the ability to remove the pancreatic tumor with a steadily decreasing operative death rate provides a basis for encouragement in developing adjuvant therapy. Perhaps resection may become one step in treatment.

To the preceding list of endocrine tumors of the pancreas might be added the carcinoid tumor, which has been reported in several patients as arising in the pancreas. It is also probable that those endocrine tumors of the pancreas currently designated as nonfunctional will subsequently be found to have an endocrine effect. All pancreatic adenocarcinomas, as well as adenocarcinomas throughout the body, may have an endocrine effect, conceivably secreting "hormones" that produce a detrimental metabolic effect leading to cachexia.

The authors of the chapter "Pancreas Transplantation in Man" have been pioneers in the field of pancreatic transplantation. Their work is distinguished by its high scientific merit and by its consistency in gradually developing the technical and biological principles. Pancreatic transplantation has much to offer in the description of the natural history of diabetes, both the juvenile- and maturity-onset types; particularly to the natural history of some of the complications of severe diabetes, such as diabetic neuropathy and the related renal complications.

I recall when all islet cell tumors were divided between "insulinomas and nonfunctioning tumors." Recognition of the multiple entities has been exciting. The accruing knowledge has stimulated and contributed to basic knowledge of GI physiology.

Certain Aspects of Intestinal Surgery

JOHN C. GOLIGHER, M.B., CH.B, CH.M, F.R.C.S.

Elective surgery for colorectal cancer in centers of excellence generally offers a five-year survival of about 50%,[1] although under less favorable circumstances, as in the records of Regional Cancer Registries, the results have seldom been nearly as good. Thus, at best roughly half of the patients are not cured. What prospects are there of improving these results? Five possibilities warrant attention.

More extensive operations.—After a limited vogue in the 1950s, so-called super radical operations were largely abandoned in America and Britain because they were followed by a higher immediate morbidity (especially in regard to sexual and bladder function), and they did not seem significantly to improve the late results.[1, 2] But a few Japanese surgeons[1, 3, 4] still practice an extended excision for rectal carcinoma, involving dissection of the internal iliac nodes, and claim enhanced survival with it (personal communications: Hajo; Takahashi and Kajatani; and Jinnai, 1982).

Adjuvant radiotherapy.—Several controlled trials of adjuvant preoperative radiotherapy in conjunction with radical operation for *rectal* cancer have mostly shown no significant long-term benefit[1, 5–8], perhaps because of inadequate dosage, generally 2,000–2,500 rad. Now, further trials of preoperative or postoperative radiotherapy are in progress,[1] using doses of 5,000–6,000 rad, and the results are awaited with interest (Schein, personal communication, 1982).

Adjuvant chemotherapy.—Adjuvant chemotherapy was also bitterly disappointing until the GITSG's controlled trial, which gave a reduced incidence of local recurrence after excision of *rectal* carcinoma when the operation was supplemented by chemotherapy, radiotherapy, or both[1] (Schein, personal communication, 1982). However, this trial has not yet run its full course, so judgment must remain suspended.

Also encouraging in its initial results has been the trial by Taylor and associates[9, 10] of continuous intrahepatic infusion with fluorouracil (5-FU) starting at the time of operation and maintained for one week thereafter. But a longer-term report on its outcome is still awaited.

More meticulous follow-up after operation, assisted by CEA monitoring and occasional second-look operations for local recurrences or metastatic disease.[1]—Martin et al.[11] have had the widest experience with this routine, but of 22 patients coming to reoperation for recurrent disease, only two survived five years, giving an improvement in the five-year survival rate of the original 300 cases monitored of less than 1%. However, they claim that with increasing experience with the system, their results are improving.

Earlier diagnosis—presymptomatic screening.—In ordinary clinical practice, by the time patients with colorectal cancer come to operation, 50% already have nodal metastases (Dukes' C cases), and in 25%–30% hepatic or other blood-borne metastases are present.[1] It is not surprising that lasting cure is achieved in only about half. One way to improve the prognosis would be somehow to change the composition of the cases to provide more in category A and B and fewer in category C or with distant metastases. Much earlier diagnosis before onset of symptoms might have that effect, although admittedly the length of time that a tumor has been present is not the only factor determining how widely it may have spread. Another very important consideration is its intrinsic malignancy.

A great aid in the conduct of screening of asymptomatic persons of "cancer age" is the routine use of the Hemoccult guaiac test for demonstrating occult blood in the feces.[12–14] Only the 4% or so of those tested who give positive responses are further investigated, which lessens greatly the burden on the medically trained staff.[14] Of 12 colorectal carcinomas detected by Hardcastle et al.[14] (personal communications, 1984) on Hemoccult screening of some 400 individuals, nine were shown on subsequent pathologic examination to be Dukes' A and three Dukes' B lesions—a much more favorable grouping than is normally encountered in practice. If the Hemoccult test could be made widely acceptable to lay people, it might greatly improve the results of treatment of colorectal cancer.

Avoidance of a permanent colostomy in the treatment of rectal cancer.—When treating a patient for carcinoma of the rectum, it is extremely gratifying if it is possible to remove the growth without having to inflict on him a permanent colostomy—always provided that the avoidance of a stoma can be accomplished without increasing the mortality or morbidity, with preservation of worthwhile anorectal function, and without lessening the prospects of ultimate cure. For most carcinomas of the upper third or half of the rectum, this ideal is readily attainable by means of the operation of anterior resection.[1] Carcinomas of the middle third or upper part of the lower third can sometimes also be dealt with satisfactorily by this operation, especially in thin female patients, but in more heavily built male subjects it is usually impossible on technical grounds.[1] If the latter are to be spared an abdominoperineal excision with permanent colostomy, some other technique of sphincter-saving resection must be employed, usually one of the following:

1. *Abdominoanal pull-through resection* (including abdominotransanal resection with endocavitary sutured coloanal anastomosis)[15, 16];

2. *Abdominosacral resection*[17, 18] (including abdominotransphincteric resection;[19]) and

3. *Extended low anterior resection with stapled colorectal or coloanal anastomosis* made with the EEA or ILS circular stapling gun.[1, 20, 21]

Because (c) is usually much easier technically than (a) or (b), it has become a great deal more popular. With the aid of the circular stapler, it is in fact possible to achieve very low colorectal anastomoses, just above the top of the anal canal, even in obese men.[1, 21] Low resection is, of course, facilitated by the fact that after the rectum is fully mobilized at operation, it straightens out and lengthens, and a lesion that lay at 5.5 cm preoperatively may rise to 7.5 cm or higher. A distal margin of clearance of 2.0–2.5 cm is now recognized to be perfectly adequate in a resection.[1, 22–24]

Results of the new breed of sphincter-saving resections for carcinomas of the middle and lower parts of the rectum.—These operations can be performed with a relatively low operative mortality (around 3%).[18, 25–30] The most common surgical complication has been sepsis in the abdominal wound or pelvis, sometimes associated with anastomotic dehiscence, which occurs in roughly 14% of cases.[16, 18, 21, 25–28]

Functional results.—Although retention of an anorectal stump 6 cm or longer certainly facilitates a rapid return to normal function,[29] recent experience with patients given anastomoses as low as 3.5–4.5 cm from the anal verge or even in the anal canal shows that as a rule they ultimately attain satisfactory control, but often only after troublesome diarrhea and some incontinence for 3–6 months.[16, 21, 27, 28]

Late results.—Earlier studies showed little difference in the five-year survival rate after sphincter-saving resection and abdominoperineal excision, respectively, for carcinomas of the mid-third,[30, 31] but no comparable evaluation of the newer breed of resections for lesions in this situation is yet available. Meanwhile, we know that the *local recurrence rate* after these operations has ranged from 2% to 3% to over 30%,[32] the latter figure being somewhat disturbing. But it must be remembered that local recurrence is not uncommon even after abdominoperineal excision, especially for low carcinomas.[1, 32] Obviously, this matter must be kept under close scrutiny.

Local excision or destruction of small, especially favorable frank carcinomas of the rectum.—Pathologic examination of rectal excision specimens shows that in 15% the growth has not yet extended outside the bowel wall or produced nodal metastases (Dukes' A lesion) and in 3% is still confined to the submucosa (a sort of Dukes' super A lesion).[1] In these cases purely local treatment would clearly have sufficed. But how reliably can the surgeon determine from his preoperative clinical examination that a tumor is in this extremely favorable pathologic state? A recent study[33] has confirmed that there is always some uncertainty, even with growths that are small (not more than 2–3 cm in diameter), not deeply or at all ulcerating, mobile on the underlying muscle coat, unassociated with palpable lymph nodes, and well or moderately well differentiated histologically on piece-biopsy. So, some errors and resulting therapeutic failures are inevitable. On the other hand, local treatment should carry virtually no immediate mortality compared to that of rectal excision, which could rise to 8%–10% in poor-risk subjects.

Perhaps purely local therapy is best reserved for the 2% or 3% of patients with very favorable carcinomas as defined above, lying within 6 cm of the anal verge, but who themselves are somewhat unfavorable candidates for major surgery. Regarding the choice of method, diathermy fulguration[1, 34, 35] and endocavitary irradiation[1, 36] are both easier to perform, but local excision has the great advantage of providing for the pathologist a specimen from which he can confirm or refute the clinical verdict of suitability for local removal.

Elective surgery for ulcerative colitis.—During the past five or six years, ileostomy and complete proctocolectomy has been gradually displaced from its premier position by operations that aim to preserve continence, particularly by the resuscitated procedure of proctocolectomy and ileoanal anastomosis combined with a pelvic ileal pouch. Recent studies[37–39] have clearly demonstrated that the addition of a pouch lessens the frequency and urgency of defecation experienced after a straight ileoanal anastomosis and affords acceptable, if not perfect, function in 80% or more of patients. A J-shaped pouch, where feasible, seems preferable to an S-shaped one, because of the occasional failure of spontaneous evacuation after the latter and the need for regular intubations[1, 40, 41] (Krause, personal communication, 1979).

Another procedure that is enjoying a mild revival is *colectomy and ileorectal anastomosis.* Keeping and using a diseased rectum is of course illogical, but it preserves absolutely normal continence, and 50%–70% of the patients in fact do very well with it.[1] There is also the risk of carcinoma arising in the retained rectal stump[1]—actually in 6% of Aylett's series of 374 cases followed up for 1–23 years.[42] Fortunately, this development can now be anticipated fairly reliably by the finding of severe epithelial dysplasia in rectal biopsies, and their performance every 6–12 months is an essential precaution.[40, 43] The development of premalignant (or malignant) changes or the failure of the operation from persistence of severe proctitis and diarrhea indicates the need for a proctectomy with either an ileostomy or an ileoanal anastomosis with ileal pouch.

In recent years better techniques for the *reservoir ileostomy* operation have much improved its results.[1, 44] The irony now is that it is difficult[5] to find suitable patients for this procedure, for most people prefer to try an ileoanal or ileorectal anastomosis, unless the rectum has already been removed by an ileostomy and complete proctocolectomy.

Emergency surgery for ulcerative colitis.—I have no doubt that the best emergency operation is an ileostomy and subtotal colectomy, which is easy to perform and preserves the rectum for subsequent consideration of all the options of elective surgery.[1]

Elective surgery for Crohn's disease.—The not infrequent recurrences after operation have led some distinguished gastroenterologists[45-48] to counsel strongly against too ready a resort to surgical intervention. But most internists discover to their chagrin that 70% or more of their patients with this condition eventually come to surgery because of dissatisfaction with chronic debilitating symptoms or the development of complications.[49] Until more effective medical therapy is developed, therefore, it seems that the surgeon will continue to play a major role in its management.

The standard operation is now *resection* for disease mainly or entirely of the small bowel; the only controversy relates to the amount of ostensibly normal bowel that should be excised proximal and distal to the diseased segment. The usual siting of recurrences, immediately proximal to the anastomosis, has suggested that they might have been prevented by removal of a larger portion of "normal" intestine at the original operation[50] (Krause, personal communication, 1979). A large uncontrolled trial[51] showed fewer recurrences after this more radical type of operation; another much smaller but controlled trial[52] failed to confirm this finding. Relevant to the issue are the data from three combined histopathologic and follow-up studies; two demonstrated no difference in the incidence of recurrence depending on whether there had been histologic evidence of disease at one or both lines of resection,[53, 54] but the third revealed a higher incidence of recurrence when the margins of resection had been diseased.[55]

My own policy in resecting for Crohn's disease has been to secure short margins of clearance, 3–5 cm long, proximally and distally, to provide "normal" tissues for the anastomosis. The resected specimen is opened immediately after removal to check by naked-eye examination that clearance on the mucosal aspect is also adequate. With this technique the recurrence rate in 98 personal cases followed up for 7–18 years was 29% at 5 years, 46% at 10 years, and 64% at 15 years.[56]

Sphincteroplasty, a minimal pyloroplasty type of operation, has recently been much promulgated for the treatment of short strictured lesions.[57, 58] It is difficult to see its advantages over a very limited resection for a single lesion of this kind, but for multiple, short, stenosed "skip" areas, a series of stricturoplasties could avoid sacrifice of a lot of bowel. Occasional fistulation might be anticipated after stricturoplasty but so far has apparently been rare (Alexander-Williams and Fornaro, personal communication, 1985). Further follow-up is obviously needed for a proper appraisal.

The most generally useful operation for disease mainly or entirely of the large bowel is *ileostomy and complete proctocolectomy.* Of course, this procedure often also means some degree of terminal ileoectomy to remove concomitant disease in the small bowel, so the resulting ileostomy frequently acts more profusely than usual. But with modern ileostomy appliances and the help of antidiarrheal drugs, such as loperamide and diphenoxylate (Lomotil), this is now seldom a serious inconvenience. For the notorious delay often encountered in the healing of the perineal wound, no regularly effective solution is yet available.[1] Various estimates have been given of the incidence of recurrence—usually just above the stoma—but in my own series of 162 cases followed up for 7–25 years (mean 15 years), the cumulative rate of recurrence has been 12% at 10 years and 20% at 20 years,[59] which is encouraging.

In about 25% of patients the rectum is spared,[1] and a colectomy and ileorectal anastomosis is an attractive proposition[59] but is followed by a high rate of recurrence (70% or more) within ten years. Nonetheless, this operation enables the patient to postpone for a time the need for an ileostomy, and no doubt it will continue to be used where possible for its temporary or occasionally lasting benefit.

A useful interim operation for acutely ill patients or those showing severe perianal disease or a rectum of dubious normality is an ileostomy and subtotal colectomy. Subsequently, according to circumstances, a proctectomy or secondary ileorectal anastomosis may be performed, or the unused rectum may be left in situ indefinitely.

Finally, it cannot be too strongly stressed that "pouch operations" (reservoir ileostomy or ileoanal anastomosis with a pelvic ileal reservoir) have absolutely no place in the treatment of Crohn's disease because of the extensive sacrifice of small bowel that would be entailed in a reoperation for recurrence. Indeed, when contemplating the use of either of these operations for what is believed to be ulcerative colitis, it is of paramount importance to make sure that the condition is not really Crohn's disease of the large bowel.

REFERENCES

1. Goligher J.C.: *Surgery of the Anus, Rectum and Colon*, ed. 5. London: Baillière-Tindall, 1984.
2. Stearns, M.W. Jr., Deddish M.R.: Five-year results of abdominopelvic lymph node dissection for carcinoma of the rectum. *Dis. Colon Rectum* 2:169, 1959.
3. Hojo K., Koyama Y.: The effectiveness of wide anatomical resection and radical lymph adenectomy for patients with rectal cancer. *Jpn. J. Surg.* 128:111, 1982.
4. Hojo K., Koyama Y.: Post-operative follow-up studies on cancer of the colon and rectum. *Am. J. Surg.* 143:293, 1982.
5. Stearns M.W. Jr., Deddish M.R., Quan S.H.Q.: Pre-operative irradiation for cancer of the rectum and rectosigmoid: preliminary review of recent experience. *Dis. Colon Rectum* 11:281, 1968.
6. Higgins G.A. Jr.: The pros and cons of irradiation treatment of colorectal cancer, in Nyhus L.M. (ed.): *Surgery Annual.* New York, Appleton-Century-Crofts, 1978.
7. Rider W.D.: Is the Miles operation really necessary for the treatment of rectal cancer? *J. Can. Assoc. Radiol.* 26:167, 1975.
8. Duncan W., Smith A.N., Freedman L.S., et al.: The evaluation of low dose pre-operative X-ray therapy in the management of operable rectal cancer: results of a randomly controlled trial: the second report of the MRC working party. *Br. J. Surg.* 71:21, 1984.
9. Taylor I., Rowling J.T., West C.: Adjuvant liver perfusion for colorectal cancer. *Br. J. Surg.* 66:833, 1979.
10. Taylor I.: Results of adjuvant cytotoxic liver perfusion in radical surgery for colorectal cancer. *Br. J. Surg.,* in press.
11. Martin E.W., Cooperman M., Carey L.C., et al.: Sixty second-look procedures indicated primarily by rise in serial CEA. *J. Surg. Res.* 28:389, 1980.
12. Greegor D.H.: Diagnosis of large bowel cancer in the asymptomatic patient. *J.A.M.A.* 201:943, 1967.
13. Greegor D.H.: Occult blood testing for detection of asymptomatic colon cancer. *Cancer* 28:131, 1971.
14. Hardcastle J.D., Balfour T.W., Amar S.S.: Screening for symptomless colorectal cancer by testing for occult blood in general practice. *Lancet* 1:791, 1980.
15. Parks A.G.: Transanal technique in low rectal anastomosis. *Proc. R. Soc. Med.* 65:975, 1972.
16. Parks A.G., Percy J.P.: Resection and sutured colo-anal anastomosis for rectal carcinoma. *Br. J. Surg.* 69:301, 1982.
17. Localio S.O., Baron B.: Abdomino-sacral resection and anastomosis for mid-rectal cancer. *Ann. Surg.* 178:540, 1973.
18. Localio S.O., Eng K., Gouge T.H., et al.: Abdominal resection for carcinoma of the mid rectum: 15 years experience. *Ann. Surg.* 383:3202, 1983.
19. Mason A.Y.: Selective surgery for carcinoma of the rectum. *Aust. N.Z. J. Surg.* 46:322, 1976.
20. Fain S.N., Patin C.S., Morgenstern L.: Use of a mechanical suturing apparatus in low colorectal anastomoses. *Arch. Surg.* 110:1079, 1975.

21. Goligher J.C., Lee P.W.R., McFie J., et al.: Experience with the Russian suture gun for rectal anastomoses. *Br. J. Surg.* 148:517, 1979.
22. Penfold C.B.:A comparison of restorative resection of carcinoma of the middle third of the rectum with abdominoperineal excision. *Aust. N.Z. J. Surg.* 44:354, 1974.
23. Manson P.N., Corman M.L., Coller J., et al.: Anastomotic recurrence after anterior resection for carcinoma: Lahey Clinic experience. *Dis. Colon Rectum* 19:1219, 1976.
24. Pollett W.G., Nicholls R.J.: The relationship between the extent of distal clearance and the survival and local recurrence rates after curative anterior resection for carcinoma of the rectum. *Ann. Surg.* 198:159, 1983.
25. Beart R.B., Kelly K.A.: Randomized prospective evaluation of the EEA stapler for colorectal anastomoses. *Am. J. Surg.* 141:43, 1981.
26. Heald R.J., Leicester R.J.: The low stapled anastomosis. *Br. J. Surg.* 68:333, 1981.
27. Thiede A., Jöstarndt L., Troidl H., et al.: Der Wert der zirkulären maschinellen Kolon-und Rektumanastomose (EEA): eine prospektive Studie an 91 Patienten. *Chirurg.* 52:30, 1981.
28. Keighley M.R.B., Matheson D.: Functional results of rectal excision and endo-anal anastomosis. *Br. J. Surg.* 67:57, 1980.
29. Goligher J.C. Functional results after sphincter-saving resections of the rectum. *Ann. R. Coll. Surg. Engl.* 8:421, 1951.
30. Waugh J.M., Turner J.C.: A study of 268 patients with carcinoma of the mid rectum treated by abdominoperineal resection with sphincter preservation. *Surg. Gynecol. Obstet.* 107:777, 1958.
31. Nicholls R.J., Ritchie J.M., Wadsworth J.K., et al.: Total excision or restorative resection for carcinoma of the middle third of the rectum. *Br. J. Surg.* 66:625, 1979.
32. Goligher J.C.: Extended low anterior resection with stapled colorectal or colo-anal anastomosis. *Ann. Chir.* In press.
33. Nicholls R.J., Mason A.Y., Morson B.C.: The clinical staging of rectal cancer. *Br. J. Surg.* 48:353, 1982.
34. Madden J.L., Kandalaft S.: Electrocoagulation in the treatment of cancer of the rectum: a continuing study. *Ann. Surg.* 174:530, 1971.
35. Crile G. Jr., Turnbull R.B. Jr.: The role of electrocoagulation in the treatment of carcinoma of the rectum. *Surg. Gynecol. Obstet.* 135:391, 1972.
36. Papillon J.: *Rectal and Anal Cancers: Conservative Treatment by Irradiation—An Alternative to Radical Surgery.* Berlin, Springer Verlag, 1982.
37. Taylor B.M., Beart R.W., Dozois R., et al.: Comparison of straight ileo-anal versus pouch anal anastomoses after colectomy and mucosal proctectomy. *Arch. Surg.* 118:696, 1983.
38. Martin L.W., Fischer J.E.: Preservation of anorectal continence following total colectomy. *Ann. Surg.* 196:517, 1982.
39. Taylor B.M., Beart R.W. Jr., Dozois R., et al.: The anorectal

ileal pouch and anastomosis: current clinical results. *Dis. Colon Rectum* 27:347, 1984.

40. Nicholls R.J., Pescatori M., Morton R.W., et al.: Restorative proctocolectomy with a three-loop ileal reservoir for ulcerative colitis and familial polyposes. *Ann. Surg.* 199:383, 1984.
41. Rothenberger D.A., Wong W.D., Buls J.G.: Restorative proctocolectomy with ileal reservoir and ileo-anal anastomosis for ulcerative colitis and familial polyposes. *Dig. Surg.* 1:19, 1984.
42. Baker W.N.W., Glass R.E., Ritchie J.K., et al.: Cancer of the rectum following colectomy and ileorectal anastomosis for ulcerative colitis. *Br. J. Surg.* 65:862, 1978.
43. Morson B.C., Pang L.S.C.: Rectal biopsy as an aid to cancer control in ulcerative colitis. *Gut* 8:423, 1967.
44. Cohen Z.: Evolution of the Kock continent reservoir ileostomy. *Can. J. Surg.* 25:509, 1982.
45. van Patter W.N., Bargen J.A., Dockerty M.B., et al.: Regional enteritis. *Gastroenterology* 26:347, 1954.
46. Cooke W.T.: Nutritional and metabolic factors in the aetiology and treatment of regional ileitis. *Ann. R. Coll. Surg. Engl.* 17:137, 1955.
47. Crohn B.B., Yarnis H.: *Regional Ileitis*, ed. 2. New York, Grune & Stratton, 1958.
48. Goodman M.J., Kirsner J.B.: The outcome of medical and surgical therapy in Crohn's disease patients suitable for primary resection and anastomosis. *Gastroenterology* 76:1140, 1979.
49. Higgins C.S., Allan R.N.: Crohn's disease of the distal ileum. *Gut* 21:933, 1980.
50. Wenckert A.: Results of surgical treatment of Crohn's disease in Sweden, in *Skandia Symposium on Regional Enteritis (Crohn's Disease)*. Stockholm, Nordiska Bokhandeln Förlag, 1971.
51. Bergman L., Krause U.: Crohn's disease: a long term study of the clinical course in 186 patients. *Scand. J. Gastroenterol.* 12:937, 1977.
52. Ewe K., Malchow H., Herfarth C.H.: Operative Radikalität und Rezidivprophylaxe mit Azulfidine bei M. Crohn: eine prospektive multizentrische Studie—erste Ergebnisse. *Langenbecks Arch. Chir.* 364:427, 1984.
53. Papaioannou N., Piris J., Lee E.C.G., et al.: The relationship between histological inflammation in the cut ends after resection of Crohn's disease and recurrence. *Gut* 20:A916, 1979.
54. Pennington L., Hamilton S.R., Baylers T.M., et al.: Surgical management of Crohn's disease: influence of disease at margin of resection. *Ann. Surg.* 192:311, 1982.
55. Wolff B.G., Beart R.B. Jr., Frydenbergh H., et al.: Importance of disease-free margins in resection of Crohn's disease. *Dis. Colon Rectum* 26(4):239, 1983.
56. Goligher J.C.: Crohn's disease: surgical treatment, in Truelove S.C., Kennedy H.J. (eds.): *Topics in Gastroenterology*, ed. 8. Oxford, Blackwell Scientific Publications, 1980.
57. Lee E.C.G., Papaioannou N.: Minimal surgery for chronic obstruction in patients with extensive or universal Crohn's disease. *Ann. R. Coll. Surg. Engl.* 64:229, 1982.
58. Alexander-Williams J., Fornaro M.: Stricturoplasty for Crohn's disease. *Scand. J. Gastroenterol.* 17(suppl. 78):496, 1982.
59. Goligher J.C.: The long-term results of excisional surgery for primary and recurrent Crohn's disease of the large intestine. *Dis. Colon Rectum* 28:51, 1985.

Index